Radiation Oncology – Principles, Precepts and Practice

Bidhu K. Mohanti • S. V. S. Deo
Jai Prakash Agarwal
Sarbani Ghosh Laskar
Ahitagni Biswas
Kumar Prabhash
Sanjoy Chatterjee • Anusheel Munshi
Editors

Radiation Oncology – Principles, Precepts and Practice

Volume II– Clinical Aspects

Second Edition

Springer

BYWORD BOOKS™

Editors
Bidhu K. Mohanti
Department of Radiation Oncology
Bagchi Sri Shankara Cancer Centre & Research Institute
Bhubaneswar, Odisha, India

Jai Prakash Agarwal
Department of Radiation Oncology
Homi Bhabha National Institute
Tata Memorial Hospital
Mumbai, Maharashtra, India

Ahitagni Biswas
Department of Radiation Oncology
All India Institute of Medical Sciences
New Delhi, Delhi, India

Sanjoy Chatterjee
Department of Radiation Oncology
Tata Medical Center
Kolkata, West Bengal, India

S. V. S. Deo
Department of Surgical Oncology
MAX Hospital, Saket
New Delhi, Delhi, India

Sarbani Ghosh Laskar
Department of Radiation Oncology
Homi Bhabha National Institute
Tata Memorial Hospital
Mumbai, Maharashtra, India

Kumar Prabhash
Department of Medical Oncology
Homi Bhabha National Institute
Tata Memorial Hospital
Mumbai, Maharashtra, India

Anusheel Munshi
Department of Radiation Oncology
BLK MAX Hospital
New Delhi, Delhi, India

ISBN 978-981-95-5170-5 ISBN 978-981-95-5171-2 (eBook)
https://doi.org/10.1007/978-981-95-5171-2

1st edition: © Elsevier 2007

Jointly published with Byword Books

This Springer imprint is published by the registered company Springer Nature Singapore Pte Ltd.
The registered company address is: 152 Beach Road, #21-01/04 Gateway East, Singapore 189721, Singapore

Co-publishing partnership between Byword Books Private Limited and Springer Nature Singapore Pte Ltd. The registered company address is 152 Beach Road, #21-01/04 Gateway East, Singapore, 189721, Singapore

Preface—Volume II

In presenting this book, Volume II of *Radiation Oncology: Principles, Precepts, and Practice*, we the editors consider it our honor and privilege to connect with the world of cancer science. This volume focuses on the clinical management of cancer using radiation therapy. Building upon the foundational principles of the discipline hitherto established in Volume I—covering the science, physics, and evolving technologies of radiation oncology—this volume II shifts the focus toward the practical, patient-centered application of radiation therapy across a diverse range of anatomical sites and cancer types.

We consider it our duty to specify the objective and context of this book. Radiation oncology is not a monolithic discipline; its clinical application must be tailored to the biological behavior, anatomical constraints, and multidisciplinary treatment goals unique to each malignancy. Globally speaking, more than 60% of all diagnosed cancer patients and nearly 40% of cancer cures are dependent upon the radiation oncology practice.

The core objective of this volume is to provide oncology students, trainees, and practicing clinicians with evidence-based, context-specific guidance on how radiation therapy can be most effectively applied for various cancers, while accounting for both curative and palliative intents.

Each chapter in this volume is structured around organ systems or tumor sites, encompassing malignancies of the head and neck, thorax, breast, gastrointestinal tract, genitourinary system, central nervous system, gynecological system, hematologic malignancies, and pediatric cancers. Within each chapter, readers will find comprehensive discussions on epidemiology, staging, prognostic factors, radiotherapy indications, treatment planning, dose regimens, organ-specific toxicity profiles, and follow-up care. Where applicable, site-specific treatment algorithms and decision trees have been included to streamline the clinical decision-making process and to help bridge the gap between theoretical knowledge and clinical practice.

This volume also reflects our commitment to multidisciplinary, patient-centered care, recognizing that radiation therapy is only one pillar of the broader cancer management paradigm. Across chapters, readers will find integrated perspectives on how radiation oncology interacts with surgical, systemic, and palliative modalities. Special emphasis has been placed on coordinated care, tumor board consensus, and shared decision-making processes, which are increasingly central to modern oncology.

This book places particular attention to clinical diversity and global applicability. Cancer care varies widely across geographic regions and economic contexts. Therefore, in addition to referencing standard guidelines and protocols from well-resourced high-income countries (HIC) settings, this volume also incorporates experiences, data, and case studies from low- and middle-income countries (LMICs). By acknowledging both the technological advantages of HICs and the ingenuity required in resource-constrained LMIC environments, we aim to ensure that this book remains relevant, adaptable, and inclusive.

Among the distinguishing features of this volume is its practical orientation, with an emphasis on general precepts of cancer care. Many chapters include insights from real-world clinical cases, highlighting nuanced decisions that radiation oncologists must make in practice—such as managing patient comorbidities, adjusting for anatomical variations, or selecting between advanced techniques like IMRT, SRS, SBRT, or brachytherapy. The role of imaging, biomarkers, and molecular profiling in refining treatment strategies is also addressed, reflecting the increasing personalization of oncologic care.

We are also mindful of the fact that clinical excellence must be coupled with compassionate patient care. Each chapter concludes with a focus on patient's quality of life, long-term survivorship, and the importance of psychosocial support. Cancer therapy can be physically and emotionally taxing, and as practitioners, we have a responsibility to address not only the disease but also the person behind the cancer diagnosis.

This volume, like its predecessor volume I, is the product of a collaborative endeavor. We are grateful to the global community of experts—radiation oncologists, medical oncologists, surgeons, pathologists, radiologists, and palliative care physicians—who contributed their knowledge, clinical wisdom, and time toward writing the 23 chapters in this book. Their collective experience has shaped a text that is as academically rigorous as it is clinically relevant.

We are deeply grateful to our publishers, Springer Nature and Byword, for their steadfast support throughout this book project of two volumes since January 2022. We extend heartfelt thanks to our editors from the publishers—Jagjeet Kaur Saini, Naren Aggarwal, and Dinesh Sinha—for their guidance and dedication. Our special appreciation goes to production editors Ejaz Ahmed, Ben Ingraham and Hemalatha Kothandaraman, whose relentless efforts were instrumental in bringing this textbook to its completion. We also acknowledge Dr. Vikas Kumar Pandey and Rahul Mehra for their consistent and invaluable day-to-day assistance during the development of this work

To our readers—whether you are medical students, radiation oncology residents, clinicians, scientists or educators—we hope that Volume II serves as a trusted companion in your clinical practice, supports your learning, and inspires your continued pursuit of excellence in patient care. We look forward to your reflections, critiques, and contributions as the field continues to evolve.

To each reader of this book, it is our hope that this volume enriches your learning and fuels your decision-making in cancer management. We eagerly welcome your thoughts, feedback, and reviews.

Bhubaneswar, Odisha, India	Bidhu K. Mohanti
New Delhi, Delhi, India	S. V. S. Deo
Mumbai, Maharashtra, India	Jai Prakash Agarwal
Mumbai, Maharashtra, India	Sarbani Ghosh Laskar
New Delhi, Delhi, India	Ahitagni Biswas
Mumbai, Maharashtra, India	Kumar Prabhash
Kolkata, West Bengal, India	Sanjoy Chatterjee
New Delhi, Delhi, India	Anusheel Munshi

04 March 2026

Contents

About the Editors

Bidhu K. Mohanti (MD) completed his residency in radiotherapy at the Postgraduate Institute of Medical Education and Research (PGIMER), Chandigarh, India; worked as faculty at Kidwai Memorial Institute of Oncology, Bangalore, and as Professor at AIIMS, New Delhi, in academic, clinical, and research areas. Currently, he is working as Emeritus Professor and Consultant in Radiation Oncology, Bagchi Sri Shankara Cancer Centre & Research Institute, Bhubaneswar, India. His clinical and basic research works are in head and neck and gastrointestinal cancers, and in palliative care. His areas of interest include the development of cancer facilities in government and private organizations. He has also been a part of the government assignment to set up the National Oncology Center at Royal Hospital, Muscat, Oman, and an expert under the IAEA, Vienna, and European Commission, Brussels, Europe. His published works cover many areas such as 200 papers in peer-reviewed national and international journals, several chapters in various books, as editor of two biomedical books, and author of a memoir.

S. V. S. Deo (MS, FACS, FRCS) completed his residency in Surgery and Surgical Oncology at AIIMS, New Delhi, and worked as Professor and Head of Department of Surgical Oncology at AIIMS, New Delhi, and at National Cancer Institute, Jhajjar, from 1995 to 2024. Currently he is the Chairman in Surgical Oncology at MAX Hospital, New Delhi. He has played a significant role in establishing the specialty of Surgical Oncology and MCh program at AIIMS, New Delhi and NCI Jhajjar. He has 34 years experience in the field of academics, research, and patient care; trained and mentored more than 200 cancer surgeons; served as advisor to Govt. of India for Cancer Control Program, Cancer Registry, and Surgical oncology training programs; published 250 articles in prestigious journals; edited 2 books; and served as President of Indian Association of Surgical Oncology (IASO), Association of Breast Surgeons of India (ABSI), and Oncology Forum, Delhi. He is member of International Advisory board of ASCO and SSO, USA.

Jai Prakash Agarwal (MD) completed his post-graduation from Tata Memorial Hospital, Mumbai. Since then he joined his alma mater as faculty in 1996 and became Professor in 2006 and subsequently as Head of the department in November 2016. Most of his work, clinical research, and scientific publications relate to head neck cancers and lung cancers in national and international journals. He is an active member of several professional societies and national committees for the development of radiation oncology facilities and access to cancer care. He has been awarded several fellowships including an honorary membership of ESTRO. He is on editorial boards on several peer-reviewed international and national scientific journals. He has been a very keen publisher of his research work, has authored and co-authored more than 400 peer-reviewed articles, and has over 6000 citations with the h-index of 37 since 2020.

Sarbani Ghosh Laskar (MD, DNB) completed her training and residency at the Tata Memorial Hospital, Mumbai. Since then, she has worked as a Senior Research Fellow for the CSIR and from 2001 working as faculty in the department of Radiation Oncology at the Tata Memorial Hospital, Mumbai. She is a recognized teacher for MD in radiation oncology. She serves as a faculty in the Head and Neck disease management group of the Institute and has a keen interest in training, quality improvement, and diverse aspects of Oncology and Radiation Oncology. She has been an expert in the multidisciplinary care of patients with head and neck cancer, with special interests in multimodality management, adjuvant therapy, surface brachytherapy, nasopharyngeal cancer, and reirradiation, to name a few areas. She has also served on Institutional Review Boards (IRB) and the Data Monitoring and Safety subunit of the IRB. She plays an active role in collaborative, multi-institutional studies, nationally and internationally. Her work has involved close collaboration with international bodies like the IAEA, ESTRO, HNCIG, etc. She has more than 85 publications in peer-reviewed journals and has authored and co-authored several textbook chapters.

Ahitagni Biswas (MD, DNB, FRCR) completed his junior residency toward MD in Radiation Oncology at All India Institute of Medical Sciences (AIIMS), New Delhi, in 2009 and subsequently did his senior residency at PGIMER Chandigarh (2009–10) and AIIMS, New Delhi (2010–12). Thereafter, he worked as a senior research associate (SRA) in neuro-oncology at AIIMS, New Delhi (2012–14) and since then as faculty in Radiation Oncology at the same institute. He cleared FRCR Clinical Oncology and MRCP Medical Oncology exams of UK in 2016 and 2017, respectively. He is currently a Professor in Radiation Oncology at AIIMS, New Delhi. He was awarded the ICMR-DHR international clinical fellowship (2024–25) at the Christie NHS Proton Beam Therapy Centre, Manchester, UK. He has 91 publications and 110 conference abstracts to his credit, which have garnered more than 1050 citations. His areas of interest include neuro-oncology, head & neck oncology, pediatric, and hematolymphoid radiation oncology.

Kumar Prabhash (MD, DM) is Professor at the Department of Medical Oncology at Tata Memorial Hospital, Mumbai. He has more than 25 years of experience in oncology. He has worked in prestigious institutes in India. He has worked at Maulana Azad Medical College, Delhi; Kidwai Memorial Institute of Oncology, Bangalore; and Tata Memorial Hospital. He has more than 400 PubMed indexed papers to his credit.

Sanjoy Chatterjee (FRCP, FRCR, FHEA) graduated from Medical College, Kolkata, with university accolades. Thereafter, he completed his residency in general medicine and was conferred the MRCP (UK) in general medicine. His super-specialty training in the UK was in clinical oncology, across centers in Dundee, Edinburgh, and Glasgow and further completed his FRCR (Clinical Oncology). He has thereafter done fellowships in prestigious institutions including the Christie Hospital, Manchester, and Royal Marsden Hospital, London. He completed his postgraduate certificate in Medical Education from the University of Dundee and was awarded the Fellowship of the Higher Education Academy of UK (FHEA). He had been practicing as a Consultant Clinical Oncologist specializing in breast and head and neck cancers. He has played an active role in setting up the services for academics and research protocols for Tata Medical Center, Kolkata. Apart from hundreds of publications in peer-reviewed indexed journals, his research endeavors include leading potentially practice changing multi-center randomized controlled trials in breast and head and neck cancers.

Anusheel Munshi (MD, DNB) is Principal Director of Radiation Oncology at the BLK MAX Hospital, New Delhi, with more than 25 years of experience in cancer care. He has worked at premier institutes across the country including at the Tata Memorial Hospital, Mumbai; All India Institute of Medical Sciences, Delhi; and the Postgraduate Institute of Medical Education and Research (PGIMER) Chandigarh, India. He has played key roles in setting up new radiation oncology facilities at Fortis Memorial Research Institute (FMRI), Gurgaon, and Manipal Hospitals, Delhi. He has published more than 150 many papers in peer-reviewed national and international journals and many of these are extensively cited. In addition, he has authored several chapters in various books, and has conducted clinical research including investigator-initiated trials in breast, brain, and lung cancers. He is reviewer for multiple international journals and member of several prestigious oncology societies.

Central Nervous System Tumours

Rakesh Jalali, Rishan Thimma Sudarsan,
Archya Dasgupta, and Debnarayan Dutta

1 Introduction

The incidence of central nervous system (CNS) tumours in India ranges from 5 to 10 per 100,000 population and accounts for 2% of all malignancies [1, 2]. Hospital-based Indian data suggests astrocytomas (38.7%) to be the most common primary tumours with the majority of astrocytomas being high-grade gliomas (59.5%). Interestingly, the median age of glial tumours was seen to be at least a decade earlier than reported in the Western population, which could be partially explained by the lower life expectancy and a higher proportion of the younger population in India [3]. However, the median age of paediatric tumours such as brainstem glioma, medulloblastoma (MB), and embryonal tumours seems to be comparable with that seen in the western population. In the paediatric age group, the most common tumour seen was astrocytoma (34.7%) followed by MB and craniopharyngioma. This was found to be comparable to data from Western countries or other Asian countries. Similar results were published from a tertiary care centre in South India reporting 15 years' experience involving 1043 patients [4]. The five most frequent tumours were astrocytoma (47.3%), MB (11.4%), craniopharyngioma (9.7%), ependymal tumours (4.8%), and nerve sheath tumours (4.1%) [5]. The standard of care for most of these brain tumours is surgery followed by radiotherapy. Chemotherapy and targeted therapy play a major role in Grades II–IV gliomas and other brain tumours. Radiotherapy, on the other hand, has evolved from conventional technique to 3D conformal, intensity-modulated radiotherapy (IMRT), stereotactic radiosurgery/radiotherapy (SRS/SRT), image-guided radiotherapy (IGRT), volumetric-modulated arc therapy (VMAT), helical tomotherapy (HT), and particle beam therapy such as passive scatter proton beam therapy (PS-PBT), image-guided intensity-modulated proton therapy (IMPT), and carbon ion therapy. This chapter addresses current status and evolving role of radiotherapy in brain tumours.

R. Jalali (✉)
Apollo Proton Cancer Centre,
Chennai, Tamil Nadu, India
e-mail: rjalali@apollohospitals.com

R. T. Sudarsan
Iswarya Hospital, Chennai, Tamil Nadu, India

A. Dasgupta
Tata Memorial Hospital, Mumbai, Maharashtra, India

D. Dutta
Amrita Institute of Medical Sciences,
Kochi, Kerala, India

2 Evolution of Modern Radiotherapy

In the past few decades, we have witnessed tremendous development in radiation therapy delivery platforms driven by technological

B. K. Mohanti et al. (eds.), *Radiation Oncology – Principles, Precepts and Practice*,
https://doi.org/10.1007/978-981-95-5171-2_1

advancements. For central nervous system (CNS) tumours, radiotherapy (RT) plays a vital role in multidisciplinary management, with target volume intricately related to several normal neural structures, demanding a high degree of conformality. Critical locations include tumours related to the brainstem, eloquent cortex, and optic structures, where adverse events can result in devastating neurological dysfunction. Due cognizance is required for structures with a well-established role in neurocognitive functioning, including the hippocampus, corpus callosum, temporal lobe, prefrontal cortex, or otherwise less understood complex interplay of diverse neural connections. Radiation techniques have evolved from 2-D to 3-D conformal and further to intensity-modulated radiotherapy (IMRT) and particle beam therapy (PBT), resulting in superior conformality for complex target volumes with complex geometrical shapes [6]. Simultaneous advancements in diagnostic imaging modalities like magnetic resonance imaging (MRI) have significantly impacted the accurate delineation of target volumes and organs at risk (OAR), more specifically in neuro-oncology management [7, 8]. MRI is preferred over other imaging techniques like computed tomography (CT) due to better soft tissue clarity, multiparametric nature, and functional sequences, and it is considered the sine qua non for the CNS radiotherapy planning process. Integration of on-board imaging to deliver IGRT has enabled in successful reduction of margins for planning target volume (PTV) and improving the accuracy and precision of treatment [9]. The traditional IGRT techniques include the cone beam computed tomography (CBCT) in conventional linear accelerators (LINAC), or megavoltage computed tomography (MVCT) in helical tomotherapy (HT). However, the volumetric-modulated arc therapy (VMAT) techniques are possible with standard LINACs and are widely used in clinical practice [10]. Another major advancement has been the development of a robotic couch with six degrees of freedom, enabling correction of rotational errors, improving treatment delivery, and using smaller PTV margins, particularly beneficial for targets in relation to the skull base, brainstem, or optic structures. In contemporary practice, most RT treatment regimens include conventionally fractionated doses spanning over approximately 5–6 weeks, with the same radiation plan undermining the temporal variations of target volumes and the OARs. Studies have demonstrated significant variations in the surgical cavities over the course of treatment, which can result in geographical miss of the target and encroachment of OARs leading to increased probabilities of toxicity [11]. The introduction of MR-LINAC in clinical practice or consideration of mid-treatment imaging forms an emerging concept of adaptive radiotherapy (ART), leading the way towards personalized radiotherapy [12, 13]. Similarly, the virtual couch shift algorithms available on certain MR-LINAC device use real-time optimization, allowing correction for set-up variations. In the recent past, proton beam therapy (PBT) has generated a lot of interest including in management of several CNS tumours. PBT has several inherent physical and biological characteristics, which utilizes delivery of little to no energy deposition distal to the target, a phenomenon known as the Bragg peak, thereby leading to zero exit dose. Evolution of technology from passive scatter towards pencil beam scanning, image guidance, and highly sophisticated physical and modern mathematical algorithms can result in literally dose painting the most complex tumour shapes with ultra-high precision including delivery of IMPT [14–18].

3 Impact of WHO 2021 Pathology Classification in Management of Brain Tumours

WHO 2021 has updated certain terminologies and has incorporated types and subtypes instead of entity and variants, and also Roman letters are replaced by Arabic numerals for grading, to show better and clearer distinction between various tumour types. Terminology such as anaplastic has been removed for better correlation, understanding and to avoid confusion among other types of tumours. Even though the classification has been relatively complex, it is imperative on the part of radiation oncologist to clinically correlate the tumour along with radiology and pathological correlation, thereby arriving at proper diagnosis, which can aid in the treatment process. It is beyond the scope of this chapter to elaborate on the entire classification, and we request the readers to refer to the actual article [19] for further clarification.

4 Imaging Protocols in Radiation Planning

With the improvement in radiation delivery techniques, accurate delineation of target volumes and organs at risk using appropriate imaging is absolutely critical. Non-contrast computed tomography (NCCT) is required for radiation planning and dose computational purposes. Typically, 2.5 mm axial CT is adequate for the majority of CNS tumours. However, thinner slices with 1–2 mm slice thickness should be considered for small volume targets, for radiosurgery planning (primary or brain metastasis), sellar/suprasellar (pituitary tumours, craniopharyngioma), skull base targets (acoustic neuroma, clival meningioma, chordoma, chondrosarcoma), orbital tumours (optic pathway glioma or meningiomas). Similarly, for larger targets like craniospinal irradiation or spinal tumours, NCCT with a 5 mm slice thickness to encompass the entire region of interest is considered adequate (separate images with thinner slice should be acquired for intracranial boost volumes). Although contrast is not essential for the majority of CNS radiotherapy, it can be considered on an individual basis for patients with contraindications for MRI, vascular lesions (cavernous angioma, meningioma), residual, or intact targets showing contrast uptake on prior imaging.

MRI is considered essential in the RT planning process, with attempts made to obtain images similar to treatment delivery. Planning MRI should be arranged close to the RT planning workflow, avoiding a long gap between MRI and radiation starting due to possible changes in the geometry of delineated (contoured) structures. Also, when treating tumours with aggressive biological behaviour like high-grade gliomas or brain metastases, the planning process should be accelerated to avoid long gaps between planning MRI and RT course delivery, in order to avoid tumour regrowth (particularly important for radiosurgery techniques where targets are usually treated with 1–2 mm margins). For intracranial targets, rigid registration of CT and MRI sequences is mostly sufficient. For the majority of CNS tumours, the basic sequences include thin slices (1–2 mm), three-dimensional fast spoiled gradient echo (3DFSPGR) and three-dimensional T2 sequences (3D T2 FLAIR/3D T2 PROPELLER), allowing accurate structural delineation of the target, OAR. Acquisition of 3D sequences allows provision of accurate reconstruction of images in all three planes, and thin slices (1–2 mm) allow more precise anatomical information (overestimation of volumes with thick slices due to volume reconstruction effects). Additional sequences should be considered on individual basis as appropriate, for example, dynamic contrast-enhanced sequences for pituitary adenomas or steady-state free precession sequences (CISS/FIESTA) for skull base lesions. Recent advances include generation of synthetic CT (pseudo-CT) for dose computation purposes from MRI avoiding the need for additional imaging in patients with CNS tumours, which is likely to be incorporated in routine clinical practice in future.

4.1 Dose Constraints

Radiation therapy from photon to particle-based therapy can be delivered via conventional or hypofractionated regimen. Some of the universally followed dose constraints for conventional and hypofractionation useful for radiation planning in brain tumours are given below in Table 1 [20].

Table 1 Common dose constraints in CNS radiotherapy

Organ	α/β (Gy)	Dose constraints (EQD2)	Toxicity
Brain	2	V60 Gy ≤3cc	Symptomatic brain necrosis
Brainstem	2	Surface D0.03cc ≤ 60 Gy Interior D0.03cc ≤ 54 Gy	Permanent cranial neuropathy/necrosis
Optic structures	2	D0.03cc ≤ 55 Gy	Optic neuropathy
Cochlea	3	D mean ≤ 45 Gy D0.03cc ≤ 32 Gy	Hearing loss Tinnitus
Cornea	3	D0.03cc ≤ 50 Gy	Ulceration/erosion
Lacrimal gland	3	D mean ≤ 25 Gy	Keratoconjunctivitis
Lens	1	D0.03cc ≤ 10 Gy	Cataract
Pituitary	2	D mean ≤ 45 Gy	Pan hypopituitarism
Hippocampi	2	D40 ≤ 7.3 Gy Mean (left) < 30 Gy	Memory loss
Retina	3	D0.03cc ≤ 45 Gy	Loss of vision
Skin	2	D0.03cc ≤ 25 Gy	Permanent alopecia

4.2 Gliomas

4.2.1 Diffusely Infiltrating Gliomas/High-Grade Gliomas (HGG)

The standard of care for glioblastoma (GBM) is surgery followed by radiotherapy with Temozolomide (TMZ) (Fig. 1) [21, 22]. The gross tumour volume for RT planning includes the T1-enhanced region with 2 cm clinical target volume and considering all relevant T2/FLAIR abnormality.

Dose and fractionation, depending upon the patient's prognosis:

- Favorable Prognosis patients: 59.4–60 Gy in 30 fractions over 6 weeks.
- Poor Prognosis patients: 35–40 Gy in 10–15 fractions over 2 weeks.

Altered radical fractionation schemes giving higher effective doses as accelerated hyperfractionated or hypofractionated regimens have not been shown to be associated with survival benefit [23, 24]. The addition radiosurgery/stereotactic radiotherapy boost also does not prolong survival. In gliomatosis cerebri, whole brain radiotherapy to doses of 45–50 Gy or more achieves disease control in a proportion of carefully selected patients [25, 26]. Various trials conducted earlier wanted to answer whether dose escalation was superior in glioblastomas. Trials included dose escalation of more than 60 Gy (66–90 Gy) with external beam radiotherapy, SRT, brachytherapy boost but did not show any improved outcomes [17, 18, 27, 28]. However, some recent data revealed moderate dose escalation up to 66 Gy was associated with a suggestion of improved median overall survival [29, 30]. Some early data suggested PBT is superior to conventional radiotherapy in improving outcomes with median survival of 45.9 versus 29.7 months, with a median follow-up of 62.1 months [31]. A recent NRG-BN001 is underway to show the efficacy of photon versus proton dose escalation compared to the standard dose radiation therapy, where dosage of up to 75 Gy both in photon and proton arms were used. Group 1 results with Dose Intense (DI) IMRT showed median overall survival of 18.7 months versus 16.3 months with standard dose RT (statistically not significant) [32]. Number of cycles of adjuvant temozolomide that has to be given still remains a debate, as to whether six or twelve cycles are enough. Results from the CATNON trial comparing concurrent and adjuvant TMZ with RT in non codeleted anaplastic gliomas showed that, adjuvant and not concurrent TMZ, especially in IDH mutant patients was associated with significant survival benefit with a median overall survival of 82.3 months versus 46.9 months (with and without adjuvant TMZ) respectively [33]. Hence, one can consider the usage of 12 cycles of adjuvant temozolomide in IDH mutant tumours extrapolating the same.

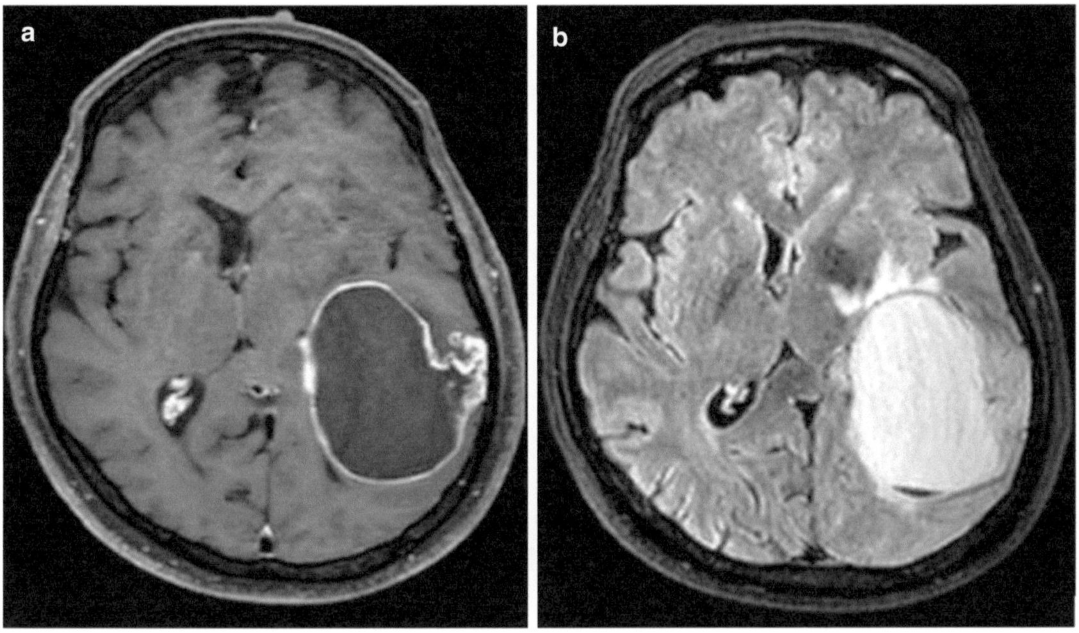

Fig. 1 MRI image showing high-grade glioma (Glioblastoma), (**a**) contrast, (**b**) FLAIR image

4.2.2 Role of Lymphopenia in Brain Tumours

One of the niche areas during treatment of brain tumours is the association of radiotherapy with body's immune system. Radiotherapy has been shown to be associated with lymphopenia, and host immunosuppression, thereby leading to inferior outcomes for high grade gliomas and other types of tumours [34, 35]. Correction of lymphopenia is complex and may range from depletion of regulatory T-cell population, shifting of bone marrow derived suppressor cells including macrophages away from immunosuppressive phenotypes to altered systemic therapy and usage of cytokines that stimulate lymphocyte proliferation and other pathways. Recent data suggest that female sex, baseline absolute lymphocyte count and whole brain dose receiving V25 were the most significant prognostic indicators for Grade 3 lymphopenia, which may be associated with decreased overall survival. PBT, by virtue of its reduced dosage to nearby structures, leads to sparing of circulating lymphocyte population, thereby resulting in reduced Grade 3 lymphopenia (14% vs 39%) and may potentially improve outcomes also [36]. Data for mature results of this intervention is awaited.

4.2.3 Role of Subventricular Zonal Irradiation

Glioblastoma progenitor or stem cells residing in the stem-cell niche in the subventricular zones (SVZ) and subgranular zones (SGZ) are known to be associated with initiation or promotion of tumourigenesis. They can also migrate throughout the brain, resulting in disease progression. Numerous studies have analysed the pros and cons of irradiating the SVZ/SGZ including local control against the potential side effects including neurocognitive deficits and potential repair of normal brain tissues post treatment. So far, studies done showed mixed results in overall survival or local control; however, it did show that tumours that are close to the ventricles or extending onto contralateral SVZ are associated with inferior local control and overall survival [37–40].

4.2.4 Diffusely Intermediate Low/ Lower Grade Gliomas (LGG)

Management options for these tumours have ranged from observation to a biopsy for histological confirmation to aggressive radical resections followed by adjuvant radiotherapy with or without additional chemotherapy. Hence, the goal of treatment for patients with these tumours include prolonging overall and progression-free survival and minimizing morbidity. Recent clinical and molecular insights are helping shape more evidence based optimal management in this group of patients. Molecular markers have been incorporated in the recent WHO classification of CNS tumour updates [19]. Surgery alone may not be curative in patients with diffuse intermediate-low grade glioma, and additional treatment may be required**.** Factors to consider when selecting patients for immediate postoperative therapy include the presence of tumour-related symptoms and risk factors, which include age ≥ 40 years, large preoperative tumour size (e.g. ≥5 cm), incomplete resection, astrocytic histology, elevated MIB-1 index (>3%), and absence of a 1p/19q-codeletion [41]. Alkylating chemotherapy using the PCV regimen initially and TMZ more recently has assumed a firm place in the treatment of patients with low grade gliomas. The RTOG 9802 trial comparing RT alone or RT followed by six cycles of PCV chemotherapy showed that the PFS at 10 years was 51% in the group that received radiation therapy plus chemotherapy versus 21% in the group that received radiation therapy alone; the corresponding rates of overall survival at 10 years were 60% and 40% respectively [42].

This management approach has been particularly adopted as per evidence gathered from two large cooperative group trials (RTOG 9402 and RTOG 0424 studies). RTOG 9402 was a phase III trial of chemo-radiotherapy for patients with Grade 3 oligodendroglioma has shown favourable results with PCV plus RT versus RT alone with median PFS of 9.8 versus 2.9 years and median OS of 13.2 versus 7.3 years respectively [43]. RTOG 0424 investigated hazardous high risk LGG (LGG) treated with TMZ and RT, and results were contrasted with those of historic controls. The 3-year OS rate was 73.5%, which was significantly improved compared to that of historical control of 54%. Five- and 10-year OS were 60.9% and 34.6%, respectively [44]. CODEL was a phase III Intergroup study of TMZ alone versus radiotherapy with concomitant and adjuvant TMZ versus radiotherapy with adjuvant PCV chemotherapy in patients with 1p/19q co-deleted anaplastic glioma or low-grade glioma (Fig. 2). TMZ alone treated patients experienced shorter PFS, OS, and time to death from progression versus those treated with RT or RT + TMZ. Based on initial reports the TMZ alone arm was closed, also the RT alone arm was closed based on reports of RTOG 9402 trial. CODEL is currently ongoing as a two-arm comparison of RT + adjuvant PCV versus RT + concomitant/adjuvant TMZ [45]. It is to be noted that a majority of Grade 3 oligodendroglioma are in young age group, those with IDH-mutant 1p/19q codeleted (codel) histology, would show improved survival and tumor control when adjuvant PCV+RT is delivered compared to the standard TMZ+RT.

Radiation Dose 54–59.4 Gy in 30–33 fractions with concurrent TMZ followed by 6-12 monthly adjuvant TMZ cycles. However, emerging interest is in giving 54–55.8 Gy in 31 fractions in co-deleted Grade 3 oligodendroglioma.

Role of PBT in low-grade gliomas are well noted, with the fact that it spares normal brain tissue and other organs at risk. Studies have shown that PBT is superior in reducing dose to developing brain tissue resulting in acceptable toxicities, without compromising on disease control, thereby preserving neurocognitive function and quality of life [46, 47]. Prospective data from a series involving adult LGG with a median follow-up of 5.1 years showed OS at 1, 3, and 5 years were 100%, 95%, and 84%, respectively, and corresponding PFS at 1, 3, and 5 years were 100%, 85%, and 40% [48]. A recent randomized NRG-BN005 trial is assessing PBT in comparison to IMRT in preservation of cognitive outcomes as measured by Clinical Trial Battery Composite (CTB-COMP) score which is calculated from the Hopkins Verbal learning test [49].

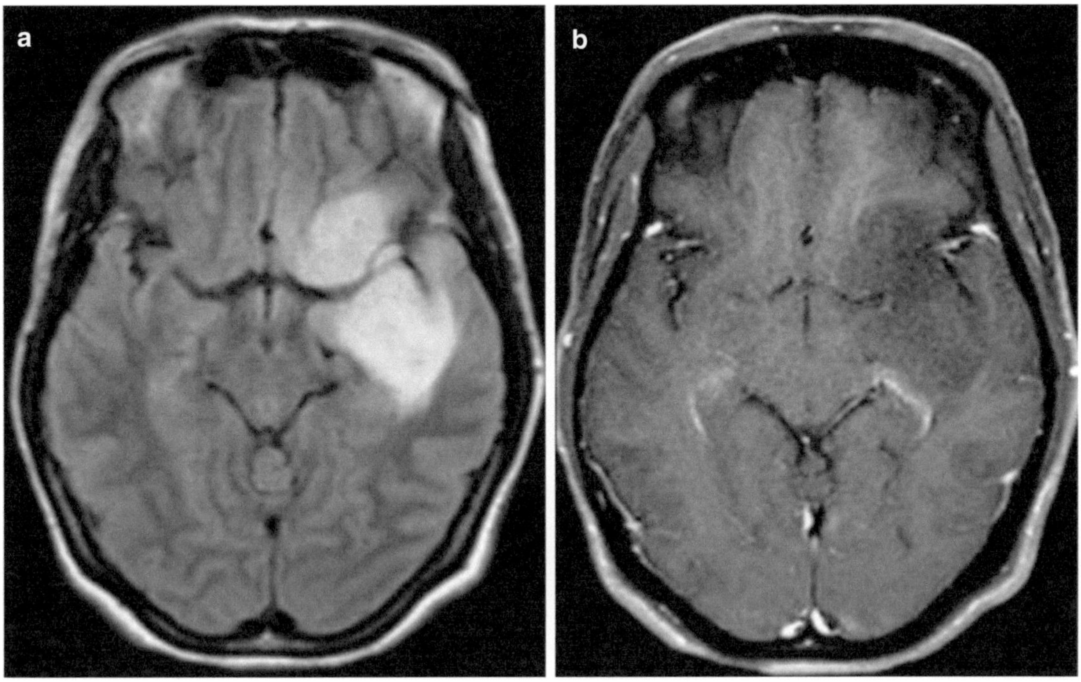

Fig. 2 MRI image showing low-grade glioma, (**a**) FLAIR, (**b**) contrast (no enhancement)

4.2.5 Diffuse Midline Gliomas

Brain stem gliomas are usually not amenable to radical surgical resection, and hence if a biopsy is feasible, it is advisable to proceed with the same followed by RT (Fig. 3). Role of TMZ was analysed in various trials in diffuse midline gliomas, however, did not improve outcomes compared to RT alone. The prognosis remains poor even if treated with various RT modalities reinforcing the aggressiveness of these tumours [50, 51]. Molecular analyses are being investigated, as these tumours are more prone for H3K27M alterations, where a prospective trial is ongoing, assessing the benefits of selective Dopamine receptor agonist (DRD2), ONC 201. Preliminary results from the ONC-201 study shows favourable clinical and radiological outcomes compared to historical cohorts [52]. Trials such as ONC 206, CAR-T cell and oncolytic viruses are underway for further hope in the future.

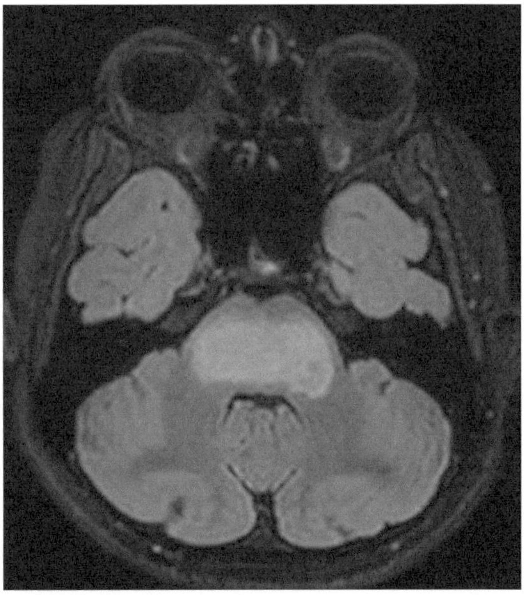

Fig. 3 MRI image showing brain stem glioma (diffuse midline glioma) (T2 FLAIR)

4.2.6 Hemispheric Gliomas

The recent WHO 2021 classification [19] considers this as a specific entity, which comprise of H3F3A G34R mutant gliomas, that most frequently involved the parietal lobe (Fig. 4), more frequently presented as hemorrhagic tumour at

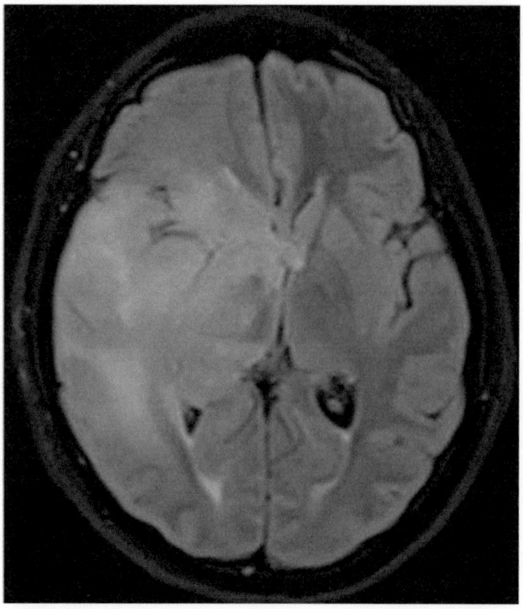

Fig. 4 T2 FLAIR image showing hemispheric glioma (H3F3A G34R/V mutant)

diagnosis, less frequently demonstrated contrast-enhancement and necrosis, displayed ADC restriction with less expression of OLIG2 [53]. TERT promoter mutations were lacking in these tumours in contrary to IDH wildtype glioblastomas, while MGMT promoter methylation were more frequent in these tumours. They comprise of 1% of all gliomas but in 15% of high-grade gliomas in adolescents and young adults. Treatment paradigm is same as that of high-grade gliomas, however, has better prognosis than H3K27M counterpart; and remains to be seen in randomized controlled trials [54].

5 Radiotherapy for Paediatric CNS Tumours

5.1 Embryonal Tumours

The classification and nomenclature of embryonal tumours have witnessed paradigm shifts in the recent WHO editions for classifying CNS tumours. Medulloblastoma is one of the common malignant brain tumours in the paediatric age group and is encountered less frequently in the adolescent and adult age groups (Fig. 5). Groundbreaking research in the past two decades has unfolded the underlying molecular pathogenesis of medulloblastoma, with the identification of distinct molecular subgroups, with distinct genomic profile, demographics, and clinical outcomes. The 2012 consensus considered four molecular subgroups as wingless (WNT), sonic hedgehog (SHH), Group 3, and Group 4 [55]. Given the stark differences in biological behaviour, the recent WHO classifications have acknowledged the molecular information in defining medulloblastoma. While ongoing clinical trials are exploring risk-adapted treatment strategies to find the optimal balance between cure and treatment-related adverse effects incorporating molecular information, we discuss the current standard treatment protocols in medulloblastoma. Maximal safe resection is the first line of treatment, which helps establish tissue diagnosis and reversal of neurological symptoms. Staging investigations with appropriately scheduled (<48 h or >2 weeks from surgery) post-operative MRI brain (to detect residual disease) and spine (>2 weeks from surgery to avoid false-positive findings) to detect macroscopic disease spread (if not undertaken pre-operatively), and cerebrospinal fluid (CSF) studies (cytology and biochemistry) to detect microscopic disease is required to decide further adjuvant therapy. Any one of the factors such as age < 3 years, residual tumour >1.5 cm^2, or metastatic disease is considered a high-risk disease, while the absence of all three is treated as standard-risk or average-risk medulloblastoma [56, 57]. Currently, there are well-established adverse prognostic impact features such as large cell anaplastic (LCA) histology, TP53 mutation in SHH subgroup, MYC amplification in Group 3, or loss of chromosome 11 in Group 4 medulloblastoma each feature needs to be treated as high-risk disease [58].

Craniospinal irradiation (CSI) forms the cornerstone of medulloblastoma management. Reduced-dose CSI 23.4 Gy in 13 fractions and boost to primary tumour bed (TB) to a dose of 30.6 Gy in 17 fractions is considered in average-risk medulloblastoma [57]. Following completion of RT, patients are treated with 6–8 cycles of

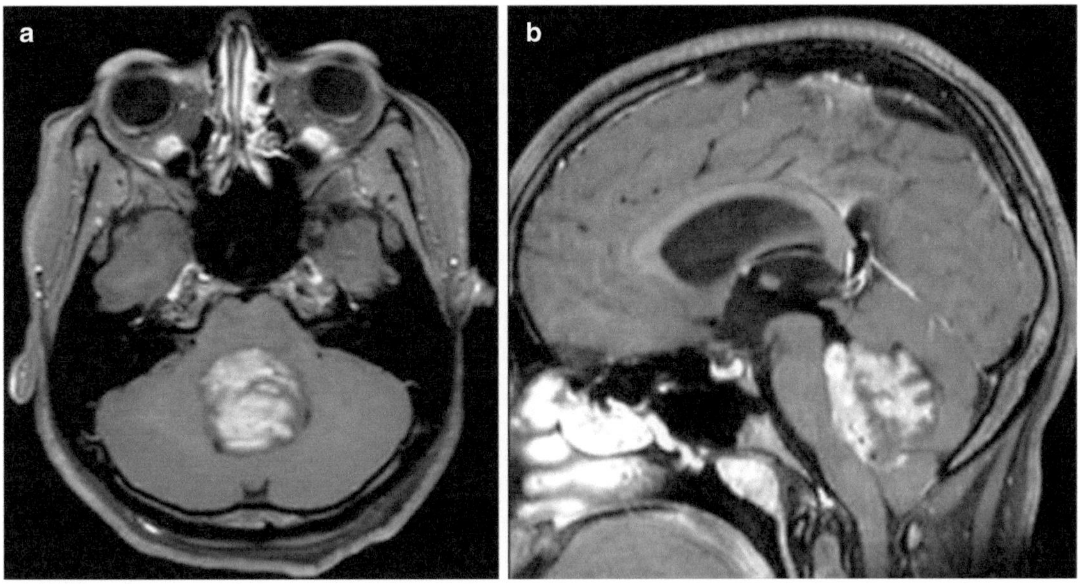

Fig. 5 MRI image showing medulloblastoma in T1C sequences (**a** axial, **b** sagittal)

adjuvant chemotherapy with cisplatin, lomustine, vincristine or cisplatin, cyclophosphamide, and vincristine. The ACNS 0331 trial demonstrated the safety of reduction of boost volume (tumor bed volume instead of posterior fossa) for average-risk medulloblastoma. In the same study, the reduction of CSI dose to 18 Gy was associated with higher failure rates precluding the use of such dose in generalized average-risk medulloblastoma [59]. However, the role of reduced dose CSI (15–18 Gy) with chemotherapy is being investigated in average-risk WNT-driven medulloblastoma, which is associated with excellent long-term outcomes. The latest published FORWNT trial shows that omission of CSI is associated with high risk of neuraxial failure, and hence, the second study, FOR-WNT2 is underway to address the role of reduced dose CSI in medulloblastomas [60, 61]. In post-pubertal children (>15 years) and adults, chemotherapy sparing approach can be considered in average-risk medulloblastoma due to poor compliance to chemotherapy. Standard dose CSI with 35–36 Gy in 20–21 fractions followed by tumor bed (TB) boost of 18–19.8 Gy in 10–11 fractions is used in such setting. A similar dose of RT (CSI 35–36 Gy and TB boost) is given for high-risk medulloblastoma followed to 6–8 cycles of chemotherapy as mentioned previously. In patients with disseminated leptomeningeal disease, higher dose of CSI 39.4–40 Gy in 22–24 fractions followed by boost of 14.4 Gy in 8 fractions and a boost of 5.4–9 Gy in 3–5 fractions to other significant metastatic sites is often considered. Concurrent chemotherapy with carboplatin along with CSI in given high-risk disease (metastatic disease or LCA histology). Results of a randomized controlled trial using concurrent carboplatin from the Children's Oncology Group (COG) and an Indian study had shown improvement of 5-year event-free survival by 19% in high-risk Group 3 medulloblastoma [62, 63]. Children less than 3 years of age, can be treated with pre-radiation chemotherapy, to avoid the detrimental effects on premature neural tissue; however, care must be taken to see that too much delay in implementing radiotherapy is also detrimental, and must be jointly decided as per multidisciplinary board discussion. One can also consider the usage of modern intensity modulated proton beam therapy to avoid side effects to nearby organs at risk. Radiation sparing approaches with the use of high-dose myeloablative chemotherapy with autologous hematopoietic stem-cell rescue (avoiding RT until progression or for residual disease or reduced volume) is practiced by several groups, which need appropriate facilities for such intensive regimens.

As discussed, craniospinal irradiation forms a crucial part of treatment for embryonal tumours or less frequently in other malignancies with CSF dissemination treated with radical intent (e.g., ependymoma, germ cell tumours). Delineation of target volume for CSI is critical, with special attention needed to encompass all the CSF spaces, including the cribriform plate, inferior temporal aspect, sella, skull base, spinal nerve roots, the lower limit of thecal sac [64]. The technical delivery of CSI is often challenging due to the length of the target volumes as well as appropriate PTV margins. Depending upon availability and expertise, CSI treatment delivery can be considered using 3D conformal, IMRT, Helical Tomotherapy, VMAT, or proton beam therapy (Fig. 6) [65–67]. When multiple fields are used to encompass the entire target (particularly for 3D conformal techniques), including cranial-spinal field geometry, it is important to consider strategies to mitigate the effect of dosimetric uncertainties at the field junctions using techniques like moving junction. Appropriate delivery of CSI with good quality control is absolutely essential for therapeutic success as protocol deviations have shown higher incidences of failures [68].

One of the landmark studies regarding PBT versus photon therapy in MBs tried to assess the intellectual outcomes associated with treatment of CSI with PBT and photon therapy. In this study, longitudinal intelligence data from 79 patients were examined over the years 2007–2018. PBT showed superior intellectual outcomes in terms of global intelligence quotient (IQ), perceptual reasoning, working memory, verbal reasoning compared to photon group, with no difference in processing speed in both the arms [69]. Similarly, another study assessed 125 patients and demonstrated favourable outcomes in both intelligence and processing speed with PBT compared to photon therapy [70]. Other tox-

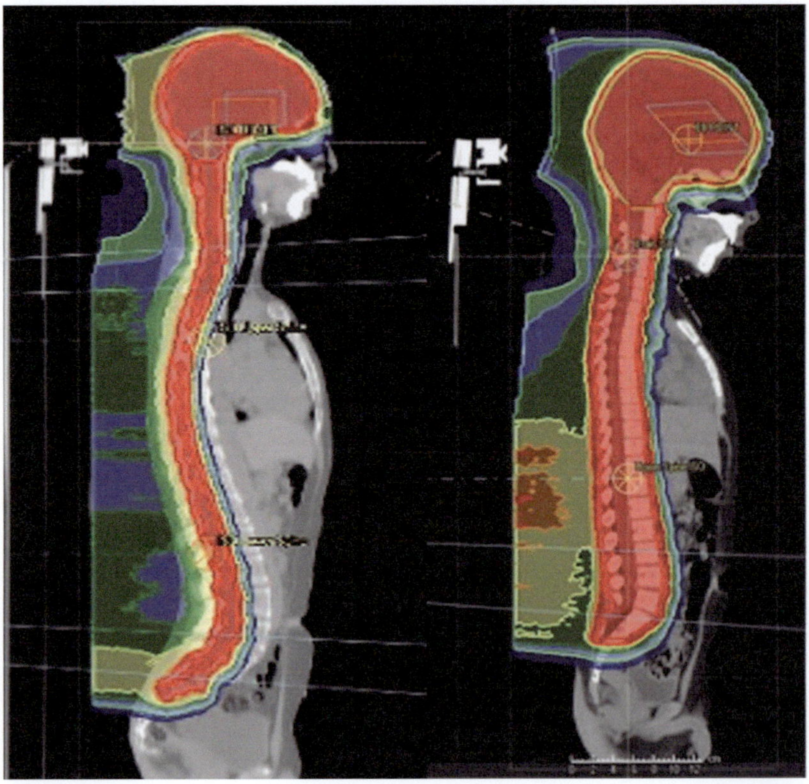

Fig. 6 Dose distribution of paediatric CSI with intensity modulated proton therapy (IMPT) in an adult and paediatric patient

icities such as haematological toxicity with reduction in lymphopenia and thrombocytopenia was seen with PBT compared to conventional RT [71]. Risk of second malignant neoplasms (SMN) were also less with PBT compared to conventional RT with crude rate of SMN being 5.2% versus 7.5%, respectively [72–74].

Other embryonal tumours are encountered less frequently, including atypical teratoid/ rhabdoid tumour (ATRT), embryonal tumour with multilayered rosettes (ETMR) (Fig. 7), CNS neuroblastoma FOXR2-activated, CNS tumour with BCOR internal tandem duplication, CNS embryonal tumour. Given the rarity of the rarity of these disease entities, there is a lack of consensus on standard treatment protocols with varied practice across different institutions utilizing different regimens of chemotherapy and radiation. Multi-institutional clinical trials are mandated in the future to develop optimal strategies. ETMR and ATRT are associated with poor prognosis with median survival ranging between 1 and 2 years with the of these tumours are seen in young children <3 years. Despite younger age group, in many institutions, these tumours are often treated

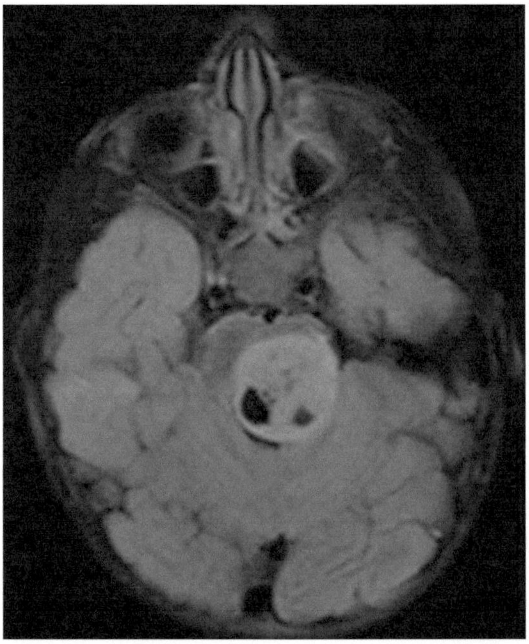

Fig. 7 T2 FLAIR image showing ETMR in posterior fossa embryonal tumor

with RT, since adverse effects of RT are less likely to make a clinical impact due to lack of long-term survivors. In the infantile age group, chemotherapy and focal RT to the resection site can be considered. Otherwise, in children >3 year, standard dose CSI of 35–36 Gy followed by boost of 18–19.8 Gy to the primary tumour bed is considered, followed by adjuvant chemotherapy. The ACNS0333 trial by the COG reported 4-year overall survival of 43% in AT/RT using 2 cycles of induction chemotherapy (methotrexate, vincristine, etoposide, cyclophosphamide, cisplatin) followed by 3 cycles of high-dose myeloablative chemotherapy with carboplatin and thiotepa with autologous stem-cell rescue and focal RT (50.4 Gy in <3 years and 54 Gy otherwise) [75].

5.2 Paediatric Gliomas

Paediatric gliomas include a diverse spectrum of tumours including circumscribed gliomas (pilocytic astrocytoma, high-grade astrocytoma with piloid features, subependymal giant cell astrocytoma, etc.), diffuse low-grade glioma (diffuse astrocytoma MYB or MYBL1-altered, diffuse low-grade glioma MAPK pathway-altered, etc.) or high-grade gliomas (diffuse midline glioma H3 K27-altered, diffuse hemispheric glioma H3 G34-mutant, diffuse high-glioma H3-wildtype and IDH-wildtype, infant-type hemispheric glioma) as per 2021 WHO classification. For paediatric gliomas, it is essential to elicit appropriate history and perform a detailed clinical examination to find syndromic associations like neurofibromatosis type 1 (NF 1), constitutional mismatch repair deficiency (CMMRD), Li-Fraumeni syndrome, etc.

Paediatric low-grade glioma (PLGG) is mostly driven by the activation of the RAS/ MAPK pathway, with BRAF-KIAA 1549 fusion seen in pilocytic astrocytoma associated with good prognosis (Fig. 8), BRAF V600E mutations in pleomorphic xanthoastrocytoma (PXA), ganglioglioma, a minority of pilocytic astrocytoma having relatively worse clinical outcomes [76]. Other less common genetic alterations in PLGG include

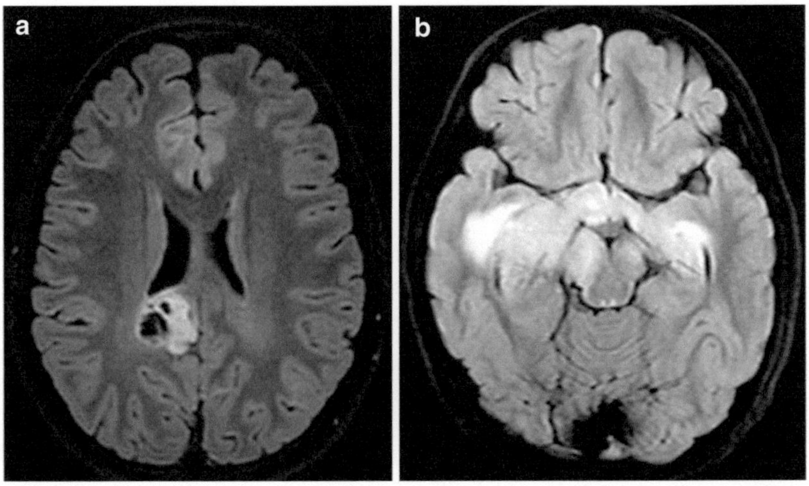

Fig. 8 T2 FLAIR images showing a small pilocytic astrocytoma (**a**) and large optic-chiasmatic pilocytic astrocytoma (**b**)

FGFR alterations, ALK, ROS, NTRK, and PDGFB fusions. Given the young age at diagnosis and excellent long-term survival, decision regarding radiation needs to be carefully considered and discussed on multidisciplinary tumour boards. Circumscribed gliomas with BRAF fusions can be observed following gross total resection, monitored with annual imaging surveillance. Subtotal resection, disease recurrence, absence of BRAF fusions need discussion on an individual basis for initiation of further therapy. Radiation is an effective modality to improve the control rates in PLGG. Conformal RT using IMRT/ VMAT techniques are used with smaller CTV margins (5 mm) to the residual/ recurrent disease and tumour bed to deliver doses of 50.4–54 Gy over 28–30 fractions. In a group of 117 patients with pilocytic astrocytoma treated with RT (upfront or progression after primary chemotherapy), 10-year progression-free survival and overall survival were 70% and 97%, respectively [77]. No benefit in tumour control was demonstrated with doses higher than 50.4 Gy. The use of daily image guidance enables using smaller PTV margins (2–3 mm) with robotic 6D couch should be used when possible. Since a majority of the patients will be controlled for disease, PBT may be preferred when feasible to reduce radiation spillage to the OARs. In infants and younger children, chemotherapy with low-grade glioma regimens using vincristine, carboplatin (VC), thioguanine, procarbazine, lomustine, vincristine (TPCV), or single-agent vinblastine can be considered [78, 79]. With the understanding of molecular pathways, the role of targeted therapy with the use of BRAF and MEK inhibitors is emerging, particularly for relapsed PLGG [80, 81].

High-grade gliomas (HGG) in the paediatric and adolescent age group are often contributed by histone alterations associated with a dismal prognosis. Due to difficult locations of diffuse midline gliomas not feasible for major tumour debulking, radiation is the mainstay of treatment following biopsy to obtain a histopathological and molecular diagnosis. 3D conformal or IMRT techniques using wider CTV margins (10–20 mm) beyond the gross tumour is considered to deliver 55.8–59.4 Gy in 31–33 fractions. Although the benefit of chemotherapy is debatable for these tumours, concurrent and adjuvant TMZ should be considered as per adult high-grade glioma protocols till further evidence are available. Other p-HGG are treated similarly like their adult counterparts with radiation and TMZ, and due cognizance is to be given to limit higher doses to optic structures or brainstem (D_{max} < 56–57 Gy). Diffuse intrinsic pontine gliomas (DIPG) are diagnosed using clinico-radiological criteria with the presence of cranial nerve palsies, motor tract signs, and on radiological >50% involvement of axial diameter of pons, exophytic growth into prepontine cistern. Radiotherapy using 3D conformal or IMRT techniques to deliver 54Gy in 30 fractions often leads to clinical improvement, although the prognosis continues to be universally poor. Several studies have demonstrated the absence of benefit of chemotherapy in DIPG and can be omitted from treatment protocols.

5.3 Ependymomas

Ependymomas (Fig. 9) are more commonly seen in the paediatric age group compared to adults. The location of ependymomas can include both brain (supratentorial and infratentorial) and spine and can be Grades 1–3. With insights from molecular pathology, several distinct ependymoma subtypes have been identified, with genetic alterations-ZFTA fusion-positive supratentorial and post fossa ependymoma, subtype PFA associated with aggressive biological behaviour. Radiation is indicated in ependymomas with subtotal resection or higher grade ependymomas (including subtypes with poor prognosis). Conformal techniques to deliver doses of 54–59.4 Gy in 30–33 fractions (higher dose for higher grades) to the tumour bed, residual disease with 5–10 mm are used. A recent series including a large cohort of 179 children with grade 2/3 intracranial ependymomas treated with PBT reported 3-year local control and overall survival of 85% and 90%, respectively [82]. In the recent WHO classification, myxopapillary ependymomas (MPE) are typically located in the conus medullaris; the grading was revised to be considered Grade 2 ependymomas. For MPE with gross total excision or near-total excision, radiation can be avoided in the majority, with patients monitored with serial imaging and reserved as a salvage therapy during further progression. Other grade 2/3 spinal ependymomas should be offered focal radiation to a dose of 50.4–54 Gy in 28–30 fractions, giving due respect to spinal cord tolerance. Following treatment completion, a majority of ependymomas encounter local recurrence, which can be treated with a repeat course of reirradiation, provided a sufficient interval from the first of RT (>2 years). In a cohort of 55 patients with recurrent ependymoma, reirradiation (surgery in 84%) provided promising outcomes with 3-year progression-free survival and overall survival of 40% and 51%, respectively [83]. Craniospinal reirradiation in the recurrent setting can be considered in carefully selected patients with disseminated disease or in the presence of features with a higher chance of metastatic relapse (1q gain for PFA ependymomas).

5.4 Germ Cell Tumours

Intracranial germ cell tumours (ICGCT) form the most common extragonadal location for germ cell tumours, more commonly seen in the paedi-

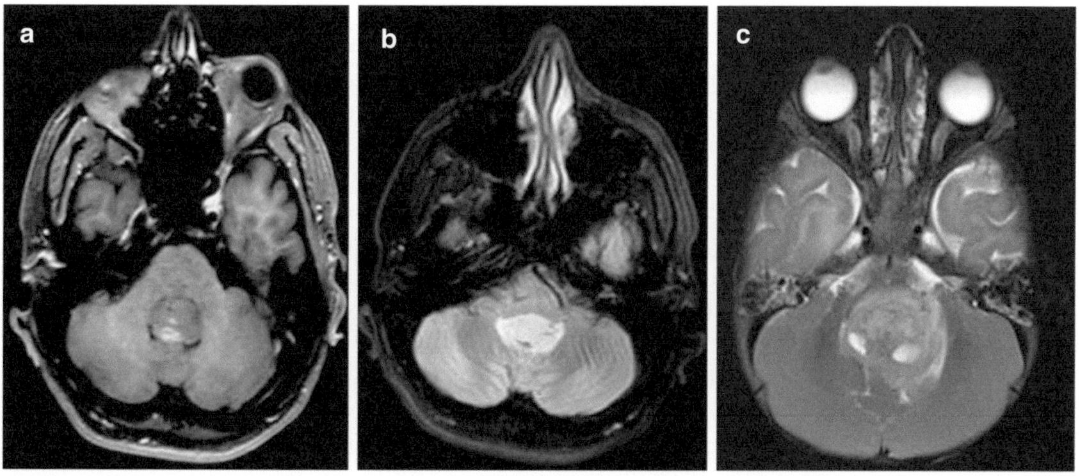

Fig. 9 MRI image showing ependyoma (**a** contrast, **b** FLAIR, **c** T2)

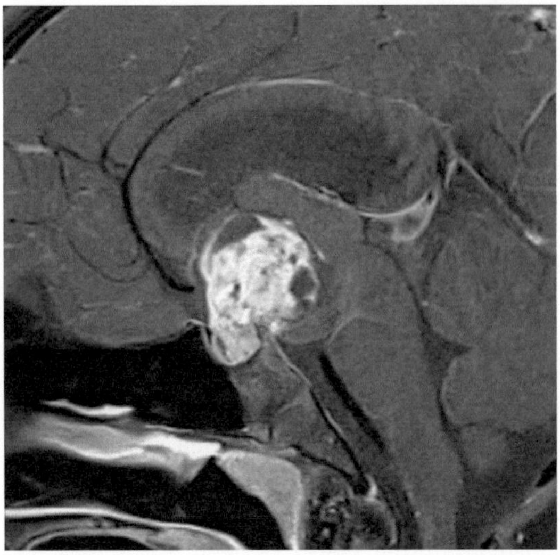

Fig. 10 T1 contrast image showing mixed germ cell tumour (sagittal)

atric and adolescent age group, constituting <1% of primary CNS tumours. The ICGCT are classified as germinoma (with 5-year survival >90%) and non-germinomatous germ cell tumours (NGGCT) (Fig. 10), which can have components of embryonal carcinoma, yolk sac tumour, choriocarcinoma, or teratoma (5-year survival 50%–90%) [84]. Common locations include pineal (approximately 50%), suprasellar, bifocal (pineal and suprasellar), and basal ganglia. ICGCT is diagnosed using radiological, biochemical criteria (tumour markers beta-HCG and AFP in CSF and serum), and histopathology. Contrast-enhanced sagittal screening of the entire spine should be considered mandatory in all patients before initiation of therapy. The current treatment paradigms include the use of chemotherapy with regimens having cisplatin/ carboplatin, cyclophosphamide/ ifosfamide, and etoposide. For localised germinomas, treatment protocols include 4 cycles of chemotherapy followed by 24–25 Gy of whole ventricular irradiation (WVI), and boost to the primary site to deliver a total dose of 40 Gy (using fraction size of 1.67–1.8 Gy). Conformal RT techniques with IMRT, VMAT should be considered in all patients to reduce normal tissue doses, with recent emerging reports of encouraging results using proton beam therapy [85]. In the recently reported ACNS1123 trial, a response-based RT was used for localized germinomas, with consideration of 18 Gy WVI and 12 Gy to tumour bed for complete responders to 4 cycles of carboplatin and etoposide chemotherapy [86]. With the trial failing to demonstrate non-inferiority with 3-year progression-free survival of 86.5%, future studies are warranted to explore alternative de-escalation strategies. For NGGCT, treatment includes 6 cycles of chemotherapy followed by CSI 30–35 Gy and the tumour bed boosted to a total dose of 54 Gy. In the recently published results from a pooled analysis of several clinical trials, metastatic relapses presenting within the first year were the most common pattern of recurrence encountered for NGGCT [87].

6 Skull Base Tumours

Skull base tumours represent a diverse spectrum of histological entities like chordoma, chondrosarcoma, meningioma, acoustic neuroma, craniopharyngioma, pituitary tumours, osteosarcoma, or other subcranial tumours with upward extension to skull base like sinonasal carcinoma, nasopharyngeal carcinoma, adenoid cystic carcinoma, etc. The management of tumours is often challenging due to its relation with critical structures like brainstem, cranial nerves, neural foramina, cavernous sinus, precluding complete surgical debulking as well as technical challenges. Radiation delivery also needs to be precise for skull base tumours mandating strict immobilization techniques, IMRT/VMAT techniques with daily image guidance, and the use of 6D couch whenever available. Dedicated MRI protocols should be adopted in the routine workflow using 3D sequences, and consideration of additional sequences like CISS/FIESTA provide merit in planning process. In this section, we will limit our discussion to skull base chordomas and chondrosarcomas, with other CNS tumours discussed in respective sections. Intracranial chordomas and chondrosarcomas are mostly seen in relation to the clivus. Chordomas usually represent more aggressive biology, with higher rates of relapses (local recurrence seen in the majority of patients).

Chondrosarcomas have relatively better clinical outcomes, which is further dependent on the variants, low grade and high grade or mesenchymal variants. Following surgical resection, RT is considered for most tumours due to subtotal resection in the majority and high-grade histology. Typically doses higher than 70 Gy needs to be considered for chordomas (76–78 Gy), limiting Dmax to the brainstem surface (<66–70 Gy, as reported by different series); and 70–72 Gy for high-grade chondrosarcomas. Adequate delivery of higher dose has resulted in 5-year local control of 50%–80%, with <10% > Grade 2 toxicities of temporal necrosis or brainstem necrosis, and 20%–50% cranial neuropathies (resulting from tumour also) [88]. For centres not equipped with 6D couch or robust image guidance protocols need to consider tighter constraints for brainstem PRV (<60–63 Gy) or ideally should consider referral to an appropriate facility. There has been a significant body of literature reporting promising outcomes with the use of proton beam therapy or heavy ion therapy, enabling delivery of higher biological doses resulting from better conformality resulting in skull base tumours a foremost indication for such high-end therapies. Encouraging results from our own experience have been published in treating these tumours using modern image guided pencil beam scanning proton beam therapy [89].

7 Benign Brain Tumours

7.1 Meningiomas

Meningiomas are the most common primary intracranial tumours, of which most are classified as WHO Grade I, with a minority being classified as WHO Grade II or III based on the local invasiveness and cellular features of atypia. For symptomatic and growing tumours, surgery is the primary treatment modality, which can achieve long-term tumour control, and in many cases can be curative. However, despite surgical advances, not all are amenable to surgical resection in view of proximity to critical neurovascular structures or tumour consistency. Furthermore, even if meningiomas are completely resected, recurrences can still occur. Due to this fact, radiotherapy have always had a clear role in the management of meningiomas to achieve a durable long-term control. Meningiomas are classified according to the WHO classifications based on their histological appearance, divided into 15 subtypes, and on various aggressiveness criteria (mitoses, necrosis, and cellular aspect). Majority of the meningiomas (around 80%) are grade I benign tumours [90], while atypical Grade II includes 4%–15% of meningiomas and malignant Grade III account for 1%–3% of cases. Recent WHO 2021 classification has not recommended any modification in existing histology and grading of these tumours. High-grade meningiomas are notorious for recurrence, and despite this, our understanding of genomic profiling in these tumours remains incomplete. Genomic profiling varies with grades of meningiomas, notorious being chromosome 22q loss associated with Neurofibromatosis-2 (NF-2). In addition, low-grade meningiomas are noted to have AKT1 and 3, PIK3CA, TERT, and SMO are also associated with proto-oncogenic pathways downstream. However, high-grade meningiomas are noted to have NF-2 mutations mainly, with other mutations like loss of chromosome 18q and loss of CDKN2A/2B in case of Grade 2 and in case of Grade 3 meningiomas, significant mutations other than NF-2 with clinical implications are yet to be identified. Even in cases of non-NF-2, 25% of the patients with chromosome 22q loss might exhibit cryptic NF-2 inactivating events. Also, TERT mutations are associated with reduced survival in meningiomas [91–93]. Loss of H3K27me3 is also found to be associated with increased risk of recurrence in meningioma [94].

Radiotherapy (RT) has always been an integral part in the multimodal management of meningiomas. Numerous studies have showed significant role of radiotherapy in local control and reducing recurrences in large meningiomas, either sub optimally excised or as the only treatment in inoperable tumours. RT has also become a first-line option for some meningiomas, particularly skull base lesions encasing vasculo-nervous structures such as the optic nerve sheath or the cavernous sinus. Technological advancements in precise delivery of modern conformal radiotherapy like stereotactic RT, IMRT and PBT aided in optimal dose delivery and reduction of normal tissue damage (Fig. 11). The role of RT, indications and guidelines for energy, dose and fractionation of RT for meningioma are relatively lacking due to lack of phase III randomized controlled trials. Available evidence for adjuvant or upfront radiotherapy for meningioma is based on large retrospective studies or non-randomized prospective studies showing excellent local control rates with stereotactic radiosurgery (SRS) and fractionated external beam radiotherapy (EBRT). Among various large studies, a review of nearly 50 studies involving more than 4500 patients by Mehta et al., showed merits and demerits of various forms of radiotherapy. SRS showed 5-year recurrence free survival of 75%–100%, while fractionated radiotherapy showed these figures to the tune of 80%–100% [95].

7.1.1 Grade I Meningiomas

Gross total resection of these lesions is required especially in Simpson Grades 1–3 tumours. Definitive RT can be considered if the tumours

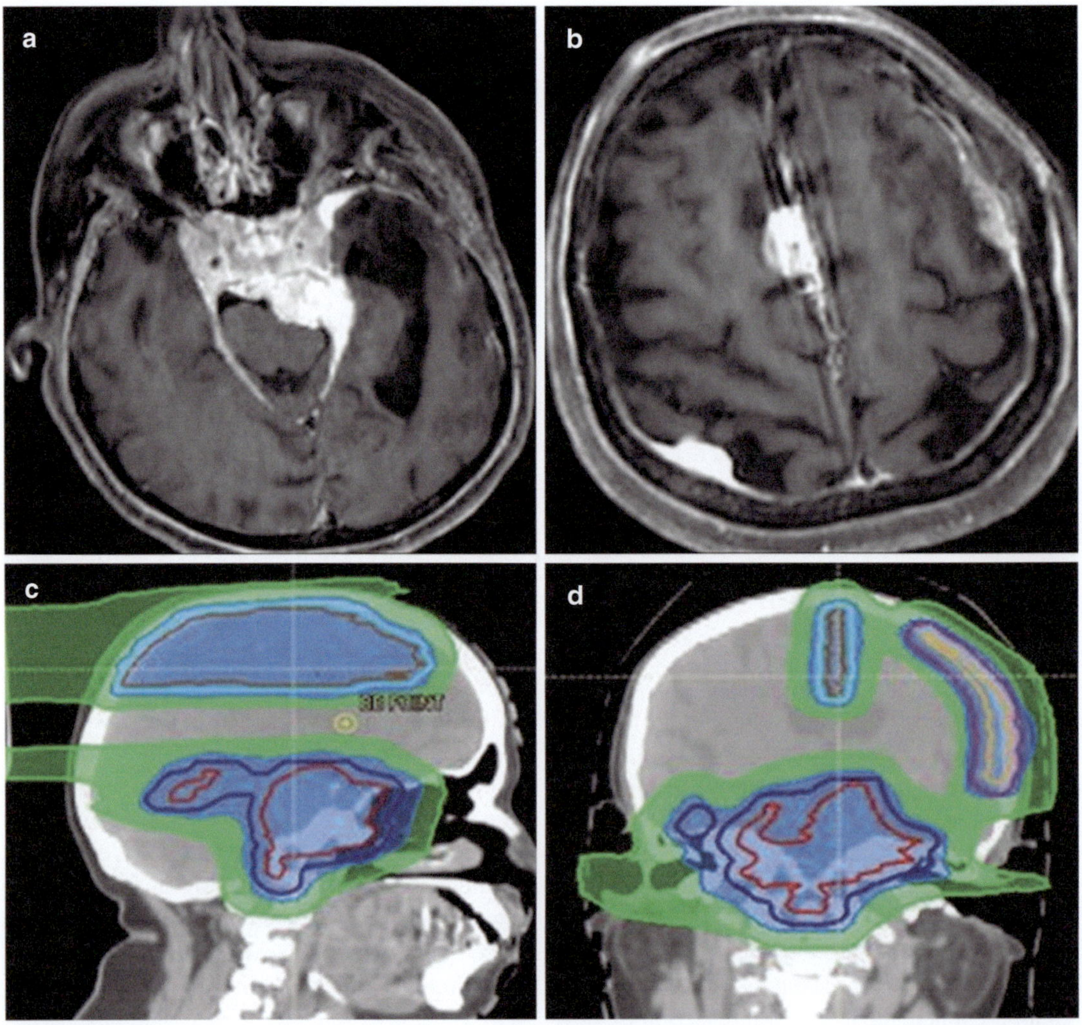

Fig. 11 T1 contrast showing skull base meningioma (**a**), parietal region meningioma (**b**), sagittal and coronal dose distribution (**c** and **d**) with IMPT

are very small, surgically difficult, or challenging locations such as optic nerve sheath meningiomas or cavernous sinus meningiomas, if unwilling or not fit for surgical resection, and as per patient or physician preferences [96–100]. In a meta-analysis, SRS was compared with observation in incidentally detected meningiomas, 16 studies were analysed, and risk of progression were significantly reduced with upfront SRS compared to observation; with absence of calcification, T2W hyperintensity, larger initial size in MRI and younger age were predictors of rapid tumour growth and should be considered for early intervention [101].

In case of gross total resection (GTR), excellent survival is noted, however, in cases of subtotal resection (STR), adjuvant RT is indicated as the results are suboptimal if left untreated. Adjuvant RT increases survival, with rates ranging from 80% to 100%, and nearly upto 98% in patients treated after 1980 [102–108]. In summary, SRS/SRT can be considered as an alternative to surgery in small sized tumours especially less than 2.5 cm in diameter or not close to critical structures; and fractionated EBRT to be considered if the tumours are more than 3 cm in diameter or located to critical structures along with initial tumour size and perilesional edema, so as to guide the treatment appropriately [109]. Doses considered are usually 50–54 Gy in 25–30 fractions for fractionated and 14–16 Gy in one fraction (SRS) or 21–27 Gy in 3–5 fractions for hypofractionated radiotherapy (SRT) for Grade I meningiomas.

7.1.2 Grade II Meningiomas

Atypical meningiomas (AM) are much less common compared to Grade I meningiomas; and comprise 15%–25% of all meningiomas. However, the risk of recurrence is significantly higher, with a seven to eightfold increased risk in 3–5 years, and only 40%–60% are disease-free at 10 years. Surgical resection is the treatment of choice, with GTR to be attempted/intended with the evolving role of adjuvant RT in these tumours. According to the SEER database in 2012, the role of adjuvant RT was reviewed in higher grade meningiomas, with EBRT not showing any survival benefit, however, further literature analysis showed adjuvant RT improving local control (LC) in STR but did not have an impact on OS [110–112]. An Indian study analyzed the impact of timing of RT on outcomes in 86 patients with atypical meningiomas with RT being delivered either as early adjuvant or as salvage RT. 51 patients were considered for early adjuvant RT, whereas 30 patients were considered for salvage RT. Twelve of 30 (40%) patients recurred/progressed after salvage RT, compared to 6 of 51 (12%) patients after early adjuvant RT ($p = 0.003$). Post-RT 5-year progression-free survival (PFS) was significantly better for early adjuvant RT compared to salvage RT (69% vs 28%, log-rank $p < 0.001$), supporting the fact that early adjuvant RT significantly reduce the risk of local recurrence/progression compared to initial observation in AM. Also, salvage RT was not found to be as effective as early adjuvant RT in AM [113].

The role of PBT in AM was analysed in a single institution review, where 22 patients were analysed between 2005 and 2013. The 5-year LC was 87.5% versus 50% following a radiation dose of more than 60 Gy (RBE) compared to less than or equal to 60 Gy (RBE), respectively. Also, fractionated PT was associated with favourable tumour control rates in these tumours [114, 115]. Studies such as PANAMA [116] and NRG 0539 are underway to assess the role of RT, including PT compared to observation in these intermediate risk meningiomas. However, whether early adjuvant radiotherapy reduces the risk of tumour recurrence when compared to observation is still a matter of debate. ROAM (Radiation therapy vs Observation following surgical resection of AM) is a multi-institutional randomised controlled trial been undertaken by the NHS, that aims to address this very important scenario. This study aims to determine clinical practice and treatment modality, thereby generating high-quality data in the case of AM and results are awaited [117]. Doses considered are usually 50–60 Gy in 25–33 fractions based on institute protocol.

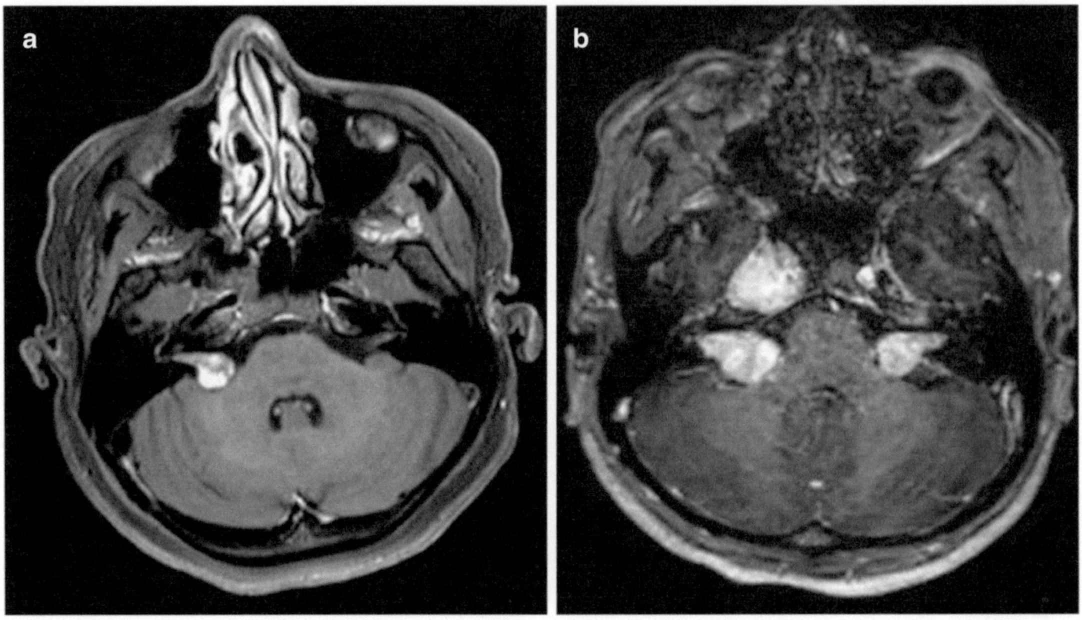

Fig. 12 T1 contrast image showing small vestibular schwannoma (**a**) and multiple NF-2 associated schwannoma and meningioma (**b**)

7.1.3 Grade III Meningiomas

Malignant meningiomas (MM) are uncommon when compared to Grades I and II meningiomas and comprise only about 5% of meningiomas. These tumours are associated with aggressive biological clinical behaviour, with surgical resection being the treatment of choice, and GTR to be attempted whenever feasible. These tumours have a strong tendency to recur locally and, in some cases, can metastasize distally to the lungs, lymph nodes, and bones. These tumours are always treated with adjuvant RT, with doses 59.4–60 Gy or more being considered in routine clinical practice. Also, there is no proven role of upfront systemic chemotherapy or targeted therapy in these tumours and are usually associated with suboptimal outcomes despite aggressive multimodal management. Doses considered are usually 59.4–60 Gy in 30–33 fractions.

7.2 Vestibular Schwannoma

Incidence of vestibular schwannoma (VS), also called acoustic neuroma, has increased in recent times mostly due to incidental diagnosis of asymptomatic lesions with widespread use of MRI and improved awareness. Most of them are sporadic while 15%–20% are associated with Neurofibromatosis 2 (NF-2) (Fig. 12). Treatment options include surveillance for asymptomatic small tumours in elderly, stereotactic or fractionated radiation therapy either with photons or with PBT; and surgical excision.

7.2.1 Surgical Excision

There has been a major paradigm shift in the objectives of surgery from complete resection to preservation of long-term functional and neurological outcomes. It is accepted that subtotal resection followed by observation or SRS, particularly for a large VS, can achieve long-term tumour control with improved nerve preservation [118, 119]. In Koos Grade IV, surgery is considered as the primary treatment to remove a symptomatic lesion or potentially life-threatening mass effect over the brainstem. Surgery may also be considered for smaller tumours, if cystic degeneration is present. The choice of surgical approach depends on hearing status, tumour characteristics, patient's preferences, and surgeon's expertise. Intra-operative monitoring of

Table 2 Studies comparing SRS with fSRT in vestibular schwannoma

Author, year	Dose (Gy)	*n*	Tumour control (%)	Hearing preservation (%)	Facial nerve preservation (%)
Andrews, 2001 [129]	SRS: 12	69	98	33	98
	fSRT: 50 in 25 fractions	56	97	81	98
Meijer, 2003 [130]	SRS: 10–12.5	49	100	75	93
	fSRT: 20–25 in 5 fractions	80	94	61	97
Collen, 2011 [131]	SRS: 11–14	78	95	82	83
	fSRT: 30–40 in 10 fractions 50 in 25 fractions	31 10	95	59	97
Kopp, 2011 [132]	SRS: 12	68	99	85	93
	fSRT: 54 in 30 fractions	47	98	79	96
Puataweepong, 2013 [133]	SRS: 12	39	95	75	99
	fSRT: 25–50 in 5–25 fractions	79	100	87	99
Anderson, 2014 [134]	SRS: 12 (9.7–16)	48	97	60	98
	fSRT: 20 in 5 50.4 in 28 fractions	37 19	90.5 100	63 44	100 100
Combs, 2015 [135]	SRS: 13 (10–20)	67	95	86	97
	fSRT: 57.6 in 32 fractions	67	95	84	99

facial and cochlear nerves is vital. Conventional brainstem auditory evoked potential (BAEP) method and novel methods such as auditory evoked dorsal cochlear nucleus action potential (AEDNAP) monitoring and facial nerve root exit zone–elicited compound muscle action potential (FREMAP) monitoring are in use. Positive predictive factors for preservation of serviceable hearing post microsurgery are tumour size <1 cm and good preoperative hearing function. An MRI is recommended 6–12 months post-surgery to document the extent of tumour removal and helps in subsequent follow-ups.

7.2.2 Radiotherapy

The first non-invasive treatment option for VS was SRS with Gamma knife, which had further evolved into LINAC-based SRS, SRS-dedicated machines like Cyberknife, fractionated stereotactic radiotherapy (fSRT), and conventional radiotherapy. PBT is also an option with high long-term tumour control rates and encouraging outcomes in terms of preserved neurological function [120–125].

Fractionated Stereotactic Radiotherapy (fSRT) is given either hypofractionated in doses greater than 2.5 Gy per fraction (5 Gy × 5 daily; 3 Gy × 10 daily; 6 Gy × 3) or conventionally fractionated in 1.8–2.0 Gy/day to a dose of 50–50.4 Gy. There were six non-randomized studies comparing single fraction SRS (9.7–16 Gy) versus fractionated RT reporting no difference in outcomes (Table 2). When the 5-year tumour control rates were pooled, there was still no statistically significant difference, with a hazard ratio (HR) of 1.66 (95% CI 0.81, 3.42), $p = 0.17$ [126]. Care should be taken when treating tumours more than 3 cm with SRS/fSRT as marginal miss might result in recurrence, and hence one can consider conventional fractionated radiotherapy in such cases. Conventional RT can be either used as single agent modality or as adjuvant therapy to subtotal resection. Encouraging results were seen with studies showing local control rate of 94% at 15 years in case of adjuvant setting, and 86% in case of primary modality of treatment [127]. When compared to SRS, fractionated RT had equivalent or superior hearing preservation rates of around 63%–94% [128–135]. Fractionated proton beam therapy has also shown encouraging results with excellent local control, minimal cranial nerve toxicities, and improved rates of hearing preservation as comparable with SRS/FSRT [136].

7.3 Pituitary Adenoma

Pituitary tumours account for 10%–15% of all primary cerebral tumours and are the most common cause of sellar–suprasellar masses. There is a female predilection, with most cases occurring in the 45–55-year age range. Most common pituitary tumour is pituitary adenoma (PA) (Fig. 13), which accounts for around 10% of all intracranial tumours. The classic tumour predisposition syndromes include multiple endocrine neoplasia type 1 (MEN1) and type 4 (MEN4) syndromes, Carney complex, and McCune-Albright syndrome. Neurofibromatosis type 1 (NF1), DICER1 syndrome, and SDHx mutations have all been linked to pituitary tumours. Mitotic count and Ki-67 labelling index are strongly suggested to assist in detecting clinically aggressive adenomas [137, 138]. Historically, an invasive tumour with a high mitotic index −1-labelling index more than 3% and significant nuclear immunostaining for p53 was classified as an 'atypical adenoma'. Atypical adenoma was removed from the WHO classification, and new entities were added, such as pituitary blastoma, which appears to be a paediatric and DICER1-specific malignancy [138, 139].

7.3.1 Fractionated Radiation Therapy

There are prospective and retrospective series with large number of patients and long-term follow-up with conventional fractionated radiation therapy. Hence, conventional fraction is considered the standard of care and results of stereotactic radiosurgery are evaluated on the light of results obtained by these studies with long-term outcome data. Long-term results following conventional RT is published in the literature are shown in Table 3 [140–146]. Overall actuarial PFS is 80%–90% at 10 years and 75%–90% at 20 years [147]. Largest series of patients (n = 411) with pituitary adenomas treated with conventional fractionated radiotherapy from the Royal Marsden Hospital reported a 10-year PFS of 92% and a 20-year PFS of 88% [140]. In secretory tumours, normalization of hormone functions are the most important indicator regarding response to treatment. Fractionated irradiation leads to normalization of excess pituitary hormone secretion in a proportion of patients; however, there is delay in response following treatment. For acromegaly, RT achieves normalization of GH/IGF-I levels in 30%–50% of patients at 5–10 years, and in 75% of patients at 15 years, after treatment. Normalization of

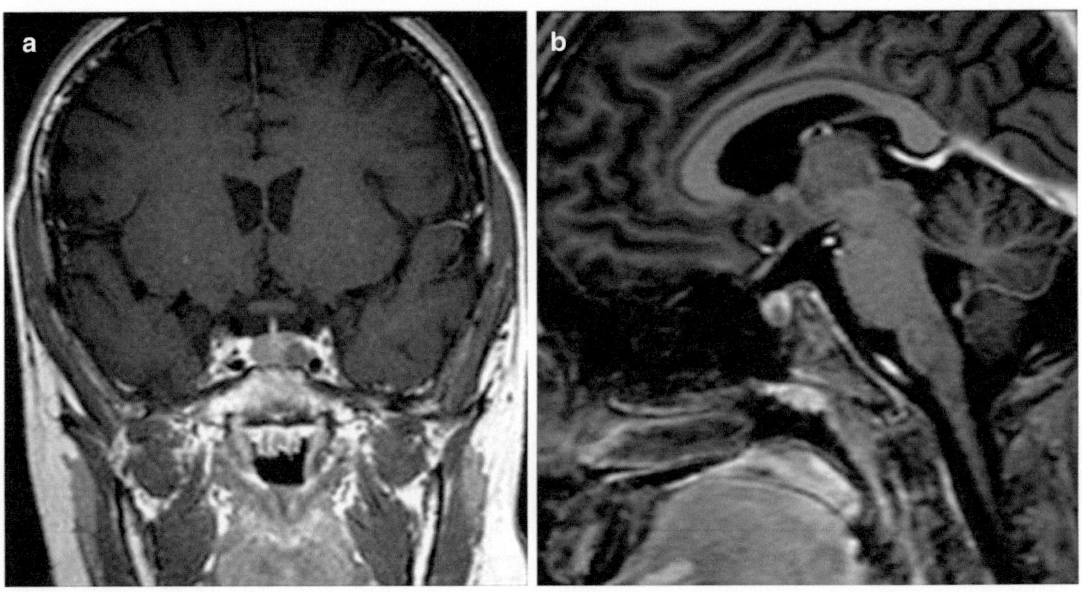

Fig. 13 MRI images of T1 contrast showing pituitary adenoma in coronal (**a**) and sagittal (**b**) sections

Table 3 Results after conventional fractionated radiotherapy in pituitary adenomas

Author (year)	*N*	FU (years)	Outcome
Brada et al. (1993) [140]	411	10.8	PFS: 94% at 10 years and 88% at 20 years Optic atrophy: 30 pt. at 10 years
Minniti et al. (2005) [141]	45	12	PFS: 52% at 10 years Hipo-pit: 45 patients at 10 years
Langsenlehner et al. (2007) [142]	87	15	PFS: 93% at 15 years Hipo-pit: 88% at 10 years
Minniti et al. (2007) [143]	40	9	PFS: 78% at 5 years and 84% at 10 years Hipo-pit: 62 patients at 10 years
Rim et al. (2011) [144]	60	5.6	PFS: 96% at 10 years and 66% at 10 years Hipo-pit: 76 patients
Kim et al. (2016) [145]	73	8	PFS: 98% at 10 years
Patt et al. (2016) [146]	36	4.9	PFS: 89% at 5 years Hipo-pit: 33 patients

GH is related to pre-treatment GH level and time to achieve 50% reduction in GH levels. In Cushing's disease, usually urinary free cortisol (UFC) is reduced to 50% of the pre-treatment levels after an interval of 6–12 months, and plasma cortisol after around 12 months. The median time to cortisol level normalization is around 24 months [143]. At 8 years median follow up, tumour control rate is 97% and hormone control rates is 74%. In prolactimona, radiation therapy is used only in case of failed surgery of medical therapy. 10-year tumour and hormone control rates are 90% and 50% respectively [148].

Toxicity of RT with total treatment doses of 45–50 Gy with daily fraction sizes of <2 Gy is low. Hypopituitarism is the most common long-term complication following RT, reported to occur in 30%–60% of patients by 10 years after treatment [140]. After RT, GH secretion being affected most frequently, followed by gonadotrophins, ACTH, and then TSH. Hypopituitarism also depends upon the mean dose to pituitary stalk. Incidence of optic neuropathy resulting in visual deficit following conventional RT is 1%–3%. Pituitary disease is associated with increased mortality, principally due to vascular disease. An increased incidence of stroke (relative to the general population) in patients treated with RT for both non-functioning and functioning pituitary adenomas has been reported. However, the impact of RT, surgery, hormonal imbalance, metabolic disturbances and the multi-factorial effect of these factors were not clear [149], suggesting that untreated hormone deficiency may be a significant factor in the pathogenesis of stroke in patients treated for pituitary adenoma, rather than or in addition to treatment with radiotherapy. Cumulative incidence of second malignancies (gliomas and meningiomas) following radiotherapy for pituitary adenomas in retrospective case series is 2% at 20 years. Large retrospective study of patients received radiotherapy for pituitary and sellar lesions has shown a relative risk of 3.34 (95% confidence interval 1.06–10.6) for development of malignant brain tumours and 4.06 (95% confidence interval 1.51–10.9) for development of meningiomas in comparison with patients who did not receive radiotherapy. Secondary malignant neoplasms rates are relatively higher in younger age patients, which can be significantly reduced with modern PBT.

7.3.2 Nonfunctioning Adenomas

Nonfunctioning pituitary adenomas (NFPA),, the most common type of macroadenoma, are characterized by a loss of visual acuity, restriction of the visual field abnormalities, and, in certain cases, hypopituitarism in variable degrees [150, 151]. Non-functioning adenomas account for around 30% of all pituitary adenomas and often extend beyond the sella turcica [152–157].

7.3.3 Functioning Adenomas

Prolactinomas are the most frequent pituitary tumours, with microadenomas accounting for the great majority of cases in women. In women, amenorrhea, galactorrhea, and infertility are common symptoms, whereas in men, libido loss, infertility, impotence, gynecomastia, and visual abnormalities are common. Although a negative MRI can be detected in women with microadenomas, it can assist confirm the diagnosis. Restoration of sexual and reproductive function, normalization of prolactin levels, management of galactorrhea, and decrease in neurologic symptoms are all goals of therapy. Observation, medical therapy, surgery, and irradiation are all alternatives for treatment. Acromegaly is a rare disorder, having an incidence of 60/1000,000. Multiple organs have metabolic and functional changes because of GH hypersecretion (e.g., cardiovascular, musculoskeletal, and respiratory dysfunction).

Cushing disease is caused by an anterior pituitary ACTH-secreting adenoma, which accounts for 70%–80% of ACTH-dependent Cushing syndrome cases in adults. The diagnosis is frequently delayed because to the numerous nonspecific symptoms and signs. This condition is more frequent in women and is a heterogeneous disorder. It is related to higher morbidity and age-corrected mortality. Truncal obesity, hirsutism, acne, easy bruisability, abdominal striae, buffalo hump, muscular weakness, and moon facies are some of the clinical symptoms. Menstrual abnormalities, gonadal dysfunction, hypertension, diabetes mellitus, and osteoporosis are common in these people. Untreated or incompletely treated hypercortisolism is linked to a high rate of morbidity and death, with a median survival time of around 5 years.

7.3.4 Role of RT

Incomplete resection of a large NFPA, cavernous sinus invasion, recurring or progressing malignancies, inoperable symptomatic or potentially symptomatic tumours, or refractory secreting tumours are also common indications for RT. RT for Pituitary adenomas has advanced from two-dimensional (2D) treatment to three-dimensional (3D) treatment, intensity modulated radiation, and stereotactic therapies, with either fractionated stereotactic radiotherapy (fSRT) or stereotactic radiosurgery (SRS). Sophisticated RT methods can offer a steeper dose gradient, enabling for greater tumour control and fewer long-term RT-induced adverse effects by providing a larger dosage to the tumour while minimizing the radiation to surrounding essential structures. In general, at 5 years, both forms of RT (fractionated RT and SRS) control the tumour in around 90% of patients. As of now, there is no evidence that distinguishes between these two techniques in terms of efficacy or safety. A meta-analysis of eight trials found that fractionated RT and SRS have similar outcomes [158]. Few retrospective studies have suggested that SRS is more efficacious in functional adenoma than fractionated RT, but both are similarly effective in NFPA [159]. SRS may be considered for treatment in tumours located at least 2 mm away from optic structures, or cavernous sinus involvement, or persistent high serum hormone levels postoperatively, but it currently only offers the time advantage of treatment in a single session versus a longer 5 weeks course of fractionated RT. When the optic pathway is involved or closely apposed, or when the lesion is big (diameter >3 cm) and the risk of radio necrosis with SRS is considerable, fractionated RT is favoured over SRS.

The objective of therapy in a functional PA is to establish radiological control while also reducing endocrine over secretion, in comparison to NFPA, in which, SRS dose of 13–14 Gy is sufficient for long-term tumour suppression and tolerable neurological damage, and in case of functioning PA, a larger dose of SRS (16–25 Gy) is usually necessary. A multicenter retrospective study of NFPA found that SRS doses of less than 12 Gy were linked with poor outcomes, although doses of more than 20 Gy did not give extra tumour control when compared to doses of 12–20 Gy [155]. SRS is effective in achieving 5-year tumour control rate of 90%–100% in NFPA. Hypopituitarism is the most commonly reported toxicity after SRS with a 5-year incidence of increasing pituitary deficits ranging from 10% to 40% in different studies [160]. Risk of radiation related optic neuropathy is less than 3% if the maximum point dose to optic apparatus is 8–10 Gy, but significantly increases after 12 Gy [161].

In conventional fractionated radiation treatment at 1.8 Gy per fraction, adequate RT doses for NFPA and functional PA are 45–50.4 Gy and 50.4–54 Gy, respectively [162]. Local control with conventional RT can range from 80% to 94% for functioning adenomas and from 75% to 90% for non-functioning adenomas after 20 years (Table 3) [163]. After 5–10 years of RT for acromegaly, nearly half of the patients' GH/IGF-1 levels normalize [164]. Within 3 years of fractionated RT, biochemical control in Cushing's can be demonstrated in 50%–80% of patients [159]. After 5–10 years, around a third of individuals with prolactinomas respond to RT, with prolactin levels returning to normal. Hypopituitarism is the most documented late toxicity of RT. Hypopituitarism can be detected in 30%–50% of individuals following 5 years of conventional RT at doses of 45–50.4 Gy at 1.8 Gy per fraction. The reported incidence of vision loss due to radiation-induced optic neuropathy ranges from 0% to 6% (2% with an RT dosage of 45 Gy in a daily fraction of 1.8 Gy). Cerebrovascular accidents (CVA) have also been reported to be on the rise. Another long-term consequence of RT is radiation-induced second cancers [143].

During RT planning, T1w MRI images obtained postoperatively are particularly useful in target delineation. T2w MRI is not commonly utilized to measure brain parenchyma infiltration and perilesional edema. GTV refers to any lesion that may be seen on an MRI; except in the intracavernous region of aggressive adenoma to account for probable microscopic dissemination, CTV margin is rarely indicated. For setup uncertainties, a 3–5 mm margin is added to PTV. Off-late, PBT has been utilized in these tumours with 3-year CR of 54% with Cushing's disease, 63% for Nelsons, 26% for acromegaly and 22% for prolactinomas [165].

7.4 Craniopharyngioma

Craniopharyngioma most commonly present in children between 5 and 14 years of age and in adults between 50 and 75 years The tumor typically arises in the sellar/supra-sellar region. Two histological types exist, namely adamantinomatous and the squamous-papillary types. Beta-catenin gene mutations have been identified in the adamantinomatous subtype and activating mutations in *BRAF* (V600E) is seen in the papillary

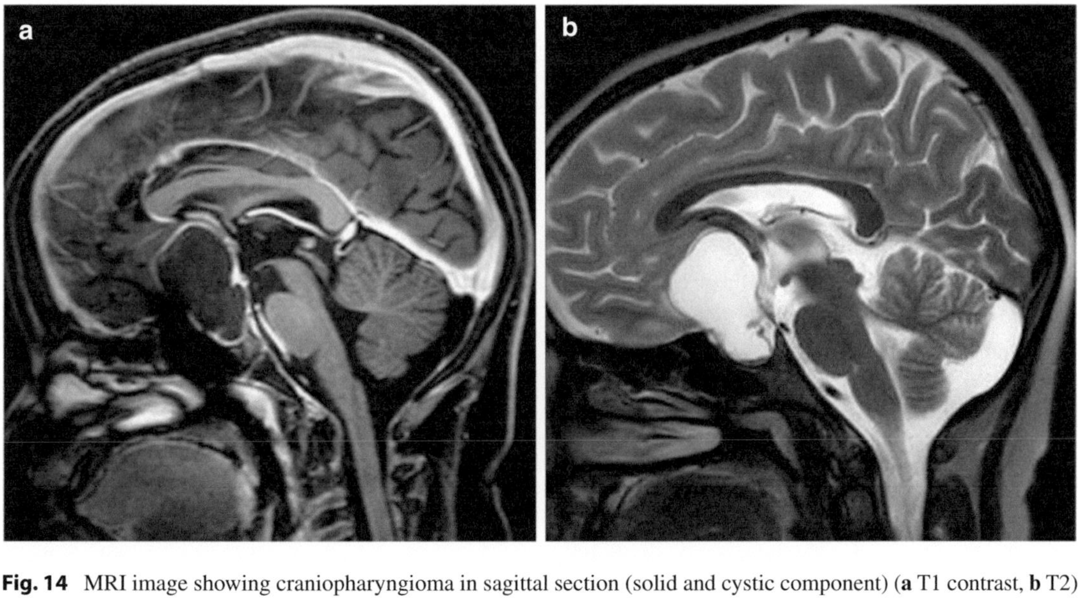

Fig. 14 MRI image showing craniopharyngioma in sagittal section (solid and cystic component) (**a** T1 contrast, **b** T2)

variant [166]. The more common adamantinomatous craniopharyngioma (Fig. 14) is similar to adamantinoma of the jaw which occurs in children. Papillary craniopharyngiomas occur in adults, are typically solid, do not calcify, do not have the characteristic 'motor oil' cyst fluid, and usually are better circumscribed lesions that are less distinctive microscopically lacking the peripheral palisades, stellate reticulum, wet keratin, and cholesterol clefts. Both types manifest cytokeratin and epithelial membrane antigen positivity, as seen with other epithelial tumours. Patients with craniopharyngioma frequently exhibits hypothalamic–pituitary axis dysfunction, including growth hormone deficiency (GHD), adrenocortical insufficiency, central hypothyroidism, hypogonadism, precocious puberty, hyperprolactinemia, central diabetes insipidus, and hypothalamic obesity [167]. Endocrine evaluation should include the assessment of anterior and posterior pituitary functions. Signs and symptoms indicative for hypopituitarism including Diabetes insipidus should be assessed.

7.4.1 Treatment

Surgery is the first-line approach to the treatment of craniopharyngiomas. Surgery can be complete resection, subtotal resection alone or subtotal resection or biopsy followed by post-operative radiotherapy. Aggressive surgery with gross total resection (GTR) of the tumour, however, may result in significant and devastating peri- and post-operative morbidity especially after resection of tumours invading the hypothalamus [167]. Sub total or partial resection of the tumour to reduce pressure effects on adjacent like the optic pathways or to re-establish circulation of the cerebrospinal fluid with or without subsequent radiotherapy is an alternative approach. Subtotal resection carries a mortality of only 1%. Sub total or partial resection followed by radiotherapy has local control and survival rates as comparable to those achieved with complete resection. Dose of 50.4–54 Gy in 28–30 fractions are delivered to the post-operative residual tumours. Surgical decompression is essential as tumour responds slowly to radiotherapy. Risk of visual impairment is low with this dose. Surgery and radiotherapy are the cornerstones in therapeutic management of craniopharyngioma. Radical excision is associated with a risk of mortality or morbidity particularly as hypothalamic damage, visual deterioration, and endocrine complication. Initially, hypophyseal stalk tumours were considered radioresistant. Carpenter et al. in Philadelphia was the first to publish systematic study on radiotherapy of craniopharyngioma [168]. In 1950 Kramer et al. reported on the experience at the Royal Marsden Hospital and the National Hospital for Nervous Diseases in London which was very important for changing the view on treatment for craniopharyngioma [169]. They introduced the policy of combining surgery, not intended to be radical, with radiotherapy with a relatively high dose of radiation begun immediately after operation. Though they included only 10 patients, their results were remarkably good. Hetelekidis et al. in 1993 assessed the long-term impact of various treatments in childhood craniopharyngioma. All patients in the radiotherapy and surgery plus radiotherapy groups were treated with megavoltage radiation with a median dose of 5464 cGy. With median follow up of 10-year actuarial freedom from progression for the surgery group was 31% compared with 100% for patients treated with radiation therapy only (log rank p = 0.0 1), and 86% for patients treated with surgery plus radiotherapy at diagnosis (p = 0.001) [170]. Excellent long-term outcome of conventional radiotherapy was found in many retrospective series which reported 10 and 20 years progression-free survival up to 95% and 54% [171–176]. With the advent of conformal/intensity modulated radiation therapy, excellent adjustment of treatment portals to tumour site and sparing of normal tissue became possible and various studies showed excellent tumour control rates with IMRT.

The results of fractionated RT in the era of CT-based treatment planning with or without MRI fusion show high control rates (92.0%–100.0%) in mostly shorter follow-up studies. Modern imaging, utilizing CT simulation with MRI fusion has allowed for better delineation of intracranial tumour volume. This has allowed for expansion of the GTV by 5 mm to cover microscopic disease (CTV) with an additional expansion margin of

3 mm to account for daily setup (PTV). There is a possibility of increase in cystic component after RT. Proton therapy have the potential to reduce integral dose and preserve cognitive functions by sparing hippocampus, dentate gyrus region. Optic neuropathies can occur from radiotherapy and are dose-related. However, no evidence of optic neuritis or optic necrosis has been reported when these structures are treated with 54 Gy in conventional fractionation schedule. Hypothalamic-pituitary dysfunction can result from radiation doses needed to control craniopharyngiomas. This complication can take months to years to develop. In modern radiation techniques, neurocognitive function remains stable through 5 years of follow-up [177]. One report has revealed that worse neurocognitive outcomes were associated with ages <7 years, hydrocephalus, large cystic tumours, extensive surgery, and diabetes insipidus. Vascular complications are rare after RT; however, incidence of Moyamoya disease is reported. Patients with neurofibromatosis type 1 are more susceptible to Moyamoya disease. Radiation-induced malignancies after the treatment of craniopharyngiomas are exceedingly rare following conventional fractionated RT [170, 172, 178, 179].

Kobayashi et al. in 2009 published long-term results of 100 consecutive cases treated with gamma knife. A total of 98 of 107 patients were followed up for a mean of 65.5 months after radio surgery. Results showed that complete response was 19.4%, partial response was 67.4%, tumour control rate 79.6% and progression rate was 20.4%. He concluded that stereotactic gamma knife radio surgery is safe and effective as adjuvant or boost therapy for residual and/or recurrent craniopharyngiomas after surgical removal, and has acceptable side effects [180–182]. Lee et al. reported results obtained in 16 patients treated using Cyber Knife for residual recurrent craniopharyngioma. Tumour shrinkage was achieved in 7 of these 11 patients and tumour control in another 3 patients. The overall tumour control was achieved in 91% of patients without complications [183]. Compared with photon therapy, PBT offers a better opportunity to preserve IQ scores in patients with craniopharyngioma. In a review of 40 paediatric craniopharyngioma patients who received PBT, the 5-year local control and overall survival rates were 100% [184]. Other modalities used in the treatment of craniopharyngioma have included intralesional bleomycin and radioactive colloid instillation for cystic tumours. There are different series reporting on the intracavitary application of different β-ray emitting isotopes such as Rhenium186, Yttrium 90, or Phosphorus 32, which has a range of few millimetres. Response rate and cyst control were achieved in more than 80% of case. Tumours with a solid component, however, are insufficiently controlled [185, 186].

7.5 Primary CNS Lymphoma

Primary central nervous system lymphoma (PCNSL) is a rare tumour in elderly and more common in immunocompromised patients. PCNSL is a radiosensitive tumour. Historically, radiation therapy (RT) was the sole modality of therapy for PCNSL [187, 188]. Management paradigm for PCNSL has over the years evolved from radical radiotherapy alone to combined modality treatment with high dose methotrexate (HDMTX) based induction chemotherapy followed by WBRT and consolidation chemotherapy [189–192]. Radiation therapy in PCNSL primarily as consolidation after induction chemotherapy, as radical intent in situation when patient not suitable for high dose MTX and as salvage RT after recurrence.

There are three phase III randomized trials testing the role of radiation therapy as consolidation therapy [193–195]. The SG-I trial was one of the first randomized trials that looked into the role of WBRT versus observation following induction therapy with high dose methotrexate (HDMTX). MATRix trial and the PRECIS trial compared WBRT to ASCT after induction HD MTX based regimens demonstrated contrasting results in terms of 2-year progression free survival (IELSG-32, MATRix trial demonstrated an improvement in WBRT arm as opposed to ASCT arm, while the PRECIS trial demonstrated an improved PFS in ASCT arm compared to the WBRT arm) [195].

Whole brain radiation therapy (WBRT) was the first effective treatment for PCNSL. WBRT induces rapid but transitory remissions, improving the median survival to 12–18 months [187] Prospective phase-II clinical trials (RTOG-8315) used 60 Gy radiation dose (40 GyWBRT & 20 Gy boost). Complete remission rate was 39%, but 1 and 2 years OS was only 45% and 25% respectively [196]. In WBRT (41 Gy and 9 Gy boost) with high-dose steroids in elderly patients (≥70 years of age) with newly diagnosed PCNSL, response rate was 42% but OS was dismal [188]. These studies demonstrated that RT alone is active, but not effective in achieving long-term remissions in patients with PCNSL.

7.5.1 Current Potential Indications for WBRT in PCNSL

1. Consolidation in patients who have achieved a complete response (CR) to induction chemotherapy;
2. *De-novo* therapy in patients who cannot receive high dose methotrexate based chemotherapy;
3. Salvage treatment in patients with refractory or relapsed disease.

7.5.2 Radiotherapy Dose Schedule

Radiotherapy dose schedule in PCNSL is still an unresolved issue and there is no consensus among the cooperative groups [193–195, 197]. In DeAngelis protocol doses of around 45 Gy have been shown to decrease the risk of progression or relapse after chemotherapy at the cost of significant neurotoxicity. Various fractionation strategies and dose schedule is considered to reduce the risk of neurocognitive deficits [198, 199]. Radiation dose reduction to 23.4 Gy by Morris et al. and 36 Gy by Ferreri et al. did not find any benefit of increasing the dose beyond 36 Gy [189, 200]. Biswas et al's study at AIIMS ($n = 22$) receiving similar reduced dose RT (23.4 Gy) regimen had inferior clinical outcome [201]. Majority of the cooperative groups commonly use doses between 23.4 and 36 Gy with or without boost (boost only in partial responders). The present recommendation is WBRT with a total dose of 36 Gy in 1.8 Gy per fraction schedule. Boost is considered in partial responders with a dose of 9 Gy at 1.8 Gy per fraction. However, in patients with compromised health status and limited lesion(s) in the brain, focal RT covering the lesion area(s) can be safely delivered.

7.6 Brain Metastases

Brain metastases have become increasingly relevant to oncologic management as advances in systemic therapy promote extracranial disease control (Fig. 15). In addition, the management of brain metastases is becoming more specific to the primary tumour type [202]. Management poses unique challenges because of the blood–brain barrier thus limiting the effect of chemotherapeutic medications. Management of brain metastases depends on various factors like the performance status of the patient, pathology of the primary tumour, status of systemic disease, number of brain metastases, site of disease, and intracranial pressure status (mass effect) [203].

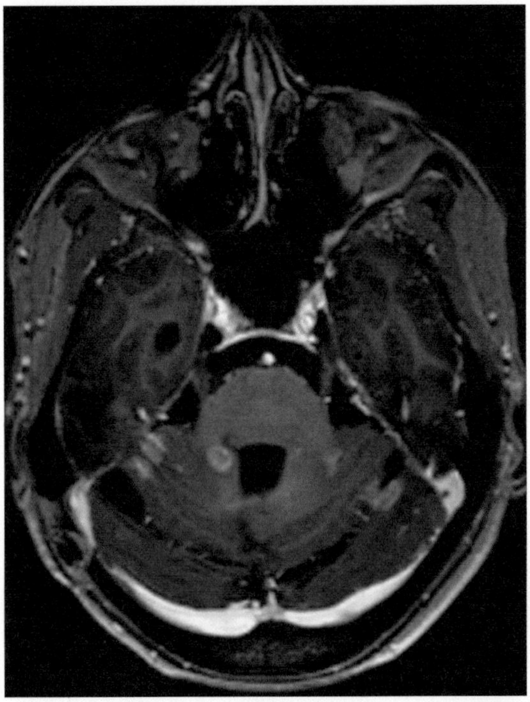

Fig. 15 MRI showing small multiple brain lesions in cerebellum

7.6.1 Treatment Modalities

The common treatment modalities in brain metastasis are whole brain radiation therapy, surgery and SRS (Table 4) [204].

Table 4 Treatment modalities in brain metastases

Multiple brain metastases	WBRT
Oligo-brain metastases with controlled primary	SRS/SRT
If large brain metastasis causing raised intracranial pressure with midline shift	Surgery followed by adjuvant RT
Progressive systemic disease and poor performance status	Best supportive care

7.6.2 Radiation Therapy Modality-Evidence

There are multi-centric randomized studies (Table 5) with different radiation schedule in brain metastasis [205–211]. There is level I evidence for role of SRS in 1–4 brain metastasis and in post-operative SRS.

7.6.3 Hippocampal Avoidance WBRT (HA-WBRT)

HA-WBRT protected the hippocampal neural stem cells from injury in WBRT (Fig. 16) thus helping in memory preservation. In a phase III trial published by Brown et al. in JCO 2020, HA WBRT plus Memantine has lower risk of deterioration in exec-

Table 5 RCTs in brain metastases with various radiation dose schedules

Author	Study	Design	Results
Patchell et al. NEJM 1990 [205]	Phase III RCT 54 patients	Surgery plus WBRT vs WBRT alone in solitary brain met	Surgery reduced local recurrence (52% vs 20%) and improved median survival (40 vs 15 weeks)
EORTC 22952–26001 Kocher et al. JCO 2011 [206]	Phase III study 359 patients	Adjuvant WBRT vs observation after surgery/SRS in 1–3 brain mets	WBRT decreased 2 years distant brain failure (27% vs 59%) No difference in OS (WBRT vs Obs) 10.7 vs 10.9 months Median time to PS > 2 9.5 vs 10 months
Patchell et al. JAMA, 1998 [207]	Phase III RCT 95 patients	Surgery followed by WBRT vs surgery alone in single brain met	WBRT reduced in brain failure (anywhere 18% vs 70%; local 10% vs 46%); likelihood of neurological death (14% vs 44%) No effect on OS (48 vs 43 weeks)
QUARTZ study Mulvenna et al. Lancet 2016 [208]	Phase III non inferiority study 538 patients NSCLC with brain mets unsuitable for resection or SRS	Optimal supportive care vs WBRT(20 Gy/5 Fr)	No difference in MS (8.5 vs 9.2 weeks) OS (48 vs 43 weeks)
Brown et al. Lancet, 2017 [209]	Phase III RCT 194 patients with 1–4 mets and resection of one brain lesion	Post op SRS vs WBRT	No difference in OS (MS 11.8 months vs 11.5 months) Less neurocognitive decline with SRS (54% vs 86%) and better QOL Less time to intracranial failure with SRS (6.4 months vs 27.5 months)
Aoyama et al. JAMA, 2006 [210]	Phase III RCT 132 patients with 1–4 brain mets	SRS + WBRT vs SRS alone	No difference in OS (SRS alone 8 months vs 7.5 in SRS + WBRT) Distant brain control (24% in SRS alone and 53% in SRS + WBRT)
Mahajan et al. Lancet, 2017 [211]	Phase III RCT 132 patients with complete resection of 1–3 brain mets	Post op SRS vs observation	One year local control (72% in SRS group vs 43% in observation group) Similar median OS

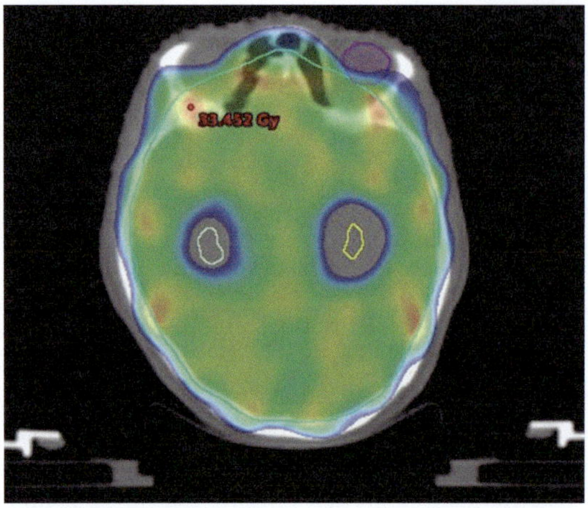

Fig. 16 Dose distribution of hippocampal sparing WBRT (HA-WBRT) with VMAT technique

utive functions at 4 months and learning, memory at 6 months. There was no significant difference in OS, toxicity or intracranial PFS [212–214].

7.6.4 Indication for HA-WBRT

- >4 brain lesions
- Oligo brain metastasis with extra-cranial progression and good PS
- Oligo brain metastasis with poor PS
- SRS in special histology—SCLC, Melanoma, SCC, adenocarcinoma
- SRS in molecular subtypes

7.6.5 ASTRO 2022 Guideline

The American Society for Radiation Oncology (ASTRO) has updated its 2012 guideline on the use of radiation therapy to treat patients with brain metastases, reflecting recent research developments [215].

Intact/Unresected Brain Metastases

- 1–4 brain metastases and good performance status (ECOG 0–2), stereotactic radiosurgery (SRS) is recommended.
- 5–10 brain metastases and good performance status, SRS is conditionally recommended. For patients with tumours exerting mass effect and/or larger size, surgical resection is suggested.
- Symptomatic brain metastases: upfront local therapy (radiation and/or surgery) is strongly recommended.
- Asymptomatic brain metastases eligible for CNS-directed systemic therapy, local therapy may be deferred in only definitive condition after multi-disciplinary decision.
- Brain metastasis with favourable prognosis: ineligible for surgery and/or SRS (multiple lesions, leptomeningeal involvement), whole brain radiation therapy (WBRT) is recommended as a primary treatment. Hippocampal avoidance is recommended when appropriate to preserve memory function, (along with memantine).
- Routine adjuvant WBRT added to SRS is not recommended.
- Poor prognosis and brain metastases: WBRT may not improve outcomes compared to supportive care alone. Palliative/supportive care or hospice, or short-course WBRT for symptomatic brain metastases.
- SRS indication is driven by (1) number of brain metastases, (2) total tumour volume, (3) tumour location, (4) age, and (5) extracranial disease status.

Resected Brain Metastases

- Radiation therapy is recommended for all patients following resection of brain metastases to improve intracranial control. For patients with limited brain metastases after resection, post-operative SRS is recommended over WBRT to preserve the patient's neurocognitive function and quality of life [207].
- SRS prior to brain metastasis resection is conditionally recommended.

7.6.6 Dosage Schedule

Though multiple dose schedules have been tried for WBRT, a dose of 30 Gy in 10 daily fractions or 20 Gy in five fractions is usually the standard protocol. Dose schedules in SRS/SRT is dependent on size of the lesion and location. Dose schedules vary from 15 to 30 Gy in 1–5 fractions. Shaw et al. in the RTOG 9005 study done to determine the maximum tolerated single dose (SRS) for patients. with previously treated primary brain tumours and recurrent brain metastases showed that doses for tumours with diameter 0–2 cm, 2.1–3 cm, and 3.1–4 cm were 24 Gy, 18 Gy, and 15 Gy, respectively [216].

7.6.7 Leptomeningeal Disease (LMD)

In one National Cancer Database (NCDB) analysis of 519 patients treated for LMD from any histology from 2005 to 2014 by Hyun et al., 52 patients were treated with RT alone, 88 patients were treated with RT + CT, 232 patients were treated with CT alone, and 147 patients were treated with BSC [217]. Of the patient's that received RT, 85% were treated with WBRT, 14% with focal brain RT (FBRT), and 1% with WBRT and focal spine RT (FSRT). Median OS for the entire cohort was 3 months (2.7–3.3 months). Treated patients exhibited a higher median OS compared to BSC; and patients treated with CT + RT revealed the highest median OS of 5 months (3.5–6.5 months) followed by patients treated with RT alone who had a median OS of 3 months (1.7–4.3 months). Leptomeningeal involvement is considered as a poor prognostic parameter. However, patients with good performance status and normal CSF levels had a more favourable prognosis upon active treatment. Recent phase 2 randomized controlled trial comparing proton CSI to photon involved field radiotherapy for solid tumours with leptomeningeal metastases showed that proton CSI showed improved PFS compared to the other arm, and also showing significant OS benefit with comparable Grade 3 toxicities [218].

7.6.8 Re-radiation in Brain Metastasis

Though reirradiation in brain metastases after prior WBRT has its own limitations, Scharp et al. showed that re-WBRT (20 Gy/10 Fr) was tolerated well with the main side effects being fatigue, erythema, focal alopecia [219]. Median survival was 2.8 months since the end of the re-WBRT with good performance status at the start of the re-irradiation being a key indicator for longer survival. Logie et al. created a re-RT score wherein 1 point was assigned for each of the following poor prognostic factors: SCLC; presence of extracranial metastases; KPS <80, interval between radiation therapy courses <9 months; and uncontrolled primary [220]. The sum ranged from 0 to 5. Re RT score of 1–2 should be taken up for re RT; score of 4–5 may consider BSC while a score of 3 entails a risk versus benefit discussion and treatment tailored accordingly. Post SRS recurrence in other lobe or 'out of field' recurrences in preserved performance status patients are treated with common practice.

7.6.9 Complications of RT in Brain Metastasis

Local control depends upon the peripheral dose. Dose delivered and tumour volume determines the toxicities and mentioned in Table 6.

Table 6 Common toxicities after brain RT

Acute toxicities (within 6 weeks of RT)	Fatigue, radiation-induced alopecia, dermatitis, nausea and vomiting, decreased appetite, cerebral edema
Early delayed toxicities (6 weeks to 3 months)	Fatigue, somnolence, neurocognitive deficits such as decline in memory, and other general or focal neurologic symptoms
Late toxicity (>3 months)	Neurocognitive dysfunction, leukoencephalopathy, radiation necrosis, hypothalamic-pituitary axis dysfunction, Vasculopathies, second malignant neoplasms, gonadal toxicity

8 Quality of Life in Brain Tumours

Quality of life is an important endpoint in the treatment of brain tumours. In high-grade gliomas, survival benefit is questionable after radiation and chemotherapy is limited to few months. Hence, in such cases, quality of life becomes an important end point to evaluate the efficacy of the treatment. On the other hand, benign brain tumours and low-grade malignant tumours have excellent progression free and overall survival, and in view of being highly curable tumours, preservation of normal functions and quality of life becomes critical in such situations. Important outcome parameters of treatment include long-term survivorship, job or placement opportunity, normal social life and psychological well-being after treatment. Brain tumours cause wide range of neurocognitive deficits, which significantly affect patients' daily functions and quality of life [221, 222]. Radiation therapy for brain tumours is known to have an impact on neuropsychological functions, emotional functions and quality of life [223–225]. Prospective randomized studies with conventional fractionation radiation therapy have shown that high precision radiation therapy preserves neurocognitive function [177, 214]. Prospective studies on proton therapy also have shown to have better dosimetric parameters compared with photon therapy and have better preservation of cognitive function and quality of life. Modern intensity modulated proton beam therapy have shown to improve quality of life by preserving critical structures, which cannot be achieved with other modalities of radiotherapy [69, 226, 227]. Quality of life is evaluated by questionnaire-based methods such as European Organization for the Research and Treatment of Cancer Quality of Life Questionnaire (EORTC) (QLQ-30) and Specific Brain Cancer module (BN 20) for quality of life and FACT Br. Common neuropsychological evaluation for cognitive evaluation, are NIMHANS Neuropsychology Battery (2004) and Wechsler Memory Scale-III (WMS); Emotional Processing Scale (EPS) for evaluation of emotional processing, Hospital Anxiety and Depression Scale (HADS) for measuring anxiety and depressive symptoms. Functional independence measurement and functional activity measurement system (FIMFAM) and BARTHEL's scoring system is used for Activities of Daily Living. QOL function depends upon many patient and disease related factors such as socioeconomic factors, educational status, disease control status and treatment related toxicities. Neurocognitive evaluation and quality of life assessment should be made part of as routine protocol in clinical practice.

9 Conclusion

Primary intracranial neoplasms range from benign to malignant tumours which, when compared to other tumours, may not be common, but still are very common in daily practice. Treatment options include surgical resection, histopathological evaluation followed by adjuvant radiotherapy with or without chemotherapy in case of malignant brain tumours and in most of the benign tumours depending upon the clinical scenario. Radiation therapy ranges from conventional photon-based radiotherapy to particle-based radiotherapy, to maintain tumour control, spare the critical structures and preserve quality of life. For these patients, post-therapy physiotherapy and rehabilitation are equally important. Continued long-term follow-up and novel treatment approaches are needed to improve the management of these brain tumours.

Percepts Box

1. Incidence of CNS tumours in India ranges from 5 to 10 per 100,000 population, with majority being high-grade gliomas in adults and astrocytomas in paediatric age group.
2. The standard of care for most of these brain tumours is surgery followed by radiotherapy. Chemotherapy and targeted therapy plays a major role in Grades II–IV gliomas and other brain tumours.
3. Radiotherapy has evolved from conventional and 3D-CRT to high end techniques such as IMRT, VMAT, SRS/SRT, HT, and PBT.
4. WHO 2021 classification has made certain changes, and the onus is on the radiation oncologist to correlate them using clinical, radiological, and pathological details to arrive at proper diagnosis and further management.
5. Radiation therapy from photon to particle based therapy can be delivered via conventional or hypofractionated regimen. Same has been mentioned above in tables.
6. The standard of care for glioblastoma (GBM) is surgery followed by radiotherapy with Temozolomide and then with adjuvant temozolomide. Second line treatment usually involves resurgery, reirradiation, systemic therapy such as bevacizumab, irinotecan, and lomustine.
7. Management for LGG have ranged from observation to a biopsy for histological confirmation to aggressive radical resections followed by adjuvant radiotherapy with or without additional chemotherapy.
8. Brain stem gliomas are usually not amenable to radical surgical resection, and hence if a biopsy is feasible, it is advisable to proceed with the same followed by RT. H3K27M alterations are usually present in these tumours being named as diffuse midline gliomas. ONC-201 has shown favourable clinical and radiological outcomes in preliminary analysis in these tumours.
9. Hemispheric gliomas (G34R/V) belong to recent WHO classification tumours, and treatment is similar to that of high-grade gliomas but has better prognosis than H3K27M counterpart.
10. Management of MB have changed from histopathology to molecular correlation, with CSI being the core part of treatment protocol. Recent evidence has supported the use of daily carboplatin in Group 3 MB. Usage of Modern proton beam therapy will be very beneficial in these tumours.
11. CSI is integral part of treatment in other embryonal tumours such as ependymomas, ATRT, ETMR, BCOR and other rare tumours.
12. Low-grade paediatric gliomas are usually treated with surgery, and then further management based on histopathology and molecular evaluation. Radiotherapy plays a major role in these tumours. Decision regarding observation versus treatment has to be carefully based on clinical, radiological, and pathological correlation.
13. High-grade paediatric gliomas are similar to that of adults, except for the fact that they are more prone to have histone mutations, and thereby guarded prognosis.
14. Intracranial germ cell tumours are usually classified into germinomatous and nongerminomatous, with whole ventricular radiotherapy playing a major role in the former and CSI in the latter. Both involves surgical resection, tumour marker correlation in both CSF and serum, and chemotherapy as per ACNS protocol.
15. Management of skull base tumours are usually challenging, in view of subto-

(continued)

tal resection, close proximity to critical structures, with radiotherapy being given taking into account the organs at risk. IMPT have shown encouraging results in treatment of these skull base tumours.

16. Benign tumours such as meningiomas are usually treated with surgical resection and histopathological correlation, with Grades 2 and 3 tumours are usually considered for adjuvant radiotherapy.
17. Vestibular schwannomas are treated based on symptomatology. Treatment paradigm ranges from observation to conventional fractionated radiotherapy, SRS/SRT, and surgical resection in tumours with impending brainstem compression.
18. Pituitary adenomas are usually managed with surgery and medical management, with radiotherapy being considered in situations such as large tumours, cavernous sinus invasion, recurrence, and refractory/secreting tumours.
19. Management of Craniopharyngiomas are based on surgical resection, however, aggressive surgery with gross total resection may result in significant peri- and postoperative sequelae, and hence treatment has to be carefully tailored based on the tumour and surgical decompression. Radiotherapy forms an integral part of treatment in these tumours and can be treated with fractionated, stereotactic radiotherapy or with modern proton beam therapy.
20. Primary CNS lymphoma are rare tumours, with systemic therapy being the main backbone of treatment, and radiotherapy is usually considered after partial response and in patients less than 60 years of age. Neurological deficits are more seen in patients treated with radiotherapy more than 60 years of age.
21. Treatment of brain metastases differ significantly, with common treatment modalities being WBRT, hippocampal sparing WBRT, SRS/SRT, and surgical resection.
22. CNS tumours are not only treated based on the type of these tumours, but also depends on quality of life, which must be considered before proceeding with the treatment of these tumours. Functional preservation should be given precedence in this modern era in the treatment of brain tumours.

Multiple Choice Questions

1. Recent WHO 2021 classification has incorporated what changes of the following?
   (a) Entity and variants
   (b) Types and subtypes
   (c) Hierarchy and sub hierarchy
   (d) Roman letters and Devanagiri
2. 3 years old child presented with history of early morning headache and projectile vomiting. Family has come to the outpatient clinic, and you suspect a brain lesion. Which is the ideal imaging you should order further?
   (a) MRI Brain (contrast)
   (b) MRI Brain with whole spine screening (contrast)
   (c) CT Brain (Contrast)
   (d) CT Brain with whole spine screening (Contrast)
3. 78-years-old gentleman, diagnosed with a lesion in the left parietal lobe. MRI was suspicious of high-grade glioma. Partial excision of lesion was done, and histopathology was reported as Glioblastoma, Grade 4. Post-surgery, patient was in poor performance status (PS 3). You explain to the family the need for chemoradiation and explain to them that you will proceed with one of the following.
   (a) 59.4 Gy–60 Gy in 30–33 fractions
   (b) 54–55.8 Gy in 30–31 fractions
   (c) 40 Gy in 15 fractions
   (d) Will not treat at all

4. ONC-201 is useful in which of the following scenario?
   (a) H3F3A G34 R/V mutations
   (b) BRAF V600E mutations
   (c) H3K27me3 mutations
   (d) H3K27M alterations
5. Oligodendroglioma can be diagnosed, but must be confirmed with the following.
   (a) IDH mutant
   (b) ATRX retained
   (c) 1p19q codeletion
   (d) None of the above
6. BRAF V600E mutation can be present in all except
   (a) Pleomorphic xanthoastrocytoma
   (b) Ganglioglioma
   (c) Epithelioid glioblastoma
   (d) Neurocytoma
7. Daily carboplatin has to be considered in which subgroup of medulloblastoma?
   (a) WNT
   (b) SHH
   (c) Group 3
   (d) Group 4
8. Vismodegib and Sonidegib is useful in which subgroup of medulloblastoma?
   (a) WNT
   (b) SHH
   (c) Group 3
   (d) Group 4
9. Craniospinal irradiation must be considered in newly diagnosed localized tumours of the following except?
   (a) Medulloblastoma
   (b) Ependymoma
   (c) Atypical teratoid rhabdoid tumour
   (d) High grade neuroepithelial tumour with BCOR positivity
10. Extra-neuraxial spread can be seen in the following except
    (a) SHH type medulloblastoma
    (b) Malignant meningioma
    (c) Pilocytic astrocytoma
    (d) CNS lymphoma
11. Serum elevation of AFP/HCG in an otherwise reported pure germinomatous tumour should infer which of the following?
    (a) No need to interfere. False value. Proceed with treatment as planned
    (b) Be cautious. Observe. However, proceed as per germinomatous tumour
    (c) Should evaluate further. Examine genitalia and check for any further chances of extracranial source
    (d) Proceed as per non-germinomatous tumour treatment
12. Conventional dosage for non-functioning pituitary adenoma is
    (a) 45 Gy in 25 fractions
    (b) 50.4 Gy in 28 fractions
    (c) 54 Gy in 30 fractions
    (d) 59.4 Gy in 33 fractions
13. BRAF V600E/MEK inhibitors are
    (a) Vismodegib and Sonidegib
    (b) Dabrafenib and Trametinib
    (c) Dabrafenib and Lorlatinib
    (d) Sunitinib and Dasatinib
14. 45 years old female diagnosed with Carcinoma of left breast, presented with headache and giddiness. MRI evaluation showed multiple lesions (5–6 in number), largest being 2 cm involving the parietal lobes and single lesion in cerebellum. PET-CT reveals small lesions in lung and liver. Patient otherwise is in excellent performance status. Patient has been referred for radiotherapy to brain. Ideal treatment paradigm will be as follows.
    (a) Whole brain radiotherapy
    (b) Hippocampal sparing whole brain radiotherapy
    (c) Observation
    (d) Stereotactic radiotherapy to all the lesions
15. 6 years old boy, presented with sudden onset visual deterioration; MRI revealed opticochiasmatic lesion. Biopsy was done which was reported as Pilocytic astrocytoma. Patient has been referred for radiotherapy. Optimal management will be which of the following.
    (a) Observation
    (b) Proceed with radiotherapy
    (c) Examine clinically, evaluate for genetic syndromes
    (d) Do BRAF fusion/V600E testing. Proceed with targeted therapy if positive

Answer Key

1. (b)
2. (b)
3. (c)
4. (d)
5. (c)
6. (d)
7. (c)
8. (b)
9. (c)
10. (c)
11. (c)
12. (a)
13. (b)
14. (b)
15. (c)

References

1. Yeole BB. Trends in the brain cancer incidence in India. Asian Pac J Cancer Prev. 2008;9(2):267–70.
2. Dasgupta A, Gupta T, Jalali R. Indian data on central nervous tumors: a summary of published work. South Asian J Cancer. 2016;05(03):147–53.
3. Jalali R, Datta D. Prospective analysis of incidence of central nervous tumors presenting in a tertiary cancer hospital from India. J Neuro-Oncol. 2008;87(1):111–4.
4. Asirvatham JR, Deepti AN, Chyne R, MSN P, Chacko AG, Rajshekhar V, et al. Pediatric tumors of the central nervous system: a retrospective study of 1,043 cases from a tertiary care center in South India. Childs Nerv Syst. 2011;27(8):1257–63.
5. Bray F, Ferlay J, Soerjomataram I, Siegel RL, Torre LA, Jemal A. Global cancer statistics 2018: GLOBOCAN estimates of incidence and mortality worldwide for 36 cancers in 185 countries. CA Cancer J Clin. 2018;68(6):394–424.
6. Garibaldi C, Jereczek-Fossa BA, Marvaso G, Dicuonzo S, Rojas DP, Cattani F, et al. Recent advances in radiation oncology. Ecancermedicalscience. 2017;11:785.
7. Sabeghi P, Zarand P, Zargham S, Golestany B, et al. Advances in Neuro-Oncological Imaging: An Update on Diagnostic Approach to Brain Tumors. Cancers (Basel). 2024;16:576. https://doi.org/10.3390/cancers16030576.
8. Pereira GC, Traughber M, Muzic RF. The role of imaging in radiation therapy planning: past, present, and future. Biomed Res Int. 2014;2014:231090.
9. Jaffray DA. Image-guided radiotherapy: from current concept to future perspectives. Nat Rev Clin Oncol. 2012;9(12):688–99.
10. Teoh M, Clark CH, Wood K, Whitaker S, Nisbet A. Volumetric modulated arc therapy: a review of current literature and clinical use in practice. Br J Radiol. 2011;84(1007):967–96.
11. Stewart J, Sahgal A, Lee Y, Soliman H, Tseng CL, Detsky J, et al. Quantitating interfraction target dynamics during concurrent chemoradiation for glioblastoma: a prospective serial imaging study. Int J Radiat Oncol Biol Phys. 2021;109(3):736–46.
12. Baumann M, Krause M, Overgaard J, Debus J, Bentzen SM, Daartz J, et al. Radiation oncology in the era of precision medicine. Nat Rev Cancer. 2016;16(4):234–49.
13. Brock KK. Adaptive radiotherapy: moving into the future. Semin Radiat Oncol. 2019;29(3):181–4.
14. Tsang DS, Murray L, Ramaswamy V, Zapotocky M, Tabori U, Bartels U, et al. Craniospinal irradiation as part of re-irradiation for children with recurrent intracranial ependymoma. Neuro-Oncology. 2019;21(4):547–57.
15. Chilukuri S, Burela N, Uppuluri R, Indumathi D, Nangia S, Panda PK, et al. Preliminary experience of treating children and Young adults with image-guided proton beam therapy in India. JCO Glob Oncol. 2020;6:1736–45.
16. Jalali R, Sudarsan RT. Advances in radiation therapy in malignant brain tumors. Int J Neurooncol. 2021;4(3):208.
17. Cardinale R, Won M, Choucair A, Gillin M, Chakravarti A, Schultz C, et al. A phase II trial of accelerated radiotherapy using weekly stereotactic conformal boost for supratentorial glioblastoma multiforme: RTOG 0023. Int J Radiat Oncol Biol Phys. 2006;65(5):1422–8.
18. Badiyan SN, Markovina S, Simpson JR, Robinson CG, DeWees T, Tran DD, et al. Radiation therapy dose escalation for glioblastoma multiforme in the era of temozolomide. Int J Radiat Oncol Biol Phys. 2014;90(4):877–85.
19. Louis DN, Perry A, Wesseling P, Brat DJ, Cree IA, Figarella-Branger D, et al. The 2021 WHO classification of tumors of the central nervous system: a summary. Neuro-Oncology. 2021;23(8):1231–51.
20. Combs SE, Baumert BG, Bendszus M, Bozzao A, Brada M, Fariselli L, et al. ESTRO ACROP guideline for target volume delineation of skull base tumors. Radiother Oncol. 2021;156:80–94.
21. Stupp R, Hegi ME, Mason WP, van den Bent MJ, Taphoorn MJB, Janzer RC, et al. Effects of radiotherapy with concomitant and adjuvant temozolomide versus radiotherapy alone on survival in glioblastoma in a randomised phase III study: 5-year analysis of the EORTC-NCIC trial. Lancet Oncol. 2009;10(5):459–66.
22. Cabrera AR, Kirkpatrick JP, Fiveash JB, Shih HA, Koay EJ, Lutz S, et al. Radiation therapy for glioblastoma: executive summary of an American Society for Radiation Oncology evidence-based clinical practice guideline. Pract Radiat Oncol. 2016;6(4):217–25.

23. Hasegawa M, Niibe H, Mitsuhashi N, Yamakawa M, Kato S, Furuta M, et al. Hyperfractionated and hypofractionated radiation therapy for human malignant glioma xenograft in nude mice. Jpn J Cancer Res Gann. 1995;86(9):879–84.
24. Hingorani M, Colley WP, Dixit S, Beavis AM. Hypofractionated radiotherapy for glioblastoma: strategy for poor-risk patients or hope for the future? Br J Radiol. 2012;85(1017):e770–81.
25. Rajz GG, Nass D, Talianski E, Pfeffer R, Spiegelmann R, Cohen ZR. Presentation patterns and outcome of gliomatosis cerebri. Oncol Lett. 2012;3(1):209–13.
26. Ranjan S, Warren KE. Gliomatosis cerebri: current understanding and controversies. Front Oncol. 2017;7:165. Available from: https://www.frontiersin.org/article/10.3389/fonc.2017.00165.
27. Chan JL, Lee SW, Fraass BA, Normolle DP, Greenberg HS, Junck LR, et al. Survival and failure patterns of high-grade gliomas after three-dimensional conformal radiotherapy. J Clin Oncol Off J Am Soc Clin Oncol. 2002;20(6):1635–42.
28. Laperriere NJ, Leung PM, McKenzie S, Milosevic M, Wong S, Glen J, et al. Randomized study of brachytherapy in the initial management of patients with malignant astrocytoma. Int J Radiat Oncol Biol Phys. 1998;41(5):1005–11.
29. Shieh LT, Guo HR, Ho CH, Lin LC, Chang CH, Ho SY. Survival of glioblastoma treated with a moderately escalated radiation dose—results of a retrospective analysis. PLoS One. 2020;15(5):e0233188.
30. Zschaeck S, Wust P, Graf R, Misch M, Onken J, Ghadjar P, et al. Locally dose-escalated radiotherapy may improve intracranial local control and overall survival among patients with glioblastoma. Radiat Oncol. 2018;13(1):251.
31. Jhaveri J, Cheng E, Tian S, Buchwald Z, Chowdhary M, Liu Y, et al. Proton vs. photon radiation therapy for primary gliomas: an analysis of the National Cancer Data Base. Front Oncol. 2018;8:440. Available from: https://www.frontiersin.org/article/10.3389/fonc.2018.00440.
32. NRG Oncology. NRG-BN001 photon IMRT treatment group displays no significant survival difference between arms for patients with glioblastoma, proton treatment group still accruing [Internet]. NRG. [cited 2022 May 1]. Available from: http://www.nrgoncology.org/Home/News/Post/nrg-bn001-photon-imrt-treatment-group-displays-no-significant-survival-difference-between-arms-for-patients-with-glioblastoma-proton-treatment-group-still-accruing.
33. van den Bent MJ, Tesileanu CMS, Wick W, Sanson M, Brandes AA, Clement PM, et al. Adjuvant and concurrent temozolomide for 1p/19q non-co-deleted anaplastic glioma (CATNON; EORTC study 26053-22054): second interim analysis of a randomised, open-label, phase 3 study. Lancet Oncol. 2021;22(6):813–23.
34. Kleinberg L, Sloan L, Grossman S, Lim M. Radiotherapy, lymphopenia, and host immune capacity in glioblastoma: a potentially actionable toxicity associated with reduced efficacy of radiotherapy. Neurosurgery. 2019;85(4):441–53.
35. Grossman SA, Ye X, Lesser G, Sloan A, Carraway H, Desideri S, et al. Immunosuppression in patients with high-grade gliomas treated with radiation and temozolomide. Clin Cancer Res Off J Am Assoc Cancer Res. 2011;17(16):5473–80.
36. Mohan R, Liu AY, Brown PD, Mahajan A, Dinh J, Chung C, et al. Proton therapy reduces the likelihood of high-grade radiation-induced lymphopenia in glioblastoma patients: phase II randomized study of protons vs photons. Neuro-Oncology. 2021;23(2):284–94.
37. Gupta T, Nair V, Paul SN, Kannan S, Moiyadi A, Epari S, et al. Can irradiation of potential cancer stem-cell niche in the subventricular zone influence survival in patients with newly diagnosed glioblastoma? J Neuro-Oncol. 2012;109(1):195–203.
38. Bender K, Träger M, Wahner H, Onken J, Scheel M, Beck M, et al. What is the role of the subventricular zone in radiotherapy of glioblastoma patients? Radiother Oncol. 2021;158:138–45.
39. Capilla-Gonzalez V, Bonsu JM, Redmond KJ, Garcia-Verdugo JM, Quiñones-Hinojosa A. Implications of irradiating the subventricular zone stem cell niche. Stem Cell Res. 2016;16(2):387–96.
40. Khalifa J, Tensaouti F, Lusque A, Plas B, Lotterie JA, Benouaich-Amiel A, et al. Subventricular zones: new key targets for glioblastoma treatment. Radiat Oncol. 2017;12(1):67.
41. Pignatti F, van den Bent M, Curran D, Debruyne C, Sylvester R, Therasse P, et al. Prognostic factors for survival in adult patients with cerebral low-grade glioma. J Clin Oncol Off J Am Soc Clin Oncol. 2002;20(8):2076–84.
42. Buckner JC, Shaw EG, Pugh SL, Chakravarti A, Gilbert MR, Barger GR, et al. Radiation plus procarbazine, CCNU, and vincristine in low-grade glioma. N Engl J Med. 2016;374(14):1344–55.
43. Lassman A, Won M, Gregory Cairncross J, Shaw E, Ashby L, Souhami L, et al. ACTR-13. Final results with chemoradiotherapy for anaplastic oligodendroglial tumors from NRG oncology/RTOG 9402. Neuro-Oncology. 2019;21(Suppl 6):vi15.
44. Fisher BJ, Pugh SL, Macdonald DR, Chakravatri A, Lesser GJ, Fox S, et al. Phase 2 study of a temozolomide-based chemoradiation therapy regimen for high-risk, low-grade gliomas: long-term results of radiation therapy oncology group 0424. Int J Radiat Oncol Biol Phys. 2020;107(4):720–5.
45. Lassman AB, Cloughesy TF. Early results from the CODEL trial for anaplastic oligodendrogliomas: is temozolomide futile? Neuro-Oncology. 2021;23(3):347–9.
46. Indelicato DJ, Rotondo RL, Uezono H, Sandler ES, Aldana PR, Ranalli NJ, et al. Outcomes following proton therapy for pediatric low-grade glioma. Int J Radiat Oncol Biol Phys. 2019;104(1):149–56.

47. Thurin E, Nyström PW, Smits A, Werlenius K, Bäck A, Liljegren A, et al. Proton therapy for low-grade gliomas in adults: a systematic review. Clin Neurol Neurosurg. 2018;174:233–8.
48. Shih HA, Sherman JC, Nachtigall LB, Colvin MK, Fullerton BC, Daartz J, et al. Proton therapy for low-grade gliomas: results from a prospective trial. Cancer. 2015;121(10):1712–9.
49. Protocol [Internet]. [cited 2022 May 1]. Available from: https://www.nrgoncology.org/Clinical-Trials/Protocol/nrg-bn005?filter=nrg-bn005.
50. Jalali R, Raut N, Arora B, Gupta T, Dutta D, Munshi A, et al. Prospective evaluation of radiotherapy with concurrent and adjuvant temozolomide in children with newly diagnosed diffuse intrinsic pontine glioma. Int J Radiat Oncol Biol Phys. 2010;77(1):113–8.
51. Rizzo D, Scalzone M, Ruggiero A, Maurizi P, Attinà G, Mastrangelo S, et al. Temozolomide in the treatment of newly diagnosed diffuse brainstem glioma in children: a broken promise? J Chemother. 2015;27(2):106–10.
52. Chi AS, Tarapore RS, Hall MD, Shonka N, Gardner S, Umemura Y, et al. Pediatric and adult H3 K27M-mutant diffuse midline glioma treated with the selective DRD2 antagonist ONC201. J Neuro-Oncol. 2019;145(1):97–105.
53. Picart T, Barritault M, Poncet D, Berner LP, Izquierdo C, Tabouret E, et al. Characteristics of diffuse hemispheric gliomas, H3 G34-mutant in adults. Neuro-Oncol Adv. 2021;3(1):vdab061.
54. Roux A, Pallud J, Saffroy R, Edjlali-Goujon M, Debily MA, Boddaert N, et al. High-grade gliomas in adolescents and young adults highlight histomolecular differences from their adult and pediatric counterparts. Neuro-Oncology. 2020;22(8):1190–202.
55. Taylor MD, Northcott PA, Korshunov A, Remke M, Cho YJ, Clifford SC, et al. Molecular subgroups of medulloblastoma: the current consensus. Acta Neuropathol. 2012;123(4):465–72.
56. Gupta T, Shirsat N, Jalali R. Molecular subgrouping of medulloblastoma: impact upon research and clinical practice. Curr Pediatr Rev. 2015;11(2):106–19.
57. Gupta T, Sarkar C, Rajshekhar V, Chatterjee S, Shirsat N, Muzumdar D, et al. Indian Society of Neuro-Oncology consensus guidelines for the contemporary management of medulloblastoma. Neurol India. 2017;65(2):315–32.
58. Ramaswamy V, Remke M, Bouffet E, Bailey S, Clifford SC, Doz F, et al. Risk stratification of childhood medulloblastoma in the molecular era: the current consensus. Acta Neuropathol. 2016;131(6):821–31.
59. Michalski JM, Janss AJ, Vezina LG, Smith KS, Billups CA, Burger PC, et al. Children's oncology group phase III trial of reduced-dose and reduced-volume radiotherapy with chemotherapy for newly diagnosed average-risk Medulloblastoma. J Clin Oncol Off J Am Soc Clin Oncol. 2021;39(24):2685–97.
60. Gupta T, Pervez S, Dasgupta A, Chatterjee A, Epari S, Chinnaswamy G, et al. Omission of upfront craniospinal irradiation in patients with low-risk WNT-pathway medulloblastoma is associated with unacceptably high risk of neuraxial failure. Clin Cancer Res. 2022;28:OF1–6.
61. Tata Memorial Centre. Focal radiotherapy plus low dose craniospinal irradiation followed by adjuvant chemotherapy in WNT subgroup medulloblastoma [Internet]. 2021 Oct [cited 2022 Jul 31]. Report No.: NCT04474964. Available from: https://clinicaltrials.gov/ct2/show/NCT04474964.
62. Leary SES, Packer RJ, Li Y, Billups CA, Smith KS, Jaju A, et al. Efficacy of carboplatin and Isotretinoin in children with high-risk Medulloblastoma: a randomized clinical trial from the children's oncology group. JAMA Oncol. 2021;7(9):1313–21.
63. Gupta T, Sinha S, Chinnaswamy G, Vora T, Prasad M, Bhat V, et al. Safety and efficacy of concurrent carboplatin during full-dose craniospinal irradiation for high-risk/metastatic medulloblastoma in a resource-limited setting. Pediatr Blood Cancer. 2021;68(5):e28925.
64. Ajithkumar T, Horan G, Padovani L, Thorp N, Timmermann B, Alapetite C, et al. SIOPE—brain tumor group consensus guideline on craniospinal target volume delineation for high-precision radiotherapy. Radiother Oncol. 2018;128(2):192–7.
65. Sharma DS, Gupta T, Jalali R, Master Z, Phurailatpam RD, Sarin R. High-precision radiotherapy for craniospinal irradiation: evaluation of three-dimensional conformal radiotherapy, intensity-modulated radiation therapy and helical TomoTherapy. Br J Radiol. 2009;82(984):1000–9.
66. Noufal M, Sharma S, Krishnan G, Sawant M, Gaikwad U, Jalali R. Robustly optimized hybrid intensity-modulated proton therapy for craniospinal irradiation. J Cancer Res Ther. 2021;0(0):0.
67. Yock TI, Yeap BY, Ebb DH, Weyman E, Eaton BR, Sherry NA, et al. Long-term toxic effects of proton radiotherapy for paediatric medulloblastoma: a phase 2 single-arm study. Lancet Oncol. 2016;17(3):287–98.
68. Miralbell R, Bleher A, Huguenin P, Ries G, Kann R, Mirimanoff RO, et al. Pediatric medulloblastoma: radiation treatment technique and patterns of failure. Int J Radiat Oncol Biol Phys. 1997;37(3):523–9.
69. Kahalley LS, Peterson R, Ris MD, Janzen L, Okcu MF, Grosshans DR, et al. Superior intellectual outcomes after proton radiotherapy compared with photon radiotherapy for pediatric medulloblastoma. J Clin Oncol Off J Am Soc Clin Oncol. 2020;38(5):454–61.
70. Gross JP, Powell S, Zelko F, Hartsell W, Goldman S, Fangusaro J, et al. Improved neuropsychological outcomes following proton therapy relative to X-ray therapy for pediatric brain tumor patients. Neuro-Oncology. 2019;21(7):934–43.
71. Liu KX, Ioakeim-Ioannidou M, Susko MS, Rao AD, Yeap BY, Snijders AM, et al. A multi-institu-

tional comparative analysis of proton and photon therapy-induced hematologic toxicity in patients with medulloblastoma. Int J Radiat Oncol Biol Phys. 2021;109(3):726–35.
72. Xiang M, Chang DT, Pollom EL. Second cancer risk after primary cancer treatment with three-dimensional conformal, intensity-modulated, or proton beam radiation therapy. Cancer. 2020;126(15):3560–8.
73. Chilukuri S, Jalali R. Risk of second malignancy after modern conformal and proton beam radiotherapy-minimizing risks, improving survivorshipInstructions to authors and other literary works of fiction. Indian J Cancer. 2018;55(4):316–7.
74. Gaikwad U, Noufal MP, Sylvia J, Reddy AK, Panda PK, Chilukuri S, et al. Encouraging early outcomes with image guided pencil beam proton therapy for cranio-spinal irradiation: first report from India. Radiat Oncol. 2022;17(1):115.
75. Reddy AT, Strother DR, Judkins AR, Burger PC, Pollack IF, Krailo MD, et al. Efficacy of high-dose chemotherapy and three-dimensional conformal radiation for atypical Teratoid/Rhabdoid tumor: a report from the children's oncology group trial ACNS0333. J Clin Oncol Off J Am Soc Clin Oncol. 2020;38(11):1175–85.
76. Ryall S, Zapotocky M, Fukuoka K, Nobre L, Guerreiro Stucklin A, Bennett J, et al. Integrated molecular and clinical analysis of 1,000 pediatric low-grade gliomas. Cancer Cell. 2020;37(4):569–583.e5.
77. Müller K, Gnekow A, Falkenstein F, Scheiderbauer J, Zwiener I, Pietsch T, et al. Radiotherapy in pediatric pilocytic astrocytomas. A subgroup analysis within the prospective multicenter study HIT-LGG 1996 by the German Society of Pediatric Oncology and Hematology (GPOH). Strahlenther Onkol Organ Dtsch Rontgengesellschaft Al. 2013;189(8):647–55.
78. Lassaletta A, Zapotocky M, Mistry M, Ramaswamy V, Honnorat M, Krishnatry R, et al. Therapeutic and prognostic implications of BRAF V600E in pediatric low-grade gliomas. J Clin Oncol Off J Am Soc Clin Oncol. 2017;35(25):2934–41.
79. de Blank P, Bandopadhayay P, Haas-Kogan D, Fouladi M, Fangusaro J. Management of pediatric low-grade glioma. Curr Opin Pediatr. 2019;31(1):21–7.
80. Hargrave DR, Bouffet E, Tabori U, Broniscer A, Cohen KJ, Hansford JR, et al. Efficacy and safety of Dabrafenib in pediatric patients with BRAF V600 mutation-positive relapsed or refractory low-grade glioma: results from a phase I/IIa study. Clin Cancer Res. 2019;25(24):7303–11.
81. Wen PY, Stein A, van den Bent M, De Greve J, Wick A, de Vos FYFL, et al. Dabrafenib plus trametinib in patients with BRAFV600E-mutant low-grade and high-grade glioma (ROAR): a multicentre, open-label, single-arm, phase 2, basket trial. Lancet Oncol. 2022;23(1):53–64.
82. Indelicato DJ, Bradley JA, Rotondo RL, Nanda RH, Logie N, Sandler ES, et al. Outcomes following proton therapy for pediatric ependymoma. Acta Oncol. 2018;57(5):644–8.
83. Gupta T, Maitre M, Gupta P, Krishnatry R, Chatterjee A, Moiyadi A, et al. Extent of re-excision, sequence/timing of salvage re-irradiation, and disease-free interval impact upon clinical outcomes in recurrent/progressive ependymoma. J Neuro-Oncol. 2020;147(2):405–15.
84. Frappaz D, Dhall G, Murray MJ, Goldman S, Faure Conter C, Allen J, et al. EANO, SNO and Euracan consensus review on the current management and future development of intracranial germ cell tumors in adolescents and young adults. Neuro-Oncology. 2022;24(4):516–27.
85. Sudarsan RT, Chilukuri S, Padannayil NM, Panda PK, Jalali R. Introduction of proton beam therapy in intracranial germ cell tumors in India. Indian Pediatr. 2021;58(2):182–3.
86. Bartels U, Onar-Thomas A, Patel SK, Shaw D, Fangusaro J, Dhall G, et al. Phase II trial of response-based radiation therapy for patients with localized Germinoma: a children's oncology group study. Neuro-Oncology. 2022;24(6):974–83.
87. Fonseca A, Faure-Conter C, Murray MJ, Fangusaro J, Bailey S, Goldman S, et al. Pattern of treatment failures in central nervous system non-germinomatous germ cell tumors (CNS-NGGCT): a pooled analysis of clinical trials. Neuro-Oncology. 2022;24:noac057.
88. Palmer JD, Gamez ME, Ranta K, Ruiz-Garcia H, Peterson JL, Blakaj DM, et al. Radiation therapy strategies for skull-base malignancies. J Neuro-Oncol. 2020;150(3):445–62.
89. Tonse R, Chilikuri S, Shamurailatpam D, Jalali R. Introduction of image-guided pencil beam for skull base tumors in India: a report of two cases and a brief review of the literature. Neurol India. 2020;68(1):42.
90. Banerjee J, Pääkkö E, Harila M, Herva R, Tuominen J, Koivula A, et al. Radiation-induced meningiomas: a shadow in the success story of childhood leukemia. Neuro-Oncology. 2009;11(5):543–9.
91. Barresi V, Simbolo M, Fioravanzo A, Piredda ML, Caffo M, Ghimenton C, et al. Molecular profiling of 22 primary atypical Meningiomas shows the prognostic significance of 18q heterozygous loss and CDKN2A/B homozygous deletion on recurrence-free survival. Cancer. 2021;13(4):903.
92. Bi WL, Greenwald NF, Abedalthagafi M, Wala J, Gibson WJ, Agarwalla PK, et al. Genomic landscape of high-grade meningiomas. NPJ Genom Med. 2017;2:15.
93. Spiegl-Kreinecker S, Lötsch D, Neumayer K, Kastler L, Gojo J, Pirker C, et al. TERT promoter mutations are associated with poor prognosis and cell immortalization in meningioma. Neuro-Oncology. 2018;20(12):1584–93.

94. Nassiri F, Wang JZ, Singh O, Karimi S, Dalcourt T, Ijad N, et al. Loss of H3K27me3 in meningiomas. Neuro-Oncology. 2021;23(8):1282–91.
95. Rogers L, Mehta M. Role of radiation therapy in treating intracranial meningiomas. Neurosurg Focus. 2007;23(4):E4.
96. Adeberg S, Hartmann C, Welzel T, Rieken S, Habermehl D, von Deimling A, et al. Long-term outcome after radiotherapy in patients with atypical and malignant meningiomas—clinical results in 85 patients treated in a single institution leading to optimized guidelines for early radiation therapy. Int J Radiat Oncol Biol Phys. 2012;83(3):859–64.
97. Compter I, Zaugg K, Houben RMA, Dings JTA, Bosmans G, Buescher C, et al. High symptom improvement and local tumor control using stereotactic radiotherapy when given early after diagnosis of meningioma. A multicentre study. Strahlenther Onkol. 2012;188(10):887–93.
98. Jalali R, Loughrey C, Baumert B, Perks J, Warrington AP, Traish D, et al. High precision focused irradiation in the form of fractionated stereotactic conformal radiotherapy (SCRT) for benign meningiomas predominantly in the skull base location. Clin Oncol. 2002;14(2):103–9.
99. Maclean J, Fersht N, Bremner F, Stacey C, Sivabalasingham S, Short S. Meningioma causing visual impairment: outcomes and toxicity after intensity modulated radiation therapy. Int J Radiat Oncol Biol Phys. 2013;85(4):e179–86.
100. Pirzkall A, Debus J, Haering P, Rhein B, Grosser KH, Höss A, et al. Intensity modulated radiotherapy (IMRT) for recurrent, residual, or untreated skull-base meningiomas: preliminary clinical experience. Int J Radiat Oncol Biol Phys. 2003;55(2):362–72.
101. Zhang C, Zhang H. Stereotactic radiosurgery versus observation for treating incidental meningiomas: a systematic review and meta-analysis. Turk Neurosurg. 2021;31(2):151–60.
102. Adegbite AB, Khan MI, Paine KW, Tan LK. The recurrence of intracranial meningiomas after surgical treatment. J Neurosurg. 1983;58(1):51–6.
103. Barbaro NM, Gutin PH, Wilson CB, Sheline GE, Boldrey EB, Wara WM. Radiation therapy in the treatment of partially resected meningiomas. Neurosurgery. 1987;20(4):525–8.
104. Condra KS, Buatti JM, Mendenhall WM, Friedman WA, Marcus RB, Rhoton AL. Benign meningiomas: primary treatment selection affects survival. Int J Radiat Oncol Biol Phys. 1997;39(2):427–36.
105. Goldsmith BJ, Wara WM, Wilson CB, Larson DA. Postoperative irradiation for subtotally resected meningiomas. A retrospective analysis of 140 patients treated from 1967 to 1990. J Neurosurg. 1994;80(2):195–201.
106. Mirimanoff RO, Dosoretz DE, Linggood RM, Ojemann RG, Martuza RL. Meningioma: analysis of recurrence and progression following neurosurgical resection. J Neurosurg. 1985;62(1):18–24.
107. Soyuer S, Chang EL, Selek U, Shi W, Maor MH, DeMonte F. Radiotherapy after surgery for benign cerebral meningioma. Radiother Oncol. 2004;71(1):85–90.
108. Taylor BW, Marcus RB, Friedman WA, Ballinger WE, Million RR. The meningioma controversy: postoperative radiation therapy. Int J Radiat Oncol Biol Phys. 1988;15(2):299–304.
109. Rogers L, Barani I, Chamberlain M, Kaley TJ, McDermott M, Raizer J, et al. Meningiomas: knowledge base, treatment outcomes, and uncertainties. A RANO review. J Neurosurg. 2015;122(1):4–23.
110. Kaur G, Sayegh ET, Larson A, Bloch O, Madden M, Sun MZ, et al. Adjuvant radiotherapy for atypical and malignant meningiomas: a systematic review. Neuro-Oncology. 2014;16(5):628–36.
111. Stessin AM, Schwartz A, Judanin G, Pannullo SC, Boockvar JA, Schwartz TH, et al. Does adjuvant external-beam radiotherapy improve outcomes for nonbenign meningiomas? A surveillance, epidemiology, and end results (SEER)-based analysis. J Neurosurg. 2012;117(4):669–75.
112. Wang C, Kaprealian TB, Suh JH, Kubicky CD, Ciporen JN, Chen Y, et al. Overall survival benefit associated with adjuvant radiotherapy in WHO grade II meningioma. Neuro-Oncology. 2017;19(9):1263–70.
113. Pant S, Tonse R, Kannan S, Moiyadi A, Shetty P, Epari S, et al. Impact of timing of radiation therapy on outcomes in atypical meningioma: a clinical audit. Pract Radiat Oncol. 2018;8(5):e275–84.
114. Halasz LM, Bussière MR, Dennis ER, Niemierko A, Chapman PH, Loeffler JS, et al. Proton stereotactic radiosurgery for the treatment of benign meningiomas. Int J Radiat Oncol Biol Phys. 2011;81(5):1428–35.
115. Henzel M, Gross MW, Hamm K, Surber G, Kleinert G, Failing T, et al. Significant tumor volume reduction of MENINGIOMAS after stereotactic radiotherapy. Neurosurgery. 2006;59(6):1188–94.
116. Krause M. Proton dose escalation for patients with atypical or anaplastic meningiomas [Internet]. clinicaltrials.gov; 2021 [cited 2022 May 1]. Report No.: NCT02978677. Available from: https://clinicaltrials.gov/ct2/show/NCT02978677.
117. Jenkinson MD, Javadpour M, Haylock BJ, Young B, Gillard H, Vinten J, et al. The ROAM/EORTC-1308 trial: radiation versus observation following surgical resection of atypical meningioma: study protocol for a randomised controlled trial. Trials. 2015;16:519.
118. Kemink JL, Langman AW, Niparko JK, Graham MD. Operative management of acoustic neuromas: the priority of neurologic function over complete resection. Otolaryngol-Head Neck Surg. 1991;104(1):96–9.
119. Sughrue ME, Kaur R, Rutkowski MJ, Kane AJ, Kaur G, Yang I, et al. Extent of resection and the long-term durability of vestibular schwannoma surgery. J Neurosurg. 2011;114(5):1218–23.

120. Weber DC, Chan AW, Bussiere MR, Harsh GR, Ancukiewicz M, Barker FG, et al. Proton beam radiosurgery for vestibular schwannoma: tumor control and cranial nerve toxicity. Neurosurgery. 2003;53(3):577–86. discussion 586–8.
121. Foote RL, Coffey RJ, Swanson JW, Harner SG, Beatty CW, Kline RW, et al. Stereotactic radiosurgery using the gamma knife for acoustic neuromas. Int J Radiat Oncol Biol Phys. 1995;32(4):1153–60.
122. Kondziolka D, Lunsford LD, McLaughlin MR, Flickinger JC. Long-term outcomes after radiosurgery for acoustic neuromas. N Engl J Med. 1998;339(20):1426–33.
123. Hasegawa T, Kida Y, Kato T, Iizuka H, Kuramitsu S, Yamamoto T. Long-term safety and efficacy of stereotactic radiosurgery for vestibular schwannomas: evaluation of 440 patients more than 10 years after treatment with gamma knife surgery. J Neurosurg. 2013;118(3):557–65.
124. Breivik CN, Nilsen RM, Myrseth E, Pedersen PH, Varughese JK, Chaudhry AA, et al. Conservative management or gamma knife radiosurgery for vestibular schwannoma: tumor growth, symptoms, and quality of life. Neurosurgery. 2013;73(1):48–56. discussion 56–7.
125. Boari N, Bailo M, Gagliardi F, Franzin A, Gemma M, del Vecchio A, et al. Gamma knife radiosurgery for vestibular schwannoma: clinical results at long-term follow-up in a series of 379 patients. J Neurosurg. 2014;121(Suppl 2):123–42.
126. Tsao MN, Sahgal A, Xu W, De Salles A, Hayashi M, Levivier M, et al. Stereotactic radiosurgery for vestibular schwannoma: international stereotactic radiosurgery society (ISRS) practice guideline. J Radiosurg SBRT. 2017;5(1):5–24.
127. Murphy ES, Suh JH. Radiotherapy for vestibular schwannomas: a critical review. Int J Radiat Oncol Biol Phys. 2011;79(4):985–97.
128. Thomas C, Di Maio S, Ma R, Vollans E, Chu C, Clark B, et al. Hearing preservation following fractionated stereotactic radiotherapy for vestibular schwannomas: prognostic implications of cochlear dose. J Neurosurg. 2007;107(5):917–26.
129. Andrews DW, Suarez O, Goldman HW, Downes MB, Bednarz G, Corn BW, et al. Stereotactic radiosurgery and fractionated stereotactic radiotherapy for the treatment of acoustic schwannomas: comparative observations of 125 patients treated at one institution. Int J Radiat Oncol Biol Phys. 2001;50(5):1265–78.
130. Meijer OWM, Vandertop WP, Baayen JC, Slotman BJ. Single-fraction vs. fractionated linac-based stereotactic radiosurgery for vestibular schwannoma: a single-institution study. Int J Radiat Oncol Biol Phys. 2003;56(5):1390–6.
131. Collen C, Ampe B, Gevaert T, Moens M, Linthout N, De Ridder M, et al. Single fraction versus fractionated linac-based stereotactic radiotherapy for vestibular schwannoma: a single-institution experience. Int J Radiat Oncol Biol Phys. 2011;81(4):e503–9.
132. Kopp C, Fauser C, Müller A, Astner ST, Jacob V, Lumenta C, et al. Stereotactic fractionated radiotherapy and LINAC radiosurgery in the treatment of vestibular Schwannoma—report about both stereotactic methods from a single institution. Int J Radiat Oncol Biol Phys. 2011;80(5):1485–91.
133. Puataweepong P, Dhanachai M, Hansasuta A, Saetia K, Dangprasert S, Sitathanee C, et al. Clinical outcomes of intracranial nonvestibular Schwannomas treated with LinacBased stereotactic radiosurgery and radiotherapy. Asian Pac J Cancer Prev. 2016;17(7):3271–6.
134. Anderson BM, Khuntia D, Bentzen SM, Geye HM, Hayes LL, Kuo JS, et al. Single institution experience treating 104 vestibular schwannomas with fractionated stereotactic radiation therapy or stereotactic radiosurgery. J Neuro-Oncol. 2014;116(1):187–93.
135. Combs SE, Engelhard C, Kopp C, Wiedenmann N, Schramm O, Prokic V, et al. Long-term outcome after highly advanced single-dose or fractionated radiotherapy in patients with vestibular schwannomas—pooled results from 3 large German centers. Radiother Oncol. 2015;114(3):378–83.
136. Barnes CJ, Bush DA, Grove RI, Loredo LN, Slater JD. Fractionated proton beam therapy for acoustic neuromas: tumor control and hearing preservation. Int J Part Ther. 2018;4(4):28–36.
137. Mete O, Lopes MB. Overview of the 2017 WHO classification of pituitary tumors. Endocr Pathol. 2017;28(3):228–43.
138. Lopes MBS. The 2017 World Health Organization classification of tumors of the pituitary gland: a summary. Acta Neuropathol. 2017;134(4):521–35.
139. Micko ASG, Wöhrer A, Höftberger R, Vila G, Marosi C, Knosp E, et al. MGMT and MSH6 immunoexpression for functioning pituitary macroadenomas. Pituitary. 2017;20(6):643–53.
140. Brada M, Rajan B, Traish D, Ashley S, Holmes-Sellors PJ, Nussey S, et al. The long-term efficacy of conservative surgery and radiotherapy in the control of pituitary adenomas. Clin Endocrinol. 1993;38(6):571–8.
141. Minniti G, Jaffrain-Rea ML, Osti M, Esposito V, Santoro A, Solda F, et al. The long-term efficacy of conventional radiotherapy in patients with GH-secreting pituitary adenomas. Clin Endocrinol. 2005;62(2):210–6.
142. Langsenlehner T, Stiegler C, Quehenberger F, Feigl GC, Jakse G, Mokry M, et al. Long-term follow-up of patients with pituitary macroadenomas after postoperative radiation therapy: analysis of tumor control and functional outcome. Strahlenther Onkol. 2007;183(5):241–7.
143. Minniti G, Osti M, Jaffrain-Rea ML, Esposito V, Cantore G, Maurizi Enrici R. Long-term follow-up results of postoperative radiation therapy for Cushing's disease. J Neuro-Oncol. 2007;84(1):79–84.
144. Rim CH, Yang DS, Park YJ, Yoon WS, Lee JA, Kim CY. Radiotherapy for pituitary adenomas: long-

term outcome and complications. Radiat Oncol J. 2011;29(3):156–63.

145. Kim MY, Kim JH, Oh YK, Kim E. Long-term outcomes of surgery and radiotherapy for secreting and non-secreting pituitary adenoma. Radiat Oncol J. 2016;34(2):121–7.
146. Patt H, Jalali R, Yerawar C, Khare S, Gupta T, Goel A, et al. High-precision conformal fractionated radiotherapy is effective in achieving remission in patients with acromegaly after failed Transsphenoidal surgery. Endocr Pract. 2016;22(2):162–72.
147. Minniti G, Gilbert DC, Brada M. Modern techniques for pituitary radiotherapy. Rev Endocr Metab Disord. 2009;10(2):135–44.
148. Tsagarakis S, Grossman A, Plowman PN, Jones AE, Touzel R, Rees LH, et al. Megavoltage pituitary irradiation in the management of prolactinomas: long-term follow-up. Clin Endocrinol. 1991;34(5):399–406.
149. Erfurth EM, Bülow B, Svahn-Tapper G, Norrving B, Odh K, Mikoczy Z, et al. Risk factors for cerebrovascular deaths in patients operated and irradiated for pituitary tumors. J Clin Endocrinol Metab. 2002;87(11):4892–9.
150. Snyder PJ. Clinically nonfunctioning pituitary adenomas. Endocrinol Metab Clin N Am. 1993;22(1):163–75.
151. Wang H, Sun W, Fu Z, Si Z, Zhu Y, Zhai G, et al. The pattern of visual impairment in patients with pituitary adenoma. J Int Med Res. 2008;36(5):1064–9.
152. Park KJ, Kano H, Parry PV, Niranjan A, Flickinger JC, Lunsford LD, et al. Long-term outcomes after gamma knife stereotactic radiosurgery for nonfunctional pituitary adenomas. Neurosurgery. 2011;69(6):1188–99.
153. Gopalan R, Schlesinger D, Vance ML, Laws E, Sheehan J. Long-term outcomes after gamma knife radiosurgery for patients with a nonfunctioning pituitary adenoma. Neurosurgery. 2011;69(2):284–93.
154. Iwata H, Sato K, Tatewaki K, Yokota N, Inoue M, Baba Y, et al. Hypofractionated stereotactic radiotherapy with CyberKnife for nonfunctioning pituitary adenoma: high local control with low toxicity. Neuro-Oncology. 2011;13(8):916–22.
155. Sheehan JP, Starke RM, Mathieu D, Young B, Sneed PK, Chiang VL, et al. Gamma knife radiosurgery for the management of nonfunctioning pituitary adenomas: a multicenter study. J Neurosurg. 2013;119(2):446–56.
156. Lee CC, Kano H, Yang HC, Xu Z, Yen CP, Chung WY, et al. Initial gamma knife radiosurgery for nonfunctioning pituitary adenomas: clinical article. J Neurosurg. 2014;120(3):647–54.
157. Bir SC, Murray RD, Ambekar S, Bollam P, Nanda A. Clinical and radiologic outcome of gamma knife radiosurgery on nonfunctioning pituitary adenomas. J Neurol Surg Part B Skull Base. 2015;76(5):351–7.
158. Li X, Li Y, Cao Y, Li P, Liang B, Sun J, et al. Safety and efficacy of fractionated stereotactic radiotherapy and stereotactic radiosurgery for treatment of pituitary adenomas: a systematic review and meta-analysis. J Neurol Sci. 2017;372:110–6.
159. Scheick S, Amdur RJ, Kirwan JM, Morris CG, Mendenhall WM, Roper S, et al. Long-term outcome after fractionated radiotherapy for pituitary adenoma: the curse of the secretory tumor. Am J Clin Oncol Off J Am Soc Clin Oncol. 2016;39(1):49–54.
160. Minniti G, Flickinger J. The risk/benefit ratio of radiotherapy in pituitary tumors. Best Pract Res Clin Endocrinol Metab. 2019;33(2):101269.
161. Pollock BE, Link MJ, Leavitt JA, Stafford SL. Dose-volume analysis of radiation-induced optic neuropathy after single-fraction stereotactic radiosurgery. Neurosurgery. 2014;75(4):456–60. discussion 460
162. Loeffler JS, Shih HA. Radiation therapy in the management of pituitary adenomas. J Clin Endocrinol Metab. 2011;96(7):1992–2003.
163. Sebastian P, Balakrishnan R, Yadav B, John S. Outcome of radiotherapy for pituitary adenomas. Rep Pract Oncol Radiother. 2016;21(5):466–72.
164. Biermasz NR, Dulken HV, Roelfsema F. Postoperative radiotherapy in acromegaly is effective in reducing GH concentration to safe levels. Clin Endocrinol. 2000;53(3):321–7.
165. Wattson DA, Tanguturi SK, Spiegel DY, Niemierko A, Biller BMK, Nachtigall LB, et al. Outcomes of proton therapy for patients with functional pituitary adenomas. Int J Radiat Oncol Biol Phys. 2014;90(3):532–9.
166. Lin D, Zhao W, Yang J, Wang H, Zhang H. Integrative analysis of biomarkers and mechanisms in adamantinomatous craniopharyngioma. Front Genet. 2022;13:830793.
167. Jensterle M, Jazbinsek S, Bosnjak R, Popovic M, Zaletel LZ, Vesnaver TV, et al. Advances in the management of craniopharyngioma in children and adults. Radiol Oncol. 2019;53(4):388–96.
168. Roderick E, Karavitaki N, Wass JAH. Craniopharyngiomas. Historical aspects of their management. Hormones (Athens). 2008;7(3):271–4.
169. Kramer S, McKissock W, Concannon JP. Craniopharyngiomas: treatment by combined surgery and radiation therapy. J Neurosurg. 1961;18(2):217–26.
170. Hetelekidis S, Barnes PD, Tao ML, Fischer EG, Schneider L, Scott RM, et al. 20-year experience in childhood craniopharyngioma. Int J Radiat Oncol Biol Phys. 1993;27(2):189–95. Available from: https://pubmed.ncbi.nlm.nih.gov/8407391/.
171. Merchant TE, Kiehna EN, Sanford RA, Mulhern RK, Thompson SJ, Wilson MW, et al. Craniopharyngioma: the St. Jude children's research hospital experience 1984–2001. Int J Radiat Oncol Biol Phys. 2002;53(3):533–42.
172. Merchant TE, Kun LE, Hua CH, Wu S, Xiong X, Sanford RA, et al. Disease control after reduced volume conformal and intensity modulated radiation therapy for childhood craniopharyngioma. Int J Radiat Oncol. 2013;85(4):e187–92.

173. Karavitaki N, Cudlip S, Adams CBT, Wass JAH. Craniopharyngiomas. Endocr Rev. 2006;27(4):371–97.
174. Stripp DCH, Maity A, Janss AJ, Belasco JB, Tochner ZA, Goldwein JW, et al. Surgery with or without radiation therapy in the management of craniopharyngiomas in children and young adults. Int J Radiat Oncol Biol Phys. 2004;58(3):714–20.
175. Lin LL, Naqa IE, Leonard JR, Park TS, Hollander AS, Michalski JM, et al. Long-term outcome in children treated for craniopharyngioma with and without radiotherapy. J Neurosurg Pediatr. 2008;1(2):126–30.
176. Scott M, Hetelekidis S, Barnes PD, Goumnerova L, Tarbell NJ. Surgery, radiation, and combination therapy in the treatment of childhood Craniopharyngioma—a 20-year experience. Pediatr Neurosurg. 1994;21(1):75–81.
177. Jalali R, Gupta T, Goda JS, Goswami S, Shah N, Dutta D, et al. Efficacy of stereotactic conformal radiotherapy vs conventional radiotherapy on benign and low-grade brain tumors. JAMA Oncol. 2017;3(10):1368–76.
178. Minniti G, Saran F, Traish D, Soomal R, Sardell S, Gonsalves A, et al. Fractionated stereotactic conformal radiotherapy following conservative surgery in the control of craniopharyngiomas. Radiother Oncol. 2007;82(1):90–5.
179. Combs SE, Thilmann C, Huber PE, Hoess A, Debus J, Schulz-Ertner D. Achievement of long-term local control in patients with craniopharyngiomas using high precision stereotactic radiotherapy. Cancer. 2007;109(11):2308–14.
180. Kobayashi T, Tsugawa T, Hatano M, Hashizume C, Mori Y, Shibamoto Y. Gamma knife radiosurgery of craniopharyngioma: results of 30 cases treated at Nagoya radiosurgery center. Nagoya J Med Sci. 2015;77(3):447–54.
181. Hashizume C, Mori Y, Kobayashi T, Shibamoto Y, Nagai A, Hayashi N. Stereotactic radiotherapy using Novalis for craniopharyngioma adjacent to optic pathways. J Neuro-Oncol. 2010;98(2):239–47.
182. Conti A, Pontoriero A, Ghetti I, Senger C, Vajkoczy P, Pergolizzi S, et al. Benefits of image-guided stereotactic hypofractionated radiation therapy as adjuvant treatment of craniopharyngiomas. A review. Childs Nerv Syst. 2019;35(1):53–61.
183. Lee M, Kalani MYS, Cheshier S, Gibbs IC, Adler JR, Chang SD. Radiation therapy and CyberKnife radiosurgery in the management of craniopharyngiomas. Neurosurg Focus. 2008;24(5):E4.
184. Li P, Wang J, Axier A, Zhou K, Yun J, Wang H, et al. Proton therapy for craniopharyngioma in adults: a protocol for systematic review and meta-analysis. BMJ Open. 2021;11(6):e046043.
185. Voges J, Sturm V, Lehrke R, Treuer H, Gauss C, Berthold F. Cystic craniopharyngioma: long-term results after Intracavitary irradiation with stereotactically applied colloidal β-emitting radioactive sources. Neurosurgery. 1997;40(2):263–70.
186. Hasegawa T, Kondziolka D, Hadjipanayis CG, Lunsford LD. Management of cystic craniopharyngiomas with phosphorus-32 intracavitary irradiation. Neurosurgery. 2004;54(4):813–22.
187. Nelson DF. Radiotherapy in the treatment of primary central nervous system lymphoma (PCNSL). J Neuro-Oncol. 1999;43(3):241–7.
188. Laack NN, Ballman KV, Brown PB, O'Neill BP. North central cancer treatment group. Whole-brain radiotherapy and high-dose methylprednisolone for elderly patients with primary central nervous system lymphoma: results of north central cancer treatment group (NCCTG) 96-73-51. Int J Radiat Oncol Biol Phys. 2006;65(5):1429–39.
189. Ferreri AJM, Verona C, Politi LS, Chiara A, Perna L, Villa E, et al. Consolidation radiotherapy in primary central nervous system lymphomas: impact on outcome of different fields and doses in patients in complete remission after upfront chemotherapy. Int J Radiat Oncol Biol Phys. 2011;80(1):169–75.
190. DeAngelis LM, Seiferheld W, Schold SC, Fisher B, Schultz CJ. Combination chemotherapy and radiotherapy for primary central nervous system lymphoma: radiation therapy oncology group study 93-10. J Clin Oncol Off J Am Soc Clin Oncol. 2002;20(24):4643–8.
191. Shibamoto Y, Hayabuchi N, Hiratsuka J, Tokumaru S, Shirato H, Sougawa M, et al. Is whole-brain irradiation necessary for primary central nervous system lymphoma? Patterns of recurrence after partial-brain irradiation. Cancer. 2003;97(1):128–33.
192. Koh HK, Kim IH, Kim TM, Lim DH, Oh D, Cho JH, et al. Role of radiation therapy in primary central nervous system lymphoma: KROG 14–20 Collaborative Study of Brain and Lymphoma Committee. J Neuro-Oncol. 2017;135(3):629–38.
193. Houillier C, Taillandier L, Dureau S, Lamy T, Laadhari M, Chinot O, et al. Radiotherapy or autologous stem-cell transplantation for primary CNS lymphoma in patients 60 years of age and younger: results of the intergroup ANOCEF-GOELAMS randomized phase II PRECIS study. J Clin Oncol Off J Am Soc Clin Oncol. 2019;37(10):823–33.
194. Thiel E, Korfel A, Martus P, Kanz L, Griesinger F, Rauch M, et al. High-dose methotrexate with or without whole brain radiotherapy for primary CNS lymphoma (G-PCNSL-SG-1): a phase 3, randomised, non-inferiority trial. Lancet Oncol. 2010;11(11):1036–47.
195. Ferreri AJM, Cwynarski K, Pulczynski E, Fox CP, Schorb E, La Rosée P, et al. Whole-brain radiotherapy or autologous stem-cell transplantation as consolidation strategies after high-dose methotrexate-based chemoimmunotherapy in patients with primary CNS lymphoma: results of the second randomisation of the international Extranodal lymphoma study Group-32 phase 2 trial. Lancet Haematol. 2017;4(11):e510–23.
196. Nelson DF, Martz KL, Bonner H, Nelson JS, Newall J, Kerman HD, et al. Non-Hodgkin's lymphoma

of the brain: can high dose, large volume radiation therapy improve survival? Report on a prospective trial by the radiation therapy oncology group (RTOG): RTOG 8315. Int J Radiat Oncol Biol Phys. 1992;23(1):9–17.
197. Fisher B, Seiferheld W, Schultz C, DeAngelis L, Nelson D, Schold SC, et al. Secondary analysis of radiation therapy oncology group study (RTOG) 9310: an intergroup phase II combined modality treatment of primary central nervous system lymphoma. J Neuro-Oncol. 2005;74(2):201–5.
198. Correa DD, Rocco-Donovan M, DeAngelis LM, Dolgoff-Kaspar R, Iwamoto F, Yahalom J, et al. Prospective cognitive follow-up in primary CNS lymphoma patients treated with chemotherapy and reduced-dose radiotherapy. J Neuro-Oncol. 2009;91(3):315–21.
199. Doolittle ND, Korfel A, Lubow MA, Schorb E, Schlegel U, Rogowski S, et al. Long-term cognitive function, neuroimaging, and quality of life in primary CNS lymphoma. Neurology. 2013;81(1):84–92.
200. Morris PG, Correa DD, Yahalom J, Raizer JJ, Schiff D, Grant B, et al. Rituximab, methotrexate, procarbazine, and vincristine followed by consolidation reduced-dose whole-brain radiotherapy and cytarabine in newly diagnosed primary CNS lymphoma: final results and long-term outcome. J Clin Oncol Off J Am Soc Clin Oncol. 2013;31(31):3971–9.
201. Adhikari N, Biswas A, Gogia A, Sahoo RK, Garg A, Nehra A, et al. A prospective phase II trial of response adapted whole brain radiotherapy after high dose methotrexate based chemotherapy in patients with newly diagnosed primary central nervous system lymphoma-analysis of acute toxicity profile and early clinical outcome. J Neuro-Oncol. 2018;139(1):153–66.
202. Johnson JD, Young B. Demographics of brain metastasis. Neurosurg Clin N Am. 1996;7(3):337–44.
203. Lin X, DeAngelis LM. Treatment of brain metastases. J Clin Oncol Off J Am Soc Clin Oncol. 2015;33(30):3475–84.
204. Moravan MJ, Fecci PE, Anders CK, Clarke JM, Salama AKS, Adamson JD, et al. Current multidisciplinary management of brain metastases. Cancer. 2020;126(7):1390–406.
205. Patchell RA, Tibbs PA, Walsh JW, Dempsey RJ, Maruyama Y, Kryscio RJ, et al. A randomized trial of surgery in the treatment of single metastases to the brain. N Engl J Med. 1990;322(8):494–500.
206. Kocher M, Soffietti R, Abacioglu U, Villà S, Fauchon F, Baumert BG, et al. Adjuvant whole-brain radiotherapy versus observation after radiosurgery or surgical resection of one to three cerebral metastases: results of the EORTC 22952-26001 study. J Clin Oncol Off J Am Soc Clin Oncol. 2011;29(2):134–41.
207. Patchell RA, Tibbs PA, Regine WF, Dempsey RJ, Mohiuddin M, Kryscio RJ, et al. Postoperative radiotherapy in the treatment of single metastases to the brain: a randomized trial. JAMA. 1998;280(17):1485–9.
208. Mulvenna P, Nankivell M, Barton R, Faivre-Finn C, Wilson P, McColl E, et al. Dexamethasone and supportive care with or without whole brain radiotherapy in treating patients with non-small cell lung cancer with brain metastases unsuitable for resection or stereotactic radiotherapy (QUARTZ): results from a phase 3, non-inferiority, randomised trial. Lancet Lond Engl. 2016;388(10055):2004–14.
209. Brown PD, Ballman KV, Cerhan JH, Anderson SK, Carrero XW, Whitton AC, et al. Postoperative stereotactic radiosurgery compared with whole brain radiotherapy for resected metastatic brain disease (NCCTG N107C/CEC·3): a multicentre, randomised, controlled, phase 3 trial. Lancet Oncol. 2017;18(8):1049–60.
210. Aoyama H, Shirato H, Tago M, Nakagawa K, Toyoda T, Hatano K, et al. Stereotactic radiosurgery plus whole-brain radiation therapy vs stereotactic radiosurgery alone for treatment of brain metastases: a randomized controlled trial. JAMA. 2006;295(21):2483–91.
211. Mahajan A, Ahmed S, McAleer MF, Weinberg JS, Li J, Brown P, et al. Post-operative stereotactic radiosurgery versus observation for completely resected brain metastases: a single-centre, randomised, controlled, phase 3 trial. Lancet Oncol. 2017;18(8):1040–8.
212. Brown PD, Gondi V, Pugh S, Tome WA, Wefel JS, Armstrong TS, et al. Hippocampal avoidance during whole-brain radiotherapy plus memantine for patients with brain metastases: phase III trial NRG oncology CC001. J Clin Oncol Off J Am Soc Clin Oncol. 2020;38(10):1019–29.
213. Gondi V, Pugh SL, Tome WA, Caine C, Corn B, Kanner A, et al. Preservation of memory with conformal avoidance of the hippocampal neural stem-cell compartment during whole-brain radiotherapy for brain metastases (RTOG 0933): a phase II multi-institutional trial. J Clin Oncol Off J Am Soc Clin Oncol. 2014;32(34):3810–6.
214. Goda JS, Dutta D, Krishna U, Goswami S, Kothavade V, Kannan S, et al. Hippocampal radiotherapy dose constraints for predicting long-term neurocognitive outcomes: mature data from a prospective trial in young patients with brain tumors. Neuro-Oncology. 2020;22(11):1677–85.
215. Vogelbaum MA, Brown PD, Messersmith H, Brastianos PK, Burri S, Cahill D, et al. Treatment for brain metastases: ASCO-SNO-ASTRO guideline. J Clin Oncol. 2022;40(5):492–516.
216. Shaw E, Scott C, Souhami L, Dinapoli R, Kline R, Loeffler J, et al. Single dose radiosurgical treatment of recurrent previously irradiated primary brain tumors and brain metastases: final report of RTOG protocol 90-05. Int J Radiat Oncol Biol Phys. 2000;47(2):291–8.
217. Hyun JW, Jeong IH, Joung A, Cho HJ, Kim SH, Kim HJ. Leptomeningeal metastasis: clinical experience of 519 cases. Eur J Cancer. 2016;56:107–14.

218. Yang JT, Wijetunga NA, Pentsova E, Wolden SL, Young RJ, Correa D, et al. Phase II randomized study comparing proton craniospinal irradiation with photon involved-field radiotherapy for patients with solid tumor leptomeningeal metastasis. J Clin Oncol. 2022;40(16_suppl):2000.
219. Scharp M, Hauswald H, Bischof M, Debus J, Combs SE. Re-irradiation in the treatment of patients with cerebral metastases of solid tumors: retrospective analysis. Radiat Oncol Lond Engl. 2014;9:4.
220. Logie N, Jimenez RB, Pulenzas N, Linden K, Ciafone D, Ghosh S, et al. Estimating prognosis at the time of repeat whole brain radiation therapy for multiple brain metastases: the reirradiation score. Adv Radiat Oncol. 2017;2(3):381–90.
221. Zucchella C, Capone A, Codella V, De Nunzio AM, Vecchione C, Sandrini G, et al. Cognitive rehabilitation for early post-surgery inpatients affected by primary brain tumor: a randomized, controlled trial. J Neuro-Oncol. 2013;114(1):93–100.
222. Veretennikoff K, Walker D, Biggs V, Robinson G. Changes in cognition and decision making capacity following brain tumour resection: illustrated with two cases. Brain Sci. 2017;7(10):122.
223. Haldbo-Classen L, Amidi A, Wu LM, Lukacova S, von Oettingen G, Gottrup H, et al. Long-term cognitive dysfunction after radiation therapy for primary brain tumors. Acta Oncol. 2019;58(5):745–52.
224. Budrukkar A, Jalali R, Dutta D, Sarin R, Devlekar R, Parab S, et al. Prospective assessment of quality of life in adult patients with primary brain tumors in routine neurooncology practice. J Neuro-Oncol. 2009;95(3):413–9.
225. Jalali R, Dutta D. Factors influencing quality of life in adult patients with primary brain tumors. Neuro-Oncology. 2012;14(Suppl 4):iv8–16.
226. Langegård U, Fransson P, Bjork-Eriksson T, Johansson B, Ohlsson-Nevo E, Sjövall K, et al. Health-related quality of life in patients with primary brain tumors during and three months after treatment with proton beam therapy. Tech Innov Patient Support Radiat Oncol. 2021;17:5–17.
227. Dutz A, Agolli L, Bütof R, Valentini C, Baumann M, Lühr A, et al. Neurocognitive function and quality of life after proton beam therapy for brain tumour patients. Radiother Oncol. 2020;143:108–16.

Online Links

IDH mutation in glioma: molecular mechanisms and potential therapeutic targets. https://www.nature.com/articles/s41416-020-0814-x.

Importance of molecular profile in CNS tumours. https://www.youtube.com/watch?v=fEcni2qxnlc.

Indian Society of Neuro-Oncology consensus guidelines for the contemporary management of medulloblastoma. https://www.neurologyindia.com/article.asp?issn=0028-3886;year=2017;volume=65;issue=2;spage=315;epage=332;aulast=Gupta.

Introductory video on proton beam therapy. https://www.youtube.com/watch?v=4EH0fUyp0LM.

Second interim analysis of CATNON trial. https://www.thelancet.com/journals/lanonc/article/PIIS1470-2045(21)00090-5/fulltext#%20.

The 2021 WHO Classification of tumours of the central nervous system: a summary. https://academic.oup.com/neuro-oncology/article/23/8/1231/6311214.

Orbital and Ocular Tumors

Santosh G. Honavar, P. Vijay Anand Reddy, Rolika Bansal, Raksha Rao, Shilpa K. Reddy, and Kirti R. Mohanty

1 Introduction

Ocular oncology encompasses the diagnosis and management of a spectrum of benign and malignant tumors arising from the eyelids, ocular surface, uvea, retina, orbit, and adnexal structures. The clinicians need to be able to differentiate between benign and malignant tumors and triage the management. An accurate diagnosis and timely referral to ocular oncologists is mandatory for appropriate management and optimal outcome. Considering the wide spectrum of presentations, a tailored management approach must be adopted for each patient. Sequential management includes appropriate clinical diagnosis, radiological investigations, surgery with incisional or excisional biopsy, histopathological confirmation, and histopathology-guided adjuvant therapy as appropriate. Treatment modalities include observation, medical management, surgery, chemotherapy, immunotherapy, and radiotherapy.

The advent of radiotherapy has brought in a revolution; however, ionizing radiation can also damage the adjacent structures. To prevent collateral damage and to provide an ideal dose, it is mandatory to have a good understanding of the types of ionizing radiation, the optimal dose of radiation required by individual tumors, the current modes of delivery and the selection of ideal protocols. Aesthetic requirements, psychological aspects, and rehabilitation should also be duly considered while approaching these tumors. With the advances in technology over the past few decades, ocular oncology has evolved in unimaginable ways, which has helped in timely accurate diagnosis, cost-effective treatment modalities, expedited management, and gratifying outcomes.

In this chapter, we shall be providing an overview of the spectrum of tumors of the eyelid, ocular surface, intraocular structures, orbit and adnexa, and their preferred management approaches.

2 Tumors of the Eyelid

2.1 Keratoacanthoma

Keratoacanthoma is an aggressive periocular lesion that is considered as a variant of

S. G. Honavar (✉) · R. Bansal
Department of Oculoplasty and Ocular Oncology, Centre for Sight,
Banjara Hills, Hyderabad, Telangana, India

P. Vijay Anand Reddy · S. K. Reddy · K. R. Mohanty
Department of Radiation Oncology, Apollo Hospitals, Jubilee Hills, Hyderabad, Telangana, India
e-mail: Cancercare@drvijayanandreddy.com

R. Rao
Department of Orbit, Ocular Oncology and Oculoplasty, Narayana Nethralaya,
Bangalore, Karnataka, India

B. K. Mohanti et al. (eds.), *Radiation Oncology – Principles, Precepts and Practice*,
https://doi.org/10.1007/978-981-95-5171-2_2

psueudoepitheliomatous hyperplasia or a borderline tumor between benign and malignant squamous cell carcinoma (SCC) [1]. These lesions have a rapid onset and progression; however, smaller lesions (0.5–2.0 cm) may regress spontaneously [2]. The presence of multiple lesions necessitates a detailed evaluation to rule out associated systemic neoplasms and possible syndromic presentations (Ferguson-Smith syndrome or Muir-Torre syndrome). These lesions are characterized by elevated margins with a central umbilication or crater. The differential diagnosis includes basal cell carcinoma (nodulo-ulcerative type), invasive SCC and other adnexal tumors. The larger lesions are treated by excision with frozen-section guided margin control. Intralesional injections of chemotherapeutic agents (5-fluorouracil, imiquimod, bleomycin, methotrexate), immunotherapy, cryotherapy, or corticosteroids have also been tried with limited success [3, 4].

Radiotherapy with combined external beam photon and electron therapy is effective in cases with recurrent or single large periocular lesions where surgery may be morbid. A margin of 1.0–1.5 cm can be covered around the lesion. Although a dose in the range of 26–30 Gy has shown good results [5], the authors prefer 40–42 Gy at 200 cGy per fraction in cases with keratoacanthoma.

2.2 Squamous Cell Carcinoma

Around 5%–10% of periocular cutaneous tumors are SCC—the second most common cancer of the eyelids in India. These tumors can arise either de novo or from premalignant lesions, including actinic keratosis, Bowen's disease, or in association with xeroderma pigmentosa or even albinism [6]. Xeroderma pigmentosa patients are younger, with multiple and recurrent cutaneous lesions in the eyelids and other parts of the body [7]. These lesions are sessile or elevated, erythematous with indurated borders and with a scaly surface. The lower eyelid is most commonly involved. The lesions frequently ulcerate (Fig. 1), become friable, and tend to bleed on touch. Often secondary infection occurs at the central part of the necrotic lesion. SCC of the eyelid shows neurotrophism and regional lymph node metastasis. Histopathologically, the tumor consists of nests of squamous epithelial cells arising from the epidermis and extending into the dermis. These cells with eosinophilic cytoplasm can also contain keratin pearls.

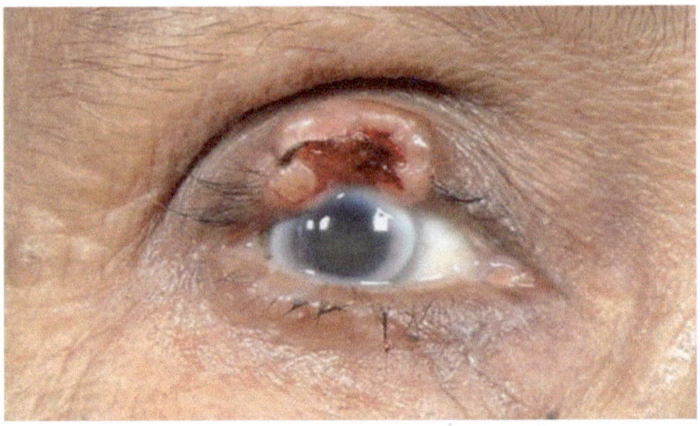

Fig. 1 External image of a 72-year-old male with an elevated nodulo-ulcerative lesion involving the right upper eyelid (approximately 20 × 10 × 6 mm), extending beyond the tarsus, with central ulceration, intrinsic vascularity, indurated borders, loss of eyelashes and erythema—a typical squamous cell carcinoma

Ideal treatment remains complete excision with intra-operative frozen section margin control. Other treatment options are radiation, cryotherapy, and intralesional interferon [8–10]. In early stages of SCC, the likelihood of cure is similar after surgery or radiotherapy [11]. Interstitial brachytherapy is an effective and established method for periocular invasive SCC with the advantage of excellent local tumor control, and cosmesis. It has the advantage of sudden dose fall off, thereby preserving critical structures (like crystalline lens). Single-plane high-dose rate (HDR) brachytherapy can be planned with a dose of 45 Gy in five fractions twice daily to the CTV, with a margin of 1 cm around the primary lesion.

Radiation to these regions can be safely delivered with an orthovoltage energy beam or electrons, along with a protective shield between the eyelid and conjunctiva, with a dose ranging from 5600 to 6000 cGy. Radiation may be especially useful in cases with perineural invasion as an adjuvant therapy [12]. Metastasis to regional lymph nodes, such as pre-auricular lymph nodes, parotid lymph nodes, or cervical lymph nodes can be managed with radical neck dissection and adjuvant radiotherapy.

Periocular SCC lesions are often aggressive with prognosis correlating to high rates of local recurrence and metastasis. Exenteration or immunotherapy is reserved for cases with radiological evidence of orbital invasion [13]. Post-exenteration adjuvant radiotherapy is indicated in cases with positive margins, lymph nodal involvement and perineural invasion. CTV includes the entire orbit/tumor bed, tracing the involved nerve to the skull base and cavernous sinus. Oncologists should be careful while including critical structures such as superior orbital fissure, inferior orbital fissure, supraorbital foramen, infra-orbital groove, and foramen, after proper evaluation of preoperative scans.

2.3 Basal Cell Carcinoma

Basal cell carcinoma (BCC) is the most common malignant tumor of the periocular skin in Western countries, arising mostly in the lower eyelid (65%) (Fig. 2a) followed by medial canthus (15%) and upper eyelid (15%) [2]. It is relatively less common in India. Exposure to ultraviolet (UV) radiation is the most important risk factor along with the association of several genetic syndromes including Gorlin-Goltz syndrome and xeroderma pigmentosa. It characteristically presents as a well-circumscribed, pearly, waxy, or translucent tumor with telangiectasia at the margins (Fig. 2b).

The most common clinical types of BCC are nodular and nodular-ulcerative. Other varieties include pigmented, cystic, superficial and morpheaform BCC. Histo-pathologically, the tumor cells consist of nests of well-differentiated basal cells arranged in a palisading pattern. Eyelid BCC includes slow-growing lesions with a low incidence of metastasis and mortality; however, advanced BCC can invade the orbit, nasal cavity, and paranasal sinuses [14].

Excision biopsy with margin control by frozen section offers a long-term cure in BCC [15, 16]. Cryotherapy has also been used for smaller lesions with comparable outcomes. Topical application of 5% Imiquimod offers an excellent alternative treatment for small periocular BCC. However, radiation therapy is an attractive option for cases when surgical excision may result in loss of function or unacceptable cosmesis. This is particularly relevant to lesions affecting the inner canthus. Radiation in such cases may be delivered as either photon, electron, or proton beam or by interstitial brachytherapy technique. Radiotherapy is indicated in palliative settings as well [17].

In cases with orbital invasion or positive margins post-exenteration, adjuvant radiation therapy is delivered [18]. Proton therapy is a recent

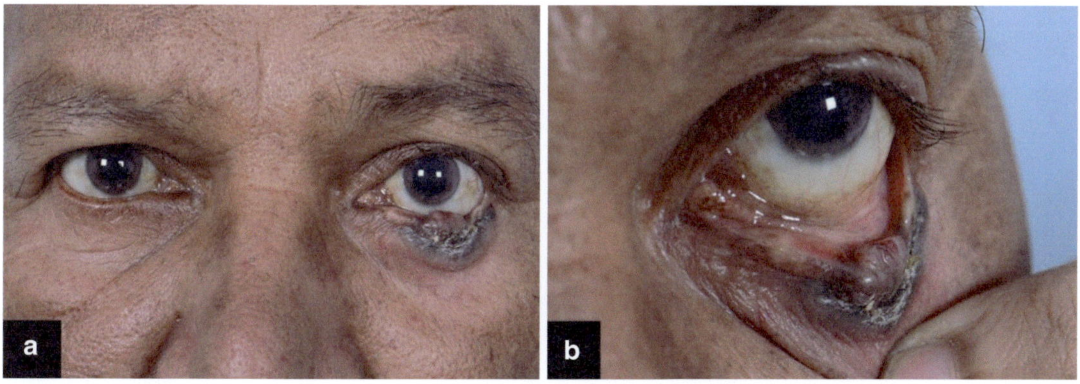

Fig. 2 (**a**) External image of a 68-year-old male with a diffuse, pigmented lesion involving the left lower eyelid with ulcerated surface and erythematous surrounding region (20 × 9 × 5 mm). (**b**) Higher magnification image with traction on the lower eyelid shows loss of lower eyelid architecture, thickening of the lower eyelid margin, and prominent vascularity, along with loss of lashes. This was a pigmented basal cell carcinoma

advance. Interstitial brachytherapy is very effective with the advantage of short duration of treatment and steep dose gradient thereby decreasing collateral damage to adjacent structures. Care must be taken to avoid damage to the tarsal plate while placing the needles in the eyelids. The preferred dose is in the range of 3–4 Gy per fraction twice daily, 6 h apart for 12–15 fractions.

2.4 Sebaceous Gland Carcinoma

Sebaceous gland carcinoma (SGC) of the eyelid and periocular structures can arise from the meibomian glands, Zeis glands of the cilia, glands of the eyebrows, caruncle, and glands of the fine hair follicles on the skin of the eyelid. Due to the abundance of sebaceous glands in the periocular region, 75% of all SGCs occur in this area. In the Western countries, SGC has been reported to account for approximately 2%–7% of all eyelid malignancies [19]. In contrast, several studies from Asian countries, have reported that SGC accounts for up to 30%–60% of malignant eyelid neoplasms and is the most common malignant eyelid neoplasm in these regions [20].

Eyelid SGC presents either as a solitary nodule (Fig. 3a, b) or diffuse eyelid thickening (Fig. 4), which is often misinterpreted as chronic blepharitis. The latter presentation leads to a delay in accurate diagnosis and treatment, leading to an unfavorable prognosis. The tumor typically causes distortion of the posterior eyelid margin, obliteration of meibomian gland orifices, loss of cilia, with surrounding telangiectasia and sometimes ulceration in advanced cases. Even though there are no variations in clinical features of different age groups, the older age group tend to have higher rates of local tumor recurrence whereas the younger patients tend to have higher mortality rates [21]. Up to 35% of the patients can have a pagetoid spread on histopathology.

Etiological factors leading to SGC are not well-established. SGC is associated with Muir-Torre syndrome, a rare autosomal dominant disorder characterized by neoplasms of the sebaceous glands and visceral malignancies that is caused by mutation of DNA mismatch repair genes, leading to the propagation of genetic defects within replicating cells and predisposition to tumor formation.

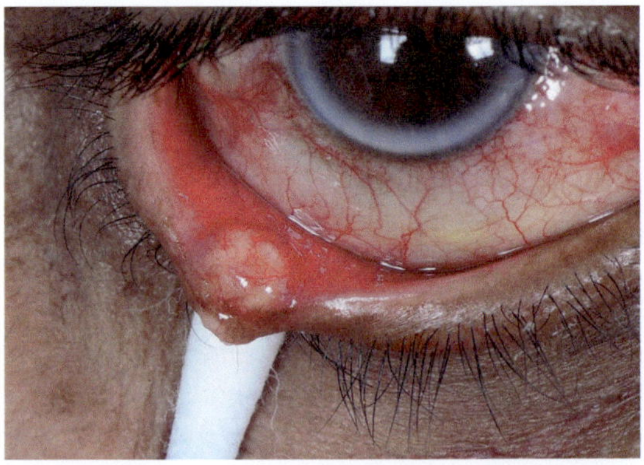

Fig. 4 A High magnification image of a small, whitish lesion 5 × 4 × 4 mm in size, involving the lower eyelid and the posterior lamella with conjunctival congestion, thickened eyelid margin, erythematous surface, and the loss of eyelashes. The diagnosis was sebaceous gland carcinoma

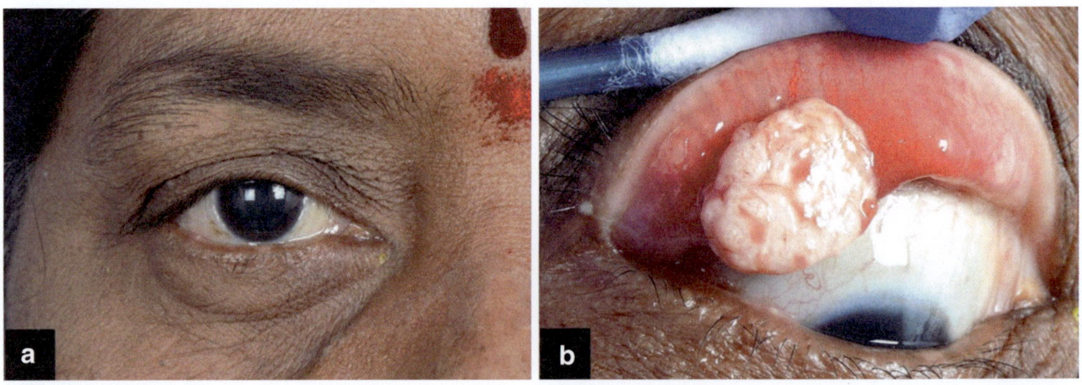

Fig. 3 (**a**) External image of the right eye of a 55-year-old female with mild fullness of the right upper eyelid. (**b**) On upper eyelid eversion, a well-defined, whitish, lobulated, elevated mass (8 × 8 × 4 mm) was seen with surrounding conjunctival erythema. The features are suggestive of a sebaceous gland carcinoma

Histopathologically, the tumor consists of malignant proliferation of sebaceous cells with vacuolated cytoplasm owing to the presence of lipids.

Standard treatment for SGC of eyelids consists of wide local excision with 4-mm clinically clear margins with intra-operative frozen-section margin control. When a pagetoid conjunctival spread is suspected, a 17-site conjunctival map biopsy, as described by Putterman, is performed to determine the extent, followed by a definitive surgical planning. Cryotherapy is a useful adjunctive treatment for pagetoid extension of SGC. Topical mitomycin-C has been tried for pagetoid spread with variable success [22]. Systemic chemotherapy as a neoadjuvant treatment in advanced periocular SGC is evolving, with good results seen with cisplatin/carboplatin and 5-fluorouracil. This helps to down-stage the disease and make eye salvaging surgery feasible in a patient where orbital exenteration would be otherwise imminent.

Orbital exenteration is considered in a diffuse pagetoid tumor or with orbital extension. Radiation therapy is considered mostly as an alternative to surgical treatment in patients who may be poor surgical candidates [23] or as an adjuvant measure. Radiotherapy with doses in the range of 6000–6600 cGy is considered optimal. CTV includes the entire orbit with superior orbital fissure, inferior orbital fissure, supraorbital foramen, cavernous sinus, infra orbital groove, and foramen, after proper evaluation of pre-treatment baseline extent of the tumor.

In these tumors, after the surgical excision, adjuvant brachytherapy is often warranted to achieve higher local control. In our study at Tata Memorial Centre, Mumbai high dose rate-interstitial brachytherapy (HDR-ISBT) was utilized to avoid postoperative external beam radiotherapy. Implant volume encompassed primary tumor with 3-5 mm margin for placing the catheters, a dental compound individualized conformer was used during dose delivery to reduce exposure to underlying ocular structures. Treatment protocol consisted of a total dose of 21-49 Gy, delivered in 7-14 fractions at 3-3.5 Gy per fraction, with two fractions administered daily, separated by a 6-8-hour interval. The eyelid and eye function were preserved in 89% and 5-year disease-free survival was 83% [24].

Considering the high local and regional recurrence rate, post-exenteration loco-regional adjuvant radiotherapy has proven to be effective in some case reports with locally advanced SGC with margin involvement, perineural, or lymphovascular invasion or positive lymph nodes [25]. Ipsilateral parotid and submandibular lymph nodes are common sites of regional spread. Radical neck dissection may be necessary in patients with locoregional metastases.

2.5 Malignant Melanoma

Eyelid melanoma appears as a variably pigmented mass that can ulcerate. It can occur as lentigo maligna melanoma (premalignant lesion—lentigo maligna/melanotic freckle of Hutchinson), superficial spreading melanoma, or nodular melanoma. The lesion is more common in Caucasians. They can be located at the lower eyelid (most common site), upper eyelid, outer canthus, or inner canthus. Surgical excision with intra-operative frozen section margin control is the standard primary treatment option for melanoma-in-situ or smaller lesions. If the lesion is too large with an orbital component, an orbital exenteration may be planned. Melanoma is considered as a relatively radioresistant tumor; however, the role of radiotherapy in the management of these lesions cannot be ignored. Radiotherapy has proven to be effective as an adjuvant treatment in recent times and it's role remains underutilized and controversial due to low survival benefit [26, 27].

According to National Comprehensive Cancer Network (NCCN) 2023, the treatment for stages 0, IA, and IB (<0.76 mm thick) is wide local excision (5-10 mm margins). For stages IA, IB, and II (>0.75 mm thick), sentinel lymph node (SLN) biopsy is recommended with wide local excision. Melanomas >2.0 mm thick should have 20 mm margins. However, this large a margin is not feasible in the eyelids without compromising on the functional integrity of the eye. Patients in stage III with a positive SLN biopsy or clinically positive nodes should be considered for baseline imaging for further staging. These patients should undergo excision and complete lymph node dissection, followed by observation or interferon alpha as adjuvant therapy. Radiation therapy to the nodal basin in some patients can also be considered specially with extra-nodal extension or multiple node positivity. Patients with stage IV disease should undergo biopsy for genetic testing and PET-CT scan. Treatment can include limited resection, systemic chemotherapy/immunotherapy, radiation therapy, and consideration for clinical trials.

3 Tumors of the Conjunctiva

3.1 Conjunctival Epithelial Tumors

Conjunctival epithelial tumors include a wide spectrum of conjunctival and corneal squamous cell proliferation including benign squamous papilloma, keratoacanthoma, hereditary benign intraepithelial dyskeratosis, intraepithelial neoplasia, and malignant SCC. Ocular surface squamous neoplasia is an umbrella term for premalignant and malignant epithelial tumors on the eye, including mild, moderate, and severe dysplasia, conjunctival intraepithelial neoplasia (CIN) and invasive SCC. CIN is squamous neoplasia that extends through the entire thickness of the conjunctival epithelium, but is confined to the epithelium, not invading beyond the basement membrane. On the other hand, invasive SCC has gross or microscopic invasion into the adjacent tissue.

Invasive conjunctival SCC typically presents in the elderly between 60 and 80 years of age. Younger patients with conjunctival SCC often have underlying risk factors like immunodeficiency, human papilloma virus (HPV) infection, or xeroderma pigmentosa, with the inability to repair DNA alterations [28]. The exact pathogenesis of conjunctival SCC is unknown but it most commonly occurs in areas with high ultraviolet exposure. Patients with human immunodeficiency virus (HIV) and other immunodeficiency diseases are reported to have multifocal, bilateral, recurrent, and more aggressive tumors. There is also a relationship of conjunctival SCC with heavy cigarette smoking [2].

Clinically, conjunctival SCC typically manifests in the limbal area as a placoid lesion with a gelatinous or papillomatous surface, occasionally forming a nodular mass (Fig. 5a). A clinical variant of this tumor, called diffuse conjunctival SCC, appears flat and gelatinous in a horizontal growth pattern with diffuse thickening of the conjunctiva and corneal surface. This can be mistaken as chronic conjunctivitis, leading to a delay in diagnosis and treatment. Invasive SCC is associated with characteristic findings such as feeder vessels, intrinsic vascularity, keratin, and sometimes surface inflammation. The tumor may extend into the sclera and can have intraocular or orbital extension in advanced cases. Rarely, metastasis to regional lymph nodes and distant sites can occur, particularly in immune-deficient patients. The mucoepidermoid variant of SCC tends to be more aggressive with an increased capacity for local invasion.

Topical chemotherapy (mitomycin-C and 5-fluorouracil) and topical immunotherapy (topical or injection interferon alpha-2b) are preferable over surgical intervention for potentially compliant patients, dexterous in placing eye drops, for small tumors and large unresectable tumors [29–31]. The "no touch" technique involves tumor removal without directly touching the mass and only manipulating the surrounding normal conjunctival tissue. A 4-mm wide margin is ensured while excising these lesions, followed by double freeze-thaw cryotherapy to the resected conjunctival edges. The corneal epithelial component is excised by the alcohol-assisted keratoepitheliectomy technique. Conjunctival reconstruction is done by conjunctival advancement or sliding flaps, or with the use of amniotic membrane grafts. Primary (clinically proven) or secondary (histopathologically proven) plaque brachytherapy has turned out to be highly effective in lesions with corneal stromal/scleral/corneo-scleral invasion or limited intraocular extension in ensuring excellent local tumor control with vision salvage (Fig. 5b) [32–34].

Plaque brachytherapy with isotopes such as Ruthenium-106, Strontium-90 or Iodine-125, has been used to control residual microscopic tumors following surgical resection of conjunctival SCC with apex dose ranging from 50 to 80 Gy. The tumor dimensions are important in plaque config-

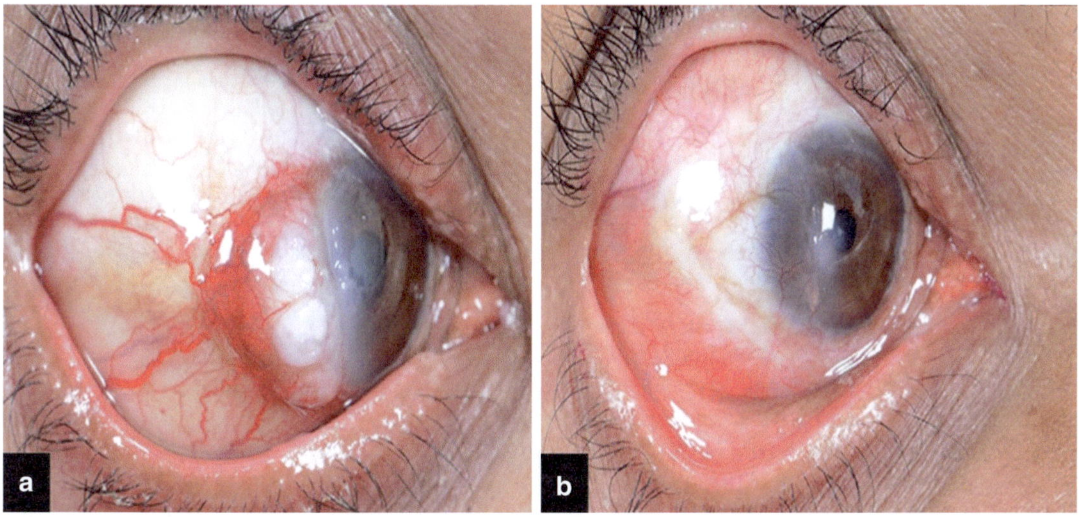

Fig. 5 (**a**) A 38-year-old male presented with a whitish conjunctival lesion temporally from 7 to 12 o'clock along with stromal edema at the cornea edge, dilated feeder episcleral vessels, conjunctival congestion suggestive of ocular surface squamous neoplasia with a corneo-scleral invasion. (**b**) Excision and primary plaque brachytherapy was performed which led to complete local tumor control at a final follow-up of 6 years

uration and seed orientation. The plaque size varies from 13 to 22 mm in diameter. The plaque is sutured directly to the tumor bed. Ruthenium-106 and Strontium-90 are beta emitters. Iodine-125 that emits gamma rays may have its own advantages and disadvantages because of its deep penetration property. Exenteration is reserved for advanced cases with clinical and radiological evidence of orbital invasion [35].

Indian study using plaque brachytherapy for conjunctival tumors is rare, because of lack of availability of plaques containing the β emitters, the ideal treatment technique with the advantage of treating only a few millimetres of tissue while sparing the underlying normal eye. A small study from Tata Memorial Centre, Mumbai used Strontium-90 brachytherapy in early invasive conjunctival malignancies as an adjunct to surgery in primary and recurrent settings. The 5-year results showed optimal disease control and ocular functional outcomes in more than 90% of the treated patients [36].

External beam radiotherapy (EBRT) with photons is indicated in post-exenteration cases with positive or close margins, perineural invasion and optic nerve with positive cut margin. CTV is the entire orbital cavity with orbital apex along with optic canal coverage with a dose in the range of 60–66 Gy in 30–33 fractions.

3.2 Conjunctival Melanocytic Tumors

The conjunctival melanocytic tumors include nevus, racial melanosis, primary acquired melanosis, and melanoma. Conjunctival primary acquired melanosis (PAM) refers to an acquired conjunctival pigmentation that is flat and non-cystic, and which does not resemble either a nevus or complexion-associated melanosis (CAM). Conjunctival melanoma is a malignant lesion that arises either de novo or from a pre-existing PAM or a nevus. The presentation is generally in middle-aged or elderly individuals and it appears as a pigmented or fleshy, elevated conjunctival mass with a lobulated surface. The most frequent location of melanoma is the bulbar conjunctiva, although the forniceal or palpebral conjunctiva are occasionally the site of origin (Fig. 6) or contiguous extension. Conjunctival melanoma can be amelanotic, and the diagnosis is confirmed on histopathology.

Conjunctival melanoma can metastasize to preauricular and submandibular lymph nodes and carries the potential for remote hematogenous spread to the brain, liver, skin, and bone. Therefore, complete baseline systemic evaluation by liver imaging (CT, MRI, or ultrasound), brain

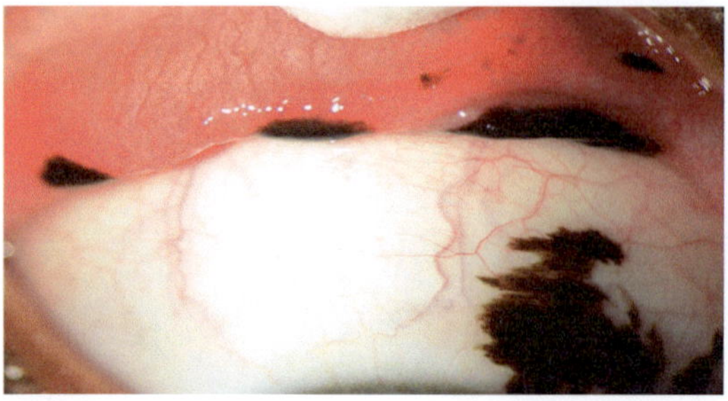

Fig. 6 Evidence of forniceal involvement in a case of conjunctival melanoma seen on double eversion of the upper eyelid

Table 1 CTV volumes and doses for different types of lymphoma

	ENMZL	Follicular NHL	DLBCL
Dose	24–30 Gy	30–36 Gy	36–40 Gy
CTV	GTV + 0.5 cm	Entire globe	Entire orbit with SOF/IOF and optic canal

CTV clinical target volume, *GTV* gross tumor volume, *ENMZL* extranodal marginal zone lymphoma, *NHL* non-Hodgkin lymphoma, *DLBCL* diffuse large B-cell lymphoma

MRI, and chest CT or PET-CT scan should be considered under an oncologist's guidance.

Malignant melanoma is managed by complete excisional biopsy using the traditional "no-touch" technique with surface reconstruction. Primary or secondary plaque brachytherapy is highly effective in invasive conjunctival melanomas or recurrent lesions, with excellent outcomes, therefore replacing radical measures such as enucleation [37]. Plaque brachytherapy is frequently done with Ruthenium-106, Strontium-90, and Iodine-125 with a dose of 10,000 cGy over the tumor bed. Iodine-based plaque brachytherapy is more frequently used in invasive lesions due to deeper penetration of gamma rays.

Treatment of diffuse growth patterns and involvement of non-bulbar conjunctiva can be challenging. In cases with extensive palpebral, forniceal, conjunctival, or caruncular involvement, an alternative to extensive surgical treatment or exenteration is proton beam irradiation. Patients with locoregional spread or advanced disease undergoing surgery for primary lesion should also be offered sentinel lymph node biopsy or neck dissection. Distant metastasis should ideally be dealt with by immunotherapy with or without local therapy for palliative care.

3.3 Conjunctival Lymphoid Tumors

Conjunctival lymphoma occurs due to abnormal clonal proliferation of the normally occurring lymphoid tissue. The lymphoid proliferation includes benign reactive lymphoid hyperplasia (BRLH), atypical lymphoid hyperplasia, and lymphoma. Clinically, a lymphoid tumor presents as a well-circumscribed or diffuse, slightly elevated fleshy salmon-colored mass deep to the epithelium, frequently located in the forniceal or bulbar conjunctiva. Conjunctival lymphoma is most commonly the B-cell non-Hodgkin lymphoma (NHL) type, which could either present as an isolated lesion or as a manifestation of generalized systemic disease. Other subtypes include extranodal marginal zone lymphoma (ENMZL), follicular lymphoma, diffuse large B-cell lymphoma (DLBCL), and mantle cell lymphoma. Whole-body PET-CT should be performed to rule out any disseminated or systemic disease. Bone marrow aspiration and biopsy are also required for staging lymphoma.

For localized, less aggressive, indolent lymphoma, EBRT remains the treatment of choice. The CTV (Table 1) includes only the gross tumor volume (GTV) with a 0.5 cm margin for ENMZL and the entire globe for a follicular NHL. Good local tumor control can be achieved by 24–30 Gy for ENMZL and 30–36 Gy at 180–200 cGy per fraction for a low-grade follicular NHL. Aggressive DLBCL of the conjunctiva should receive chemotherapy followed by radiotherapy to the entire orbit, covering the supraorbital fissure (SOF), inferior orbital fissure (IOF) and the optic canal (Fig. 7).

In case of disseminated disease, systemic therapy with combination chemotherapy for NHL with Rituximab or single-agent Rituximab can be opted as per the grade of the lymphoma. Radiotherapy to the affected orbit may be planned after systemic chemotherapy.

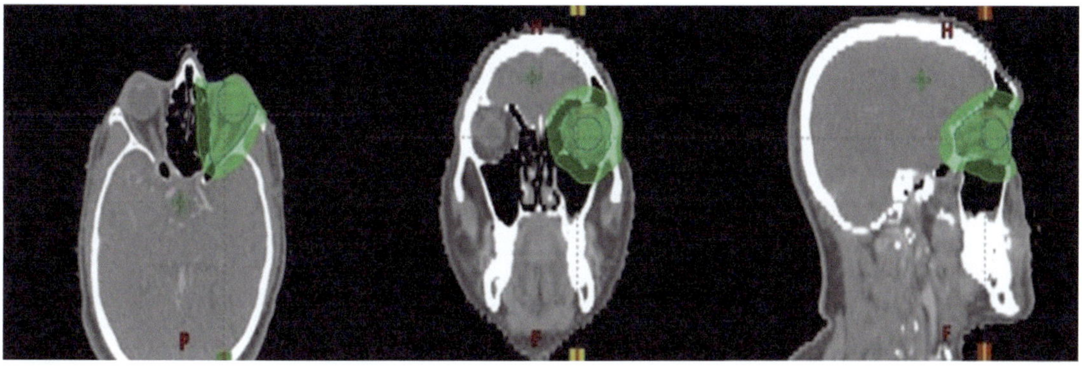

Fig. 7 Planning CT scan of head and neck showing dose distribution for diffuse large B-cell lymphoma of the left bulbar conjunctiva in axial, coronal, and sagittal sections (left to right), respectively

4 Tumors of the Orbit

4.1 Cavernous Hemangioma

Cavernous hemangioma is the most common benign primary tumor of the orbit in adults. Generally, the patient remains asymptomatic until adulthood. It is usually solitary, unilateral, and tends to produce a relatively stationary or slowly progressive proptosis (Fig. 8a) and is rarely associated with other vascular abnormalities. The resultant globe compression may lead to hyperopia, choroidal striae, and visual field defects, especially when located near the orbital apex. It is almost always intraconal (Fig. 8b), although extraconal lesions, intramuscular and intraosseous cavernous hemangiomas are also seen.

Radiological localization of the lesion is mandatory for surgical planning and further intervention. Anterior lesions or lesions unlikely to cause functional deficit should be excised completely [38]. For posterior lesions, orbitotomy with cryo-assisted tumor delivery can be performed and the minimally invasive transconjunctival approaches provides an excellent aesthetic postoperative outcome with minimal functional deficit [39, 40]. The smaller orbital apical lesions not causing any functional deficit can be left alone for observation. However, surgically non-accessible, posterior lesions with functional deficit may be treated with EBRT with a dose ranging from 45.0 to 50.4 Gy at 1.8–2.0 Gy per fraction, with excellent outcomes and vision salvage [41].

4.2 Optic Nerve Glioma

Optic nerve glioma (ONG) is the most common optic nerve tumor arising either from the optic nerve matter or the surrounding sheath [42]. It can be of two types: benign pilocytic astrocytoma (juvenile) or malignant glioblastoma of adulthood [43]. The benign variant occurs in the first decade of life as a unilateral lesion with higher female predominance. Most of these cases have an association with neurofibromatosis type 1 (NF-1) which has a favorable prognosis. Nearly, 10%–70% of patients with ONG are associated with NF-1, whereas 8%–31% of cases with NF-1 have ONG [42, 44]. A broad spectrum of presentation includes painless and progressive proptosis, visual acuity loss, visual field loss, motility restriction, compressive features, including optic nerve atrophy, dissociated vertical nystagmus, central retinal vein occlusion (CRVO) and even neovascular glaucoma [42]. When chiasmal gliomas occur, they are associated with endocrinal disturbances.

Rarely, malignant lesions present in varying age groups from the second to eighth decade with no gender predilection. These cases have an involvement of the anterior visual system. They

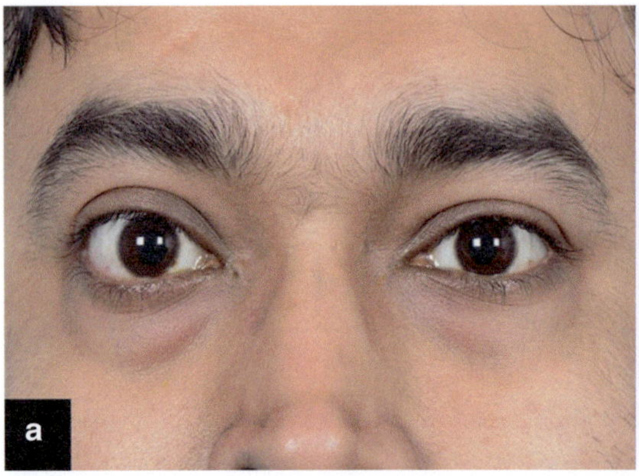

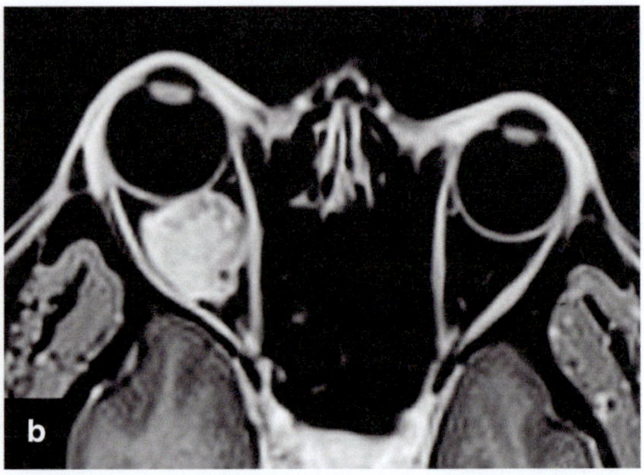

Fig. 8 (**a**) A 33-year-old male presented with 3 mm axial proptosis of the right eye along with mild lower eyelid fullness and a best corrected visual acuity of 6/6 in OU. (**b**) Magnetic Resonance Imaging (MRI) fat-suppressed T2 axial sections showing a well-defined intra-conal, iso-to-hyper intense lesion, abutting the globe posteriorly without involvement of the adjacent structures, suggestive of an orbital cavernous hemangioma

present with progressive visual loss and neurologic deficit. Histologically these lesions have cellular pleomorphism, hyperchromaticity and scattered mitosis [44, 45].

Early diagnosis and appropriate management help halt or alter the rate of disease progression in ONG. Posterior progression with chiasmal involvement leads to bilateral blindness and higher mortality. Radiologically, a combination of CT and MRI is required to assess the optic nerve involvement, posterior extent, and intracranial extension to other regions such as the optic chiasm and hypothalamus. Biopsy can be performed to avoid misdiagnosis in situations where the clinical presentation and/or imaging are atypical [42]. Biopsy, if performed, should be from an area of the tumor with potentially no or minimal visual morbidity and by an experienced orbital surgeon.

Multiple treatment strategies exist, including surveillance, chemotherapy, radiation therapy, surgery, or a combination of therapies. In patients with no visual deterioration, observation with regular follow-up for clinical and radiological assessment is preferred [43]. In younger children (<2 years) with progressive disease, chemotherapy is used as bridge therapy untill they grow to the age of 24 months. A combination of chemotherapeutic agents such as vincristine and carboplatin has been the most common first-line therapy in ONG. Other chemotherapy regimens include cisplatin, etoposide and single-agent temozolomide. Radiotherapy should be considered in children above the age of 2 years if progressing while on chemotherapy and in adults with preservable vision.

Radiation therapy has resulted in 10-year survival rates ranging from 40% to 93% [46]. Stereotactic radiotherapy (SRT) is preferred over conventional techniques of radiation. A margin of 2–3 mm over GTV is sufficient to achieve the ideal planning target volume (PTV) (Fig. 9). A dose in the range of 5000–5400 cGy is prescribed. Preferably, pulse dose of steroid should be administered during radiotherapy for neuroprotection. Proton therapy is always a better option due to its unique properties of Bragg-peak where the dose falls rapidly beyond the target. Surgery is considered the last choice of treatment, due to the high risk of blindness and damage to the affected eye. It is considered in cases with disfiguring proptosis, enlarging and/or expanding tumor or a combination of both or where the tumor is confined to a single optic nerve with no useful vision, and/or for cosmetic rehabilitation. Targeted therapies are also being explored for ONG [43].

4.3 Optic Nerve Sheath Meningioma

Optic nerve sheath meningioma (ONSM) is a slowly progressive rare benign tumor of the anterior visual pathway arising from the meningoepi-

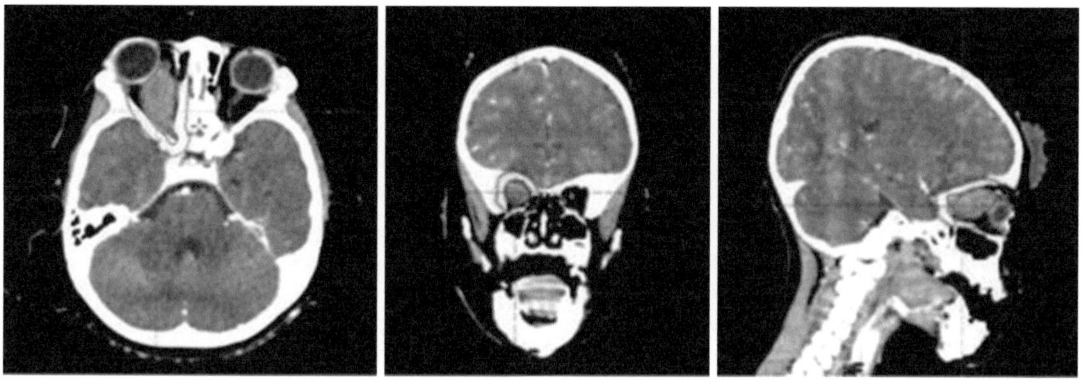

Fig. 9 Contrast-enhanced CT scan with axial, coronal and sagittal sections (left to right) respectively showing a fusiform growth of the right optic nerve with optic canal widening, suggestive of an optic nerve glioma. A margin of 3 mm is given around the gross lesion to form GTV (red) and PTV (purple). The dose is prescribed to the PTV

thelial cap cells of the arachnoid villi. It constitutes 2% of orbital tumors and 1%–2% of meningiomas and is the second most common tumor of the optic nerve after ONG [47, 48]. There is female predominance, especially in the middle-age group [38]. The clinical presentation is usually painless visual loss, progressive proptosis, with optic disc edema or atrophy. These lesions can cause a high level of morbidity due to the compressive effect on the pial vasculature leading to irreversible visual loss. A characteristic sign of this disease is the presence of a retinochoroidal (opto-ciliary) shunt vessels at the disc margin.

Intra-canalicular meningiomas can cause optic neuritis and glaucoma as well. They appear typically as fusiform or round lesions around a well-defined normal optic nerve, rarely with foci of calcification. Timely clinico-radiological assessment and regular follow-up help in identifying disease progression. Diagnosis is mostly by radiology to differentiate between ONG and ONSM (Table 2). Gallium-68-DOTA-NOC uptake is typically seen in meningioma. A biopsy is rarely advocated in clinic-radiologically atypical cases to confirm the diagnosis.

When asymptomatic, these lesions are left to be observed with regular follow-up. Visual disturbances occur late in the disease when the tumor compresses the optic nerve at the optic canal [38]. Surgical intervention may lead to vision loss. Fractionated SRT is preferred with vision preservation in >80% of cases [49]. Therefore, fractionated SRT is the preferred treatment modality in cases requiring therapeutic intervention [50] with a dose ranging from 50.4 to 54.0 Gy for conventional fractionation as most of ONSM are low grade. Sparing the normal structures like retina, lacrimal gland and lens with great accuracy is essential. Usually, a margin of 3–5 mm for daily setup variation should be added as PTV around GTV. Proton therapy can also be considered whenever feasible.

Table 2 Radiological differentiation of ONG and ONSM

	CT with contrast	MRI with contrast	Gallium DOTANOC
ONG	Enlargement of the optic nerve and optic canal Fusiform or exophytic mass. The optic nerve may be elongated with kinking or buckling	Heterogeneous enhancement may present with solid and cystic component	Uptake absent
ONSM	CT shows tram-track appearance on axial sections and doughnut sign on coronal sections	Homogenous enhancement with tubular, fusiform, or exophytic lesion	Uptake present

ONG optic nerve glioma, *ONSM* Optic nerve sheath meningioma

4.4 Orbital Rhabdomyosarcoma

Orbital rhabdomyosarcoma (RMS) is the most common primary orbital malignant tumor of childhood with a mean age at diagnosis of 8–10 years [38]. The presenting features include proptosis, globe displacement, ptosis, conjunctival and eyelid swelling, palpable orbital mass and pain. Often the patients are misdiagnosed, considering their rarity, therefore, a detailed clinical assessment with radiological investigations is required to rule out this aggressive possibility. This aggressive neoplasm can invade orbital bone and even extend into the cranial cavity.

The management of orbital RMS has evolved over the last two decades. Multimodal management including a combination of surgery, irradiation, and chemotherapy has shown good results. Metastasis most commonly occurs to the lung and bone via hematogenous dissemination. Prognosis and treatment depend upon the histology (type of RMS—Embryonal, Pleomorphic, Alveolar, Undifferentiated, Anaplastic), the extent of surgery (biopsy only, excision with R0, R1) and site (favorable or unfavorable, orbit comes under favorable site) and the stage. Intergroup Rhabdomyosarcoma Study (IRS) Group V recommends a specific chemotherapy regimen in combination with radiation based on the tumor staging. An incisional biopsy is first performed to establish a histopathological diagnosis, followed by chemotherapy consisting of a combination of vincristine (V), actinomycin-D (A), etoposide (E), cyclophosphamide (C)/ifosfamide (I) [51–53]. Broadly, the management depends on the stage of the disease and excision (Table 3). However, based on their experience, the authors suggest that every patient should be considered for adjuvant radiation and chemotherapy irrespective of the extent of excision.

For R1 resection, chemotherapy (VA) is recommended. In case of incomplete excision, chemotherapy followed by radiotherapy is considered wherein radiotherapy is sandwiched between chemotherapy. Usually, radiotherapy is planned for the third week of treatment initiation. For a locally advanced disease, where only biopsy is possible, multidrug chemotherapy (VAC/IE) with radiotherapy sandwiched between it, is the recommended line of treatment [52].

Table 3 Treatment options as per the extent of surgery

Surgery	Chemotherapy	Radiation
Complete removal (R0)	No treatment	No treatment
Incomplete removal (R1)	VA or VAC	±RT
Biopsy only	VAC/IE	RT

V vincristine, *A* actinomycin-D, *E* etoposide, *C* cyclophosphamide, *I* ifosfamide, *RT* radiotherapy

CTV for radiation therapy has two schools of thought. One covers the GTV consisting of pre-chemotherapy tumor volume with a margin and the other covers the entire orbit including all the fissures, supraorbital notch, infraorbital foramen, optic canal, and the ipsilateral cavernous sinus. It also includes bony erosion or pterygopalatine fossa, while sparing the lens, cornea and lacrimal gland (if not involved) (Fig. 10). The dose of RT is approximately 45–50.4 Gy at 180 cGy per fraction. For gross disease, the dose can be increased up to 60 Gy while respecting normal tissue dose limits with adaptive radiotherapy.

Despite meticulous treatment a local recurrence rate of 18% has been observed with metastasis in 6% and death in 3% of cases [54, 55]. For locally recurrent lesions, interstitial brachytherapy is a reasonable option. Orbital exenteration is reserved for refractory cases.

4.5 Adenoid Cystic Carcinoma of the Lacrimal Gland

Adenoid cystic carcinoma of the lacrimal gland is the most common malignant epithelial neoplasm of the lacrimal gland accounting for >60% of tumors in this category. The age at diagnosis (mean age 40 years) has a bimodal pattern, with patients generally belonging to the first to second decade or the sixth to seventh decade. Typical features include progressive proptosis and downward displacement of the eye. Periocular pain is frequently reported due to perineural invasion by the tumor. Imaging is mandatory to localize the lesion and the association of the adjacent structures. The presence of bony

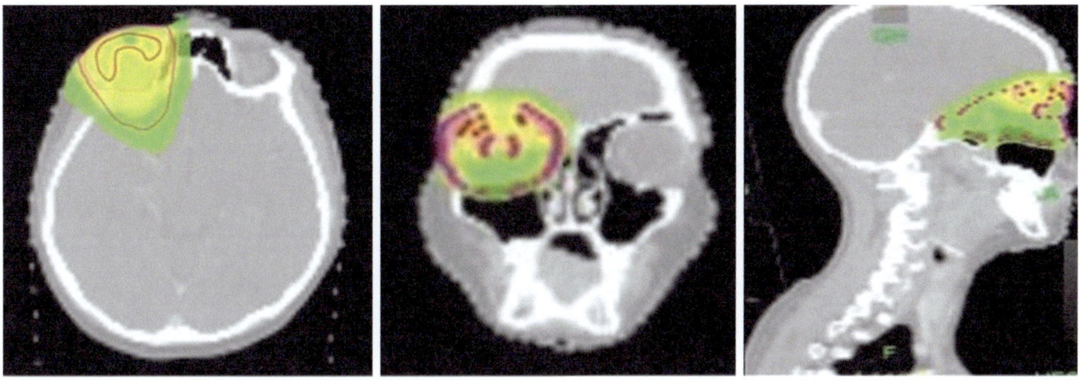

Fig. 10 CT scan of head and neck axial, coronal and sagittal (left to right) respectively showing rhabdomyosarcoma of the right orbit with dose of 46 Gy covering the PTV (green). Special care has been taken to ensure coverage of the superior orbital fissure, inferior orbital fissure, supraorbital notch, infraorbital foramen, pterygopalatine fossa, optic canal. Yellow zone marks the boost volume for a dose upto 60 Gy

erosions on radiology shows the aggressive nature of the disease. Histopathologically, the tumor is characterized by solid areas or cords of bland-appearing malignant epithelial cells. Adenoid cystic carcinoma of the lacrimal gland has been subdivided into several histopathologic subtypes, namely cribriform, sclerosing, basaloid, comedocarcinoma, and tubular types [56].

Small lesions that are well-circumscribed can be excised completely without breaching the capsule. However, larger and diffuse lesions are subjected to a trans-arcus marginalis or trans-septal incisional biopsy with histopathology-guided neoadjuvant chemotherapy, en-bloc excision, extended-field radiotherapy and adjuvant chemotherapy (Fig. 11) [57]. The decision for exenteration depends on the involvement of the orbital apex and extension beyond the orbit. Removal of bone is usually avoided. Tumor going beyond the periosteal fossa of the lacrimal gland with invasion of nearby structures, large size with perineural invasion, and basaloid type carries poor prognosis. In cases of advanced tumors, with a high risk of recurrence, neoadjuvant intra-arterial or intravenous chemotherapy with cisplatin and doxorubicin have been used followed by exenteration and irradiation. For adjuvant radiotherapy, CTV includes the entire bony orbit along with superior and inferior orbital fissures, orbital apex, ipsilateral cavernous sinus as well as pterygopalatine fossa.

In case of intact orbit, CTV for 46 Gy should include pre-surgery/pre-chemotherapy tumor bed with residual disease plus bony erosion (if present) with margin, to cover superior and inferior orbital fissures, orbital apex, ipsilateral cavernous sinus, and pterygopalatine fossa. The dose to the tumor bed ranges from 60 to 66 Gy. In cases where minimal residual tumor remains after surgical intervention, interstitial brachytherapy can be planned at the same sitting pre-operatively (Fig. 12) [25].

Neoadjuvant intra-arterial chemotherapy or even plaque brachytherapy can reduce the size of the tumor [58, 59].

4.6 Lacrimal Gland Adenocarcinoma

Lacrimal gland adenocarcinoma is known to carry a dismal prognosis with fatality up to 60%–80%. If properly managed, the results can be far better. The tumor tends to have perineural infiltration and bone invasion, making it difficult to achieve surgically clear margins. Ipsilateral preauricular and cervical lymph nodal metastasis are also seen. Furthermore, distant metastasis occurs in about half of the patients. The rarity of this cancer makes it difficult to study the efficacy of various therapeutic modalities. En-bloc excision is a good option for small lesions with less extensive involvement. Orbital exenteration is the

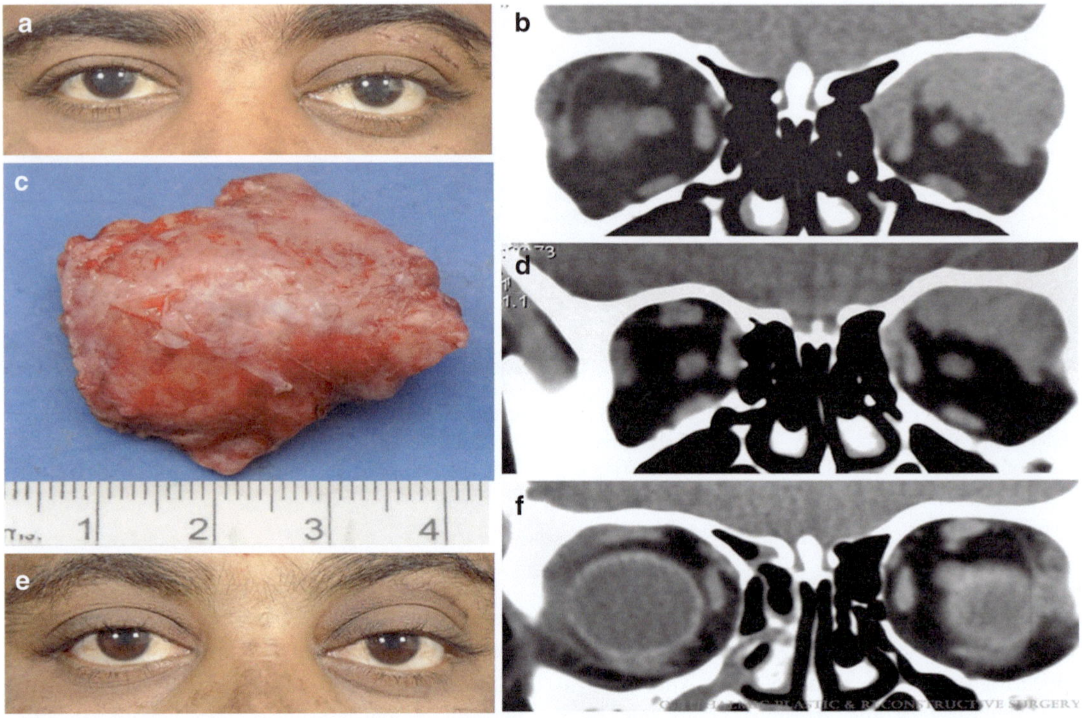

Fig. 11 (**a**) A 40-year-old man with adenoid cystic carcinoma of the lacrimal gland in the left orbit. (**b**) Computed tomography (coronal plane) showed pretreatment appearance of the lacrimal gland tumor. (**c**) Following neoadjuvant chemotherapy, the well-circumscribed tumor was excised en bloc along with overlying periosteum. (**d**) CT scan shows 30%–40% reduction in tumor following post-neoadjuvant chemotherapy pre-operatively. (**e**) At a follow-up of 3 years, the patient is doing well with no local tumor recurrence. (**f**) CT scan confirms the clinical findings with no recurrence [57]

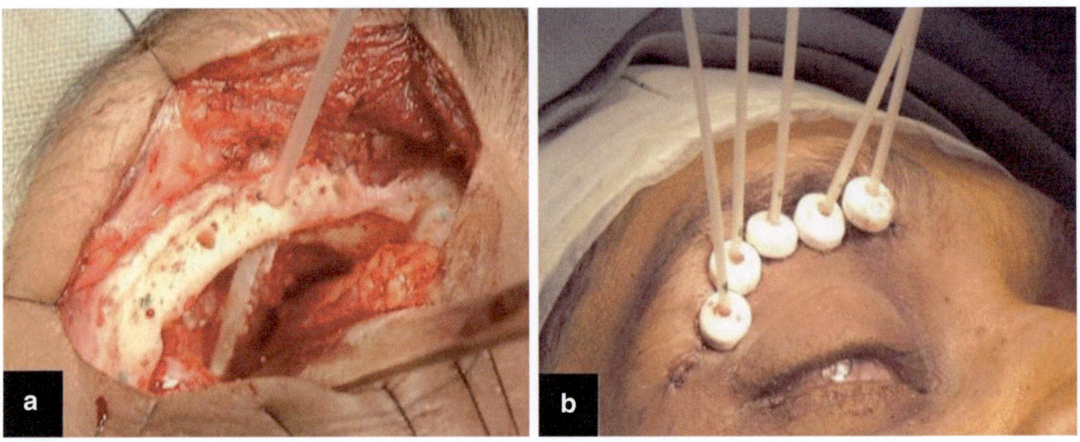

Fig. 12 (**a**) Intra-operative image showing surgical insertion of interstitial tubes with accurate spacing based on pre-excision tumor location. (**b**) Stop buttons are placed for securing the tubes in position for the procedure where the source guide wires are attached to the machine

widely accepted form of treatment in extensive cases. Neoadjuvant chemotherapy by the intra-arterial route or as systemic therapy has also been tried as a part of multimodal management [59]. Chemotherapy agents like Carboplatin and Paclitaxel have shown good response. Adjuvant radiotherapy for lacrimal gland carcinomas is indicated in all cases because of perineural invasion, bone invasion and difficulty in achieving clear microscopic margins.

EBRT of approximately 60–66 Gy covers the tumor bed/pre-chemotherapy volume along with a margin to include the adjacent bony invasion, ipsilateral pre-auricular and cervical lymph nodal areas, if clinically or radiologically positive and a dose of 46 Gy to cover the entire orbit, superior and inferior orbital fissure, ipsilateral cavernous sinus, pterygopalatine fossa and orbital apex [25]. Interstitial brachytherapy with Iridium-192 as a boost pre-operatively followed by delivery of 46–50 Gy through an external beam is very promising to deliver the desired total dose of radiation, keeping the dose constraints for normal structures within normal limits. This method is also an effective alternative for small recurrences with or without EBRT.

4.7 Orbital Lymphoma

Orbital lymphoproliferative lesions range from benign reactive lymphoid hyperplasia to atypical lymphoid hyperplasia and malignant lymphomas. These lesions can involve the conjunctiva, eyelids, lacrimal glands, extraocular muscles, orbital soft tissue, or lacrimal sac, either individually or in combination. Lymphomas of the ocular adnexa constitute approximately 8%–10% of all extranodal lymphomas. Orbital lymphoma is a malignant orbital neoplasm that occurs in the middle-aged and the elderly. It is most commonly unilateral, although bilateral involvement is also known. Orbital lymphomas most often cause proptosis. It may present as an enlarged lacrimal gland, an enlarged extraocular muscle, or as a diffuse extraconal lesion.

Most orbital lymphomas are primary tumors and are usually the NHL B-cell type [38]. The most common primary lymphoma subtype is the low-grade malignant ENMZL of the MALT type (mucosa-associated lymphoid tissue). In isolated orbital presentation, systemic lymphoma may eventually develop in one-third by 10 years, whereas only about 5% of patients with NHL develop ocular adnexal involvement. The diagnosis is based on excisional or incisional biopsy followed by histopathological confirmation with a vital role of immunohistochemistry. Based on the classification of the tumor, further management is done with radiotherapy, chemotherapy, and even alternative therapies like immunotherapy [60, 61].

Systemic evaluation is mandatory in these patients with regular follow-up. Systemic involvement advocates chemotherapy as the treatment option. In the absence of systemic lymphoma, small and well-circumscribed lesions are amenable to local radiation with low-dose radiotherapy of 24–30 Gy offering excellent local tumor control with a prolonged regression [62, 63]. In a low-grade follicular NHL, the entire orbit should be covered along with supra- and infraorbital fissures, the pterygopalatine fossa, and the orbital apex in the radiation field with a dose ranging from 30 to 36 Gy.

4.8 Orbital Metastatic Tumors

Metastasis to the orbit occurs mainly by the hematogenous route. The primary tumor causing metastasis to the orbit depends on age. In adults, the most common primary tumors metastasizing to the orbit are carcinomas of the breast, prostate gland, lung, and gastrointestinal tract. Rarely, cutaneous and uveal melanoma can metastasize to the orbit. In children, orbital metastases occur from adrenal neuroblastoma, Wilms tumor, and Ewing tumor [2]. The presenting features of orbital metastasis depend on the exact location of the tumor in the orbit and the type of primary neoplasm. Some of these lesions are confined to the extraocular muscles while others occur as solitary intraconal or extraconal masses producing rapidly progressive proptosis, pain, diplopia, ptosis, and eyelid swelling. Enophthalmos is seen in tumors that cause fibrosis of the orbital tissues, namely the scirrhous carcinoma of the breast and stomach. A thorough history, systemic examination and whole-body imaging are undertaken to diagnose the primary tumor. After an excisional or incisional biopsy, histopathology-guided adjuvant treatment is to be done with chemotherapy, radiation or hormone-based therapy as per the systemic evaluation by the oncologist.

Individualized treatment should be planned, considering disease extent and life expectancy with the primary goal of maintaining life, eye and vision salvage, in that order. EBRT has been effective in controlling the disease and preservation of vision, with the doses ranging from 20 to 40 Gy. The largest published data by Rosset et al., assessed 88 eyes of choroidal (not orbital) metastases treated with EBRT with a median dose of 35.5 Gy (range 20–53 Gy) in 10–30 fractions [64].

Our experience with high-end technology of SBRT (stereotactic body radiotherapy) with higher doses of 3000 cGy in five fractions (2 Gy equivalent to 52 Gy) has shown excellent local control with prompt recovery of vision (Fig. 13). During SBRT or EBRT simulation, the immobilization device should be cut at the eye portion and the patient should receive instructions to keep eyes open and the gaze fixed at a point on the roof. The same process should be repeated during simulation scan and treatment.

Plaque brachytherapy is usually reserved for solitary intraocular metastasis. Key factors to consider for plaque brachytherapy include the size and thickness of the lesion, the distance of the lesion from the optic nerve, and the distance of the lesion from the foveola. Wills Eye Hospital studied about 36 patients who received plaque brachytherapy either as primary or as salvage treatment (after EBRT). A mean dose to the apex and the base of tumor was 68.8 and 235.6 Gy, respectively [65].

5 Intraocular Tumors

5.1 Uveal Melanoma

Uveal melanoma is the most common primary intraocular malignant tumor in adults. It most commonly involves the choroid (90%), followed by the ciliary body (6%), or iris (4%). Caucasians are more commonly affected as compared to any other race. The tumor is detected usually in the sixth decade, although a wide variation in age is noted. Uveal melanomas can develop de novo, or from a preexisting choroidal nevus, or in the region of melanocytosis in congenital ocular/oculodermal melanocytosis.

Choroidal melanoma generally manifests with symptoms of varying degrees of visual loss, photopsia, floaters, and visual field loss. The presence of dilated episcleral vessels over the tumor region is an important sign. Choroidal melanoma can present as a sessile, pigmented or non-pigmented (atypical) lesion with a dome, mushroom, or diffuse configuration (Fig. 14a). Orange pigment may be present overlying the tumor along with dilated retinal vessels, exudative retinal detachment, and sub-retinal fluid. The diagnosis of choroidal melanoma can be solely based on ophthalmoscopic examination. However, multi-modal ancillary imaging by autofluorescence, ultrasonography, fluorescein angiography, indocyanine-green angiography, and optical coherence tomography help in defining the characteristics of the tumor.

Fine-needle aspiration biopsy is used in cases with atypical presentation for confirming the diagnosis, or for cytogenetic analysis of the tumor. Histopathologically the tumor develops from the melanocytes of the uvea that are derived from the neural crest cells. Younger and middle-aged adults present with small basal dimensions of melanoma with lower tumor-related metastasis and mortality. The presence of cataract, secondary glaucoma and extraocular extension carries a grave prognosis [66].

The management of melanoma depends primarily on the tumor size and location. It is clinically grouped into three sizes based on the tumor thickness and base diameter, including small (1.5–2.4 mm in apical height and 5–16 mm in basal diameter), medium (2.5–10 mm in apical height and ≤16 mm in basal diameter) [67]. For every millimetre increase in the melanoma thickness the risk of metastasis increases by 5% [68]. For small and medium lesions, transpupillary thermotherapy, plaque radiotherapy, charged particle irradiation or local resection can be performed based on the tumor location and accompanying features.

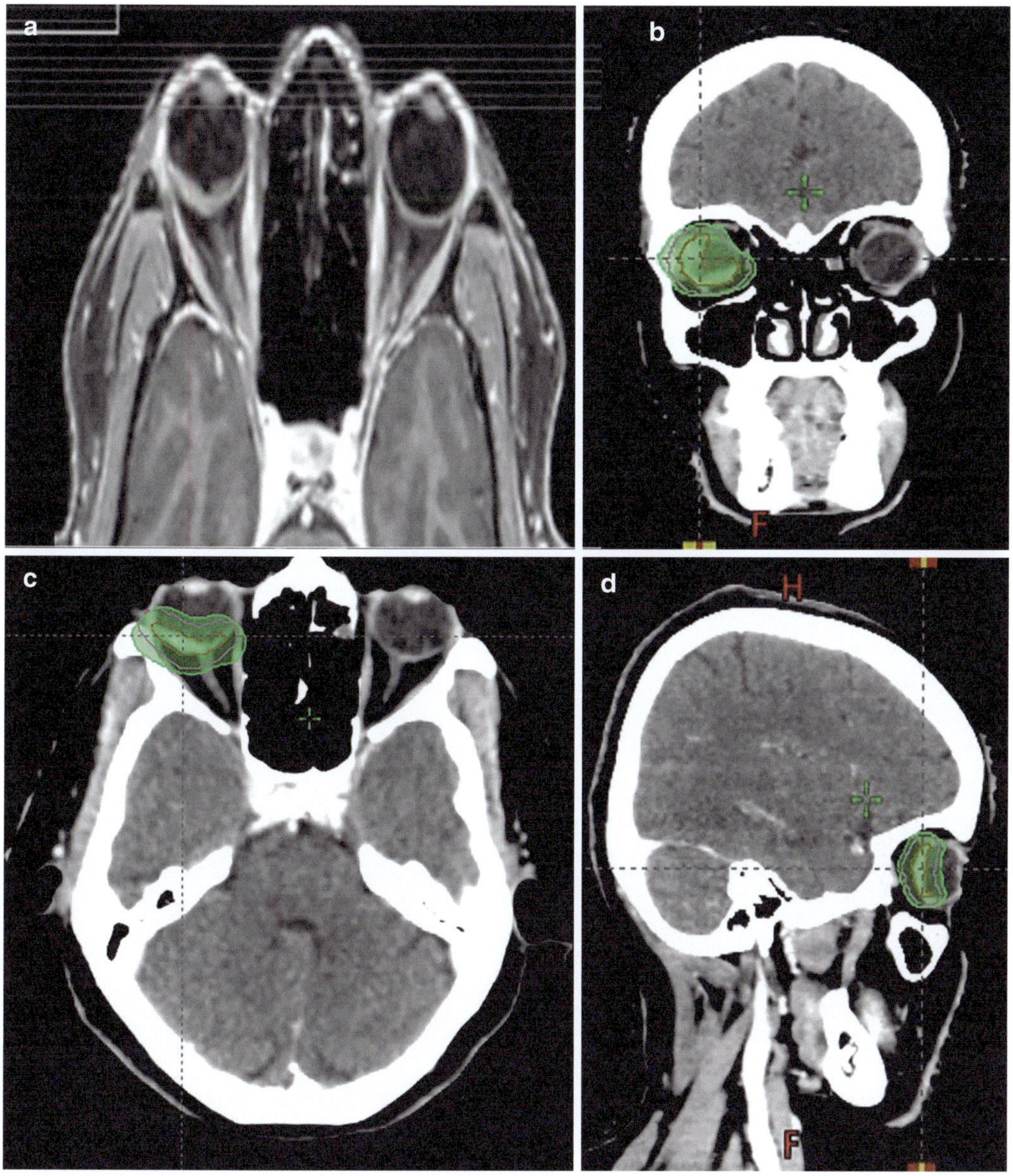

Fig. 13 (**a**) Contrast-enhanced MRI of the brain demonstrating choroidal thickening with enhancement in posterior aspect of right eye, consistent with choroidal metastasis in a patient with breast carcinoma as the primary malignancy. Images (**b–d**): Treatment planning CT images illustrating target delineation (image "**c**" shows the choroidal thickening) and dose coverage of the choroidal metastatic lesion planned for stereotactic radiation therapy

Whenever visual preservation is feasible, radiation should be delivered ideally in the form of plaque brachytherapy. Plaque brachytherapy can be used in patients with melanoma of apical height 2.5–10 mm and maximum basal tumor diameter of 16 mm. The most commonly used plaque radiation worldwide is I-125, followed by Ru-106 (Fig. 14b) [69, 70]. I-125 emits gamma rays which have a range sufficient for tumors up to 8–10 mm thickness, while Ru-106 is appropriate for a tumor thickness of 6 mm (Fig. 15). The dose used is in the range of 7000–10,000 cGy. For large tumors enucleation is necessary, and for tumors with orbital extension, orbital exentera-

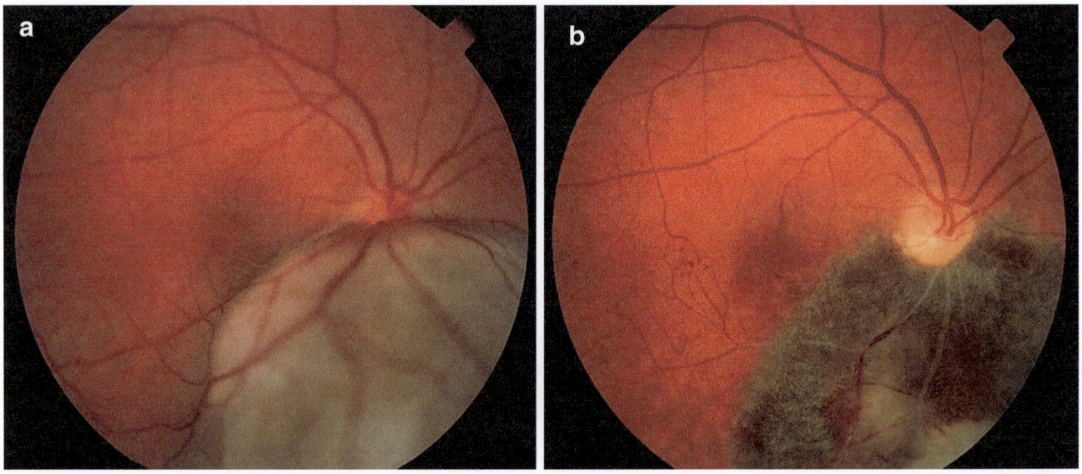

Fig. 14 (**a**) A large, elevated, choroidal brownish pigmented lesion seen from 3 to 7 o'clock in the right eye causing retinal detachment, with surrounding sub-retinal fluid, dilated retinal vessels, orange pigmentation on surface and obscuring the lower one-third of the optic disc. It was diagnosed to be a choroidal melanoma. (**b**) After treatment with Ruthenium-106 plaque brachytherapy (notch plaque), the lesion scarred well with resolved subretinal fluid and improvement in visual acuity

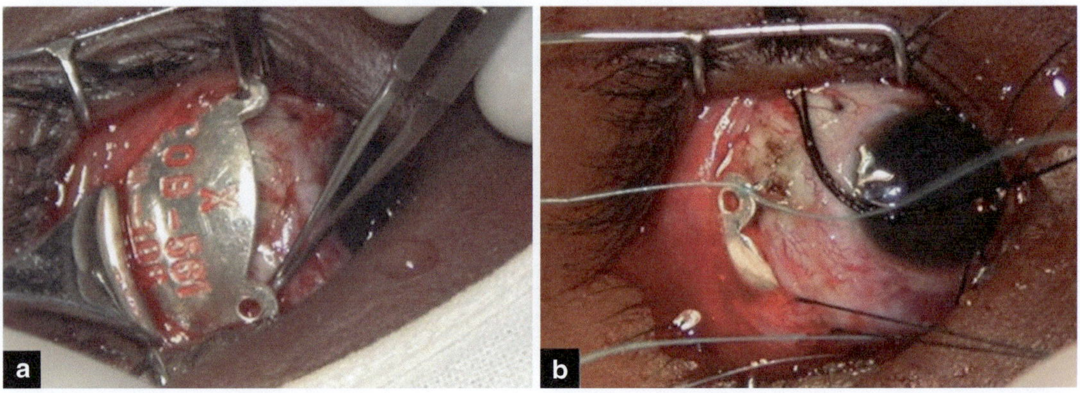

Fig. 15 (**a**) Intra-operative picture of a Ruthenium-106 plaque being placed for the treatment of choroid melanoma. (**b**) The plaque is secured by suturing to the sclera and is centered over the target area in order to provide optimal apex dose to the lesion

tion is performed. Patients with uveal melanoma are at risk for metastatic disease to the liver, lung, and skin. Systemic monitoring with physical examination, liver function tests twice yearly, chest radiographs and liver imaging using MRI or ultrasonography annually is advised [66]. Tumors close to or contiguous with the optic disc, referred to as parapapillary or peripapillary, were once considered for enucleation, and have now become suitable for organ preservation with the advent of notch plaque or proton beam external radiotherapy.

Even large tumors and lesions of the iris and ciliary body may be treated with proton beam therapy where a homogenous higher tumor dose is delivered with a sharp dose fall off, thereby sparing the optic nerve. SRT with linear accelerator has shown good results for tumors <12 mm in thickness and diameter <16 mm [71, 72]. A dose of 50 Gy delivered in five fractions over five consecutive days is the preferred schedule for SRT. Postoperative radiotherapy is also offered for positive margins. Conventional dose fractionation for 6000–7000 cGy is appropriate.

5.2 Choroidal Hemangioma

Hemangiomas of the choroid occur in two forms, circumscribed and diffuse. Circumscribed choroidal hemangiomas (CCH) are solitary benign vascular tumors which are congenital in origin. On the other hand, diffuse choroidal hemangiomas (DCH) are usually a part of variable systemic manifestations of Sturge-Weber syndrome. Although CCH is believed to be present since birth, it is generally detected in the second or the third decade when it starts producing visual symptoms. It presents with a reddish-orange hue to the fundus (Fig. 16a). It can enlarge to involve the fovea, or produce subretinal fluid to cause macular detachment.

A DCH, on the other hand, causes an exudative retinal detachment with macular involvement. Long standing fluid in the macular region can result in photoreceptor cell loss and cystoid degeneration of the sensory retina causing permanent visual damage. The treatment options for a symptomatic choroidal hemangioma include transpupillary thermotherapy, photodynamic therapy, plaque brachytherapy, EBRT or proton beam radiotherapy. Plaque radiotherapy (dose range 30–35 Gy) is the most commonly performed procedure for choroidal hemangioma as it is most effective in retaining good vision in patients with sub-macular tumors. As plaque may not be able to cover the entire tumor, it may not be ideal for larger DCH than CCH. In juxtapapillary CCH treated by plaque brachytherapy, the risk of radiation papillopathy is more due to close proximity of the optic nerve head. Stability in the size of the tumor, regression of the subretinal fluid and resolution of symptoms can be achieved in a majority of the patients (Fig. 16b).

Low-dose EBRT of around 24–30 Gy can also achieve good results in treating DCH and juxtapapillary CCH with minimal side-effects. EBRT absorbs the exudates associated with DCH even at fractionated doses of 24–30 Gy [73]. It improves visual acuity in 80% of the cases. Disadvantages of EBRT are slow absorption of SRF, recurrence or persistence of exudative retinal detachment. Proton beam Therapy with a dose of 20 Cobalt Gray Equivalent is very effective with minimal side effects [74]. SRT to CCH in single fraction 12 Gy is also an effective treatment option [75].

5.3 Retinoblastoma

Retinoblastoma is the most common intraocular malignancy in children. Its average age of diagnosis is 18 months, and the classic presentation is a white reflex in the eye. It results from a genetic mutation in chromosome 13 and can be hereditary or non-hereditary presenting as either unilateral or bilateral. The diagnosis of the tumor and its grouping is based on clinical examination, along with ocular imaging in suspected orbital

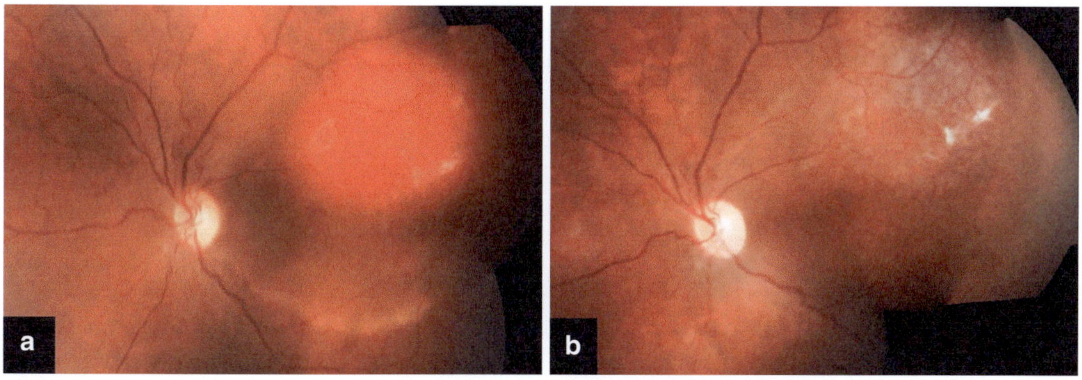

Fig. 16 (**a**) A reddish, elevated, choroidal lesion approximately 8 × 6 × 3 mm in size located along the superior arcade in the left eye, just touching the macular region with surrounding sub-retinal fluid. It was diagnosed to be a choroidal hemangioma. (**b**) Plaque brachytherapy was performed and the lesion regressed very well at a final follow-up of 5-years with resolution of sub-retinal fluid and gain of visual acuity

invasion. Orbital retinoblastoma, although rare in developed nations, continues to pose a major challenge in developing nations [76]. Retinoblastoma typically manifests as a unifocal or multifocal, well-circumscribed, dome-shaped retinal mass with dilated retinal vessels. Although initially transparent and difficult to visualize, it grows to become opaque and white. When small, the tumor is entirely intraretinal. As it enlarges, it grows in a three-dimensional plane, extending towards the vitreous cavity (endophytic) or away from it (exophytic).

Treatment options for retinoblastoma depend on the tumor grouping, staging, location, laterality, retinal seeding, vitreous seeding, and status of the opposite eye [77]. Focal therapy (cryotherapy or transpupillary thermotherapy) alone for smaller tumors (<3 mm in diameter and height) located in visually non-crucial areas is the preferred treatment [78].

EBRT played a major role in the 1990s before the introduction of chemoreduction. EBRT led to the development of second cancers in and around the treatment site and also caused orbital hypoplasia. Thus, chemoreduction by intravenous chemotherapy (IVC) gained popularity [79]. Chemoreduction with standard-dose of six cycles of chemotherapeutic agents like vincristine, carboplatin, etoposide and sequential aggressive focal therapy is recommended for larger tumors and those located in visually crucial areas [80].

Intra-arterial chemotherapy (IAC) can be used upfront in unilateral retinoblastoma or eyes with useful vision [81]. Commonly single drug melphalan is used or a triple-drug therapy with a combination of topotecan, melphalan and carboplatin is delivered through the ophthalmic artery. Although IAC is being widely used, IVC continues to be the primary mode of management in bilateral retinoblastoma. Periocular chemotherapy and intravitreal chemotherapy (IVit) are mainly used to achieve regression of vitreous seeds [82–85].

Retinoblastoma is a radiosensitive tumor. Focal radiation in the form of plaque brachytherapy achieves excellent tumor control, especially in eyes with sub-optimal response to chemoreduction and focal therapy [86]. Management of recurrent retinoblastoma can be challenging. The recurrence of vitreous seeds alone is managed by IVit chemotherapy. Small recurrences are treated with focal therapy consisting of thermotherapy or cryotherapy. Larger recurrences, those with localized vitreous and/or subretinal seeds, can be typically treated with plaque radiotherapy or IAC. Extensive recurrences are generally treated with three or more cycles of standard or high-dose IVC, IAC, or even enucleation [87]. Enucleation is reserved for advanced retinoblastoma or treatment-resistant eyes. The presence of histo-pathological risk factors advocates initiation of adjuvant chemotherapy [88]. High-dose adjuvant chemotherapy and orbital EBRT are considered for patients with extra-scleral infiltration, extra-ocular extension, and optic nerve extension to transection [89]. In cases where chemotherapy has failed and enucleation needs to be avoided to provide some useful vision for the child, EBRT is very rarely recommended.

Orbital retinoblastoma (Fig. 17) (International Staging, Stage 3A or 3B with regional nodal metastasis) is currently managed by multimodal treatment. Orbital exenteration alone is unlikely to achieve complete surgical clearance, EBRT does not prevent systemic metastasis, and chemotherapy alone may not eradicate the residual orbital disease. Neoadjuvant high-dose chemotherapy for 3 to 6 cycles is hence indicated to downstage the disease, and enucleation or exenteration is then performed depending on the extent of the residual disease. This is followed by

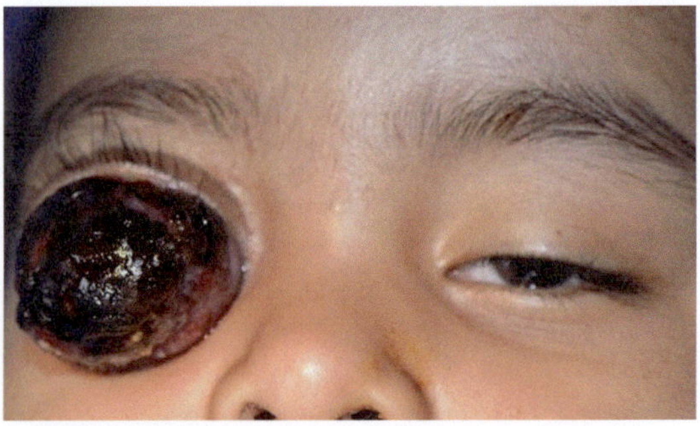

Fig. 17 A 2-year-3-months old child presented with a large fungating mass protruding out of the right orbit, indicating orbital retinoblastoma

radiation therapy to the orbit, followed by an adjuvant course of high-dose chemotherapy [76, 90]. For hematogenous or central nervous system metastasis (International Staging, stage 4), palliative therapy can be considered.

The dose of EBRT ranges from 3600 to 4600 cGy depending on dose per fractionation, daily or alternate day schedule and residual gross or microscopic disease. CTV for intact eyes with useful vision should cover the entire retina up to ora serrata and at least 1 cm of the optic nerve, at the same time sparing the lens, cornea and lacrimal gland (Fig. 18). With intensity-modulated radiation therapy (IMRT) and Arc therapy, the lacrimal gland mean dose can be kept below 3500 cGy, to reduce the chance of xerophthalmia. Bony orbit should be contoured and care should be taken to reduce the dose over it to reduce the possibility of orbital hypoplasia. Proton therapy has the edge over photons in sparring bony orbit. For patients receiving EBRT to orbit after enucleation with high-risk features, CTV should include the entire orbit along with superior and inferior orbital fissures, orbital apex and ipsilateral cavernous sinus (CVS).

5.4 Intraocular Lymphoma

Intraocular lymphomas are a form of extranodal lymphomas and are of two types: vitreoretinal and uveal. Both are primarily NHL, B-cell type. The most common intraocular lymphoma is the pri-

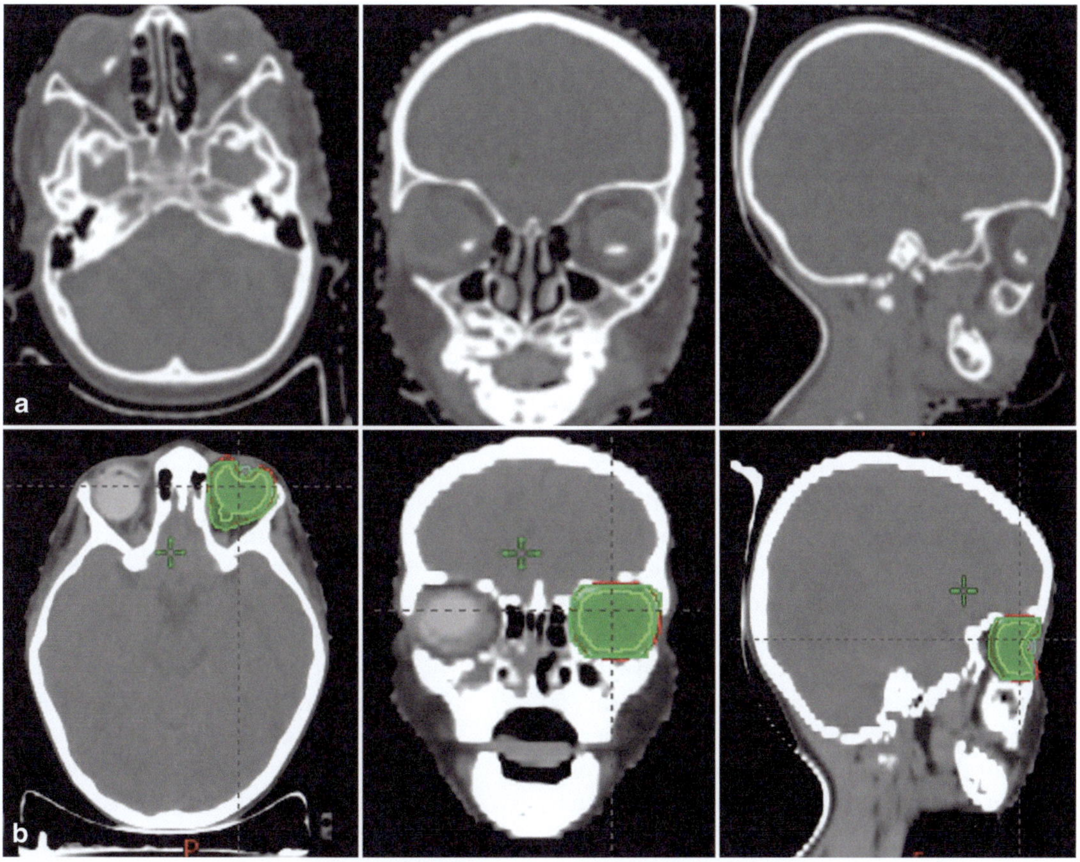

Fig. 18 (**a**) Axial, coronal, and sagittal CT images (left to right) demonstrating bilateral retinal calcifications in a child with bilateral intraocular retinoblastoma. (**b**) Corresponding axial, coronal, and sagittal treatment planning CT images (left to right) showing dose distribution achieved with conformal radiotherapy using volumetric arc therapy (VMAT)

mary vitreoretinal lymphoma (PVRL). It can be an extension of the primary CNS lymphoma (PCNSL), involving the brain and the cerebrospinal fluid. Most commonly, it presents as uveitis and is frequently bilateral. Multiple subretinal yellow infiltrates are typically seen in this form of high-grade lymphoma, belonging to the subtype DLBCL. In contrast, the primary uveal lymphomas are low-grade B-cell lymphomas. Uveal lymphomas are characterized by amelanotic, solitary or multifocal, uveal stromal lesions in one or both eyes. Secondary vitreoretinal and choroidal lymphomas occur in patients with disseminated disease.

Intraocular lymphoma may occur independently, prior to or subsequent to a primary CNS lymphoma. Given the rarity of the tumor, the optimal treatment regimen is unclear. Systemic evaluation is mandatory. For uveal lymphomas without systemic involvement, EBRT has proven to achieve high regression rates [91]. Radiation therapy has been used with desirable control after 30–40 Gy given exclusively to both eyes in the absence of CNS disease [92].

In the presence of systemic lymphoma, systemic chemotherapy is advised. Methotrexate and cytosine arabinoside are most commonly used, given their ability to cross the blood-brain barrier. Progression leading to intracranial involvement is seen in 60%–85% of the cases. For vitreoretinal lymphoma with CNS involvement, ocular and CNS irradiation is most effective [93, 94]. Intrathecal and intraocular methotrexate/rituximab also achieve a very good response. Our experience with the use of VMAT radiotherapy technique combinded with Image guidance as the sole modality for primary intraocular lymphoma has been encouraging with long-term local control in elderly patients. CTV includes the entire globe or a part of the globe, sparing the lacrimal gland and in some cases lens depending on the location of the gross tumor. In recent years, intravenous/intrathecal and intra-vitreal chemotherapy are combined to improve local control. In patients with recurrent disease, progressive disease and CNS involvement, the modern techniques of focal radiotherapy increase the disease control and survival [95].

6 Conclusion

A clear understanding of the possible differential diagnosis and variable clinical presentations of the orbital and ocular tumors is mandatory for oncologists. A logical approach includes accurate timely clinical diagnosis with radiological imaging, protocol-based planning, systemic evaluation, neoadjuvant treatment as appropriate, meticulous surgical intervention, histopathological confirmation, and adjuvant therapy. This aids in optimizing the outcome, thus minimizing morbidity and mortality with adequate aesthetic and functional outcomes.

Percepts Box

1. Ophthalmic oncology is a specialized branch of ophthalmology that deals with eye tumors, both benign and malignant.
2. Worldwide, the most common ocular cancers are retinoblastoma and melanoma. In India, the most common tumor is retinoblastoma.
3. Tumors of eyelid: Common eyelid lesions, like squamous papilloma, is benign. A thorough clinical assessment should be done to distinguish them from serious condition that may require referral to specialist. Most common malignant lesion in eyelid is basal cell carcinoma, other malignant conditions includes squamous cell carcinoma, sebaceous carcinoma, keranthoma, and malignant melanoma.
4. Tumors of conjunctiva: Conjunctival tumors encompass a broad range of diagnosis like benign conjunctival choristomas. Important malignant lesions include conjunctival epithelial tumors, conjunctival melanocytic tumors and conjunctival lymphoid tumors. Conjunctival tumors are rarely seen in children. Management includes exci-

(continued)

sion biopsy and cryotherapy with "no touch" technique with or without adjuvant treatment. Plaque brachytherapy is highly efficient. Systemic therapy and targeted therapy can be used in lymphomas.
5. Tumors of orbit: Comprise of heterogeneous group ranging from benign lesions-like orbital desmoid tumors, orbital teratomatous cyst, capillary hemangioma, lymphangioma, cavernous hemangioma, orbital varix, orbital neurofibroam and optic nerve sheath meningioma to malignant lesions like—optic nerve glioma, orbital rhabdomyosarcoma, adenoid cystic carcinoma of lacrimal gland, orbital lymphomaand orbital metastatic tumors. Treatment depends upon the nature of disease, location, and associated symptoms.
6. Intraocular tumors includes uveal melanoma, choroidal hemangioma, retinoblastoma, intraocular lymphoma, paraneoplastic retinopathy and age-related macular degeneration.
7. Retinoblastoma—most common primary intraocular malignancy of childhood, which can be heritable or non-heritable. It typically presents as leucoria in child less than 3 years. Diagnosis is based on clinical findings, ophthalmologic examination, and imaging. Classification is based on ICRB. Treatment options includes globe and vision sparing therapies.
8. Post-radiotherapy ocular complications are dose-dependent.

Multiple Choice Questions

1. What is volume of orbit?
   (a) 20 cc
   (b) 30 cc
   (c) 40 cc
   (d) 50 cc
2. How many extraocular muscles originate from Annulus of Zinn?
   (a) 1
   (b) 2
   (c) 3
   (d) 4
3. What is the most common eye tumor in India?
   (a) Melanoma
   (b) Retinoblastoma
   (c) Ocular surface squamous neoplasia
   (d) Keratoacanthoma
4. Most common site for basal cell carcinoma is
   (a) Medial canthus
   (b) Lateral canthus
   (c) Upper eyelid
   (d) Lower eyelid
5. A 25 years male from China presented with diffuse eyelid swelling. On examination there was distortion of the posterior lid margin, blockage of meibomian gland orifices, loss of cilia, with surrounding telangiectasia. Histopathology revealed pagetoid spread. What is the standard treatment of this condition?
   (a) Wide local excision with frozen section
   (b) Topical chemotherapy
   (c) Systemic chemotherapy
   (d) Radiotherapy
6. Middle-aged female presented to ophthalmology OPD with visual loss, progressive proptosis, with optic disc edema or atrophy. On examination, there is presence of a retinochoroidal shunt vessel at the disc margin. MRI orbit revealed fusiform to round lesion

around a well-defined normal intracanalicular part of optic nerve. What is the diagnosis?
   (a) Orbital neurofibroma
   (b) Optic nerve glioma
   (c) Optic nerve sheath meningioma
   (d) Orbital schwannoma
7. How many patients presenting with primary orbital lymphoma would eventually develop systemic lymphoma
   (a) One-half
   (b) One-third
   (c) One-fourth
   (d) Two-third
8. Most common site for uveal melanomas?
   (a) Choroid
   (b) Ciliary body
   (c) Iris
   (d) Lens
9. According to ICRB, discrete tumor with subretinal fluid, present or past, without seeding, involving up to one-quarter of the retina, local fine vitreous seeding present close to discrete tumor or local subretinal seeding <3 mm (2 DD) from the tumor are classified as what Group of Retinoblastoma
   (a) Group A
   (b) Group B
   (c) Group C
   (d) Group D
10. What is indication for external beam radiotherapy for patient with Retinoblastoma?
   (a) Unifocal tumors
   (b) Tumors that respond to chemotherapy
   (c) Tumor away from macula or optic nerve with preserved vision
   (d) Vitreous seeding that do not respond to systemic chemotherapy

Answer Key

1. (b)
2. (d)
3. (b)
4. (d)
5. (a)
6. (c)
7. (b)
8. (a)
9. (c)
10. (d)

References

1. Donaldson MJ, Sullivan TJ, Whitehead KJ, Williamson RM. Periocular keratoacanthoma: clinical features, pathology, and management. Ophthalmology. 2003;110(7):1403–7.
2. Shields JA, Shields CL. Eyelid, conjunctival, and orbital tumors: an atlas and textbook. Lippincott Williams & Wilkins; 2008. p. 872.
3. Bergin DJ, Lapins NA, Deffer TA. Intralesional 5-fluorouracil for keratoacanthoma of the eyelid. Ophthalmic Plast Reconstr Surg. 1986;2(4):201–4.
4. Urosevic M, Dummer R. Role of imiquimod in skin cancer treatment. Am J Clin Dermatol. 2004;5(6):453–8.
5. Veness MJ. The important role of radiotherapy in patients with non-melanoma skin cancer and other cutaneous entities. J Med Imaging Radiat Oncol. 2008;52(3):278–86.
6. Lagler CNP, Freitag SK. Management of periocular actinic keratosis: a review of practice patterns among ophthalmic plastic surgeons. Ophthalmic Plast Reconstr Surg. 2012;28(4):277–81.
7. Goyal JL, Rao VA, Srinivasan R, Agrawal K. Oculocutaneous manifestations in xeroderma pigmentosa. Br J Ophthalmol. 1994;78(4):295–7.
8. Doxanas MT, Iliff WJ, Iliff NT, Green WR. Squamous cell carcinoma of the eyelids. Ophthalmology. 1987;94(5):538–41.
9. Sullivan TJ. Topical therapies for periorbital cutaneous malignancies: indications and treatment regimens. Curr Opin Ophthalmol. 2012;23(5):439–42.
10. Cook BE, Bartley GB. Treatment options and future prospects for the management of eyelid malignancies: an evidence-based update. Ophthalmology. 2001;108(11):2088–98. quiz 2099–100, 2121.
11. Mendenhall W, Million R, Mancuso A. Carcinoma of skin. In: Million RR, Cassisi NJ, editors. Management of head and neck cancer: multidisciplinary approach. 2nd ed. Philadelphia: JB Lippincott; 1994. p. 643–91.
12. Jackson JE, Dickie GJ, Wiltshire KL, Keller J, Tripcony L, Poulsen MG, et al. Radiotherapy for perineural invasion in cutaneous head and neck carcinomas: toward a risk-adapted treatment approach. Head Neck. 2009;31(5):604–10.
13. Demirci H, Elner VM, Demirci FY, Robinson DR, Chinnaiyan A, Schlachter D, et al. Immunotherapy for conjunctival squamous cell carcinoma with orbital extension. Ophthalmology. 2021;128(5):801–4.
14. Payne JW, Duke JR, Butner R, Eifrig DE. Basal cell carcinoma of the eyelids. A long-term follow-up study. Arch Ophthalmol. 1969;81(4):553–8.
15. Gayre GS, Hybarger CP, Mannor G, Meecham W, Delfanti JB, Mizono GS, et al. Outcomes of exci-

sion of 1750 eyelid and periocular skin basal cell and squamous cell carcinomas by modified en face frozen section margin-controlled technique. Int Ophthalmol Clin. 2009;49(4):97–110.

16. Levin F, Khalil M, McCormick SA, Della Rocca D, Maher E, Della Rocca RC. Excision of periocular basal cell carcinoma with stereoscopic microdissection of surgical margins for frozen-section control: report of 200 cases. Arch Ophthalmol. 2009;127(8):1011–5.
17. Fitzpatrick PJ, Thompson GA, Easterbrook WM, Gallie BL, Payne DG. Basal and squamous cell carcinoma of the eyelids and their treatment by radiotherapy. Int J Radiat Oncol Biol Phys. 1984;10(4):449–54.
18. Leibovitch I, McNab A, Sullivan T, Davis G, Selva D. Orbital invasion by periocular basal cell carcinoma. Ophthalmology. 2005;112(4):717–23.
19. Shields JA, Demirci H, Marr BP, Eagle RC, Shields CL. Sebaceous carcinoma of the ocular region: a review. Surv Ophthalmol. 2005;50(2):103–22.
20. Kaliki S, Ayyar A, Dave TV, Ali MJ, Mishra DK, Naik MN. Sebaceous gland carcinoma of the eyelid: clinicopathological features and outcome in Asian Indians. Eye (Lond). 2015;29(7):958–63.
21. Kaliki S, Morawala A, Krishnamurthy A, Divya Jajapuram S, Mohamed A. Sebaceous gland carcinoma: influence of age at presentation on outcomes. Ophthalmic Plast Reconstr Surg. 2021;37(4):341–5.
22. Murthy R, Honavar SG, Burman S, Vemuganti GK, Naik MN, Reddy VAP. Neoadjuvant chemotherapy in the management of sebaceous gland carcinoma of the eyelid with regional lymph node metastasis. Ophthalmic Plast Reconstr Surg. 2005;21(4):307–9.
23. Shields JA, Demirci H, Marr BP, Eagle RC, Shields CL. Sebaceous carcinoma of the eyelids: personal experience with 60 cases. Ophthalmology. 2004;111(12):2151–7.
24. Laskar SG, Kumar A, Sharma P, Budrukkar A, et al. Brachytherapy for eyelid cancers: Re-defining outcomes and esthetics in rare histologies. J Contemp Brachytherapy. 2025;17:174–82. https://doi.org/10.5114/jcb.2025.152540.
25. Huang YH, Chang TH, Chou TW, Liu MT, Pi CP, Huang CC, et al. Adjuvant radiotherapy for sebaceous carcinoma of the eyelid after orbital exenteration. Ther Radiol Oncol. 2019;3:21. Available from: https://tro.amegroups.org/article/view/5120.
26. Shi W. Radiation therapy for melanoma. In: Ward WH, Farma JM, editors. Cutaneous melanoma: etiology and therapy. Brisbane: Codon Publications; 2017. Available from: http://www.ncbi.nlm.nih.gov/books/NBK481863/.
27. Lazarevic D, Ramelyte E, Dummer R, Imhof L. Radiotherapy in periocular cutaneous malignancies: a retrospective study. Dermatology. 2019;235(3):234–9.
28. Scott IU, Karp CL, Nuovo GJ. Human papillomavirus 16 and 18 expression in conjunctival intraepithelial neoplasia. Ophthalmology. 2002;109(3):542–7.
29. Karp CL, Galor A, Chhabra S, Barnes SD, Alfonso EC. Subconjunctival/perilesional recombinant interferon α2b for ocular surface squamous neoplasia: a 10-year review. Ophthalmology. 2010;117(12):2241–6.
30. Shah SU, Kaliki S, Kim HJ, Lally SE, Shields JA, Shields CL. Topical interferon alfa-2b for management of ocular surface squamous neoplasia in 23 cases: outcomes based on American Joint Committee on Cancer classification. Arch Ophthalmol. 2012;130(2):159–64.
31. Shields CL, Kaliki S, Kim HJ, Al-Dahmash S, Shah SU, Lally SE, et al. Interferon for ocular surface squamous neoplasia in 81 cases: outcomes based on the American Joint Committee on Cancer classification. Cornea. 2013;32(3):248–56.
32. Shields JA, Shields CL, Gunduz K, Eagle RC. The 1998 Pan American Lecture. Intraocular invasion of conjunctival squamous cell carcinoma in five patients. Ophthalmic Plast Reconstr Surg. 1999;15(3):153–60.
33. Arepalli S, Kaliki S, Shields CL, Emrich J, Komarnicky L, Shields JA. Plaque radiotherapy in the management of scleral-invasive conjunctival squamous cell carcinoma: an analysis of 15 eyes. JAMA Ophthalmol. 2014;132(6):691–6.
34. Rao R, Honavar SG, Lahane S, Mulay K, Reddy VP. Histopathology-guided management of ocular surface squamous neoplasia with corneal stromal or scleral invasion using ruthenium-106 plaque brachytherapy. Br J Ophthalmol. 2023;107(5):621–6.
35. Shields JA, Shields CL, De Potter P. Surgical management of conjunctival tumors. The 1994 Lynn B. McMahan Lecture. Arch Ophthalmol. 1997;115(6):808–15.
36. Laskar S, Gurram L, Laskar SG, Chaudhari S, Khanna N, Upreti R. Superficial ocular malignancies treated with strontium-90 brachytherapy: long term outcomes. J Contemp Brachytherapy. 2015;7:369–73. https://doi.org/10.5114/jcb.2014.55003.
37. Walsh-Conway N, Conway RM. Plaque brachytherapy for the management of ocular surface malignancies with corneoscleral invasion. Clin Experiment Ophthalmol. 2009;37(6):577–83.
38. Shields JA, Shields CL, Scartozzi R. Survey of 1264 patients with orbital tumors and simulating lesions: the 2002 Montgomery Lecture, part 1. Ophthalmology. 2004;111(5):997–1008.
39. Gdal-On M, Gelfand YA. Surgical outcome of transconjunctival cryosurgical extraction of orbital cavernous hemangioma. Ophthalmic Surg Lasers. 1998;29(12):969–73.
40. Cho KJ, Paik JS, Yang SW. Surgical outcomes of transconjunctival anterior orbitotomy for intraconal orbital cavernous hemangioma. Korean J Ophthalmol. 2010;24(5):274–8.
41. Ratnayake GS, McNab AA, Dally MJ, Zajarski C, Senthi S, Ruben JD. Fractionated stereotactic radiotherapy for cavernous venous malformations of the orbital apex. Ophthalmic Plast Reconstr Surg. 2019;35(4):322–5.
42. Miller NR. Primary tumours of the optic nerve and its sheath. Eye. 2004;18(11):1026–37.

43. Nair AG, Pathak RS, Iyer VR, Gandhi RA. Optic nerve glioma: an update. Int Ophthalmol. 2014;34(4):999–1005.
44. Cummings TJ, Provenzale JM, Hunter SB, Friedman AH, Klintworth GK, Bigner SH, et al. Gliomas of the optic nerve: histological, immunohistochemical (MIB-1 and p53), and MRI analysis. Acta Neuropathol. 2000;99(5):563–70.
45. Brodovsky S, ten Hove MW, Pinkerton RM, Ludwin SK, Smith RM. An enhancing optic nerve lesion: malignant glioma of adulthood. Can J Ophthalmol. 1997;32(6):409–13.
46. Pierce SM, Barnes PD, Loeffler JS, McGinn C, Tarbell NJ. Definitive radiation therapy in the management of symptomatic patients with optic glioma. Survival and long-term effects. Cancer. 1990;65(1):45–52.
47. Eddleman CS, Liu JK. Optic nerve sheath meningioma: current diagnosis and treatment. Neurosurg Focus. 2007;23(5):E4.
48. Douglas VP, Douglas KAA, Cestari DM. Optic nerve sheath meningioma. Curr Opin Ophthalmol. 2020;31(6):455–61.
49. Bloch O, Sun M, Kaur G, Barani IJ, Parsa AT. Fractionated radiotherapy for optic nerve sheath meningiomas. J Clin Neurosci. 2012;19(9):1210–5.
50. Turbin RE, Thompson CR, Kennerdell JS, Cockerham KP, Kupersmith MJ. A long-term visual outcome comparison in patients with optic nerve sheath meningioma managed with observation, surgery, radiotherapy, or surgery and radiotherapy. Ophthalmology. 2002;109(5):890–9; discussion 899–900.
51. Crist WM, Anderson JR, Meza JL, Fryer C, Raney RB, Ruymann FB, et al. Intergroup rhabdomyosarcoma study-IV: results for patients with nonmetastatic disease. J Clin Oncol. 2001;19(12):3091–102.
52. Raney RB, Anderson JR, Barr FG, Donaldson SS, Pappo AS, Qualman SJ, et al. Rhabdomyosarcoma and undifferentiated sarcoma in the first two decades of life: a selective review of intergroup rhabdomyosarcoma study group experience and rationale for Intergroup Rhabdomyosarcoma Study V. J Pediatr Hematol Oncol. 2001;23(4):215–20.
53. Perry JD, Patel BCK. Orbital Rhabdomyosarcoma. In: Patel BC, Singh AD (eds), *Clinical Ophthalmic Oncology*. Springer, Cham. 2025. https://doi.org/10.1007/978-3-031-95179-4_19.
54. Shields CL, Shields JA, Honavar SG, Demirci H. Primary ophthalmic rhabdomyosarcoma in 33 patients. Trans Am Ophthalmol Soc. 2001;99:133–42. discussion 142–3.
55. Shields CL, Shields JA, Honavar SG, Demirci H. Clinical spectrum of primary ophthalmic rhabdomyosarcoma. Ophthalmology. 2001;108(12):2284–92.
56. Shields JA, Shields CL, Epstein JA, Scartozzi R, Eagle RC. Review: primary epithelial malignancies of the lacrimal gland: the 2003 Ramon L. Font lecture. Ophthalmic Plast Reconstr Surg. 2004;20(1):10–21.
57. Manjandavida FP, Honavar SG, Murthy R, Das S, Vemuganti GK, Mulay K, et al. Does multimodal treatment improve eye and life salvage in adenoid cystic carcinoma of the lacrimal gland? Ophthalmic Plast Reconstr Surg. 2022;38(4):348–54.
58. Shields JA, Shields CL, Freire JE, Brady LW, Komarnicky L. Plaque radiotherapy for selected orbital malignancies: preliminary observations: the 2002 Montgomery Lecture, part 2. Ophthalmic Plast Reconstr Surg. 2003;19(2):91–5.
59. Tse DT, Benedetto PW, Tse BC, Feuer WJ. Neoadjuvant intra-arterial cytoreductive chemotherapy for lacrimal gland adenoid cystic carcinoma: a long-term follow-up study of a trimodal strategy. Am J Ophthalmol. 2022;240:239–51.
60. Campo E, Swerdlow SH, Harris NL, Pileri S, Stein H, Jaffe ES. The 2008 WHO classification of lymphoid neoplasms and beyond: evolving concepts and practical applications. Blood. 2011;117(19):5019–32.
61. Tuncer S, Tanyıldız B, Basaran M, Buyukbabani N, Dogan O. Systemic rituximab immunotherapy in the management of primary ocular adnexal lymphoma: single institution experience. Curr Eye Res. 2015;40(8):780–5.
62. Uno T, Isobe K, Shikama N, Nishikawa A, Oguchi M, Ueno N, et al. Radiotherapy for extranodal, marginal zone, B-cell lymphoma of mucosa-associated lymphoid tissue originating in the ocular adnexa: a multiinstitutional, retrospective review of 50 patients. Cancer. 2003;98(4):865–71.
63. Woolf DK, Kuhan H, Shoffren O, Akinnawo EM, Sivagurunathan B, Boyce H, et al. Outcomes of primary lymphoma of the ocular adnexa (orbital lymphoma) treated with radiotherapy. Clin Oncol (R Coll Radiol). 2015;27(3):153–9.
64. Rosset A, Zografos L, Coucke P, Monney M, Mirimanoff RO. Radiotherapy of choroidal metastases. Radiother Oncol. 1998;46(3):263–8.
65. Shields CL, Shields JA, De Potter P, Quaranta M, Freire J, Brady LW, et al. Plaque radiotherapy for the management of uveal metastasis. Arch Ophthalmol. 1997;115(2):203–9.
66. Shields CL, Kaliki S, Furuta M, Mashayekhi A, Shields JA. Clinical spectrum and prognosis of uveal melanoma based on age at presentation in 8,033 cases. Retina. 2012;32(7):1363–72.
67. Damato B, Coupland SE. A reappraisal of the significance of largest basal diameter of posterior uveal melanoma. Eye. 2009;23(12):2152–62.
68. Shields CL, Furuta M, Thangappan A, Nagori S, Mashayekhi A, Lally DR, et al. Metastasis of uveal melanoma millimeter-by-millimeter in 8033 consecutive eyes. Arch Ophthalmol. 2009;127(8):989–98.
69. Melia BM, Abramson DH, Albert DM, Boldt HC, Earle JD, Hanson WF, et al. Collaborative ocular melanoma study (COMS) randomized trial of I-125 brachytherapy for medium choroidal melanoma. I. Visual acuity after 3 years COMS report no. 16. Ophthalmology. 2001;108(2):348–66.
70. Collaborative Ocular Melanoma Study Group. Accuracy of diagnosis of choroidal melanomas in the

Collaborative Ocular Melanoma Study. COMS report no. 1. Arch Ophthalmol. 1990;108(9):1268–73.
71. Muller K, Nowak PJCM, de Pan C, Marijnissen JP, Paridaens DA, Levendag P, et al. Effectiveness of fractionated stereotactic radiotherapy for uveal melanoma. Int J Radiat Oncol Biol Phys. 2005;63(1):116–22.
72. Muller K, Naus N, Nowak PJCM, Schmitz PIM, de Pan C, van Santen CA, et al. Fractionated stereotactic radiotherapy for uveal melanoma, late clinical results. Radiother Oncol. 2012;102(2):219–24.
73. Randon M, Lévy-Gabriel C, Abbas R, Dendale R, Lumbroso L, Desjardins L, et al. Results of external beam radiotherapy for diffuse choroidal hemangiomas in Sturge-Weber syndrome. Eye (Lond). 2018;32(6):1067–73.
74. Levy-Gabriel C, Rouic LLL, Plancher C, Dendale R, Delacroix S, Asselain B, et al. Long-term results of low-dose proton beam therapy for circumscribed choroidal hemangiomas. Retina. 2009;29(2):170–5.
75. Agarwal A, Raghavan V, Rathnadevi R, Rishi P. Treatment of circumscribed choroidal hemangioma using CyberKnife: a viable alternative. Indian J Ophthalmol. 2019;67(5):704–6.
76. Honavar SG, Manjandavida FP, Reddy VAP. Orbital retinoblastoma: an update. Indian J Ophthalmol. 2017;65(6):435–42.
77. Ancona-Lezama D, Dalvin LA, Shields CL. Modern treatment of retinoblastoma: a 2020 review. Indian J Ophthalmol. 2020;68(11):2356–65.
78. Shields CL, Santos MC, Diniz W, Gündüz K, Mercado G, Cater JR, et al. Thermotherapy for retinoblastoma. Arch Ophthalmol. 1999;117(7):885–93.
79. Shields CL, Kaliki S, Rojanaporn D, Al-Dahmash S, Bianciotto CG, Shields JA. Intravenous and intra-arterial chemotherapy for retinoblastoma: what have we learned? Curr Opin Ophthalmol. 2012;23(3):202–9.
80. Shields CL, Honavar SG, Meadows AT, Shields JA, Demirci H, Singh A, et al. Chemoreduction plus focal therapy for retinoblastoma: factors predictive of need for treatment with external beam radiotherapy or enucleation. Am J Ophthalmol. 2002;133(5):657–64.
81. Manjandavida FP, Stathopoulos C, Zhang J, Honavar SG, Shields CL. Intra-arterial chemotherapy in retinoblastoma—a paradigm change. Indian J Ophthalmol. 2019;67(6):740–54.
82. Manjandavida FP, Shields CL. The role of intravitreal chemotherapy for retinoblastoma. Indian J Ophthalmol. 2015;63(2):141–5.
83. Ueda M, Tanabe J, Inomata M, Kaneko A, Kimura T. Study on conservative treatment of retinoblastoma—effect of intravitreal injection of melphalan on the rabbit retina. Nippon Ganka Gakkai Zasshi. 1995;99(11):1230–5.
84. Ericson L, Karlberg B, Rosengren BH. Trials of intravitreal injections of chemotherapeutic agents in rabbits. Acta Ophthalmol. 1964;42(4):721–6.
85. Rao R, Honavar SG, Sharma V, Reddy VAP. Intravitreal topotecan in the management of refractory and recurrent vitreous seeds in retinoblastoma. Br J Ophthalmol. 2018;102(4):490–5.
86. Shields CL, Shields JA, De Potter P, Hernandez C, Brady LW. Plaque radiotherapy for retinoblastoma. Int Ophthalmol Clin. 1993;33(3):107–18.
87. Shields CL, Honavar SG, Shields JA, Demirci H, Meadows AT, Naduvilath TJ. Factors predictive of recurrence of retinal tumors, vitreous seeds, and subretinal seeds following chemoreduction for retinoblastoma. Arch Ophthalmol. 2002;120(4):460–4.
88. Gupta R, Vemuganti GK, Reddy VAP, Honavar SG. Histopathologic risk factors in retinoblastoma in India. Arch Pathol Lab Med. 2009;133(8):1210–4.
89. Honavar SG, Singh AD, Shields CL, Meadows AT, Demirci H, Cater J, et al. Postenucleation adjuvant therapy in high-risk retinoblastoma. Arch Ophthalmol. 2002;120(7):923–31.
90. Kaliki S, Palkonda VAR. Management of retinoblastoma with extraocular tumour extension. Community Eye Health. 2018;31(101):18–9.
91. Mashayekhi A, Hasanreisoglu M, Shields CL, Shields JA. External beam radiation for choroidal lymphoma: efficacy and complications. Retina. 2016;36(10):2006–12.
92. Peterson K, Gordon KB, Heinemann MH, DeAngelis LM. The clinical spectrum of ocular lymphoma. Cancer. 1993;72(3):843–9.
93. Teckie S, Yahalom J. Primary intraocular lymphoma: treatment outcomes with ocular radiation therapy alone. Leuk Lymphoma. 2014;55(4):795–801.
94. Jahnke K, Korfel A, Komm J, Bechrakis NE, Stein H, Thiel E, et al. Intraocular lymphoma 2000–2005: results of a retrospective multicentre trial. Graefes Arch Clin Exp Ophthalmol. 2006;244(6):663–9.
95. Zhao XY, Cheng TT, Meng LH, Zhang WF, Chen YX. Clinical features, diagnosis, management and prognosis of primary intraocular lymphoma. Front Oncol. 2022;12:808511. https://doi.org/10.3389/fonc.2022.808511.

Online Links

American Academy of Ophthalmology. Plaque brachytherapy: radiating positivity. https://www.aao.org/education/annual-meeting-video/plaque-brachytherapy-radiating-positivity.

A summary on Retinoblastoma. https://www.youtube.com/watch?v=TxPC7W6_o44.

Head and Neck Cancers

Sarbani Ghosh Laskar, Anuj Kumar,
Shwetabh Sinha, Yoke Lim Soong,
Ahitagni Biswas, Sushmita Ghoshal, Amit Bahl,
Vanita Noronha, Alok Thakkar,
and Bidhu K. Mohanti

1 Introduction

Head and neck cancers (HNC) constitute a significant global public health challenge and represent the sixth most common group of cancers worldwide. They account for approximately 900,000 new cases and over 400,000 deaths annually (Global Cancer Observatory, International Agency for Research on Cancer, World Health Organization). Cancers arising in the head and neck region are heterogeneous, with squamous cell carcinoma being the most common histology. The most significant risk factors are tobacco and alcohol consumption, while viral etiologies such as human papillomavirus and Epstein-Barr virus have emerged as important contributors in specific subsites. Diagnostic and therapeutic modalities have evolved over the years, including minimally invasive surgeries, advanced radiation therapy (RT) techniques, and targeted therapy. Early stage cancers are associated with an excellent prognosis; however, most head and neck cancers present in locally advanced stages, particularly in Low- and Middle-Income Countries (LMIC). A multidisciplinary approach is thus essential for their management to maximize outcomes with minimum morbidity. This chapter deals with cardinal aspects of head and neck cancers, including epidemiology, risk factors, diagnosis, and contemporary management strategies.

S. G. Laskar (✉) · A. Kumar · S. Sinha
Department of Radiation Oncology, Tata Memorial Centre, Homi Bhabha National Institute, Mumbai, Maharashtra, India

Y. L. Soong
Radiation Oncology National Cancer Centre, Singapore, Singapore
e-mail: soong.yoke.lim@singhealth.com.sg

A. Biswas
Department of Radiation Oncology, All India Institute of Medical Sciences, New Delhi, Delhi, India

S. Ghoshal · A. Bahl
Radiation Oncology, PGIMER, Chandigarh, India

V. Noronha
Medical Oncology, TMH, Mumbai, India

A. Thakkar
Head & Neck Cancer Surgery, Medanta Hospital, NOIDA, U.P., India

B. K. Mohanti
Department of Radiation Oncology, Bagchi Sri Shankara Cancer Centre & Research Institute, Bhubaneswar, Odisha, India

2 Incidence and Epidemiology

Head and neck cancers vary in different parts of the world depending upon the subsite and histology. Figure 1 shows the anatomy of the head and neck region and Fig. 2 illustrates the anatomical subsites of the head and neck. About 90% of head and neck cancers are squamous cell carcinomas with a significant male preponderance. Head and

B. K. Mohanti et al. (eds.), *Radiation Oncology – Principles, Precepts and Practice*,
https://doi.org/10.1007/978-981-95-5171-2_3

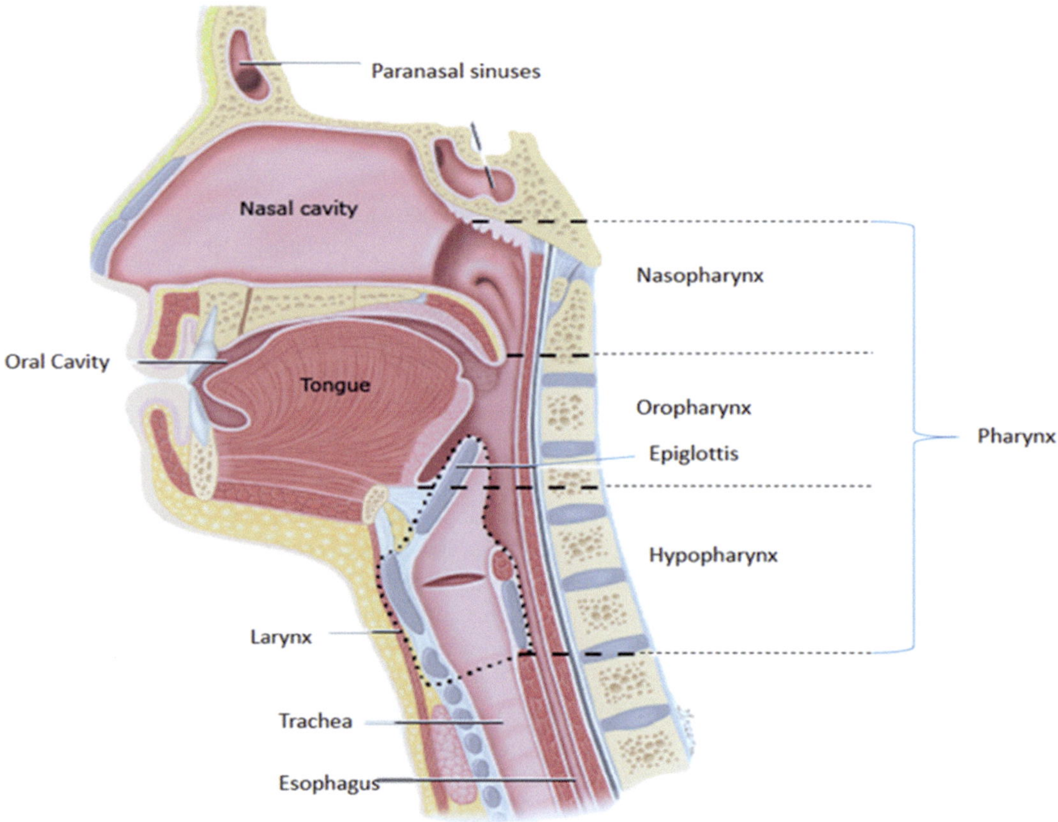

Fig. 1 Anatomy of head and neck

neck cancers account for approximately 3% of all cancers in the United States and 4% in Europe [1]. In contrast, in India, they constitute a substantial proportion of the overall cancer burden. India has a distinct profile compared to western countries, predominantly attributed to differences in lifestyle and cultural habits [2]. Oral cancer is a serious health issue in India in the young and adult population. Lip and oral cavity cancers, India's second most common, comprise about 10.3% of all cancers. It is also the most common cancer in the Indian male population (16.2%), the fourth most common in females (4.6%) and the third most common cause of cancer-related deaths in India (8.8%). The lower gingivobuccal complex is the most common site for oral cancer in the Indian subcontinent largely due to the widespread practice of chewing tobacco [3].

Oropharyngeal cancers are less common as compared to oral cancers in countries such as India. The most frequent histology is SCC, and the incidence rates are twice as high in men compared to women. Over the years, a shift has occurred in the incidence of human papillomavirus (HPV)–associated oropharyngeal cancers, especially in western countries [4]. Patients with HPV-positive oro-pharyngeal squamous cell carcinoma (OPSCC) tend to be younger with better performance status and prognosis [5]. In its eighth edition, the American Joint Committee for Cancer (AJCC) has staged HPV positive and negative cancers separately. De-escalation strategies in treating HPV positive oropharyngeal cancers have recently gained popularity, and various ongoing randomized trials are underway [6–8]. It is noteworthy that the incidence of HPV-negative tobacco-driven OPSCC remains high in countries like India.

Laryngeal cancers are more common than hypopharyngeal cancers. The majority of

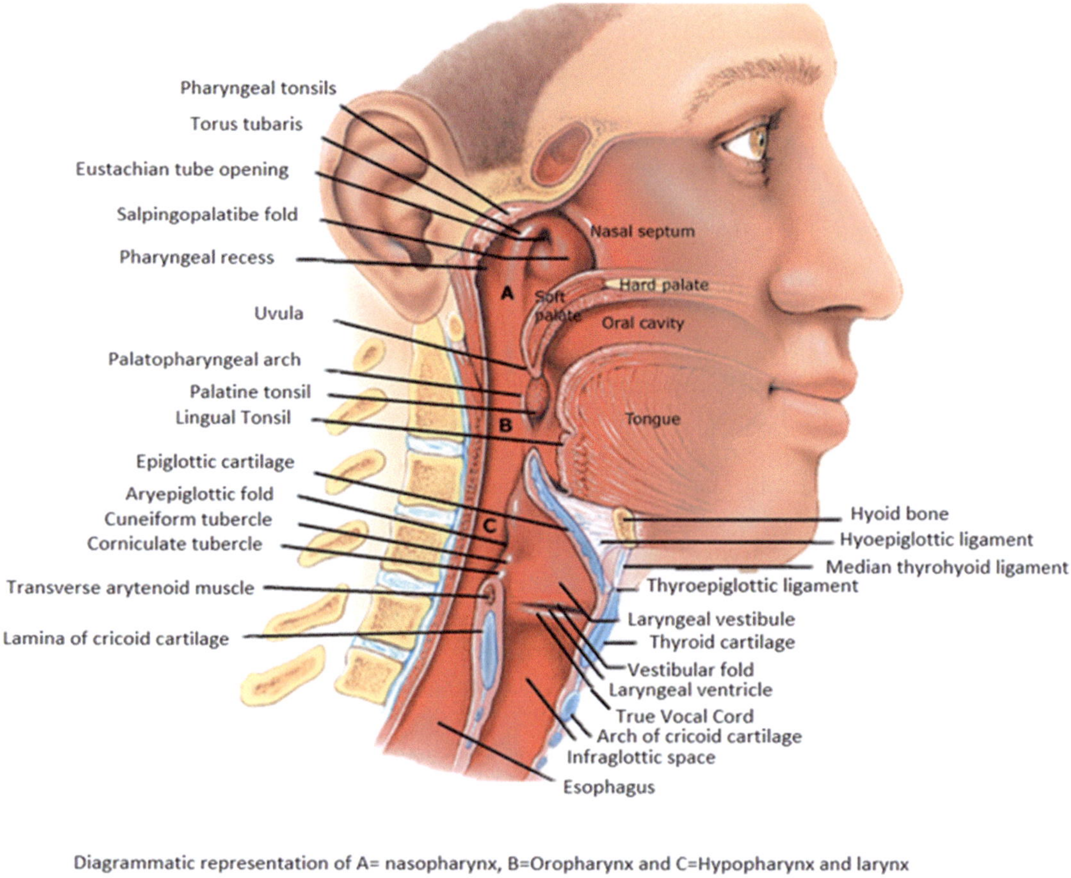

Fig. 2 Diagrammatic representation of A = Nasopharynx, B = Oropharynx and C = Hypopharynx and Larynx

individuals diagnosed with laryngeal cancer are older than 50. Approximately 95% of all laryngeal cancers are SCCs. Glottic cancers represent about two-thirds of the laryngeal cancers in the west. Supraglottic cancers are more common in the Indian subcontinent. Hypopharyngeal tumours are most commonly encountered within the pyriform sinuses (65%), followed by the posterior pharyngeal wall (25–35%) and post cricoid region. More than 95% of all hypopharyngeal malignancies are SCCs, and often poorly differentiated [9].

Nasopharyngeal cancers (NPC) have marked geographic variation, present with a bimodal age distribution and are three times more common in men than women. NPCs can be non-endemic or endemic and have a high incidence in southern China, including Hong Kong. Genetic, ethnic, and environmental factors play a role in the aetiology of the disease. In India, these cancers are common in the North-Eastern population [10]. Paranasal sinus tumours account for about 3–4% of all head and neck malignancies. Most sinonasal malignancies are diagnosed in Caucasians, with a 2:1 male predominance occurring in the sixth or seventh decade of life. The maxillary sinus is the commonly affected site, followed by the nasal cavity and ethmoid sinuses [11].

Salivary gland tumours account for 6 to 8% of head and neck cancers. Salivary gland cancers are divided into epithelial, nonepithelial, or mesenchymal lesions. Epithelial-derived salivary malignancies are far more common than nonepithelial. The parotid gland is the most frequent site of salivary gland tumours (80–85%). Approximately 20–25% of parotid gland tumours are malignant. Mucoepidermoid carcinoma (MEC) and Adenoid Cystic carcinoma comprise

Table 1 GLOBOCAN 2020 data on head and neck cancers

Site	India	New cases (%)	Deaths (%)	World	New cases (%)	Deaths (%)
Lip, oral cavity	135,929	10.3	8.8	377,713	2	1.8
Larynx	34,687	2.6	2.5	184,615	0.96	1
Nasopharynx	5697	0.43	0.49	133,354	0.69	0.8
Oropharynx	20,617	1.6	1.5	98,412	0.51	0.48
Hypopharynx	28,489	2.2	1.3	84,254	0.44	0.39
Salivary glands	7850	0.59	0.60	53,583	0.28	0.23
Thyroid	20,432	1.5	0.57	586,202	3	0.44

50% of all malignant salivary gland tumours [12]. Thyroid cancer has an increased incidence in high-income countries. India has also seen a rise in incidence, particularly among the younger population. Papillary and follicular cancers are differentiated cancers. Anaplastic (undifferentiated) cancers appear to arise from differentiated cancers. Medullary thyroid cancer (MTC) arises from the parafollicular or C cells of the thyroid gland, which are primarily sporadic; however, one-fourth of them are familial [13].

Table 1 lists the GLOBOCAN 2020 data of the incidence and deaths among the major subsites of head and neck cancers in India compared to the world

3 Risk Factors

The primary risk factors for most head and neck cancers are tobacco and alcohol consumption. Combined use of tobacco and alcohol markedly increases the risk compared with either exposure alone. Ill-fitting dentures, viral infections, high-risk sexual behaviour, etc., also increase the risk. Persistent infection with high risk HPV, especially HPV16, is a significant risk factor for oropharyngeal cancers. The predominantly affected areas are the tonsillar region and the base of the tongue. Environmental exposure (asbestos, cement, wood dust and perchloroethylene) has a role in laryngeal cancers. Plummer–Vinson syndrome, with chronic malnutrition and anemia, is a risk factor for post-cricoid cancer.

Epstein Barr virus infection, salt-preserved fish and genetic predisposition increase the risk of nasopharyngeal cancers. Paranasal tumours are associated with occupational exposure (including leather, textile, wood dust and formaldehyde), air pollution, tobacco smoke, and certain viruses. Although risk factors are not well defined for salivary cancers, RT exposure, smoking and viral infections have shown some association. Previous radiation exposure, iodine deficiency, family history and female gender are common risk factors for differentiated thyroid cancers [14].

4 Genetic and Familial Factors

Hereditary conditions like Fanconi Anaemia, Li-Fraumeni Syndrome, Xeroderma Pigmentosum and Ataxia-Telangiectasia are associated with head and neck cancers. Genetic susceptibility, in conjunction with Epstein–Barr virus infection and environmental factors, plays an important etiologic role in nasopharyngeal carcinoma Certain HLA (human leukocyte antigen) haplotypes are associated with NPC. NPC has a link with genetic polymorphisms, such as CYP2A6 (cytochrome P450 2A6). Comparative genomic hybridization studies have demonstrated alterations in multiple chromosomes, such as deletion of regions at 14q, 16p, 1p, and amplification of 12q and 4q. Loss of heterozygosity and tumour suppressor gene alterations involving chromosome 14q have been reported in nasopharyngeal carcinoma. Salivary duct carcinoma is characterized by androgen receptor positivity and may demonstrate HER2 overexpression. Rare actionable alterations such as NTRK fusions have also been described. Mutations or rearrangements in the genes encoding the proteins in the mitogen-activated protein kinase (MAPK) pathway have a role in differentiated thyroid cancers. Point mutations of the *RAS* oncogene are seen in approximately 40% of follicular cancers. PAX8-PPAR gamma 1 gene rearrangement is also seen in follicular cancers. Follicular thyroid cancer is also seen as part of familial neoplastic syndromes, such as Cowden syndrome (PTEN), Carney complex type 1 (PRKAR1alpha), or Werner syndrome (WRN). 30% of medullary thyroid carcinomas are attributed to autosomal dominant germline mutations, and several syndromes such as Gardner's syndrome and Cowden's disease are associated with papillary thyroid carcinoma [15].

5 Tobacco and Head and Neck Cancers

Tobacco is a causative factor for over 20 types or subtypes of cancer and kills more than 8 million people yearly. Tobacco consumption in any form increases the incidence of head and neck cancers. 70 to 80% of head and neck cancers are linked to tobacco use. Approximately 70–80% of head and neck squamous cell carcinomas worldwide are attributable to tobacco use, with significant variation by subsite and geography. According to the Global Adult Tobacco Survey, the tobacco consumption rate among adults in India is 34.6% and is higher in males (47.9%) than females (20.7%) [16]. The risk for HNSCC in smokers is approximately ten times higher than that of never-smokers. Tobacco is consumed in smoked, chewed or applied forms. Smokeless tobacco is equally hazardous and contains over 3000 chemicals and at least 28 known carcinogens. Cancers of the gingivobuccal complex are widespread in Indians due to the habitual placement of smokeless tobacco products in the gingivobuccal sulcus. Tobacco also synergises with alcohol and can augment the incidence of head and neck cancers [17].

6 Screening

Currently, there is no evidence for population-based screening in head and neck cancers. There is no effective screening program in western countries as well. However, screening for oral cavity cancers has been reported in various studies. A landmark cluster-randomized trial from Kerala (Sankaranarayanan et al.) involving 96,517 participants demonstrated a 27% reduction in oral cancer mortality among high-risk individuals undergoing visual oral examination. In this study, participants were randomized to three rounds of oral visual inspection done by trained health workers at 3-year intervals and a control group. The study identified subsets of patients with the highest risks who derive the maximum benefit. In contrast, screening studies from the United States have demonstrated low positive predictive value, with malignancy detected in only a small proportion of individuals with abnormal screening findings. Ancillary methods include toluidine blue supravital staining, brush cytology, light-based techniques and autofluorescence.

There is no role in screening for oropharyngeal cancers. For nasopharyngeal cancers, there is no data from RCTs or CCTs to determine the efficacy of screening for nasopharyngeal cancer (Cochrane Database, 2015). In nasopharyngeal cancers, plasma or serum EBV copy numbers play a role in screening, prognosis and early relapse detection. In endemic regions, observational studies suggest that EBV-based screening strategies may facilitate earlier detection; however, no level I evidence supports routine population-based screening. Screening has not been described for salivary gland tumours due to its rarity and no established familial aetiology. Primary prevention is vital for specific head and neck cancers, including oral cancers. Public awareness of smoking and alcohol cessation should be encouraged. Chemoprevention remains investigational, with no agent demonstrating consistent survival benefit, even in premalignant lesions [18–22].

7 Clinical Presentation

Tobacco-related cancers of the oral cavity, larynx and hypopharynx are most commonly diagnosed in the fifth to sixth decade of life, although age at presentation varies by subsite and aetiology. Patients with oral tongue and floor of mouth cancers are likely to present with early symptoms, including a non-healing ulcer, pain or bleeding. One of the presenting symptoms, otalgia, often resulting from referred pain mediated by cranial nerves IX and X due to perineural involvement or deep infiltration. Presentation of oropharyngeal cancers can differ based on the HPV status. Non--HPV-mediated tobacco-related cancers are typically seen in elderly patients. Pain in throat and more so while swallowing food or drinking liquid are commonly experienced symptoms. However, HPV-related cancers occur in the younger population and present with a small primary and large neck nodal mass.

Dysphagia and voice changes are common presenting symptoms in patients with laryngeal cancers. Supraglottic tumours may present with referred otalgia due to shared sensory innervation via the vagus nerve. Asymptomatic primary lesions may also present as a neck mass, particularly in the supraglottis. Hypopharyngeal tumours tend to present late, with most of them presenting with locally advanced disease. Symptoms occur when the tumour reaches considerable size or invades surrounding structures, including progressive dysphagia, neck mass, odynophagia, and otalgia.

Nasopharyngeal cancers present as neck mass or with symptoms related to the primary tumour. Involvement of cranial nerves III, IV, V, and VI due to superior extension of the tumour into the skull base can cause neurological symptoms including headache, diplopia, or facial numbness. Bilateral lymph nodal involvement is expected because the nasopharynx is in the midline. Many of these symptoms are inconspicuous and nonspecific; the painless, enlarged lymph nodes are frequently beneath the sternocleidomastoid muscle and remain unnoticed until they reach a significant size. Lymph node metastases are seen in 75–90% of cases at presentation and are bilateral in over 50%. Distant metastases are found in 5–11% of patients at initial presentation.

For paranasal sinus tumours, the most common symptoms include facial or dental pain, nasal obstruction, and epistaxis. Symptoms and signs depend upon the involved site and extent of the disease. Most patients present in locally advanced stages. A classic triad of facial asymmetry, malar prominence, palpable/visible tumour in the oral cavity and visible intranasal tumour occurs in 40–60% of patients with advanced disease. Differentiated thyroid cancers present as incidental nodules during routine physical examination or imaging. Symptoms of pain, dysphagia, dyspnoea and signs such as voice change, stridor, or rapid growth of a neck mass in the background of a known thyroid nodule should all increase suspicion of thyroid malignancy.

Weight loss and nutritional compromise are commonly seen in head and neck cancer patients. Assessment of the patient's comorbidities and a history of tobacco and alcohol consumption are vital parts of the evaluation. Comorbidities can impact diagnosis, selection of treatment, and prognosis. Distant metastases are uncommon at

Table 2 Common clinical manifestations of head and neck cancers

Oral cavity cancer	Oropharynx	Larynx and hypopharynx	Nasal cavity and PNS	Nasopharyngeal cancer
Non-healing ulcer Growth Bleeding from the lesion Trismus Local Pain/otalgia Neck mass	Growth Dysphagia Odynophagia Throat pain Otalgia Hot potato voice Neck swelling	Hoarseness Throat pain Dysphagia Odynophagia Stridor Dyspnoea Local pain/otalgia Neck swelling	Nasal obstruction Epistaxis Proptosis Trismus Neurological symptoms; headache and cranial nerve deficits	Painless neck swelling Epistaxis Nasal obstruction Aural symptoms Headache, Cranial Nerve deficits (CN III, V, VI, IX, X, XII) Neurological symptoms; diplopia

presentation in most HNCs; higher rates of metastases may be seen in nasopharyngeal, HPV-positive oropharyngeal and hypopharyngeal cancers. Some of the common clinical manifestations of head and neck cancers are given in Table 2.

8 Evaluation and Workup

8.1 History

A detailed history is critical for the initial evaluation of head and neck cancers. This includes documentation of comorbidities, addictions, environmental exposures, lifestyle, medical and family history, including any prior malignancy. Duration, progression, and rate of symptom progression are critical in differentiating indolent from aggressive disease. Detailed disease-related information is essential and should be documented properly before the initiation of planned treatment.

8.2 Physical Examination

Baseline performance status and nutritional assessment are of high importance before commencing therapy. The extent of the primary tumour and the neck nodes are documented, including size, number, and neck node levels involved. For oral cancers, operability is assessed. Fixity to underlying structures, extensive skin oedema, skull base, hyoid infiltration, and carotid involvement are some features that make the tumour inoperable. Small oropharyngeal primary with a large cystic neck node point more towards HPV-related cancer. Cranial nerve examination is essential in cases of nasopharyngeal and paranasal sinus tumours. Hopkins examination and fiberoptic laryngoscopy (FOL) are done for laryngeal cancers. Figure 3 shows the normal anatomical structure seen on FOL. Figure 4 shows lesion in pyriform fossa on FOL.

Upper GI endoscopy is done for hypopharyngeal cancers, especially when the postcricoid area is involved. Speech and swallowing evaluation is a vital aspect for tumours involving the laryngopharynx to assess the functionality of the larynx or for any symptoms of penetration or aspiration.

8.3 Endoscopy and Biopsy

After physical examination, the next step is endoscopy for not directly visible lesions. Endoscopy (rigid/flexible) is used to map the extent of the primary disease and, at times, rule out the existence of a synchronous primary. If the endoscopic evaluation is inadequate, then examination under anaesthesia (EUA) is performed. Biopsy of the

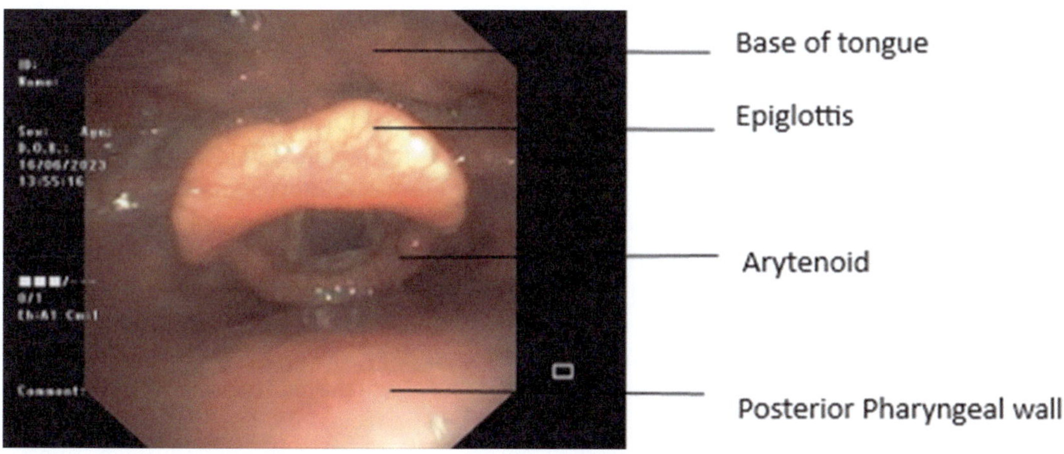

Fig. 3 FOL showing normal structures as labelled. (Courtesy: Dr Shubham Jain, Manipal Hospital, Delhi)

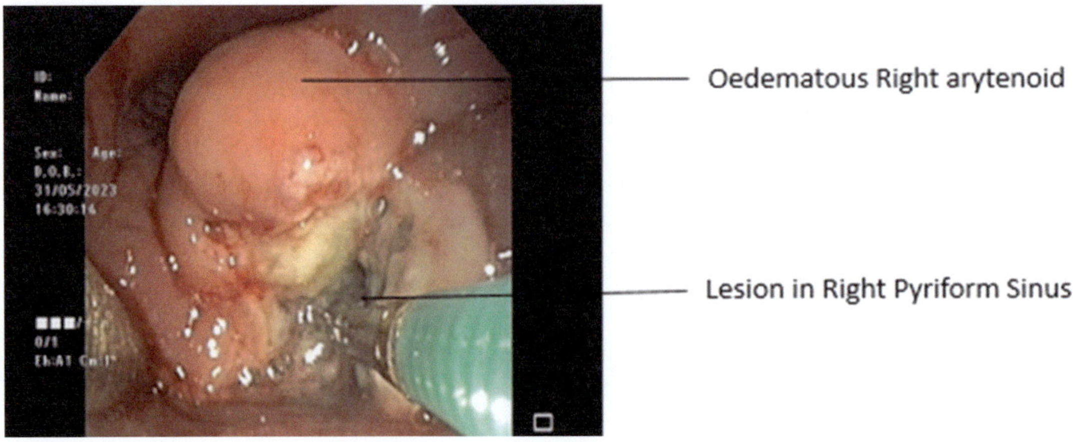

Fig. 4 FOL showing lesion in right pyriform sinus. (Courtesy: Dr Shubham Jain, Manipal Hospital, Delhi)

lesion for histological confirmation, histological subtype, and grade would confirm the HNC diagnosis. Histological diagnosis is also established by methods like fine needle aspiration cytology (FNAC), especially in cases of cervical adenopathy. Comprehensive immunohistochemistry may be limited on FNAC samples; tissue biopsy is preferred when extensive IHC or molecular testing is required. Assessment of HPV status in oropharyngeal cancers is carried out using p16, a surrogate marker. Epstein-Barr Virus (EBV) detection by Epstein-Barr encoding region in-situ hybridization (EBER-ISH) in tissue or measurement of EBV titres in blood is done for nasopharyngeal cancers. In cases of metastatic cervical lymphadenopathy from an unknown primary, HPV (p16) and EBV (EBER-ISH) testing aid in identifying a likely oropharyngeal or nasopharyngeal origin and guide treatment planning.

8.4 Imaging

Imaging is an essential component of evaluation in head and neck cancers, including early-stage disease, for accurate staging and treatment planning. Imaging features are essential for prognostication, assessing the locoregional extent, and evaluating residual/recurrent disease. Imaging with guided biopsies is indispensable before planning radiation therapy. The leading imaging modalities used in head and neck cancers include CT, MRI, USG and PET/CT, which guide diagnosis, staging, treatment planning, response evaluation, and follow-up.

MRI is generally preferred for soft-tissue dominant suprahyoid subsites, while CT is often favored for evaluating cartilaginous and bony structures in the infrahyoid neck. A contrast-enhanced CT scan is the imaging modality for buccal mucosa, gingiva-buccal sulcus, RMT, laryngeal and hypopharyngeal cancers. Contrast-enhanced multidetector tomography (MDCT) has the advantages of speed of scanning and the use of the 'puffed cheek' technique for imaging gingivobuccal and Retromolar trigone (RMT) cancers. CT is most specific for detecting cortical mandibular erosion, while MRI is superior for assessing marrow invasion. CT also has a complementary role in evaluating paranasal sinuses and skull base. However, the use of CT is limited in assessing perineural spread, dural involvement and marrow infiltration.

MRI is the preferred modality for imaging in the nasopharynx, oropharynx, base of tongue, anterior tongue, hard palate, salivary glands and paranasal sinuses, owing to its superiority over CT. Both non-contrast and post gadolinium scans are essential. MRI is more accurate in delineating the soft tissue extension, skull base invasion, intracranial extension, cavernous sinus extension, and perineural spread. Paravertebral space invasion and distinguishing the primary tumour from retropharyngeal lymphadenopathy can be assessed by MRI as a problem-solving modality [23–25].

FDG PET-CT is one of the imaging techniques which has gained popularity over the last few years. PET is a functional imaging modality and assesses the metabolic status of tumours. It is valuable for response assessment in the post-treatment setting due to its high negative predictive value. PET also has a role in radiotherapy planning, evaluating an unknown primary and detecting second primary cancers. It is the best modality for metastatic workup in locally advanced disease, N2, N3 nodes, advanced T stage, nasopharyngeal and hypopharyngeal cancers, all of these with a high propensity for distant metastasis. PET-CT is superior for detecting nodal and distant metastases but has limited spatial resolution for detailed assessment of primary tumour extent. PET-CT also has been proven to be superior to CT and MRI in differentiating post-radiation effects from residual/recurrent disease with sensitivities ranging from 88% to 100% and specificities ranging from 77% to 100% and is the imaging modality of choice for post-therapy surveillance [26].

Modern imaging modalities demonstrate comparable diagnostic accuracy in evaluating the clinically N0 neck.

CT and MRI have similar sensitivity and specificity in assessing cervical nodal metastasis. Ultrasound is mainly used to detect lymph nodes, especially in early cancers. Guided FNAC is done in cases of suspicious cervical adenopathy, which is associated with a high sensitivity/specificity. A 5–10-MHz linear transducer is used for diagnostic sonography. Ultrasound also has a role in the evaluation of thyroid nodules.

Imaging helps to determine the operability status of various head and neck cancers. Critical criteria for inoperability are involvement of skull base, encasement of internal carotid artery and infiltration of prevertebral fascia. The advanced T stage is classified as T4a and T4b, where T4a indicates advanced but resectable disease while T4b is mostly unresectable. The three major T4b issues common to all head and neck cancers are carotid artery invasion, mediastinal invasion and prevertebral fascial infiltration. Circumferential involvement of the artery at more than 270° by the tumour on imaging indicates an inability to strip the vessel off the tumour. In contrast, circumferential contact at less than 180° suggests a high likelihood of peeling the vessel off the tumour.

During treatment planning for radiation therapy, imaging done at the time of initial diagnosis is registered with the RT simulation scans for accurate tumour delineation. After-treatment completion, response assessment again requires a single or combination of imaging modalities depending on individual subsites. Thus, imaging in head and neck cancers is of utmost importance at all phases of treatment, starting from diagnosis to routine follow-up.

9 Pathology

A tissue biopsy of the primary tumour is necessary to obtain a histological diagnosis. The majority of head and neck cancers are squamous cell carcinomas. For oral cavity cancers, squamous cell carcinoma (SCC) is the most common histology in the oral cavity (90%). Over 90% of oropharyngeal cancers are also of squamous histology. Testing for HPV is essential to obtain a complete diagnosis for oropharyngeal cancers. p16 is a surrogate marker for the diagnosis of HPV status and is used for staging as per AJCC 8th edition. There are various tests to determine the presence of HPV. These are carried out in fresh frozen or formalin-fixed paraffin-embedded (FFPE) tissue. The polymerase chain reaction (PCR) test, which detects HPV DNA has high sensitivity and is cost-effective. However, PCR cannot determine viral load. ISH has a high specificity but the test has a low sensitivity and is technically challenging. RT-PCR detecting E6/E7 mRNA can determine active infection; however, this procedure is costly. P16 has a high sensitivity (95%) and moderate specificity (85%). False positivity of p16 in non-HPV-driven tumours remains a recognized limitation.

Smoking-related (HPV-negative) tumours are well-to-moderately differentiated with keratinizing morphology. HPV-related (HPV-positive) cancers are mostly poorly differentiated, non-keratinizing or basaloid morphology, although overlap exists. HPV-related OPC diagnosis can be challenging when the primary is very small.

For laryngeal and hypopharyngeal tumours, squamous histology is commonly seen. The 8th edition of AJCC has incorporated significant changes in the staging based on histology. The incorporation of DOI has brought changes in the T staging in oral cavity cancers. For oropharyngeal cancers, the stage is different for HPV positive and HPV negative tumours. For nasopharyngeal cancers, T2 tumours were earlier denoted only as parapharyngeal extension. Presently T2 includes parapharyngeal extension medial and lateral pterygoid muscles. For nodal staging, incorporating extranodal extension has led to upstaging of tumours.

Verrucous carcinoma is a well-differentiated squamous cell carcinoma with minimal cytologic atypia. The surface characteristically shows papillary fronds with prominent hyperkeratosis. Its benign appearance makes the diagnosis difficult, leading to delays in treatment. Figure 5 shows verrucous carcinoma of larynx.

According to the World Health Organization (2017), nasopharyngeal carcinoma is classified into keratinizing squamous cell carcinoma and non-keratinizing carcinoma (differentiated and undifferentiated), the latter being strongly associated with EBV. Sinonasal malignant tumours are varied, complex and rare. The many overlapping histopathological features make the diagnosis of these tumours challenging. Sinonasal tumours are unique as they show diverse differentiation from epithelial and mesenchymal to neuroectodermal and haematolymphoid. There is also a higher probability of having a non-squamous carcinoma with unusual biological behaviour. Some of them, like esthesioneuroblastomas, have good outcomes. Melanomas, small cell neuroendocrine tumours and sinonasal undifferentiated carcinoma have a higher chance of distant metastasis. Some round cell tumours such as embryonal rhabdomyosarcoma, lymphoma or plasmacytoma require non-surgical protocols. Hence, it is vital to atvtain a histological diagnosis before further management.

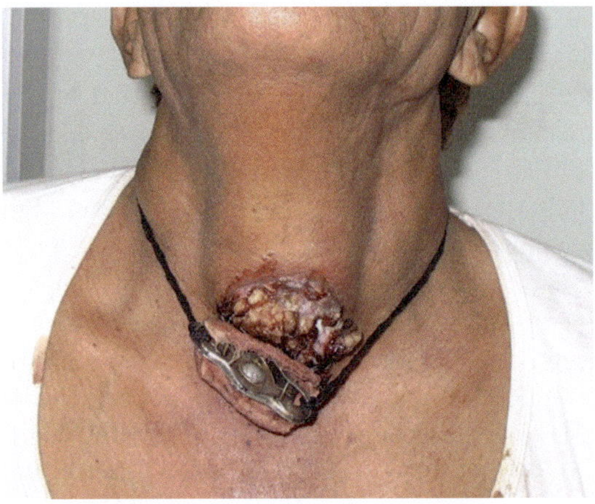

Fig. 5 Verrucous carcinoma of the Larynx. (Courtesy: Dr Anusheel Munshi, Radiation Oncology, BLK Max Hospital, New Delhi)

Salivary gland tumours arise from the progenitor cells in the ductal system of the glands. The majority of the salivary glands are benign. Pleomorphic adenoma is the most common benign tumour. Salivary gland cancers can be broadly divided into epithelial, nonepithelial, or mesenchymal lesions. Epithelial-derived salivary malignancies are far more common than those that are nonepithelial. The majority, 70%, have been shown to arise from the parotid gland, 8% from the submandibular gland, and 22% from seromucinous glands in the upper aerodigestive tract. Tumours arising from the main ducts are mainly epithelial and highly malignant, while those developing from the terminal ducts have epithelial and myoepithelial components and behave less aggressively. Among the malignant tumours, the most common are MEC, ACC and adenocarcinoma.

Thyroid cancers can be differentiated or undifferentiated. Differentiated thyroid carcinomas arise from the follicular cell of the thyroid gland. They are less aggressive and have a better prognosis than poorly differentiated thyroid carcinomas. DTCs comprise more than 90% of all thyroid carcinomas and include papillary thyroid carcinoma (PTC), FTC, Hurthle cell carcinoma

(HCC), and their respective variants. Medullary thyroid carcinoma arises from parafollicular C cells derived from ultimobranchial body neural crest cells derived from the fourth branchial pouch. MTCs secrete calcitonin and carcinoembryonic antigen (CEA) used in post-treatment surveillance. Approximately 50% of sporadic MTCs arise from somatic RET (RE-arranged during Transfection) oncogene mutations. Nearly all hereditary MTCs arise from autosomal dominant RET germline mutations.

Immunohistochemistry is essential in knowing the intricate details of a tumour. Incorporating tumour markers and genetic testing helps clinch diagnosis in tumours with uncommon histology. A systematic approach using ancillary techniques such as immunohistochemistry, cytogenetics and molecular pathology help in the differential diagnosis.

10 Principles

Treatment for head and neck cancer includes surgery, radiotherapy and chemotherapy, either as single or combined modality.

10.1 General Guidelines

Stage I/II disease is usually managed with a single modality (Surgery or Radiotherapy). Stage III and IV disease typically require multimodality treatment, including surgery followed by adjuvant radiotherapy or concurrent chemoradiotherapy, depending on site, resectability, and risk factors.

10.2 Selection of Modality

The selection of a modality depends on the site of the tumour. When different modalities are available, the one with equivalent oncologic outcomes and superior functional preservation should be preferred. Table 3 shows comparison of surgery versus radiotherapy in head and neck cancers.

Table 3 Comparing surgery vs radiotherapy in head and neck cancers

Surgery is preferred when	Radiotherapy is preferred when
Sites where surgery is not morbid (cosmetically and functionally)	Severe impairment of function/cosmesis with surgery, e.g. base tongue, the glottis
Lesions involving or close to the bone—to prevent radionecrosis	Surgery is technically tricky with high morbidity and poor results, e.g. nasopharyngeal carcinoma.
Young patients—possibility of a subsequent second primary	Patient refuses surgery
Presence of submucous fibrosis (SMF)	High risk of surgery
	Alternative to planned surgery

10.3 Assessment of Resectability

Tumour involvement of the following structures is considered technically unresectable:

- Erosion of pterygoid plates, sphenoid bone, widening of foramen ovale
- Extension to superior nasopharynx or deep extension into Eustachian tube or lateral nasopharyngeal wall
- Encasement of the internal carotid artery, defined radiologically as a tumour surrounding the carotids >270°
- Involvement of mediastinal structures
- Involvement of prevertebral fascia or cervical vertebrae

10.4 Principles of Resection

En-bloc resection of the primary tumour with adequate margins is crucial. A gross surgical margin of 1–1.5 cm is typically aimed for, with a pathological clear margin defined as ≥5 mm. Evaluation of the third dimension, the base, should be taken into account before excision. Close margin is less than 5 mm. Frozen section confirmation for margins may be done if the facility is available.

10.5 Management of Neck

Selective neck dissection (SND) is performed, for levels of neck nodes, depending on the site and the draining lymph nodes. Selective neck dissection typically includes levels I–III for oral cavity cancers and levels II–IV for oropharyngeal, laryngeal, and hypopharyngeal cancers. In clinically involved neck disease (cN+), modified radical neck dissection (Levels I–V) is performed. Radical neck dissection is rarely indicated. Internal jugular vein (IJV), sternocleidomastoid muscle or spinal accessory nerve is sacrificed only when involved by tumour. The contralateral neck should be addressed when the probability of contralateral metastases is high, tumours crossing or reaching the midline or with extensive nodal disease.

10.6 Reconstruction

Minor defects are closed with local flaps, with free flaps preferred over pedicled flaps. Segmental bony defects are optimally reconstructed using vascularized osseous free flaps. Primary closure/local flap/split-thickness skin grafting (STSG)/healing by secondary intention according to the site involved for mucosal defects. A pedicled flap may be considered for repairing a pharyngeal mucosal defect. For soft tissue loss, free flap (free radial artery forearm flap, anterolateral thigh flap, lateral arm flap)/pedicled flap, for example, pectoralis major myocutaneous (PMMC) flap can be used. A free fibula/scapula/iliac crest is utilized for skeletal defects for reconstruction. PMMC flap can be considered in select posterior mandibular defects.

Repair with an obturator may be considered for palatal defects, except for those crossing the midline or extending superiorly up to the orbital floor.

10.7 Principles of Radiotherapy

Radiotherapy can be used as a definitive treatment instead of surgery for organ preservation or as an adjuvant treatment with or without chemotherapy for long-term disease control following surgery. Radiotherapy can be delivered as external beam radiotherapy (EBRT) or brachytherapy. Factors while considering patients for radical treatment in head and neck cancers is shown in Table 4.

Table 4 Factors to consider when selecting patients for radical treatment in head and neck cancers

Patient related	Tumour related	Others
Age	Organ function, e.g.: Speech and swallowing status	Social support
Life expectancy	Stage at presentation	Cessation of ill habits
Performance status	Site and extent of the disease	
Comorbidities	Proximity to normal tissues and critical structures	
	Expected survival outcomes and toxicities	

10.8 Definitive Radiotherapy

Definitive radiotherapy is widely used in managing head and neck cancer where surgical resection may result in a significant functional or cosmetic deficit, especially in cancers of the oropharynx, larynx and hypopharynx. In cancer of the nasopharynx, radiotherapy is the only curative local treatment to eradicate the disease and is used in all stages of presentations except for distant metastasis. It is often combined with concurrent chemotherapy for locally advanced head and neck cancer to offer a better chance of cure. Table 5 shows commonly used radiotherapy schedules for head and neck cancers.

10.9 Post-operative Radiotherapy (PORT)

Indications of radiotherapy vary as per different subsites in the head and neck region. It can be classified for primary and for nodes separately. For primary, indications include:

Table 5 Commonly used definitive radiotherapy schedules

T1/T2 Glottic carcinoma
Definitive radiotherapy
50–52.5 Gy in 16 fractions over 3 weeks (For T1 disease)
55 Gy in 20 fractions over 4 weeks (for T1 and T2 disease)
63–66 Gy in 28–30 fractions over 5.5–6 week (for T1 and T2 disease)
Radiotherapy of oropharynx/hypopharynx/larynx/oral cavity
Definitive radiotherapy
SIB technique:
High risk PTV: 66 Gy in 30 fractions over 6 weeks
Intermediate risk PTV: 60 Gy in 30 fractions over 6 weeks
Low risk PTV: 54 Gy in 30 fractions over 6 weeks
High risk volume includes gross primary disease as well as grossly involved nodes
Intermediate risk volume includes nodal regions at high risk of involvement
Low risk volume includes nodal regions at low risk of involvement
Sequential technique:
Total dose: 70 Gy in 35 fractions over 7 weeks
Phase I: 46 Gy in 23 fractions to primary disease and involved nodes plus elective nodal volumes
Phase II: Cone down up to 60 to primary disease and involved nodes plus nodal volumes at high risk of subclinical disease
Phase III: Boost up to 70 Gy to primary disease and involved nodes
Post-operative radiotherapy:
60–66 Gy in 30–33 fractions over 6–6.5 weeks
Concurrent Chemotherapy:
Cisplatin 100 mg/m^2 IV every three weeks × 3 (Days 1, 22 and 43 during RT) (level I evidence)
40 mg/m^2 weekly with hydration and antiemetic prophylaxis
A cumulative dose of 200 mg/m^2 should be achieved (level IIB evidence)

- T3/T4 lesions
- DOI >1 cm
- Deep infiltrative tumour
- High-grade tumour
- Lymphovascular and perineural invasion
- Positive or close margin after curative resection

  For lymph nodes, some of the indications are

- Bulky nodal disease, N2/N3
- Extra nodal extension

10.10 Additional Adverse Pathological Factors

- Perineural invasion (PNI)
- Lymphovascular emboli (LVE)
- Early nodal metastasis (N1 disease)

10.11 Post-operative CRT

- Microscopically positive resection margins
- Lymph node extracapsular extension (ECE)

11 Neck Levels and Contouring of Neck Levels

Table 6 shows cervical nodes and their boundaries for contouring as per latest guidelines. Figure 6 shows the diagrammatic representation of neck node levels.

11.1 The Organs at Risk (OARs)

Due to the proximity of several organs at risk (OAR) to the intended treatment volume, treatment planning for head and neck cancer is challenging. It is important to delineate and set constraints to the important OARs in the head and neck region in an attempt to limit the normal tissue toxicities. Some of the OARs that are commonly delineated is given in Table 7 with constraints as per QUANTEC (Quantitative Analyses of Normal Tissue Effects in the Clinic)

11.2 Brachytherapy

Brachytherapy is a form of radiation therapy wherein the source is placed directly in the tumour tissue. Interstitial brachytherapy can be an alternative to EBRT for selected head and

Table 6 Cervical nodes and their boundaries for contouring as per latest guidelines

Nodal level	Cranial	Caudal	Medial	Lateral	Anterior	Posterior
Ia (Submental)	Mylohyoid	Platysma	NA	Medial edge of anterior belly of digastric	Symphysis menti	Body of hyoid bone/ mylo hyoid muscle
Ib (Submandibular)	Cranial edge of submandibular gland: anteriorly mylohyoid	Caudal edge of submandibular gland, alternatively plane through caudal edge of hyoid bone or mandible, whichever is caudal	Lateral edge of anterior belly of digastric (cranially), posterior belly of digastric (caudally)	Medial aspect (innerside) of mandible down to caudal edge/ platysma m. (caudal)/ medial pterygoid m. (posteriorly)	Symphysis menti	Posterior edge of submandibular gland (caudally)/posterior belly of digastric m. (cranially)
II (upper jugular group)	Caudal edge of the lateral process of C1	Caudal edge of the lateral process of C1	Medial edge of internal carotid artery (ICA)/ scalenius muscle	Caudal edge of the lateral process of C1	Posterior edge of the submandibular gland/ posterior edge of posterior belly of digastric m	Posterior edge of sternocleidomastoid m
III (middle jugular group)	Caudal edge of the body of the hyoid bone	Caudal edge of the body of the hyoid bone	Caudal edge of the body of the hyoid bone	Deep (medial) surface of sternocleidomastoid m	Deep (medial) surface of sternocleidomastoid m	Posterior edge of sternocleidomastoid m
IVa (lower jugular group)	Caudal edge of cricoid cartilage	2 cm cranial to sternal manubrium	Medial edge of common carotid artery/lateral edge of thyroid gland/ scalenius mm. (cranially)/medial edge of sternocleidomastoid m. (caudally)	Medial edge of common carotid artery/lateral edge of thyroid gland/ scalenius mm. (cranially)/medial edge of sternocleidomastoid m. (caudally)	Anterior edge of sternocleidomastoid m. (cranially)/body of sternocleidomastoid m. (caudally)	Posterior edge of sternocleidomastoid m. (cranially)/scalenius mm. (caudally)
IVb (medial supraclavicular group)	Caudal border of level IVa (2 cm cranial to sternal manubrium)	Cranial edge of sternal manubrium	Lateral border of level VI (pre-tracheal component)/medial edge of common carotid artery	Lateral edge of scalenius m.	Deep surface of sternocleidomastoid m./ deep aspect of clavicle	Deep surface of sternocleidomastoid m./ deep aspect of clavicle
Va, b (posterior triangle group)	Cranial edge of the body of hyoid bone	Plane just below transverse cervical vessels	Levator scapulae m./ scalenius m. (caudally)	Levator scapulae m./ scalenius m. (caudally)	Posterior edge of sternocleidomastoid m	Posterior edge of sternocleidomastoid m
Vc (lateral supraclavicular group)	Plane just below transverse cervical vessels (caudal border of level V)	2 cm cranial to sternal manubrium, i.e. caudal border of level IVa	Anterior border of trapezius m. (cranially)/±1 cm anterior to serratus anterior m. (caudally)	Trapezius m (cranially)/ clavicle (caudally)	Skin	Anterior border of trapezius m. (cranially)/±1 cm anterior to serratus anterior m. (caudally)

VIa (anterior jugular nodes)	Caudal edge of the hyoid bone or caudal edge of the sub-mandibular gland, whichever is more caudal	Caudal edge of the hyoid bone or caudal edge of the sub-mandibular gland, whichever is more caudal	NA	Anterior edges of both sternocleidomastoid mm	Caudal edge of the hyoid bone or caudal edge of the sub--mandibular gland, whichever is more caudal	Anterior aspect of the infrahyoid (strap) mm
VIb	Caudal edge of the thyroid cartilage	Cranial edge of the sternal manubrium	Lateral aspect of trachea & oesophagus (caudally)	Common carotid artery on both sides	Posterior aspect of infrahyoid (strap) mm	Anterior aspect of larynx, thyroid gland and trachea (pre--laryngeal and pre--tracheal nodes)/ pre-vertebral m. (right side)/esophagus (left side)
VIIa (retro-pharyngeal node)	Upper edge of body of c1/hard palate	Cranial edge of the body of the hyoid bone	A line parallel to the lateral edge of the longus capiti muscle	Medial edge of the internal carotid artery	Posterior edge of the superior or middle pharyngeal constrictor muscle	Longus capitis m. and longus colli m
VIIb (retrostyloid)	Base of skull (jugular foramen)	Caudal edge of the lateral process of C1 (upper limit of level II)	Posterior edge of prestyloid para--pharyngeal space	Posterior edge of prestyloid para--pharyngeal space	Posterior edge of prestyloid para--pharyngeal space	Posterior edge of prestyloid para--pharyngeal space
VIII (parotid)	Zygomatic arch, external auditory canal	Angle of the mandible	Styloid process and styloid muscle	SMAS layer in sub-cutaneous tissue	Posterior edge of mandidular ramus & posterior edge of masseter m. (laterally) medial pterygoid muscle (medially)	Anterior edge of sternocleidomastoid m. (laterally), posterior belly of digastric m. (medially)
IX (bucco-facial group)	Caudal edge of the orbit	Caudal edge of the orbit	Buccinator muscle	SMAS layer in sub-cutaneous tissue	SMAS layer in sub-cutaneous tissue	Anterior edge of masseter m. & corpus adiposum buccae (bichat's fat pad)
Xa (retroauricular nodes)	Cranial edge of external auditory canal	Tip of the mastoid	Splenius capitis m. (caudally)/temporal bone (cranially)	Sub-cutaneous tissue	Anterior edge of the mastoid (caudally)/ posterior edge of the external auditory canal (cranially)	Anterior border of occipital nodes—posterior edge of sternocleidomastoid muscle
Xb (suboccipital nodes)	External occipital protuberance	Cranial border of level V	Splenius capitis muscle	Sub-cutaneous tissue	Posterior edge of sternocleidomastoid muscle	Anterior (lateral) edge of trapezius muscle

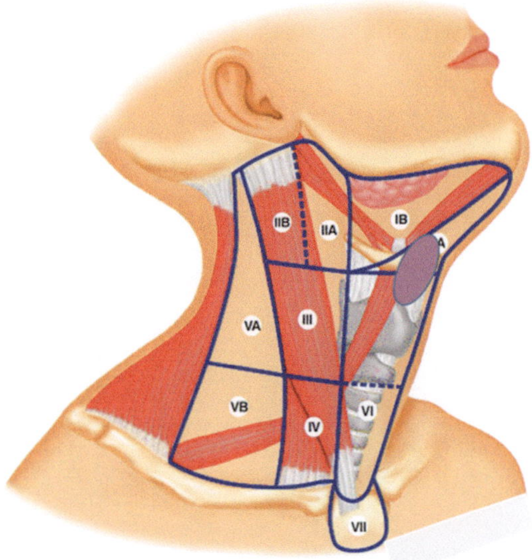

Fig. 6 Diagrammatic representation of neck node levels

Table 7 OARs with constraints in head and neck cancers

OAR	Constraints
Brainstem	Dmax $\leq$54 Gy
Spinal Cord	Dmax $\leq$50 Gy
Optic Chiasm	Dmax $\leq$54 Gy
Dose to b/l optic nerves	Dmax $\leq$54 Gy
Temporal lobe	Dmax $\leq$70 Gy, V65 $\leq$1%
I/L Parotid	Dmean <26 Gy
C/L Parotid	Dmean <20 Gy
Mandible	Dmax <70 Gy, V75 <1%

neck cancers. It can be applied as a definitive treatment for early disease or as a 'boost' in combination with EBRT to escalate the local dose to the tumour site. It can also be an effective salvage option for small burden persistent or recurrent disease. However, there are no randomized trials performed so far, practice is guided by GEC-ESTRO recommendations that have been established through expert panel consensus. Some of the indications are

- Small (preferable <3 cm) tumours
- Lesions away from the bone
- N0 nodal status
- Superficial lesions
- Recurrent tumours

Figure 7 gives an example of a case of carcinoma of the lip that can be considered for brachytherapy.

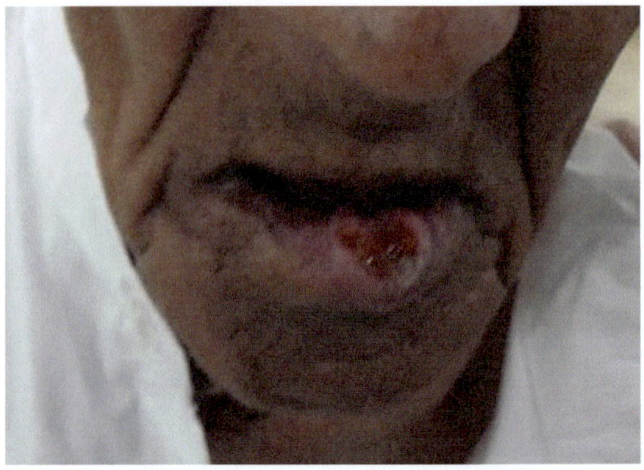

Fig. 7 Carcinoma of lower lip cT1 cN0 M0

11.3 Chemotherapy

Systemic therapy is an integral component in the management of locally advanced, recurrent, and metastatic head and neck cancers and is used in the definitive concurrent, adjuvant, and palliative settings. Platinum-based chemotherapy, most commonly cisplatin, remains the backbone of concurrent chemoradiotherapy, administered either three-weekly (100 mg/m²) or weekly (30–40 mg/m²). In patients ineligible for cisplatin, carboplatin or epidermal growth factor receptor (EGFR) targeted therapy may be considered. Immune checkpoint inhibitors targeting the PD-1 pathway have become standard in the recurrent or metastatic setting, particularly in platinum-refractory disease. Their use in the neoadjuvant, definitive, or adjuvant settings in combination with radiotherapy remains investigational and is currently limited to clinical trials.

11.4 Follow-Up

After completing the planned treatment, the patient is advised to come for a routine follow-up. Most recurrences occur in the first 24 months; hence, meticulous follow-up is warranted in the first two years. PETCT scan is the imaging modality of choice due to its high negative predictive value. It is done 10–12 weeks after treatment completion to avoid false-positive results. MRI may be indicated depending on the disease's origin and nature, especially in nasopharyngeal and PNS tumours. Follow-up should be done every 2–3 months in the first two years, six-monthly for the next three years and annually after that. A thorough head and neck examination for assessing locoregional control and late sequelae of treatment is carried out at each follow-up. Imaging is not indicated on a routine basis during follow-ups and is done only in cases of clinical suspicion. Serum T3, T4 & TSH every 6–12 months for all patients receiving neck irradiation.

11.5 Rehabilitation

Patients should be strictly instructed to continue care even after the completion of planned treatment. Some of the post-therapy counselling measures include abstinence from tobacco/alcohol, maintaining oral hygiene, shoulder physiotherapy in all cases of neck dissections, bite guide prosthesis following mandibulectomy, jaw stretching exercises to prevent post-operative trismus, speech and swallow rehabilitation, etc. are some of the critical aspects. A good life style routine, balanced meal, and physical exercises are essential steps to restore health.

11.6 Site-Specific Management

11.6.1 Oral Cavity

Oral cavity extends anteriorly from the skin-vermillion border of lips to junction of the hard and soft palate superiorly, and to the line of circumvallate papillae of the tongue inferiorly. Oral cavity and oropharynx are demarcated by anterior tonsillar pillars and glossotonsillar folds (Fig. 8).

11.7 Oral Cavity Subsites

- Oral tongue (Anterior 2/3rd)
- Mucosal lip
- Buccal mucosa
- Alveolar ridge
- Retromolar trigone

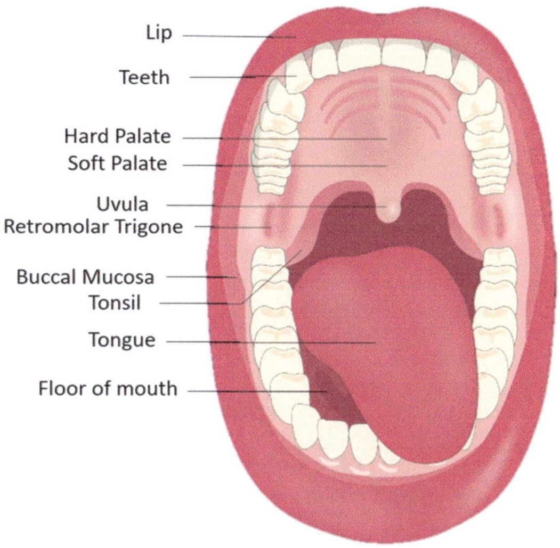

Fig. 8 Anatomy of oral cavity

- Floor of mouth
- Hard palate

11.8 TNM Staging of Oral Cancers

Table 8 gives the T staging of oral cancers

Table 9 gives the N staging of oral cancers

Table 10 shows the stage grouping of oral cancers

12 Diagnostic Workup

12.1 History and Physical Examination

History of smoking and alcohol, leukoplakia/erythroplakia [27] should be noted. Local examination includes visual inspection of the tumour, size, location, extent, bleeding, skin and bone involvement, fistula, pain at local site/radiation to ear/head. Halitosis may indicate anaerobic infection or necrotic tumour growth. Acute trismus indicates pterygoid muscle involvement, whereas chronic trismus indicates submucous fibrosis. Tongue movement restriction indicates extrinsic muscle involvement. Loss of sensation over the mental area indicates the inferior alveolar nerve

Table 8 T staging (AJCC 8th edition)

TX	Primary tumour cannot be assessed
Tis	Carcinoma in situ
T1	Tumour ≤2 cm, ≤5 mm DOI
T2	Tumour ≤2 cm, DOI >5 mm and ≤10 mm, or tumour >2 cm but ≤4 cm, and ≤10 mm DOI
T3	Tumour >4 cm or any tumour >10 mm DOI
T4a	Moderately advanced local disease: Tumour invades adjacent structures only (e.g. through cortical bone of the mandible or maxilla, or involves the maxillary sinus or skin of the face)
T4b	Very advanced local disease: Tumour invades masticator space, pterygoid plates, or skull base and/or encases internal carotid artery

Table 9 N staging (AJCC 8th edition)

Regional lymph nodes (N)	
NX	Regional lymph nodes cannot be assessed
N0	No regional lymph node metastasis
N1	Metastasis in a single ipsilateral lymph node, ≤3 cm in greatest dimension and ENE-negative
N2a	Metastasis in single ipsilateral or contralateral lymph node ≤3 cm in greatest dimension and ENE positive; or metastasis in single ipsilateral lymph node more than 3 cm but not more than 6 cm in greatest dimension and ENE-negative
N2b	Metastasis in multiple ipsilateral lymph nodes, none more than 6 cm in greatest dimension and ENE negative
N2c	Metastasis in bilateral or contralateral lymph nodes, none more than 6 cm in greatest dimension and ENE-negative
N3a	Metastasis in a lymph node >6 cm in greatest dimension and ENE-negative
N3b	Metastasis in a single ipsilateral lymph node >3 cm in greatest dimension and ENE-positive; or metastasis in multiple ipsilateral, contralateral, or bilateral lymph nodes, with any ENE-positive

Table 10 Stage grouping of oral cavity cancers

	N0	N1	N2	N3	M1
T1	Stage I				
T2	Stage II				
T3		Stage III			Stage IVC
T4a			Stage IVA		
T4b				Stage IVB	

in mandible involvement. Figure 9 shows squamous cell carcinoma of the anterior tongue (right lateral side)

Indirect laryngoscopy should be done to identify extension to base of tongue/synchronous lesions in larynx/hypopharynx. Systematic neck nodal examination should be done. Dental evaluation is essential to identify the need for extraction, simultaneously nutritionist review and speech and swallow evaluation should be done prior to starting radiotherapy.

13 Imaging

13.1 CT Imaging

Diagnostic imaging should be done with puffed cheek for gingivobuccal and RMT cancers. The software should allow isotropic coronal, sagittal and oblique reformations.

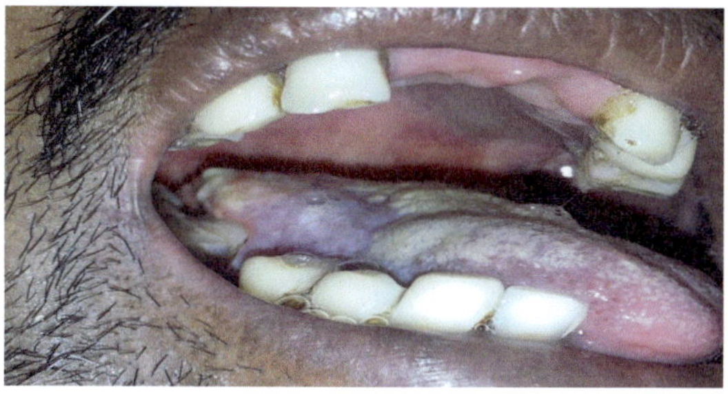

Fig. 9 Squamous cell carcinoma of the anterior tongue (right lateral side). (Courtesy: Dr Anusheel Munshi, Radiation Oncology, Manipal Hospital, Delhi)

13.2 MR Imaging

An optimal MR imaging protocol must include post gadolinium T1W sequences. Sequences are acquired at 4-mm thickness with a 1-mm intersection gap. Non-contrast T1W sequences demonstrate cortical erosion and marrow invasion. Contrast-enhanced T1W sequences demonstrate marrow invasion, perineural spread, soft tissue extent, tumour thickness, and best demonstrate necrosis in nodes. T2W sequences depict extrinsic muscle and FOM involvement as well as nodes. STIR images have high sensitivity for visualizing nodes but with reduced specificity. Diffusion-Weighted images are of added value, particularly in sub-centimetre metastatic nodes.

13.3 PET CECT

PET scan is not routinely indicated in oral cancers but may be considered for patients with stages III-IV disease with an extensive primary or heavy nodal burden. PET is sensitive in detecting distant metastasis (DM) or synchronous primary malignancies. The high negative predictive value of PET is utilised for response assessment after radical treatment completion [26, 28].

14 Pathology

Pathological examination plays a central role in diagnosis, staging, prognostication, and guiding adjuvant treatment in oral cavity cancers. The post-operative histopathology should mention the type of histology, grade, size, location and epicentre of the tumour, adjacent structure invasion, margin status, depth of invasion, PNI, lymphovascular space invasion (LVSI), the pattern of invasion, which are factors that can essentially determine the prognosis and need for adjuvant treatment [29]. An adequate surgical resection should have at least 5 mm margins around the tumour. The incorporation of Depth of invasion (DOI) in AJCC 8th edition has made it mandatory for all reports to provide DOI status rather than just tumour thickness. Depth of invasion, a vital prognosticator, is defined as the extent of cancer growth into the tissue beneath an epithelial surface [30–33].

Some of the other adverse factors are PNI, LVI and WPOI. PNI is defined as tumour cells within any layer of the nerve sheath or tumour in the perineural space that involves at least one-third of the nerve circumference [34, 35]. LVI is defined as the presence of tumour cells within an endothelial-lined space. Penetration of tumour cells into lymphovascular spaces through the endothelial cell layer has a role in tumour metastasis [36–38]. WPOI describes how cancer infiltrates tissue at the tumour/host interface and ranges from a broad pushing front of the tumour (good prognosis) to infiltrative satellite islands of the tumour (worse prognosis) [35, 39, 40].

15 Treatment Algorithm

Early stage oral cavity cancers are treated with single modality therapy, while advanced stages are managed with a multimodality approach [41]. Surgery is the preferred modality for resectable oral cavity cancers; except early lesions on the lip, angle of mouth and hard palate. Resectable cancers are generally treated with surgery ± post-operative radiotherapy/chemoradiotherapy. The overall management of oral cancers is given in the Fig. 10.

The decision regarding adjuvant therapy is usually based on the evaluation of stage and histopathological risk factors. Locally advanced tumours involving the masticator space, encasing the carotids or infiltrating the prevertebral mus-

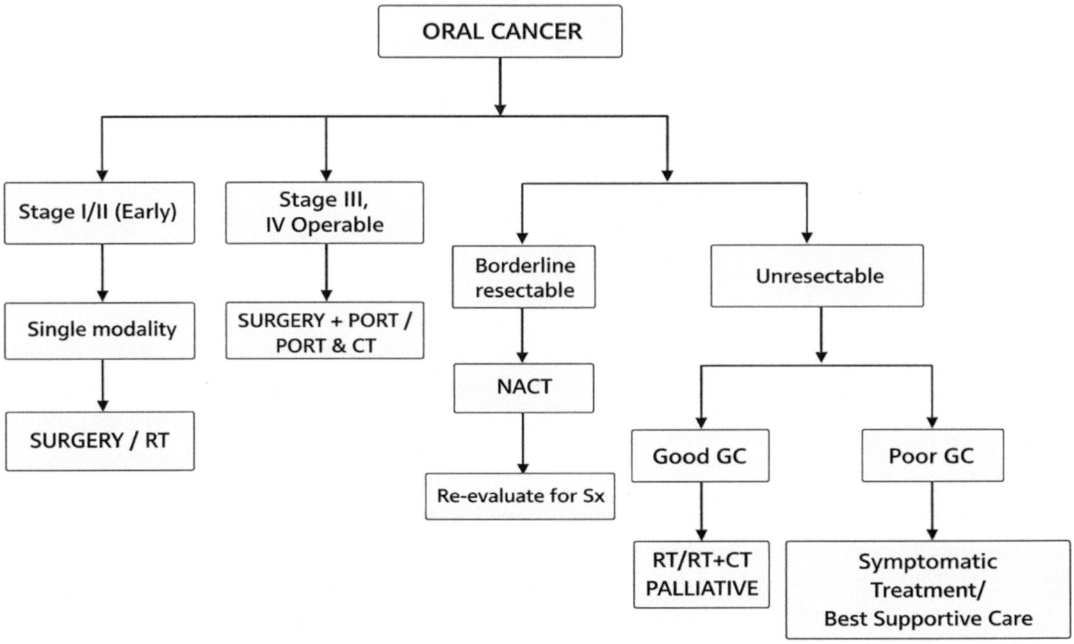

Fig. 10 Management of oral cancers

cles are generally unresectable. They are usually managed with chemo-radiotherapy, or in some instances, neoadjuvant chemotherapy may be used to shrink the tumour and attempt curative surgery. Systemic therapy is an integral component in the management of locally advanced, recurrent, and metastatic head and neck cancers and is used in the definitive concurrent, adjuvant, and palliative settings. Platinum-based chemotherapy, most commonly cisplatin, remains the backbone of concurrent chemoradiotherapy, administered either three-weekly (100 mg/m^2) or weekly (30–40 mg/m^2). In patients ineligible for cisplatin, carboplatin or epidermal growth factor receptor (EGFR)–targeted therapy may be considered. Immune checkpoint inhibitors targeting the PD-1 pathway have become standard in the recurrent or metastatic setting, particularly in platinum-refractory disease. Their use in the neoadjuvant, definitive, or adjuvant settings in combination with radiotherapy remains investigational and is currently limited to clinical trials.

16 Surgery

Initial surgical resection is the standard of care for oral cancers [42]. Achieving negative surgical margins is critical, and if feasible, repeat resection of positive margin is preferred [43, 44]. Close surgical margins are defined as within 5 mm. Early-stage OC-SCC can be resected without significant functional or cosmetic deficits. Locally advanced cancers require glossectomy, maxillectomy or mandibulectomy. Reconstruction is done with grafts or flaps to overcome considerable speech and swallowing deficits. Standard transoral or open approaches are used, and minimally invasive surgery with transoral laser or robotic surgery is done for very early cancers.

Mandibulectomy is performed as per the location and extent of involvement of the primary tumour. Marginal mandibulectomy is done when the lesion is close to the mandible, with limited superficial bony erosion and limited periosteal invasion. Segmental Mandibulectomy is performed with gross mandibular invasion, prior radiotherapy, edentulous mandible, gross paramandibular disease and when a margin of 1 cm is not possible. Hemimandibulectomy, which involves removal of the mandible symphysis to the condyle on one side, results in significant cosmetic and functional loss [45]. Reconstruction is performed with a composite osteomyocutaneous flap. Criteria for inoperability include fixed node, involvement of base of skull, extensive soft tissue reaching zygoma and root of tongue involvement (inseparable from hyoid) [46].

Ipsilateral elective neck dissection should be performed for patients with node-negative SCC of the oral cavity [47]. An adequate dissection should include at least 18 lymph nodes. For T1 lip and hard palate cancer, lymph node dissection may be omitted, as the risk of metastasis is low. The clinically node-negative neck should undergo level I to level III lymph node dissection due to the high incidence of occult nodal metastases [48]. Patients with primary tumours crossing the midline should be managed with bilateral neck dissection. An ipsilateral therapeutic selective neck dissection for a clinically node-positive (cN+) neck should include nodal levels Ia, Ib, IIa, IIb, III, and IV. In patients with a cN+ contralateral neck, contralateral neck dissection should be performed [49].

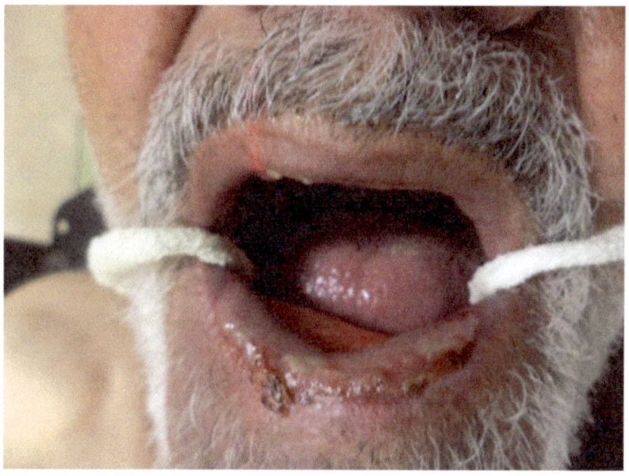

Fig. 11 Squamous cell carcinoma of the lower lip

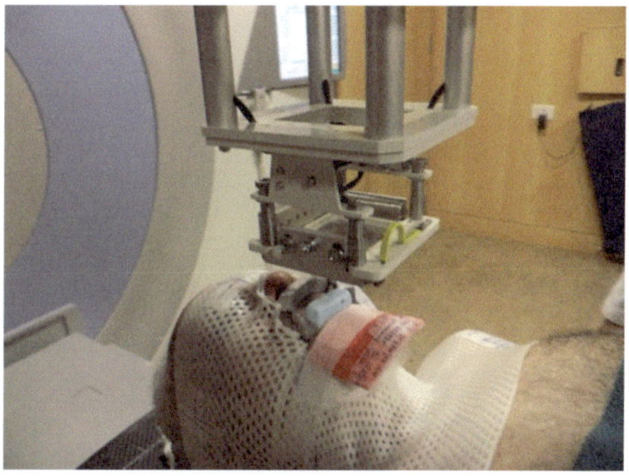

Fig. 12 The patient was treated by electron therapy with use of a bolus. Note the shielding measures taken to protect the adjacent structures. (Courtesy: Dr Anusheel Munshi, Radiation Oncology, Manipal Hospital, Delhi)

17 Radiation Therapy Planning

In oral cancers, external beam radiation therapy is predominantly used in the adjuvant setting to primary site and unilateral or bilateral neck nodes. Patients should be simulated in supine position with arms by the side using thermoplastic mask and neck extended. Wire should be placed over scar. Intraoral prosthesis (IOP) should be used for oral tongue cancer and hard palate tumours to reduce dose to superior and inferior structures, respectively. RT planning CT should be performed using slice thickness of 3mm from vertex to carina. Dental evaluation should be done before starting radiotherapy. Figure 11 shows squamous cell carcinoma of the lower lip. Figure 12 shows the patient was treated by electron therapy with use of a bolus.

Table 11 shows target volume delineation for radical and adjuvant radiotherapy. Table 12 shows approach to neck nodal levels. Adjuvant RT enhances locoregional control for cases with unfavourable pathological features. Typical indications include T3/T4, Close/positive margins, DOI > 5 mm, high grade, PNI, LVE, or node-positive disease with perinodal extension. PORT should start in about 4–6 weeks after surgery. Adjuvant concurrent chemoradiotherapy (CT-RT) is reserved for patients with extranodal extension or positive surgical margins. For nonoperative cases, definitive chemoradiation is a feasible and viable

Table 11 Target volume delineation for radical and adjuvant radiotherapy

Intent	Target volumes	Definition and description
Radical	GTV	Primary disease + Gross nodes
	CTV	GTV + 1 cm margin including potential site of spread + neck nodal stations
	PTV	As per institutional protocol
Adjuvant	CTV66 (if needed)	Region of microscopically positive margin or ECE
	CTV60	Postoperative bed + involved nodal region
	CTV 54	Elective nodal region
	PTV	As per institutional protocol

Table 12 Shows approach to neck nodal levels

Nodal category (AJCC 8th edition)	Ipsilateral neck levels to be included	Contralateral neck levels to be included[a]
N0-1	I, II, III, IVA, IX	I, II, III, IVA
N2a-b	I, II, III, IVA, VA & B, IX	I, II, III, IVA
N2c	According to N category on each side	According to N category on each side
N3	I, II, III, IVA, VA & B, VIIB, IX	I, II, III, IVA

[a]Unilateral treatment is recommended for N1-N2a laterized tumours of buccal mucosa, lateral floor of mouth and upper and lower alveolus. It could be considered for N0-1 lateral border of tongue not approaching midline by less than 1 cm

Level IX to be included in tumours of the buccal mucosa

Level IVB should be included in case of involvement of level IVA

Level V can be omitted if levels I and II is only involved

Level VIIB should be included in case of bulky involvement of upper part of level II

approach. Primary radiotherapy can be performed when surgery is technically challenging (e.g. Stage IVB) with high morbidity, the patient refuses surgery and medically inoperable disease [50–53].

Brachytherapy Interstitial implant can be used alone or in combination with EBRT for the treatment of oral tongue, floor of mouth, or buccal mucosa. For tumour thickness <1 cm, a single-plane implant is adequate; otherwise, a double-plane or volumetric implant is used. Surface mould brachytherapy can be used for select superficial (<1 cm depth) or recurrent superficial lesions of the hard palate [54–58].

18 Chemotherapy

Chemotherapy is indicated in adjuvant setting when there is a margin-positive disease and lymph nodes with perinodal extension [59–63]. Neoadjuvant chemotherapy has a role in mandibular preservation [64].

When surgically unresectable, some of the indications for giving neo-adjuvant chemotherapy are:

1. Buccal mucosa primary, with diffuse margins and peritumoural oedema going up to or above the level of the zygomatic arch and without any satellite nodules.
2. Tongue primary {anterior 2/3rds} with the tumour extending up to or below the level of the hyoid bone.
3. Extension of tumour of anterior two-thirds of the oral tongue to the vallecula.
4. Extension of tumour into the high infratemporal fossa, as defined by the extension of the tumour above an axial plane passing at the level of the sigmoid notch.
5. Extensive skin infiltration [46].

In the palliative setting, either a 3-drug regimen or oral metronomic chemotherapy (OMCT) is indicated [65–67].

18.1 Biotherapy

Targeted agents, in particular, epidermal growth factor receptor (EGFR) inhibitors like Cetuximab, have a potential role in head and neck cancers. However, the benefit of adding cetuximab to radiation for the treatment of locoregionally advanced SCC head and neck cancer has been shown primarily in cancers of the oropharynx and laryngopharynx. Role in oral cavity cancers has not been adequately studied in phase III randomized trials. The initial promise of Cetuximab (Bonner, 2006) to replace platinum-based chemotherapy has not been fulfilled [68].

18.2 Toxicities

Acute toxicities of radiotherapy include skin reaction, mucositis, loss of taste, xerostomia, thrush, dermatitis, dysphagia and odynophagia.

Figure 13 gives a representation of acute dermatitis that occurs as a side effect of radiation therapy

Chronic toxicity includes skin and soft tissue atrophy and fibrosis, xerostomia, lifelong need for fluoride prophylaxis, risk for dental caries, lymphedema, trismus and osteoradionecrosis. Figure 14 gives an example of osteoradionecrosis of the mandible that occurs as a long-term complication.

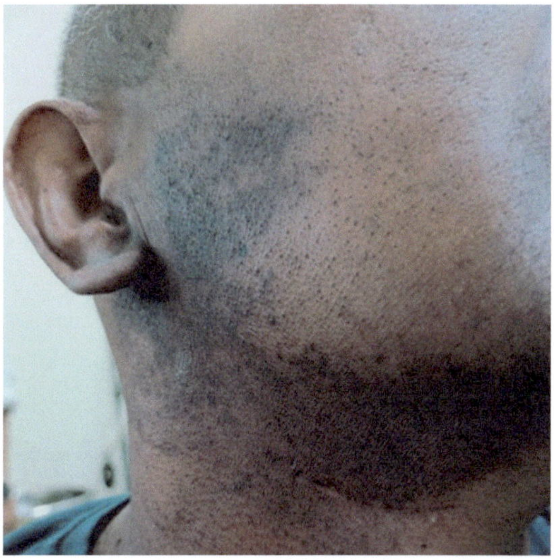

Fig. 13 Grade 1 acute dermatitis. (Courtesy: Dr Anusheel Munshi, Radiation Oncology, Manipal Hospital, Delhi)

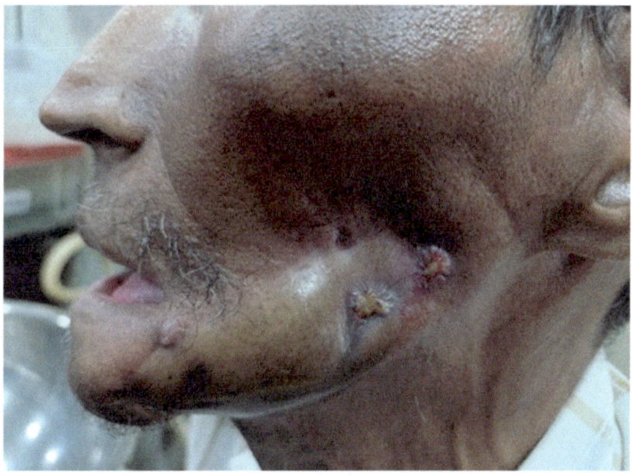

Fig. 14 Osteoradionecrosis of the mandible. (Courtesy: Dr Anusheel Munshi, Radiation Oncology, Manipal Hospital, Delhi)

18.3 Oropharyngeal Cancer

Oropharyngeal cancer (OPC) arises in soft palate, uvula, base of tongue, vallecular, tonsillar region and lateral pharyngeal wall and posterior oropharyngeal wall.

Oropharyngeal cancers can be caused by various factors, including human papillomavirus (HPV) infection. HPV-positive oropharyngeal cancer is more common in younger patients, nonsmokers and those with no or light alcohol consumption history. On the other hand, HPV-negative oropharyngeal cancers are more commonly associated with traditional risk factors such as tobacco and heavy alcohol use. They may be more aggressive and less responsive to treatment, resulting in poorer outcomes and prognosis. Table 13 gives the differences between HPV positive and HPV negative oropharyngeal cancers.

The AJCC, 8th edition, has divided staging of oropharyngeal cancers as per the HPV status of the tumour. Tables 14 and 15 give the T staging, and Tables 16, 17 and 18 gives the clinical and pathological nodal staging of HPV-negative and -positive oropharyngeal cancers, respectively. Tables 19 and 20 give the stage grouping of both groups.

Table 13 Differences between HPV-positive and HPV--negative oropharyngeal cancers

	HPV-positive	HPV-negative
Incidence	Increasing incidence	Decreasing incidence
Risk factors	Sexual behaviour Possible association with marijuana use	Tobacco, alcohol, poor oral hygiene
Sex ratio	Male predominance (≈3:1)	Male predominance (≈3:1)
Age	Younger age group	Older age group
Performance status	Better	Variable
Anatomical site	Tonsil, BOT	Multiple oropharyngeal subsites
Histology	Non-keratinising	Keratinising
Stage	T1–2 primary with advanced nodal disease	Variable stage at presentation
Treatment	Better tolerance & outcomes	Variable
Second primary malignancies	Lower risk	Higher risk
	Late recurrences	Usually within the first 2 years
	Isolated Lung, brain mets	DM usually with LRF

18.4 HPV-Negative Oropharyngeal Cancers

Table 14 Primary tumour (T)

TX	Primary tumour cannot be assessed
T0	No evidence of primary tumour
Tis	Carcinoma in situ
T1	Tumour ≤2 cm in greatest dimension
T2	Tumour >2 cm but not >4 cm in greatest dimension
T3	Tumour >4 cm in greatest dimension or extension to lingual surface of epiglottis
T4a	Moderately advanced local disease Tumour invades the larynx, deep/extrinsic muscle of the tongue, medial pterygoid, hard palate or mandible
T4b	Very advanced local disease Tumour invades the lateral pterygoid muscles, pterygoid plates, lateral nasopharynx, or skull base, or encases internal carotid artery

18.5 HPV-Positive Oropharyngeal Cancers

Table 15 Primary Tumor(T) staging for HPV +ve (Positive) oropharyngeal cancer

TX	Primary tumour cannot be assessed
T0	No evidence of primary tumour
Tis	Carcinoma in situ
T1	Tumour ≤2 cm in greatest dimension
T2	Tumour >2 cm but not >4 cm in greatest dimension
T3	Tumour >4 cm in greatest dimension or extension to lingual surface of epiglottis
T4	Moderately advanced local diseaseTumour invades the larynx, extrinsic muscle of the tongue, medial pterygoid, hard palate, mandible or beyond

Table 16 Nodal staging (HPV-negative oropharyngeal cancer)

NX	Regional lymph nodes cannot be assessed
N0	No regional lymph node metastasis
N1	Metastasis in a single ipsilateral lymph node, ≤3 cm in greatest dimension and ENE-negative
N2a	Metastasis in single ipsilateral or contralateral lymph node ≤3 cm in greatest dimension and ENE positive; or metastasis in single ipsilateral lymph node more than 3 cm but not more than 6 cm in greatest dimension and ENE-negative
N2b	Metastasis in multiple ipsilateral lymph nodes, none more than 6 cm in greatest dimension and ENE-negative
N2c	Metastasis in bilateral or contralateral lymph nodes, none more than 6 cm in greatest dimension and ENE-negative
N3a	Metastasis in a lymph node >6 cm in greatest dimension and ENE-negative
N3b	Metastasis in a single ipsilateral lymph node >3 cm in greatest dimension and ENE-positive; or metastasis in multiple ipsilateral, contralateral, or bilateral lymph nodes, with any ENE-positive

Table 17 Clinical nodal staging (HPV-positive oropharyngeal cancer)

NX	Regional lymph nodes cannot be assessed
N0	No regional lymph node metastasis
N1	One or more ipsilateral lymph nodes, none larger than 6 cm
N2	Contralateral or bilateral lymph nodes, none larger than 6 cm
N3	Lymph nodes larger than 6 cm

Table 18 Pathological nodal staging (HPV-positive oropharyngeal cancer)

NX	Regional lymph nodes cannot be assessed
N0	No regional lymph node metastasis
pN1	Metastasis in 4 or fewer lymph nodes
pN2	Metastasis in more than 4 lymph nodes

Table 19 Stage grouping for HPV-negative cancers

	T1	T2	T3	T4a	T4b
N0	I	II	III	IVA	IVB
N1	III	III	III	IVA	IVB
N2	IVA	IVA	IVA	IVA	IVB
N3	IVB	IVB	IVB	IVB	IVB

Table 20 Stage grouping for HPV-positive cancers (Note: Stage IV is only when distant metastasis)

	T1	T2	T3	T4
N0	I	II	II	III
N1	II	II	II	III
N2	II	II	II	III
N3	III	III	III	III

19 Diagnostic Workup

19.1 History and Physical Examination

The most common presentation of oropharyngeal cancer is painless neck swelling. Other symptoms include otalgia, dysphagia, odynophagia, restricted tongue mobility (involvement of extrinsic tongue muscles), trismus (medial pterygoid invasion) and a hot potato voice (oropharyngeal mass lesions). Referred otalgia occurs via the glossopharyngeal nerve (cranial nerve IX).

HPV-negative cancers are associated with tobacco use. Alcohol consumption has a synergistic effect with tobacco [69]. On the other hand, HPV-positive cancers can be associated with high-risk sexual behaviour, including multiple sexual partners [70]. Following an inspection, palpation of subsites like BOT is essential to understand the extent of involvement and infiltration of the anterior tongue. A dental exam, neurologic exam and indirect laryngoscopy are important.

Core biopsy of the primary lesion should include p16 IHC. The entire oral cavity and oropharynx should be inspected. The tongue should be assessed for bulk, and deviation on protrusion. Inability to protrude the tongue may indicate deep musculature involvement. The oral tongue should be palpated to assess submucosal involvement. Although difficult, palpation of the soft palate should be attempted. A local anaesthetic may be used due to tide over the difficulty due to gag reflex. Bilateral neck palpation from cranial to caudal extent (level I–V) including the parotid, preauricular region and the supraclavicular fossa is an important component of physical examination to detect lymphadenopathy. Speech and swallow evaluation should be done to assess the voice quality and severity of dysphagia.

Figure 15 shows the primary lesion of a patient with early oropharyngeal cancer.

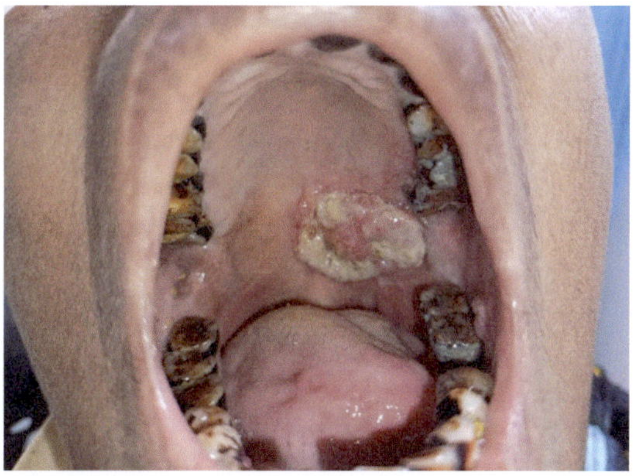

Fig. 15 Early lesion of the soft palate. (Courtesy: Dr Anusheel Munshi, Radiation Oncology, Manipal Hospital, Delhi)

19.2 Pathology

Over 90% of the oropharyngeal cancers are squamous cancers. Variants such as papillary SCC, spindle cell (sarcomatoid) SCC and others may occur. HPV-negative cancers are mostly well-to-moderately differentiated with keratinizing morphology, whereas HPV-positive cancers are more likely to be poorly differentiated with non-keratinizing or basaloid morphology [71]. Immunostaining for p16 is used as a surrogate marker for HPV-associated OPC, with a lower cost than other methods of detection. HPV DNA is detected by methods such as fluorescence in situ hybridization (FISH). Immunohistochemistry for p16 is more sensitive but less specific than HPV DNA–based testing. HPV viral oncoproteins E6 and E7 bind p53 and Rb, respectively, followed by loss of tumour suppression. Establishing the diagnosis for HPV-related OPC can also be challenging if the primary is very small with minimal mucosal changes. A superficial biopsy may miss a small viable tumour [72].

20 Treatment De-escalation in HPV-Positive Oropharyngeal Cancers [73]

In view of favourable outcomes for HPV positive oropharyngeal cancers, many treatment de-escalation approaches have been used in these tumours.

These include

1. *De-intensification of Systemic Therapy*

Compared with the standard cisplatin regimen, de intensification using cetuximab has not shown benefit in terms of reduced toxicity in such patients. Instead, such approaches have shown detriment in terms of tumour control. Cisplatin and radiotherapy should be used as the standard of care for HPV-positive low-risk patients who are able to tolerate cisplatin [74–77].

2. *De-intensification of Radiotherapy*

Researchers have tested reduced dose radiotherapy in such patients [78, 79]. Other approaches include reduced volume (unilateral RT, avoidance of RT to primary site after minimally invasive surgery) [80].

3. *De-intensification of Surgery/Adjuvant Therapy*

Surgical deintensification approaches have also been used in HPV-positive oropharyngeal cancer. Minimally invasive surgery like Trans Oral Robotic Surgery (TORS) has been proposed [81–83]. Other approaches include omission of adjuvant RT after surgery and omission of post-operative concurrent chemotherapy in patients being planned for RT

However, as of now, none of the de-escalation approaches have become standard of care.

21 Treatment Algorithm

Early-stage oropharyngeal cancers can be treated with surgery or radiation therapy. Lesions amenable to transoral resection are treated with this approach combined with neck dissection. Ideal cases include well-lateralized primaries with the minimal nodal burden (without extranodal extension) in medically fit patients with adequate mouth opening. Well-selected cases may be treated with surgery followed by adjuvant radiation as per surgical specimen risk factors. Minimally invasive transoral robotic surgery (TORS) for early T1, T2 is evolving as a safe practice when patient selection is done properly. Patients with locally advanced cancers are treated with definitive chemoradiation as surgery is associated with significant morbidity. The Fig. 16 shows the management of oropharyngeal cancers.

21.1 Radiation Therapy

RT is indicated for definitive treatment of OPC or in postoperative setting. In definitive setting, standard dose is 70 Gy/35 fractions/7 weeks or 66 Gy/30 fractions/6 weeks. Dose to the elective neck is typically 56 Gy in 35 fractions or 54 Gy in 30 fractions, respectively. Definitive radiation is administered with concurrent cisplatin, which

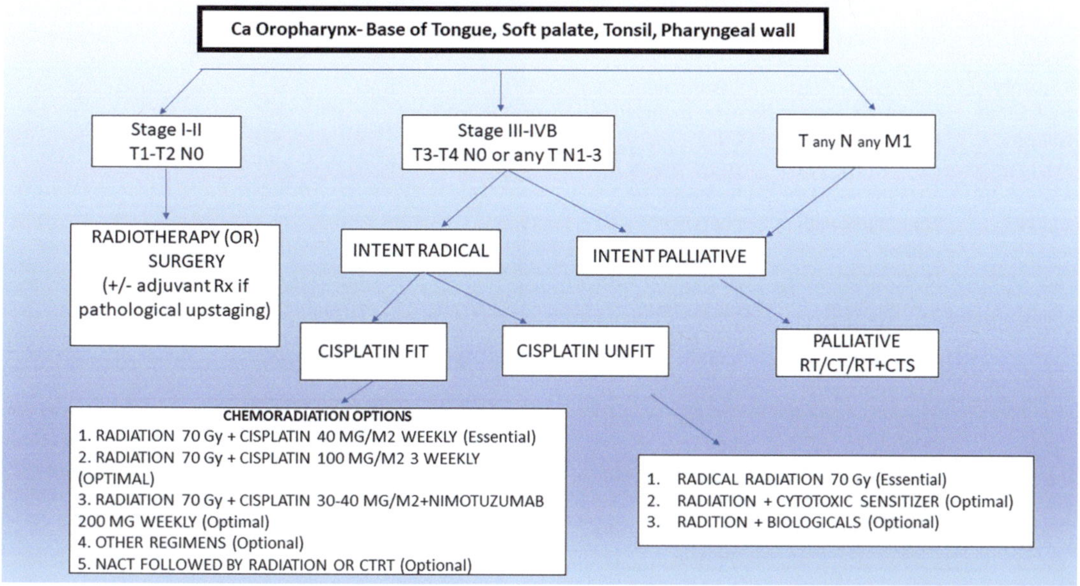

Fig. 16 Management of oropharyngeal cancers

may be administered 3 weekly (100 mg/m^2) or weekly (40 mg/m^2) [72]. Cisplatin ineligible patients can be treated with concurrent cetuximab (400 mg/m^2 loading dose 1 week before RT followed by 250 mg/m^2 weekly maintenance).

21.2 Radiotherapy Planning

Patients should be simulated in supine position with arms by the side using thermoplastic mask and neck extended. RT planning CT should be performed using slice thickness of 3 mm from vertex to carina. Dental evaluation should be done before starting radiotherapy. IMRT is the modality of choice for definitive radiation of oropharyngeal cancers [84]. Gross tumour volume (GTVp and GTVn) includes the disease noted during examination and radiology. A margin of 5 mm is generated around the GTV to create the CTV (HR-CTV or CTVP1). This volume is then edited from air, bone and other uninvolved structures. An additional CTV can be created which is another 10 mm expansion of GTVp (IR-CTV or CTVP2) [61]. Elective nodal irradiation is mostly recommended for levels II–IV bilaterally [85, 86]. Table 21 shows neck levels to be included in carcinoma oropharynx. In well lateralised early node negative tonsillar cancers, the contralateral elective neck radiation may be omitted in highly selective cases [87]. The PTV is generally a 3–5 mm isotropic expansion around the CTV as per institutional protocol.

21.3 Chemotherapy

Concurrent cisplatin is standard for eligible patients receiving definitive RT for stage III to IVB disease. Cisplatin dosage is 100 mg/m^2 every 3 weeks or 40 mg/m^2 weekly concurrent with RT. Cetuximab given concurrently with RT may be considered for cisplatin-ineligible candidates, however, it is associated with inferior outcomes without a meaningful reduction in overall toxicity compared to cisplatin in eligible patients. In patients planned for induction chemotherapy, the most common regimen consists of cisplatin, 5-FU, and docetaxel (TPF) every 3 weeks for 3 cycles [88, 89]. However in the Indian subcontinent, a sizable proportion of the patients with OPC will not be medically fit for TPF regimen

Table 21 It shows neck levels to be included in carcinoma oropharynx

Nodal Category (AJCC 8th edition)	Ipsilateral neck to be included in CTV	Contralateral neck to be included in CTV[a]
N0-1 (in level II, III and IV)	(Ib)[b], II, III, IVa, VIIa for posterior pharyngeal wall tumour	II, III, IVa, VIIa for posterior pharyngeal wall tumour
N2a-b	Ib, II, III, IVa, Va, b, VIIa, VIIb	II, III, IVa, VIIa for posterior pharyngeal wall tumour
N2c	According to N category on each side	According to N category on each side
N3	Ib, II, III, IVa, Va, b, VIIa, VIIb	II, III, IVa, VIIa for posterior pharyngeal wall tumour

[a]Unilateral treatment is recommended for N0-N2a tonsil fossa tumour not infiltrating the soft palate nor the base of tongue; and discussed for N2b patients
[b]Any tumour with extension to the oral cavity (e.g. retromolar trigone, mobile tongue, inferior gum, oral side of anterior tonsillar pillar) and/or in case of anterior involvement of level II

and the alternative induction regimens in this context is a doublet of cisplatin or carboplatin with 5-fluorouracil or paclitaxel.

21.4 Clinical Outcome

Treatment outcomes depend on various factors including intrinsic tumour biology, HPV status, subsite of the primary tumour, mode of treatment, age of the patient, performance status and comorbidities. In a retrospective analysis of 720 patients with stage III or IV OPSCC, enrolled in the RTOG 0129 trial, the authors classified patients as having a low, intermediate or high risk of death on the basis of four factors: HPV status, pack-years of tobacco smoking, tumour stage and nodal stage [4]. The HPV positivity rate was 63.8% in this study. These patients had better 3-year rates of OS (82.4%) compared to patients with HPV-negative tumours (57.1%, $P < 0.001$). In the IMRT era, there has been a significant improvement in locoregional tumour control with a simultaneous decrease in severe treatment related toxicities. In the largest study of IMRT for 776 patients with OPC from MDACC, the 5-year rates of OS and LRC were 84% and 90%, respectively [90].

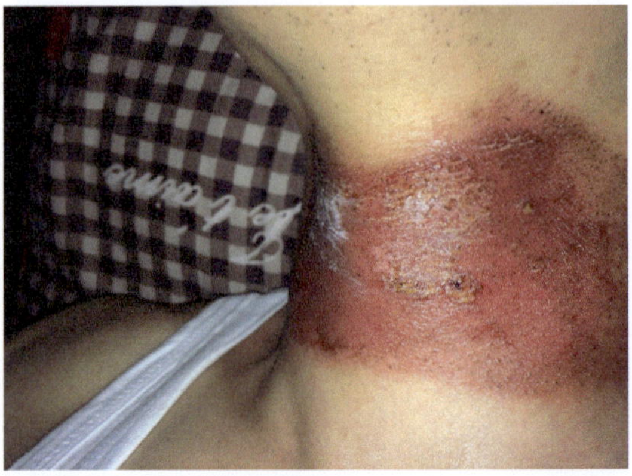

Fig. 17 Skin reactions in the neck region in a case of CA Glottis immediately after radiotherapy conclusion (Dose in this case was 55 Gy/20 fractions/4 weeks). (Courtesy: Dr Anusheel Munshi, Radiation Oncology, Manipal Hospital, Delhi)

21.5 Toxicities

Acute toxicities include skin reactions (dermatitis) (Fig. 17), mucositis, dysphagia, odynophagia and aspiration, xerostomia. Late toxicities include dysphagia, xerostomia, neck fibrosis, trismus, osteoradionecrosis and hypothyroidism

22 Laryngeal and Hypopharyngeal Cancers

22.1 Subsites of Larynx

The larynx is divided into three sites
Supraglottis:
- Epiglottis
- Aryepiglottic Folds
- Arytenoids
- False vocal cords
- Laryngeal Ventricle

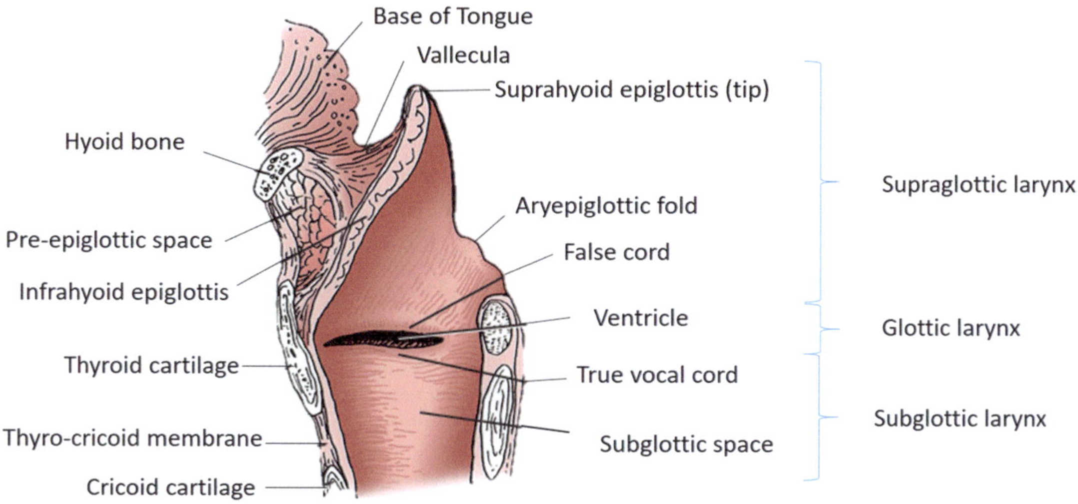

Fig. 18 Anatomy of Larynx

Glottis
- True vocal cords
- Anterior Commissure
- Inter-arytenoid area (Posterior Commissure)

Subglottis
- Region extending from the inferior border of the vocal cords to the lower border of the cricoid cartilage

Subsites of Hypopharynx (Fig. 18)
- Pyriform sinus
- Posterior pharyngeal wall
- Postcricoid region

22.2 Staging of Laryngeal Cancers

The T staging of supraglottic, glottic, subglottic and hypopharyngeal cancers are shown in Tables 22, 23, 24 and 25. The nodal staging is represented in Table 26 and stage grouping in Table 27.

23 Diagnostic Workup

23.1 History and Physical Examination

The history should include the smoking status, alcohol consumption and comorbidities. Patients with laryngeal and hypopharyngeal cancers have poor oral intake with weight loss and malnutrition. Dysphonia, dysphagia, dyspnoea or hemoptysis are the common presenting symptoms. Hoarseness is usually the first sign of glottic cancer. Symptoms depend on the size of the tumour, location and patient-related factors. Laryngopharyngeal cancers may also present as neck nodal mass. Patients may have referred ear pain or odynophagia due to vagus nerve involvement. Speech and swallow evaluation is vital to assess functionality of the larynx.

Physical examination should include a thorough head and neck examination with complete visualization of the oral cavity, oropharynx, larynx and hypopharynx. In addition, palpation of the neck should be performed to assess lymphadenopathy. Laryngoscopy is essential to assess the extent of the primary and for biopsy. Specific attention should be given to assess for vocal cord mobility, airway patency, and extent of tumour spread. Clinicians should note the relationship of lesions to specific subsites of the supraglottis, glottis and subglottis. Involvement of the aryepiglottic folds, postcricoid region, arytenoid processes, valleculae and subglottis are particularly important as they may guide treatment options and have impact on staging [91]. Further diagnostic workup in laryngeal lesions is guided by subsite involvement and extent of lesion spread.

Table 22 T staging for supraglottic cancers

TX	Primary tumour cannot be assessed
T0	No evidence of primary tumour
Tis	Carcinoma in situ
T1	Tumour limited to one subsite of the supraglottis with normal vocal fold mobility
T2	Tumour invades mucosa of more than one adjacent subsite of the supraglottis or glottis or region outside the supraglottis (e.g. mucosa of base of tongue, vallecula, medial wall of pyriform sinus) without fixation of the larynx
T3	Tumour limited to the larynx with vocal fold fixation and/or invades any of the following: postcricoid area, preepiglottic tissues, paraglottic space, and/or inner cortex of thyroid cartilage
T4a	Moderately advanced local disease. Tumour invades through the thyroid cartilage and/or invades tissues beyond the larynx (e.g. trachea, soft tissues of neck, including deep extrinsic muscle of the tongue, strap muscles, thyroid or oesophagus)
T4b	Very advanced local disease. Tumour invades prevertebral space, encases carotid artery or invades mediastinal structures

Table 23 T staging of glottic cancers

TX	Primary tumour cannot be assessed
T0	No evidence of primary tumour
Tis	Carcinoma in situ
T1	Tumour limited to the vocal fold(s) (may involve anterior posterior commissure) with normal mobility
T1a	Tumour limited to one vocal fold
T1b	Tumour involves both vocal folds
T2	Tumour extends to the supraglottis and/or subglottis, and/or with impaired vocal fold mobility
T3	Tumour limited to the larynx with vocal fold fixation and/or invasion of paraglottic space and/or inner cortex of the thyroid cartilage
T4a	Moderately advanced local disease. Tumour invades the outer cortex of the thyroid cartilage and/or invades tissues beyond the larynx (e.g. trachea, soft tissues of the neck, including deep extrinsic muscle of the tongue, strap muscles, thyroid or oesophagus)
T4b	Very advanced local disease. Tumour invades prevertebral space, encases carotid artery or invades mediastinal structures (Continued)

Table 24 T staging of subglottic cancers

TX	Primary tumour cannot be assessed
T0	No evidence of primary tumour
Tis	Carcinoma in situ
T1	Tumour limited to the subglottis
T2	Tumour extends to the vocal cord(s) with normal or impaired mobility
T3	Tumour limited to the larynx with vocal fold fixation
T4a	Moderately advanced local disease. Tumour invades cricoid or thyroid cartilage and/or invades tissues beyond the larynx (e.g. trachea, soft tissues of the neck including deep extrinsic muscles of the tongue, strap muscles, thyroid or oesophagus)
T4b	Very advanced local disease. Tumour invades prevertebral space, encases carotid artery or invades mediastinal structures

Table 25 T staging of hypopharyngeal cancers

TX	Primary tumour cannot be assessed
T0	No evidence of primary tumour
Tis	Carcinoma in situ
T1	Tumour limited to one subsite of the hypopharynx and ≤6.2 cm in greatest dimension
T2	Tumour invades more than one subsite of the hypopharynx or an adjacent site, or measures >2 cm but not >4 cm in greatest dimension without fixation of the hemilarynx or extension to the oesophagus
T3	Tumour >4 cm in greatest dimension or with fixation of the hemilarynx or extension to the oesophagus
T4a	Moderately advanced local disease. Tumour invades thyroid/cricoid cartilage, hyoid bone, thyroid gland, oesophagus, or central compartment soft tissue
T4b	Very advanced local disease. Tumour invades prevertebral fascia, encases carotid artery, or involves mediastinal structure

23.2 Imaging

Thin-cut computed tomography (CT) of the neck with contrast is the standard investigation of choice. It assesses extent of disease, preepiglottic

Table 26 Nodal staging of laryngeal and hypopharyngeal cancers

NX	Regional lymph nodes cannot be assessed
N0	No regional lymph node metastasis
N1	Metastasis in a single ipsilateral lymph node, ≤3 cm in greatest dimension
N2	Metastasis in a single ipsilateral lymph node >3 cm but not >6 cm in greatest dimension; or in multiple ipsilateral lymph nodes, none >6 cm in greatest dimension; or in bilateral or contralateral lymph nodes, none >6 cm in greatest dimension
N2a	Metastasis in a single ipsilateral lymph node >3 cm but not >6 cm in greatest dimension
N2b	Metastasis in multiple ipsilateral lymph nodes, none >6 cm in greatest dimension
N2c	Metastasis in bilateral or contralateral lymph nodes, none >6 cm in greatest dimension
N3	Metastasis in a lymph node >6 cm in greatest dimension

Table 27 Stage grouping of laryngeal and hypopharyngeal cancers

	T1	T2	T3	T4a	T4b
N0	I	II	III	IVA	IVB
N1	III	III	III	IVA	IVB
N2	IVA	IVA	IVA	IVA	IVB
N3	IVB	IVB	IVB	IVB	IVB

and paraglottic involvement, extralaryngeal spread, thyroid cartilage involvement, and lymphadenopathy. MRI is preferred for evaluation of soft tissue extent but susceptible to motion artefacts. Special attention should be given to involvement of the preepiglottic and paraglottic spaces, as well as that of the cricoid and thyroid cartilages. PETCT should be considered when there is heavy nodal burden and having a high suspicion of distant metastasis.

23.3 Treatment

Figures 19, 20, 21, 22, 23 and 24 give an overview of the overall management of laryngeal and hypopharyngeal cancers.

23.4 Treatment Algorithm

Key endpoints guiding treatment decisions in laryngeal cancers include local disease control, cause-specific survival and overall survival. Surgery and RT are equally effective options for disease control for early cancers. The standard of care for laryngeal cancers has evolved over the decades with the advent of organ preservation strategies [92]. Organ preservation should be attempted if the larynx is functional [93].

23.5 Surgery

Tumours not fit for organ conservation due to gross cartilage erosion or dysfunctional larynx are managed with a total laryngectomy. Total laryngectomy includes removal of the larynx and reconstruction of the pharynx. The downsides of total laryngectomy are loss of natural voice, alteration in deglutition and a permanent tracheostomy. It carries significant morbidity with deterioration of quality of life. For patients treated with a primary surgical approach, elective neck dissection of bilateral levels II to IV is warranted for most patients with locally advanced laryngeal cancers.

Voice-preserving options for supraglottic tumours are:

Supraglottic Laryngectomy (SGL): Swallow- and voice-preserving surgery may be used for tumours of the epiglottis, single arytenoid, ary-epiglottic fold, or false cord. Hyoid bone, epiglottis, superior half of thyroid cartilage, AE folds and false cords to arytenoids are resected.
Supracricoid partial laryngectomy-cricohyoidoepiglottopexy (SCPL–CHEP): Entails resection of both true and false cords, paraglottic space, preepiglottic space, epiglottis and thyroid cartilage. Reconstruction includes suturing of cricoid to hyoid, cricohyoidopexy.

In glottic cancers, modern surgical techniques like endoscopic resection are often used. Endoscopic procedures include mucosal stripping, and CO2 laser (Transoral Laser Microsurgery). Voice preserving options like

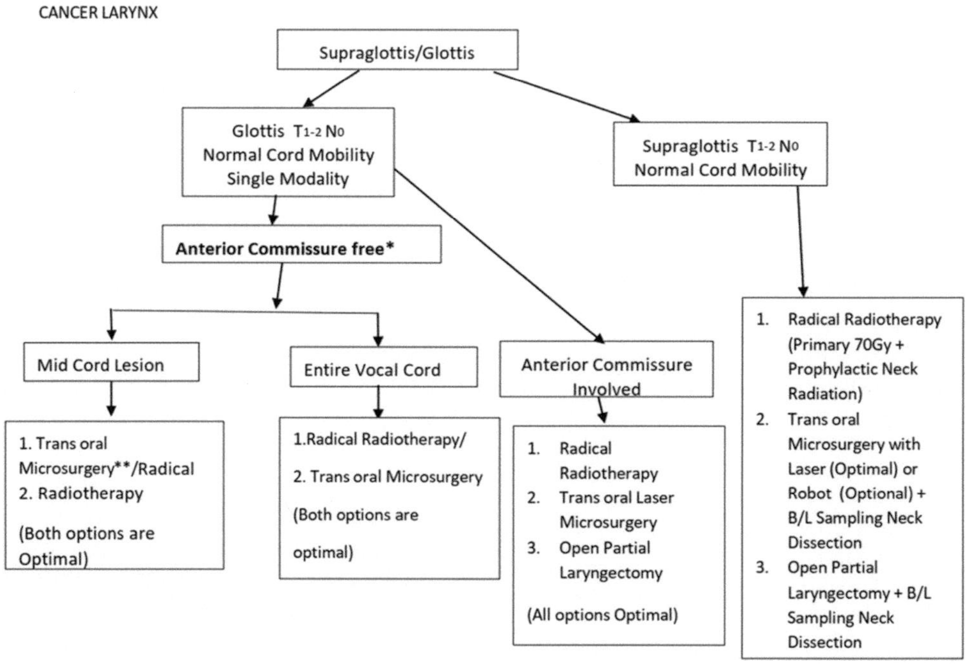

Fig. 19 Management of early supraglottic/glottic cancers

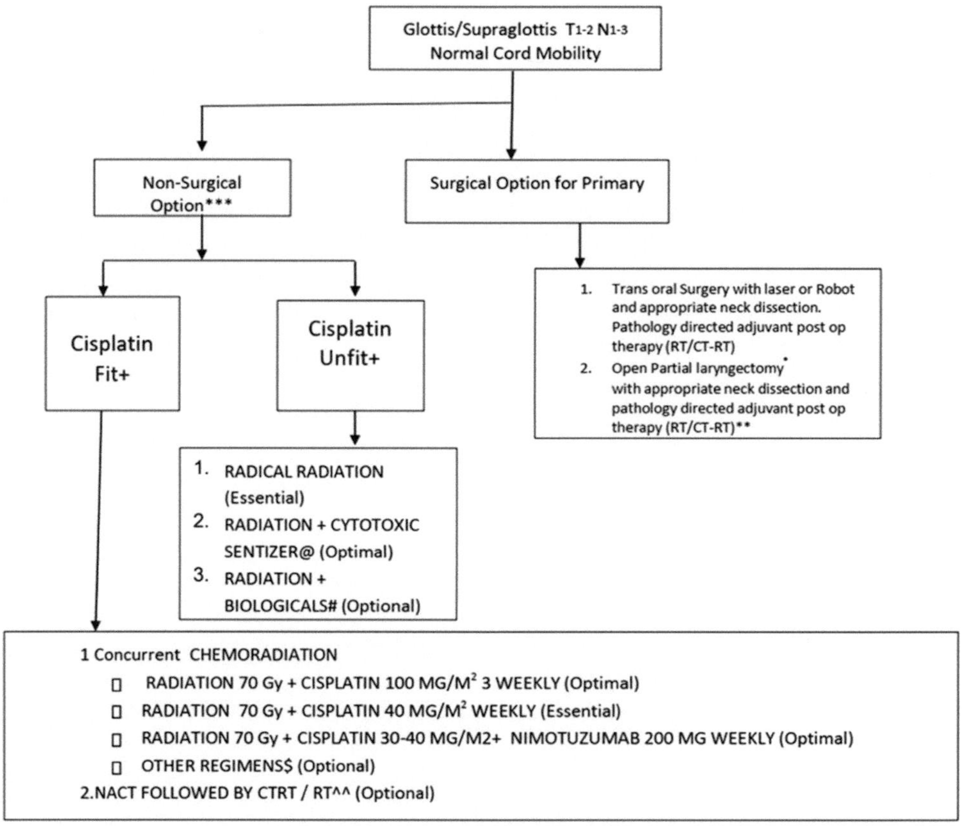

Fig. 20 Management of early laryngeal cancers with advanced nodal disease

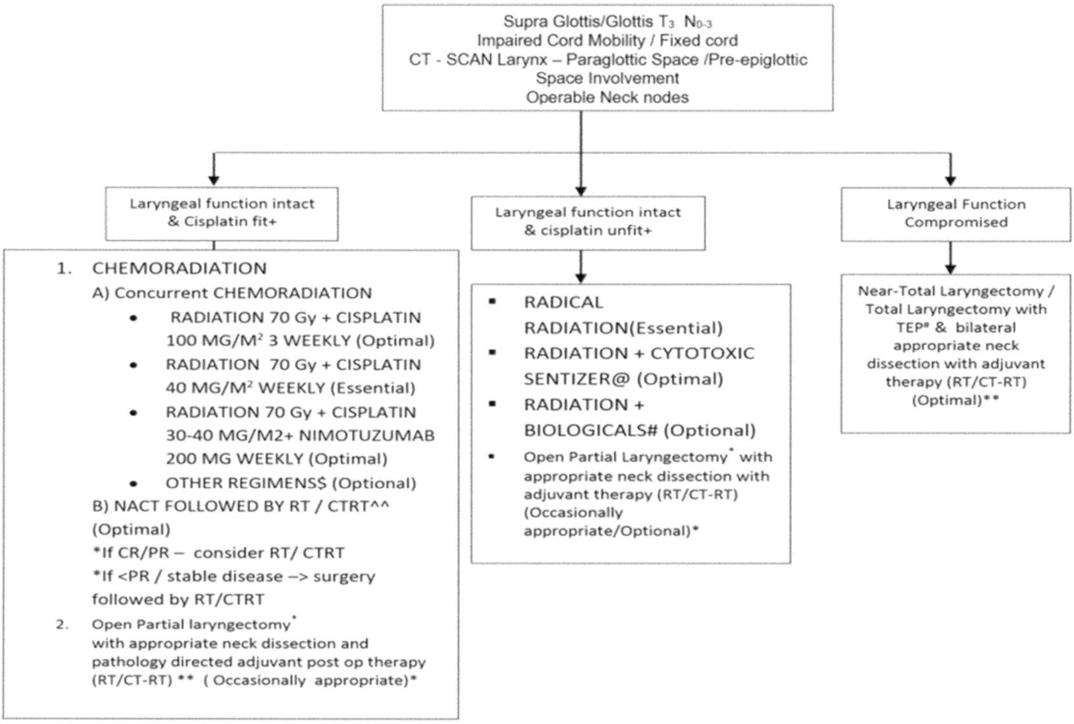

Fig. 21 Management of locally advanced laryngeal cancers

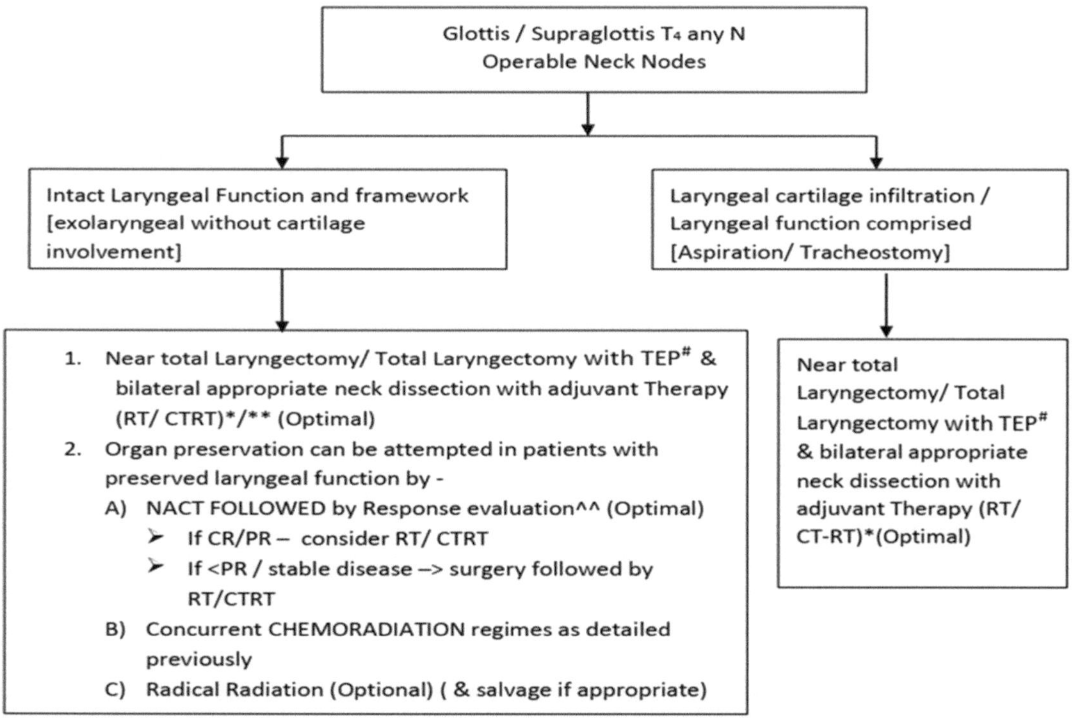

Fig. 22 Management of locally advanced laryngeal cancer with operable neck nodes

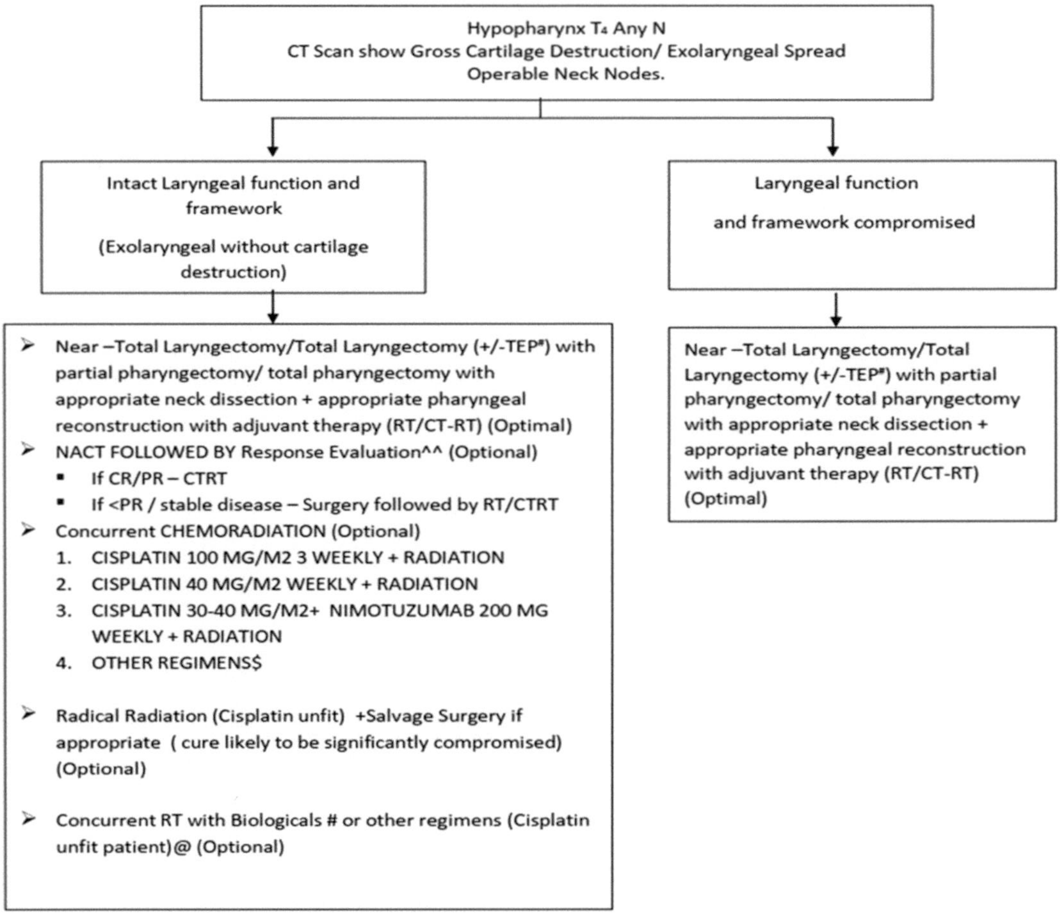

Fig. 23 Management of locally advanced hypopharyngeal cancer with operable neck node

Vertical hemilaryngectomy and SCPL–CHEP are also practised.

23.6 Radiation Therapy

Early-stage laryngeal cancers are typically treated with RT alone. Nodal basins are typically not electively included in RT volumes in early stage glottic cancers unless supraglottic involvement is suspected, making the risk of occult nodal metastasis higher. For T1N0 glottic cancers, accelerated hypofractionation has been shown to improve local control compared to standard fractionation. Hence, the recommended dose is 62.5 Gy/25 fractions (2.25 Gy/fx) or 55 Gy in 20 fractions over 4 weeks [94]. Tables 28 and 29 show neck nodes to be included in laryngeal and hypopharyngeal tumours.

23.7 EBRT Planning

Patients should be simulated in supine position with arms by the side using thermoplastic mask and neck slightly hyperextended. Bolus may be used for early glottis cancer and in case of involvement of anterior commissure. RT planning CT should be performed using slice thickness of 3 mm from vertex to carina, for early glottis tumours 1mm slice thickness is preferred. Dental evaluation should be done before starting radiotherapy

Larynx preservation strategies are utilised for locally advanced disease based on organ func-

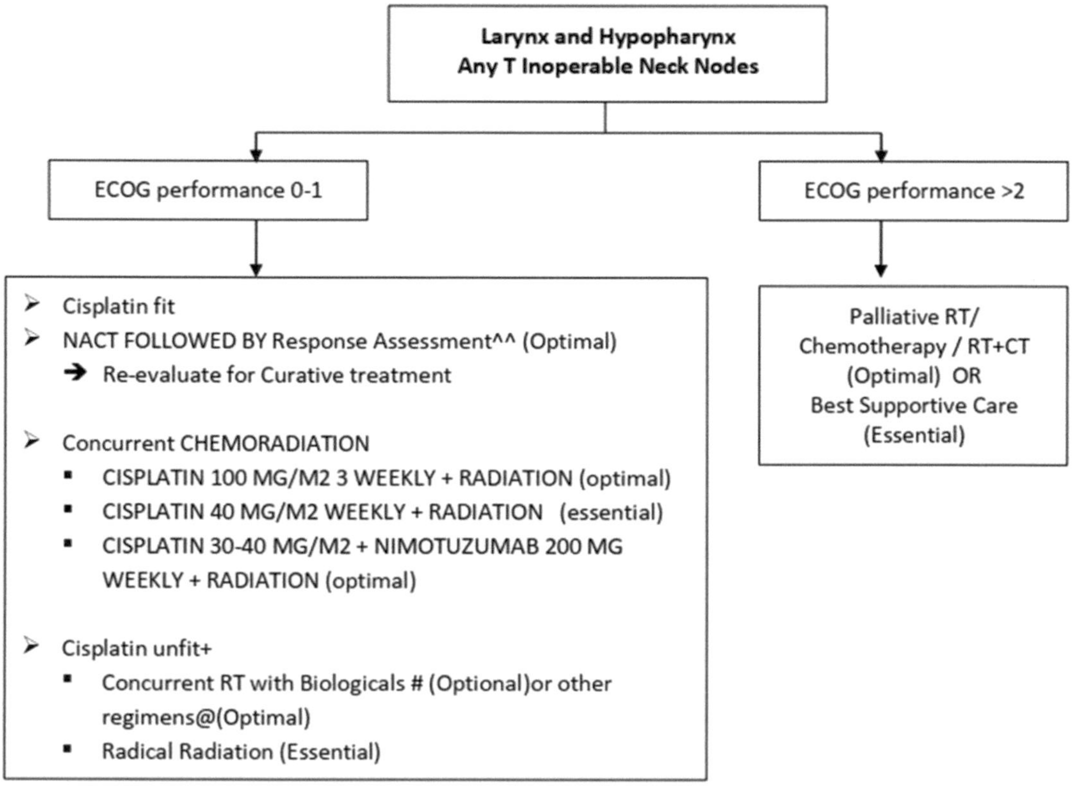

Fig. 24 Management of laryngeal and hypopharyngeal cancer with inoperable neck node

tion. Tables 28, 29, 30 and 31 show target and nodal delineation in carcinoma larynx and hypopharynx. Bilateral neck nodal irradiation is also warranted as per the extent of the primary tumour and involvement of lymph nodes. Radical doses of 70 Gy/35 fractions with concurrent chemotherapy are practised. Elective nodal irradiation is administered to an equivalent dose of 56 Gy/35 fractions [95].

23.8 Chemotherapy

Concurrent chemotherapy is not routinely given for an early-stage disease. In locally advanced disease, concurrent cisplatin is the standard of care, given as three weekly doses of 100 mg/m^2 or 40 mg/m^2 weekly. Cetuximab can be used for non-platinum candidates, with a loading dose of 400 mg/m^2 1 week before RT followed by 250 mg/m^2 weekly during RT. Induction chemotherapy is utilised for select patients with a bulky primary disease with exolaryngeal spread without gross cartilage erosion [96–98]. Three drug regimen of docetaxel, cisplatin, and 5-fluorouracil (TPF) every 3 weeks is preferred for induction [88, 89].

23.9 Toxicity

Acute toxicities include radiation dermatitis, dysphagia, mucositis, hoarseness, xerostomia, odynophagia and aspiration.

Late toxicities include dysphagia, oesophageal stricture, aspiration, hoarseness, hearing loss, renal insufficiency, neck fibrosis and hypothyroidism.

Table 28 Target volumes for radical and adjuvant radiotherapy for laryngeal tumours

Intent	Target volumes	Definition and description
Early glottis laryngeal tumour	GTV	Gross disease
	CTV	Entire larynx or involved hemilarynx, including the anterior commissure and arytenoid region, as per institutional practice.
	PTV	CTV with appropriate margins as per institutional protocol, accounting for setup uncertainty and organ motion (typically 3–5 mm).
For advanced tumours		
Radical	GTV	Primary disease and gross nodes
	CTV	GTV with an appropriate margin to encompass the involved hypopharyngeal subsite and adjacent high-risk mucosal and submucosal regions, including laryngeal extension if present.
	PTV	As per institutional protocol
Adjuvant	CTV 66(if needed)	Post-operative bed + positive margin/ECE
	CTV 60	Post-operative bed + stoma + involved nodes
	CTV 54	Elective nodal station

Table 29 Target volumes for radical radiotherapy for hypopharyngeal tumours

Target volumes	Definition and description
GTV	Gross disease and nodes
CTV high	GTV + 1 cm margin, to include entire hypopharynx and larynx and involved nodal station
CTV low	Elective nodal station
PTV	As per institutional protocol

Table 30 Selection of neck nodal levels for hypopharyngeal tumours

Nodal category (AJCC 8th edition)	Ipsilateral neck levels to be included	Contralateral neck levels to be included[a]
N0	II, III, IVa, VIIa for posterior pharyngeal wall tumours, VI for apex pyriform sinus, post cricoid and/or pharyngeal extension	II, III, IVa, VIIa for posterior pharyngeal wall tumour, VI for oesophageal extension
N1, N2a-b	Ib, II, III, IVa, Va, b, VIIa, VIIb, VI for apex pyriform sinus, post cricoid and/or pharyngeal extension, and/or possibly N2b	II, III, IVa, VIIa for posterior pharyngeal wall tumour, VI for oesophageal extension
N2c	According to N category on each side	According to N category on each side
N3	Ib, II, III, IVa, Va, b, VIIa, VIIb, VI	II, III, IVa, VIIa for posterior pharyngeal wall tumour, VI for oesophageal extension

[a]Unilateral neck treatment for small tumour of the lateral wall of pyriform sinus

Level IIb can be omitted if no cervical lymph nodes involvement on the same side

Level IVb should be included in case of involvement of level IVa

Level VIIb should be included in case of bulky involvement of the upper part of level II

24 Nasopharyngeal Cancers

24.1 Anatomy

The nasopharynx is a cuboidal chamber located behind the nasal cavity with the following boundaries:

Anteriorly: Communicates with nasal cavities via posterior choanae.

Inferiorly: Communicates with the oropharynx at the soft palate

Lateral walls: Openings of the eustachian tube, torus tubarius, pharyngeal recess

Roof: Formed by the basilar portions of the sphenoid, basiocciput and the anterior arch of atlas vertebra.

Posterior wall: Superior pharyngeal constrictor muscle, pharyngo-basilar fascia and buccopharyngeal fascia.

24.2 Staging of Nasopharyngeal Cancers

Tables 32 and 33 represent the T and N staging of nasopharyngeal cancers with Table 34 showing the various stage groups

Table 31 Selection of neck nodal levels for laryngeal tumours

Nodal category (AJCC 8th edition)	Ipsilateral neck levels to be included	Contralateral neck levels to be included
N0-1	II, III, IVa, VI for transglottic or subglottic extension	II, III, IVa, VI for transglottic or subglottic extension
N2a-b	II, III, IVa, Va, b, VI for transglottic or subglottic extension	II, III, IVa, VI for transglottic or subglottic extension
N2c	According to N category on each side	According to N category on each side
N3	Ib, II, III, IVa, Va, b, VIIb, VI	II, III, IVa, VI for transglottic or subglottic extension

Level IIb could be omitted if no cervical lymph nodes involvement on the same side

Level Ib should be included in case of anterior involvement of level II

Level IVb should be included in case of involvement of level IVa

Level VIIb should be included in case of bulky involvement of upper part of level II

Table 32 Primary T staging (AJCC 8th edition)

TX	Primary tumour cannot be assessed
T0	No evidence of primary tumour
T1	Tumour confined to the nasopharynx or tumour extends to the oropharynx and/or nasal cavity without parapharyngeal extension
T2	Tumour with parapharyngeal extension, adjacent soft tissue involvement (medial pterygoid, lateral pterygoid, prevertebral muscles)
T3	Tumour involves bony structures of skull base and/or paranasal sinuses
T4	Tumour with intracranial extension and/or involvement of cranial nerves, hypopharynx, orbit or with extensive soft tissue involvement (beyond the lateral surface of the lateral pterygoid muscle, parotid gland)

Etiologic factors can be genetic, viral, environmental, salted fish intake and nitrosamines.

Table 33 Neck nodal staging (AJCC 8th edition)

NX	Regional lymph nodes cannot be assessed
N0	No regional lymph node metastasis
N1	Unilateral metastasis in cervical lymph node(s), ≤6 cm in greatest dimension, above caudal border of cricoid cartilage, and/or unilateral or bilateral retropharyngeal lymph nodes, ≤6 cm in greatest dimension
N2	Bilateral metastasis in cervical lymph node(s), ≤6 cm in greatest dimension, above the caudal border of cricoid cartilages
N3	Metastasis in lymph nodes >6 cm and/or to below the caudal border of cricoid cartilage

24.3 Screening

There are no established screening protocols for nasopharyngeal carcinoma. Some screening methods have been studied in endemic areas. These include IgA to EBV viral capsid antigen and circulating plasma EBV DNA [22].

24.4 History and Physical Examination

Nasopharyngeal cancers are endemic and non-endemic. These tumours have a bimodal age distribution (15–25 years and 50–59 years). Presentation at advanced stages due to paucity of symptoms. There is a high predilection for nodal and distant metastasis.

The most common presentation is a painless neck mass. Other common symptoms are epistaxis, headache, diplopia, or facial numbness. Diplopia occurs due to local invasion, with CN VI often compressed first. Jacod's triad of vision loss, ophthalmoplegia and trigeminal neuralgia results from cavernous sinus invasion. Dysphagia, hoarseness, Horner's syndrome, and CN XI deficits can occur from lateral RPN compression on CNs IX to XII or from invasion into the jugular foramen.

Table 34 Stage grouping of nasopharyngeal cancers

	T1	T2	T3	T4	M1
N0	I	II	III	IVA	IVB
N1	II	II	III	IVA	IVB
N2	III	III	III	IVA	IVB
N3	IVA	IVA	IVA	IVA	IVB

24.5 Patterns of Spread

Besides local infiltration into adjacent areas, including bone, nasopharygeal cancer is known for lymph node metastasis. Lymphatic spread happens though three specific routes of lymphatic drainage. (1) The retropharyngeal nodes (2) Jugulodigastric nodes (Level II) (3) Deep posterior cervical nodes (Level V) to other cervical nodal regions. Hematogenous Dissemination can happen at presentation can happen in 3% to 6% of the cases and during the disease course in 18% to 50% of cases. The rate of distant metastasis is highest in patients with advanced neck node metastasis, especially with low-neck involvement. The distant metastatis are most common in bone (bone > lungs > liver).

25 Pathology

25.1 WHO Classification

- Type 1 (I)—Keratinizing Squamous Cell Carcinoma
- Type 2a (II)—Non-Keratinizing Differentiated Carcinoma
- Type 2b (III)—Non-Keratinizing Undifferentiated Carcinoma—Favourable Prognosis
- Basaloid squamous carcinoma—Very rare, poor survival (10% 5 years survival)

Plasma EBV DNA titres have overall prognostic significance in nasopharyngeal cancers.

26 Staging Workup

Staging workup for nasopharyngeal cancer includes endoscopic examination and biopsy. Blood investigations including complete blood counts, renal, liver function tests, and viral markers should be done. Urine pregnancy test needs to be done for women of reproductive age. Other investigations include MRI face, PNS and Neck, PETCECT and Plasma EBV titres (Baseline and response assessment). Finally, it is also advisable to do dental prophylaxis, audiometry and visual examination, endocrine evaluation and nutritional counselling.

26.1 Imaging

In nasopharyngeal cancers, imaging is done prior to induction chemotherapy and for response. *MRI* is essential to assess the local extent of the disease and PETCECT for nodal assessment and to rule out any distant metastasis. MRI has better soft tissue contrast for muscles, nerves and parapharyngeal fat pad.

Disadvantages of *CT* include difficulty in demarcate the tumour, as nasopharyngeal tumours (unlike other H&N tumours) do not show contrast enhancement. Further CT cannot differentiate hyperplastic lymphoid tissue obliterating the pharyngeal recess. CT scan is useful for RT simulation planning.

PETCT is emerging as a preferred tool for assessing local as well as distant disease, especially for T3–4 or node-positive patients.

Table 35 Overview of management of nasopharyngeal cancers

T1N0M0	T2N0M0	T1-T2N1M0, T3-T4N0/N+ M0	Oligometastatic M1 disease	Widely metastatic disease
Definitive RT to nasopharynx and elective RT to the neck	Definitive RT +/- concurrent systemic therapy	3 cycles of NACT f/b CTRT	Systemic therapy f/b CTRT based on response	Good PS: Systemic therapy, RT if CR/near CR Poor PS: Best supportive care

26.2 Treatment Algorithm (NCCN 2022)

Table 35 shows a broad overview of the management of nasopharyngeal cancers

27 Treatment Modalities

27.1 Surgery

There is no role in upfront setting. Surgery can be used as a salvage option in select patients. Persistent nodal disease after primary therapy or nodal recurrence may be treated with neck dissection.

27.2 Radiation

Patients should be simulated in supine position with arms by the side using thermoplastic mask and neck extended. RT planning CT should be performed using slice thickness of 3 mm from vertex to carina. Dental evaluation should be done before starting radiotherapy.

T1N0M0 tumours are generally treated with RT alone. T2N0M0 tumours are treated with concurrent CTRT. Stage III to stage IV tumours are treated with induction chemotherapy followed by concurrent chemoradiation.

27.3 Doses for RT

- High Risk: 70 Gy/35 #@ 2 Gy/# (69.96 Gy/33# @2.12 Gy/# is an accepted alternative)
- Intermediate Risk: 63 Gy/35 # @1.8 Gy/# (60 Gy/33# @ 1.82 Gy/# is an acceptable alternative)
- Low Risk: 56 Gy/35 # @1.6 Gy/fraction (54 Gy/33# @ 1.64 Gy/# is an acceptable alternative)

IG-IMRT Technique should be practised for all patients [99].

28 EBRT Planning

28.1 Risk Volumes (Primary) [100]

The primary volumes are contoured as per the international guideline for the delineation of the clinical target volumes for nasopharyngeal carcinoma published in 2017. Table 36 gives the high and intermediate risk volumes for primary target delineation.

29 Risk Volumes

29.1 Risk Volumes (Nodal)

High Risk: GTV-N + 5–10 mm margin.

Intermediate Risk: All cases: bilateral retropharyngeal, levels II, III and Va.

Cervical node positive cases: One level below involved level(s) ± level IB. Table shows neck nodes to be included. Selection of nodal target volumes for nasopharyngeal cancers is shown in Table 37.

29.2 Organs at Risk

The nasopharynx is situated close to various critical structures in the skull base. Hence, it is important to carefully delineate the OARs and achieve constraints to reduce toxicities. Some of the important OARs and their dose constraints are given in Table 38.

Table 36 High and intermediate risk volume for nasopharyngeal cancers

HIGH DOSE CLINICAL TARGET VOLUME (CTVP1)	
Margin from GTVp	GTVp + 5 mm (±whole NP)
Minimal margin if tumour in close proximity to critical OARs	GTVp + 1 mm
INTERMEDIATE DOSE CLINICAL TARGET VOLUME (CTVP2)	
Nasal cavity—Posterior Part	At least 5 mm from choana
Maxillary sinuses—Posterior part	At least 5 mm from posterior wall
Posterior ethmoid sinus	Include vomer
Skull base	Cover foramina ovale, rotundum, lacerum & petrous tip
Cavernous sinus	If T3–4 (involved side only)
Pterygoid fossa, Parapharyngeal spaces	+
Sphenoid Sinus	Inferior 1/2 if T1–2; whole if T3–4
Clivus	1/3 if no invasion; whole if invasion
Minimal margin if tumour in close proximity to critical OARs	2 mm

Table 37 Selection of nodal target volumes for nasopharyngeal cancers

Nodal category (AJCC 8th edition)	Ipsilateral neck levels to be included	Contralateral neck levels to be included
N0	II–V, VIIa, VIIb	II–V, VIIa, VIIb
N1,2	II–V, VIIa, VIIb	II–V, VIIa, VIIb
N3	II–IVb, Va, b, c, VIIa, VIIb	II–IVb, Va, b, c, VIIa, VIIb

Levels IV and Vb could be omitted for patients with no cervical lymph nodes involvement on the same side

Level Ib in case of disease involvement of the submandibular gland, and/or involvement of structures that drain to level Ib as the first echelon site, and/or level II involvement (adenopathy >2 cm and/or with extra-nodal extension suspicion)

Level IVb in case of levels III–IVa involvement

Level Vc in case of level Va, b involvement

Table 38 The various OARs with constraints based on the priorities 1 and 2 parameters

Priority 1 Parameters	
Brain stem	DMax ≤54 Gy
Spinal cord	DMax ≤45 Gy
Optic chiasm	DMax ≤54 Gy
B/L optic nerves	DMax ≤54 Gy
GTVp & GTVn	100% of GTV ≥95% of prescription dose
High-dose PTV—minimum dose	95% of PTV ≥ 95% of prescription dose
Priority 2 Parameters	
High-dose PTV—maximum dose	<107% outside PTV
Intermediate-dose PTV—minimum dose	95% of PTV ≥95% of prescription dose
Temporal lobe	1cc volume <65 Gy

29.3 Chemotherapy

Induction chemotherapy reduces tumour load of loco-regional disease before start of RT and early use of chemotherapy can eradicate micrometastases. Induction chemotherapy consists of 3 weekly cisplatin (80 mg/m^2 day 1) and gemcitabine (1 g/m^2 days 1 and 8); other induction regimens include TPF (docetaxel, cisplatin, and 5-FU) and cisplatin with 5-FU [101–104]. Cisplatin is given concurrently with RT as 100 mg/m^2 bolus at weeks 1, 4 and 7 or 40 mg/m^2 weekly.

29.4 Toxicity

Acute toxicities include dermatitis, mucositis, xerostomia, dysphagia, odynophagia, nausea and weight loss. Late toxicities include hearing loss, dental caries, trismus, brainstem necrosis, optic neuritis, endocrinopath and cranial nerve palsies.

29.5 Outcomes

Based on SEER data, the 5-year survival rate is 81% for localized, 73% for regional and 48% for distant metastatic disease.

30 Nasal Cavity and Paranasal Sinuses (PNS): Sino-Nasal Cancers

30.1 PNS Anatomy

The anterior group of PNS includes anterior ethmoid, maxillary and frontal sinuses. The posterior group includes sphenoid and posterior ethmoid sinuses.

30.2 History and Physical Examination

It is well known that sino-nasal cancers are heterogenous in tumor origin and natural history of disease spread. A diagnostic nasal endoscopy and oral cavity examination is an important initial investigation. In view of the location of disease, ophthalmic and cranial nerves examination is also important. Most patients present with nasal obstruction, epistaxis, proptosis, headache and visual impairment (Fig. 25).

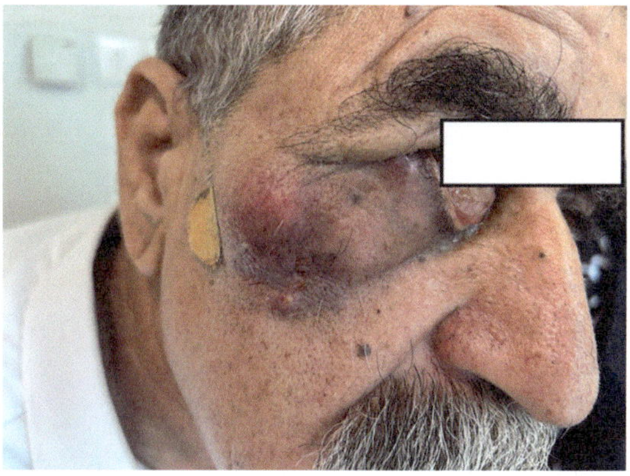

Fig. 25 A case of Ca Maxilla with involvement of the orbit (causing conjuvtival chemosis) along with infratemporal fossa involvement. (Courtesy: Dr Anusheel Munshi, Radiation Oncology, Manipal Hospital, Delhi)

30.3 Imaging

Contrast enhanced CT scan with bone algorithm with thin section reformatting in coronal and sagittal plane is important. The scan should assess involvement of orbit, pterygopalatine fossa, infratemporal fossa, skull base and nodal involvement. MRI provides better delineation of intracranial involvement, differentiate inflammatory changes from tumour, and assess perineural spread. PETCT can be considered to rule out distant metastasis: in advanced stages, high grade malignancies, multiple low-level neck nodes, and in response evaluation.

30.4 Pathology

These cancers can arise from epithelial, glandular, neural, skeletal or lymphoid tissues resulting in a spectrum of histopathological diagnosis. WHO- 44 gives an exhaustive malignant histologies involving the paranasal sinuses. Table 39 mentions some of the salient differences with various histologies of paranasal tumours.

30.5 Treatment of the Neck

For negative nodes, the option of observation of neck versus ENI is Controversial. Suggested Indications for ENI include T3-T4-Maxillary sinus and nasal cavity SCC, SNUC Histology and Kadish stage C and/or Hyams grade III/IV esthesioneuroblastoma (levels II–III, VIIa)

For positive nodes N+, U/L neck irradiation should be considered if not crossing mid-line & without C/L neck involvement. Consider Level IV B—if level IVa is involved. Also, we can consider Level VIIB irradiation if Bulky level II nodes are present.

30.6 Surgery

Surgery is the treatment of choice for almost all sinonasal malignancies. The goal of surgery is to achieve en bloc resection of all involved bone and soft tissue with clear margins while maximizing the cosmetic and functional outcome.

Surgical approaches for early-stage disease include midfacial degloving, lateral rhinotomy,

Table 39 Important histologies of paranasal sinus tumours

	Squamous cell carcinoma	Adenocarcinoma	Adenoidcystic carcinoma
How common?	MC-60–80%	10–20%	6–18%
Site predilection	Maxillary	Ethmoid	Maxillary
Subtypes	MDSCC/ PDSCC-nonkeratinizing-sinuses WDSCC-keratinising-nasal cavity	Intestinal type(ITAC)-MC Non-intestinal type	Type of Salivary gland type carcinomas (which include Adenoid cystic/ Mucoepidermoid/Acinic cell etc.)
Presentation and loco regional extent	85%-present as T3/T4 N+ at presentation-10–15%	Majority present as T3/T4 LN- uncommon	Slow growth, locally aggressive LN-uncommon Neurotropism—PNI/V2/V3/Vidian nerve involvement
Distant metastasis	Uncommon	Uncommon	Delayed recurrences esp Distant Mets over time (vs SCC—faster growth)—requires long f/u, MC-Lung
Outcomes	5y OS-60–64%	5y OS-70%	5y OS-35%, 10y OS-10%

	Neuroendocrine tumours	
	SNUC, NEC and small cell carcinoma	Esthesioneuroblastoma (Olfactory neuroblastoma)
How common?	Rare	<5%
Presentation and loco regional extent	Aggressive, extensive local tissue infiltration 80–90% present as T4 50% with orbital/skull base involvement N+-10–30%	Arises from cribriform plate Neuroectodermal derivation from olfactory epithelium Bimodal age distribution (11–20 years, 51–60 years) N+ lt;5%
Distant metastasis	M+ - 25–30% (Lungs/bone)	Uncommon
Outcomes	SNUC-5y OS- 43–60% (with CTRT), 20% (with surgery) SNEC- 5y OS <30%	5y OS- 60–80%

endoscopic transnasal approach and medial maxillectomy with ethmoidal clearance.

Surgical approaches for late-stage disease include total maxillectomy with ethmoidectomy, combined craniofacial approach for lesions reaching/involving the cribriform plate and orbital exenteration if eye is involved.

Unresectable tumours include those tumours with gross infiltration of infratemporal fossa, Pterygoplatine fissure involvement, involvement of dura and intra-cerebral extension of squamous carcinoma, cavernous sinus involvement, involvement of sphenoid, extensive soft tissue and skin infiltration and bilateral orbital involvement

30.7 Radiation Therapy

Indications of radical radiation therapy includes:

- Unresectable tumours (T4b and some T4a)
- Absolute: Involvement of cavernous sinus, internal carotid artery, bilateral orbit and extensive cerebral involvement
- Relative: Gross infiltration of ITF, pterygopalatine fissure involvement, extensive soft tissue and skin infiltration

Indications for adjuvant RT indications includes those with T3–T4 tumours, presence of PNI/LVE, Positive lymph nodes in pathology, adenoid cystic histology, involvement of adjacent structures like dura and brain.

Adjuvant CT-RT is reserved for positive margins and ENE.

30.8 EBRT Planning

Patients should be simulated in supine position with arms by the side using thermoplastic mask and neck extended. RT planning CT should be performed using slice thickness of 3 mm from vertex to carina (Fig. 26).

Target Volume Delineation

Target volume delineation for gross disease, CTV high and low is enlisted in Table 40, neck nodal levels are enlisted in Table 41.

30.9 Chemotherapy

NACT can be considered for Borderline resectable/technically unresectable tumours. These include tumours with Pterygoid plate involvement, ITF involvement and involvement of orbit reaching up to anterior cranial fossa. Typical regimens include two cycles of chemotherapy with platinum + taxane or platinum + taxane + 5FU for SCC. For SNEC/high-grade esthesioneuroblastoma/SNUC with neuroendocrine-2# Platinum + etoposide.

30.10 Follow-Up

Proper follow-up of these tumours is important. Besides clinical examination, one can consider fibreoptic nasoendoscopy and Imaging at follow up.

Post Adjuvant treatment, a Baseline post-treatment-(MRI preferred) scan is done 2–3 months after completion of treatment. Post Definitive treatment, a FDG PET-CT is done at 10 weeks (± MRI if suspicious findings). Follow-up imaging with MRI recommended annually for at least 2 years, thereafter when symptomatic.

Other tests include thyroid function test every 6 months if neck has been irradiated, dental evaluation, nutritional evaluation, ophthalmological and ENT evaluation as required and endocrine evaluation as required.

Follow up schedule counselled to the patient would be every 3 months for 2 years, 6 months until 5 years and yearly thereafter.

30.11 Esthesioneuroblastoma

Esthesioneuroblastoma is also known as olfactory neuroblastoma/esthesioneurocytoma

The site of origin is the olfactory region and these tumours have a neural crest origin. There is a unique bimodal age distribution (Male: Female: 2:1). These tumours constitute 3% of all intra nasal neoplasms. Sometimes the tumours are mistaken for small round cell tumours

a b c

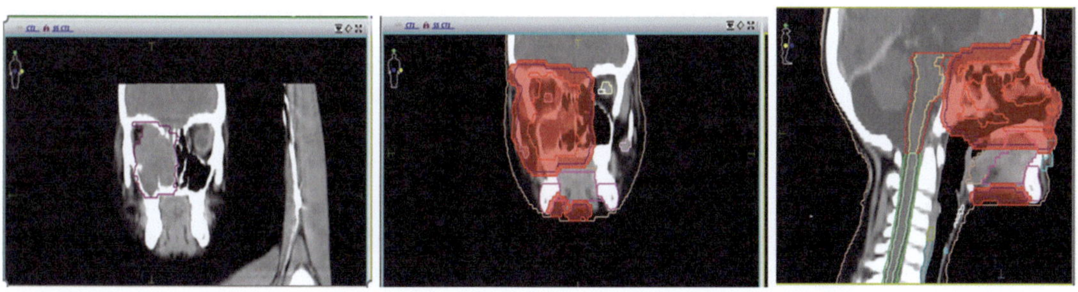

Fig. 26 PNS tumor (right side)- RT planning: A. contouring, B. dose plan (coronal), C. dose plan (sagittal). Note: gross infiltration of right orbit [courtesy: Dr. Ahitagni Biswas, AIIMS, Delhi)

Table 40 Suggested target volumes for gross, high- and low-risk regions

Target volumes	Definition and description	
GTV	All gross disease on physical examination and imaging	
CTV high	Should encompass the gross tumour volume with 3–5 mm margin. In adjuvant, setting positive margin and extranodal extension should be included in high-risk volume	
CTV low	Encompass areas with high risk of microscopic tumour spread from GTV. Variation in CTV can be depending upon site and case, proposed limits are shown below:	
	Ethmoid	Maxillary
	Sup—If cribriform not resected, should be included for maxillary sinus tumour If cribriform plate resected include 10 mm superior to cribriform plate or encompass initial GTV	
	Inf—Inferior turbinate, encompass 10 mm around GTV and exclude hard palate if possible	Inf—Inferior margin of maxilla and hard palate, should encompass 10 mm around GTV
	Lateral—the nasal cavity, ethmoid sinuses, and the ipsilateral maxillary sinus and when indicated the volume should extend to the rectus muscle	Lateral—medial aspect should be the nasal septum, unless violation of midline structures occurs
	Posteriorly—include the sphenoid sinus. The retropharyngeal lymph nodes should be encompassed if the tumour extended close to the nasopharynx or if there are metastatic neck nodes from an ethmoidal carcinoma	Posteriorly—the pterygopalatine and the infratemporal fossa should be included, paying special attention to encompass the masticator space and the infraorbital fissure
PTV	CTV + 3–5 mm margin as per institutional protocol	

Table 41 Selective nodal target for nasal and paranasal sinuses cancers

Site	Nodal category (AJCC 8th edition)	Ipsilateral neck levels to be included	Contralateral neck levels to be included[a]
Maxillary sinus	N0	Ib–III, VIIa, IX	Ib–III, VIIa
	N1-3	Ib–V, VIIa, IX	Ib–V, VIIa
Ethmoid sinus	N0	–	–
	N1–3	Ib–V, VIIa	Ib–V, VIIa
Nasal cavity	N0	Ib–III, VIIa, IX for anterior third nasal cavity involvement	Ib–III, VIIa
	N1–3	Ib–V, VIIa, IX for anterior third nasal cavity involvement	Ib–V, VIIa

[a]Unilateral irradiation for maxillary sinuses and nasal cavity cancers not crossing the mid-line without contralateral neck involvement

Prophylactic neck irradiation for T3-T4 squamous cell carcinoma and sinonasal undifferentiated carcinoma (SNUC)

Level IVb should be included in case of involvement of level IVa

Level VIIb should be included in case of bulky involvement of the upper part of level II

Prophylactic neck irradiation for Kadish stage ≥C and/or Hyams grade III/IV esthesioneuroblastoma (levels II–III, VIIa)

Table 42 gives the T staging of maxillary sinus tumours, and Table 43 shows the principles of management of paranasal sinus tumours.

Kadish Staging

Group A: lesions are limited to the nasal cavity

Group B: lesions involve the nasal cavity and paranasal sinuses

Group C: lesions extend beyond the nasal cavity and paranasal sinuses

Group D: for tumours with regional (cervical lymph node) or distant metastasis

Table 42 T staging for maxillary sinus cancers

T1	Tumour limited to the maxillary sinus mucosa with no erosion or destruction of bone
T2	Tumour causing bone erosion or destruction, including extension into the hard palate and/or middle nasal meatus, except extension to the posterior wall of the maxillary sinus and pterygoid plates
T3	Tumour invades any of the following: bone of the posterior wall of the maxillary sinus, subcutaneous tissues, floor or medial wall of the orbit, pterygoid fossa, or ethmoid sinuses
T4a	Moderately advanced local disease Tumour invades anterior orbital contents, skin of cheek, pterygoid plates, infratemporal fossa, cribriform plate, sphenoid or frontal sinuses
T4b	Very advanced local disease Tumour invades any of the following: orbital apex, dura, brain, middle cranial fossa, cranial nerves other than maxillary division of trigeminal nerve (V2), nasopharynx or clivus

Table 43 Principles of management

T1 and T2	*Single modality*: Surgery (Preferred) Definitive RT (Unfit/Unwilling for surgery)
T3 and T4a	*Combined modality*: Surgery + Adj RT +/- CT Concomitant chemoradiotherapy
T4b	*PS-0-1* CTRT especially in radio- and chemo sensitive tumours—SNUC, SNEC, SmCC, high grade ENB Surgery in favourable histologies (adenoid cystic/low grade adenocarcinoma) in limited dura/brain involvement *PS ≥2* Palliative RT Best Supportive care

31 Salivary Glands

31.1 Anatomy

The major salivary glands are the paired parotids, submandibular and sublingual glands (Fig. 27). In addition, there are many minor salivary glands. These are small accessory glands scattered throughout the upper aero digestive tract in palate, buccal mucosa, base of tongue, pharynx, trachea, cheek, lip, gingiva, floor of mouth, tonsil, paranasal sinuses, nasal cavity and nasopharynx.

Salivary glands can be classified as serous, mucous or seromucous; on the basis of type of fluid secretion from the glands. Parotid gland is the largest salivary gland, predominantly serous and divided into superficial and deep lobes in relation to ramus of mandible. It drains by the parotid duct into the mouth at the level of the second upper molar tooth. The submandibular gland produces both serous fluid and mucus, drains by the submandibular duct (Whartons duct) that opens alongside the fraenum of the tongue, and is crossed by the lingual nerve. Around 70% of saliva in the oral cavity is produced by the submandibular glands. The sublingual gland with mostly mucous secretions, lies in the floor of the mouth into which it drains directly by a series of short ducts. About 5% of saliva in oral cavity is produced by these glands.

31.2 Risk Factors

There are no definite risk factors related to alcohol or smoking. Prior history of radiation exposure (especially Mucoepidermoid cancer and Warthin's tumour) can be a risk factor in some cases.

31.3 History and Physical Examination

These tumours present as swelling in front/below the ear (parotid), and as a lump or swelling below the jaw (submandibular). A rapidly enlarging swelling suggests a malignant aetiology. Pain can indicate involvement of deep structures. Examination should involve a thorough evaluation of the local swelling as well as cranial nerve examination.

Table 44 gives the various benign and malignant salivary gland neoplasms, and Table 45 gives the stratification of salivary gland carcinomas based on aggressiveness as per the WHO 2017 criteria.

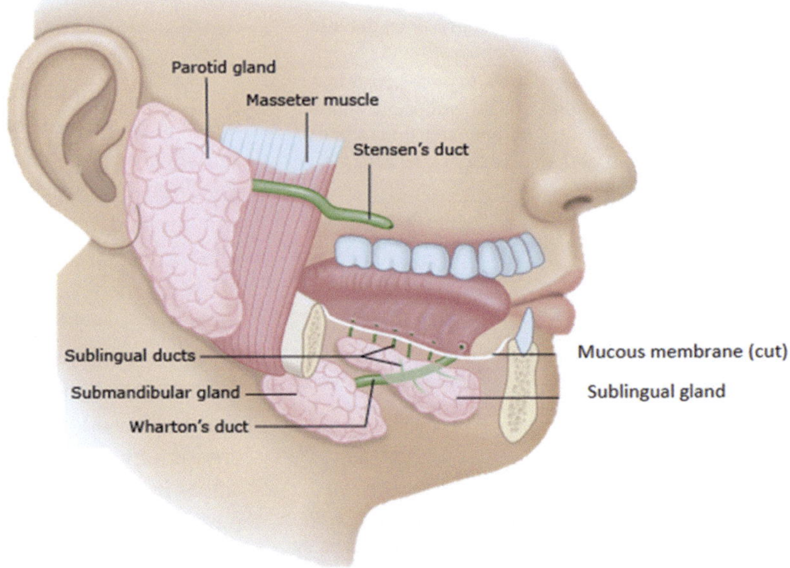

Fig. 27 Anatomy of salivary glands

Table 44 Pathology

Benign	Malignant
Pleomorphic adenoma (mixed tumour)	Adenoid cystic carcinoma
Warthin's tumour	Adenocarcinoma (NOS)
Oncocytoma	Acinic cell carcinoma
Other adenomas	Mucoepidermoid carcinoma
Basal cell adenoma	Malignant mixed tumour
Canalicular adenoma	Squamous cell carcinoma
Ductal papilloma	Other carcinomas

32 Treatment Paradigm

32.1 Surgery

Surgical resection of the primary tumour is the standard of care for all resectable salivary gland tumours. Enucleation shouldn't be done, and tumour spillage should be avoided. Preservation of cranial nerves should be attempted. Microscopic margins are preferred over facial nerve sacrifice, although not at the expense of residual gross disease. Nerve grafting can be considered for reconstruction of sacrificed cranial nerve. For all locations and histologies, clinically node-positive neck should be dissected. For parotid tumours, elective nodal dissection of levels II to III, and possibly IV, may be recommended and is surgeon-dependent based on risk factors (size, stage, grade, histology, location). For submandibular tumours, elective dissection of levels I to III, again surgeon dependent. For parotid tumours, levels I and V may be at risk only if levels II to IV are involved.

32.2 Indications of Radiation

- Gross residual disease
- Microscopically positive or close (<5 mm) surgical margins
- Large tumours (T3 or T4 disease) requiring radical resection
- Tumour spillage during operation
- High tumour grade
- Involvement of skin, bone, nerve (gross invasion or extensive PNI)
- Tumour extension beyond the capsule of the gland with periglandular and soft tissue invasion
- Lymph node metastases
- Recurrent cancer (including benign histology such as recurrent pleomorphic adenoma)

Table 45 Stratification of salivary gland carcinomas

Low aggression	High aggression
Acinic cell carcinoma	Adenoid cystic carcinoma Tubular/cribriform pattern predominant solid pattern 30%
(Mammary analogue) Secretory carcinoma	Poorly differentiated carcinoma: Neuroendocrine and non-neuroendocrine Undifferentiated carcinoma Large-cell neuroendocrine carcinoma Small-cell neuroendocrine carcinoma
Mucoepidermoid carcinoma Low grade Intermediate grade	Mucoepidermoid carcinoma High grade
Polymorphous adenocarcinoma Classic Cribriform	Polymorphous adenocarcinoma High grade
Epithelial-myoepithelial carcinoma	
(Hyalinizing) Clear cell carcinoma	
Basal cell adenocarcinoma	
Sebaceous adenocarcinoma	Lymphoepithelial carcinoma
Intraductal carcinoma Low grade High grade	(Conventional) Salivary duct carcinoma
Adenocarcinoma, NOS Low grade	Adenocarcinoma, NOS High grad
Myoepithelial carcinoma	
Oncocytic carcinoma	Carcinosarcoma
Carcinoma ex pleomorphic adenoma—risk is determined by the type of carcinoma and extent of invasion	

Based on WHO 2017 [105]

32.3 Dose

Typically, 60 Gy to primary site and 54 Gy to elective neck (if included) is recommended for these tumours. Treatment of ipsilateral neck for pathologically node-positive disease is required, and elective nodal coverage should be considered for pT3–4, high-grade, facial nerve deficits or recurrent disease.

32.4 Chemotherapy

Use of chemotherapy has been reported in small case series. There is no frank benefit of concurrent chemotherapy in curative setting (ref). Chemotherapy alone for advanced/metastatic/recurrent disease showed modest response.

Palliative: For patients with progressive symptomatic disease or pressure up on vital structures. Response rates 15–50% lasting for 6–9 months.

Multidrug regimens: CAP regimen: Cyclophosphamide 500 mg/m^2, Adriamycin 50 mg/m^2, Cisplatin 50 mg/m^2 q28 days have shown good response.

Single agents: Cisplatin alone has shown 20% response rate for locoregional and 7% for distant disease. Paclitaxel can also be used except in adenoid cystic carcinoma. In adenoid cystic carcinoma: single agent vinorelbine, mitoxantrone, epirubicin can be used.

32.5 Complications

Post-surgery complications include facial nerve paresis. The risk of temporary paresis can range from 8–38%. With proper selectin of cases, the risk of permanent paresis is <1%.

Salivary fistulae is another complication, which can often be distressing.

Neuromas of greater auricular nerve can occur post-surgery. Finally, Frey's syndrome (gustatory sweating—local facial sweating and flushing during meals) is a known complication post-surgery in salivary gland tumours.

Post RT complications can be classified as short term and long term. Short-term side effects of radiotherapy include skin erythema, mucositis, dysphagia, desquamation and mucosal ulcers

Long-term side effects of radiotherapy include permanent taste impairment, subcutaneous fibrosis, xerostomia, trismus, chronic otitis externa or media, hearing loss-conductive of sensori-neural, otomastoiditis, dry-eye syndrome, nasolacrimal duct obstruction, cataract, retinopathy, bone necrosisand temporal lobe necrosis.

33 Thyroid Cancers

33.1 Anatomy

Average adult thyroid gland measures about 5 × 5 cm and weighs 10–20 g. Thyroid gland consists of numerous lobules comprising individual follicles that forms structural and functional units of the gland. Each follicle consists of single layer of cuboidal epithelium comprising thyroid follicular cells surrounding a central lumen containing colloid rich in thyroglobulin (Tg). Approximately 10% of cells are para-follicular cells, derived from neural-crest containing calcitonin granules.

33.2 Physiology

The thyroid secretes two hormones: Thyroxine: 93% (3, 5, 3′, 5′ iodothyronine or T_4) and triiodothyronine: 7% (3, 5, 3′ iodothyronine or T_3). T_4 is eventually converted to T_3 in tissues and T_3 is 4 times more active than T_4. Secretion is controlled by TSH secreted by ant pituitary, which in turn is controlled by TRH from hypothalamus.

33.3 Risk Factors

Family history, previous radiation exposure particularly during childhood, female preponderance and Iodine deficiency can all be considered risk factors for thyroid neoplasms. Approximately 85% of RT-induced thyroid cancers are well-differentiated PTC. MEN2, an autosomal-dominant syndrome in which mutations in the RET proto-oncogene cause development of MTC.

33.4 History and Physical Examination

Thyroid neoplasms commonly present as a palpable nodule. Hoarseness in patients generally indicates involvement of recurrent laryngeal nerve. Anaplastic Carcinoma of Thyroid generally presents as rapidly enlarging neck mass. Thyroid cancer is of four main types: papillary (PTC), follicular (FTC), medullary (MTC), and anaplastic (ATC). Overall, papillary and follicular types together are called Differentiated Thyroid Cancers (DTC). Table 46 shows pathological classification of thyroid tumours. Classification based on ability to concentrate radio-active iodine (RAI) is shown in Table 47.

Tables 48 and 49 show the T staging and N staging of thyroid cancers, respectively.

Based on prognosis, thyroid cancers are classified into favourable and unfavourable which is shown in Table 50. Risk stratification is shown in Table 51.

34 Radioactive Iodine Therapy

RAIT is defined as the systemic administration of 131-sodium or potassium iodide (^{131}I) for selective irradiation of thyroid remnants, microscopic

Table 46 Pathological classification

Follicular epithelial cells	Para follicular cell origin
A. *Differentiated thyroid cancers* 1. *Papillary and its variants (80–90%)* Classic Papillary microcarcinoma Encapsulated variant Follicular variant Aggressive variants Diffuse sclerosing/tall cell/ columnar cell 2. *Follicular cancers (15–30%)* Classic Hurthle cell	*Medullary carcinoma*
B. *Poorly differentiated—Insular*	
C. *Undifferentiated—Anaplastic*	

Table 47 Classification based on ability to concentrate RAI

Usually concentrate RAI	Frequently do not concentrate RAI	Never concentrate RAI
Classical papillary carcinoma Encapsulated papillary Ca Follicular variant Follicular Ca	Tall cell/ columnar call Hurthle cell Insular Ca	Anaplastic thyroid carcinoma Medullary Ca

Table 48 T staging of thyroid cancers

Tx	Primary tumour cannot be assessed
T0	No evidence of primary tumour
T1	Tumour ≤2 cm in greatest dimension limited to the thyroid *T1a*: Tumour ≤1 cm in greatest dimension limited to the thyroid *T1b*: Tumour >1 cm but ≤2 cm in greatest dimension limited to the thyroid
T2	Tumour >2 cm but ≤4 cm in greatest dimension limited to the thyroid
T3	Tumour >4 cm limited to the thyroid or gross extrathyroidal extension invading only strap muscles *T3a**: Tumour >4 cm limited to the thyroid *T3b**: Gross extrathyroidal extension invading only strap muscles (sternohyoid, sternothyroid, thyrohyoid or omohyoid muscles) from a tumour of any size
T4	Includes gross extrathyroidal extension into major neck structures *T4a*: Gross extrathyroidal extension invading subcutaneous soft tissues, larynx, trachea, oesophagus or recurrent laryngeal nerve from a tumour of any size *T4b*: Gross extrathyroidal extension invading prevertebral fascia or encasing carotid artery or mediastinal vessels from a tumour of any size

DTC or other non-resectable or incompletely resectable DTC, or both purposes.

35 Recommendation of I-131 Usage (ATA 2015 Guidelines)

For low risk, I 131 is not routinely recommended (weak recommendation, low quality evidence).

Table 49 Nodal staging

NX	Regional lymph nodes cannot be assessed
N0	No evidence of regional lymph node metastasis *N0a**: One or more cytologic or histologically confirmed benign lymph nodes *N0b**: No radiologic or clinical evidence of locoregional lymph node metastasis
N1	*N1a**: Metastasis to level VI or VII (pretracheal, paratracheal, prelaryngeal/ Delphian or upper mediastinal) lymph nodes; this can be unilateral or bilateral disease *N1b**: Metastasis to unilateral, bilateral or contralateral lateral neck lymph nodes (levels I, II, III, IV or V) or retropharyngeal lymph nodes

Table 50 Favourable and unfavourable prognosis [106]

Variable	Favourable	Unfavourable
Age	15–44 years	≥45 years
Gender	Female	Male
Family history	Absent	Present
Tumour size	≤4 cm	>4 cm
Focality/ laterality	Unifocal/ Unilateral	Multifocal/ bilateral
Extrathyroid extension	Organ confined	Extrathyroid extension
Histologic grade	Low grade	High grade
Lymph node metastases	Absent	Present
Distant metastases	Absent	Present
RAI concentration	Concentrate RAI	Inability to concentrate RAI

For intermediate risk, I 131 should be considered (weak recommendation, low quality evidence). However, for high risk, I 131 is routinely recommended (strong recommendation, moderate quality evidence).

36 TSH Suppression Recommendation (ATA 2015 Guidelines)

Low risk: 0.5 to 2 Mu/L (Weak recommendation, low quality evidence).

Intermediate risk: 0.1 to 0.5 Mu/L (Weak recommendation, low quality evidence).

Table 51 Risk stratification

Low risk	Intermediate risk	High risk
No local or distant metastases All macroscopic tumour has been resected There is no tumour invasion of locoregional tissues or structures The tumour does not have aggressive histology or vascular invasion If ^{131}I is given, there is no ^{131}I uptake outside the thyroid bed on the first RxWBS	Microscopic invasion of tumour into the perithyroidal soft tissues at initial surgery Cervical lymph node metastases or ^{131}I uptake outside the thyroid bed on the RxWBS done after thyroid remnant ablation Tumour with aggressive histology or vascular invasion	Macroscopic tumour invasion Incomplete tumour resection Distant metastases Thyroglobulinemia out of proportion to what is seen on the posttreatment scan

High risk: <0.1 Mu/L (Strong recommendation, moderate quality evidence).

37 Adjuvant External RT in Thyroid Cancers

37.1 American Thyroid Association (ATA) and British Thyroid Association (BTA) Guidelines for Adjuvant EBRT in DTC

37.1.1 ATA

ATA supports the use of EBRT when post-surgery status shows aero-digestive infiltration (trachea and/or esophagus) in DTC neoplasms. In these situations, RAIT is combined with EBRT. In locally advanced inoperable anaplastic or medullary types (ATC, MTC), role of EBRT should be considered because of lack of radio-iodine concentration. In recent years, systemic and targeted therapy have evolved for management of ATC and MTC.

37.1.2 BTA

EBRT can be considered for gross residual/unresectable disease or when there is high risk of locoregional recurrence and disease is unlikely to be controlled by surgery and/or RAI, particularly in older patients or those with invasive pT4 disease.

37.2 Carcinoma of Unknown Primary (CUP)

Carcinoma of Unknown Primary is defined is defined as the presence of histologically confirmed metastatic cancer in a patient where a detailed medical history, complete physical examination or investigations fail to identify a primary site. Majority of CUP in relation to HNC presents as unilateral or bilateral neck nodes, and accounts for 2–5% of all HN malignancies [107].

37.3 Risk Factors

General risk factors for head and neck cancers are also risk factors for CUP, including tobacco, alcohol, HPV and EBV infections.

37.4 History and Physical Examination

A history of nativity and occupation should be documented. Tobacco and alcohol use, high-risk sexual behaviour and h/o previous malignancy should be probed.

37.5 Diagnostic Workup

A complete upper aerodigestive tract evaluation of mucosal sites at risk (oral cavity, nasopharynx, oropharynx, hypopharynx and larynx is mandatory.

FNAC or Biopsy should be taken from suspicious neck mass and oral-oropharyngeal areas. Random biopsies are no longer preferred. FOL may be complemented with advanced visualization techniques, like narrow-band imaging. HPV testing for level II and level III nodes should be considered. EBV testing for HPV-negative metastasis should be done.

37.6 Imaging

Initial imaging investigation of choice for workup is a CECT Neck. PET-CT should be the next diagnostic step if primary is not evident on clinical examination or CECT. PET detection rate of primary tumour is around 30% in patients with HNCUP.

37.7 Surgical Procedures

If primary is identified during operative upper aerodigestive tract evaluation, advanced techniques like transoral resection may be performed to achieve a negative surgical margin. Tissue specimens from suspected primary should be submitted entirely for histologic examination.

Resection specimens should be anatomically oriented by the surgeon, with evaluation of margins.

Intraoperative frozen section may be performed to confirm the presence of tumour prior to resection.

37.8 Role of Tonsillectomy

(a) Unilateral Lymphadenopathy
  - Ipsilateral palatine tonsillectomy is preferred.
  - If primary still not identified, ipsilateral lingual tonsillectomy may be performed.
  - Bilateral palatine tonsillectomy may be done according to clinical suspicion.

(b) Bilateral lymphadenopathy
  - Unilateral lingual tonsillectomy may be performed on the side with the greater nodal burden.
  - Contralateral lingual tonsillectomy if the ipsilateral procedure fails to identify a primary.
  - Bilateral palatine tonsillectomy after bilateral lingual tonsillectomy to be avoided.

37.9 Pathology

- Most common pathology of HNCUP is SCC (75%) followed by adenocarcinoma and undifferentiated carcinoma.

38 Treatment Paradigm in HNCPU

38.1 Surgery

For unilateral, small-volume neck disease either definitive surgery or RT are reasonable options. For small-volume bilateral neck disease without ENE, options include definitive surgery (with or without adjuvant therapy) or radiotherapy (with or without concurrent chemotherapy)

For large-volume bilateral neck disease and/or ENE, consider definitive chemoradiotherapy. If extensive bilateral neck dissection is contemplated, there shall be an increased likelihood of trimodality therapy.

Levels IIA, III, and IV should be dissected in suspected oropharyngeal primary. Additional levels can be considered depending upon the extent of the disease.

38.2 Radiation

Patients should be simulated in supine position with arms by the side using thermoplastic mask and neck extended. RT planning CT should be performed using slice thickness of 3mm from vertex to carina. Dental evaluation should be done before starting radiotherapy. Following points to be considered during target delineation:

- Gross nodal disease, neck regions at risk of containing microscopic disease and the anatomic mucosal regions at risk of harbouring the occult primary is ideally treated.

- Unilateral nodal treatment is controversial.
- For HPV related tumours: Gross node(s) are treated with consideration of coverage of putative primary sites in the ipsilateral tonsillar bed, ipsilateral soft palate and the mucosa of the entire base of tongue.
- In occult nasopharyngeal primary, the mucosal radiation can be considered to the nasopharynx. Nodal volumes should include bilateral levels II-V, including retropharyngeal nodes.
- Ipsilateral multiple nodes without ENE, should ideally receive bilateral treatment.
- Patients treated with primary radiotherapy for N3 and/or bilateral nodal involvement and/or clinical and/or radiologic evidence of ENE require bilateral neck treatment.

38.3 Dose

For definitive radiotherapy, Definitive: 70 Gy/35 # is considered for RT to the gross disease and 56 to 63 Gy/35 # to mucosal sites at risk and uninvolved neck. In the adjuvant, setting a dose of 60 Gy/30 # to the post-operative bed and pathologically involved nodal levels, and 54 Gy/30 # to the uninvolved neck is considered appropriate.

38.4 Chemotherapy

- Concurrent administration of cisplatin with definitive radiotherapy should be offered to patients with a suspected mucosal primary SCC in the presence of nodal disease.

38.5 Recurrent Cancers and Reirradiation

Nearly one-third of the head and neck cancer patients, after definitive treatment develop a locoregional recurrence. Rate of development of second primary: 1% per year. Reirradiation is one of the most challenging decision-making processes. Recurrent or second primary tumours have varied tumour characteristics. Patients also present with various comorbidities and previous treatment-related sequelae [108] Re-irradiation is a well established treatment approach for recurrent and second tumor HNC. Re-irradiation is feasible as combined approach with surgery and/ or chemotherapy for disease control or, palliative RT for growth restrain and symptom relief measure in advanced inoperable disease.

Table 52 Prognostic factors for recurrent head and neck cancers

Patient related	Treatment related	Disease related
Performance status	Surgically resectable	Stage of recurrent disease
Life expectancy	Time interval since last irradiation	Smaller volumes demonstrate better outcomes
Comorbidities	Received chemo or not	Second Primary Tumours vs. recurrence
Baseline organ function	Previous volumes treated	Location-Benefit more for larynx and nasopharynx
Previous treatment sequalae	Dose received Target and OARS	

38.6 Risk Factors

Common risk factors for recurrent cancers include continued lifestyle, including continuation of tobacco use. Biological parameters such as radioresistance can also play a role. Phenomena such as field cancerization too can lead to recurrent tumours. Finally, improper, inadequate in the initial treatment course delivered earlier can also be important risk factors. Prognostic factors for recurrent head and neck cancers are shown in Table 52.

38.7 ACR Appropriateness Criteria [87]

The following are the ACR appropriateness criteria for re-irradiation(re-RT) in head and neck cancers. Careful restaging evaluation is a must. PETCECT can be done in addition to CT/MRI. Comorbidities, Life expectancy, performance status, speech and swallowing function, nutritional status, severity of current symptoms, sequelae of previous treatment should be well documented. There is a greater likelihood of local control with at least 50–60 Gy in irradiation at once daily standard fractionation. For addition of Chemotherapy, the likely benefit should be estimated for an individual case. Reirradiation should be done at centres with multi-disciplinary approach and a skilled oncology team. Preferably, advanced radiation techniques should be used for reirradiation.

38.8 Principles of Reirradiation

The goal of therapy has to be curative. Patients should have a reasonable life expectancy. Generally, reirradiation is not considered before 1 year of the last course. Whenever possible, it is desirable to give a dose greater than 50 Gy. Previous radiotherapy dose should be calculated as EQD2 for the record, to be combined with re-irradiation dose schedule. Elective nodal irradiation is not recommended in reirradiation. It is very important to take into account the tolerance of surrounding critical structures.

38.9 Refining Patient Selection for Reirradiation as per MIRI (Multi-institutional Reirradiation)

Table 53 gives the Recursive Partitioning Analysis (RPA) classification for patient selection in reirradiation of head and neck cancers.

Table 53 Recursive partitioning analysis (RPA) classification [109]

RPA 1	Interval ≥2 years from prior RT, resected recurrence/second primary, no organ dysfunction
RPA 2	Interval ≥2 years with unresected disease OR interval < 2 years with no organ dysfunction
RPA 3	Interval <2 years with organ dysfunction, irrespective of resection status

38.10 Overall Survival as per RPA Class

RPA Class 1: ~61.9% (2-year OS)
RPA Class 2: ~40% (2-year OS)
RPA Class 3: ~16.8% (2-year OS)

38.11 Organs at Risk

In radiation planning for recurrent head and neck tumours, OAR's need to be given stringent constraints. The risks include myelopathy in spinal cord, brainstem necrosis, temporal lobe necrosis, cataract, painful red eye and retinopathy. Finally, ORN of mandible is an important complication that needs to be avoided.

38.12 Osteoradionecrosis of the Mandible

Radionecrosis of the mandible after re-irradiation is always a known treatment-related risk. For patient who has received earlier dose >50 Gy, and would be planned for reirradiation dose EQD2 equivalent to 50-60 Gy. Before re-irradiation course, the oro-dental and mandible bone status should be carefully assessed, including mandible x-ray and CT scan, and oro-dental prophylaxis should be prescribed as a routine practice. Modern techniques like IMRT, VMAT, SBRT and proton therapy have reduced the incidence of radionecrosis.

38.13 Carotid Blowout [110]

Carotid blowout syndrome (CBS) results from necrosis and disruption of the carotid arterial wall, most commonly following surgery and/or reirradiation for head and neck cancers. Although uncommon, it is a life-threatening complication. CBS is classified into three types: Type I (Threatened): Carotid artery exposure identified on clinical examination or imaging (e.g., perivascular air, adjacent abscess, tumour, or fistula). Type II (Impending): Self-limited "sentinel bleeding" episodes that may temporarily respond to pressure or wound packing. Type III (Acute): Frank carotid rupture with massive hemorrhage, often rapidly fatal, particularly outside a hospital setting. It is well known the risk of CBS with modern re-irradiation techniques is less than 3-5%, yet it is recognised as a life-threatening event with high mortality and neurologic deficits. Re-irradiation dose to the carotid volume is to be carefully planned for sparing the structure as much as possible.

38.14 Recent Advances in the Management of Head and Neck Cancers

Recent years have witnessed a paradigm shift in the management of head and neck cancers, especially recurrent/ metastatic disease, driven by advances in systemic therapy and radiation therapy technology. Immunotherapy, particularly immune checkpoint inhibitors targeting the PD-1/PD-L1 axis, has emerged as a standard of care in recurrent and metastatic settings and is increasingly being explored in locally advanced disease, including peri-operative, definitive and recurrent/ metastatic treatment strategies [111, 112]. Parallel progress in molecular profiling has expanded the role of targeted therapies, enabling biomarker-driven treatment in selected subgroups such as salivary gland malignancies, thyroid cancers, and rare head and neck tumours with actionable genetic alterations. Also, with the wider use of more conformal radiotherapy techniques, the area of hypo fractionated radiotherapy [113] is re-emerging, whether it be with conventional treatment volumes or stereotactic body radiotherapy. This emanates from the fact that it is possible to spare better without compromising disease outcomes. In radiation oncology, particle therapy, most notably proton therapy, has gained prominence for its ability to deliver highly conformal dose distributions while minimizing exposure to adjacent critical structures, thereby reducing toxicity and improving functional outcomes, particularly in complex anatomical sites and re-irradiation scenarios [114]. Collectively, these developments underscore the transition toward precision-based, individualized treatment approaches in head and neck oncology, with the dual goals of optimizing oncological outcomes and preserving quality of life.

Percepts Box

1. Head and neck cancers are the sixth most common cancers worldwide. Substantial geographic variations are heavily influenced by key risk factors which include tobacco products, alcohol consumption and virus like Epstein Barr virus and HPV.
2. Clinical presentation—Initial symptoms and subsequent staging depend upon the site of the primary tumour.
3. Diagnostic evaluation—To develop an optimal treatment plan, proper staging of primary tumour, regional lymph nodes and distant metastases is required. Physical examination, imaging, examination under anaesthesia and biopsy aid in staging.
4. Treatment of head and neck cancers need a multidisciplinary approach including surgeons, medical oncologist, radiation oncologist, dentist, pathologist and rehabilitation therapist.
5. Clinical factors that influence the treatment includes tumour site and stage, the functional outcomes and morbidity, performance status and co-morbidities.
6. Early-stage diseases are generally managed by either surgery or radiotherapy alone, except for patients with high-risk features. Advanced stage patients need multimodality approach.
7. Locally recurrent or metastatic are managed mostly by palliative systemic therapy and/or supportive care. Immunotherapy can be used in selected

(continued)

patients. Patients with disease confined to head and neck may be benefited from surgical or radiation salvage and/or reirradiation.
8. Post-treatment evaluation and surveillance are an essential part of patient care.

Multiple Choice Questions

1. The Intergroup 0099 trial in Nasopharyngeal Cancer compared:
   (a) CTRT to NACT+CTRT
   (b) CTRT+ Adjuvant CT to RT alone
   (c) NACT+CTRT to NACT+RT
   (d) NACT+RT to CTRT
2. The 5Rs which form the basis for fractionation in Radiotherapy are:
   (a) Repair, Reassortment, Reoxygenation, Repopulation and Inherent Radiosensitivity
   (b) Repair, Regrowth, Reallignment, Renewal, Reassortment
   (c) Inherent Radiosensitivity, Regrowth, Redistribution, Reduction, Renewal
   (d) None of the above
3. Conventional Fractionation is:
   (a) 1.8–2G y/fraction, 5 fractions per week
   (b) 2.1–2.2 Gy/fraction, 5 fractions per week
   (c) 12 Gy/week, 6 fractions/week
   (d) 3 Gy/fraction, 5 fractions per week, for 2 week
4. The trial that evaluated various altered fractionation schedules in Head and Neck radiotherapy is
   (a) RTOG 9003
   (b) BCCA 9113
   (c) Oro 9301
   (d) RTOG 9111
5. As per the MARCH analysis, the gain in overall survival with the use of hyperfractionated radiotherapy is
   (a) 8.2%
   (b) 2%
   (c) 1.7%
   (d) 3.4%
6. According to the MACH-NC, the gain in survival with the use of concurrent chemoradiotherapy is
   (a) 8%
   (b) 5%
   (c) 3.2%
   (d) None of the above
7. Almost _____% of head and neck cancers express EGFR
   (a) 80–100
   (b) 30–50
   (c) 40–50
   (d) 10–15
8. The most effective anti-EGFR molecule in Head and Neck cancers is
   (a) Cilengitide
   (b) Geftinib
   (c) Cetuximab
   (d) Erlotinib
9. Irreversible Xerostomia occurs when the entire salivary apparatus receives a total dose
   (a) Above 30 Gy
   (b) 6 Gy
   (c) 15 Gy
   (d) 26 Gy
10. The optimal dose for adjuvant radiotherapy in the absence of extracapsular spread and positive cut margins is:
   (a) >54 Gy
   (b) 50 Gy
   (c) 46–50 Gy
   (d) 63 Gy

Answer Key

1. (b)
2. (a)
3. (a)
4. (a)
5. (a)
6. (a)
7. (a)
8. (c)
9. (a)
10. (a)

References

1. Sung H, Ferlay J, Siegel RL, et al. Global cancer statistics 2020: GLOBOCAN estimates of incidence and mortality worldwide for 36 cancers in 185 countries. CA A Cancer J Clin. 2021;71(3):209–49. https://doi.org/10.3322/caac.21660.
2. Prabhash K, Babu G, Chaturvedi P, et al. Indian clinical practice consensus guidelines for the management of squamous cell carcinoma of head and neck. Indian J Cancer. 2020;57(5):1. https://doi.org/10.4103/0019-509X.278971.
3. Dandekar M, Tuljapurkar V, Dhar H, Panwar A, DCruz AK. Head and neck cancers in India. J Surg Oncol. 2017;115(5):555–63. https://doi.org/10.1002/jso.24545.
4. Ang KK, Harris J, Wheeler R, et al. Human papillomavirus and survival of patients with oropharyngeal cancer. N Engl J Med. 2010;363(1):24–35. https://doi.org/10.1056/NEJMoa0912217.
5. Laskar S, Swain M. HPV positive oropharyngeal cancer and treatment deintensification: how pertinent is it? J Can Res Ther. 2015;11(1):6. https://doi.org/10.4103/0973-1482.151445.
6. Kalra B, Sinha S, Laskar SG. De-escalation in HPV: near yet elusive. JCO. 2021;39(24):2733–4. https://doi.org/10.1200/JCO.21.00635.
7. Gress DM, Edge SB, Greene FL, et al. Principles of cancer staging. In: Amin MB, Edge SB, Greene FL, editors. AJCC cancer staging manual. Springer; 2017. p. 3–30. https://doi.org/10.1007/978-3-319-40618-3_1.
8. Amin MB, Greene FL, Edge SB, et al. The Eighth Edition AJCC Cancer Staging Manual: continuing to build a bridge from a population-based to a more "personalized" approach to cancer staging. CA Cancer J Clin. 2017;67(2):93–9. https://doi.org/10.3322/caac.21388.
9. Baugnon KL, Beitler JJ. Pitfalls in the staging of cancer of the laryngeal squamous cell carcinoma. Neuroimag Clin N Am. 2013;23(1):81–105. https://doi.org/10.1016/j.nic.2012.08.008.
10. Wong KCW, Hui EP, Lo KW, et al. Nasopharyngeal carcinoma: an evolving paradigm. Nat Rev Clin Oncol. 2021;18(11):679–95. https://doi.org/10.1038/s41571-021-00524-x.
11. Laskar SG, Pai P, Sinha S, et al. Intensity-modulated radiation therapy for nasal cavity and paranasal sinus tumors: experience from a single institute. Head Neck. 2021;43(7):2045–57. https://doi.org/10.1002/hed.26669.
12. Akbaba S, Rühle A, Rothhaar S, et al. Treatment outcomes of elderly salivary gland cancer patients undergoing radiotherapy – results from a large multicenter analysis. Radiother Oncol. 2021;156:266–74. https://doi.org/10.1016/j.radonc.2020.12.024.
13. Haugen BR, Alexander EK, Bible KC, et al. 2015 American Thyroid Association Management guidelines for adult patients with thyroid nodules and differentiated thyroid cancer: the American Thyroid Association Guidelines Task Force on Thyroid Nodules and Differentiated Thyroid Cancer. Thyroid. 2016;26(1):1–133. https://doi.org/10.1089/thy.2015.0020.
14. Dhull AK, Atri R, Dhankhar R, Chauhan AK, Kaushal V. Major risk factors in head and neck cancer: a retrospective analysis of 12-year experiences. World J Oncol. 2018;9(3):80–4. https://doi.org/10.14740/wjon1104w.
15. Riaz N, Morris LG, Lee W, Chan TA. Unraveling the molecular genetics of head and neck cancer through genome-wide approaches. Genes Dis. 2014;1(1):75–86. https://doi.org/10.1016/j.gendis.2014.07.002.
16. Bhawna G. Burden of smoked and smokeless tobacco consumption in India - results from the Global adult Tobacco Survey India (GATS-India)- 2009-201. Asian Pac J Cancer Prev. 2013;14(5):3323–9. https://doi.org/10.7314/apjcp.2013.14.5.3323. PMID: 23803124.
17. Osazuwa-Peters N, Adjei Boakye E, Chen BY, Tobo BB, Varvares MA. Association between head and neck squamous cell carcinoma survival, smoking at diagnosis, and marital status. JAMA Otolaryngol Head Neck Surg. 2017;9 https://doi.org/10.1001/jamaoto.2017.1880.
18. Sankaranarayanan R, Ramadas K, Thara S, et al. Long term effect of visual screening on oral cancer incidence and mortality in a randomized trial in Kerala, India. Oral Oncol. 2013;49(4):314–21. https://doi.org/10.1016/j.oraloncology.2012.11.004.
19. Cheung LC, Ramadas K, Muwonge R, et al. Risk-based selection of individuals for oral cancer screening. JCO. 2021;39(6):663–74. https://doi.org/10.1200/JCO.20.02855.
20. D'Cruz AK, Vaish R. Risk-based oral cancer screening – lessons to be learnt. Nat Rev Clin Oncol. 2021;18(8):471–2. https://doi.org/10.1038/s41571-021-00511-2.
21. Sankaranarayanan R, Ramadas K, Thomas G, et al. Effect of screening on oral cancer mortality in Kerala, India: a cluster-randomised controlled trial. Lancet. 2005;365(9475):1927–33. https://doi.org/10.1016/S0140-6736(05)66658-5.
22. Yang S, Wu S, Zhou J, Chen XY. Screening for nasopharyngeal cancer. Cochrane ENT Group. Cochrane Database Syst Rev. 2015;2015(11) https://doi.org/10.1002/14651858.CD008423.pub2.
23. Arya S, Chaukar D, Pai P. Imaging in oral cancers. Indian J Radiol Imaging. 2012;22(03):195–208. https://doi.org/10.4103/0971-3026.107182.
24. Joshi VM, Wadhwa V, Mukherji SK. Imaging in laryngeal cancers. Indian J Radiol Imaging. 2012;22(03):209–26. https://doi.org/10.4103/0971-3026.107183.
25. Hui WJ, Zhao J, Hong LZ, et al. Comparison of CT and MRI in diagnosis of laryngeal carcinoma with anterior vocal commissure involvement. Sci

Rep. 2016;6(1):30353. https://doi.org/10.1038/srep30353.
26. Huellner MW. PET/MR in head and neck cancer – an update. Semin Nucl Med. 2021;51(1):26–38. https://doi.org/10.1053/j.semnuclmed.2020.07.006.
27. Lodi G, Franchini R, Warnakulasuriya S, et al. Interventions for treating oral leukoplakia to prevent oral cancer. Cochrane Oral Health Group. Cochrane Database Syst Rev. 2016;2016(7) https://doi.org/10.1002/14651858.CD001829.pub4.
28. Mehanna H, Wong WL, McConkey CC, et al. PET-CT surveillance versus neck dissection in advanced head and neck cancer. N Engl J Med. 2016;374(15):1444–54. https://doi.org/10.1056/NEJMoa1514493.
29. Lin NC, Hsu JT, Tsai KY. Survival and clinicopathological characteristics of different histological grades of oral cavity squamous cell carcinoma: A single-center retrospective study. Sapkota D. PLoS One. 2020;15(8):e0238103. https://doi.org/10.1371/journal.pone.0238103.
30. Ebrahimi A, Gil Z, Amit M, et al. Depth of invasion alone as an indication for postoperative radiotherapy in small oral squamous cell carcinomas: an international collaborative study. Head Neck. 2019;41(6):1935–42. https://doi.org/10.1002/hed.25633.
31. D'Cruz AK, Dhar H, Vaish R, et al. Depth of invasion in early oral cancers – is it an independent prognostic factor? Eur J Surg Oncol. 2021;47(8):1940–6. https://doi.org/10.1016/j.ejso.2021.03.243.
32. Almangush A, Bello IO, Keski-Säntti H, et al. Depth of invasion, tumor budding, and worst pattern of invasion: prognostic indicators in early-stage oral tongue cancer. Head Neck. 2014;36(6):811–8. https://doi.org/10.1002/hed.23380.
33. Zanoni DK, Patel SG. New AJCC: how does it impact oral cancers? Oral Oncol. 2020;104:104607. https://doi.org/10.1016/j.oraloncology.2020.104607.
34. Ko HC, Gupta V, Mourad WF, et al. A contouring guide for head and neck cancers with perineural invasion. Pract Radiat Oncol. 2014;4(6):e247–58. https://doi.org/10.1016/j.prro.2014.02.001.
35. Cracchiolo JR, Xu B, Migliacci JC, et al. Patterns of recurrence in oral tongue cancer with perineural invasion. Head Neck. 2018;40(6):1287–95. https://doi.org/10.1002/hed.25110.
36. Cassidy RJ, Switchenko JM, Jegadeesh N, et al. Association of lymphovascular space invasion with locoregional failure and survival in patients with node-negative oral tongue cancers. JAMA Otolaryngol Head Neck Surg. 2017;143(4):382. https://doi.org/10.1001/jamaoto.2016.3795.
37. Huang S, Zhu Y, Cai H, Zhang Y, Hou J. Impact of lymphovascular invasion in oral squamous cell carcinoma: a meta-analysis. Oral Surg Oral Med Oral Pathol Oral Radiol. 2021;131(3):319–328.e1. https://doi.org/10.1016/j.oooo.2020.10.026.
38. Michikawa C, Uzawa N, Kayamori K, et al. Clinical significance of lymphatic and blood vessel invasion in oral tongue squamous cell carcinomas. Oral Oncol. 2012;48(4):320–4. https://doi.org/10.1016/j.oraloncology.2011.11.014.
39. Nair D, Mair M, Singhvi H, et al. Perineural invasion: Independent prognostic factor in oral cancer that warrants adjuvant treatment. Head Neck. 2018;29 https://doi.org/10.1002/hed.25170.
40. Yang X, Tian X, Wu K, et al. Prognostic impact of perineural invasion in early stage oral tongue squamous cell carcinoma: results from a prospective randomized trial. Surg Oncol. 2018;27(2):123–8. https://doi.org/10.1016/j.suronc.2018.02.005.
41. Kumar A, Sinha S, Laskar S. Intensification of adjuvant treatment in early oral cancers. Ann Oncol Res Ther. 2021;1(1):3. https://doi.org/10.4103/aort.aort_15_21.
42. Kerawala C, Roques T, Jeannon JP, Bisase B. Oral cavity and lip cancer: United Kingdom National Multidisciplinary Guidelines. J Laryngol Otol. 2016;130(S2):S83–9. https://doi.org/10.1017/S0022215116000499.
43. Bulbul MG, Tarabichi O, Sethi RK, Parikh AS, Varvares MA. Does clearance of positive margins improve local control in oral cavity cancer? A meta-analysis. Otolaryngol Head Neck Surg. 2019;161(2):235–44. https://doi.org/10.1177/0194599819839006.
44. Mishra A, Malik A, Datta S, et al. Defining optimum surgical margins in buccoalveolar squamous cell carcinoma. Eur J Surg Oncol. 2019;45(6):1033–8. https://doi.org/10.1016/j.ejso.2019.01.224.
45. Ma H, Van Dessel J, Shujaat S, et al. Long-term functional outcomes of vascularized fibular and iliac flap for mandibular reconstruction: a systematic review and meta-analysis. J Plast Reconstruct Aesth Surg. 2021;74(2):247–58. https://doi.org/10.1016/j.bjps.2020.10.094.
46. Patil VM, Prabhash K, Noronha V, et al. Neoadjuvant chemotherapy followed by surgery in very locally advanced technically unresectable oral cavity cancers. Oral Oncol. 2014;50(10):1000–4. https://doi.org/10.1016/j.oraloncology.2014.07.015.
47. D'Cruz AK, Vaish R, Kapre N, et al. Elective versus therapeutic neck dissection in node-negative oral cancer. N Engl J Med. 2015;373(6):521–9. https://doi.org/10.1056/NEJMoa1506007.
48. Biau J, Lapeyre M, Troussier I, et al. Selection of lymph node target volumes for definitive head and neck radiation therapy: a 2019 update. Radiother Oncol. 2019;134:1–9. https://doi.org/10.1016/j.radonc.2019.01.018.
49. Koyfman SA, Ismaila N, Crook D, et al. Management of the neck in squamous cell carcinoma of the oral cavity and oropharynx: ASCO clinical practice guideline. JCO. 2019;37(20):1753–74. https://doi.org/10.1200/JCO.18.01921.

50. Peters LJ, Goepfert H, Ang KK, et al. Evaluation of the dose for postoperative radiation therapy of head and neck cancer: first report of a prospective randomized trial. Int J Radiat Oncol Biol Phys. 1993;26(1):3–11. https://doi.org/10.1016/0360-3016(93)90167-T.
51. Ang KK, Foote RL, Klotch DW. Randomized trial addressing risk features and time factors of surgery plus radiotherapy in advanced head-and-neck cancer. Int J Radiat Oncol Biol Phys. 2001;51(3):8.
52. Rosenthal DI, Mohamed ASR, Garden AS, et al. Final report of a prospective randomized trial to evaluate the dose-response relationship for postoperative radiation therapy and pathologic risk groups in patients with head and neck cancer. Int J Radiat Oncol Biol Phys. 2017;98(5):1002–11. https://doi.org/10.1016/j.ijrobp.2017.02.218.
53. Torrecillas V, Shepherd HM, Francis S, et al. Adjuvant radiation for T1-2N1 oral cavity cancer survival outcomes and utilization treatment trends: Analysis of the SEER database. Oral Oncol. 2018;85:1–7. https://doi.org/10.1016/j.oraloncology.2018.07.019.
54. Mazeron JJ, Ardiet JM, Haie-Méder C, et al. GEC-ESTRO recommendations for brachytherapy for head and neck squamous cell carcinomas. Radiother Oncol. 2009;91(2):150–6. https://doi.org/10.1016/j.radonc.2009.01.005.
55. Kovács G, Martinez-Monge R, Budrukkar A, et al. GEC-ESTRO ACROP recommendations for head & neck brachytherapy in squamous cell carcinomas: 1st update – improvement by cross sectional imaging based treatment planning and stepping source technology. Radiother Oncol. 2017;122(2):248–54. https://doi.org/10.1016/j.radonc.2016.10.008.
56. Budrukkar A, Dasgupta A, Pandit P, et al. Clinical outcomes with high-dose-rate surface mould brachytherapy for intra-oral and skin malignancies involving head and neck region. JCB. 2017;3:242–50. https://doi.org/10.5114/jcb.2017.66773.
57. García-Consuegra A, Gimeno Morales M, Cambeiro M, et al. Dose volume histogram constraints in patients with head and neck cancer treated with surgery and adjuvant HDR brachytherapy: a proposal of the head and neck and skin GEC ESTRO Working group. Radiother Oncol. 2021;154:128–34. https://doi.org/10.1016/j.radonc.2020.09.015.
58. Kumar A, Chopra S, Mahantshetty U, Reddy VA. Brachytherapy in India: learning from the past and looking into the future. Brachytherapy. 2020;19(6):861–73. https://doi.org/10.1016/j.brachy.2020.08.019.
59. Bernier J, Ozsahin M, Lefèbvre JL, Maingon P, Cognetti F, van Glabbeke M. Postoperative irradiation with or without concomitant chemotherapy for locally advanced head and neck cancer. N Engl J Med. 2004:8.
60. Cooper JS, Pajak TF, Forastiere AA, et al. Postoperative concurrent radiotherapy and chemotherapy for high-risk squamous-cell carcinoma of the head and neck. N Engl J Med. 2004;350(19):1937–44. https://doi.org/10.1056/NEJMoa032646.
61. Cooper JS, Zhang Q, Pajak TF, et al. Long-term follow-up of the RTOG 9501/Intergroup Phase III Trial: postoperative concurrent radiation therapy and chemotherapy in high-risk squamous cell carcinoma of the head and neck. Int J Radiat Oncol Biol Phys. 2012;84(5):1198–205. https://doi.org/10.1016/j.ijrobp.2012.05.008.
62. Agarwal JP, Kane S, Ghosh-Laskar S, et al. Extranodal extension in resected oral cavity squamous cell carcinoma: more to it than meets the eye. Laryngoscope. 2019;129(5):1130–6. https://doi.org/10.1002/lary.27508.
63. Trifiletti DM, Smith A, Mitra N, et al. Beyond positive margins and extracapsular extension: evaluating the utilization and clinical impact of postoperative chemoradiotherapy in resected locally advanced head and neck cancer. JCO. 2017;35(14):1550–60. https://doi.org/10.1200/JCO.2016.68.2336.
64. Chaukar D, Prabash K, Rane P, et al. Prospective Phase II open-label randomized controlled trial to compare mandibular preservation in upfront surgery with neoadjuvant chemotherapy followed by surgery in operable oral cavity cancer. JCO. 2022;40(3):272–81. https://doi.org/10.1200/JCO.21.00179.
65. Sultania M, Imaduddin M, Deo S, et al. Role of metronomic therapy for advanced oral cancers and predictors of response: multi-institutional feasibility study. Head Neck. 2022;44(1):104–12. https://doi.org/10.1002/hed.26904.
66. Patil V, Noronha V, Dhumal SB, et al. Low-cost oral metronomic chemotherapy versus intravenous cisplatin in patients with recurrent, metastatic, inoperable head and neck carcinoma: an open-label, parallel-group, non-inferiority, randomised, phase 3 trial. Lancet Glob Health. 2020;8(9):e1213–22. https://doi.org/10.1016/S2214-109X(20)30275-8.
67. Banavali S, Vaidya A, Prabhash K, Pai P. Oral metronomic scheduling of anticancer therapy-based treatment compared to existing standard of care in locally advanced oral squamous cell cancers: a matched-pair analysis. Indian J Cancer. 2013;50(2):135. https://doi.org/10.4103/0019-509X.117024.
68. Krishnamurthy S, Ahmed I, Bhise R, Mohanti BK, Sharma A, Rieckmann T, Paterson C, Bonomo P. The dogma of Cetuximab and Radiotherapy in head and neck cancer - A dawn to dusk journey. Clin Transl Radiat Oncol. 2022;34:75-81. https://doi.org/10.1016/j.ctro.2022.03.009.
69. Vaish R, Bajpai J. Alcohol and cancer: waiting for the storm to pass or dancing in the rains! Indian J Med Paediatr Oncol. 2020;41(04):473–5. https://doi.org/10.4103/ijmpo.ijmpo_91_20.
70. Margalit DN, Karam SD, Chua MLK, Anderson C, Kimple RJ. Four influential clinical trials in human papilloma virus-associated oropharynx cancer. Int J Radiat Oncol Biol Phys. 2020;106(5):893–9. https://doi.org/10.1016/j.ijrobp.2019.12.015.

71. Nair D, Mair M, Singh A, D'Cruz A. Prevalence and impact of human papillomavirus on head and neck cancers: review of Indian studies. Indian J Surg Oncol. 2018;9(4):568–75. https://doi.org/10.1007/s13193-018-0813-z.
72. Kiyota N, Tahara M, Mizusawa J, et al. Weekly cisplatin plus radiation for postoperative head and neck cancer (JCOG1008): a multicenter, noninferiority, Phase II/III Randomized Controlled Trial. JCO:2022:JCO.21.01293. https://doi.org/10.1200/JCO.21.01293.
73. Economopoulou P, Kotsantis I, Psyrri A. De-escalating strategies in HPV-associated head and neck squamous cell carcinoma. Viruses. 2021;13(9):1787. https://doi.org/10.3390/v13091787.
74. Gillison ML, Trotti AM, Harris J, et al. Radiotherapy plus cetuximab or cisplatin in human papillomavirus-positive oropharyngeal cancer (NRG Oncology RTOG 1016): a randomised, multicentre, non-inferiority trial. Lancet. 2019;393(10166):40–50. https://doi.org/10.1016/S0140-6736(18)32779-X.
75. Mehanna H, Robinson M, Hartley A, et al. Radiotherapy plus cisplatin or cetuximab in low-risk human papillomavirus-positive oropharyngeal cancer (De-ESCALaTE HPV): an open-label randomised controlled phase 3 trial. Lancet. 2019;393(10166):51–60. https://doi.org/10.1016/S0140-6736(18)32752-1.
76. Rischin D, King M, Kenny L, et al. Randomized trial of radiation therapy with weekly cisplatin or cetuximab in low-risk HPV-associated oropharyngeal cancer (TROG 12.01) – a Trans-Tasman radiation oncology group study. Int J Radiat Oncol Biol Phys. 2021;111(4):876–86. https://doi.org/10.1016/j.ijrobp.2021.04.015.
77. Chera BS, Amdur RJ, Green R, et al. Phase II Trial of de-intensified chemoradiotherapy for human papillomavirus–associated oropharyngeal squamous cell carcinoma. JCO. 2019;37(29):2661–9. https://doi.org/10.1200/JCO.19.01007.
78. Yom SS, Torres-Saavedra P, Caudell JJ, et al. Reduced-dose radiation therapy for HPV-associated oropharyngeal carcinoma (NRG oncology HN002). J Clin Oncol. 39(9):19.
79. Marur S, Li S, Cmelak AJ, et al. E1308: Phase II Trial of induction chemotherapy followed by reduced-dose radiation and weekly cetuximab in patients with HPV-associated resectable squamous cell carcinoma of the oropharynx – ECOG-ACRIN Cancer Research Group. JCO. 2017;35(5):490–7. https://doi.org/10.1200/JCO.2016.68.3300.
80. Swisher-McClure S, Lukens JN, Aggarwal C, et al. A Phase 2 Trial of alternative volumes of oropharyngeal irradiation for de-intensification (AVOID): omission of the resected primary tumor bed after transoral robotic surgery for Human Papilloma Virus–related squamous cell carcinoma of the oropharynx. Int J Radiat Oncol Biol Phys. 2020;106(4):725–32. https://doi.org/10.1016/j.ijrobp.2019.11.021.
81. Nichols AC, Theurer J, Prisman E, et al. Radiotherapy versus transoral robotic surgery and neck dissection for oropharyngeal squamous cell carcinoma (ORATOR): an open-label, phase 2, randomised trial. Lancet Oncol. 2019;20(10):1349–59. https://doi.org/10.1016/S1470-2045(19)30410-3.
82. Nichols AC, Theurer J, Prisman E, et al. Randomized trial of radiotherapy versus transoral robotic surgery for oropharyngeal squamous cell carcinoma: long-term results of the ORATOR trial. JCO. 2022;40(8):866–75. https://doi.org/10.1200/JCO.21.01961.
83. Palma DA, Prisman E, Berthelet E, et al. Assessment of Toxic effects and survival in treatment deescalation with radiotherapy vs transoral surgery for HPV-associated oropharyngeal squamous cell carcinoma: the ORATOR2 Phase 2 Randomized Clinical Trial. JAMA Oncol. 2022; https://doi.org/10.1001/jamaoncol.2022.0615.
84. Nutting CM, Morden JP, Harrington KJ, et al. Parotid-sparing intensity modulated versus conventional radiotherapy in head and neck cancer (PARSPORT): a phase 3 multicentre randomised controlled trial. Lancet Oncol. 2011;12(2):127–36. https://doi.org/10.1016/S1470-2045(10)70290-4.
85. Chao KSC, Wippold FJ, Ozyigit G, Tran BN, Dempsey JF. Determination and delineation of nodal target volumes for head-and-neck cancer based on patterns of failure in patients receiving definitive and postoperative IMRT. Int J Radiat Oncol Biol Phys. 2002;53(5):1174–84. https://doi.org/10.1016/S0360-3016(02)02881-X.
86. Grégoire V, Ang K, Budach W, et al. Delineation of the neck node levels for head and neck tumors: a 2013 update. DAHANCA, EORTC, HKNPCSG, NCIC CTG, NCRI, RTOG, TROG consensus guidelines. Radiother Oncol. 2014;110(1):172–81. https://doi.org/10.1016/j.radonc.2013.10.010.
87. Yeung AR, Garg MK, Lawson J, et al. ACR appropriateness criteria® ipsilateral radiation for squamous cell carcinoma of the tonsil. Head Neck. 2012;34(5):613–6. https://doi.org/10.1002/hed.21993.
88. Vermorken JB, Remenar E, van Herpen C, et al. Cisplatin, fluorouracil, and docetaxel in unresectable head and neck cancer. N Engl J Med. 2007;357(17):1695–704. https://doi.org/10.1056/NEJMoa071028.
89. Posner MR, Hershock DM, Blajman CR, et al. Cisplatin and fluorouracil alone or with docetaxel in head and neck cancer. N Engl J Med. 2007;357(17):1705–15. https://doi.org/10.1056/NEJMoa070956.
90. Garden AS, Dong L, Morrison WH, et al. Patterns of disease recurrence following treatment of oropharyngeal cancer with intensity modulated radiation therapy. Int J Radiat Oncol Biol Phys. 2013;85(4):941–7. https://doi.org/10.1016/j.ijrobp.2012.08.004.
91. Sinha S, Agarwal JP, Mahajan A, et al. Implications of limited exolaryngeal disease and cricoarytenoid

joint involvement in organ conservation protocols for laryngopharyngeal cancers: results from a prospective study. Head Neck. 2021;43(4):1289–99. https://doi.org/10.1002/hed.26593.
92. Pignon JP, Bourhis J, Domenge C, Designé L. Chemotherapy added to locoregional treatment for head and neck squamous-cell carcinoma: three meta-analyses of updated individual data. Lancet. 2000;355:7.
93. Forastiere AA, Goepfert H, Maor M, et al. Concurrent chemotherapy and radiotherapy for organ preservation in advanced laryngeal cancer. N Engl J Med. 2003;349(22):2091–8. https://doi.org/10.1056/NEJMoa031317.
94. Yamazaki H, Nishiyama K, Tanaka E, Koizumi M, Chatani M. Radiotherapy for early glottic carcinoma (T1N0M0): results of prospective randomized study of radiation fraction size and overall treatment time. Int J Radiat Oncol Biol Phys. 2006;64(1):77–82. https://doi.org/10.1016/j.ijrobp.2005.06.014.
95. Laskar SG, Sinha S, Singh M, et al. Post-cricoid and upper oesophagus cancers treated with organ preservation using intensity-modulated image-guided radiotherapy: a Phase II prospective study of outcomes, toxicity and quality of life. Clin Oncol. 2022;34(4):220–9. https://doi.org/10.1016/j.clon.2021.11.012.
96. Lefebvre JL, Andry G, Chevalier D, et al. Laryngeal preservation with induction chemotherapy for hypopharyngeal squamous cell carcinoma: 10-year results of EORTC trial 24891. Ann Oncol. 2012;23(10):2708–14. https://doi.org/10.1093/annonc/mds065.
97. Cohen EEW, Karrison TG, Kocherginsky M, et al. Phase III Randomized Trial of induction chemotherapy in patients with N2 or N3 locally advanced head and neck cancer. JCO. 2014;32(25):2735–43. https://doi.org/10.1200/JCO.2013.54.6309.
98. Haddad R, O'Neill A, Rabinowits G, et al. Induction chemotherapy followed by concurrent chemoradiotherapy (sequential chemoradiotherapy) versus concurrent chemoradiotherapy alone in locally advanced head and neck cancer (PARADIGM): a randomised phase 3 trial. Lancet Oncol. 2013;14(3):257–64. https://doi.org/10.1016/S1470-2045(13)70011-1.
99. Peng G, Wang T, Yu YK, et al. A prospective, randomized study comparing outcomes and toxicities of intensity-modulated radiotherapy vs. conventional two-dimensional radiotherapy for the treatment of nasopharyngeal carcinoma. Radiother Oncol. 2012;104(3):286–93. https://doi.org/10.1016/j.radonc.2012.08.013.
100. Lee AW, Ng WT, Pan JJ, et al. International guideline for the delineation of the clinical target volumes (CTV) for nasopharyngeal carcinoma. Radiother Oncol. 2018;126(1):25–36. https://doi.org/10.1016/j.radonc.2017.10.032.
101. Sun XS, Michel C, Babin E, et al. Approach to oligometastatic disease in head and neck cancer, on behalf of the GORTEC. Future Oncol. 2018;14(9):877–89. https://doi.org/10.2217/fon-2017-0468.
102. Tan TH, Soon YY, Cheo T, et al. Induction chemotherapy for locally advanced nasopharyngeal carcinoma treated with concurrent chemoradiation: a systematic review and meta-analysis. Radiother Oncol. 2018;129(1):10–7. https://doi.org/10.1016/j.radonc.2018.02.027.
103. Zhang Y, Chen L, Hu GQ, et al. Gemcitabine and cisplatin induction chemotherapy in nasopharyngeal carcinoma. N Engl J Med. 2019;381(12):1124–35. https://doi.org/10.1056/NEJMoa1905287.
104. Ghosh-Laskar S, Pilar A, Johnny C, et al. Clinical outcomes for nasopharyngeal cancer with intracranial extension after taxane-based induction chemotherapy and concurrent chemo-radiotherapy in the modern era. World J Otorhinolaryngol Head Neck Surg. 2020;6(1):25–33. https://doi.org/10.1016/j.wjorl.2020.02.003.
105. Geiger JL, Ismaila N, Beadle B, et al. Management of salivary gland malignancy: ASCO guideline. JCO. 2021;39(17):1909–41. https://doi.org/10.1200/JCO.21.00449.
106. Bible KC, Kebebew E, Brierley J, et al. 2021 American Thyroid Association Guidelines for Management of Patients with Anaplastic Thyroid Cancer: American Thyroid Association Anaplastic Thyroid Cancer Guidelines Task Force. Thyroid. 2021;31(3):337–86. https://doi.org/10.1089/thy.2020.0944.
107. Maghami E, Ismaila N, Alvarez A, et al. Diagnosis and management of squamous cell carcinoma of unknown primary in the head and neck: ASCO guideline. JCO. 2020;38(22):2570–96. https://doi.org/10.1200/JCO.20.00275.
108. Ho AS, Kraus DH, Ganly I, Lee NY, Shah JP, Morris LGT. Decision making in the management of recurrent head and neck cancer: salvage options for recurrent head and neck cancer. Head Neck. 2014;36(1):144–51. https://doi.org/10.1002/hed.23227.
109. Ward MC, Riaz N, Caudell JJ, et al. Refining patient selection for reirradiation of head and neck squamous carcinoma in the IMRT era: a multi-institution Cohort Study by the MIRI collaborative. Int J Radiat Oncol Biol Phys. 2018;100(3):586–94. https://doi.org/10.1016/j.ijrobp.2017.06.012.
110. Suárez C, Fernández-Alvarez V, Hamoir M, et al. Carotid blowout syndrome: modern trends in management. CMAR. 2018;10:5617–28. https://doi.org/10.2147/CMAR.S180164.
111. Uppaluri R, Haddad RI, Tao Y, Le Tourneau C, Lee NY, Westra W et al. KEYNOTE-689 Investigators. Neoadjuvant and Adjuvant Pembrolizumab in Locally Advanced Head and Neck Cancer. N Engl J Med. 2025;393:37–50.
112. Burtness B, Harrington KJ, Greil R, Soulières D, Tahara M, de Castro G Jr et al. KEYNOTE-048 Investigators. Pembrolizumab alone or with che-

motherapy versus cetuximab with chemotherapy for recurrent or metastatic squamous cell carcinoma of the head and neck (KEYNOTE-048): a randomised, open-label, phase 3 study. Lancet. 2019 Nov 23;394:1915–1928.
113. Bentzen SM, Rosenblatt E, Gupta T, Agarwal JP, Ghosh Laskar S, Bhasker S, et al. Randomized Controlled Trial of Hypofractionated vs. Normofractionated Accelerated Radiation Therapy with or without Cisplatin for Locally Advanced Head and Neck Squamous Cell Carcinoma (HYPNO). Int J Radiat Oncol Biol Phys. 2023;117(4):e2.
114. Frank SJ, Busse PM, Lee JJ, Rosenthal DI, Hernandez M, Swanson DM et al et al University of Texas MD Anderson Cancer Center Clinical Trial Consortium. Proton versus photon radiotherapy for patients with oropharyngeal cancer in the USA: a multicentre, randomised, open-label, non-inferiority phase 3 trial. Lancet. 2025;11:S0140-6736(25)01962–2.

Online Links

https://www.youtube.com/watch?v=hvhKhMcfxY4
https://www.youtube.com/watch?v=tDdau-4kvCg
https://www.youtube.com/watch?v=t4urLOZ2WVc
https://www.youtube.com/watch?v=dWj5-sc8Wpo
https://www.youtube.com/watch?v=E1HrCVdOViU
OAR of H&N. https://www.thegreenjournal.com/article/S0167-8140(15)00401-6/fulltext

Skin Cancer

Saikat Das and Anusheel Munshi

1 Introduction

Due to the general aging population and the fashion trend of sun exposure, nonmelanoma skin cancer (NMSC) is rising [1]. The management of NMSC is difficult and necessitates a multidisciplinary team (i.e., pathologists, dermatologists, medical oncologists, surgeons, and radiation oncologists) [2]. There are situations when surgery is not an option or will cause unacceptable functional morbidity. In such cases, radiation therapy (RT) may be a preferred tissue-preserving option. Whether used alone or in combination with other treatments, RT has been shown to be quite effective in terms of cosmetic results and local control. Contact hypofractionated RT, brachytherapy, and electronic brachytherapy are all promising new treatments. However, rigorous, randomized trials are missing, explaining the disparity in dose, fractionation, and technique recommendations. Therefore, it is essential that interdisciplinary teams better understand RT modalities, benefits, and drawbacks. This chapter will provide the role and indications for RT in patients with NMSC.

S. Das (✉)
Department of Radiation Oncology,
All India Institute of Medical Sciences Bhopal,
Bhopal, Madhya Pradesh, India
e-mail: Saikat.radiotherapy@aiimsbhopal.edu.in

A. Munshi (✉)
Department of Radiation Oncology,
BLK Max Hospital, New Delhi, Delhi, India

2 Anatomy

The skin is the largest organ of the human body and the incidence of skin malignancies is reported separately from other neoplasms in various registries of the world. Skin is a complex organ in which precisely regulated cellular and molecular interactions govern many crucial responses to our environment. The skin is divided into two distinct parts, the superficial part, the epidermis and the deep part, the dermis. The epidermis is a stratified epithelium whose cells become flattened as they mature and rise to the surface. Melanocytes within the epidermis are cells responsible for the production of a brown pigment (melanin). This pigment also represents an important endogenous screen against harmful ultraviolet rays. Squamous epithelial cells are major sites for the biosynthesis of soluble molecules (cytokines) important in the functional regulation of adjacent epidermal cells. Langerhans cells are dendritic histiocytic cells that take up and process antigenic signals and communicate this information to lymphoid cells. The dermis is composed of dense connective tissue containing many blood vessels, lymphatic vessels, and nerves. The dermis of the skin is connected to the underlying deep fascia or bones by the superficial fascia, otherwise known as subcutaneous tissue. The appendages of the skin are the nails, hair follicles, sebaceous glands, and sweat glands.

B. K. Mohanti et al. (eds.), *Radiation Oncology – Principles, Precepts and Practice*,
https://doi.org/10.1007/978-981-95-5171-2_4

3 Epidemiology

The incidence of the skin cancers is sporadic in various parts of the world. The majority of skin cancers are either basal cell carcinoma (BCC) or squamous cell carcinoma (SCC), the so-called nonmelanomatous skin cancers (NMSC). The nonmelanoma skin cancer is commonest in all parts of the world, with Australia reporting the highest burden of age-standardised rate, 37.0 per 100,00 population [1, 2]. Basal and squamous cell carcinoma, or nonmelanoma skin cancers, are the most common malignancies in the United States, with more cases than all other cancers combined [3, 4]. When comparing the two, basal cell carcinoma is four to five times more common than squamous cell carcinoma.

Skin cancers commonly occur due to the exposure to the actinic radiation and ultraviolet radiation especially in melanin deficient skin of the white people. In India, the documented incidence of skin cancer is not complete and accounts for less than 1% of all cancers [5]. The incidence of melanomatous skin lesions all over the world is 30–40 times less common than basal and squamous cell carcinomas. However as stated above, the exact incidence is not available in the Indian context. The most comprehensive epidemiological study has been reported from Australia, and 4.6% of persons aged 20–69 years in Queensland had skin cancer (commonly BCC), and 40% of the surveyed population had solar keratosis [6]. Melanoma accounts for 1.7% of global cancer diagnoses and is the fifth most common cancer in the United States. Melanoma incidence is rising in developed, predominantly fair-skinned countries, growing over 320% in the United States since 1975.

4 Etiology/Risk Factors

Three main types of skin cancers include

(a) Basal cell carcinoma (BCC)
(b) Squamous cell carcinoma (SCC)
(c) Melanoma

BCC and SCC are the most common forms of skin cancer and together are referred to as nonmelanoma skin cancers (NMSC). Other malignant disorders of skin include

- Cutaneous T-cell lymphomas (e.g., mycosis fungoides)
- Kaposi sarcoma
- Merkel cell carcinoma
- Extramammary Paget disease
- Apocrine skin carcinoma
- Cutaneous metastasis from various primary sites

In majority of skin cancers, the etiology is clear. Various etiologic agents have been attributed to skin cancers. The solar radiation, especially actinic and ionizing component, are detrimental to the skin. Melanin usually protects the skin from ·the damaging effect of the ultraviolet radiation. The exposure to ultraviolet radiation also increases the risk of skin cancer. There are three types of ultraviolet radiation, that is, UV-A, UV-B, and UV-C. The UV-B radiation falls in the range of 290–320 nm spectrum and has carcinogenic potential. The majority of skin cancers (BCC and SCC) occur over the sun exposed areas of the body. Chemical carcinogens including hydrocarbons also play a role in the etiology of skin cancer (Table 1).

Melanoma is most common in white, older men, with an average age of diagnosis of 65. The main risk factor is outdoor UV exposure. Indoor tanning beds, immunosuppression, family history and rare congenital diseases, moles, and obesity also contribute to the disease.

Table 1 Risk factors for non-melanoma skin cancers

UV radiation exposure/sunlight/tanning beds
History of sunburns
Light complexion and eye color
Family history or personal history of BCC, SCC, actinic keratosis, familial dysplastic nevus syndrome, or atypical nevi
Chronic cutaneous inflammation (long standing ulcers)
Immune suppression (including organ transplant patients)
Environmental exposure (arsenic/therapeutic radiation)

Table 2 Investigations for nonmelanoma skin cancer (NMSC)

1	Histology/cytology (skin scrape, punch biopsy, excision biopsy)
2	FNAC of enlarged lymph nodes
3	Imaging in high risk sites to delineate deep extent and bone or cartilage involvement (CT/MRI/PET CT)

5 Diagnositic Workup (NMSC)

A comprehensive clinical history and detailed physical examination is critical for the evaluation of skin cancer. The draining lymph node basins should be thoroughly palpated. Tissue biopsy (e.g., shave, punch, or excisional) remains the standard of care for diagnosing nonmelanoma skin cancers (Table 2). Biopsies should include the deep reticular dermis for adequate evaluation of invasive disease. Clinicians need to be aware of the false negative rates of the sampling error with punch and shave biopsies. A more aggressive histologic subtype may be missed in 10%–20% of cases [7].

6 Management Principles

Skin being a visible site with low metastatic potential, most patients of nonmelanomatous skin cancers present with early disease. Management is guided by stage of disease and cosmetic aspects. Factors deciding the approach to management of skin cancer include lesion location, size and extent, stage of disease, histology subtype age/performance status of patient. Whenever a carcinoma of the sweat gland or sebaceous gland is suspected, preference should be given to surgical removal. Surgery often is indicated for the treatment of carcinomas that have recurred after previous adequate or inadequate therapy of various kinds. In the treatment of nodal metastases from primary lesions of skin, a radical dissection of the lymph nodes is the logical therapeutic approach, since radiation therapy is likely to achieve a poor control.

7 Management Modalities

7.1 Mohs Micrographic Surgery

It is a form of tumor excision that involves progressive radial sectioning. It incorporates real-time examination of the resection margins until adequate uninvolved margins have been achieved. The goal is to achieve the narrowest margins necessary to avoid tumor recurrence while maximally preserving cosmesis. However, because the technique removes tumor growing in contiguity, it may miss noncontiguous in-transit cutaneous micrometastases. Hence, some practitioners remove an additional margin of skin in high-risk lesions, even after the Mohs surgical procedure has confirmed uninvolved margins [8]. In small case series, Mohs surgery has been associated with a lower local recurrence rate than the other local modalities [9, 10]. However, there are no randomized trials allowing direct comparison.

7.2 Curettage and Electrodesiccation (C&D)

Electrodessication and curettage, requires local anesthesia, uses mechanical debridement and electrocoagulation to denature and remove visible tumor. Given its destructive properties, electrodessication and curettage does not allow for histologic margin assessment. In addition, it leaves an open wound that is left to heal by secondary intention, which can result in an unsightly, hypopigmented scar. C&D should be reserved for lesions located in non–hair-bearing areas, as post-operative alopecia can result. It is a good method for treating tumors in older patients for whom a prolonged or extensive surgical procedure might be more difficult. In general, C&D can be used either for SCCs or BCCs, however, it is more commonly used for BCCs. The C&D is simplest form of treatment for superficial cutaneous lesions, but whenever there is suspicion of deeper invasion in SCCs or BCCs (morphea form) this technique is not suitable. Sites such as forehead, ear, eyes, nose, or face commonly recur, therefore, this technique is not advocated in these areas. The cosmetic results are surprisingly good in curettage and dessication. Also, because neoplastic cells can extend down hair follicles, this superficial destructive treatment can lead to incomplete removal and an increased recurrence rate [11]. Hence, the proper technique of curettage scraping and electrodessication to a distance of 2–4 mm into the normal appearing tissue should be practiced. If there is any doubt as to the diagnosis, a prior biopsy should be taken. This technique is based on the difference in the consistency between the tumor and the surrounding normal tissue. Cure rates with this technique range from 77% to 97% [11]. In low-risk basal cell carcinoma and squamous cell carcinoma lesions, C&D has shown similar 5-year recurrence rates of 3%–9% compared to surgical excision [12, 13].

7.3 Topical Agents, Photodynamic Therapy, or Cryotherapy

"Superficial" or "shallow" nonmelanoma skin cancer (NMSC) lesions are defined as being contained to the epidermis and superficial papillary dermis [14]. Three categories of treatment options for these lesions exist, including topical agents, photodynamic therapy, or cryotherapy. Among topical therapies, imiquimod 5% is a novel immune modifier, capable of inducing local production of cytokines. It has been used successfully in a number of NMSCs, including Bowen's disease and Basal cell carcinoma. The drug 5-fluorouracil has been used in the treatment of actinic keratoses as well as BCCs. Topical tazarotene gel (0.05%) has been reported to treat Bowenoid papulosis of the genitalia [5]. Topical agents promote apoptosis of malignant skin cells by means of inhibition of DNA synthesis and activation of the cell-mediated immune response. These therapies are highly effective in the treatment of superficial, low-risk basal cell carcinoma and squamous cell carcinoma lesions, with 5-year recurrence rates ranging from 10% to 16% [15, 16].

Laser Surgery The CO_2 laser is an infrared laser beam and when the beam is focused, it is used to vaporize cutaneous lesions such as basal cell carcinomas, superficial SCC, and nonmalignant conditions like solar keratosis [17]. The laser can also be used along with curettage.

Liquid Nitrogen Cryosurgery Cryotherapy, usually with liquid nitrogen, is a non-invasive procedure. The twice repeated I-min freeze and thaw cycle necessary for cryotherapy leaves a wound for 3–4 weeks. They often heal with a fairly acceptable scar and sometimes with not much more change than hypopigmentation. This procedure can be performed easily at the bed side. However, this method does not provide tissue for histopathological study. It is easier to treat wider margins with cryotherapy than it is with excision or C&D. Optimally administered cryosurgery is a good treatment for superficial BCCs and SCCs. The favorable sites include ears, face, neck, eyelids, and trunk.

7.4 Radiation Therapy in NMSC

Radiation therapy has the advantage of being painless and it provides minimal morbidity and excellent healing. Radiation therapy is usually indicated in the treatment of lesions on the face (nose, lip, eyelid, and canthus) where surgery is either technically difficult or likely to yield poor cosmesis. Radiotherapy is not generally satisfactory once tumor has invaded underlying bone or cartilage. General principles of radiation therapy (1) the dose should be calculated at the depth (not the surface) of the tumor. (2) Basal cell carcinoma usually requires the same dose as squamous cell cancer. (3) The energy of the beam is selected, so that the dose to the base of the lesion is not less than 50% of that to the surface.

7.5 Indications for Radiotherapy in NMSC

(a) Preferred for lesions that would require reconstructive surgery, where irradiation

may be considered to produce better cosmesis, e.g., nose, upper and lower eyelid (preferably avoid the middle third of the upper eyelid), the lip and lesions involving the commissure of mouth, the nasolabial sulcus, lesions arising in the pre and post auricular areas and the ear
(b) Large superficial lesions
(c) Older patients
(d) Patients who refuse or are unfit for surgery (RT does not need anaesthesia)
(e) Post-surgery: for incomplete/marginal excision, perineural invasion

Radiotherapy should be used with caution in the following circumstances as some skin sites tolerate radiotherapy poorly:

(a) Sites of previous burns
(b) Sites of prior radiotherapy
(c) Fragile "tissue-paper" skin after steroids
(d) Areas of vascular insufficiency
(e) Middle third of the upper eyelid
(f) The skin of the back overlying the spine (this being an area of skin placed under pressure, leading to compromised healing, and late skin necrosis)
(g) The skin overlying the shin and malleoli of the lower leg (the skin is under tension, and there may be impaired healing)

RT is contraindicated for genetic conditions predisposing to skin cancer (e.g., basal cell nevus syndrome) and relatively contraindicated for patients with connective tissue diseases (e.g., scleroderma).

In patients with squamous cell or basal cell carcinoma of the skin, clinically uninvolved regional nodes are not irradiated electively.

8 Simulation: All Skin Cancers (NMSC and Melanomas)

Informed consent is obtained. Patients are treated in a position that best suits the location of the lesion. Immobilization is achieved as appropriate. Low energy photons or electrons are used. Generally, lesions around the eye, ear, nose, and those with an irregular border will require a customized lead cut-out, necessitating a prior mold room appointment. All other areas are treated as "mark on set" using standard lead cutouts to shield the nontarget areas using the appropriate thickness of lead.

The eye requires special protection when eyelids are treated. A spatula (if one eyelid involved) or a lead contact eye shield (if both eyelids involved) is inserted under local anaesthetic (LA) to protect the cornea, the lens and uninvolved eyelid (with spatula). Patients' will require an eye pad for 2–3 h after the procedure until the LA effect is reversed and corneal reflex restored. Ensure that patient has an escort, as he/she may not be able to drive back. The nasal septum and gum are respectively shielded when lower nose and lip are treated. Wax or aluminum is used to cover the lead shield to absorb electron backscatter.

9 Target Volumes

(a) All patients are examined under a bright light with a magnifying glass.
(b) Squamous cell carcinoma [SCC]: Planning target volume (PTV) = Gross tumor volume (GTV) + 1 cm margin all around laterally and 5 mm or more deep according to clinician's discretion. NB consider electrons for tumor thickness over 5 mm and if the tumor is attached to bone or cartilage or is up against bone, discuss with physics.
(c) Basal cell carcinoma [BCC]: PTV = GTV + 0.5 cm margin laterally (1 cm if morphoeic, large, or poorly defined) and 0.5 cm deep margin. If on mobile skin, a 0.25 cm deep margin is adequate.
(d) For electron therapy, an additional 0.5 cm margin is required laterally to account for penumbra of the electrons.
(e) Clinical photographs are taken for record, clearly indicating the site, extent of lesion and orientation of the photograph.
(f) For extensive perineural invasion, clinically evident perineural involvement, or involve-

ment of named nerves (particularly in the head and neck region), consider including the course of the local nerves proximally.

(g) In the setting of clinically evident perineural invasion (PNI) (or if grossly radiographically involved) for head and neck CSCCs, comprehensive coverage of involved cranial nerve pathways in addition to proximal local nerves should be considered.

- RT is contraindicated for genetic conditions predisposing to skin cancer (e.g., basal cell nevus)

9.1 Energy/Modality

Aim to cover PTV with the 90% isodose, both laterally and at depth.

Low energy photons or electrons are used depending on depth, site, size, and availability. Avoid electrons near eyes (lateral scatter) and for field sizes <4 cm. If the external auditory meatus is included in the electron field, a wax block should be used to avoid funneling effect on the eardrum. Try and avoid superficial X-rays over cartilage and bone due to risk of radionecrosis (absorption by photoelectric effect).

When using electrons, discuss "build-up" (bolus) requirements with physicist, to bring the skin dose to 90% or more, and encompass the target depth with the 90% isodose.

Photons of low voltage deliver almost 100% to the skin, and so do not require "build-up."

The depth dose characteristics of the beam depend on energy and field size

9.2 Dose Prescription

Prescriptions are applied doses (D_{max}) for photons, and to the 100% isodose for electrons (follow ICRU guidelines). Doses depend upon lesion size, histology, and patient characteristics (Table 3). For small and favorable location skin cancers, hypofractionated RT is commonly used. Protracted fractionation should be utilized for poorly vascularized or cartilaginous areas and can be associated with improved cosmetic results in such situations.

Table 3 Dose schedule options for basal cell carcinoma and squamous cell carcinoma

Indication	Dose
Small tumors where cosmesis is relatively unimportant	18 Gy/1#
For small lesions ≤4 cm diameter but not when over cartilage	32.5 Gy/5#/1 week
Target size up to 5–6 cm diameter; this can be given as alternate day fractions over a 3 week period if patient access to hospital is limited, or in the elderly	40.5 Gy/9#/2–3 weeks
Target < 6 cm, in areas of poor radiation tolerance	55 Gy/20#/4 weeks
Target is between 4 and 6 cm diameter and not in an area of poor radiation tolerance	50 Gy/15#/3 weeks
Target > 6 cm in areas of poor radiation tolerance	60 Gy/30#/6 weeks

10 Basal Cell and Squamous Cell Carcinoma (NMSC)

BCC is at least three times more common than SCC in non-immunocompromised patients. It usually occurs on sun-exposed areas of skin, with the nose being the most common site. Although there are many different clinical presentations for BCC, the most characteristic type is the asymptomatic nodular or nodular ulcerative lesion that is elevated from the surrounding skin, has a pearly quality, and contains telangiectatic vessels [18]. BCCs are composed of non-keratinizing cells derived from the basal cell layer of the epidermis. They are slow growing and rarely metastasize. BCC has a tendency to be locally destructive and can result in serious deforming damage if left untreated or if local recurrences cannot be completely excised (Fig. 1).

High-risk areas for tumor recurrence after initial treatment include the central face (e.g., periorbital region, eyelids, nasolabial fold, or nose-cheek angle), postauricular region, pinna, ear canal, forehead, and scalp [19]. Morpheaform type is a specific BCC subtype. This subtype typically appears as a scar-like, firm plaque. Because of indistinct clinical tumor margins, morphea form type is difficult to treat adequately with traditional treatments [20]. BCCs often have a char-

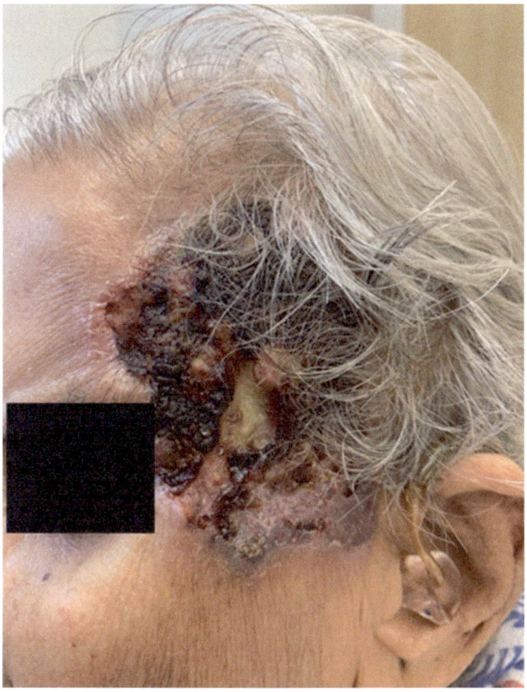

Fig. 1 Basal cell carcinoma of the outer canthus of the left eye. (Courtesy: Anusheel Munshi, Head, Radiation Oncology, Manipal Hospital, Delhi)

acteristic mutation in the PTCH1 tumor suppressor gene, although the mechanism of carcinogenesis is not clear [21].

Basal cell carcinomas and squamous cell carcinomas share some of the same high-risk features, including poorly defined borders, recurrent lesion, immunosuppressed patient, site of prior radiotherapy, perineural involvement, and aggressive histologic subtype. Aggressive histologic subtypes for basal cell carcinoma include morpheaform, basosquamous, sclerosing, mixed infiltrative, or micronodular. These are more likely to recur than nodular basal cell carcinoma; superficial basal cell carcinoma; and nonaggressive subtypes such as keratotic variant, infundibulocystic variant, and fibroepithelioma of Pinkus.

Squamous cell carcinoma is the other variant in NMSC (Fig. 2). Aggressive histologic subtypes for squamous cell carcinoma include adenoid (acantholytic), adenosquamous, desmoplastic (showing mucin production), or metaplastic (carcinosarcomatous). These subtypes can

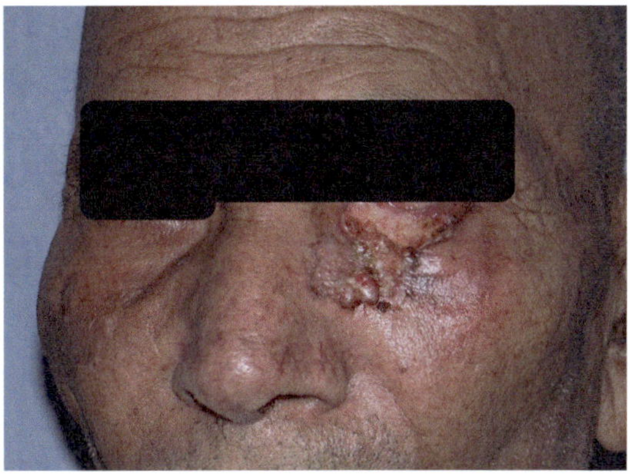

Fig. 2 Squamous cell carcinoma of the eyelid. (Courtesy: Dr. SVS Deo, Head, Department of Surgical Oncology, IRCH, AIIMS, New Delhi)

have very high recurrence rates ranging from 20% to 80%.

In addition, the size and location criteria for high-risk basal cell carcinoma/squamous cell carcinoma lesions include tumor size greater than or equal to 20 mm in the trunk or extremities. Further, these lesions can also develop in background of genetic syndromes (Fig. 3).

As already stated, the primary goals of treatment of NMSC is the complete removal of the tumor and the maximal preservation of function and cosmesis. Treatment decisions should be preferably customized to account for the particular patient and disease factors, incorporating the patient's preference wherever possible. Risk stratification is an important part of the evaluation process (Table 4). For low-risk NMSC, single modality treatment with an appropriate local treatment modality is sufficient. This can be surgical approach, radiation therapy approach or any of the local approached described in previous section. If a surgical approach is chosen, then it is only in margin positive cases (with challenges in revising margins) that additional radiotherapy is needed.

For high risk NMSC radiation therapy is often required even after surgical approach. For patient not suitable for surgical approached, RT alone with or without systemic therapy should be considered.

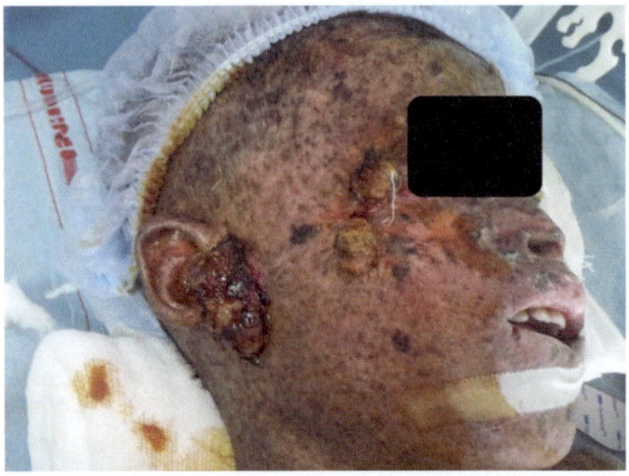

Fig. 3 Basal cell carcinoma and squamous cell carcinoma (mixed type) in a case of xeroderma pigmentosum. (Courtesy: Dr. SVS Deo, Head, Department of Surgical Oncology, IRCH, AIIMS, New Delhi)

Table 4 Classifying low-risk and igh-risk basal and squamous cell carcinoma

Characteristic	Low-risk	High-risk
Location		
Trunk and extremities	Any lesion <2 cm	Any lesion ≥2 cm
Forehead, scalp, cheeks, neck, pretibia	Any lesion <1 cm	Any lesion ≥1 cm
Genitalia, hands, feet, mask area of face	N/A	Any sized lesion
Site of prior radiation therapy	No	Yes
Borders	Well-defined	Ill defined
Primary vs. recurrent	Primary	Recurrent
Aggressive histologic subtypes (for SCC)	No	Yes
Perineural involvement/ neurologic symptoms	No	Yes
Immunosuppression	No	Yes
Chronic inflammation in skin	No	Yes
Rapidly growing	No	Yes
Poorly differentiated	No	Yes
Depth of invasion ≥ 2 mm	No	Yes
Clark level IV or V	No	Yes
Lymphovascular invasion	No	Yes

11 Systemic Therapy

Concurrent systemic therapy with RT can be considered for some cases of local, high-risk/very-high-risk CSCC in case of positive margins. It is unclear which systemic therapies are appropriate for localized disease in the context of concomitant RT. Some systemic therapy options for use with RT include cisplatin or epidermal growth factor receptor (EGFR) inhibitors (e.g., cetuximab, erlotinib, or gefitinib) Cisplatin + 5-fluorouracil (5-FU) and carboplatin ± paclitaxel. For complicated cases of locally advanced disease in which curative surgery and curative RT are not feasible, multidisciplinary consultation is recommended to consider systemic therapy alone. In a landmark, multicenter, phase II trial (ERIVANCE study), oral vismodegib resulted in 43% and 30% response rates in basal cell carcinoma patients with locally advanced and metastatic disease, respectively [22]. Similarly, sonidegib has shown promising results in advanced cases of basal cell carcinoma [23]. However, both of these drugs are not very well tolerated, with 30%–32% of patients experiencing mild adverse effects (e.g., muscle spasms, alopecia, taste disturbance, weight loss, and fatigue).

Table 5 present the outcomes in primary low-risk and high-risk basal and squamous cell carcinomas.

Table 5 Recurrence rates and outcomes with different treatment modalities (in primary NMSC)

Treatment modality	5-Year recurrence rate
Standard surgical excision	4%–10% BCC; 8% SCC
Radiation therapy	15%
Low-risk lesions post standard surgical excision	2%–5% BCC; 8%–10% SCC
Electrodessication and curettage	3%–9% BCC/ SCC
Radiation therapy	5%–15% BCC/ SCC
Superficial, low-risk lesions topical 5-FU or imiquimod	10%–15% BCC/ SCC
Photodynamic therapy	5%–20% BCC/ SCC
Cryotherapy	1%–10% BCC/ SCC
High-risk lesions post Mohs micrographic surgery	1% BCC; 3%–5% SCC

Special Clinical Situations These may require different approaches to the treatment of lesions. Lesions over cartilage or bone are typically excised, but in some cases, they may be treated with radiation using electron beam or Iridium-192 plaque. However, radiation failure or necrosis can occur, which may require surgical removal and skin grafting for optimal cosmetic results. Lesions invading bone or cartilage are usually treated with surgery, as radiation may cause radiation chondritis and osteoradionecrosis. Meanwhile, lesions on the eyelid may result in poor cosmesis and a defect in the eyelid if surgically removed. In these cases, judicious use of radiotherapy can provide satisfactory results. For small lesions, a radiation dose of 3500–4500 cGy in 5–10 fractions may be sufficient, while larger lesions may require a dose of 5000–6000 cGy in 20–30 fractions, with appropriate shielding of the cornea and lens. Surface application (mould therapy) used to be common, but it has been largely replaced by electron beam therapy (Fig. 4).

Interstitial brachytherapy is now more feasible than in the past due to advances in technology. Miniaturized sources like iridium-192 can be applied via thin guides and needles, making it a viable option for lesions involving the face, orifices such as the nose and ears, and the periorbital region.

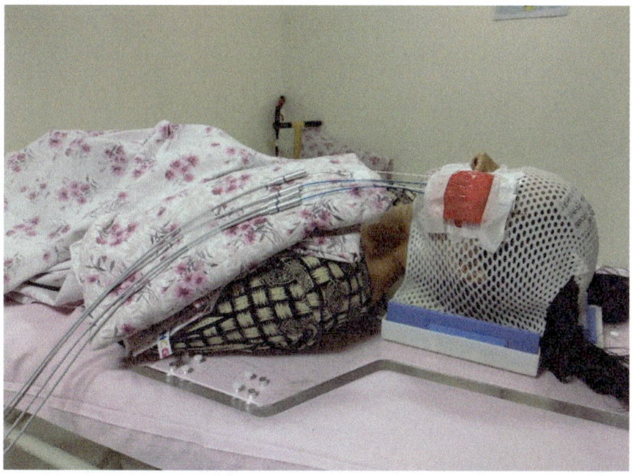

Fig. 4 A patient treated with surface mold for basal cell ca postop with close margin about a cm below the outer canthus with mold brachytherapy. (Contributed by Dr. Manur Gururajachar Janaki, Professor, Department of Radiation Oncology, Ramaiah Medical College, RUAS, Bangalore)

12 Acute and Late Radiation Reactions (RTOG)

Acute Reactions (Skin)

Grade 0 No change over baseline.

Grade I Follicular faint or dull erythema, epilation, dry desquamation, decreased sweating.

Grade II Tender or bright erythema, patchy moist desquamation/moderate edema.

Grade III Confluent, moist desquamation other than skin folds, pitting edema (Fig. 5).

Grade IV Ulceration, hemorrhage, necrosis.

Late Reaction (Skin)

Grade 0 None.

Grade I Slight atrophy, pigmentation change, some hair loss.

Grade II Patchy atrophy, moderate telangiectasia, patchy hair loss.

Grade Ill Marked atrophy, gross telangicetasia, total hair loss.

Grade IV Ulceration/bone exposed.

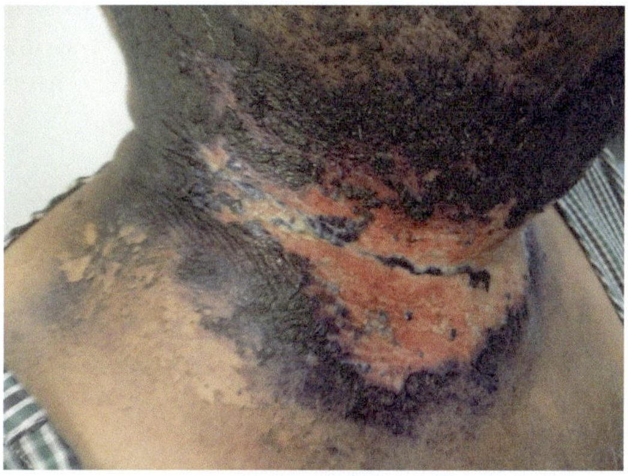

Fig. 5 Moist confluent skin reaction in a patient with head and neck cancer. (Such reactions are rare in the present megavoltage beam era)

13 Prognosis and Outcome

Prognosis for skin carcinomas (NMSC) is generally favorable compared to other types of cancer, with factors such as location, cause, and size affecting the outcome. Squamous cell carcinoma on the lower lip, for instance, has a relatively low incidence of metastasis at 10%–20%. However, carcinomas that develop in areas such as burn scars, chronic ulcers, or from exposure to high doses of ionizing radiation are typically less differentiated and have a higher incidence of metastasis at 20%–30%.

The presence of metastatic adenopathy also worsens the prognosis of squamous cell carcinomas. Recurrences following inadequate treatment have the worst prognosis. Delay in presentation or unsuccessful treatment may lead to extensive advanced carcinoma of the skin, which can be difficult and frustrating to treat. For selected patients, a combination of wide surgical excision, reconstructive procedures, and radiotherapy may be beneficial, but such treatments may not be suitable for very elderly patients.

Patients who have developed skin cancer are at higher risk for developing additional skin tumors, so continued surveillance is necessary at 6-month or annual intervals. Patients can also perform self-examinations of their skin regularly, using a full-length mirror, hand-held mirror, and a well-lit room. To examine hard-to-see areas, such as the back, scalp, and buttocks, patients may need assistance from a spouse, relative, or friend.

14 Melanoma

Melanoma is a type of skin cancer that arises from melanocytes and nevus cells, which migrate from the neuroectoderm to the skin during the embryonic period. Melanoma can develop from pre-existing nevi or spontaneously (Fig. 6). Although it accounts for only 3% of all primary cutaneous malignancies, melanomas are responsible for the majority of deaths attributed to skin malignancies.

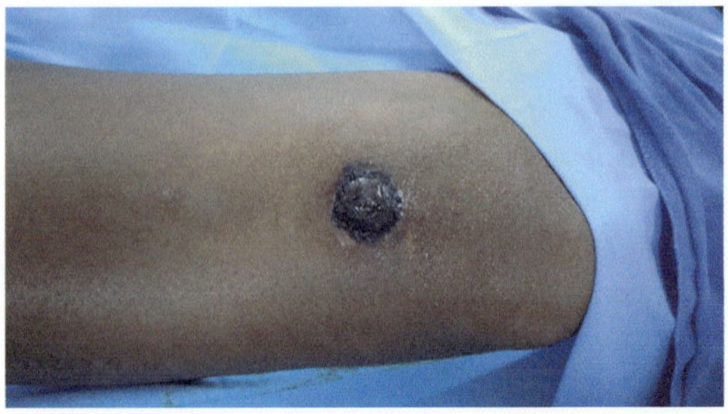

Fig. 6 Melanoma. (Courtesy: Dr. SVS Deo, Head, Department of Surgical Oncology, IRCH, AIIMS, New Delhi)

The incidence of melanoma has been increasing during the last two decades, and with increased awareness, patients with small early lesions are being diagnosed more often. Risk factors for melanoma include skin type, prior melanoma, multiple clinically atypical moles, multiple dysplastic nevi, positive family history of melanoma, and rarely, inherited genetic mutations [24]. Melanoma metastasizes through the regional lymphatics and through the hematogenous route to various organs, including the liver, lung, gut, skin, and brain. Melanoma can occur anywhere on the cutaneous surface, but it is more common on the trunk and extremities [25]. There are several clinical types of cutaneous melanomas, including superficial spreading melanoma (SSM), nodular melanoma (NM), lentigo maligna melanoma (LMM), acral lentiginous melanoma (ALM), and amelanotic melanoma. Besides cutaneous regions, melanomas can also occur in areas such as the mucose. Mucosal melanomas most often occur in the head and neck sinuses and oral cavity, anorectum, vulva, and vagina, but can arise in any of the mucosal membranes lining the gastrointestinal and urogenital tracts.

14.1 Presentation and Outcomes

The outcome of melanoma depends on the stage at presentation. Generally, 80% of patients with melanoma initially present with localized disease, 15% with regional disease, and 5% with distant metastatic disease. Table 6 presents the outcomes with skin melanoma.

In addition to patient-specific factors of age and gender, tumor specific factors of Breslow

Table 6 Outcomes of skin melanoma

Thickness (mm)	Disease status	Outcomes (5 year survival)
<1.0	Localized	More than 90%
>1.0	Localized	50%–90%
Any thickness	Regional nodes involved	25%–60%
Any thickness	Metastatic disease	20%–25%

Table 7 Melanoma lesion thickness (mm) and the corresponding surgical margin required (cm)

Thickness (mm)	Surgical margins (cm)
In situ	0.5–1.0
<1.0	1.0
1.0–2.0 mm	1.0–2.0
2.0–4.0 mm	2.0
>4 mm	2.0

tumor thickness, ulceration, and mitotic rate were found to be the three most important characteristics independently predictive of outcome by multivariate analysis among patients with nodal metastases (stage III), the clinical nodal status (nonpalpable vs. palpable) and the number of metastatic nodes are the most important predictors of survival. For patients with clinically positive nodes, prognostic factors include number of positive nodes, extranodal extension, primary tumor ulceration, and patient age. Among patients with distant metastatic melanoma (stage IV), the site of metastases is the most significant predictor of outcome. The three risk categories recognized by the AJCC are skin, soft tissue, and remote nodes (M1a); visceral-pulmonary (M1b); and visceral-nonpulmonary (M1c).

15 Management of Melanoma

15.1 Surgery for Melanoma

Wide local excision has remained the primary mode of therapy for melanoma. For melanomas 1.0 mm or less, wide excision with a 1-cm margin is recommended. Wide excision with a 1- to 2-cm margin is recommended for melanomas measuring 1.01 to 2 mm in thickness. For melanomas measuring more than 2 mm in thickness, wide excision with 2-cm margins is recommended (category 1) [26]. SLNB should generally be discussed and offered for patients with higher risk stage IB (>1 mm thick or 0.76–1.0 mm thick with ulceration or mitotic rate $\geq 1/mm^2$) or stage II melanoma.

The current recommendations for surgical margins for excision of stages I and II primary melanomas are that excision should include full thickness of normal skin surrounding the lesion, including the subcutaneous fat. Fascial (deep fascia) excision should be performed for moderate and high-risk melanomas, that is, those of more than 1.5 mm depth (Table 7). For thin lesions, less than 0.76 mm depth, fascial excision is not necessary. Deeper lesions require wide local excision and skin graft coverage.

The management of metastatic lymphadenopathy is crucial to achieving positive treatment outcomes in patients with cutaneous melanoma. Surgical removal of affected lymph nodes in the neck, axilla, and groin is the most effective means of achieving local control. Therefore, any suspicious or palpable lymph nodes in the region of the melanoma should be assessed with aspiration cytology. For patients with isolated metastasis in the liver, lungs, or brain, surgical removal can offer good palliation and improved survival. Patients presenting with a suspicious pigmented lesion optimally should undergo an excisional biopsy (elliptical, punch, or saucerization), preferably with 1- to 3-mm negative margins. Excisional biopsy may be inappropriate for certain sites (including the face, palmar surface of the hand, sole of the foot, ear). In these cases, a full-thickness incisional or punch biopsy of the clinically thickest portion of the lesion is an acceptable option. Comparative genomic hybridization (CGH) or fluorescence in situ hybridization (FISH) may be helpful in detecting the presence of selected gene mutations for histologically equivocal lesions.

SLNB is an important staging tool. While SLNB itself has not been shown to improve disease-specific survival (DSS), it is associated with improved regional nodal disease control [27]. A positive SLNB would upstage a patient to stage III. Although surgical excision remains the

Table 8 Local radiotherapy dose schedules in melanoma

Radical radiotherapy	Adjuvant radiotherapy
Indication: Considered as a treatment option for MIS, LM-type (i.e., high-CSD) in medically inoperable patients or those in whom surgical morbidity of complete resection would be prohibitive	Indication: Select cases of high-risk melanoma based on a combination of risk factors for local recurrence
64–70 Gy/32–35#/6–7 weeks	60–66 Gy/30–33# 6–7 weeks
50–57.5 Gy/20–23 #4–5 weeks	48 Gy/20#/4 weeks
35 Gy/5#/1 week for fields <3 cm in diameter	30 Gy/5#/2 weeks (twice per week or every other day)
32 Gy/4# (once per week)	

MIS melanoma in situ, *LM* Lentigo maligna, *CSD* cumulative sun damage

standard of care for in situ melanoma, it is sometimes not feasible due to comorbidity or cosmetically sensitive tumor location. Topical imiquimod has emerged as a treatment option, especially for lentigo maligna [28].

15.2 Radiation Therapy for Melanoma

Radiation therapy for Melanoma can be definitive, adjuvant or palliative. Table 8 gives the dose schedules commonly used in definitive and adjuvant settings.

Adjuvant radiotherapy is usually not considered for adequately operated melanoma. However, RT should be used in patients with close or positive margins if repeat surgery cannot be done. Locoregional radiotherapy in node positive disease improved locoregional recurrence but its impact on improving survival is not well established [29]. Risk factors for regional recurrence include gross and/or histologic extracapsular extension of melanoma in clinically (macroscopic) involved node (s), ≥2 cervical or axillary nodes, ≥3 inguinofemoral nodes. Also, ≥3 cm cervical or axillary node, and/or ≥4 cm inguinofemoral node are considered high risk features. For palliative radiotherapy, the dose fractionation schedules remain the same as for other sites.

16 Adjuvant Systemic Therapy

For adjuvant treatment of melanoma in patients rendered free of disease by surgery, traditional systemic therapy approaches have proven to be ineffective. Adjuvant treatment outside of a clinical trial is not recommended for patients with stages I/II disease. For patients with resected advanced melanoma, adjuvant interferon alfa (IFN alfa), particularly high-dose IFN alfa, has been widely used in patients with melanoma for many years. IFN alfa has been supplanted, however, by targeted therapy and immune checkpoint inhibitor options based on results from recent and ongoing prospective randomized trials. There have been a number of prospective randomized trials suggesting that immune checkpoint inhibitor and BRAF-targeted therapy are effective options for adjuvant treatment. Systemic therapy is generally considered for Stage IIIA and above [30, 31]. Risk of toxicity is the other major consideration when deciding whether a patient with stage III disease should receive adjuvant therapy. Although anti-PD-1 agents and BRAF/MEK inhibitor therapy are associated with lower rates of toxicity than historical adjuvant therapy options (i.e., IFN alfa, biochemotherapy), grades 3–4 AEs (all cause) were observed in 25%–41% of patients treated in adjuvant trials.

17 Regional Therapy: Isolated Limb Perfusion and Infusion

For patients with regionally recurrent melanoma not suitable for local or topical therapy, regional administration of cytotoxic chemotherapy with either isolated limb perfusion (ILP) or isolated limb infusion (ILI) is designed to administer high doses to an affected extremity while avoiding toxicities associated with systemic drug exposure. These approaches also allow delivery of chemotherapy under hyperthermic conditions, suggested by some studies to improve efficacy of cytotoxic agents.

18 Systemic Therapy in Melanoma

Several targeted therapies have been developed for patients with melanoma harboring specific mutations. Patients with metastatic melanoma with activating mutations of *BRAF*, an intracellular signaling kinase in the mitogen activated protein kinase (MAPK) pathway, have been shown to be likely to respond to BRAF inhibitors. Likewise, patients with metastatic melanoma with activating mutations in *KIT*, a receptor tyrosine kinase, have been shown to be more likely to respond to Imatinib, a tyrosine kinase inhibitor, compared with patients without activating *KIT* [32–34].

19 Systemic Therapy for Stage IV Melanoma

With the recent development of new medicines that have shown greater success than conventional chemotherapy, the treatment landscape for metastatic melanoma is fast evolving [35]. Vemurafenib, dabrafenib, and ipilimumab, members of the first generation of new targeted and immunotherapy medicines, have dramatically outperformed standard therapies in terms of response rates and outcomes [36]. Thus, a number of phase II and phase III trials exploring novel immunotherapies, targeted treatments, and combination regimens are currently active or have recently ended with notable outcomes. In previously untreated patients with untreatable stage III or IV melanoma, nivolumab/ipilimumab combination therapy is linked with improved overall response rate (ORR), PFS, and OS compared to single-agent ipilimumab, at the cost of dramatically higher toxicity [37, 38]. In patients who had not previously received treatment and who had AJCC seventh Edition stage IIIC or stage IV illness, BRAF/MEK inhibitor combination therapy was associated with improved response rate, PFS, and OS compared to BRAF inhibitor monotherapy [39]. Second and emerging third generations of effective agents and combination regimens are now available for treatment of advanced unresectable or metastatic melanoma [40–42]. For patients who experience progression of melanoma during or shortly after adjuvant or first-line therapy, consider second-line agents if not used first line and if from a different class. For patients who progressed on single-agent anti-PD-1 checkpoint immunotherapy, anti-PD-1/ipilimumab or BRAF/MEK inhibitor combination therapy or ipilimumab monotherapy are reasonable treatment options.

20 Cutaneous Lymphomas

Cutaneous lymphomas are rare in oncology practice, but can manifest as skin infiltrations in T cell lymphoproliferative disorders, Hodgkin's disease, or leukemia [43, 44]. The most common form of cutaneous T cell lymphoma is mycosis fungoides (MF), which progresses slowly through three clinical phases: the erythematous patch or premycotic phase, the infiltrated plaque in the mycotic phase, and the tumor or fungoid phase. Biopsies of advanced lesions are necessary to confirm the diagnosis, since all three phases may occur simultaneously in a single patient.

MF is named for the mushroom-like appearance of its cutaneous tumours, and is characterized by an upper dermal infiltration of mononuclear cells and histiocytes, some of which exhibit atypia with hyperchromatic nuclei. The malignant mycosis cell, also known as the "Sezary cell," is a T cell with a large nucleus and minimal cytoplasm. MF may present with nonspecific cutaneous manifestations that persist for an average of 5–10 years, but it becomes progressive and covers wide areas of the body during the plaque phase. Generalized erythroderma, which involves most of the skin surface, is associated with skin thickening, severe itching, and bleeding.

MF can also spread to peripheral blood and lymph nodes, and patients with evidence of more than 5% mycosis cells in the blood are diagnosed with "Sezary syndrome." Visceral involvement, which occurs frequently in the terminal stages of the disease, may affect almost every organ, with bone marrow, lung, spleen, and liver being the most common sites. Infection due to breakdown of the skin barrier is the most common cause of death, with progressive dissemination in the blood and organs also contributing. More details about Cutaneous Lymphomas and Total Skin Electron Therapy (TSET) can be found in chapter "Molecular Biology and Genetics in Radiation Oncology Practice", Vol 1 (Special Techniques: Total Body Irradiation, T-SET, IORT, Hyperthermia).

21 Kaposi's Sarcoma

Aggressive disseminated Kaposi's sarcoma and Kaposi's sarcoma with systemic B symptoms can be treated with combination chemotherapy, while cytoreductive therapy is necessary for specific organ dysfunction, such as pulmonary disease. Painful lesions, tumor-associated edema, and cosmetic disfigurement require palliative radiotherapy or chemotherapy. For fibrosarcoma, surgical excision is the preferred treatment, but growth restraint palliative therapy can be useful for inoperable or recurrent inoperable growths. Langerhans' cell histiocytosis (Histiocytosis-X) lesions with surrounding soft tissue mass can be treated with radiation therapy using a dose of 300 cGy × I or 150 cGy × 2. Radiation therapy is also recommended for deeply invasive keratoacanthoma lesions, with a recommended dose of 25 Gy given in five daily fractions.

In conclusion, the overall incidence of skin cancers is rising. It is therefore imperative for the practicing radiation oncologist, surgical oncologist, plastic surgeon, and medical oncologist to be knowledgeable about the prevention, diagnosis, staging, and treatment of both basal and squamous cell carcinoma. Skin carcinomas are frequently occurring and treatable conditions. The goal of treatment is to achieve local control while also prioritizing cosmetic outcome and patient comfort. Radiation therapy may be recommended in cases where preserving normal tissue is crucial for functional or cosmetic reasons The basis of nonmelanoma skin cancer manage-

Percepts Box

1. The majority of skin cancers are either basal cell carcinoma (BCC) or squamous cell carcinoma (SCC). BCC is thrice as common as SCC. Melanomas are 30–40 times less common.
2. Risk factors for nonmelanomatous skin cancers (NMSC) include exposure to UV rays, history of sunburn, light complexion, family history, chronic infection among others.
3. BCC occurs most commonly on the nose, grows slow, rarely metastasize and are locally destructive. Recurrence is more likely with aggressive histologies like morpheaform, basosquamous, sclerosing, mixed infiltrative, or micronodular.
4. SCC recurrence is also seen in aggressive histologies like adenoid (acantholytic), adenosquamous, desmoplastic, or metaplastic, with a recurrence rate of 20%–80%.
5. Systemic therapy in NMSC is given in high-risk cases like positive margins.
6. Local therapy such as Moh's micrographic surgery, curettage and electrodessication, cryotherapy, topical applications. Liquid nitrogen are treatment option in early stages.
7. Radiation therapy is usually indicated in the treatment of lesions on the face (nose, lip, eyelid, canthus) where surgery is either technically difficult or likely to yield poor cosmesis, large superficial lesions, older patients, patients who refuse, or are unfit for surgery (RT avoids anaesthesia), post-surgery: for incomplete/marginal excision, perineural invasion.
8. Dose and fractionation can vary from 18 to 60 Gy, as a single or fractionated regimen depending on the size and sensitivity to radiation.

(continued)

9. Melanoma arises from melanocytes and nevus cells. It's most commonly seen on the trunk and extremities. Mucosal melanomas most often occur in the head and neck sinuses and oral cavity, anorectum, vulva, and vagina.
10. Most common cutaneous melanomas include superficial spreading melanoma (SSM), nodular melanoma (NM), lentigo maligna melanoma (LMM), acral lentiginous melanoma (ALM), and amelanotic melanoma.
11. Wide local excision has remained the primary mode of therapy for melanoma, margins depend on the size of the lesion.
12. Radiation therapy for Melanoma can be definitive, adjuvant, or palliative. Dose can vary between 30 and 60 Gy depending on the indication.
13. Systemic therapy, like BRAF inhibitors or IFN-alpha, are generally considered for Stage IIIA and above.
14. Cutaneous lymphomas are rare in oncology, but can be seen in T cell lymphoproliferative disorders, Hodgkin's disease, or leukemia,
15. The most common form of cutaneous T cell lymphoma is mycosis fungoides (MF), which progresses slowly through three clinical phases: the premycotic phase, the mycotic phase, and the tumor phase.
16. Aggressive disseminated Kaposi's sarcoma and Kaposi's sarcoma with systemic B symptoms can be treated with combination chemotherapy, while cytoreductive therapy is necessary for specific organ dysfunction, such as pulmonary disease.

ment is determining whether the lesion is low risk or high risk. High-risk lesions should be adequately worked up, treated, and followed up to ensure prevention of recurrence and prolonged survival outcomes.

Multiple Choice Questions

1. The most common cancer of the skin is
   (a) Basal cell carcinoma
   (b) Squamous cell carcinoma
   (c) Melanoma
   (d) Kaposi sarcoma
2. Range of carcinogenic UV-B radiation
   (a) 270–300 nm
   (b) 180–270 nm
   (c) 290–320 nm
   (d) 320–350 nm
3. All of the following are true about Curettage and Electrodessication except
   (a) Does not allow histologic margin assessment
   (b) Used preferably in non-hair bearing areas
   (c) Open wound healed by secondary indentation
   (d) No anesthesia needed
4. All of these are true for RT in NMSC except
   (a) Dose for BCC and SCC are the same
   (b) Beam energy chosen is such that the dose to the base of the lesion is not less than 50% of that to the surface
   (c) Dose is calculated at the depth of the tumor
   (d) Dose is calculated at the surface of the tumor
5. All of the following are indications for RT in NMSC except
   (a) Young Patients
   (b) Cosmetic preservation
   (c) Patients unfit for surgery
   (d) Perineural invasion
6. All of the following statements are true about BCC except
   (a) Locally destructive
   (b) Arise from the basal cell layer
   (c) Rapidly growing
   (d) Most commonly seen on the nose
7. RT dose preferred for a lesion >6 cm in areas of poor radiation tolerance is
   (a) 60 Gy/30 fractions/6 weeks
   (b) 18 Gy/single fraction
   (c) 55 Gy/20 fractions/4 weeks
   (d) 32.5 Gy/5 fractions/1 week

8. Surgical margin for a melanoma lesion measuring 3 mm in thickness is
   (a) 0.5–1.0 cm
   (b) 1.0–1.5 cm
   (c) 1.5–2.0 cm
   (d) >2.0 cm
9. High risk features for regional recurrence in melanoma include all of the following except
   (a) 1 cm axillary node
   (b) ≥4 cm inguinofemoral node
   (c) Nodal ECE
   (d) None of the above
10. Cutaneous lymphomas can manifest as skin infiltrations in all except
   (a) HL
   (b) NHL
   (c) Mycosis fungoides
   (d) Leukemia

Answer Key

1. (a)
2. (c)
3. (d)
4. (d)
5. (a)
6. (c)
7. (a)
8. (d)
9. (d)
10. (a)

References

1. Hu W, Fang L, Ni R, et al. Changing trends in the disease burden of non-melanoma skin cancer globally from 1990 to 2019 and its predicted level in 25 years. BMC Cancer. 2022;22:836. https://doi.org/10.1186/s12885-022-09940-3.
2. Ciążyńska M, Kamińska-Winciorek G, Lange D, et al. The incidence and clinical analysis of non-melanoma skin cancer. Sci Rep. 2021;11:4337.
3. https://www.nccn.org/professionals/physician_gls/pdf/squamous.pdf. Accessed March 2023.
4. Rogers HW, Weinstock MA, Harris AR, et al. Incidence estimate of nonmelanoma skin cancer in the United States, 2006. Arch Dermatol. 2010;146:283–7.
5. Panda S. Nonmelanoma skin cancer in India: current scenario. Indian J Dermatol. 2010;55(4):373–8.
6. Green A, Battistutta D, Hart V, Leslie D, Weedon D. Skin cancer in a subtropical Australian population: incidence and lack of association with occupation. The Nambour Study Group. Am J Epidemiol. 1996;144(11):1034–40.
7. Wolberink EA, Pasch MC, Zeiler M, van Erp PE, Gerritsen MJ. High discordance between punch biopsy and excision in establishing basal cell carcinoma subtype: analysis of 500 cases. J Eur Acad Dermatol Venereol. 2013;27:985–9.
8. Motley R, Kersey P, Lawrence C, et al. Multiprofessional guidelines for the management of the patient with primary cutaneous squamous cell carcinoma. Br J Dermatol. 2002;146(1):18–25.
9. Rowe DE, Carroll RJ, Day CL. Prognostic factors for local recurrence, metastasis, and survival rates in squamous cell carcinoma of the skin, ear, and lip. Implications for treatment modality selection. J Am Acad Dermatol. 1992;26(6):976–90.
10. Brodland DG, Zitelli JA. Surgical margins for excision of primary cutaneous squamous cell carcinoma. J Am Acad Dermatol. 1992;27(2 Pt 1):241–8.
11. Lewin JM, Carucci JA. Advances in the management of basal cell carcinoma. F1000Prime Rep. 2015;7:53.
12. Barlow JO, Zalla MJ, Kyle A, DiCaudo DJ, Lim KK, Yiannias JA. Treatment of basal cell carcinoma with curettage alone. J Am Acad Dermatol. 2006;54:1039–45.
13. Werlinger KD, Upton G, Moore AY. Recurrence rates of primary nonmelanoma skin cancers treated by surgical excision compared to electrodesiccation-curettage in a private dermatological practice. Dermatologic Surg. 2002;28:1138–42. discussion 1142.
14. National Comprehensive Cancer Network. National clinical practice guidelines in oncology: basal cell skin cancer (version I.2017). Available at: https://www.nccn.org/profession-als/physician_gls/pdf/nmsc.pdf. Accessed 14 Aug 2017.
15. Bath-Hextall F, Ozolins M, Armstrong SJ, et al. Surgery versus Imiquimod for Nodular Superficial basal cell carcinoma (SINS) study group. Surgical excision versus imiquimod 5% cream for nodular and superficial basal-cell carcinoma (SINS): a multicentre, non-inferiority, randomised con- trolled trial. Lancet Oncol. 2014;15:96–105.
16. Arits AH, Mosterd K, Essers BA, et al. Photodynamic therapy versus topical imiquimod versus topical fluorouracil for treatment of superficial basal-cell carcinoma: a single blind, non-inferiority, randomised controlled trial. Lancet Oncol. 2013;14:647–54.
17. Wheeland RG, Bailin PL, Ratz RL, et al. Carbon dioxide laser vasporization and curettage in the treatment of large or multiple superficial basal carcinomas. J Dermatol Surg Oncol. 1987;13:119.
18. Spiller WF, Spiltcr RF. Treatment of basal cell carcinoma by curettage and electrodesication. J Am Acad Dertmatol. 1984;11:808.
19. Dubin N, Kopf AW. Multivariate risk score for recurrence of cutaneous basal cell carcinomas. Arch Dermatol. 1983;119(5):373–7.

20. Wagner RF, Casciato DA. Skin cancers. In: Casciato DA, Lowitz BB, editors. Manual of clinical oncology. 4th ed. Lippincott, Williams, and Wilkins; 2000. p. 336–73.
21. Reszko A, Aasi SZ, Wilson LD, et al. Cancer of the skin. In: DeVita Jr VT, Lawrence TS, Rosenberg SA, editors. Cancer: principles and practice of oncology. 9th ed. Lippincott Williams & Wilkins; 2011. p. 1610–3.
22. Sekulic A, Migden MR, Oro AE, et al. Efficacy and safety of vismodegib in advanced basal-cell carcinoma. N Engl J Med. 2012;366:2171–9.
23. Migden MR, Guminski A, Gutzmer R, et al. Treatment with two different doses of sonidegib in patients with locally advanced or metastatic basal cell carcinoma (BOLT): a multicentre, randomised, double-blind phase 2 trial. Lancet Oncol. 2015;16:716–28.
24. Evans RD, Kopf AW, Lew RA, et al. Risk factors for the development of malignant melanoma—I: review of case-control studies. J Dermatol Surg Oncol. 1988;14:393–408.
25. Breslow A. Thickness, cross sectional areas and depth of invasion in the prognosis of cutaneous melanoma. Ann Surg. 1970;172:902–8.
26. Haigh PI, DiFronzo LA, McCready DR. Optimal excision margins for primary cutaneous melanoma: a systematic review and meta-analysis. Can J Surg. 2003;46:419–26.
27. Multicenter Selective Lymphadenectomy Trials Study Group, Crystal JS, Thompson JF, Hyngstrom J, Caracò C, Zager JS, Jahkola T, Bowles TL, Pennacchioli E, Beitsch PD, Hoekstra HJ, Moncrieff M, Ingvar C, van Akkooi A, Sabel MS, Levine EA, Agnese D, Henderson M, Dummer R, Neves RI, Rossi CR, Kane JM 3rd, Trocha S, Wright F, Byrd DR, Matter M, Hsueh EC, MacKenzie-Ross A, Kelley M, Terheyden P, Huston TL, Wayne JD, Neuman H, Smithers BM, Ariyan CE, Desai D, Gershenwald JE, Schneebaum S, Gesierich A, Jacobs LK, Lewis JM, McMasters KM, O'Donoghue C, van der Westhuizen A, Sardi A, Barth R, Barone R, McKinnon JG, Slingluff CL, Farma JM, Schultz E, Scheri RP, Vidal-Sicart S, Molina M, Testori AAE, Foshag LJ, Van Kreuningen L, Wang HJ, Sim MS, Scolyer RA, Elashoff DE, Cochran AJ, Faries MB. Therapeutic value of sentinel lymph node biopsy in patients with melanoma: a randomized clinical trial. JAMA Surg. 2022;157(9):835–42. https://doi.org/10.1001/jamasurg.2022.2055. Erratum in: JAMA Surg. 2022;157(9):859. PMID: 35921122; PMCID: PMC9475390.
28. Cotter MA, McKenna JK, Bowen GM. Treatment of lentigo maligna with imiquimod before staged excision. Dermatologic Surg. 2008;34:147–51, 248–64.
29. Henderson MA, Burmeister BH, Ainslie J, et al. Adjuvant lymph-node field radiotherapy versus observation only in patients with melanoma at high risk of further lymph-node field relapse after lymphadenectomy (ANZMTG 01.02/TROG 02.01): 6-year follow-up of a phase 3, randomized controlled trial. Lancet Oncol. 2015;16:1049–60.
30. Eggermont AM, Chiarion-Sileni V, Grob JJ, et al. Adjuvant ipilimumab versus placebo after complete resection of high-risk stage III melanoma (EORTC 18071): a randomised, double-blind, phase 3 trial. Lancet Oncol. 2015;16:522–30.
31. Eggermont AM, Chiarion-Sileni V, Grob JJ, et al. Prolonged survival in stage III melanoma with Ipilimumab adjuvant therapy. N Engl J Med. 2016;375:1845–55.
32. Davies H, Bignell GR, Cox C, et al. Mutations of the BRAF gene in human cancer. Nature. 2002;417:949–54.
33. Long GV, Menzies AM, Nagrial AM, et al. Prognostic and clinicopathologic associations of oncogenic BRAF in metastatic melanoma. J Clin Oncol. 2011;29:1239–46.
34. Dhillon AS, Hagan S, Rath O, Kolch W. MAP kinase signaling pathways in cancer. Oncogene. 2007;26:3279–90.
35. Flaherty LE, Othus M, Atkins MB, et al. Southwest Oncology Group S0008: a phase III trial of high-dose interferon Alfa-2b versus cisplatin, vinblastine, and dacarbazine, plus interleukin-2 and interferon in patients with high-risk melanoma--an intergroup study of cancer and leukemia Group B, Children's Oncology Group, Eastern Cooperative Oncology Group, and Southwest Oncology Group. J Clin Oncol. 2014;32:3771–8.
36. Maio M, Lewis K, Demidov L, et al. Adjuvant vemurafenib in resected, BRAF(V600) mutation-positive melanoma (BRIM8): a randomised, doubleblind, placebo-controlled, multicentre, phase 3 trial. Lancet Oncol. 2018;19:510–20.
37. Larkin J, Chiarion-Sileni V, Gonzalez R, et al. Combined nivolumab and ipilimumab or monotherapy in untreated melanoma. N Engl J Med. 2015;373:23–34.
38. Hodi FS, Chesney J, Pavlick AC, et al. Combined nivolumab and ipilimumab versus ipilimumab alone in patients with advanced melanoma: 2-year overall survival outcomes in a multicentre, randomised, controlled, phase 2 trial. Lancet Oncol. 2016;17:1558–68.
39. Long GV, Stroyakovskiy D, Gogas H, et al. Dabrafenib and trametinib versus dabrafenib and placebo for Val600 BRAF-mutant melanoma: a multicentre, double-blind, phase 3 randomised controlled trial. Lancet. 2015;386:444–51.
40. Ribas A, Puzanov I, Dummer R, et al. Pembrolizumab versus investigator-choice chemotherapy for ipilimumab-refractory melanoma (KEYNOTE-002): a randomised, controlled, phase 2 trial. Lancet Oncol. 2015;16:908–18.
41. Long GV, Stroyakovskiy D, Gogas H, et al. Combined BRAF and MEK inhibition versus BRAF inhibition alone in melanoma. N Engl J Med. 2014;371:1877–88. Available at: http://www.ncbi.nlm.nih.gov/pubmed/25265492.
42. Larkin J, Del Vecchio M, Ascierto PA, et al. Vemurafenib in patients with BRAF(V600) mutated

metastatic melanoma: an open-label, multicentre, safety study. Lancet Oncol. 2014;15:436–44.
43. Gibson F, Hanly A, Fisher R, Wyant WA, Wu M, Collard M, Alani RM. Epigenetics and cutaneous neoplasms: from mechanism to therapy. Epigenomics. 2023;15:167–87. https://doi.org/10.2217/epi-2023-0016. Epub ahead of print. PMID: 37020393.
44. Titou H, Bouhamidi A. Epidemiology and prognostic factors of 114 patients with mycosis fungoides in a Moroccan cohort: a 29-year review. Clin Exp Med. 2023;23:3751–8. https://doi.org/10.1007/s10238-023-01056-7. Epub ahead of print. PMID: 37029872.

Online Links

Cutaneous SCC contouring. https://econtour.org/cases/133.

https://www.sciencedirect.com/science/article/pii/S0167814018300355.

https://www.youtube.com/watch?v=5UUdX-45nNc.

https://www.youtube.com/watch?v=g-z7IG_-Coo.

https://www.youtube.com/watch?v=HLCNB5d9otA.

Breast Cancer

Anusheel Munshi, Sanjoy Chatterjee, Nuran Bese, Sudeep Gupta, S. V. S. Deo, Ashutosh Mishra, Vikas Kumar Pandey, and Sudhir Raj Silwal

1 Introduction

Breast cancer is the most common malignant neoplasm afflicting women in developed and developing countries [1]. Worldwide, there were be about 2.1 million newly diagnosed female breast cancer cases in 2018, accounting for almost 1 in 4 cancer cases among women [2]. The disease is the most frequently diagnosed cancer in the vast majority of the countries. It is also the sixth leading cause of cancer death in over 100 countries [3]. In India, breast cancer has overtaken cervical cancer as the leading cause of death in women. Breast cancer is a heterogeneous disease with varied biologic potential. While surgery is the oldest treatment method, radiotherapy, chemotherapy, endocrine treatment, targeted treatments, and immunotherapy have evolved and convincingly established their role in managing this disease over the past few decades [4–7]. Present day management of breast cancer, therefore, requires an integrated multimodality multidisciplinary approach.

A. Munshi (✉)
Department of Radiation Oncology, BLK MAX Hospital, New Delhi, Delhi, India

S. Chatterjee
Department of Radiation Oncology, Tata Medical Center, Kolkata, West Bengal, India

N. Bese
Department of Clinical Senology, MAA Acibadem University, Research Institute of Senology, Istanbul, Turkey

S. Gupta
Department of Medical Oncology, TMH, Mumbai, India

S. V. S. Deo
Department of Surgical Oncology, MAX Hospital, Saket, New Delhi, Delhi, India

A. Mishra
Department of Surgical Oncology, AIIMS, New Delhi, Delhi, India

V. K. Pandey
Department of Radiation Oncology, Cancer Care Manitoba, Winnipeg, Canada

S. R. Silwal
Department of Radiation Oncology, Bhaktapur Cancer Hospital, Bhaktapur, Nepal

2 Anatomy

The breast is essentially made up of two components: fatty tissue and glandular (milk-producing) tissue. The ratio of these two components depends on age and can vary between individuals. The decrease of estrogen levels related to the onset of menopause makes the relative amount of fatty tissue increase as the glandular tissue diminishes. The breast skin is rich in blood supply and lymphatics. The subdermal plexus that supplies the breast skin is also in communication with deeper underlying vessels that supply the breast parenchyma. The blood supply is derived from the internal mammary perforators, the thoracoacromial artery, the vessels to serratus anterior, the

B. K. Mohanti et al. (eds.), *Radiation Oncology – Principles, Precepts and Practice*,
https://doi.org/10.1007/978-981-95-5171-2_5

Fig. 1 Cross-sectional anatomical diagram of the human breast showing the internal arrangement of the skin, subcutaneous fat, lobules, lactiferous ducts and sinuses, nipple, areola, Cooper's (suspensory) ligaments, pectoralis major muscle, pectoral fascia, rib, and thoracic wall

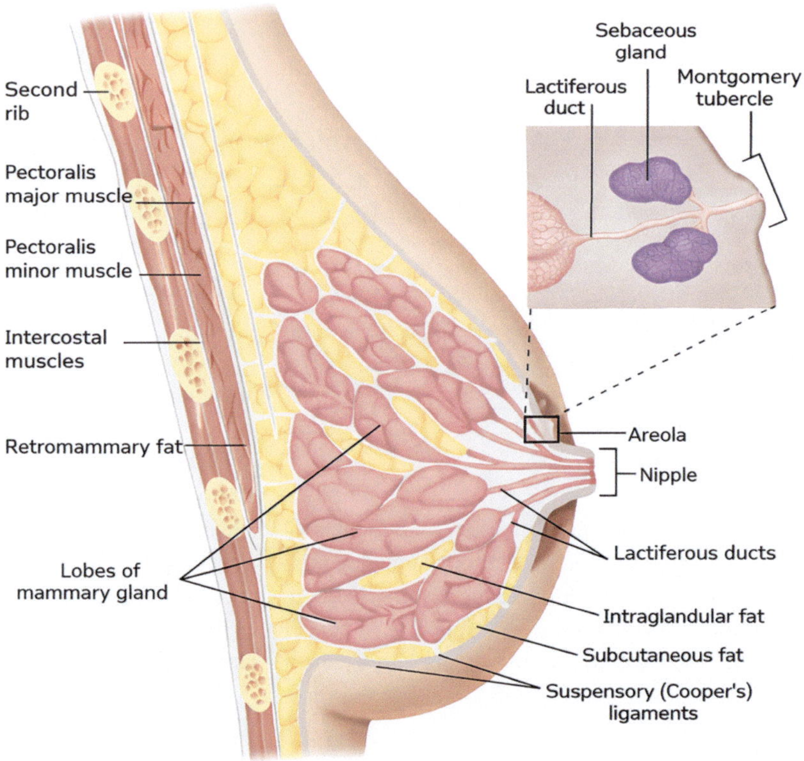

lateral thoracic artery and the terminal branches of the third to eighth intercostal perforators. This rich blood supply ensuring the viability of the skin flaps even after complex surgeries. Sensory innervation of the breast is from the thoracic intercostal nerves T3-T5. From the lower fibers of the cervical plexus, the supraclavicular nerves also provide innervation to the upper and lateral portions of the breast. The breast base rests over the pectoralis major muscle between the second and sixth ribs (Fig. 1). The gland itself is anchored to the fascia of pectoralis major fascia by suspensory ligaments. Because they are not rigid or taut, they allow for the proper natural motion of the breast. However, over some time and with increasing age, the ligaments relax, resulting in breast ptosis. Extending obliquely up to the medial wall of the axilla is the tail of Spence. The breast lies over the musculature that encases the chest wall. The muscles involved include the pectoralis major, serratus anterior, external oblique, and rectus abdominal fascia.

3 Epidemiological Aspects and Risk Factors

As per Globocan 2020, the global breast cancer incidence in 2020 was 2,261,419 (11.7% of all new cancers) [8]. Breast cancer contributed to 684,996 deaths (6.9% of all cancer deaths). By the end of 2020, there were 7.8 million women alive who had been diagnosed with breast cancer in the past 5 years, making it the world's most prevalent cancer. As per Globocan, India saw 1,324,413 new cancer cases and 851,678 cancer deaths in 2020. In 2020, there were a total of 178,361 new cancer cases in India (13.5% of all new cancer cases), with 90,408 deaths (10% of all cancer-related deaths) related to breast cancer in the same year. The 5-year prevalence (across all ages) was 459,271.

The median age of presentation for invasive breast cancer in the Western population is 61 years [9]. Recent reports from India suggest that most patients present a decade earlier [10].

Differing median ages at breast cancer onset among countries have been attributed to the different shapes of the underlying population pyramids (more younger population in countries such as India) and/or to low breast cancer incidence rates in older women in these low/middle-income countries.

Breast cancer has been ranked the number one cancer among Indian females with an age-adjusted rate as high as 25.8 per 100,000 women and mortality 12.7 per 100,000 women. The age adjusted incidence rate of carcinoma of the breast was found as high as 41 per 100,000 women for Delhi, followed by Chennai (37.9), Bangalore (34.4) and Thiruvananthapuram District (33.7).

The western population has nearly similar incidence in white and black women. However, the mortality rates are higher among the black race. Some studies indicate that the reason for this is the weak socioeconomic status of the black population. This contributes to Black women not having the same access to healthcare, with consequent effects on preventive care, cancer detection, and treatment.

In India, the highest burden of breast cancer has been observed in metropolitan cities. In recent years, there is an increase in the trend of incidence of breast cancer, whereas cervix uteri cancer is on the decline [11].

Across the world, breast cancer mortality has changed little from the 1930s through to the 1970s. Improvements in survival began in the 1980s in countries with early detection programmes combined with different modes of treatment to eradicate invasive diseases.

3.1 Breast Cancer Risk Factors

Most of the established risk factors are linked to estrogens. Breast cancer risk is increased by early menarche, late menopause, high concentrations of endogenous oestradiol, oral contraceptives, hormonal replacement therapy, alcohol, previous radiation exposure, and the presence of obesity [12, 13].

Hereditary and genetic factors, including a personal or family history of breast or ovarian cancer and inherited mutations (in BRCA1, BRCA2, and other breast cancer susceptibility genes), account for 5%–10% of breast cancer cases [14]. Breast cancer risk is reduced by breastfeeding and physical activity by childbearing (greater protection for early first birth and multiparity).

Table 1 Breast cancer risk factors

Nonmodifiable risk factors	Modifiable risk factors
Increasing age	Physical inactivity
Female gender	Obesity
Presence of genetic mutations (BRCA1, BRCA2 and others)	Hormonal replacement therapy (oestrogen/progesterone)
Early menarche, late menopause	First pregnancy after 30, lack of breast feeding
Dense breasts	Alcohol intake
Strong family history of Breast/Ovarian cancer	Smoking
Prior thoracic radiotherapy	
Diethylstilbestrol (DES) use	

Breast cancer is a noncommunicable disease. While some cancers such as cervical cancer and oral cancer are linked to infection-related causes, such as human papillomavirus (HPV), there are no known bacterial or viral infections related to the etiology of breast cancer. The risk factors related to breast cancer have been summarized in Table 1. However, approximately 50% of breast cancers develop in women with no identifiable breast cancer risk factors other than gender (female) and age (over 45 years).

4 Clinical Symptoms and Signs

In resourceful establishment, most patients present with abnormal mammogram. Early-stage breast cancer patients mostly present with a painless breast lump. Locally advanced breast cancer may present with skin changes in breast- edema or dimpling or thickening, axillary adenopathy and bloody nipple discharge. Symptoms of metastatic breast cancer depend on the organ involved. The breast mass is classically described on palpation as hard, fixed, mostly single lesion with

Table 2 Symptoms and signs of breast cancer

A breast lump or swelling
Redness, dimpling, pitting, or any other alteration in the skin of the breast
Change in the appearance of nipple or areola
Alteration in size, shape or appearance of the breast
Abnormal discharge from the nipple

irregular borders. Signs and symptoms of breast cancer are enumerated in Table 2.

It t is to be noted that there can be multiple etiologies for a breast lump. Further, nearly 90% of breast lumps are non-cancerous. The benign causes of breast lumps include fibroadenomas, fibrosis, and simple cysts, ductal or lobular hyperplasia, lobular carcinoma in situ (LCIS), adenosis, fibroadenomas, phyllodes tumors, intraductal papillomas, granular cell tumors, fat necrosis and oil cysts, mastitis duct ectasia, other non-cancerous breast conditions.

4.1 Pathology

Invasive carcinomas are a heterogeneous group of tumors differentiated into histological subtypes. Of these, infiltrating ductal carcinoma (IDC) is, by far, the most common subtype accounting for 70%–80% of all invasive lesions. IDC is further sub-classified as either well-differentiated (grade 1), moderately differentiated (grade 2), or poorly differentiated (grade 3). This is based on (a) Nuclear pleomorphism (b) Glandular/Tubule formation (c) Mitotic rate (per 10 HPF).

The utility of ER, PR and HER2/neu is well accepted for IDC. In contrast, the use of molecular markers in DCIS is still debated.

Ductal Carcinoma in situ (DCIS) is characterized by malignant proliferation of cells in ducts without invasion of the basement membrane. DCIS is mainly an incidental finding on mammography and rarely presents as mass. DCIS is further classified into low and intermediate grade (papillary, cribriform, and solid) and high grade (cribriform) based on architecture, cytological features and cell necrosis [15].

Invasive ductal carcinoma has various histologic patterns

- Invasive ductal carcinoma is the most common type accounting for 70%–80% of invasive breast cancers. Biopsy reveals duct-like structures in desmoplastic stroma. IDC is classified into three grades based on architectural and cytological features- Well-differentiated (Grade-I), moderately differentiated (Grade-II) and poorly differentiated (Grade-III).
- Invasive lobular carcinoma- second most common type accounting for 5%–10% of invasive cancers. They characteristically grow in a single file pattern; cells may exhibit signet ring morphology. No duct formation due to lack of E-cadherin.
- Other histologies
  - Tubular
  - Mucinous
  - Medullary
  - Tubulo-lobular
  - Micropappliary
  - Metaplastic
  - Adenoid cystic
  - Secretory
  - Apocrine

4.2 Molecular Classification

Based on immunohistochemistry and proliferation index breast cancer is classified as per Table 3.

4.3 Stage & Stage Group

4.3.1 Staging (AJCC 8 Breast Cancer Staging) [16]

Clinical Staging

Primary Tumor (cT)

- *TX*: primary tumor cannot be assessed
- *T0*: no evidence of primary tumor
- *Tis (DCIS)**: Ductal carcinoma in situ
- *Tis (Paget)*: Paget disease of nipple is NOT associated with invasive carcinoma and/or carcinoma in situ (DCIS) in the underlying breast parenchyma. Carcinoma in the breast

Table 3 Molecular classification of breast tumors

	Luminal A	Luminal B	Her2 rich	Basal-like
Clinical	50% of invasive breast cancer	20% of invasive breast cancer	15% of invasive breast cancer	15% of invasive breast cancer
IHC	(ER+, PR+, HER 2-) or (ER+, PR-, HER 2-) CK 8/18+	(ER + PR-, HER 2 +) or (ER – PR+, HER 2 +) or (ER + PR+, HER 2 +) CK 8/18+	ER-, PR- HER 2+	ER-, PR-, HER 2-, CK5/6+
Biological features	Low proliferative index (Ki-67 <15%)	A higher proliferative index than luminal A (Ki-67 >15%)	Higher than luminal A/B (Ki-67 >15%)	Higher than luminal A/B (Ki-67 >15%)
Histological correlation	Tubular carcinoma, cribriform carcinoma, low grade invasive ductal Carcinoma (NOS), Classic lobular carcinoma	Invasive ductal carcinoma (NOS)	High grade invasive ductal carcinoma (NOS)	High grade invasive ductal carcinoma (NOS), metaplastic carcinoma, medullary carcinoma
5-year survival	90%	40%	30%	<5%
Response to treatment	Response to endocrine therapy. Variable response to chemotherapy	Response to endocrine therapy (lesser than Luminal A). Variable response to chemotherapy (better than luminal A)	Response to Herceptin. Response to anthracyclines	Sensitive to platinum group chemotherapy and PARP inhibitors. No response to hormonal therapy or Traztuzumab

parenchyma associated with Paget disease are categorized based on the size and characteristics of the parenchymal disease, although the presence of Paget disease should still be noted.

- *T1a*: tumor >1 mm but ≤5 mm
- *T1b*: tumor >5 mm but ≤10 mm
- *T1c*: tumor >10 mm but ≤20 mm
- *T2*: tumor >20 mm but ≤50 mm
- *T3*: tumor >50 mm
- *T4a*: extension to the chest wall (invasion or adherence to pectoralis muscle in the absence of chest wall invasion does not qualify as T4).
- *T4b*: ulceration and/or ipsilateral macroscopic satellite nodules and/or edema (including peau d'orange) of the skin that does not meet criteria for inflammatory carcinoma.
- *T4c*: both T4a and T4b.
- *T4d*: inflammatory carcinoma (involves >1/3 of the breast skin, primarily a clinical diagnosis).

*Lobular carcinoma in situ (LCIS) is a benign entity and is removed from TNM staging in AJCC 8th edition

Regional Lymph Nodes (cN)

- *cNX*: regional nodes cannot be assessed (e.g.,-previously removed)
- *cN0*: no regional lymph node metastasis (by imaging or clinical examination)
- *cN1*: metastases to movable ipsilateral Levels I, II axillary lymph node(s)
- *cN1mi***: micrometastases (approximately 200 cells, larger than 0.2 mm but none larger than 2.0 mm)
- *cN2a*: metastases in ipsilateral Levels I, II axillary lymph nodes fixed to one another (matted) or to other structures
- *cN2b*: metastases only in ipsilateral internal mammary nodes in the absence of axillary lymph node
- *cN3a*: metastases in ipsilateral infraclavicular lymph node(s)

- *cN3b*: metastases in ipsilateral internal mammary node(s) and axillary node(s)
- *cN3c*: metastases in ipsilateral supraclavicular lymph node(s)

**cN1mi is rarely used but may be useful in cases where sentinel node biopsy is performed before tumor resection, most likely in cases treated with neoadjuvant therapy

4.4 Pathological Staging

Primary Tumor (pT)

- *pTX*: cannot be assessed
- *pT0*: no evidence of primary tumor
- *pTis*: ductal carcinoma in situ, Padget disease, encapsulated papillary carcinoma, and solid papillary carcinoma
  - *pTis (DCIS)*: ductal carcinoma in situ without invasive carcinoma
  - *pTis (Paget)*: Paget disease without invasive carcinoma
- *pT1mi*: tumor ≤1 mm
- *pT1a*: tumor >1 mm but ≤5 mm
- *pT1b*: tumor >5 mm but ≤10 mm
- *pT1c*: tumor >10 mm but ≤20 mm
- *pT2*: tumor >20 mm but ≤50 mm
- *pT3*: tumor >50 mm
- *pT4a*: extension to the chest wall (not including pectoralis muscle)
- *pT4b*: edema (including peau d'orange), ulceration of skin or ipsilateral satellite skin nodules
- *pT4c*: both T4a and T4b
- *pT4d*: inflammatory carcinoma (involves >1/3 of the breast skin, primarily a clinical diagnosis)

Regional Lymph Nodes (pN)

- *pNX*: cannot be assessed
- *pN0*: no regional lymph node metastasis histologically
- *pN0(i-)*: no regional lymph node metastasis by histology or immunohistochemistry
- *pN0(i+)*: isolated tumor cells (cluster ≤0.2 mm and <200 cells)
- *pN0(mol+)*: RT-PCR positive but negative by light microscopy
- *pN1mi*: micrometastasis (tumor deposit >0.2 mm and ≤2.0 mm or ≤0.2 mm and >200 cells)
- *pN1a*: metastasis in 1–3 axillary lymph nodes with at least 1 tumor deposit >2.0 mm
- *pN1b*: metastasis in internal mammary sentinel lymph node with tumor deposit >2.0 mm
- *pN1c*: pN1a and pN1b
- *pN2a*: metastasis in 4–9 axillary lymph nodes with at least 1 tumor deposit >2.0 mm
- *pN2b*: metastasis in clinically detected internal mammary nodes with pathologically negative axillary nodes
- *pN3a*: metastasis in ≥10 axillary lymph nodes with at least 1 tumor deposit >2.0 mm or metastasis to infraclavicular lymph node
- *pN3b*: positive internal mammary node by imaging with pN1a or pN1b
- *pN3c*: metastasis in ipsilateral supraclavicular lymph node

Distant Metastasis (M)

- *M0*: no clinical or radiological evidence of distant metastases*
- *cM0(i+)*: no clinical or radiological evidence of distant metastases in the presence of tumor cells or deposits ≤0.2 mm detected microscopically or by molecular techniques in cir-

Table 4 Staging of carcinoma breast

When T is…	And N is…	And M is…	Then the stage group is…
T1	N0	M0	I
T1a	N0	M0	IA
T1b	N0	M0	IB
T1c	N0	M0	IC
T2	N0	M0	II
T2a	N0	M0	IIA
T2b	N0	M0	IIB
T1/T2	N1	M0	IIIA1
T3a	N0/N1	M0	IIIA2
T3b	N0/N1	M0	IIB
T3c	N0/N1	M0	IIIC
Any T	Any N	M1	IV
Any T	Any N	M1a	IVA
Any T	Any N	M1b	IVB

Source: From Amin MB, Edge SB. (2017). *AJCC Cancer Staging Manual* 8th Edition. Chicago, IL: American Joint Committee on Cancer culating blood, bone marrow or other non-regional nodal tissue in a patient without symptoms or signs of metastases

- *M1*: Distant metastasis detected by clinical and radiological means (cM) and/or histologically proven metastases >0.2 mm (pM)

*Note that imaging studies are not required to assign cM category. Staging in carcinoma breast is shown in Table 4.

5 Integrated Management Plan for Breast Cancer

Management of breast cancer needs a very well-integrated approach since the management in most cases is likely to include surgery, systemic treatment, and radiotherapy, in varied sequences, along with the incorporation of hormonal therapy/targeted therapies. Table 5 shows integrated management of breast cancer.

Table 5 Integrated management of breast cancer

cTNM	Systemic therapy	Sentinel node biopsy	Breast conservation	Mastectomy	Radiation
DCIS	No	Yes When invasive component >4 cm <55 years Solid component on the mammogram DCIS grades II and III	Yes When excision possible with the good cosmetic result Unifocal lesion Multifocal within 5 cm DCIS <4 cm	Sometimes When good cosmetic results not possible Multicentric DCIS >4 cm	Sometimes In patients with breast conservation
Early Breast Cancer Tumor <5 cm and <4 axilla nodes	Yes Adjuvant chemotherapy NACT to make a BCT possible in large tumors including tumours such as triple negative disease or Her-2 positive disease for tumors >2,5 cm with N0 or N1 luminal B, Triple negative or Her-2 positive disease	Always Unless US-guided fine-needle aspiration is positive	Yes When excision possible with good cosmetic result Unifocal lesion Multifocal within 5 cm Invasive Ca <5 cm	Sometimes When good cosmetic result not possible with BCT Multicentric Invasive Ca >5 cm	Sometimes In all patients with Breast conservation
Loco-regionally advanced Breast Cancer Tumor >5 cm OR > 4 axilla nodes	Yes NACT to make inoperable lesions operable	No Unreliable in this scenario	Sometimes In patients with excellent response to NACT, easily localizable disease	Yes In most patients who are operable are NACT	Yes
Metastatic Breast Cancer	Yes	No	No	Sometimes Palliative mastectomy Mastectomy in patients with oligometastasis	Sometimes Palliative RT to metastasis SBRT to oligometastasis

Therefore, it is strongly advised to discuss all patients in the Multidisciplinary Tumour Board of the hospital before starting treatment. Whilst tumour biology must take precedence in decision making, phenotypic tumour characteristics along side tumour to breast ratio is often considered before offering an appropriate treatment plan. Broadly, patients of breast cancer at presentation can be divided into three categories. (1) *Those with local (early disease, small tumors with limited nodes)* These patients should generally be considered for upfront surgery (This can be breast conservation or mastectomy, based on patient preference, tumour, logistics and other factors. Post-surgical adjuvant therapy would be guided by pathology findings. (2) *Those with advanced local/locoregional disease (tumours >3 cm, clinically positive axillary nodes, supraclavicular/ internal mammary nodes).* These patients typically are considered for neo adjuvant systemic therapies first (chemotherapy/hormonal therapy/ targeted therapy). This is followed by assessment for surgery (conservation or mastectomy based on response assessment, patient and tumor charecteristics (BRCA mutation, multicentricite etc. and patient preference) followed by radiotherapy. (3) *Those with metastatic disease*—These patients should be considered for upfront systemic therapy (chemotherapy/hormonal therapy/targeted therapy). Palliative treatment with radiotherapy or surgery should be used in appropriate cases.

6 Surgical Aspects

Surgery plays a significant role in the management of breast cancer and the field of breast surgery has witnessed a paradigm shift from the era of radical organ sacrificing procedures to era of surgical de-scalation and organ conservation. Advances in the field of systemic therapy and radiotherapy are also impacting the surgical approach to breast cancer. Surgical Interventions like breast oncoplasty and sentinel lymph node biopsy have become standard of care in the recent past.

1. *Early Breast Cancer*

Early breast cancer *(EBC)* can be defined as the disease that is confined to the breast with or without limited regional lymph node involvement. Early breast cancers are potentially curable and constitute 80%–90% of the breast cancer load in high-income countries where as EBC proportion ranges between 40% and 50% in low- and middle-income countries.

The main surgical options in EBC include breast conservation therapy (BCT) or mastectomy with or without reconstruction. Radiation therapy is an integral part of BCT and a sub set of patients are given post-mastectomy radiotherapy. The systemic treatment options include chemotherapy, endocrine therapy, and targeted therapy and clinical decisions are based on histopathology details and molecular status.

1.1 *Management of Primary Tumor*

The surgical options for primary tumor are, breast conservation surgery or modified radical mastectomy. Management options for axillary nodes include ALND, SLNB or axillary nodal irradiation.

The factors affecting the surgical decisions include:

- Tumor related factors- tumor size, location, multicentricity, tumor versus breast ratio, molecular subtypes, and overall stage.
- Patient-related factors, such as age, family history, mutation status, and willingness for breast conservation.
- The expertise of the treating surgeon.
- Available radiotherapy modality like APBI, IORT, EBRT etc.

The NSABP-06 was the first randomized trial which established the BCS with radiotherapy as the feasible option for early invasive breast cancer. The trial results didn't show any difference in OS and DFS in patients who underwent BCS with or without radiotherapy compared to those who underwent modified radical mastectomy. The rate of LRR (loco regional recurrence) was found significantly higher in patients who underwent BCS without radiation [17]. Since then, several randomized trials (MILAN 1 Study, NSABP B-17) have shown comparable long-term survival rates for breast conservation and mastectomy patients

[18–20]. Breast-conserving surgery (BCS) is now the standard surgical option for T1 and T2 unifocal cancers with good tumor versus breast size ratio. However, for large operable breast cancers, aggressive subtypes (triple-negative or HER-2 enriched) and patients with poor tumor versus breast ratio, neoadjuvant therapy (NAT) followed by surgery is the standard of care [21].

The absolute contraindications for BCS include:

- Multicentric disease not amenable for margin free resection with good cosmetic outcomes.
- Persistent positive margins.
- Diffuse microcalcifications.
- Pregnancy.
- Prior therapeutic chest wall radiation.

Relative Contraindications:

- Poor tumor breast ratio.
- Collagen vascular disease.

Optimal Margin Status

Achieving "clear" or negative margins is mandatory in BCS. Reoperations are associated with increased morbidities, delay in adjuvant treatment, cost, and burden on individual and health care facilities. The reported rates of re-excision vary from 10% to greater than 40% [23, 24].

The 2013 Society of Surgical Oncology–American Society for Radiation Oncology (SSO-ASTRO) consensus guideline on margins for BCS with whole-breast irradiation in patients with stages I and II invasive breast cancer suggest that "no ink on tumor" be considered the standard for a negative margin [22]. These margin consensuses are applied for all ages and tumor of any biology.

The SSO–ASTRO–American Society of Clinical Oncology consensus guideline (2016) on margins for BCS with whole-breast irradiation in patients with ductal carcinoma in situ (DCIS) suggested that a 2 mm margin to be considered the standard for a negative margin in these patients. The routine practice of obtaining negative margin widths wider than 2 mm is not supported by the evidence [25]. Hence, Re-excision is indicated for tumor cells on inked margin and DCIS margin is less than 2 mm. In contrary, no re-excision is needed if LCIS is present on inked margin as it is a risk factor, not the precursor of breast cancer.

Surgery for Non-palpable Breast Cancers

Various surgical techniques are described for managing screen detected non-palpable lesions, including wire guided localization (WGL), radioactive seed localization (RSL), radio occult lesion localization (ROLL), and intraoperative ultrasound. Some novel techniques like MAGSEED and RFID (Radio Frequency Identification) are also being explored for localizing the non-palpable breast lesions.

Mastectomy: There are various modifications of mastectomy. Modified radical mastectomy (MRM) is the most commonly used surgical procedure for operable breast cancer not suitable for breast conservation. The structures removed in a modified radical mastectomy are breast with pectoral fascia, nipple areola complex, part of skin and axillary lymph node dissection (ALND). For patients undergoing mastectomy for DCIS and clinically node negative patients with operable invasive cancer sentinel lymph node biopsy (SLNB) is recommended.

Other modifications of mastectomy include skin sparing and nipple areola sparing mastectomy mostly done in patients planned for whole breast reconstruction.

Postoperative radiation with breast conservation surgery improves local control and overall survival for patients with invasive breast cancer.

Ipsilateral breast tumor recurrences (IBTR) develop in and around the tumor bed in 5%–15% of cases. Pathologic data suggest that treatment of the entire breast is unnecessary as in majority of patients with negative margins the residual tumour following surgery is likely to be within 1–2 cm of the lumpectomy cavity [26–28]. This led to emergence of new concept of partial breast irradiation in selected patients with early-stage breast cancer.

1.2 Management of Axilla

Axillary node management helps in staging, prognostication and also has a therapeutic role in a subset of patients. Various options for managing axillary nodes include ALND (Axillary Lymph Node Dissection), SLNB (Sentinel Lymph Node Biopsy) and ANS (Axillary Node Sampling). ALND is considered as standard-of-care for patients with clinically positive lymph nodes and SLNB/ANS can be offered to patients with clinically node negative patients. As per current recommendations, clinical assessment of axillary nodes should include ultrasound and FNAC.

Various randomized studies [ALMANAC [29], NSABP B32 [30], ACOSOG Z0011 [31]] have established SLNB has replaced ALND for clinically node-negative axilla, thereby reducing morbidities of ALND like lymphedema, shoulder stiffness, paresthesia. Table 6 enlists landmark RCTs in the management of axilla.

For clinically positive lymph nodes, the NCCN panel recommends pathologic confirmation of malignancy using ultrasound-guided fine needle aspiration/core biopsy of suspicious lymph nodes. If positive for malignancy, complete levels I and II axillary lymph node dissection is warranted with harvesting of at least 10 lymph nodes. The level III lymph node is also dissected in case of gross disease in level II or III.

SLNB should be done with a combination of techniques (blue dye, radioactive colloid or Indocyanine green dye fluorescence) to increase the accuracy. During SLNB, if sentinel nodes are not identified, Low axillary dissection i.e. removal of fibrofatty tissue overlying the 2nd & 3rd digitation of serratus anterior below the intercostal nerve should be performed for axillary staging.

Management Approach to Axillary Nodes

Current standard of care for node positive patients is ALND and for node negative patients SLNB is recommended. If expertise for SLNB is not available, Axillary nodal sampling (ANS) could be another option in these patients.

Table 6 Landmark RCTs in the management of axilla

RCT	Population	Intervention	Mean follow-up (months)	Outcome
ALMANAC (1999–2003) [29]	$N = 1031$ Any tumor size and clinically node-negative breast cancer	ALND vs. SLNB alone (if negative) or SLNB and ALND or axillary RT (if positive)	12	Arm and shoulder morbidity and QOL: SLNB was associated with reduced arm morbidity and better QOL
NSABP B32 (1999–2004) [30]	$n = 5611$ <4 cm invasive breast cancer and clinically node-negative breast cancer	SLNB + ALND vs. SLNB alone (if negative)	96	OS: No significant difference DFS: No significant difference Axillary recurrence: No significant difference
Z0011 1999–2004 [31]	$N = 856$ T1–2 breast cancer and 1–2 metastatic nodes by SLNB. All underwent lumpectomy and whole-breast irradiation	ALND vs. no further axillary treatment	76	OS: No significant difference DFS: No significant difference
IBCSG 23–01 2001–2010 [32]	$N = 931$ <5 cm invasive breast cancer and 1 or more micrometastatic sentinel nodes	ALND vs. no further axillary treatment	60	OS: No significant difference DFS: No significant difference
AMAROS 2001–2010 [33]	$N = 4805$ T1–2 primary breast cancer and no palpable lymphadenopathy	ALND vs. axillary radiation	73	OS: No significant difference DFS: No significant difference Axillary recurrence: 0.43% ALND vs. 1.19% axillary radiation

Managing axillary nodes following neoadjuvant chemotherapy is a challenge in LMIC due limited availability of expertise for pre chemotherapy staging and localization of lymph nodes and restaging of axilla following neoadjuvant chemotherapy, making ALND the default option in majority of patients. However, SLNB can be offered to node negative patients following neoadjuvant chemotherapy if expertise is available.

Figures 2 and 3 shows axillary nodal management approach for node positive and node negative breast cancer patients as per the availability of resources and expertise.

Axillary Surgical Techniques

Two standard surgical options are available for managing axillary nodes

1. Axillary Lymph node dissection (ALND) and
2. Sentinel Lymph node biopsy (SLNB).

Levels of Axillary Lymph/Nodes

Axillary lymph nodes are divided into three levels based upon their relationship to the pectoralis minor muscle.

- Level I—Inferior and lateral to the pectoralis minor muscle
- Level II—Posterior to the pectoralis minor and
- Level III—medial to the pectoralis minor muscle and they are also known as infraclavicular nodes
- The rotter nodes or interpectoral nodes are located between the pectoralis major and minor muscle.

Axillary Lymph Node Dissection

ALND remained standard of care for managing axillary nodes for almost three quarters of the last

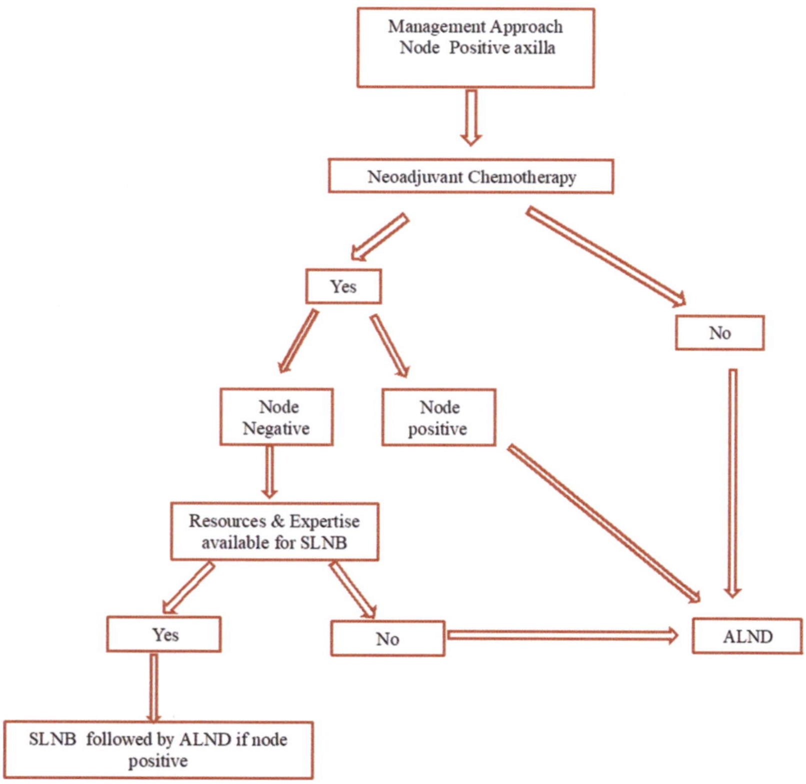

Fig. 2 Flowchart showing management approach for *node positive patients* based on the availability of resources and expertise

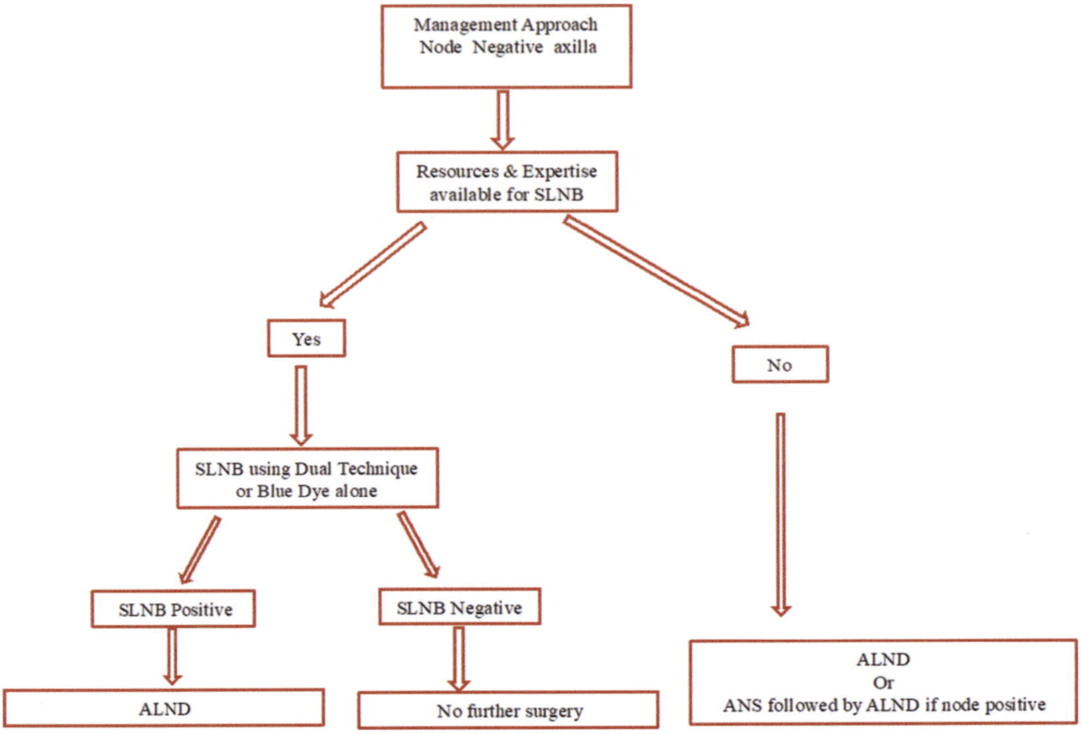

Fig. 3 Flowchart showing management approach for *node negative patients* based on the availability of resources and expertise

century. The goals of ALND are staging, prognostication and a therapeutic role in controlling axillary disease. As far as survival benefit of ALND is concerned the evidence is conflicting especially in the era of modern multimodality management. In LMICs, SLNB is still evolving and ALND is going to be the mainstay of surgical management in majority of breast cancer patients.

Indications for ALND

An axillary lymph node dissection (ALND) is performed along with mastectomy or with the lumpectomy as part of breast conserving procedure. ALND can be performed in following clinical situations.

(i) *Primary ALND*
   Clinically Node positive early stage breast cancer.
(ii) *Following Neoadjuvant Chemotherapy*
   1. In locally advanced (T4a, b, c) and inflammatory breast cancer patients.
   2. In node positive early breast cancer with residual positive nodes following neoadjuvant chemotherapy.
(iii) *Completion Axillary Lymph Node Dissection*
   1. In node positive patients presenting with incomplete axillary dissection following suboptimal surgery.
   2. Following SLNB
      (a) In patients with three or more positive, sentinel lymph nodes with T1 or T2 tumors.
      (b) In patients with any number of positive, sentinel lymph nodes with T3 tumors and or presence of extranodal extension.
      (c) In patients with any number of positive, sentinel lymph nodes who will not receive chest wall radiation following mastectomy, patient refusal or non-availability of radiation facilities and in patients undergoing partial breast irradiation.

(d) Failed SLNB procedure.
(e) Recurrence after SLNB.

Types and Modifications of ALND
Based on extent of lymph node dissection ALND can be classified in to complete ALND and levels I and II ALND. Complete axillary node dissection involves removal of all lymph nodes of levels I, II, and III, whereas in levels I and II ALND, level III nodes are spared. Complete ALND is recommended in locally advanced breast cancer with heavy nodal disease due to a higher incidence of level III involvement. A minimum of 10 lymph nodes should be harvested for optimal staging of axilla using ALND.

Complications of ALND
Apart from routine surgical morbidities like infection, haematoma and seroma, ALND can be associated with significant morbidity including lymphedema, neuropathy and shoulder dysfunction resulting in swelling of the arm, shoulder stiffness, impairment of range of movement, and paraesthesia's in the upper arm. The incidence of morbidity following ALND ranges from 10% to 50%, and can affect quality of life significantly [34]. Important risk factors for development of lymphedema include complete ALND, obesity, high axillary disease burden and post-operative radiotherapy. Prevention and rehabilitation is extremely critical for minimizing the morbidity of ALND.

Sentinel Lymph Node Biopsy (SLNB)
Sentinel lymph node biopsy (SLNB) has been developed as a step forward in the overall de-escalation strategy of surgery for breast cancer [35, 36]. Sentinel node is the first draining lymph node which receives lymph from the primary tumor and the rationale for sentinel-node biopsy is that the histology of this first draining lymph node would be representative of the status of the remaining nodes in axilla. SLNB provides surgeons with information that allows to avoid unnecessary ALND and its morbidity if the sentinel node is negative.

Different techniques of SLNB detection methods are described in literature. Blue dye and radioactive tracer guided techniques are the most widely tried and tested methods. Overall SLN identification rates range between 85% and 98% and false negative rates range between 3% and 10% depending upon the surgeon's experience, and technique used. Currently SLNB is well established in HIC and still evolving in LMIC due to various factors.

Indications for SLNB
- T1 and T2 breast cancer patients with clinically negative axillary node status.
- DCIS patients undergoing mastectomy.
- DCIS patients with suspected invasive cancer.
- Patients presenting with negative axillary lymph nodes following neo adjuvant chemotherapy.

Contraindications for SLNB
- Node positive breast cancer.
- Locally advanced and inflammatory breast cancer.
- Patients presenting with positive axillary lymph nodes following neo adjuvant chemotherapy.

6.1 SLNB Operative Techniques

Methods for SLNB Detection
Various methods have been described for SLNB detection but blue dye and radioactive tracer techniques have been validated extensively by multiple studies [37, 38].

Dye/Radiotracers Used for SLNB
- *Blue Dye*: Six different dyes have been described in literature for SLNB detection, which includes isosulfan blue, patent blue V, methylene blue, Evans blue, indigo-carmine blue, and indocyanin green. However most used dyes for SLNB detection are isosulfan blue and methylene blue.
- *Radioactive Tracer*: Five different radioactive tracers have been used in the detection of the SLNB in breast cancer patients which include technetium Tc 99 m sulfur colloid, Tc99m

albumin colloid, Tc99m dextran, Tc99m rhenium colloid, and Tc99m nanocolloid. Most widely used radioactive tracers are sulfur colloid in United States and albumin colloid in Europe.

- *Indocyanine Green (ICG)*: ICG guided sentinel node identification is emerging as a promising method. The dye is easy to use, and the lymphatic channels can be traced real time. When used alone it achieved a good identification rate of above 95%. When used in conjunction with blue dye the rates are close to 100% [39, 40].

Site, Volume, and Timing of Injection: Various sites of injection have been tried and the success rates of SLNB are comparable with peritumoral, intradermal, subdermal and sub-areolar locations. Currently single injection in sub areola location is the preferred method in most centres practicing SLNB. Generally, blue dye is injected at the time of surgery and 1–2 ml of dye is sufficient. Massage of the injection site helps in faster migration of dye in lymphatic channels. Radiotracers are typically administered by the nuclear medicine expert a day before surgery or on the day of surgery.

SLNB Using Radiotracer and Gamma Probe

A handheld gamma detection probe is held over the axilla to identify the area of highest radioactivity. Portable display screen becomes convenient for the surgical team. A small incision (3–5 cm) is made near the area of radioactivity just behind the anterior axillary fold. Level I axillary region is then evaluated with gamma probe. The first sentinel node is the node with the highest radioactivity which is known as "hot node". After removal of the node ex-vivo highest or 10 s count is recorded. All nodes whose radioactive count is 10% of the most radioactive node are considered sentinel nodes and are removed (rule of 10%).

SLNB Using Blue Dye: After the dye injection and massaging, axilla is entered through a small (3–5 cm) incision behind anterior axillary fold.

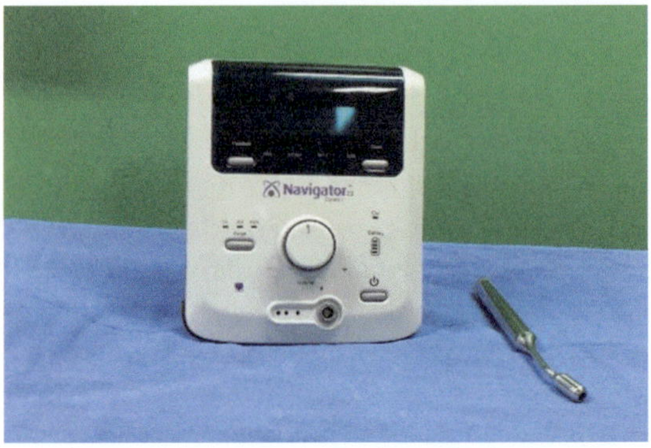

Fig. 4 Showing wireless gamma detection probe and portable display console for SLNB using radioactive tracer

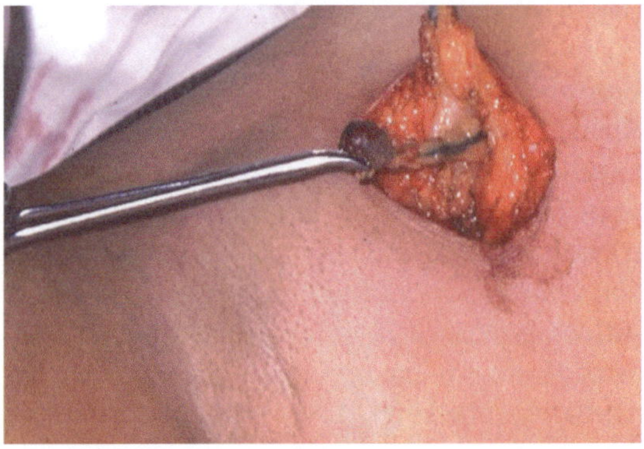

Fig. 5 Intraoperative identification of the sentinel lymph node by tracing the blue-stained lymphatic channel into the axilla until the blue-stained sentinel node is visualised

After entering subcutaneous plane surgeon should carefully watch for blue dye-filled lymphatic tract. The blue stained lymphatic is then followed in to axilla until a blue stained sentinel node is identified (Fig. 5).

The goal of SLN biopsy is to remove "hot" and/or blue nodes and/or palpable and suspicious nodes to accurately stage the axilla. Generally, number of SLN varies between 1 and 3 with a median of 2 nodes in most studies. Staging accuracy does not increase by removing more than 3–4 nodes.

Histopathology Assessment of Sentinel Lymph Nodes The basis of SLNB is to perform a focused and intensive histopathological evaluation of limited number of lymph nodes. Special expertise is needed for grossing (step sections), frozen section analysis, imprint cytology and immunohistochemistry. Nodal metastases of sentinel lymph node can be categorized as

1. Isolated tumor cells (<0.2 mm)
2. Micro-metastases (0.2–2 mm) and
3. Macro-metastases (>2 mm) based on the size of metastatic focus.

In LMIC conventional histopathology evaluation with H&E staining for identification of macrometastasis can be recommended for routine clinical use.

Complications of SLNB: The reported rates of restriction of shoulder movements, neuropathic pain, and lymphedema range between 2% and 10% following SLNB [29]. Various factors, including patient positioning, surgical technique, anatomical variations, and addition of radiation therapy can affect morbidity rates following SLNB.

Axillary Node Sampling (ANS)

Axillary Node Sampling (ANS) has been described in literature as a less invasive surgical staging tool for nodal staging prior to introduction of SLNB. The basic rationale behind ANS is sampling of high-risk lymph node stations instead of ALND in early stage node negative breast cancer patients. Various techniques of ANS are described and include as follows

- *Four Node Sampling*: Edinburgh group described four-node sample procedure in which the surgeon has to remove by inspection and palpation at least four lymph nodes from the lower axillary fat (level I).
- *Triple Node Biopsy*: In this technique lymph node from three levels - low axillary level, apex of axilla and internal mammary are removed separately. Triple node biopsy is technically more challenging than four node sampling.
- *Low Axillary Sampling*: Low axillary sampling can be performed as an alternative to SLNB for staging axilla in clinically node negative patients. In low axillary fat along with minimum of 4 lymph nodes are removed between pectoralis major anteriorly, latissimus dorsi posteriorly, serratus anterior medially and intercostobrachial nerve superiorly [41].

ANS techniques especially four node or low axillary sampling have the potential to be used as an alternative to SLNB if resources and expertise for SLNB are not available in LMIC. These are simple surgical techniques, does not require expensive resources and general surgeons can be trained easily.

Current ESMO Recommendations [21]

- SLNB is the standard of care for axillary staging in early, clinically node-negative breast cancer.
- Complete axillary dissection following positive SLNB is not needed in case of low axillary disease burden (micrometastases or 1–2 SLNs containing metastases, treated with postoperative tangential breast RT).
- Axillary radiation is a valid alternative in patients with positive SLNB, irrespective of the type of breast surgery.

Locally Advanced Breast Cancer

Locally advanced breast cancer usually treated by neoadjuvant chemotherapy followed by mastectomy. Modified Radical mastectomy is the preferred surgery for locally advanced disease particularly T4 disease. Surgery is mandatory even if the patient attains clinical complete response after NACT.

Surgery in Metastatic Breast Cancer

The goal of MBC treatment is to prolong survival, control tumour burden, reduce tumour-related symptoms, and improve quality of life.

In recent years, number of studies have been done to see the impact of elective surgical resection of the primary breast tumour before the onset

Table 7 RCTs of surgery of the primary tumor in patients with MBC

RCT	Population	Intervention in surgical arm	Mean follow-up (months)	Outcome (Sx Vs No Sx)
ECOG E2108 2011–2015 [42]	$n = 256$ MBC on systemic therapy for 4–8 months without progression	87% surgery (BCS + RT or mastectomy ± RT)	53	Median OS 54 months in both arms 3-year OS 68 versus 68% HR 1.09, 90% CI 0.80–1.49; $p = 0.63$
Austria 2011–2015 [43, 44]	$n = 90$ Stage IV breast cancer	71% mastectomy; 29% BCS + RT	37.5	Median OS 35 versus 55 months HR 0.69, 95% CI 0.36–1.33; $p = 0.27$
India 2005–2013 [45]	$n = 350$ MBC with resectable hormone receptor-positive disease, *or* Others with a partial or complete response to anthracycline-based chemotherapy	72% mastectomy; 23% BCS + RT	23	Median OS 19 versus 20.5 months 2-year OS 42 versus 43% HR 1.04, 95% CI 0.81–1.34; $p = 0.79$
Turkey MF07–01 2007–2012 [46]	$n = 274$ Stage IV breast cancer	74% mastectomy; 26% BCS + RT	40	*5-year OS 42 versus 24%* *HR 0.66, 95% CI 0.49–0.88; $p = 0.005$*

of local symptoms. Till now, four RCTs have been done to evaluate the survival effect of surgical resection of the primary lesion in metastatic breast cancer. Of four studies only one (Turkey MF07–01) showed a statistically significant difference in overall survival (OS). RCTs of surgery of the primary tumor in patients with MBC is shown in Table 7.

Over decades, improvements in systemic therapy have definitely prolonged the survival of patients with metastatic breast cancer; similarly, surgery for the primary disease may reduce the risk of symptomatic local disease and may improve survival further in select patient group.

Surgeons are also tended to perform surgical resection in patients with metastatic disease based on the following characteristics:

- *Good performance status*
- *Oligometastatic disease*
- *Long disease-free interval*
- *High likelihood of complete resection*

Still in view of currently available literature and guidelines, primary surgery is not recommended in the majority of patients with stage IV breast cancer unless it is directed towards palliation and symptom management. MBC treatment should not only pursue survival benefits but also consider quality of life and psychological needs.

7 Systemic Therapy

Systemic therapy is an essential component of treatment in patients with non-metastatic and metastatic breast cancer. History of systemic chemotherapy started following the World War II when nitrogen mustard became useful as an anticancer drug in 1950s. From 1960s and 1970s, the multi-agent chemotherapy regimens, to be delivered as adjuvant after breast surgery, were developed in USA, UK, Europe, Japan. Hormone therapy and tumor marker-based drugs became routinely used from 1980s and 1990s. Considerable progress has been made in systemic therapy in the past two decades. This is largely rooted in the conceptual recognition of breast cancer being a heterogeneous disease with at least three to four subtypes that vary in their natural histories, response to treatments, and outcomes [47, 48]. These subtypes have their biological basis in mutational profiles, gene expression programs and epigenetic modification patterns but are well approximated by routine immunohistochemical (IHC) evaluation of clinical biopsy specimens [49]. The IHC tests as a minimum should provide the marker status for prognostic and therapeutic purposes- 1. estrogen receptor (ER), 2. progesterone receptor (PR), 3. Proliferative index (Ki-67), 4. human epidermal growth recetor-2 (HER2), 5. P53. The clinically relevant IHC subtypes are estrogen and/or progesterone receptor (ER/PR) positive and HER2 (officially known as ERBB2) negative (corresponding to gene expression *intrinsic* types "luminal A" and "luminal B"), ER/PR any (positive or negative) and HER2 positive (corresponding to gene expression *intrinsic* type "HER2 like") and ER, PR, and HER2 negative [so-called triple negative breast cancer (TNBC), most of which correspond to the gene expression *intrinsic* type "basal like"].

The current systemic therapy options in breast cancer comprise of chemotherapy, endocrine therapy [selective estrogen receptor modulators (SERM) like tamoxifen, aromatase inhibitors (AI) letrozole, anastrazole, and exemestane. They also include selective estrogen receptor degraders (SERD) like fulvestrant, ovarian function suppressing agents, progestins like megesterol acetate, others], HER2 targeted therapy (monoclonal antibodies, small molecular kinase inhibitors, drug-antibody conjugates). Newer agents include immune checkpoint inhibitors, and other targeted agents [cyclin-dependent kinase 4/6 (CDK 4/6) inhibitors, phosphoinositide 3 kinase (PI3K)/Akt/mammalian target of rapamycin (mTOR) inhibitors like alpelisib and everolimus, drug antibody conjugates targeting various tumor-associated antigens and others).

The following sections briefly describe the current systemic therapy options in these subtypes in non-metastatic and metastatic disease patients. A recent retrospective analysis of a large dataset from multiple Indian institutions has suggested that outcomes in patients with operable breast cancer are comparable to those reported internationally [50].

- *Non-metastatic breast cancer*

  The most important clinical-pathological prognostic factors are tumor size, axillary lymph node status, tumor grade, proliferation and ER, PR, and HER2 status. A combination of these factors is commonly used to estimate the likely prognosis group for each patient and decide on neoadjuvant or adjuvant systemic therapy. Additionally, patient-related factors such as comorbidities, age, and competing causes of mortality are also important inputs in the adjuvant decision-making process. Simple prognostic index calculations, like the Nottingham Prognostic index scores based on the above factors can prognosticate patients into good, intermediate, and high-risk categories [51].

  Traditionally, a group of patients with locally advanced breast cancers with high tumour to breast ratio, LABC, defined variously as T3-T4 or N2-N3 disease) have been treated with neoadjuvant chemotherapy (NACT), given with neoadjuvant HER2-targeted therapy if the patient has HER2 positive disease. Such treatment aims to make such tumors resectable and/or facilitate breast-conserving treatment. However, in recent years there has been increasing use of neoadjuvant treatment even in patients with less advanced disease, driven mainly by the benefit of further risk-adapted post-neoadjuvant systemic therapy in patients with residual invasive cancer in the surgical specimen [non-achievement of complete pathological response (pCR)].

- *ER and/or PR positive and HER2 negative breast cancer*

  Patients with these tumors have a range of prognosis from excellent to good based on prognostic factors mentioned above. The decision to give chemotherapy or not in this subtype of breast cancer, especially in patients with negative node disease, is critically dependent on high quality pathology evaluation of tumors [52]. Several multi-gene assays have also been validated for use in adjuvant decision making. Almost all of these aim to select out a group of patients (mainly with node negative disease) who have such a good prognosis (long-term disease-free survival exceeding 90%–95%) with adjuvant endocrine therapy alone that additional chemotherapy is unlikely to provide meaningful additional benefit [53, 54]. However, these multi-gene tests are costly and not accessible to the vast majority of patients in most parts of the world. Based on either clinical-pathological factors or genomic assays, patients with excellent prognosis are offered endocrine therapy alone, which comprises tamoxifen for 5–10 years in premenopausal patients [55], and an aromatase inhibitor (with or without in a sequence with tamoxifen) for 5–10 years in post-menopausal patients [56]. Some premenopausal patients with high-risk disease are offered ovarian function suppression using a gonadotropin-releasing hormone (GnRH) agonist or ablation with bilateral oophorectomy [57].

Patients with less than excellent estimated prognosis by either clinical-pathological evaluation (T size ≥1–2 cm or node-positive, in some combination with grade and proliferation as measured by Ki-67) or a multi-gene test, are offered adjuvant chemotherapy if they are considered fit to receive this treatment. The chemotherapy drugs and regimens are the same as the ones used in patients with TNBC (see below).

- *ER and/or PR any, and HER2 positive breast cancer*
  HER2-targeted therapy added to chemotherapy is the most important component of adjuvant treatment in such patients. Those with ER and/or PR-positive tumors also receive adjuvant endocrine therapy as described above. The mainstay of adjuvant HER2 targeted therapy has been the HER2 targeted monoclonal antibody trastuzumab, given for 1 year, which has shown an improvement in disease-free and overall survival [58]. A recent meta-analysis has suggested that shorter durations of adjuvant trastuzumab, ranging from 9 weeks to 6 months, could be non-inferior to its 1-year use [59]. However, there are caveats to this analysis mainly related to the methodological aspects of the included randomised controlled trials. Shorter durations of adjuvant trastuzumab can be used, especially in patients with cardiac comorbidities and in those with low-risk disease. In some patients with high-risk disease, the use of HER2 targeted monoclonal antibody pertuzumab, added to trastuzumab, has been shown to result in improved disease-free survival [60] and can be considered as an option. In patients with residual invasive cancer after NACT plus HER2 targeted therapy, replacement of further trastuzumab with the drug-antibody conjugate ado-trastuzumab emtansine (T-DM1) has been shown to improve disease-free survival [61] and can be offered to the patient, if feasible.
- *Triple-negative breast cancer (TNBC)*
  Most patients with TNBC are considered to have high-risk disease and are offered adjuvant chemotherapy if the tumor size is ≥1 cm or if they have node positive disease. The standard chemotherapy is a sequence of an anthracycline regimen (such as four cycles of doxorubicin or epirubicin plus cyclophosphamide) and a taxane (paclitaxel or docetaxel). There is some evidence that dose-dense (with a shorter cycle duration of 2 weeks instead of 3 weeks) administration of anthracycline-taxane regimen may result in superior outcomes. Non-anthracycline regimens like TC (docetaxel plus cyclophosphamide X 4–6 cycles) or CMF (cyclophosphamide plus methotrexate plus 5-FU, especially in older patients) can also be used in some patients.

Neoadjuvant chemotherapy, when used, is delivered with the same drugs and regimens. One recent study in TNBC has shown that adding the immune checkpoint inhibitor pembrolizumab to neoadjuvant anthracycline-taxane-platinum chemotherapy resulted in higher pCR and event-free survival [62]. Another recent study in patients with germline BRCA 1 or BRCA 2 pathogenic/likely pathogenic mutations has shown a benefit of adding the poly (ADP-ribose) polymerase (PARP) inhibitor, olaparib, for 2 years as an adjuvant treatment, in high-risk TNBC and ER/PR positive breast cancer [63]. A third study in patients with residual invasive cancer after neoadjuvant chemotherapy has shown disease-free and overall survival benefit of adding up to 8 cycles of adjuvant capecitabine [64]. This agent is considered in many centres to be a standard treatment in this setting.

- *Metastatic breast cancer*
  - *ER and/or PR positive and HER2 negative breast cancer*
    The outcome of this subtype of metastatic breast cancer has improved in the past few years using sequential endocrine therapy with median overall survival approaching 5 years in a first-line setting. The available drugs include tamoxifen, aromatase inhibitors (anastrazole, letrozole, and exemestane), ovarian function suppressors (leuprolide acetate and goserelin), and SERD (fulvestrant). Other agents that have been used are CDK 4/6 inhibitors (palbociclib, ribociclib, and abemaciclib), PI3K inhibitor (alpelisib), mTOR inhibitor (everolimus) and progestins (megestrol acetate). CDK 4/6 inhibitors, PI3K inhibitors and mTOR inhibitors are given in combination with either an aromatase inhibitor or fulvestrant. Chemotherapy is used in patients who have large visceral disease burden requiring a rapid response or in those who have become resistant to multiple endocrine treatments. Recent reports from India have suggested that use of CDK 4/6 inhibitors shows comparable safety and efficacy as that reported in pivotal studies [65, 66].
  - *ER and/or PR any and HER2 positive breast cancer*
    The prognosis of this subtype of metastatic breast cancer has improved in the past few years with the availability of many novel HER2 targeted drugs, with median overall survival approaching 5 years in first-line setting. The available HER2 targeted drugs include monoclonal antibodies (trastuzumab, pertuzumab, and margetuximab) and small molecule kinase inhibitors (lapatinib, tucatinib, and neratinib). Both of these are given in combination with chemotherapy (sometimes endocrine therapy in ER positive disease). Drug-antibody conjugates (ado-trastuzumab emtansine and fam-trastuzumab deruxtecan-nxki) are often used as single agents.
  - *Triple-negative breast cancer*
  - The prognosis of this subtype of metastatic breast cancer continues to be poor, with median overall survival of 12–18 months after the diagnosis of metastatic disease. Chemotherapy drugs (sequential single agents or combination) are the mainstay of treatment. Available chemotherapy drugs include anthracyclines, taxanes, platinum agents, capecitabine, eribulin, vinorelbine, etc. The results of immune checkpoint inhibitors and PARP inhibitors (in patients with germline pathogenic/likely pathogenic BRCA1/BRCA2 mutation) have been modest. Sacituzumab govitecan-hziy is a novel drug-antibody conjugate, which has shown improved overall survival in patients with metastatic TNBC and has been approved for use.
    - *Surgery and local treatment of the primary tumor in patients with metastatic disease*
      An important randomized study from India established that local treatment (surgery with or without radiotherapy) of the primary tumor does not improve overall survival in patients with de novo metastatic breast cancer [67], which has subsequently been confirmed by a North American study [68]. Therefore, is is not standard practice to perform surgery in these patients.

8 Radiation Therapy: Indications and Selection

8.1 Radiotherapy after Breast Conservation

Breast conservation surgery (BCS) with radiation has been rigorously studied and validated in randomized clinical trials [17, 69–73]. Major trials have proven that there is no significant difference between BCS, when it is combined with adjuvant radiation versus mastectomy, with regard to distant metastasis and survival [17, 69–73]. It is this seminal finding that has allowed use of breast conservation among millions of appropriately selected patients. Recent update of EBCTCG in 2011 in 10,801 women from 17 randomised trials including seven new trials of radiotherapy versus no radiotherapy after breast-conserving surgery reported radiotherapy benefit outcomes similar as from earlier analysis [4, 5]. Overall, radiotherapy reduced the 10-year risk of any (i.e., loco regional or distant) first recurrence from 35.0% to 19.3% (absolute reduction 15.7%, 95% CI 13.7—17.7, $2p < 0.00001$) and reduced the 15-year risk of breast cancer death from 25.2% to 21.4% (absolute reduction 3.8%, 1.6—6.0, $2p = 0.00005$).

Nearly all patient with breast conservation need local radiotherapy. A highly select group of patients, after multidisciplinary discussions, can be avoided radiotherapy. Most of these studies have taken a select, highly favourable group of patients and demonstrated that although radiotherapy significantly reduced local recurrences, no significant difference was observed on overall survival rates [74]. Therefore in selected patients (significant comorbidities, node negative patients older than 65-y old age and tumors less than 3 cm with highly endocrine positive tumors) one could discuss the option of not offering radiotherapy. In the recent EUROPA randomised study, endocrine therapy was associated with a greater reduction in health related quality of life compared with radiotherapy at 24 months [74].

8.2 DCIS and Radiotherapy

DCIS initially accounted for approximately 2% of all breast cancers detected [75, 76]. The incidence rates have markedly increased over the past several decades because of the widespread implementation of screening mammography in the recent decades. The relationship between DCIS and invasive ductal cancer remains a subject of significant controversy, especially because not all DCIS progresses to invasive cancer [77, 78]. Specifically, DCIS that spans a diameter larger than 5 cm has been found to have a markedly increased risk for the presence of occult invasive disease [76, 79, 80]. Other such risk factors for invasion include palpable masses, high-grade histology, and cancerization of lobules [81, 82] There is no frank indication of radiotherapy after mastectomy in patients with DCIS.

Reasonable evidence exists for role of radiation therapy in DCIS patients after breast conservation. Landmark prospective randomized trials evaluate breast conservation with and without radiotherapy for maximizing local control in DCIS. These include National Surgical Adjuvant Breast and Bowel Project (NSABP) B-17 [83, 84] European Organisation for Research and Treatment of Cancer (EORTC) 10,853 [85, 86], SweDCIS, and the United Kingdom (UK), Australia, and New Zealand (UK/ANZ) trial [87–90]. An individual patient data analysis was done of these randomised trials. A total of 3729 women were eligible for analysis. Radiotherapy reduced the absolute 10-year risk of any ipsilateral breast event (i.e., either recurrent DCIS or invasive cancer) by 15.2% (SE 1.6%, 12.9% vs. 28.1% $2\ P < 0.00001$). Radiotherapy was effective regardless of the risk factors commonly used for DCIS such as age at diagnosis, extent of breast-conserving surgery, use of tamoxifen, method of DCIS detection, margin status, focality, grade, comedonecrosis, architecture, or tumor size [91].

Although adjuvant RT after lumpectomy for DCIS has been shown to improve local control in all subsets of patients, there is an ongoing debate if low risk patients can be spared radiotherapy. The inability to clearly identify a low-risk patient and the persistent risk of recurrence in follow up years after DCIS surgery makes it challenging to withhold radiotherapy from patients with DCIS and breast conservation. There is evidence that small lesion size (<2 cm), widely clear surgical margins (≥1 cm), low nuclear grade and the absence of necrosis are favourable risk factors with a risk of breast cancer recurrence after 10 years of 4%–10% in patients with all four factors, and with a very small absolute risk reduction arising from radiotherapy.

In 2009, the Eastern Cooperative Oncology Group published the results of a prospective trial of 701 women with DCIS treated with WLE alone. Surgical microscopic margins were required to be 3 mm or more. Patients were categorized into low-risk (low or intermediate histologic grade DCIS 2.5 cm or smaller) versus high-risk groups (high-grade DCIS 1 cm or smaller). Median follow-up was 6.2 years.

Although the low-risk women had acceptably low IBRT rates (6.1%) at 5 years, patients in the high-risk group had a 15.3% rate of IBTR at 5 years, suggesting that excision alone was inadequate as sole therapy in this patient subset [92].

Therefore, current evidence suggests postoperative radiotherapy after breast conserving surgery for all patients with high risk/intermediate risk DCIS following breast conservation. If the patient has very low risk factors, there should be a shared decision for the omission of radiotherapy.

8.3 Radiotherapy After Mastectomy

Even after mastectomy and systemic therapy, the occult disease may remain in the chest wall and/or regional lymph nodes. This residual disease may serve not only as a source of potentially morbid locoregional recurrence but also as an important reservoir from which distant metastases may be seeded or reseeded after the initial elimination of distant disease by sophisticated modern systemic therapies.

Historically, postoperative radiation therapy for women with breast cancer was in question as its role as effective adjuvant treatment for a few decades [93, 94]. This changed with the publication of landmark randomized trials of PMRT established the survival benefit by post-mastectomy radiotherapy [95–97]. A significant improvement was obtained on locoregional recurrences, disease-free survival, event free survival and overall survival with the addition of radiotherapy to systemic treatment. Early Breast Cancer Trialists Collaborative Group Overview metaanalysis included more than 9000 patients from randomized trials of RT after mastectomy plus varying extent of axillary surgery [4]. In this metaanalysis, PMRT was found to proportionally decrease the risk of LRR by 73% (annual odds ratio 0.28), with the 5-year risk of local recurrence of 5.8% versus 22.8% in node positive patients treated with and without PMRT. This reduction in LRR translated into a 5.4% benefit in 15-year breast cancer-specific survival and a 4.4% benefit in overall survival [4]. This data suggests that one life is saved for every four local recurrences that are prevented. Patients with 4 or more axillary lymph node metastases benefited from radiotherapy most. However, there is no evidence that radiotherapy has impact on local recurrences or overall survival rates on T1/T2 patients without axillary lymph node metastases. Ongoing trials are exploring the role of post mastectomy radiotherapy in T1/T2 N0 patients with additional adverse features (e.g., age, tumour size, grade, receptor status, Her2neu status, and lympho-vascular space invasion) [98].

Patients with 1–3 positive nodes and adequate axillary dissection present a therapeutic challenge. In the EBCTCG analysis, patients with 1–3 nodal metastasis too had survival benefit with local radiotherapy after mastectomy. However many practitioners use the presence of additional adverse factors for the decision regarding radiotherapy. These factors include triple negative disease, positive lymph node ratio >20%, presence of LVI and young patients.

The American Society of Clinical Oncology, American Society for Radiation Oncology and the Society of Surgical Oncology jointly published a focused guideline update to address the risk/beneft ratio of PMRT in patients-treated surgically with mastectomy having T1–2 tumors and 1–3 nodes positive at nodal dissection [99]. They concluded that available evidence shows PMRT reduces the risk of locoregional failure, recurrence, and breast cancer mortality in this patient population overall. However, they advised that certain subsets of patients,in view of low risk features are unlikely to have favourable risk/benefit ratio with PMRT. For these patients, the group encouraged the use of sound clinical judgment and decision-making on a case-by-case basis.

The European SUPREMO trial (Selective Use of Postoperative Radiotherapy after Mastectomy) randomizes intermediate-risk operable breast cancer (node-positive stage II tumors and node-negative tumors larger than 2 cm with adverse features [high grade or LVI]) to chest wall irradiation or observation after mastectomy (62 T). The Trans SUPREMO arm of the same trial shall address the question related to translational aspect of risk stratification related to 1–3 node positive patients. The Supremo trial was recently published. Chest-wall irradiation did not result in higher overall survival than no chest-wall irradiation among patients with intermediate-risk, early breast cancer treated with mastectomy and contemporary adjuvant systemic therapy [100].

A special situation is local radiotherapy to the reconstructed breast. In the present day, there is a wide spectrum of choices regarding reconstruction type and timings available. Many women who are candidates for autologous reconstruction have the option to wait and get reconstruction done post radiotherapy. This is aimed at avoid the side-effects of radiotherapy to the reconstruction site altogether. For women who request immediate breast reconstruction, there is emerging evidence that autologous reconstruction can tolerate radiotherapy better than was previously believed. Recent data suggests improved quality of life and cosmetic outcomes in these patients undergoing autologous reconstructions as compared with implants. It is to be noted that results of reconstruction and radiotherapy might vary depending on several factors, including radiotherapy techniques, dose or fractionation, and target volumes [101].

However, despite their higher incidence of complications, implants remain and important form of reconstruction offered to women who receive PMRT. Overall, in patients undergoing breast reconstruction of any form, evidence does not favour one schedule of radiotherapy treatment over the other. All approaches in such patients should be directed to achieve patient's oncological and reconstructive goals. Radiotherapy indications are shown in Table 8.

Table 8 Radiation therapy indications

Patients undergoing modified radical mastectomy (MRM)	Breast conserving surgery (BCS)
>5 cm tumor size	All cases Except for tumors less than 3 cm, highly HR+, N0, older than 65-y with morbidity or no access to RT
All ≥4 positive axillary nodes 1–3 with adverse prognostic factors	Preferably give a boost as well (especially in patients younger than 50 years and G3 or with extensive ductal component)
Locally advanced breast cancer (irrespective of NACT response)	
Positive margins or residual disease in postoperative bed/axilla	
Emerging evidence for stages I and II triple-negative cancer	

NACT and PMRT

With frequent use of NACT, it can become challenging to decide for the need for radiotherapy after NACT. Traditionally, the decision for recommending PMRT has been based on the initial clinical stage of disease rather than the post-chemotherapy pathology findings. Investigators at the M. D. Anderson Cancer Center retrospectively reviewed 542 patients from 1974 to 2000 who were treated with NAC, mastectomy, and PMRT and compared them to 134 patients similarly treated but without radiation. In patients presenting with clinical stage IIB or greater disease ($n = 646$), there was a significant decrease in LRR at 10 years with PMRT (11% vs 26% $P < 0.001$). An analysis of NSABP B-18/27 data also revealed that patients with any residual nodal disease after NAC have a "clinically significant" 15% risk of LRR, and therefore, may benefit from PMRT [102–105]. Postmastectomy radiation also improved cause-specific survival in patients with stage IIIB disease, clinical T4 tumors, and greater than 4 positive lymph nodes. The authors suggested that PMRT should be considered for patients in all of these subsets, regardless of their response to preoperative systemic chemotherapy [103, 104]. One of the reasons for NACT in N1 patients is to achieve response in axillary lymph node metastases and proceed with SLNB instead of axillary dissection to reduce the risk of arm edema. The role of radiotherapy in initially node positive patients who receive NACT and then are ypN0 and pyN1 is currently under investigation [106]. In the recently published NSABP- B 51 trial, a total of 1641 patients were enrolled. Patients with breast cancer with a clinical stage of T1 to T3 (tumor size, ≤2 cm to >5 cm), N1, and M0 (indicating spread to movable, ipsilateral level I and II axillary lymph nodes but no distant metastasis) who had ypN0 status after neoadjuvant chemotherapy were randomly assigned. Regional nodal irradiation did not significantly increase the invasive breast cancer recurrence–free interval, the locoregional recurrence–free interval, the distant recurrence–free interval, disease-free survival, or overall survival. Overall, the addition of adjuvant regional nodal irradiation did not decrease the risk of invasive breast cancer recurrence or death from breast cancer in patients who had negative axillary nodes after neoadjuvant chemotherapy [107]. Till further data emerges, it may be prudent to deliver regional radiotherapy in selected cases of cN1 patients that get converted to ypN0 with SLNB after NAC. Irradiation of the medial, non-dissected part of the axilla has been accepted as standard for patients who underwent axillary dissection due to ypN1 disease.

9 Simulation and Contouring

Positioning

The patient should be in the supine position for treatment with arms above the head. If supraclavicular irradiation is contemplated, the head itself may be kept straight or turned to the opposite side (if supraclavicular irradiation is contemplated). Consider using a wedge or a breast board for making the chest wall surface nearly parallel to the couch. However, keeping the patient completely supine (vacuum cushion or winged board) is also a reasonable option, especially in centers with a modern setup with MLC head and image guidance.

Simulation

1. Place lead marker/copper wire in the midaxillary line. This will of help in contouring as well as subsequent placement of tangents.
2. For breast conservation patients, place a lead marker/copper wire 1–2 cm below the ipsilateral inframammary fold. This can serve as a verification lower edge for the placement of tangents. In the case of post-mastectomy cases, place the lead marker/copper wire at the ipsilateral chest wall, 1–2 cm below the contralateral inframammary fold. Routine use of thermoplastic mask for breast conservation cases is not recommended.
3. Place copper wire all along the length of post mastectomy scar/or the scar of lumpectomy in breast conservation cases.
4. A circumferential thin copper wire all around the base of the breast (in patients with breast conservation) should be placed.
5. In an exceptional case, a thermoplastic mask may be made in patients with sagging breast to avoid inframammary fold. For pendulous breast, using prone position is another way to avoid folds in such a situation. (However, this needs a special prone breast board, also would need a wide bore CT).
6. Use of a thermoplastic mask for all post-mastectomy patients should be considered. This is also likely to provide vital bolus effect on chest wall. If thermoplastic mask not being made, then consider use of 3–5 mm universal bolus at simulation (for treatment with 6MV X- rays).
7. Many patients undergo immediate breast reconstruction (IBR) after mastectomy. Many patients who have had IBR receive PMRT to target volumes similar to conventional simulator-based whole breast irradiation. Postmastectomy radiation therapy (PMRT) contouring guidelines for target volumes in the setting of IBR are now emerging. The issue requires thorough understanding of the surgical procedures, disease stage, patterns of recurrence and radiation techniques [108].

A regular non-contrast CT with 3 mm slice thickness should be taken. A contrast CT should be taken only in special situations (e.g., treatment of internal mammary region that requires delineation of internal mammary vessels).

Contouring

Breast contouring is not a necessity as a target volume for most forward planned breast treatments. Geometry based planning to account for appropriate coverage of the breast around the index quadrant can often justify limited sparing of the low risk edges when trying to avoid unnecessary lung coverage. With the radiopaque markers for all the tangent edges in place, a medial and

Table 9 Key contouring guidelines/publications

Author/Journal	Year	Key points
ESTRO ACROP consensus guideline for target volume delineation in the setting of postmastectomy radiation therapy after implant-based immediate reconstruction for early-stage *breast* cancer, radiotherapy and oncology	2019	Describes delineation guidelines for PMRT after implant-based immediate breast reconstruction (based on an understanding of the surgical procedures, disease stage, patterns of recurrence, and radiation techniques)
ESTRO consensus guideline on target volume delineation for elective radiation therapy of early-stage breast cancer, radiotherapy, and oncology	2015	Describes delineation of CTV for breast/thoracic wall along with delineation of axillary nodal levels
Recommendations from GEC ESTRO Breast Cancer Working Group (I): Target definition and target delineation for accelerated or boost Partial Breast Irradiation using multicatheter interstitial brachytherapy after breast-conserving closed cavity surgery	2015	Achieve a reproducible and consistent definition of CTV (PTV) for Accelerated Partial Breast Irradiation (APBI) or boost irradiation after breast-conserving closed cavity surgery
Breast cancer atlas for radiation therapy planning: consensus definitions- RTOG	2015	Describes delineation of CTV for breast/thoracic wall along with delineation of axillary, internal mammary and supraclavicular nodal levels.
Breast contouring RADCOMP consortium	2016	Describes delineation of CTV for breast/thoracic wall along with delineation of axillary, internal mammary and supraclavicular nodal levels

a lateral tangent should be set to encompass the breast tissue including the area enclosed in the copper wire.

For actual contouring, appropriate guidelines such as ESTRO/RTOG/RADCOMP guidelines should be followed for breast and regional nodal irradiation [109–111], for contralateral breast and for ipsilateral breasts treated using inverse planned approaches [112]. While these guidelines represent a laudable attempt, some aspects of contouring (and implications on consequent treatment planning) remain unresolved [113]. Key contouring guidelines/publications are enlisted in Table 9.

For delineation of the cavity, one needs to contour the tumor cavity or the tumor bed. This volume needs to be given a 1–1.5 cm margin. While this volume needs to be treated at the end of whole breast radiotherapy, it is important to contour it during contouring for whole breast radiotherapy to ensure that the boost volume is also well covered in the plan for whole breast radiotherapy as well.

For breast cancer radiation therapy planning, the important OAR's include heart, lungs, and contralateral breast. Recently the trend has been toward contouring of segments of the heart, including ventricles and main coronary arteries [114]. Contouring of the liver too should be done, especially in patients with right-sided breast cancer.

For patients undergoing regional nodal irradiation, contouring of the thyroid, carotid and brachial plexus should be done.

10 Treatment Planning and Delivery

Concept of Breast Treatment Planning
Optimal coverage of ipsilateral breast with treatment isodoses must be weighed against organ at risk (OAR) dose spillage. The most critical OAR's around the breast are the ipsilateral and contralateral lungs, the contralateral breast and the heart in left sided cancers. Most importantly, one needs to minimise unnecessary low dose spillage to these OARs to avoid significant risks of lung fibrosis, second primaries and cardiac events, especially when breast irradiation remains an adjuvant concept and long-term morbidities are of importance. The brachial plexus is stationed close to the supraclavicular target area and doses must be appropriately checked to prevent unintended hotspots.

Tangential fields are used to achieve less spillage to the lungs (Fig. 6a, b). The straight posterior edge is made possible either by using half

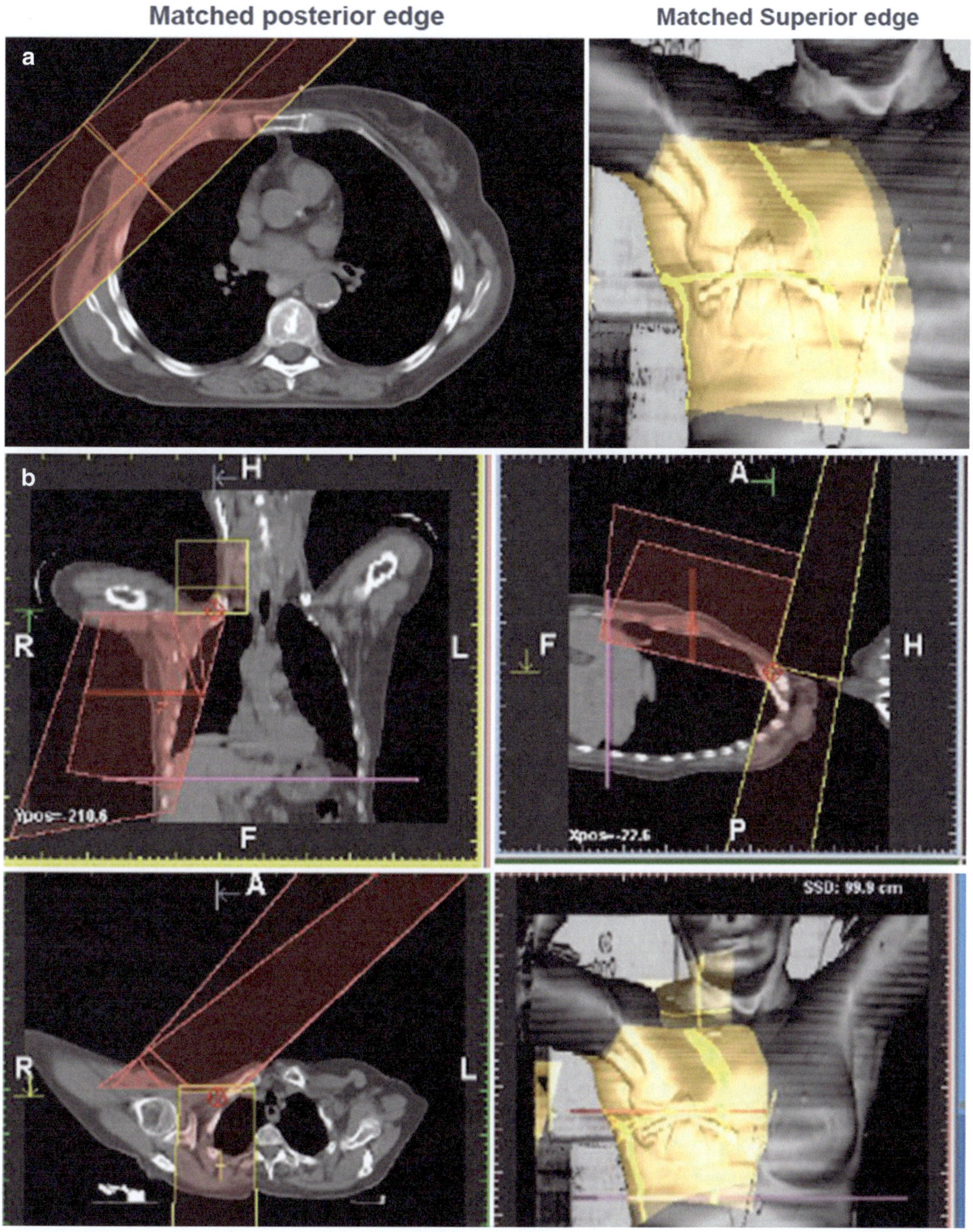

Fig. 6 Tangential fields for chest wall radiotherapy (Figure a shows the straight posterior edge matching for tangential beams, Figure b shows the matching of tangentials with the supraclavicular field, rest figures illustrate similar concepts)

beam blocks, through complex geometrical matching as described by *Lebesque JV* [115], or by multiple tangential beams.

Early radiotherapy techniques relied on clinical markings or 2 D imaging (X-rays). The emergence of CT scan imaging and dynamic multileaf collimators (MLC) enables 3 D conformal radiotherapy planning. 3 D CRT enables to see the dose distribution to the three dimensions across the breast and chest wall, thereby improving coverage of the target volume and enabling dose reduction to organs at risk. Persistent rapid advances in radiotherapy have ensured that the normal tissues get maximally spared while the tumor receives an adequate dose [116, 117]. Notably, these advances include intensity-modulated radiotherapy, image-guided radiotherapy, tomotherapy, heavy ions, and proton therapy [118]. Intensity-modulated radiation therapy (IMRT) has been frequently used in the radiotherapy of breast cancers [119–121]. However, IMRT implies several approaches or techniques rather than only one delivery technique. The best IMRT technique for breast cancer treatment has not been established. Forward planning IMRT, which employs multiple shaped beams with the same medial and lateral gantry angles, aimed to minimize hot spots has emerged as a popular technique. It needs to be noted that use of multiple gantry angles, use of large arc rotational techniques may improve the conformity of PTV, but this is at the cost of increasing dose to the contralateral breast, dose to the heart, and dose to contralateral lung [122].

For whole breast irradiation or chest wall irradiation, pragmatic options include 3 D CRT with two tangential portions, planning IMRT, inverse planning IMRT with 2–3 medial and lateral tangential beams (taking care not to enter or exit through the contralateral breast), partial tangential arcs (30-degree medial tangential arc and 30-degree lateral tangential arc) [123, 124].

Cone-beam CT can provide image guidance for treatment. Imaging with devices such as ExacTrac can have challenges in view of the obliquity of imaging and the resultant clustering of ribs in the image.

Irradiation of the internal mammary (IM) region increases the complexity of radiation planning. To spare the issue of "hot spots" the volume of IM is taken along with the breast/CW volume for integrated planning with tangential IMRT beams. For 3 D planning, use of partial wide tangents is a common technique in this scenario.

10.1 Dose and Fractionation

Radiotherapy fractionation schedules have been developed over many years based on radiobiological data, clinical experience, and resource availability. For several decades, breast conservation surgery or mastectomy patients were treated with a dosing schedule of 50 Gray in 25 fractions, using 2 Gy per fraction given over 33 days. This schedule was practical, but also meant that the patient come daily to the department for 5–6 weeks.

Hypofractionation (HFx) is defined as the delivery of larger-than-standard doses of radiation over a shorter period. The critical benefit of hypofractionation is the patient's reduction in treatment time (from 5 weeks to 3–4 weeks). Dose fractionation options in a patient with carcinoma breast after conservation or mastectomy are given in Table. Hypofractionation schedules have been tested in trials and found equivalent to standard fractionation. Recent data support the concept that hypofractionation with a modest increase in fraction size accompanied by a modest decrease in total dose is likely to result in equivalent outcomes compared with standard fractionation concerning local control and late radiation morbidity. Randomized trials that have established comparable local control and cosmetic outcomes between HFx and standard fractionation (SFx) regimens [125–127].

Standardization of Breast Radiotherapy (START) A and B trials from the United Kingdom tested various hypofractionated regimens against standard fractionation in women with node-negative and node-positive breast cancer [126, 127]. The START A trial included two different HFx schedules: 41.6 Gy delivered in 13 fractions over 5 weeks and 39 Gy delivered in 13 fractions over 5 weeks. START-A enrolled 2236 women.

Median follow-up was 9.3 years (IQR 8.0–10.0), after which 139 local-regional relapses had occurred. 10-year rates of local-regional relapse did not differ significantly between the 41.6 Gy and 50 Gy regimen groups (6.3%, 95% CI 4.7–8.5 vs 7.4%, 5.5–10.0; hazard ratio [HR] 0.91, 95% CI 0.59–1.38; $p = 0.65$) or the 39 Gy (8.8%, 95% CI 6.7–11.4) and 50 Gy regimen groups (HR 1.18, 95% CI 0.79–1.76; $p = 0.41$). *I*n START-A, moderate or marked breast induration, telangiectasia, and breast oedema were significantly less common normal tissue effects in the 39 Gy group than in the 50 Gy group. Normal tissue effects did not differ significantly between 41.6 Gy and 50 Gy groups. START-B enrolled 2215 women. Median follow-up was 9.9 years (IQR 7.5–10.1), after which 95 local-regional relapses had occurred. The proportion of patients with local-regional relapse at 10 years did not differ significantly between the 40 Gy group (4.3%, 95% CI 3.2–5.9) and the 50 Gy group (5.5%, 95% CI 4.2–7.2; HR 0.77, 95% CI 0.51–1.16; $p = 0.21$). In START-B, breast shrinkage, telangiectasia, and breast oedema were significantly less common normal tissue effects in the 40 Gy group than in the 50 Gy group [128]. In contrast, the 39 Gy HFx group demonstrated a significantly higher local recurrence rate (5.2%). The START B trial compared SFx to aHFx regimen of 40 Gy delivered in 15 fractions over 3 weeks. With a median followup of 6 years, the HFx group demonstrated a lower but not statistically significant recurrence rate (2.2%) compared with the SFx arm [129]. The trial found no detectable difference in local-regional control between the two arms of the study. Interestingly, both photographic scored assessment of change in breast appearance and patient assessed quality of life questionnaires of late tissue effects revealed better results for the experimental arm [130, 131]. Importantly, data from India confirms the benefits of moderate hypofractionation in the unscreened population with safet and benefits as reported by the START trialists [132].

The UK prospective randomized clinical trial tested 5.7 Gy and 6.0 Gy fractions of whole breast radiotherapy in terms of late normal tissue responses and tumor control (FAST trial) [133]. It randomized 915 women 50 years old or older with node-negative tumors following breast conservation surgery to receive whole-breast radiotherapy delivered using 3D dosimetry to a total dose of 50 Gy in 25 fractions (control) versus 28.5 or 30 Gy in 5 once-weekly fractions of 5.7 or 6.0 Gy and no tumor bed boost. At 10 years, there was no significant difference in normal tissue effects (NTE) rates after 28.5 Gy/5 fr compared with 50 Gy/25 fr, but NTE were higher after 30 Gy/5 fr. Results confirm the published 3-year findings that a once-weekly 5-fr schedule of whole-breast radiotherapy can be identified that appears to be radiobiologically comparable for NTE to a conventionally fractionated regimen. With 9.9 years median follow-up, 11 ipsilateral breast cancer events (50 Gy: 3; 30 Gy: 4; 28.5 Gy: 4) and 96 deaths (50 Gy: 30; 30 Gy: 33; 28.5 Gy: 33) have occurred [134].

The FAST Forward trial tested two five fraction regimens (26Gy/5#/1wk and 27Gy/5#/1wk) over a week against standard 3 weekly treatment(40Gy/5#/3 weeks) [135]. Total of 1361 patients were assigned to the 40 Gy schedule, 1367 to the 27 Gy schedule, and 1368 to the 26 Gy schedule. At a median follow-up of 71.5 months, 26 Gy in five fractions over 1 week was non-inferior to the standard of 40 Gy in 15 fractions over 3 weeks for local tumour control, and was as safe in terms of normal tissue effects up to 5 years for patients prescribed adjuvant local radiotherapy after primary surgery for early-stage breast cancer. These results are being validated by the HYPORT Adjuvant trialists, who are not only doing a multicentre indian study comparing 26 Gy in 5 fractions over 5 days versus the standard 40Gy in 15 fractions over 3 week, but also addressing the safety and feasibility of a simultaneous integrated boost to the tumour bed to confirm whether even in high risk cases a genuine five fraction solution is safely effective [136]. Dose fractionation options in patients of carcinoma breast is shown in Table 10. Dose-volume constraints for RT planning in Carcinoma breast is enlisted in Table 11.

Table 10 Dose fractionation options in patients of carcinoma breast

Breast conservation			
	Whole breast and boost	*SCF and axilla (if needed)*	*Comments*
1	50Gy/25#/5 weeks+ boost 15Gy/6#/5 days	50Gy/25#/5 weeks	Duration 5 weeks,
2	40Gy/15#/3 weeks + boost 12.5Gy/5#/5 days	40Gy/15#/3 weeks	Duration 4 weeks.
4	45Gy/20#/4 weeks+ boost 12.5Gy/5#/5 days	45Gy/20#/4 weeks	Duration 5 weeks
5.	40Gy/15#/3 weeks with SIB of 48Gy/15#/3 weeks to the tumor bed	40Gy/15#/3 weeks	Duration 3 weeks
6.	26Gy/5#/1 week (with a SIB of 30-32 Gy)	NA	Duration 1 week Limited evidence for regional RT (SFC/IMC/Axilla)with this fractionation
Mastectomy			
	Chest wall	*SCF and axilla (if needed)*	*Comments*
1	50Gy/25#/5 weeks	50Gy/25#/5 weeks	Duration 5 weeks.
2	45Gy/20#/4 weeks	45Gy/20#/4 weeks	Duration 4 weeks
3	40Gy/15#/3 weeks	40Gy/15#/3 weeks	Duration 3 weeks No robust evidence for extended field RT (IMC/Axilla)with this fractionation

SIB Simultaneous Integrated Boost

Table 11 Dose-volume constraints for RT planning in carcinoma breast

Structure	Category	Constraint	Ref
Target volume		95% of isodose covers 100% PTV The maximum dose to PTV not to exceed prescription dose by >10%	RTOG0319
Heart	Mean dose	<2.5Gy (left sided) <0.5Gy (right sided)	Derby et al.
Heart	Coronary vessel mean dose		
Lung	Ipsilateral V 30	<15%	RTOG0319
Lung	Ipsilateral V 20	<30%	285
Contralateral lung	5% of the prescribed dose	<10%	RTOG0319
Contralateral breast	Mean dose	<1Gy	RTOG0319

10.2 Boost After Breast Conservation

The scientific rationale for giving a boost is the greater likelihood of tumor cells in or adjacent to the tumor bed and the greater incidence of recurrent disease in this zone. While a boost is recommended in all patients with breast conservation, it is especially necessary in younger patients (<50 years). Typically, boost is given sequentially after whole breast radiotherapy. However, modern approaches include giving simultaneous integrated boost (SIB), to further reduce treatment time [137–140].

In the larger EORTC randomized trial [139], patients were randomly assigned to receive or not receive a 16 Gy boost after 50 Gy of whole breast radiation treatment [140]. 2657 patients were randomly assigned to receive no radiation boost and 2661 patients randomly assigned to receive a radiation boost. Median follow-up was 17.2 years (IQR 13.0–19.0). 20-year overall survival was 59.7% (99% CI 56.3–63.0) in the boost group versus 61.1% (57.6–64.3) in the no boost group, hazard ratio (HR) 1.05 (99% CI 0.92–1.19, $p = 0.323$). The 20-year cumulative incidence of ipsilateral breast tumour recurrence was 16.4% (99% CI 14.1–18.8) in the no boost group versus 12.0%

(9.8–14.4) in the boost group. The cumulative incidence of severe fibrosis at 20 years was 1.8% (99% CI 1.1–2.5) in the no boost group versus 5.2% (99% CI 3.9–6.4) in the boost group ($p < 0.0001$). *Overall,* a radiation boost after whole-breast irradiation has no effect on long-term overall survival, but can improve local control, with the largest absolute benefit in young patients, although it increases the risk of moderate to severe fibrosis. The extra radiation dose can be avoided in most patients older than age 60 years.

A subgroup analysis of the EORTC boost trial assessed the outcome of 251 patients with R1 resection who were randomized to receive either a 10 Gy or a 26 Gy boost. There was no statistically significant difference in local control or survival between the lower and the higher boost dose group. Fibrosis occurred significantly more often after 26 Gy [141]. The "Young Boost Trial" (34,NCT00212121) was started in 2004 in the Netherlands, Germany, and France to evaluate the need for a further increase of the boost dose from 16 to 26 Gy for patients up to 50 years of age. In 2011, after including more than 2000 patients, the estimated local recurrence rate at 4 years remains 2%, far below the results obtained in the previous EORTC trials despite the much younger age population investigated [142].

Conflicting evidence exists whether an extra boost dose can mitigate the effects of a positive surgical margin. As such, it may be advisable to get any positive margin to be reexcised. In patients with focal positive margin and challenges in reexcision higher boost dose (16 Gy/8#/1.5 weeks or 20Gy/8#/1.5 weeks) can be considered [143, 144].

10.3 Regional Nodal Irradiation

Most guidelines recommend giving radiotherapy to the supraclavicular lymphatics (level 4) and level 3 lymphatics in patients with four or more positive axillary nodes. SCF radiotherapy can also be used in patients with 1 or more positive nodes with additional factors such as T3 tumors, Grade 3 pathology, extranodal extension (ENE), or lymphovascular involvement (LVI). Regional nodal irradiation in breast cancer trails are enlisted in Table 12.

Whenever a decision for axillary irradiation is made, it is essential not to irradiate the dissected portion of the axilla since this significantly increases the risk of lymphedema. The exception to this rule would be a patient whose axillary disease has been left behind during surgery.

One of the recent randomized studies Intergroup/NCIC-CTG MA.20 (2000–7), studied the role of regional nodal irradiation in patients of early breast cancer [145]. This was randomized multicenter trial of 1832 patients with high-risk node-negative or node-positive, treated with BCS and adjuvant chemo and endocrine therapy. Patients were randomized to whole breast RT (50 Gy/25 fx ± boost) or whole breast RT with regional nodal irradiation (45 Gy/25 fx) to internal mammary, SCLV, and axillary apex. The median follow-up was 9.5 years. At the 10-year follow-up, there was no significant between-group difference in survival, with a rate of 82.8% in the nodal-irradiation group and 81.8% in the control group (hazard ratio, 0.91; 95% confidence interval [CI], 0.72 to 1.13; $P = 0.38$). The rates of disease-free survival were 82.0% in the nodal-irradiation group and 77.0% in the control group (hazard ratio, 0.76; 95% CI, 0.61 to 0.94; $P = 0.01$). Patients in the nodal-irradiation group had higher rates of grade 2 or greater acute pneumonitis (1.2% vs. 0.2%, $P = 0.01$) and lymphedema (8.4% vs. 4.5%, $P = 0.001$).

EORTC 22922/10925 randomized. 4004 women, intermediate-risk disease; BCT 76%, mastectomy 24% to internal mammary and medial supraclavicular to 50 Gy / 25 fr versus no radiotherapy to regional nodes (260). The updated outcomes of this trial did show an overall survival advantage with the use of RNI [146].

A French trial of 1334 women with positive axillary LN or medial tumors (LN negative) were randomized to the Chest wall and supraclavicular fossa (50 Gy) with or without IMN irradiation (50 Gy to first 5 IC spaces at 3 cm depth). At a median follow-up of 8.6 years, there was no difference in DFS ($P = 0.35$) or OS ($P = 0.8$) [150]. A second trial randomized 263/270 patients of stage I-II treated with BCS and two field tangent techniques, randomized to include

Table 12 Regional nodal irradiation in breast cancer

Study	Comparison/Randomization arms	Local recurrence	Regional recurrence	DFS	OS	Comments
MA 20 study [148]	WBI vs WBI + RNI *Inclusion criteria*: Patients with BCS and SLNB/ALND and who had positive axillary lymph nodes or negative axillary nodes with high-risk features(primary tumor 5 cm or more or 2 cm or more with fewer than 10 axillary nodes removed and at least one of the following: Grade 3 histologic categorization, estrogen-receptor (ER) negativity, or lymphovascular invasion.	WBI- 4.1% WBI + RNI-3.6%	WBI- 2.5% WBI + RNI-0.5%	WBI- 77% WBI + RNI- 82%	WBI- 81.8% WBI + RNI- 82.8%	Addition of RNI to WBI did not improve OS but reduced the rate of breast-cancer recurrence
EORTC 22922/10925 study (15 year result) [149]	WBI/PMRT VS WBI/PMRT with RNI *Inclusion criteria*: Women up to 75 years of age, stage I–III breast cancer with a primary tumour located centrally or in the medial quadrants of the breast irrespective of axillary involvement, or a primary tumour located in the external quadrants combined with axillary lymph node involvement	WBI/PMRT- 6.6% WBI/PMRT+ RNI-6.4%	WBI/PMRT- 5% WBI/PMRT+RNI-3.2%	WBI/PMRT- 59.9% WBI/ PMRT+RNI- 60.8%	WBI/PMRT- 70.9% WBI/PMRT+RNI- 73.1%	The 15-year results show a significant reduction of breast cancer mortality and any breast cancer recurrence by IM-MS irradiation in stages I–III breast cancer. No difference in OS

French study [150]	CW + MS-LN VS CW+ MS + IMN-LN *Inclusion criteria*: Patients with positive axillary nodes or a medial/central tumor with or without axillary lymph node involvement, tumor size larger than 1 cm, age <75 years, ≥70% KPS	MS-LN-9.8% MS + IMN-LN-9.2%	MS-LN-3.8% MS + IMN-LN-5.3%	MS-LN-49.9% MS + IMN-LN-53.2%	MS-LN-59.3% MS + IMN-LN-62.6%	Median follow-up of 11.3 years. No benefit could be demonstrated for IMN irradiation
Nordic study [151]	Ipsilateral parasternal area + internal mammary chain (IMC-RT)- Ipsilateral parasternal area (no IMC-RT) *Inclusion criteria*: 270 patients with unilateral stage I or II invasive breast cancer treated by segmental resection, axillary dissection and radiation	Not stated	Not stated	Not stated	Not stated	No difference in OS
Danish study (population based) [152]	Right-sided breast cancer allocated to IMNI vs left-sided breast cancer allocated to no IMNI, naturally allocated population-based cohort study. *Inclusion criteria*: Patients treated with RT after surgery for unilateral node-positive breast cancer	IMNI-1.9% No IMNI- 1.4%	IMNI-0.7% No IMNI-0.9%	IMNI-72.6% No IMNI-70.3%	IMNI- 79.1% No IMNI-76.6%	IMNI increased overall survival in patients with early-stage node-positive breast cancer.

WBI Whole breast irradiation, *RNI* Regional nodal irradiation, *IMNI* Internal Mammary Nodal irradiation, *CW* Chest wall, *MS-LN* Medial supraclavicular, *IMN-LN* Internal mammary lymph node the IMN in the tangent fields or not. With a median follow up of 2.7 years, no difference in pneumonitis (18% vs. 14%) or recurrence rates were seen. There was no difference in toxicity, but follow up was too short for commenting on recurrences [147].

Overall, the issue of including IMN during RNI for breast cancer has been debated for a long time. For patients with initial IMN involvement, the volume of IMN should be included in RT planning, irrespective of systemic therapy response. In patients with no frank IMN involvement, many guidelines have included extended field RT including IM chain for patients with 4 or more axillary lymph node involvement or patients with large inner quadrant lesions. For patients with 1–3 axillary lymph node positivity or lymph node-negative patients, the decision should be given on an individual basis, considering the presence of multiple adverse factors, such as LVI, tumors more than 2 cm, medial tumors, medial central tumours and adverse biology.

10.4 Axillary Radiotherapy

Axillary irradiation is a rational alternative to ALND in clinically N0 axilla as irradiation achieves comparable local tumor control with less morbidity. The available data suggest that axillary irradiation yields low axillary recurrence rates in cN0 with early-stage breast cancer patients comparable to ALND, but with less morbidity. EORTC Trial 10,981–22,023 (AMAROS: "After Mapping of the Axilla, Radiotherapy Or Surgery") investigated the role of completion axillary dissection versus radiotherapy to axilla after a positive sentinel lymph node biopsy in patients with T1–T2 (<3 cm) clinically N0. As per institutional protocol, patients with 4+ lymph nodes on axillary dissection are allowed axillary RT [153, 154]. The outcome did not suggest any difference in DFS or OS. There were lower rates of lymphedema in the axillary radiotherapy arm as compared to axillary surgery arm [155]. The OTOASAR trial yielded similar outcomes. The overall regional nodal management is provided in Table 13.

Table 13 Regional nodal management

S. no	Clnical/pathological situation	Suggested management
1	cN0 and pN0(S.N.)	No further nodal treatment
2	cN0 and pN+ (S.N.) with no other risk factors	Management options Complete ALND and RT non-resected part of axilla OR RT to axilla level 1–2
3	cN0 and pN+(S.N.) with additional risk factors	Management options Complete ALND and RT non-resected part of axilla OR RT axilla L1–4
4	cN+ (no NACT)	ALND and RT to the non-resected part of axilla
5	cN+ and ycN0 and ypN+(S.N.)	Management options ALND and RT to the non-resected part of axilla OR RT to axilla L 1–4
6	cN+ and ycN0 and ypN0(S.N.)	RT to the non-resected part of axilla

Note: Use of IMC nodal irradiation can be considered in situations 3–6

S.N Sentinel node, *cN+* clinically Node positive, *ycN+* clinically node positive after neo adjuvant chemo, *pN+* pathologically nodal positive, *ALND* Axillary lymph node dissection, *IMC* internal mammary chain, *NACT* Neo adjuvant chemotherapy

10.5 Accelerated Partial Breast Irradiation (APBI)

The conventional treatment for early breast cancer includes postoperative radiotherapy to the whole breast. Whole-breast radiotherapy is usually delivered daily over 5–7 weeks. Despite the efficacy of this schedule, there are logistical issues related to the long course of RT (time commitment, travel distances, limited radiotherapy resources, fears or treating physician's bias) [156–162]. Accelerated partial-breast irradiation (APBI) typically delivers a larger daily dose of radiation once or twice daily to the tumor bed region and completing treatment in 1 week. The rationale for APBI is twofold (1) Pathology data indicating that most of the microscopic cell spread is clustered around the primary tumour only [163, 164] (2) Recurrence patterns after breast conservation suggest that at least 80% of the early failures after BCT are in the same quadrant as the original primary tumor (67%–85%) [69, 164].

APBI advantages over whole breast irradiation include (1) shortened treatment time (from 5 weeks to 1 week) (2) decreased radiation dose to uninvolved portions of the breast and surrounding normal organs such as the heart and lungs [158–162, 165–171].

Selection criteria for APBI patients is given in Table 14.

A comparison of APBI techniques is given in Table 15.

Multicatheter Interstitial Brachytherapy (MIB) predates other forms of APBI by nearly a decade. Intra operative multicatheter per operative interstitial brachytherapy placement is shown in Fig. 7. X-ray based planning and CT based planning in interstitial brachytherapy of breast is shown in Fig. 8a, b.

Several trials [171–180], with over 5 years of followup (median 5.25–11.1 years), demonstrated control rates similar to those reported for WBI with good cosmesis. The Hungarian trial [180] was a phase III compared WBRT with APBI using HDR implants or electrons (normal fractionation) in 258 women with margin negative, early stage breast cancers. At 5 years, the actuarial rate of local recurrence (around 5%) was not statistically different between the two arms. The rate of good-to-excellent cosmesis was 77.6% in the combined PBI group. Patients treated with MIB APBI had an improved cosmesis, rated as good-to-excellent cosmesis, compared to limited-field external-beam PBI, 81.2% versus 70.0%.

Table 14 APBI selection Criteria

Age	More than 40 years
Tumour size	Upto 3 cm
Histology	Infiltrating ductal carcinoma
Cut margins	Free
EIC	Negative
Node	Negative

Note ER- PR- patient, Her2 positive patients or Triple negative patients are generally not taken for APBI

The most popular form of ABPI currently used in the United States is the Mammosite.

This was developed to simplify the brachytherapy procedure. Figure 9 shows mammosite placed in postoperative cavity. Multiple small, single-institution experiences have been published with good results in low-risk, highly selected patients with MammoSite. The most extensive study of this treatment modality to date is the American Society of Breast Surgeons MammoSite Registry Trial, which has now reported 5-year actuarial [181] rates of ipsilateral breast tumor recurrence (IBTR) of 3.8% and good-excellent cosmesis of 90.6%. The technique is being explored in the NSABP/RTOG-0413 phase III trial [165].

IORT is used to deliver a single fraction (one-time treatment) in the operating room during BCS. A randomized controlled trial evaluating IORT APBI with WBI is the TARGIT A trial. The initial results were published in 2010 and updated subsequently [182, 183]. A total of 2232 patients were randomly allocated to WBRT or IORT (20 Gy with 50 kV Intrabeam). According to conventional imaging, patients aged 45 years or older with unifocal invasive ductal carcinoma were eligible. With a median followup of 2 years, the estimated 4-year local recurrence rate was 0.95% in the WBRT group and 1.2% in the TARGIT group ($p < 0.41$). Neither complication nor toxicity rates differed between the two groups. The latest update was published in Lancet 2020 [175]. In this analysis, the local failure rate in the TARGIT group was 2.11% vs. 0.95% in the WBI arm. The absolute difference was 1.16%, within the predefined non-inferiority margin of 2.50 percentile. TARGIT-IORT has similar long-term local tumor control and cancer survical outcomes with lower mortality than WBI.

The ELIOT trial addressed the issue of single fraction intraoperative radiotherapy by electrons. Eligible women, aged 48–75 years with an ultrasound diameter not exceeding 25 mm, clinically negative axillary lymph nodes, and who were suitable for breast-conserving surgery, were randomly assigned (1:1) to receive post-operative WBI with conventional fractionation (50 Gy given as 25 fractions of 2 Gy, plus a 10 Gy boost), or 21 Gy intra-

Table 15 APBI techniques

Technique name	Technique/method	Dose/fraction	Comments
Interstitial brachytherapy	Multiple flexible after-loading catheters placed in the breast, using a free-hand or a template-guided approach, with appropriate image guidance at placement [199, 201]. Catheters placed at 10–15 mm intervals in several planes to encompass the lumpectomy cavity. Tumor bed treated with a defined margin (typically 10–15 mm). Typically, 10–20 catheters necessary to achieve dosimetric goals [199].	For HDR brachytherapy the most common schedule is 34Gy/10# (delivered twice daily with an interval of 6 h apart)	Most common technique. However, invasive procedures require considerable training and expertise, limiting its use
Balloon based brachytherapy (Mammosite device, (MammoSite® ML and Contura® [SenoRx, Irvine, CA])	Inflatable balloon inserted into the breast cavity area per operatively. Subsequently inflated to get into contact with the postoperative cavity postoperatively, the balloon is filled with saline, and a high dose rate brachytherapy (HDR) afterloading device inserts an iridium-192 source into the center of the balloon	34Gy/10 fractions, two fractions per day) prescribed to 1 cm from balloon surface	Simple technique but cost issues and concern in irregular cavities
Balloon-based brachytherapy Strut adjusted volume implant, SAVI) (SAVI® [Strut Adjusted Volume Implant, Cianna Medical, Aliso, Viejo, CA])	Non-balloon bundled-multicatheter device	34Gy/10 fractions, 2 fractions per day) prescribed to 1 cm from balloon surface	Developed with aim of providing greater dose flexibility in treatment planning and improve conformance to the lumpectomy cavity
Intraoperative radiotherapy with electrons (ELIOT) (Liac, Mobetron_, Novac-7),	Mobile linear accelerator producing 3–12 MeV electron beams is used in combination with an electron applicator. A special applicator is used preoperatively to deliver a single fraction treatment with electrons	The applicator is placed over the surgical cavity, delivering a single fraction of 21 Gy to the tumor bed plus a 1.5–3 cm margin	Requires special equipment, A core biopsy is essential to evaluate receptor status and histopathological classification. Duration of general anesthesia is prolonged to achieve per op. SLNB results and surgical margin negativity
KV photons (TARGIT)	A special applicator is used to deliver soft 50KV X-rays. The applicator is placed intraoperatively	Delivers the dose in a single session (20 Gy to 1 mm strip abutting the applicator sphere, falling off to 5 Gy 1 cm from the surface of the sphere)	Requires special equipment, Concerns regarding dose prescription and use in irregular cavities
3D conformal external beam radiotherapy	External beam radiotherapy using multiple conformal beams	34–38 Gy given in 10 fractions, 2 # per day	Concern regarding cosmetic outcomes with this schedule

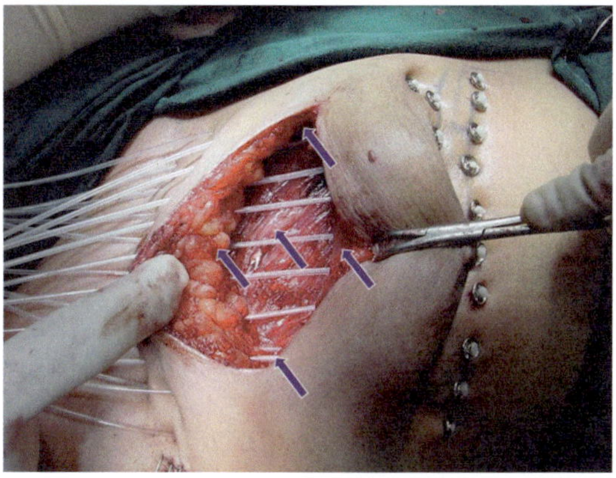

Fig. 7 Intraoperative view of multicatheter interstitial brachytherapy with two layers of catheters placed to cover the lumpectomy cavity; arrows indicate surgical clips inserted during lumpectomy for radiation planning

operative radiotherapy with electrons (ELIOT) in a single dose to the tumour bed during surgery [185–188]. Total of 1305 women were enrolled and randomly assigned: 654 to the WBI group and 651 to the ELIOT group. After a median follow-up of 12.4 years (IQR 9.7–14.7), 86 (7%) patients developed IBTR, with 70 (11%) cases in the ELIOT group and 16 (2%) in the WBI group, corresponding to an absolute excess of 54 IBTRs in the ELIOT group (HR 4.62, 95% CI 2.68–7.95, $p < 0.0001$). In the ELIOT group, the 5-year IBTR rate was 4.2% (95% CI 2.8–5.9), the 10-year rate was 8.1% (6.1–10.3), and the 15-year rate was 12.6% (9.8–15.9). In the WBI group, the 5-year IBTR rate was 0.5% (95% CI 0.1–1.3), the 10-year rate was 1.1% (0.5–2.2), and the 15-year rate was 2.4% (1.4–4.0). At final follow-up on March 11, 2019, 193 (15%) women had died from any cause, with no difference between the two groups (98 deaths in the ELIOT group vs 95 in the WBI group; HR 1.03, 95% CI 0.77–1.36, $p = 0.85$) [189]. The authors concluded that ELIOT should be offered only to selected patients at low-risk of IBTR.

Another recently developed technique for the delivery of APBI is that of external beam (3D-CRT) [189–195]. A randomised, phase 3, equivalence trial (NSABP B-39/RTOG 0413) was done in adult women (>18 years) with early-stage (0, I, or II; no evidence of distant metastases, but up to three axillary nodes could be positive) breast cancer (tumour size ≤3 cm; including all histologies and multifocal breast cancers), who had had lumpectomy with negative (i.e., no detectable cancer cells) surgical margins. Whole-breast irradiation was delivered in 25 daily fractions of 50 Gy over 5 weeks, with or without a supplemental boost to the tumour bed, and APBI was delivered as 34 Gy of brachytherapy or 38.5 Gy of external bream radiation therapy in 10 fractions, over 5 treatment days within an 8-day period [196]. Two thousand one hundred nine were assigned to the whole-breast irradiation group and 2107 were assigned to the APBI group. At a median follow-up of 10.2 years (IQR 7.5–11.5), 90 (4%) of 2089 women eligible for the primary outcome in the APBI group and 71 (3%) of 2036 women in the whole-breast irradiation group had an IBTR (HR 1.22, 90% CI 0.94–1.58). The 10-year cumulative incidence of IBTR was 4.6% (95% CI 3.7–5.7) in the APBI group versus 3.9% (3.1–5.0) in the whole-breast irradiation group. APBI did not meet the criteria for equivalence to whole-breast irradiation in controlling IBTR for breast-conserving therapy. For patients with early-stage breast cancer, the findings supported whole-breast irradiation following lumpectomy; however, with an absolute difference of less than 1% in the 10-year cumulative incidence of IBTR, APBI might be an acceptable alternative for some women.

At present, data on long-term outcomes with APBI and the best technique for its delivery are limited. Because of the rapid increase in the use of APBI, combined with a lack of sufficient randomized trial data, both the American Society for Radiation Oncology (ASTRO) and the European GEC-ESTRO Cancer Working Group has published guidelines for the implementation of APBI [197, 198]. The guidelines distinguish three categories of patients for determining suitability for APBI (Table 16).

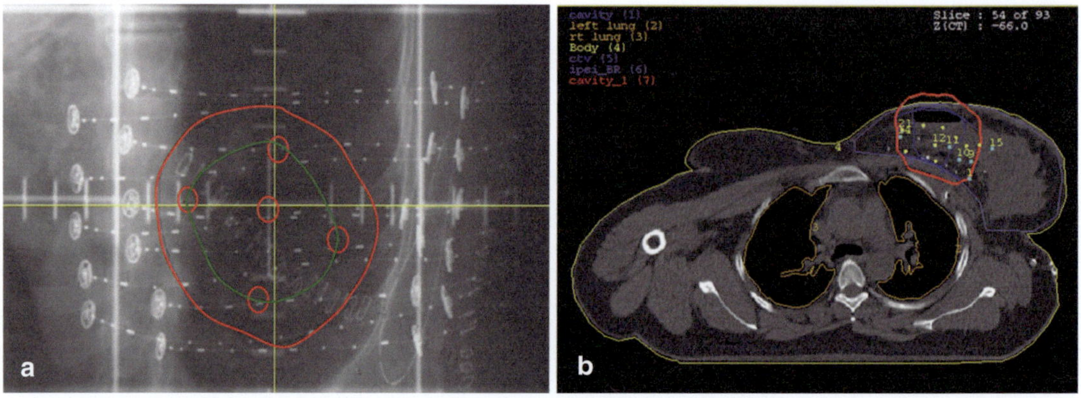

Fig. 8 (**a**) X ray based planning and (**b**) CT based planning in interstitial brachytherapy of breast

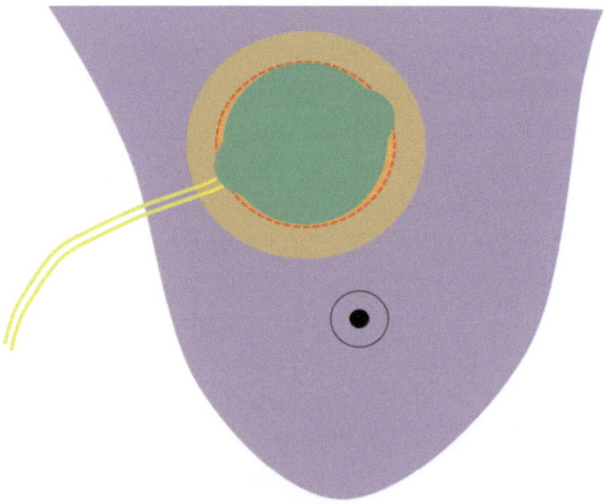

Fig. 9 Mammosite (green) placed in postoperative cavity. The outer sphere (orange) depicts the zone, beyond the edge of the cavity, typically irradiated by the mammosite

11 Radiotherapy Sequelae (Acute, Subacute, and Late), Response Assessment

Postoperative radiotherapy (RT) for breast cancer (BC) plays an important role in reducing local recurrence and death rates. However, radiotherapy for breast cancer has however also been associated with various side effects. These include skin thickening and fibrosis, pneumonitis, lymphedema, and cardiac side effects [201]. Typically, the skin changes are self-limiting [202]. These can be classified into acute (developing during RT or immediately post RT) and late effects (developing in few months to years). Acute toxicity may include fatigue, dermatitis, hyperpigmentation, desquamation, and pneumonitis. Late complications include soft tissue fibrosis, telangiectasias, pulmonary fibrosis, cardiac toxicity, rarely rib fracture and secondary malignancy. With modern megavoltage beams, such effects' incidence or severity is no longer clinically significant [202]. A recent randomised trial found that use of Mepitel film—a silicone-based polyurethane film dressing—significantly reduced the incidence of grade 2 or 3 acute radiation dermatitis in at-risk women receiving radiotherapy after surgery for breast cancer [203].

Estimates of the risk of lymphedema after breast cancer treatment vary widely from 14% to 40% [204]. Approximately, 90% of the expected cases occur during the first 24 months after treatment but the remainder occur years to decades later.

Increasingly conservative approaches to surgery and radiotherapy have driven the estimated incidence closer to the lower limits of this range [205]. Recent advances in surgery have established sentinel node biopsy as a standard procedure in appropriate cases of breast cancer, thereby lowering rates of lymphedema [206, 207]. Sentinel-node sampling techniques reduce the estimated risk of breast cancer–associated lymphedema to 6%–10% [208]. Similarly, over the years, there has been a steady decline in axillary radiotherapy use, which has contributed significantly towards declining lymphedema rates

Table 16 Selection criteria for APBI

Patient group	Risk factor	Original	Update
Suitable	*Age*	≥60 years	≥50 years
	Margins	Negative by ≥2 mm	No change.
	T stage	T1	Tis or T1
	DCIS	Not allowed	If all of the below: Screen-detected Low to intermediate nuclear grade Pathologic tumor size ≤2.5 cm Margins ≥3 mm
Cautionary	*Age*	50–59 years	40–49 years if all other criteria for "suitable" are met ≥50 if patient has at least one of the pathologic factors below and does not have any "unsuitable" factors *Pathologic factors*: Pathologic tumor size-2.1–3.0 cm Stage-T2 Close margins (<2 mm) Limited/focal LVSI Estrogen receptor negative Clinically unifocal with pathologica tumor size 2.1-3.0 cm Invasive lobular pathology Pure DCIS ≤3 cm if criteria for "suitable" not fully met EIC ≤3 cm
	Margins	Close (<2 mm)	No change
	DCIS	≤3 cm	≤3 cm and does not meet criteria for "suitable"
Unsuitable	*Age*	<50 years	<40 years 40–49 years and do not meet the criteria for cautionary
	Margins	Positive	No change
	DCIS	>3 cm	No change

[209]. With modern day surgical and radiotherapy techniques, the rates of severe lymphedema are <2%–4% [34, 205, 210, 211]. The highest rates of lymphedema of arm (>30%) have been observed in patients undergoing both complete axillary dissection as well as axillary radiotherapy [212, 213].

The pulmonary side effects are acute pneumonitis and sub-acute/late lung fibrosis [214, 215]. Decades ago, when clinical or 2 D planning was prevalent, the incidence of symptomatic radiation pneumonis post breast radiotherapy was nearly 2%–5%. However this has come down dramatically with use of 3 D and other advanced techniques. As such, pulmonary fibrosis (PF) resulting from radiotherapy often goes unrecognized. This is due to (a) low index of suspicion of the clinicians (b) traditional evaluation of patients by only a chest X ray, which can detect only gross changes. Post-radiotherapy, the severity of PF is related to the volume of the lung irradiated and the dose and fractionation schedule. The risk for acute and chronic RT-induced lung morbidity is likely to be influenced by total dose, dose per fraction and irradiated lung volume [216]. Following tight dose constraints for Lung OAR is likely to prevent radiation pneumonitis [217].

A prospective study was done on 250 breast cancer pateints referred for postoperative RT from 2007 to 2008 [218]. High-resolution computed tomography of the lungs and symptom registration were performed before RT and 3, 6, and 12 months after RT. The occurrence of Grade I rRP (radiological Radiation Pneumonitis) and Grade I cRP (clinical Radiation Pneumonitis) at 3 months was 78% and 19%. There were no reports of Grade 2 or more events. In multivariable analyses, mastectomy predicted cRP at 3 months (OR = 2.48, $p = 0.03$) at 6 months, ipsilateral lung volume receiving 20 Gray or more

(V20), V30. Mean lung dose (MLD) predicted rRP at 6 months (OR = 1.06, $p = 0.0003$).

The existing retrospective studies do not indicate any excess risks of pulmonary side effects/ pulmonary fibrosis with concurrent radiotherapy and Tamoxifen. Randomized studies are also investigating the issue [219, 220]. One such study is being led by the Tata Memorial Hospital and the preliminary results are expected soon [219].

RT to the breast also irradiates a portion of the heart poses a risk of long-term cardiac toxicity, especially in left-sided breast cancer [221, 222]. The issue of radiation risk to the heart assumes more significance in view of (1) Improved survival in breast cancer patients. (2) Utilization of other potentially cardiotoxic drugs such as herceptin and taxanes in addition to RT. Radiation predominantly acts by causing microvascular damage, which affects the myocytes and the conducting pathways of the heart [223, 224]. Cardiac irradiation can result in damage in various degrees to the heart. Their manifestations are varied, such as diffuse myocardial interstitial fibrosis, microcirculatory damage, fibrous thickening of the pericardium, valvular fibrosis, and accelerated atherosclerosis [225]. The arteries most affected after RT are the left anterior descending and the right coronary arteries [92, 226, 227]. Modern studies suggest that rates of major coronary events increased linearly with the mean dose to the heart by 7.4% per Gy (95% confidence interval, 2.9–14.5; $P < 0.001$), with no apparent threshold. The increase starts within the first 5 years after radiotherapy and continues into the third decade after radiotherapy [228].

It is well-known that RT to left-sided breast results in higher doses to the heart than right-sided cancers and thus leads to higher cardiac deaths [229]. A population-based case-control study of major coronary events (i.e., myocardial infarction, coronary revascularization, or death from ischemic heart disease) in 2168 women who underwent radiotherapy for breast cancer between 1958 and 2001 in Sweden and Denmark was conducted. The study included 963 women with major coronary events and 1205 controls. Individual patient information was obtained from hospital records Rates of major coronary events increased linearly with the mean dose to the heart by 7.4% per gray (95% confidence interval, 2.9–14.5; $P < 0.001$), with no apparent threshold. The increase started within the first 5 years after radiotherapy and continued into the third decade [228]. As an example For a 50-year-old woman with no pre-existing cardiac risk factors, radiotherapy involving a mean dose to the heart of 3Gy would increase her risk of death from ischemic heart disease before the age of 80 years from 1.9% to 2.4% (i.e., an absolute increase of about 0.5% points). It would increase her risk of having at least one acute coronary event from 4.5% to 5.4% (i.e., an absolute increase of about 0.9% points). There has been some suggestion of decreased cardiac morbidity and mortality with modern radiotherapy techniques. A study by Darby et al. suggested a definite risk of cardiac mortality in left sided breast cancer with postoperative RT [230]. However, the cardiac mortality ratio in left sided versus right-sided had gradually improved with year of treatment. Patients treated from year 1973 to 82, the risk of cardiac mortality after RT in left-sided versus right-sided at 15 years was 1.58 (95%CI 1.29–1.95); from 1983 to 92 was 1.27 (95%CI 0.99–1.63) and the patient treated between 1993 and 2001, 5–9 year follow up was 0.99 (95%CI 0.73–1.35) (300). Overgaard et al. [231] have shown no excess cardiac deaths in patients followed up for over 10 years. Danish Breast Cooperative Group has shown that newer radiotherapy techniques effectively avoid radiation-induced cardiac toxicity [232].

Critical factors to minimizing heart related morbidities and events include appropriate beam placement, judicious dose prescription, appropriate contouring of heart and cardiac substructures.

A Swedish BC cohort diagnosed from 1970 to 2003 was linked to registers of coronary angiography from 1990 to 2004, which yielded 199 patients. An increase of stenosis in mid and distal left anterior decending artery (mdLAD) and distal diagonal (dD) in irradiated left-sided BC and an association between high-risk RT and stenosis in hotspot areas for radiation indicate a direct link between radiation and location of coronary stenoses [231].

In another study, the study population consisted of 182 women treated for BC in Sweden between 1992 and 2012. All women received 3DCRT and subsequently underwent coronary angiography due to a suspected coronary event. In women receiving conventional 3DCRT for BC between 1992 and 2012, radiation doses to the LAD remained high and were associated with an increased requirement of coronary intervention in mid LAD. In this study the OR for later coronary intervention increased significantly for women receiving mid LAD dose >20 Gy [233].

It is also critical to note that cardiac toxicity after radiotherapy takes time to manifest, in some reports up to 15 years [234]. For this reason, the emphasis should be on reports with long-term data of post-radiotherapy cardiac morbidity and mortality.

There exists a small risk of secondary cancers after treatment of breast cancer. This can be related to use of radiotherapy as well as chemotherapy for breast cancer [235].

A study compared observed crude incidence rates in the entire treated population for non-metastatic breast cancer to to the expected incidence in the general population of French women 17,745 women [236]. The median follow-up since diagnosis was 13.4 years (range: 2–29 years). The 15-year cumulative incidence of second malignancies was 1.807 per 100,000 (CI 1.729–1.884). Total of 2370 s malignancies were observed during follow-up, 2010 in the radiotherapy arm and 360 in the no radiotherapy arm (relative risk [RR] 1.15 [1.03–1.28], $P = 0.0134$). Crude incidence rates were significantly higher in their cohort of treated breast cancer patients than in the general population for contralateral breast cancer sarcomas, leukaemia lung cancer and gynaecological cancer. Recently the initial results of the phase III Radiotherapy Comparative Effectiveness (RadComp) trial were reported at ASTRO 2025. The trial enrolled more than 1,200 patients and was the first randomized trial to compare photon- and proton-based radiation therapy for breast cancer. The investigators found that health-related quality of life was same with either treatment. (https://www.astro.org/news-and-publications/news-and-media-center/news-releases/2025/first-randomized-study-comparing-proton-and-photon-radiation-therapy-for-breast-cancer-finds-both-pr last accessed 6th January 2026).

An accurate prediction of radiation-induced cancer risk is complex because of the lack of long-term follow-up and epidemiological data. Several risk models have been developed to estimate secondary cancer risks but the incidence rates of radiation-induced cancer are not necessarily a linear function of dose. It is generally recommended to keep the overall mean dose to the contralateral breast <50 cGy for the entire course of radiotherapy.

12 Follow-up and Quality of Life Issues

Follow-up of breast cancer patients aims to detect early local recurrences and/or metastatic disease, evaluate treatment-related complications, and provide psychological support. Follow up of patients with early breast cancer is shown in Table 17.

Ten-year survival of early breast cancer is >65% (nearly 90% survival for local and 60% survival for regional disease). Usually, the annual hazard of recurrence peaks in the second year after diagnosis but remains at 2%–5% in years 5–20. Node-positive patients tend to have higher yearly recurrence hazards than node-negative cancers. In the first 1–2 years the risk of recurrence is higher in patients with ER-negative cancers. However after 5–8 years after diagnosis, the annual risk of recurrence drops below the level of ER positive tumours. Very late recurrences >20 years are typically associated with patients having ER/PgR-positive disease [237].

There is a lack of randomized evidence supporting any particular follow-up sequence or protocol. It is important to balance patient needs, the cost of follow-up, and the logistic issues.

There is reasonable epidemiological evidence suggesting that lifestyle factors can have an effect on the prognosis of patients with breast cancer. Regular exercise can provide a functional, psychological, and possible reduction in the risk of recurrence. Weight gain and obesity are consid-

Table 17 Follow-up of patients with early breast cancer

All patients	Thorough history, asking for symptoms and a comprehensive physical examination Mammography of existing breasts on yearly basis
Patients on aromatase inhibitors or undergoing ovarian suppression	Bone mineral density evaluation at regular intervals
Young patients, especially in cases of dense breast tissue and genetic or familial predispositions	MRI of the breast at intervals based on individual risk
Patients on tamoxifen	An annual gynecological examination by an experienced gynecologist. Routine transvaginal US not recommended (can lead to unacceptably high false-positive findings)
Note	*There is no evidence to indicate that any additional laboratory or imaging tests (e.g., blood counts, routine biochemistry tests, chest X-ray, bone scans, liver US exams, CT scans, FDG-PET-CT) or any tumor markers such as cancer antigen 15–3 (CA15–3) or carcinoembryonic antigen (CEA) produce a survival benefit*

ered adverse factors in the overall prognosis of breast cancer. Hormonal replacement therapy increases the risk of recurrence and is generally contraindicated.

For mitigating the physical, psychological and social sequelae of breast cancer treatment, specialized rehabilitation facilities and services are recommended. Lymphedema is a common issue in breast cancer patients and early initiation of physiotherapy post surgery is very important. Available data, with its limitations, confirms the safety of conceiving and pregnancy after treatment of breast cancer. Pregnancy can be considered after completion of Chemotherapy, radiotherapy and anti-HER2 therapy. Many women remain interested in future fertility after a breast cancer diagnosis, indicating that longitudinal fertility discussions are needed.The Young Women's Breast Cancer Study is a multicenter, prospective cohort of women who were diagnosed with breast cancer at age ≤40 years between 2006 and 2016. Among 130 women who attempted to become pregnant, 90 (69.2%) conceived; and, among 896 women who did not attempt to conceive, 18 (2.0%) became pregnant, with a total of 152 pregnancies resulting in 91 live births [238]. In patients with ER-positive disease, it is generally recommended to complete at least 18 months of ET.

Many patients experience depression and intense fatigue following adjuvant ChT and/or RT completion. There is a definite vacuum in addressing long-term survivorship issues (work, family, and sexuality). The most popular tools include the EORTC QLQ-BR23 and the FACIT-B. However, despite reporting the good performance for these measures, others found that current instruments do not address important specific issues such as surgery-specific conditions.

It is critical to address breast cancer patients' long-term survivorship and quality of life issues, and this should also be a focus area for follow-up clinics. The recognized tools for QOL assessment in Breast cancer include the EORTC QLQ-C30, BR 32, FACT, and SF 36. The EORTC tool is a 30-item self-administered cancer-specific questionnaire designed to measure QOL in the cancer population. The assessment comprises nine domains (physical, role, cognitive, emotional, social, fatigue, pain, nausea, and vomiting) To address the deficiencies, the EORTC quality of life study group recently updated the EORTC QLQ-BR23 and introduced the QLQ-BR45 to cover all existing gaps [239].

In a 6-month period at Tata Memorial Hospital, Mumbai, all consecutive early and locally advanced breast cancer patients treated with either BCS or mastectomy and treated with RT were analyzed [240]. One hundred and thirteen patients had mastectomy and 142 patients underwent BCS. Reliability test (Cronbach alpha) for questionnaire filling was 0.669–0.886. There was no significant difference in the quality of life in patients with BCS versus those with mastectomy. However, patients who underwent BCS had better sexual enjoyment and future perspective scores compared with mastectomy patients. There was no significant change of QOL domain scores after RT in mastectomy and BCS patients.

To summarise, quality of life in breast cancer patients improved greatly during recent years as several simple but effective interventions such as physical activity and psychosocial interventions proved to be effective. However, symptoms caused by different treatment modalities are still under estimation and need more serious attention. Pain, lymphedema, worry, sexual function especially for young patients, and the future outlooks are among issues that deserve further consideration to improve quality of life in breast cancer patients.

13 Prognosis, Results and Outcome, Survival

Prognostic factors provide information on clinical outcomes. The most important prognostic factor is the tumor stage. Other factors include age (both younger age and older age), race (blacks have a worse prognosis as compared to white), tumor morphology, histologic grade, peritumoral lymphovascular invasion, Ki-67, and receptor status (hormone receptor and Her2 overexpression). The most important predictive factors include estrogen receptor (ER), progesterone receptor (PR), and Her2neu amplification status. According to the NCI SEER database and ACS cancer facts & figures 2021, 5-year relative survival rates can be considered as follows (Table 18).

Table 18 5-year relative survival rates

Stage at diagnosis	*5 year survival*
Localized(confinedtothebreast)-	99%
Regional spread-	86%
Distant spread-	27%
Cancer subtype	*5 year survival*
HR+/Her2-	92%
HR+/Her2neu+	89%
HR-/Her2neu+	83%
HR-/Her2neu-	77%

14 Future Research Needed/ Provocative Thoughts for Research in the Given Subject

Potential new target therapies and immunotherapies especially for triple negative breast cancer should be evaluated as this is most aggressive tumour with poor prognosis. New strategises should be explored for the use of concurrent radio-immunotherapy to shorten the overall treatment time and response assessment. Approach toward personalized radiotherapy should be explored like the option of omitting radiotherapy in low risk breast cancer patients with high tumor-infiltrating cells (TILs).

15 Conclusion/Overview

Before deciding on treatment, an institutional tumor board discussion should be done for each breast cancer case. An integrated management plan of the sequence of treatment should be decided in the tumour board. Radiotherapy is a critical treatment modality for newly diagnosed, non-metastatic breast cancer patients and for palliation. Whole breast irradiation (WBI) should be offered to all women post-BCS since it improves locoregional recurrence and overall survival. APBI and hypofractionated radiotherapy should be employed whenever feasible. Radiotherapy may be considered in post-mastectomy cases based on risk factors and pathology. Ongoing research may define the safety and efficacy of radio-immunotherapy.

Precepts Box

1. Breast cancer is common cancer that requires an integrated approach of surgery, chemotherapy, radiotherapy, hormonal therapy, and targeted therapy
2. Recent trends and evidence in literature is supportive of doing breast con-

servation and avoiding complete axillary dissection in a selected group of patients
3. Chemotherapy, hormonal therapy and radiotherapy have all been proved to improve overall survival in breast cancer in indicated cases. As of today, some form of local/regional surgery is a must in all breast cancer cases
4. Neoadjuvant systemic therapy has four aims- making giant tumour suitable for conservation, achieving yp N0, and proceeding SLNB instead of AD in N1 patients making outrightly inoperable tumors operable and assessing response of tumor to therapy
5. All breast conservation cases should receive adjuvant radiotherapy unless a selected group of patients with very low risk factors, particularly with comorbitidy and no access to RT after mastectomy, is based on pathology and patient factors
6. Modern-day radiotherapy has tools that reduce doses to normal structures, including the heart. These tools should especially be used in younger patients and patients with left-sided breast cancer
7. Hypofractionated radiotherapy in the breast is strongly supported by evidence. Emerging date for regional treatment by hypofractionated radiotherapy is encouraging
8. Hormonal therapy is strongly recommended in patients with ER/PR receptor positive disease. The type of hormonal therapy and duration of hormonal therapy is to be decided on patient, tumour and related factors
9. Targeted therapy is strongly indicated in HER2 positive cases

16 Multiple Choice Questions

1. Which malignancy is the leading cause of global cancer incidence according to GLOBOCAN 2020
   (a) Lung cancer
   (b) Female breast cancer
   (c) Male breast cancer
   (d) Prostate carcinoma
2. All of the following are the protective factors for preventing breast cancer except
   (a) Breast feeding
   (b) Multiparity
   (c) Physical activity
   (d) Use of OCPs
3. Single file pattern is microscopic feature of what type of breast cancer
   (a) Tubular
   (b) Invasive ductal
   (c) Invasive lobular
   (d) Mucinous
4. Which is the most aggressive molecular subtype of breast cancer
   (a) Luminal A
   (b) Luminal B
   (c) Her2neu enriched
   (d) Triple negative breast cancer
5. All of the following structures are removed in Patey's mastectomy except:
   (a) Breast
   (b) Pectoralis minor
   (c) Axillary nodes
   (d) Pectoralis major
6. 56 years postmenopausal female patient comes to OPD with complains of lump in right breast. On clinical examination, 2 × 1 cm lump is palpable in upper outer quadrant of right breast and 1 × 1 cm fixed matted node in right axilla. No palpable nodes elsewhere. Based on clinical findings what is the tumor staging
   (a) cT1cN2M0
   (b) pT1cN2M0
   (c) cT1cN1M0
   (d) pT1cN1M0

7. A 36 years young female presents to OPD with lump in left breast. Surgical oncologist evaluated patient. Mammography was suggestive of BIRADS IVC in left breast, biopsy from lesion revealed IDC, Grade I, IHC—ER/PR positive and Her 2 neu negative. Clinically patient staged as cT1cN0 disease. Patient was planned for upfront surgery in institutional tumor board. What surgery should be offered to patient first
   (a) BCS + SLND
   (b) BCS + ALND
   (c) Mastectomy + SLND
   (d) Mastectomy + ALND
8. A postmenopausal women diagnosed with carcinoma right breast, post BCS + SLND, pT1cN0M0, ER+, Her2neu negative was referred for adjuvant RT. Due to pandemic the patient was apprehensive for frequent hospital visits. Considering this patient was offered ultrahypofractionated short course adjuvant RT of 26 Gray in five fractions. Which trial supports the above radiotherapy proposed
   (a) FAST trial
   (b) FAST forward trial
   (c) START A
   (d) START B
9. All are indications of radiotherapy post MRM except
   (a) Early breast cancer
   (b) Locally advanced breast cancer
   (c) Margin positive status post op
   (d) Nodes positive on HPR
10. Why is breast board used for positioning patient in RT planning
    (a) To make patient comfortable
    (b) Make chest wall surface parallel to couch
    (c) To make breast fall apart
    (d) To increase separation between heart and target
11. All of the following are RT contouring guidelines for breast cancer except
    (a) RTOG
    (b) ESTRO
    (c) RADCOMP
    (d) DAHANCA
12. Hypofractionated regimen with 40 Gray in 15 fraction over 3 weeks is based on which trial
    (a) START A
    (b) START B
    (c) FAST
    (d) CANADIAN TRIAL
13. What is the most commonly used technique for APBI
    (a) Interstitial
    (b) Mammosite
    (c) Intraoperative
    (d) 3D external beam based
14. All of the following are acute side effects of radiotherapy except:
    (a) Fatigue
    (b) Hyperpigmentation
    (c) Second malignancy
    (d) Desquamation
15. Which of the following is predictive factor for breast cancer treatment
    (a) Age
    (b) Hormonal status
    (c) LVI
    (d) Tumor morphology
16. According to ACS cancer facts & figures 2021, 5-year relative survival rate for metastatic breast cancer is
    (a) 57%
    (b) 37%
    (c) 27%
    (d) 17%

Answer Key

1. (b)
2. (d)
3. (c)
4. (d)
5. (d)
6. (a)
7. (a)
8. (b)
9. (a)
10. (b)
11. (d)
12. (b)

13. (a)
14. (c)
15. (b)
16. (c)

References

1. World Cancer report. International Agency for Research on Cancer 2008. Retrieved 2011-02-26.
2. Sung H, Ferlay J, Siegel RL, Laversanne M, Soerjomataram I, Jemal A, Bray F. Global cancer statistics 2020: GLOBOCAN estimates of incidence and mortality worldwide for 36 cancers in 185 countries. CA Cancer J Clin. 2021;71:209–49.
3. Sung H, Ferlay J, Siegel RL, Laversanne M, Soerjomataram I, Jemal A, et al. Global cancer statistics 2020: GLOBOCAN estimates of incidence and mortality worldwide for 36 cancers in 185 countries. CA Cancer J Clin. 2021;71:209–49.
4. Early Breast Cancer Trialists' Collaborative Group (EBCTCG). Effects of radiotherapy and surgery in early breast cancer: an overview of randomized trials. N Engl J Med. 1995;333:1444–55.
5. Early Breast Cancer Trialists Collaborative Group (EBCTCG). Effects of chemotherapy and hormonal therapy for early breast cancer on recurrence and 15 year survival: an overview of randomised trials. Lancet. 2005;365:1687–717.
6. Early Breast Cancer Trialists' Collaborative Group (EBCTCG), Clarke M, Collins R, Darby S, Davies C, Elphinstone P, Evans E, et al. Effects of radiotherapy and of differences in the extent of surgery for early breast cancer on local recurrence and 15-year survival: an overview of the randomized trials. Lancet. 2005;366:2087–106.
7. Early Breast Cancer Trialists' Collaborative Group (EBCTCG), Darby S, McGale P, Correa C, et al. Effect of radiotherapy after breast-conserving surgery on 10-year recurrence and 15-year breast cancer death: meta-analysis of individual patient data for 10,801 women in 17 randomised trials. Lancet. 2011;378:1707–16.
8. https://gco.iarc.fr/. Last accessed 5th Jan 2026
9. Bidoli E, Virdone S, Hamdi-Cherif M, Toffolutti F, Taborelli M, Panato C, Serraino D. Worldwide age at onset of female breast cancer: a 25-year population-based Cancer Registry Study. Sci Rep. 2019;9:14111.
10. Malvia S, Bagadi SA, Dubey US, Saxena S. Epidemiology of breast cancer in Indian women. Asia Pac J Clin Oncol. 2017;13:289–95.
11. Chaturvedi M, Vaitheeswaran K, Satishkumar K, et al. Time trends in breast cancer among Indian women population: an analysis of population based cancer registry data. Indian J Surg Oncol. 2015;6:427–34.
12. Breast Cancer Facts & Figures 2019–2020. American Cancer Society. Available at https://www.cancer.org/content/dam/cancer-org/research/cancer-facts-and-statistics/breast-cancer-facts-and-figures/breast-cancer-facts-and-figures-2019-2020.pdf. Last accessed 20 Mar 2022.
13. National Comprehensive Cancer Network. Breast cancer risk reduction. NCCN Clinical Practice Guidelines in Oncology. Available at https://www.nccn.org/professionals/physician_gls/pdf/breast_risk.pdf. Version 5.2021 — June 28, 2021. Last accessed 20 Mar 2022.
14. Hereditary Breast and Ovarian Cancer: Breast and Ovarian Cancer and Family History Risk Categories. Centers for Disease Control and Prevention. Available at https://www.cdc.gov/genomics/disease/breast_ovarian_cancer/. January 8, 2019. Last accessed 20 Mar 2022.
15. Agarwal I, Blanco L. WHO classification. Pathology Outlinescom website https://www.pathologyoutlines.com/topic/breastmalignantwhoclassification.html. Last accessed 20 Mar 2022.
16. Giuliano AE, Edge SB, Hortobagyi GN. Eighth edition of the AJCC Cancer staging manual: breast cancer. Ann Surg Oncol. 2018;25(7):1783–5. https://doi.org/10.1245/s10434-018-6486-6. Epub 2018 Apr 18.
17. Fisher B, Anderson S, Bryant J, et al. Twenty-year follow-up of a randomized trial comparing total mastectomy, lumpectomy, and lumpectomy plus irradiation for the treatment of invasive breast cancer. N Engl J Med. 2002;347:1233–41.
18. Veronesi U, Cascinelli N, Mariani L, Greco M, Saccozzi R, Luini A, Aguilar M, Marubini E. Twenty-year follow-up of a randomized study comparing breast-conserving surgery with radical mastectomy for early breast cancer. N Engl J Med. 2002;347(16):1227–32.
19. Wickerham DL, Costantino JP, Mamounas EP, Julian TB. The landmark surgical trials of the National Surgical Adjuvant Breast and bowel project. World J Surg. 2006;30(7):1138–46. https://doi.org/10.1007/s00268-005-0552-5.
20. Fisher B, Dignam J, Wolmark N, Mamounas E, Costantino J, Poller W, et al. Lumpectomy and radiation therapy for the treatment of intraductal breast cancer: findings from National Surgical Adjuvant Breast and Bowel Project B-17. J Clin Oncol. 1998;16(2):441–52. https://doi.org/10.1200/JCO.1998.16.2.441.
21. Cardoso F, Kyriakides S, Ohno S, Penault-Llorca F, Poortmans P, Rubio IT, et al. Early breast cancer: ESMO clinical practice guidelines for diagnosis, treatment and follow-up. Ann Oncol. 2019;30(8):1194–220. https://doi.org/10.1093/annonc/mdz173.

22. Moran MS, Schnitt SJ, Giuliano AE, Harris JR, Khan SA, Horton J, et al. Society of Surgical Oncology–American Society for Radiation Oncology consensus guideline on margins for breast-conserving surgery with whole-breast irradiation in stages I and II invasive breast cancer. Int J Radiat Oncol Biol Phys. 2014;88(3):553–64. https://doi.org/10.1016/j.ijrobp.2013.11.012.
23. Rivere AE, Chiasson KF, Corsetti RL, Fuhrman GM. An assessment of margins after lumpectomy in breast cancer management. Am Surg. 2016;82(2):156–60.
24. McCahill LE, Single RM, Aiello Bowles EJ, et al. Variability in re-excision following breast conservation surgery. JAMA. 2012;307(5):467–75.
25. Morrow M, Van Zee KJ, Solin LJ, Houssami N, Chavez-MacGregor M, Harris JR, Moran MS. Society of Surgical Oncology–American Society for Radiation Oncology–American Society of Clinical Oncology Consensus guideline on margins for breast-conserving surgery with whole-breast irradiation in ductal carcinoma in situ. Pract Radiat Oncol. 2016;6(5):287–95. https://doi.org/10.1016/j.prro.2016.06.011.
26. Fowble B, Solin LJ, Schultz DJ, Rubenstein J, Goodman RL. Breast recurrence following conservative surgery and radiation: patterns of failure, prognosis, and pathologic findings from mastectomy specimens with implications for treatment. Int J Radiat Oncol Biol Phys. 1990;19:833–42.
27. Gage I, Recht A, Gelman R, Nixon AJ, Silver B, Bornstein BA, Harris JR. Long-term outcome following breast-conserving surgery and radiation therapy. Int J Radiat Oncol Biol Phys. 1995;33:245–51.
28. Smith TE, Lee D, Turner BC, Carter D, Haffty BG. True recurrence vs. new primary ipsilateral breast tumor relapse: an analysis of clinical and pathologic differences and their implications in natural history, prognoses, and therapeutic management. Int J Radiat Oncol Biol Phys. 2000;48:1281–9.
29. Mansel RE, Fallowfield L, Kissin M, Goyal A, Newcombe RG, Dixon JM, et al. Randomized multicenter trial of sentinel node biopsy versus standard axillary treatment in operable breast cancer: the ALMANAC Trial. J Natl Cancer Inst. 2006;98(9):599–609. https://doi.org/10.1093/jnci/djj158.
30. Harlow SP, Krag DN, Julian TB, Ashikaga T, Weaver DL, Feldman SA, et al. Prerandomization surgical training for the National Surgical Adjuvant Breast and bowel project (Nsabp) B-32 trial: a randomized phase III clinical trial to compare sentinel node resection to conventional axillary dissection in clinically node-negative breast cancer. Ann Surg. 2005;241(1):48–54. https://doi.org/10.1097/01.sla.0000149429.39656.94.
31. Giuliano AE, Ballman KV, McCall L, Beitsch PD, Brennan MB, Kelemen PR, et al. Effect of axillary dissection vs no axillary dissection on 10-year overall survival among women with invasive breast cancer and sentinel node metastasis: the ACOSOG Z0011 (Alliance) randomized clinical trial. JAMA. 2017;318(10):918–26. https://doi.org/10.1001/jama.2017.11470.
32. Galimberti V, Cole BF, Zurrida S, Viale G, Luini A, Veronesi P, et al. Axillary dissection versus no axillary dissection in patients with sentinel-node micrometastases (IBCSG 23-01): a phase 3 randomised controlled trial. Lancet Oncol. 2013;14(4):297–305. https://doi.org/10.1016/S1470-2045(13)70035-4.
33. Donker M, van Tienhoven G, Straver ME, Meijnen P, van de Velde CJ, Mansel RE, et al. Radiotherapy or surgery of the axilla after a positive sentinel node in breast cancer (EORTC 10981-22023 AMAROS): a randomised, multicentre, open-label, phase 3 non-inferiority trial. Lancet Oncol. 2014;15(12):1303–10. https://doi.org/10.1016/S1470-2045(14)70460-7.
34. Rao R, Euhus D, Mayo HG, Balch C. Axillary node interventions in breast cancer: a systematic review. JAMA. 2013;310(13):1385–94.
35. Fisher CS, Margenthaler JA, Hunt KK, Schwartz T. The landmark series: axillary management in breast cancer. Ann Surg Oncol. 2020;27(3):724–9.
36. Kim T, Giuliano AE, Lyman GH. Lymphatic mapping and sentinel lymph node biopsy in early-stage breast carcinoma: a metaanalysis. Cancer. 2006;106(1):4–16.
37. Giuliano AE, Kirgan DM, Guenther JM, Morton DL. Lymphatic mapping and sentinel lymphadenectomy for breast cancer. Ann Surg. 1994;220(3):391–401.
38. Li J, Chen X, Qi M, Li Y. Sentinel lymph node biopsy mapped with methylene blue dye alone in patients with breast cancer: a systematic review and meta-analysis. PLoS One. 2018;13(9):e0204364.
39. Polom K, Murawa D, Rho Y, Nowaczyk P, Hünerbein M, Murawa P. Current trends and emerging future of indocyanine green usage in surgery and oncology: a literature review. Cancer. 2011;117(21):4812–22.
40. Reinhart MB, Huntington CR, Blair LJ, Heniford BT, Augenstein VA. Indocyanine green: historical context, current applications, and future considerations. Surg Innov. 2016;23(2):166–75.
41. Parmar V, Hawaldar R, Nadkarni MS, Badwe RA. Low axillary sampling in clinically node-negative operable breast cancer. Natl Med J India. 2009;22(5):234–6.
42. Khan SA, Zhao F, Solin LJ, et al. A randomized phase III trial of systemic therapy plus early local therapy versus systemic therapy alone in women with de novo stage IV breast cancer: a trial of the ECOG-ACRIN Research Group (E2108). J Clin Oncol. 2020;38S:ASCO #LBA2.
43. Fitzal F, Bjelic-Radisic V, Knauer M, et al. Impact of breast surgery in primary metastasized breast cancer: outcomes of the prospective randomized phase III ABCSG-28 POSYTIVE trial. Ann Surg. 2019;269:1163.

44. Bjelic-Radisic V, Fitzal F, Knauer M, et al. Primary surgery versus no surgery in synchronous metastatic breast cancer: patient-reported quality-of-life outcomes of the prospective randomized multicenter ABCSG-28 Posytive Trial. BMC Cancer. 2020;20:392.
45. Badwe R, Hawaldar R, Nair N, et al. Locoregional treatment versus no treatment of the primary tumour in metastatic breast cancer: an open-label randomised controlled trial. Lancet Oncol. 2015;16:1380.
46. Soran A, Ozmen V, Ozbas S, et al. Randomized trial comparing resection of primary tumor with no surgery in stage IV breast cancer at presentation: protocol MF07-01. Ann Surg Oncol. 2018;25:3141.
47. Perou CM, Sørlie T, Eisen MB, van de Rijn M, Jeffrey SS, Rees CA, et al. Molecular portraits of human breast tumours. Nature. 2000;406:747–52.
48. Curtis C, Shah SP, Chin SF, Turashvili G, Rueda OM, Dunning MJ, et al. The genomic and transcriptomic architecture of 2,000 breast tumours reveals novel subgroups. Nature. 2012;486:346–52.
49. Sotiriou C, Pusztai L. Gene-expression signatures in breast cancer. N Engl J Med. 2009;360:790–800.
50. https://www.nature.com/articles/s41598-020-62618-3. Last accessed 20 Mar 2022.
51. Fong Y, Evans J, Brook D, Kenkre J, Jarvis P, Gower-Thomas K. The Nottingham prognostic index: five- and ten-year data for all-cause survival within a screened population. Ann R Coll Surg Engl. 2015;97:137–9.
52. Cuzick J, Dowsett M, Pineda S, Wale C, Salter J, Quinn E, et al. Prognostic value of a combined estrogen receptor, progesterone receptor, Ki-67, and human epidermal growth factor receptor 2 immunohistochemical score and comparison with the Genomic Health recurrence score in early breast cancer. J Clin Oncol. 2011;29:4273–8.
53. Sparano JA, Gray RJ, Makower DF, Pritchard KI, Albain KS, Hayes DF, et al. Adjuvant chemotherapy guided by a 21-gene expression assay in breast cancer. N Engl J Med. 2018;379:111–21.
54. Cardoso F, van't Veer LJ, Bogaerts J, Slaets L, Viale G, et al. 70-gene signature as an aid to treatment decisions in early-stage breast cancer. N Engl J Med. 2016;25(375):717–29.
55. Davies C, Pan H, Godwin J, Gray R, Arriagada R, Raina V, Adjuvant Tamoxifen: Longer Against Shorter (ATLAS) Collaborative Group, et al. Long-term effects of continuing adjuvant tamoxifen to 10 years versus stopping at 5 years after diagnosis of oestrogen receptor-positive breast cancer: ATLAS, a randomised trial. Lancet. 2013;381:805–16.
56. Early Breast Cancer Trialists' Collaborative Group (EBCTCG). Aromatase inhibitors versus tamoxifen in early breast cancer: patient-level metaanalysis of the randomised trials. Lancet. 2015;386:1341–52.
57. Francis PA, Pagani O, Fleming GF, Walley BA, Colleoni M, Láng I, SOFT and TEXT Investigators and the International Breast Cancer Study Group, et al. Tailoring adjuvant endocrine therapy for premenopausal breast cancer. N Engl J Med. 2018;12(379):122–37.
58. Early Breast Cancer Trialists' Collaborative group (EBCTCG). Trastuzumab for early-stage, HER2-positive breast cancer: a metaanalysis of 13 864 women in seven randomised trials. Lancet Oncol. 2021;22:1139–50.
59. Gulia S, Kannan S, Badwe R, Gupta S. Evaluation of 1-year vs shorter durations of adjuvant Trastuzumab among patients with early breast cancer: an individual participant data and Trial-level meta-analysis. JAMA Netw Open. 2020;3:e2011777.
60. Piccart M, Procter M, Fumagalli D, de Azambuja E, Clark E, et al. Adjuvant Pertuzumab and Trastuzumab in early HER2-positive breast cancer in the APHINITY trial: 6 years' follow-up. J Clin Oncol. 2021;39:1448–57.
61. von Minckwitz G, Huang CS, Mano MS, Loibl S, Mamounas EP, et al. Trastuzumab Emtansine for residual invasive HER2-positive breast cancer. N Engl J Med. 2019;380:617–28.
62. Schmid P, Cortes J, Dent R, Pusztai L, McArthur H, Kümmel S, et al. VP7-2021: KEYNOTE-522: phase III study of neoadjuvant pembrolizumab + chemotherapy vs. placebo + chemotherapy, followed by adjuvant pembrolizumab vs. placebo for early-stage TNBC. Ann Oncol. 2021;32:1198–200.
63. Tutt ANJ, Garber JE, Kaufman B, Viale G, Fumagalli D, Rastogi P, et al. Adjuvant Olaparib for patients with *BRCA1*- or *BRCA2*-mutated breast cancer. N Engl J Med. 2021;384:2394–405.
64. Masuda N, Lee SJ, Ohtani S, Im YH, Lee ES, Yokota I, et al. Adjuvant Capecitabine for breast cancer after preoperative chemotherapy. N Engl J Med. 2017;376:2147–59.
65. Rath S, Elamarthi P, Parab P, Gulia S, Nandhana R, Mokal S, Kembhavi Y, Perumal P, Bajpai J, Ghosh J, Gupta S. Efficacy and safety of palbociclib and ribociclib in patients with estrogen and/or progesterone receptor positive, HER2 receptor negative metastatic breast cancer in routine clinical practice. PLoS One. 2021;16(7):e0253722.
66. Agrawal C, Goyal P, Agarwal A, Tripathi R, Dodagoudar C, Baghmar S, Sharma A, Batra U, Talwar V, Goyal S, Kumar R, Doval DC. Multicentric real world evidence with palbociclib in hormone positive HER2 negative metastatic breast cancer in Indian population. Sci Rep. 2021;11:16236.
67. Badwe R, Hawaldar R, Nair N, Kaushik R, Parmar V, Siddique S, Budrukkar A, Mittra I, Gupta S. Locoregional treatment versus no treatment of the primary tumour in metastatic breast cancer: an open-label randomised controlled trial. Lancet Oncol. 2015;16:1380–8.
68. Unger JM, Vaidya R, Albain KS, LeBlanc M, Minasian LM, Gotay CC, Henry NL, Fisch MJ, Lee SM, Blanke CD, Hershman DL. Sex differences in risk of severe adverse events in patients receiving immunotherapy, targeted therapy, or che-

motherapy in cancer clinical trials. J Clin Oncol. 2022;40(13):1474–86.
69. Veronesi U, Cascinelli N, Mariani L, et al. Twenty-year follow-up of a randomized study comparing breast-conserving surgery with radical mastectomy for early breast cancer. N Engl J Med. 2002;347:1227–32.
70. Poggi MM, Danforth DN, Sciuto LC, et al. Eighteen-year results in the treatment of early breast carcinoma with mastectomy versus breast conservation therapy: the National Cancer Institute randomized trial. Cancer. 2003;98:697–702.
71. Sarrazin D, Le MG, Arriagada R, et al. Ten-year results of a randomized trial comparing a conservative treatment to mastectomy in early breast cancer. Radiother Oncol. 1989;14:177–84.
72. Van Dongen JA, Voogd AC, Fentiman IS, et al. Long-term results of a randomized trial comparing breast-conserving therapy with mastectomy: European Organization for Research and Treatment of Cancer 10801 trial. J Natl Cancer Inst. 2000;92:1143–50.
73. Blichert-Toft M, Rose C, Andersen JA, et al. Danish randomized trial comparing breast conservation therapy with mastectomy: six years of life-table analysis. Danish Breast Cancer Cooperative Group. J Natl Cancer Inst Monogr. 1992;11:19–25.
74. Meattini I, De Santis MC, Visani L, Scorsetti M, Fozza A, Meduri B, et al. EUROPA Trial Investigators. Single-modality endocrine therapy versus radiotherapy after breast-conserving surgery in women aged 70 years and older with luminal A-like early breast cancer (EUROPA): a preplanned interim analysis of a phase 3, non-inferiority, randomised trial. Lancet Oncol. 2025 Jan;26(1):37–50
75. Rosner D, Bedwani RN, Vana J, et al. Noninvasive breast carcinoma: results of a national survey by the American College of Surgeons. Ann Surg. 1980;192:139–47.
76. Lagios MD. Duct carcinoma in situ. Pathology and treatment. Surg Clin North Am. 1990;70:853–71.
77. Silverstein MJ, Lagios MD, Martino S, et al. Outcome after localrecurrence in patients with ductal carcinoma in situ of the breast. J Clin Oncol. 1998;16:1367–73.
78. Romero L, Klein L, Ye W, et al. Outcome after invasive recurrence inpatients with ductal carcinoma in situ of the breast. Am J Surg. 2004;188:371–6.
79. Yi M, Krishnamurthy S, Kuerer HM, et al. Role of primary tumor characteristics in predicting positive sentinel lymph nodes in patients with ductal carcinoma in situ or microinvasive breast cancer. Am J Surg. 2008;196:81–7.
80. Lagios MD, Westdahl PR, Margolin FR, et al. Duct carcinoma in situ. Relationship of extent of noninvasive disease to the frequency of occult invasion, multicentricity, lymph node metastases, and short-term treatment failures. Cancer. 1982;50:1309–14.
81. King TA, Farr GH Jr, Cederbom GJ, et al. A mass on breast imaging predicts coexisting invasive carcinoma in patients with a core biopsy diagnosis of ductal carcinoma in situ. Am Surg. 2001;67:907–12.
82. Huo L, Sneige N, Hunt KK, et al. Predictors of invasion in patients with coreneedle biopsy-diagnosed ductal carcinoma in situ and recommendations for a selective approach to sentinel lymph node biopsy in ductal carcinoma in situ. Cancer. 2006;107:1760–8.
83. Fisher ER, Leeming R, Anderson S, et al. Conservative management of intraductal carcinoma (DCIS) of the breast. Collaborating NSABP investigators. J Surg Oncol. 1991;47:139–47.
84. Fisher B, Dignam J, Wolmark N, et al. Lumpectomy and radiation therapy for the treatment of intraductal breast cancer: findings from National Surgical Adjuvant Breast and Bowel Project B-17. J Clin Oncol. 1998;16:441–52.
85. Julien JP, Bijker N, Fentiman IS, et al. Radiotherapy in breast-conserving treatment for ductal carcinoma in situ: first results of the EORTC randomised phase III trial 10853. EORTC Breast Cancer Cooperative Group and EORTC Radiotherapy Group. Lancet. 2000;355:528–33.
86. Bijker N, Meijnen P, Peterse JL, et al. Breast-conserving treatment with or without radiotherapy in ductal carcinoma-in-situ: ten-year results of European Organisation for Research and Treatment of Cancer randomized phase III trial 10853–a study by the EORTC Breast Cancer Cooperative Group and EORTC Radiotherapy Group. J Clin Oncol. 2006;24:3381.
87. Houghton J, George WD, Cuzick J, et al. Radiotherapy and tamoxifen in women with completely excised ductal carcinoma in situ of the breast in the UK, Australia, and New Zealand: randomised controlled trial. Lancet. 2003;362:95–102.
88. Kerlikowske K, Molinaro A, Cha I, et al. Characteristics associated with recurrence among women with ductal carcinoma in situ treated by lumpectomy. J Natl Cancer Inst. 2003;95:1692–702.
89. Emdin SO, Granstrand B, Ringberg A, et al. SweDCIS: radiotherapy after sector resection for ductal carcinoma in situ of the breast. Results of a randomised trial in a population offered mammography screening. Acta Oncol. 2006;45:536–43.
90. Holmberg L, Garmo H, Granstrand B, et al. Absolute risk reductions for localrecurrence after postoperative radiotherapy after sector resection for ductalcarcinoma in situ of the breast. J Clin Oncol. 2008;26:1247–52.
91. Early Breast Cancer Trialists' Collaborative Group (EBCTCG), Correa C, McGale P, Taylor C, Wang Y, Clarke M, Davies C, Peto R, Bijker N, Solin L, Darby S. Overview of the randomized trials of radiotherapy in ductal carcinoma in situ of the breast. J Natl Cancer Inst Monogr. 2010;41:162–77.
92. Gyenesa G, Rutqvistb LE, Liedbergb A, Fornander T. Long-term cardiac morbidity and mortality in a randomized trial of pre- and postoperative radiation therapy versus surgery alone in primary breast cancer. Radiother Oncol. 1998;48:185–90.

93. Cuzick J, Stewart H, Peto R, et al. Overview of randomized trials comparing radical mastectomy without radiotherapy against simple mastectomy with radiotherapy in breast cancer. Cancer Treat Rep. 1987;71:7–14.
94. Early Breast Cancer Trialists' Collaborative Group. Favourable and unfavourable effects on long-term survival of radiotherapy for early breast cancer: an overview of the randomized trials. Lancet. 2000;355:1757–70.
95. Overgaard M, Hansen PS, Overgaard J, Rose C, AnderssonM, Bach F, et al. Postoperative radiotherapy in high-risk premenopausalwomen with breast cancer who receive adjuvantchemotherapy. Danish Breast Cancer Cooperative Group82b Trial. N Engl J Med. 1997;337:949–55.
96. Overgaard M, Jensen MB, Overgaard J, Hansen PS, Rose C, Andersson M, et al. Postoperative radiotherapy in high-riskpostmenopausal breast-cancer patients given adjuvanttamoxifen: Danish Breast Cancer Cooperative Group DBCG82c randomised trial. Lancet. 1999;353:1641–8.
97. Ragaz J, Jackson SM, Le N, et al. Adjuvant radiotherapy and chemotherapy in node-positive premenopausal women with breast cancer. N Engl J Med. 1997;337:956–62.
98. https://clinicaltrials.gov/ct2/show/NCT02992574.
99. Recht A, et al. Postmastectomy radiotherapy: an American Society of Clinical Oncology, American Society for Radiation Oncology, and Society of Surgical Oncology focused guideline update. Pract Radiat Oncol. 2016;6:e219–34.
100. Kunkler IH, Russell NS, Anderson N, Sainsbury R, et al. SUPREMO Trial Investigators; Sunil. Ten-year survival after postmastectomy chest-wall irradiation in breast cancer. N Engl J Med. 2025;393(18):1771–83. https://doi.org/10.1056/NEJMoa2412225.
101. Ho AY, Hu ZI, Mehrara BJ, Wilkins EG. Radiotherapy in the setting of breast reconstruction: types, techniques, and timing. Lancet Oncol. 2017;18:e742–53.
102. Fisher B, Bryant J, Wolmark N, et al. Effect of preoperative chemotherapy on the outcome of women with operable breast cancer. J Clin Oncol. 1998;16:2672–85.
103. Buchholz TA, Hunt KK, Whitman GJ, et al. Neoadjuvant chemotherapy for breast carcinoma: multidisciplinary considerations of benefits and risks. Cancer. 2003;98:1150–60.
104. Buchholz TA, Lehman CD, Harris JR, et al. Statement of the science concerning locoregional treatments after preoperative chemotherapy for breast cancer: a national cancer institute conference. J Clin Oncol. 2008;26:791–7.
105. Wolmark N, Wang J, Mamounas E, et al. Preoperative chemotherapy in patients with operable breast cancer: nine-year results from national surgical adjuvant breast and bowel project B-18. J Natl Cancer Inst Monogr. 2001;30:96–102.
106. Schlafstein A, Liu Y, Goyal S, Kahn S, Godette K, Lin J, Torres MA, Royce TJ, Patel SA. Regional nodal irradiation for clinically node-positive breast cancer patients with pathologic negative nodes after neoadjuvant chemotherapy. Clin Breast Cancer. 2022;22(2):127–35.
107. Mamounas EP, Bandos H, White JR, Julian TB, Khan AJ, Shaitelman SF, Torres MA, Vicini FA, Ganz PA, McCloskey SA, Lucas PC, Gupta N, Li XA, McCormick B, Smith B, Tendulkar RD, Kavadi VS, Matsumoto K, Seaward SA, Irvin WJ Jr, Lin JY, Mutter RW, Muanza TM, Stromberg J, Jagsi R, Weiss AC, Curran WJ Jr, Wolmark N. Omitting Regional Nodal Irradiation after Response to Neoadjuvant Chemotherapy. N Engl J Med. 2025;392(21):2113–24.
108. https://radiologyassistant.nl/breast/breast--prosthesis/breast-prosthesis-imaging. Last accessed 30 Mar 2022.
109. Loganadane G, Truong PT, Taghian AG, Tešanović D, Jiang M, Geara F, Moran MS, Belkacemi Y. Comparison of nodal target volume definition in breast cancer radiation therapy according to RTOG versus ESTRO atlases: a practical review from the TransAtlantic Radiation Oncology Network (TRONE). Int J Radiat Oncol Biol Phys. 2020;107(3):437–48.
110. https://www.astro.org/uploadedFiles/_MAIN_SITE/Affiliate/International/Content_Pieces/IESEducationalresources.pdf.
111. https://www.nrgoncology.org/About-Us/Center-for-Innovation-in-Radiation-Oncology/Breast-Cancer/RADCOMP-Breast-Atlas.
112. Duma MN. An update on regional nodal irradiation: indication, target volume delineation, and radiotherapy techniques. Breast Care (Basel). 2020;15:128–35.
113. Munshi A. Contouring for radiotherapy in carcinoma breast - why a robust uniform guideline is (nearly) impossible. J Cancer Res Ther. 2020;16:1522–3.
114. Duane F, Aznar MC, Bartlett F, Cutter DJ, Darby SC, Jagsi R, Lorenzen EL, McArdle O, McGale P, Myerson S, Rahimi K, Vivekanandan S, Warren S, Taylor CW. A cardiac contouring atlas for radiotherapy. Radiother Oncol. 2017;122:416–22.
115. Lebesque JV. Field matching in breast irradiation: an exact solution to a geometrical problem. Radiother Oncol. 1986;5:47–57.
116. Muren LP, Maurstad G, Hafslund R, Anker G, Dahl O. Cardiac and pulmonary doses and complication probabilities in standard and conformal tangential irradiation in conservative management of breast cancer. Radiother Oncol. 2002;62:173–837.
117. Reardon KA, Read PW, Morris MM, Reardon MA, Geesey C, Wijesooriya K. A comparative analysis of 3D conformal deep inspiratory-breath hold and free-breathing intensity-modulated radiation therapy for left-sided breast cancer. Med Dosim. 2013;38:190–5.

118. Freedman GM, Anderson PR, Li J, Eisenberg DF, et al. Intensity modulated radiation therapy (IMRT) decreases acute skin toxicity for women receiving radiation for breast cancer. Am J Clin Oncol. 2006;29:66–70.
119. Xie X, Ouyang S, Wang H, Yang W, Jin H, Hu B, Shen L. Dosimetric comparison of left-sided whole breast irradiation with 3D-CRT, IP-IMRT and hybrid IMRT. Oncol Rep. 2014;31:2195.
120. Yang B, Wei XD, Zhao YT, Ma CM. Dosimetric evaluation of integrated IMRT treatment of the chest wall and supraclavicular region for breast cancer after modified radical mastectomy. Med Dosim. 2014;39:185.
121. Ha B, Suh HS, Lee J, Lee KJ, Lee R, Moon BI. Long-term results of forward intensity-modulated radiation therapy for patients with early-stage breast cancerradiatoncol. Radiat Oncol J. 2013;31:191–8.
122. Abo-Madyan Y, Aziz MH, Aly MM, Schneider F, Sperk E, Clausen S, Giordano FA, Herskind C, Steil V, Wenz F, Glatting G. Second cancer risk after 3D-CRT, IMRT and VMAT for breast cancer. Radiother Oncol. 2014 Mar;110(3):471–6. https://doi.org/10.1016/j.radonc.2013.12.002. Epub 2014 Jan 17. PMID: 24444525.
123. Barnett GC, Wilkinson JS, Moody AM, et al. Randomized controlled trial of forward-planned intensity modulated radiotherapy for early breast cancer: interim results at 2 years. Int J Radiat Oncol Biol Phys. 2012;82:715–23.
124. Al-Rahbi ZS, Al Mandhari Z, Ravichandran R, et al. Dosimetric comparison of intensity modulated radiotherapy isocentric field plans and field in field (FIF) forward plans in the treatment of breast cancer. Med Phys. 2013;38:22–9.
125. Whelan T, MacKenzie R, Julian J, Levine M, Shelley W, Grimard L, et al. Randomized trial of breast irradiation schedules after lumpectomy for women with lymph node-negative breast cancer. J Natl Cancer Inst. 2002;94:1143e50.
126. START Trialists' Group, Bentzen SM, Agrawal RK, Aird EG, Barrett JM, BarrettLee PJ, et al. The UK standardisation of breast radiotherapy (START) trial A of radiotherapy hypofractionation for treatment of early breast cancer: a randomized trial. Lancet Oncol. 2008;9:331e41.
127. START Trialists' Group, Bentzen SM, Agrawal RK, Aird EG, Barrett JM, BarrettLee PJ, et al. The UK standardisation of Breast radiotherapy (START) Trial B of radiotherapy hypofractionation for treatment of early breast cancer: a randomized trial. Lancet. 2008;371(9618):1098e107.
128. Haviland JS, Owen JR, Dewar JA, Agrawal RK, Barrett J, Barrett-Lee PJ, Dobbs HJ, Hopwood P, Lawton PA, Magee BJ, Mills J, Simmons S, Sydenham MA, Venables K, Bliss JM, Yarnold JR, START Trialists' Group. The UK standardisation of breast radiotherapy (START) trials of radiotherapy hypofractionation for treatment of early breast cancer: 10-year follow-up results of two randomised controlled trials. Lancet Oncol. 2013;14:1086–94.
129. Silverstein MJ, Lagios MD. Ductal carcinoma in situ of the breast. In: Benson JR, Tuttle T, Gui G, editors. Early breast cancer: from screening to multidisciplinary management. Boca Raton: CRC Press, Taylor and Francis Group; 2013. p. 341–60.
130. Whelan TJ, Pignol JP, Levine MN, et al. Long-term results of hypofractionated radiation therapy for breast cancer. N Engl J Med. 2010;362:513–20.
131. Hopwood P, Haviland JS, Sumo G, Mills J, Bliss JM, Yarnold JR, et al. Comparison of patient-reported breast, arm, and shoulder symptoms and body image after radiotherapy for early breast cancer: 5-year follow-up in the randomized Standardisation of Breast Radiotherapy (START) trials. Lancet Oncol. 2010;11(3):231–40.
132. Chatterjee S, Arunsingh M, Agrawal S, Dabkara D, Mahata A, Arun I, Shrimali RK, Achari R, Mallick I, Ahmed R. Outcomes following a moderately hypofractionated adjuvant radiation (START B type) schedule for breast cancer in an unscreened non-Caucasian population. Clin Oncol (R Coll Radiol). 2016;28(10):e165–72. https://doi.org/10.1016/j.clon.2016.05.008. Epub 2016 Jun 28.
133. Brunt AM, Haviland JS, Sydenham M, Agrawal RK, Algurafi H, Alhasso A, Barrett-Lee P, Bliss P, Bloomfield D, Bowen J, Donovan E, Goodman A, Harnett A, Hogg M, Kumar S, Passant H, Quigley M, Sherwin L, Stewart A, Syndikus I, Tremlett J, Tsang Y, Venables K, Wheatley D, Bliss JM, Yarnold JR. Ten-year results of FAST: a randomized controlled trial of 5-fraction whole-breast radiotherapy for early breast cancer. J Clin Oncol. 2020;38(28):3261–72.
134. Agrawal RK, Alhasso A, Barrett-Lee PJ, et al. First results of the randomised UK FAST Trial of radiotherapy hypofractionation for treatment of early breast cancer (CRUKE/04/015). Radiother Oncol. 2011;100:93–100.
135. Murray Brunt A, Haviland JS, Wheatley DA, Sydenham MA, Alhasso A, Bloomfield DJ, Chan C, Churn M, Cleator S, Coles CE, Goodman A, Harnett A, Hopwood P, Kirby AM, Kirwan CC, Morris C, Nabi Z, Sawyer E, Somaiah N, Stones L, Syndikus I, Bliss JM, Yarnold JR, FAST-Forward Trial Management Group. Hypofractionated breast radiotherapy for 1 week versus 3 weeks (FAST-forward): 5-year efficacy and late normal tissue effects results from a multicentre, non-inferiority, randomised, phase 3 trial. Lancet. 2020;395:1613–26.
136. Chatterjee S, Chakraborty S, HYPORT Adjuvant Author Group. Hypofractionated radiation therapy comparing a standard radiotherapy schedule (over 3 weeks) with a novel 1-week schedule in adjuvant breast cancer: an open-label randomized controlled study (HYPORT-adjuvant)-study protocol for a multicentre, randomized phase III trial. Trials. 2020;21(1):819. https://doi.org/10.1186/

s13063-020-04751-y. PMID: 32998747; PMCID: PMC7526182.
137. Romestaing P, Lehingue Y, Carrie C, et al. Role of a 10-Gy boost in the conservative treatment of early breast cancer: results of a randomized clinical trial in Lyon, France. J Clin Oncol. 1997;15:963–8.
138. Polgar C. Electron and high-dose-rate brachytherapy boost in the conservative treatment of stage I-II breast cancer first results of the randomized Budapest boost trial. Strahlenther Onkol. 2002;178:615–23.
139. Antonini N, Jones H, Horiot JC, et al. Effect of age and radiation dose on local control after breast conserving treatment: EORTC trial 22881-10882. Radiother Oncol. 2006;82:265–71.
140. Bartelink H, Horiot JC, Poortmans PM, et al. Impact of a higher radiation dose on local control and survival in breast-conserving therapy of early breast cancer: 10-year results of the randomized boost versus no boost EORTC 22881–10882 trial. J Clin Oncol. 2007;25:3259–65.
141. Poortmans PM, Collette L, Horiot JC, et al. Impact of the boost dose of 10 Gy versus 26 Gy in patients with early stage breast cancer after a microscopically incomplete lumpectomy: 10-year results of the randomised EORTC boost trial. Radiother Oncol. 2009;90:80–5.
142. Poortmans P, Aznar M, Bartelink H. Quality indicators for breast cancer: revisiting historical evidence in the context of technology changes. Semin Radiat Oncol. 2012;22:29–39.
143. Suzuki R, Yoshida M, Oguchi M, Yoshioka Y, Tokumasu K, Osako T, Ono S, Ueno T, Miyagi Y. Efficacy of radiation boost after breast-conserving surgery for breast cancer with focally positive, tumor-exposed margins. J Radiat Res. 2020;61:440–6.
144. Sadek BT, Homayounfar G, Abi Raad RF, Niemierko A, Shenouda MN, Keruakous AR, Specht MC, Taghian AG. Is a higher boost dose of radiation necessary after breast-conserving therapy for patients with breast cancer with final close or positive margins? Breast Cancer Res Treat. 2015;154:71–9.
145. Whelan TJ, Olivotto IA, Parulekar WR, Ackerman I, Chua BH, Nabid A, Vallis KA, White JR, Rousseau P, Fortin A, Pierce LJ, Manchul L, Chafe S, Nolan MC, Craighead P, Bowen J, McCready DR, Pritchard KI, Gelmon K, Murray Y, Chapman JA, Chen BE, Levine MN, MA.20 Study Investigators. Regional nodal irradiation in early-stage breast cancer. N Engl J Med. 2015;373:307–16.
146. Kaidar-Person O, Boersma LJ, De Brouwer P, Weltens C, Kirkove C, Peignaux-Casasnovas K, Budach V, van der Leij F, Peters M, Weidner N, Rivera S, van Tienhoven G, Fourquet A, Noel G, Valli M, Guckenberger M, Koiter E, Racadot S, Abdah-Bortnyak R, Bartelink H, Struikmans H, Fortpied C, Poortmans PM; EORTC Radiation Oncology and Breast Cancer Groups. The EORTC 22922/10925 trial investigating regional nodal irradiation in stage I-III breast cancer: Outcomes according to locoregional and systemic therapies. Radiother Oncol. 2024;201:110563. https://doi.org/10.1016/j.radonc.2024.110563. Epub 2024 Sep 26. PMID: 39341505.
147. Kaija H, et al. Tangential breast irradiation with or without internal mammary chain irradiation: results of a randomized trial. Radiother Oncol. 1995;36:172–6.
148. Whelan TJ, Olivotto IA, Parulekar WR, Ackerman I, Chua BH, Nabid A, et al. Regional nodal irradiation in early-stage breast cancer. N Engl J Med. 2015;373:307–16.
149. Poortmans PM, Weltens C, Fortpied C, Kirkove C, Peignaux-Casasnovas K, Budach V. Internal mammary and medial supraclavicular lymph node chain irradiation in stage I-III breast cancer (EORTC 22922/10925): 15-year results of a randomised, phase 3 trial. Lancet Oncol. 2020;21:1602–10.
150. Hennequin C, Bossard N, Servagi-Vernat S, Maingon P, Dubois JB, Datchary J. Ten-year survival results of a randomized trial of irradiation of internal mammary nodes after mastectomy. Int J Radiat Oncol Biol Phys. 2013;86:860–6.
151. Kaija H, Maunu P. Tangential breast irradiation with or without internal mammary chain irradiation: results of a randomized trial. Radiother Oncol. 1995;36(3):172–6. https://doi.org/10.1016/0167-8140(95)01607-i.
152. Thorsen LB, Offersen BV, Danø H, Berg M, Jensen I, Pedersen AN et al. DBCG-IMN: a population-based cohort study on the effect of internal mammary node irradiation in early node-positive breast cancer. J Clin Oncol. 2016;34(4):314–20. https://doi.org/10.1200/JCO.2015.63.6456. Epub 2015 Nov 23.
153. Hurkmans CW, et al. Quality assurance of axillary radiotherapy in the EORTC AMAROS trial 10981/22023: the dummy run. Radiother Oncol. 2003;68:233–40.
154. Straver ME, et al. Sentinel node identification rate and nodal involvement in the EORTC 10981–22023 AMAROS trial. Ann Surg Oncol. 2010;17(7):1854–61.
155. Bartels SAL, Donker M, Poncet C, Sauvé N, Straver ME, van de Velde CJH, Mansel RE, Blanken C, Orzalesi L, Klinkenbijl JHG, van der Mijle HCJ, Nieuwenhuijzen GAP, Veltkamp SC, van Dalen T, Marinelli A, Rijna H, Snoj M, Bundred NJ, Merkus JWS, Belkacemi Y, Petignat P, Schinagl DAX, Coens C, van Tienhoven G, van Duijnhoven F, Rutgers EJT. Radiotherapy or Surgery of the Axilla After a Positive Sentinel Node in Breast Cancer: 10-Year Results of the Randomized Controlled EORTC 10981-22023 AMAROS Trial. J Clin Oncol. 2023;41(12):2159–2165. https://doi.org/10.1200/JCO.22.01565. Epub 2022 Nov 16. PMID: 36383926.
156. Rowell NP. Radiotherapy to the chest wall following mastectomy for nodenegative breast cancer: a systematic review. Radiother Oncol. 2009;91:23–32.

157. Vinh-Hung V, Voordeckers M, Van de Steene J, Soete G, Lamote J, Storme G. Omission of radiotherapy after breast-conserving surgery: survival impact and time trends. Radiother Oncol. 2003;67:147–58.
158. Nattinger AB. Variation in the choice of breast-conserving surgery or mastectomy: patient or physician decision making? J Clin Oncol. 2005;23:5429–31.
159. Schroen AT, Brenin DR, Kelly MD, Knaus WA, Slingluff CL Jr. Impact of patient distance to radiation therapy on mastectomy use in early-stage breast cancer patients. J Clin Oncol. 2005;23:7074–80.
160. Hershman DL, Buono D, McBride RB, Tsai WY, Joseph KA, Grann VR, et al. Surgeon characteristics and receipt of adjuvant radiotherapy in women with breast cancer. J Natl Cancer Inst. 2008;100:199–206.
161. Athas WF, Adams-Cameron M, Hunt WC, Amir-Fazli A, Key CR. Travel distance to radiation therapy and receipt of radiotherapy following breast-conserving surgery. J Natl Cancer Inst. 2000;92:269–71.
162. Fong A, Shafiq J, Saunders C, Thompson AM, Tyldesley S, Olivotto IA, et al. A comparison of surgical and radiotherapy breast cancer therapy utilization in Canada (British Columbia), Scotland (Dundee), and Australia (WesternAustralia) with models of "optimal" therapy. Breast. 2012;21:570–7.
163. Holland R, Veling SH, Mravunac M, et al. Histologic multifocality ofTis, T1-2 breast carcinomas. Implications for clinical trials of breastconserving-surgery. Cancer. 1985;56:979–90.
164. Vaidya JS, Vyas JJ, Chinoy RF, et al. Multicentricity of breast cancer: whole-organ analysis and clinical implications. Br J Cancer. 1996;74:820–4.
165. Kahán Z, et al. The risk of early and late lung sequelae after conformal radiotherapy in breast cancer patients. Int J Radiat Oncol Biol Phys. 2007;68:673–81.
166. Kwa SL, et al. Radiation pneumonitis as a function of mean lung dose: an analysis of pooled data of 540 patients. Int J Radiat Oncol Biol Phys. 1998;42:1–9.
167. Darby SC, McGale P, Taylor CW, Peto R. Long-term mortality from heart disease and lung cancer after radiotherapy for early breast cancer: prospective cohort study of about 300,000 women in US SEER cancer registries. Lancet Oncol. 2005;6:557–65.
168. Kirova YM, et al. Risk of second malignancies after adjuvant radiotherapy for breast cancer: a large-scale, single-institution review. Int J Radiat Oncol Biol Phys. 2007;68:359–63.
169. Schaapveld M, et al. Risk of new primary non-breast cancers after breast cancer treatment: a Dutch population-based study. J Clin Oncol. 2008;26:1239–46.
170. Schaapveld M, et al. The impact of adjuvant therapy on contralateral breast cancer risk and the prognostic significance of contralateral breast cancer: a population based study in The Netherlands. Breast Cancer Res Treat. 2008;110:189–97.
171. Polgár C, Major T, Fodor J, Németh G, Orosz Z, Sulyok Z, et al. High-dose-ratebrachytherapy alone versus whole breast radiotherapy with or without tumor bed boost after breast-conserving surgery: seven-year results of a comparative study. Int J Radiat Oncol Biol Phys. 2004;60:1173–81.
172. Chen PY, Vicini FA, Benitez P, Kestin LL, Wallace M, Mitchell C, et al. Long-term cosmetic results and toxicity after accelerated partial-breast irradiation: a method of radiation delivery by interstitial brachytherapy for the treatment of early-stage breast carcinoma. Cancer. 2006;106:991–9.
173. Johansson B, Karlsson L, Liljegren G, Hardell L, Persliden J. Pulse dose rate brachytherapy as the sole adjuvant radiotherapy after breast-conserving surgery of T1eT2 breast cancer: first long term results from a clinical study. Radiother Oncol. 2009;90:30–5.
174. Kaufman SA, DiPetrillo TA, Price LL, Midle JB, Wazer DE. Long-term outcome and toxicity in a phase I/II trial using high-dose-rate multicatheter interstitial brachytherapy for T1/T2 breast cancer. Brachytherapy. 2007;6:286–92.
175. Arthur DW, Winter K, Kuske RR, Bolton J, Rabinovitch R, White J, et al. A phase II trial of brachytherapy alone after lumpectomy for select breast cancer: tumor control and survival outcomes of RTOG 95-17. Int J Radiat Oncol Biol Phys. 2008;72:467–73.
176. Ott OJ, Hildebrandt G, Pötter R, Hammer J, Lotter M, Resch A, et al. Accelerated partial breast irradiation with multi-catheter brachytherapy: local control, side effects and cosmetic outcome for 274 patients. Results of the German- Austrian multi-centre trial. Radiother Oncol. 2007;82:281–6.
177. Yoshida K, Nose T, Masuda N, Yamazaki H, Kotsuma T, Yoshida M, et al. Preliminary result of accelerated partial breast irradiation after breast-conserving surgery. Breast Cancer. 2009;16:105–12.
178. Aristei C, Palumbo I, Cucciarelli F, Cavalli A, Tarducci R, Raymondi C, et al. Partial breast irradiation with interstitial high-dose-rate brachytherapy in early breast cancer: results of a phase II prospective study. Eur J Surg Oncol. 2009;35:144–50.
179. Lawenda BD, Taghian AG, Kachnic LA, Hamdi H, Smith BL, Gadd MA, et al. Dose-volume analysis of radiotherapy for T1N0 invasive breast cancer treated by local excision and partial breast irradiation by low-dose-rate interstitial implant. Int J Radiat Oncol Biol Phys. 2003;56:671–80.
180. Chao KK, Vicini FA, Wallace M, Mitchell C, Chen P, Ghilezan M, et al. Analysis of treatment efficacy, cosmesis, and toxicity using the MammoSite breast brachytherapy catheter to deliver accelerated partial-breast irradiation: the William Beaumont Hospital experience. Int J Radiat Oncol Biol Phys. 2007;69:32–40.
181. Vaidya JS, Joseph DJ, Tobias JS, et al. Targeted intraoperative radiotherapy versus whole breast

radiotherapy for breast cancer (TARGIT-A trial): an international,prospective, randomised, non-inferiority phase 3 trial. Lancet. 2010;376:91–102.
182. Vaidya J, et al. Targeted intraoperative radiotherapy for early breast cancer: TARGIT-A trial- updated analysis of local recurrence and first analysis of survival [abstract]. Cancer Res. 2012;72(Suppl. 3):S4–2.
183. Vaidya JS, Bulsara M, Wenz F, Tobias JS, Joseph D, Baum M. Targeted radiotherapy for early breast cancer. Lancet. 2018;391(10115):26–7.
184. Veronesi U, Orecchia R, Luini A, Galimberti V, Zurrida S, Intra M, et al. Intraoperative radiotherapy during breast conserving surgery: a study on 1,822 cases treated with electrons. Breast Cancer Res Treat. 2010;124:141–51.
185. Sautter-Bihl ML, Sedlmayer F, Budach W, Dunst J, Engenhart-Cabillic R, Fietkau R, et al. Intraoperative radiotherapy as accelerated partial breast irradiation for early breast cancer: beware of one-stop shops? Strahlenther Onkol. 2010;186:651e7.
186. Orecchia R. ELIOT trials in Milan: results [abstract]. Radiother Oncol. 2013;103(Suppl. 2):S4 a10.
187. Orecchia R. IORT update: what are the limits of radiation dose and volume? Radiother Oncol. 2012;103(Suppl. 1):S38.
188. Orecchia R, Veronesi U, Maisonneuve P, Galimberti VE, Lazzari R, Veronesi P, Jereczek-Fossa BA, Cattani F, Sangalli C, Luini A, Caldarella P, Venturino M, Sances D, Zurrida S, Viale G, Leonardi MC, Intra M. Intraoperative irradiation for early breast cancer (ELIOT): long-term recurrence and survival outcomes from a single-centre, randomised, phase 3 equivalence trial. Lancet Oncol. 2021;22:597–608.
189. Vicini FA, Cecchini RS, White JR, Arthur DW, Julian TB, Rabinovitch RA, Kuske RR, Ganz PA, Parda DS, Scheier MF, Winter KA, Paik S, Kuerer HM, Vallow LA, Pierce LJ, Mamounas EP, McCormick B, Costantino JP, Bear HD, Germain I, Gustafson G, Grossheim L, Petersen IA, Hudes RS, Curran WJ Jr, Bryant JL, Wolmark N. Long-term primary results of accelerated partial breast irradiation after breast-conserving surgery for early-stage breast cancer: a randomised, phase 3, equivalence trial. Lancet. 2019;394(10215):2155–64.
190. Whelan TJ, Julian JA, Berrang TS, Kim DH, Germain I, Nichol AM, Akra M, Lavertu S, Germain F, Fyles A, Trotter T, Perera FE, Balkwill S, Chafe S, McGowan T, Muanza T, Beckham WA, Chua BH, Gu CS, Levine MN, Olivotto IA, Trial RAPID, Investigators. External beam accelerated partial breast irradiation versus whole breast irradiation after breast conserving surgery in women with ductal carcinoma in situ and node-negative breast cancer (RAPID): a randomised controlled trial. Lancet. 2019;394(10215):2165–72. https://doi.org/10.1016/S0140-6736(19)32515-2.
191. Polgár C, Ott OJ, Hildebrandt G, Kauer-Dorner D, Knauerhase H, Major T, Lyczek J, Guinot JL, Dunst J, Miguelez CG, Slampa P, Allgäuer M, Lössl K, Polat B, Kovács G, Fischedick AR, Fietkau R, Resch A, Kulik A, Arribas L, Niehoff P, Guedea F, Schlamann A, Pötter R, Gall C, Uter W, Strnad V, Groupe Européen de Curiethérapie of European Society for Radiotherapy and Oncology (GEC-ESTRO). Late side-effects and cosmetic results of accelerated partial breast irradiation with interstitial brachytherapy versus whole-breast irradiation after breast-conserving surgery for low-risk invasive and in-situ carcinoma of the female breast: 5-year results of a randomised, controlled, phase 3 trial. Lancet Oncol. 2017;18(2):259–68. https://doi.org/10.1016/S1470-2045(17)30011-6.
192. Bhattacharya IS, Haviland JS, Kirby AM, Kirwan CC, Hopwood P, Yarnold JR, Bliss JM, Coles CE, IMPORT Trialists. Patient-reported outcomes over 5 years after whole- or partial-breast radiotherapy: longitudinal analysis of the IMPORT LOW (CRUK/06/003) phase III randomized controlled trial. J Clin Oncol. 2019;37(4):305–17. https://doi.org/10.1200/JCO.18.00982. Epub 2018 Dec 11. PMID: 30532984; PMCID: PMC6357225.
193. Orecchia R, Ciocca M, Tosi G, Franzetti S, Luini A, Gatti G, et al. Intraoperative electronbeamradiotherapy (ELIOT) to the breast: a need for a quality assurance programme. Breast. 2005;14:541e6.
194. Armaroli L, Barbieri E, Bertoni F, Busutti L, Cardinali M, Cartei F, et al. Breastcancer with low risk of local recurrence: partial and accelerated radiation withthree-dimensional conformal radiotherapy (3DCRT) vs. standard radiotherapyafter conserving surgery (phase IIIstudy)Version01.052007. Available from http://groups.eortc.be/radio/res/irma/synopsis_trial_irma1.pdf. Last accessed 20 June 2022.
195. Belkacemi Y, Lartigau E, Bourgier C. Standard of hypofractionated radiotherapy versusaccelerated partial breast irradiation (APBI) for breast cancer (SHARE). Available from: http://www.clinicaltrials.gov/ct2/show/NCT01247233?term¼APBIþSHARE&rank¼1. Last accessed 20 June 2022.
196. Smith BD, Arthur DW, Buchholz TA, Haffty BG, Hahn CA, Hardenbergh PH, et al. Accelerated partial breast irradiation consensus statement from the American Society for Radiation Oncology (ASTRO). Int J Radiat Oncol Biol Phys. 2009;74:987e1001.
197. Polgár C, Van Limbergen E, Pötter R, Kovács G, Polo A, Lyczek J, GEC-ESTRO breast cancer working group, et al. Patient selection for accelerated partial-breast irradiation (APBI) after breast conserving surgery: recommendations of the Groupe Européen de Curiethérapie-European Society forTherapeutic Radiology and Oncology (GEC-ESTRO) breast cancer working group based on clinical evidence. Radiother Oncol. 2009;2010:264–73. *.
198. Kuske RR Jr. Breast brachytherapy. Hematol Oncol Clin North Am. 1999;13:543–58.
199. Cuttino LW, Todor D, Arthur DW. CT-guided multi-catheter insertion technique for partial breast

brachytherapy: reliable target coverage and dose homogeneity. Brachytherapy. 2005;4:10–7.
200. Petersen C, Würschmidtf. Late toxicity of radiotherapy: a problem or a challenge for the radiation oncologist? Breast Care (Basel). 2011;6:369–74.
201. Back M, Guerrieri M, Wratten C, et al. Impact of radiation therapy on acute toxicity in breast conservation therapy for early breast cancer. Clin Oncol. 2004;16:12–6.
202. Rockson SG, Rivera KK. Estimating the population burden of lymphedema. Ann N Y Acad Sci. 2008;1131:147–54.
203. https://ascopost.com/news/january-2023/silicone--film-to-prevent-acute-radiation-dermatitis-in-patients-with-breast-cancer/?utm_source=TAP%2DEN%2D010323%2DINTL&utm_medium=email&utm_term=9f2a48d17a720dd5cc27482397c0b159. Last accessed 4 Jan 2023.
204. Wernicke AG, Goodman RL, Turner BC, et al. A 10-year follow-up of treatment outcomes in patients with early stage breast cancer and clinically negative axillary nodes treated with tangential breast irradiation following sentinel lymph node dissection or axillary clearance. Breast Cancer Res Treat. 2011;125:893–902.
205. Galimberti V, Cole BF, Zurrida S, Viale G, et al. Axillary dissection versus no axillary dissection in patients with sentinel-nodemicrometastases (IBCSG 23-01): a phase 3 randomised controlled trial.; International Breast Cancer Study Group Trial 23-01 investigators. Lancet Oncol. 2013;14:297–305.
206. Warren LE, Miller CL, Horick N, et al. The impact of radiation therapy on the risk of lymphedema after treatment for breast cancer: a prospective cohort study. Int J Radiat Oncol Biol Phys. 2014;88:565–71.
207. Hayes S, Cornish B, Newman B. Comparison of methods to diagnose lymphoedema among breast cancer survivors: 6-month follow-up. Breast Cancer Res Treat. 2005;89:221–6.
208. Warren LE, Miller CL, Horick N, Skolny MN, Jammallo LS, Sadek BT, Shenouda MN, O'Toole JA, MacDonald SM, Specht MC, Taghian AG. The impact of radiation therapy on the risk of lymphedema after treatment for breast cancer: a prospective cohort study. Int J Radiat Oncol Biol Phys. 2014;88(3):565–71. https://doi.org/10.1016/j.ijrobp.2013.11.232. Epub 2014 Jan 7. PMID: 24411624; PMCID: PMC3928974. Sávolt A, Musonda P, Mátrai Z, Polgár C, et al Optimal treatment of the axilla after positive sentinel lymph node biopsy in early invasive breast cancer.Early results of the OTOASOR trial.orvhetil. 2013;154:1934–42.
209. Bulley C, Coutts F, Blyth C, Jack W, Chetty U, Barber M, Tan CW. A morbidity screening tool for identifying fatigue, pain, upper limb dysfunction and lymphedema after breast cancer treatment: a validity study. Eur J Oncolnurs. 2014;18:218–27.
210. Bloomquist K, Karlsmark T, Christensen KB, Adamsen L. Heavy resistance training and lymphedema: prevalence of breast cancer-related lymphedema in participants of an exercise intervention utilizing heavy load resistance training. Acta Oncol. 2014;53:216–25.
211. Ugur S, Arıcı C, Yaprak M, Mescı A, Arıcı GA, Dolay K, Ozmen V. Risk factors of breast cancer-related lymphedema. Lymphat Res Biol. 2013;11:72–5.
212. Anscher MS, Peters WP, Reisenbichler H, Petros WP, Jirtle RL. Transforming growth factor beta as a predictor of liver and lung fibrosis after autologous bone marrow transplantation for advanced breast cancer. N Engl J Med. 1993;328:1592–8.
213. Bentzen SM, Skoczylas JZ, Overgaard M, Overgaard J. Radiotherapy-related lung fibrosis enhanced by tamoxifen. J Natl Cancer Inst. 1996;88:918–22.
214. Fragkandrea I, Kouloulias V, Mavridis P, et al. Radiation induced pneumonitis following whole breastradiotherapy treatment in early breast cancer patients treated with breast conserving surgery: a single institution study. Hippokratia. 2013;17:233–8.
215. Lind PA, Svane G, Gagliardi G, Svensson C. Abnormalities by pulmonary regions studied with computer tomography following local or localregional radiotherapy for breast cancer. Int J Radiat Oncol Biol Phys. 1999;43:489–96.
216. Karlsen J, Tandstad T, Sowa P, Salvesen Ø, Stenehjem JS, Lundgren S, Reidunsdatter RJ. Pneumonitis and fibrosis after breast cancer radiotherapy: occurrence and treatment-related predictors. Acta Oncol. 2021;60:1651–8.
217. Munshi A, Gupta D. Concurrent versus sequential radiotherapy and tamoxifen in breast cancer - the CONSET trial is launched. Acta Oncol. 2011;50:154–5.
218. Lingos TI, Recht A, Vicini F, Abner A, Silver B, Harris JR. Radiation pneumonitis in breast cancer patients treated with conservative surgery and radiation therapy. Int J Radiatoncolbiol Phys. 1991;21:355–60.
219. Darby S, mcgale P, Peto R, Granath F, Hall P, Akbom A. Mortality from cardiovascular disease more than 10 years after radiotherapy for breast cancer: nationwide cohort study of 90 000 Swedish women. BMJ. 2003;326:256–25.
220. Early Breast Cancer Trialists' Collaborative Group. Favourable and unfavourable effects on long-term survival of radiotherapy for early breast cancer: an overview of the randomised trials. Lancet. 2000;355:1757–0.
221. Stewart JR, Fajardo LF. Radiation-induced heart disease: clinical and experimental aspects. Radiol Clin North Am. 1971;9:511–31.
222. Stewart JR, Fajardo LF, Gillette SM. Radiation injury to the heart. Int J Radiatoncol Biol Phys. 1995;31:1205–11.
223. Fajardo LF, Stewart JR. Experimental radiation-induced heart disease. Am J Pathol. 1970;59:299–316.
224. Stewart JR, Brosius FC, Waller BF, Roberts WC. Radiation heart disease: analysis of 16 young (aged 15 to 33 years) necropsy patients who

received over 3,500 rads to the heart. Am J Med. 1981;70:519–30.
225. Bradley EW, Zook BC, Casarett GW. Coronary arteriosclerosis and atherosclerosis in fast neutron or photon irradiated dogs. Int J Radiatoncol Biol Phys. 1998;7:1103–8.
226. O'Brien PJ. Cardiac troponin is the most effective translational safety biomarker for myocardial injury in cardiotoxicity. Toxicology. 2007;245:206–18.
227. Darby SC, Ewertz M, MC gale P, bennet AM, et al. Risk of ischemic heart disease in women after radiotherapy for breast cancer. N Engl J Med. 2013;368:987–98.
228. Darby S, mcgale P, Peto R, et al. Mortality from cardiovascular disease more than 10 years after radiotherapy for breast cancer: nationwide cohort study of 90 000 Swedish women. BMJ. 2003;326:256–25.
229. Overgaard M, Hansen PS, Overgaard J, et al. Postoperative radiotherapy in high-risk premenopausal women with breast cancer who receive adjuvant chemotherapy. N Engl J Med. 1997;337:949–55.
230. Højris I, Overgaard M, Christensen JJ, et al. Morbidity and mortality of ischaemic heart disease in high-risk breast-cancer patients after adjuvant postmastectomy systemic treatment with or without radiotherapy: analysis of DBCG 82b and 82c randomised trials. Radiotherapy Committee of the Danish Breast Cancer Cooperative Group. Lancet. 1999;354:1425–30.
231. Nilsson G, Holmberg L, Garmo H, Duvernoy O, Sjögren I, Lagerqvist B, Blomqvist C. Distribution of coronary artery stenosis after radiation for breast cancer. J Clin Oncol. 2012;30(4):380–6. https://doi.org/10.1200/JCO.2011.34.5900. Epub 2011 Dec 27.
232. Munshi A. Breast cancer radiotherapy and cardiac risk: the 15-year paradox! J Cancer Res Ther. 2007;3:190–2.
233. Wennstig AK, Garmo H, Isacsson U, Gagliardi G, Rintelä N, Lagerqvist B, Holmberg L, Blomqvist C, Sund M, Nilsson G. The relationship between radiation doses to coronary arteries and location of coronary stenosis requiring intervention in breast cancer survivors. Radiat Oncol. 2019;14(1):40.
234. Brownlee Z, Garg R, Listo M, Zavitsanos P, Wazer DE, Huber KE. Late complications of radiation therapy for breast cancer: evolution in techniques and risk over time. Gland Surg. 2018;7(4):371–8. https://doi.org/10.21037/gs.2018.01.05. PMID: 30175054; PMCID: PMC6107587.
235. Abo-Madyan Y, Aziz MH, Aly MM, Schneider F, Sperk E, Clausen S, Giordano FA, Herskind C, Steil V, Wenz F, Glatting G. Second cancer risk after 3D-CRT, IMRT and VMAT for breast cancer. Radiother Oncol. 2014;110:471–6.
236. Bazire L, De Rycke Y, Asselain B, Fourquet A, Kirova YM. Risks of second malignancies after breast cancer treatment: long-term results. Cancer Radiother. 2017;21:10–5.
237. Cardoso F, Kyriakides S, Ohno S, Penault-Llorca F, Poortmans P, Rubio IT, Zackrisson S, Senkus E. Early breast cancer: ESMO clinical practice guidelines for diagnosis, treatment and follow-up†. Ann Oncol. 2019;30:1194–220.
238. Poorvu PD, Gelber SI, Zheng Y, Ruddy KJ, Tamimi RM, Peppercorn J, Schapira L, Borges VF, Come SE, Lambertini M, Rosenberg SM, Partridge AH. Pregnancy after breast cancer: results from a prospective cohort of young women with breast cancer. Cancer. 2021;127:1021–8.
239. Mokhatri-Hesari P, Montazeri A. Health-related quality of life in breast cancer patients: review of reviews from 2008 to 2018. Health Qual Life Outcomes. 2020;18:338.
240. Munshi A, Dutta D, Kakkar S, Budrukkar A, Jalali R, Sarin R, Gupta S, Parmar V, Badwe R. Comparison of early quality of life in patients treated with radiotherapy following mastectomy or breast conservation therapy: a prospective study. Radiother Oncol. 2010;97:288–93.

Online Links

IMRT in breast https://www.youtube.com/watch?v=1ISIMI5K8S8

Prone breast treatment https://www.youtube.com/watch?v=3263X1FSOTI

Germline testing in breast cancer (study from India) https://pubmed.ncbi.nlm.nih.gov/32628584

Germline testing in breast cancer (study from India) https://pubmed.ncbi.nlm.nih.gov/34601666

Contouring

Post lumpectomy with integrated boost. https://econtour.org/cases/128.

Whole Breast- Fast Forward. https://econtour.org/cases/117.

Regional nodal irradiation. https://econtour.org/cases/74.

Non-small Cell Lung Cancer

Anil Tibdewal, Amani Bhogadi, Srinivas Rathod, Jai Prakash Agarwal, Shubham Jain, and Anusheel Munshi

1 Introduction

Globally, Lung cancer is responsible for 11.7% of all cancer cases in both sexes [1]. It also ranks first among cancers causing death in both men and women, having caused 1.80 million deaths in 2020 [2]. The mortality rate of lung cancer and the case fatality rate is high. These trends are anticipated to persist for the next three to four decades.

Given the serious nature of the disease, significant efforts have been made toward lung cancer treatment. Breakthroughs include better screening procedures, progress in imaging technologies, molecular and pathological methods, alterations in surgical management, and newer radiation administration modalities. Further gains have been made by adding immunotherapy and targeted therapy in lung cancer management.

SBRT techniques, which are currently widely prevalent in operable early stage tumors and oligometastatic disease, adaptive techniques, post-systemic therapy consolidation techniques, and the new Lattice radiotherapy technology, are all examples of radiation delivery advancements.

2 Anatomy

The anatomy of the lung has increased in importance in radiation oncology as radiation delivery has shifted more toward highly conformal methods. Therefore, a more detailed understanding of thoracic anatomy is imperative for accurate target delineation and treatment design. Apart from treatment delivery, accurate staging relies on correctly understanding the anatomy of the lung and surrounding mediastinal structures.

A pair of lungs are situated on either side of the mediastinum in the thoracic cavity enclosing the central mediastinal structures. The lungs are conical, with a broad base resting on the diaphragm and an apex projective above the clavicle into the neck. There are mainly two surfaces of the lungs, the coastal surface is towards the chest wall, and the mediastinal surface is near the heart and other central mediastinal structures. Each lung is surrounded by a pleural cavity surrounded by parietal (outer) and visceral (inner) layers of

A. Tibdewal (✉) · A. Bhogadi · S. Rathod
J. P. Agarwal
Department of Radiation Oncology, Tata Memorial Hospital, Homi Bhabha National Institute, Mumbai, Maharashtra, India
e-mail: srathod@cancercare.mb.ca

S. Jain
Surgical Oncology, Fortis Flt. Lt. Rajan Dhall Hospital, Vasant Kunj, New Delhi, India
e-mail: dr.shubham.jain@gmail.com

A. Munshi
Radiation Oncology, BLK Max Hospital, New Delhi, India
e-mail: anusheel.munshi@manipalhospitals.com

B. K. Mohanti et al. (eds.), *Radiation Oncology – Principles, Precepts and Practice*,
https://doi.org/10.1007/978-981-95-5171-2_6

pleura. The lungs are freely floating and cushioned by the pleural cavity but suspended into the mediastinum by hilar structures. Each lung is divided into distinct lobes—three lobes in the right lung and two lobes in the left lung. The trachea is a central structure in the upper mediastinum, which bifurcates at the level of the carina to give rise to the right and left main bronchi. The main bronchi, in turn, divide into lobar bronchi and supply individual lobes of the lung and further divide into segments that supply individual bronchopulmonary segments, which are the functional units of the lung.

The International Association for the Study of Lung Cancer (IASLC) developed a novel lymph node map for all lymph node stations. American Joint Committee on Cancer (AJCC) incorporated this map into the staging manual. In the IASLC lymph node map, 14 lymph node levels are further grouped into intrapulmonary, hilar, and mediastinal zones. These zones have further prognostic significance and are useful in clinical practice in staging and decision-making regarding management (Figs. 1 and 2).

2.1 Epidemiological Aspects and Risk Factors

India has a population of 1.41 billion. According to the GLOBOCAN 2020 report, there were 72,510 estimated lung cancer cases in India in 2020, with 66,279 deaths [4]. The 5-year prevalence across all groups was 80,817. The crude incidence rate per 100,000 people was 5.6, the age-standardized rate (ASR) per 100,000 people was 6.9, and the cumulative risk was 0.85. Lung cancer incidence came second in men and seventh in women among the many forms of cancer, trailing only breast, cervical, and oral cavity cancer in incidence. Lung cancer had a crude incidence rate in Indian men of 8.3, an ASR of 11, and a cumulative risk of 1.36; it had a crude incidence rate in Indian women of 2.7, an ASR of 3.1, and a cumulative risk of 0.37. After breast and cervical cancer, lung cancer was India's third most common cause of cancer-related mortality.

Among Indian males, lung cancer was the leading cause of cancer mortality, and among Indian females seventh after breast, cervix, colorectal, ovary, stomach, and oral cavity cancers. It is also estimated that by 2025, lung cancer will increase to more than 1 lakh and the mortality to 92,601. It is expected that lung cancer will remain a major health problem for at least the next 30–40 years, even if there is a reduction in incidence due to smoking cessation interventions.

The prevalence of lung cancer has increased in synchrony with tobacco smoking patterns. The most significant risk factor for developing lung cancer is smoking tobacco (80–90%); occupational exposure to various carcinogenic substances is responsible for a small proportion (10–20%) of cases. In most Indian studies compared to those in the west, the smoker: nonsmoker ratios were lower. Beedis (28.4–79%), cigarettes (9.0–53.7), hookah (3.4–77.3), and mixed comprise the majority of tobacco-related items smoked in India (7.5–13.6) [5]. Peopel who smoke beedis have a relative risk of developing lung cancer of 2.64, whereas cigarettes smokers have a related risk of 2.23, with an absolute risk of tobacco use of 2.45.

Tobacco consumption is the most critical risk factor for developing lung cancer. Nearly 90% of lung cancers are attributable to cigarette smoke. Population trends of lung cancer incidence have shown a strong association with smoking behavior, which usually manifests after approximately 20 years [6]. Both the number of cigarettes smoked per day and the duration of smoking are directly proportional to the risk of lung cancer risk. An average male smoker's risk of acquiring lung cancer was assessed to be nine to 10 times higher than that of a "never smoker" in the seminal 1964 study from the U.S. Surgeon General U.S. Department of Health, Education, and Welfare [7]. Smokers who consume more than 25 cigarettes daily have a risk of at least 20 times higher. Ex-smokers who have given up smoking for more than 15 years have an 80–90% lower risk of developing lung cancer as compared to those who continue to smoke.

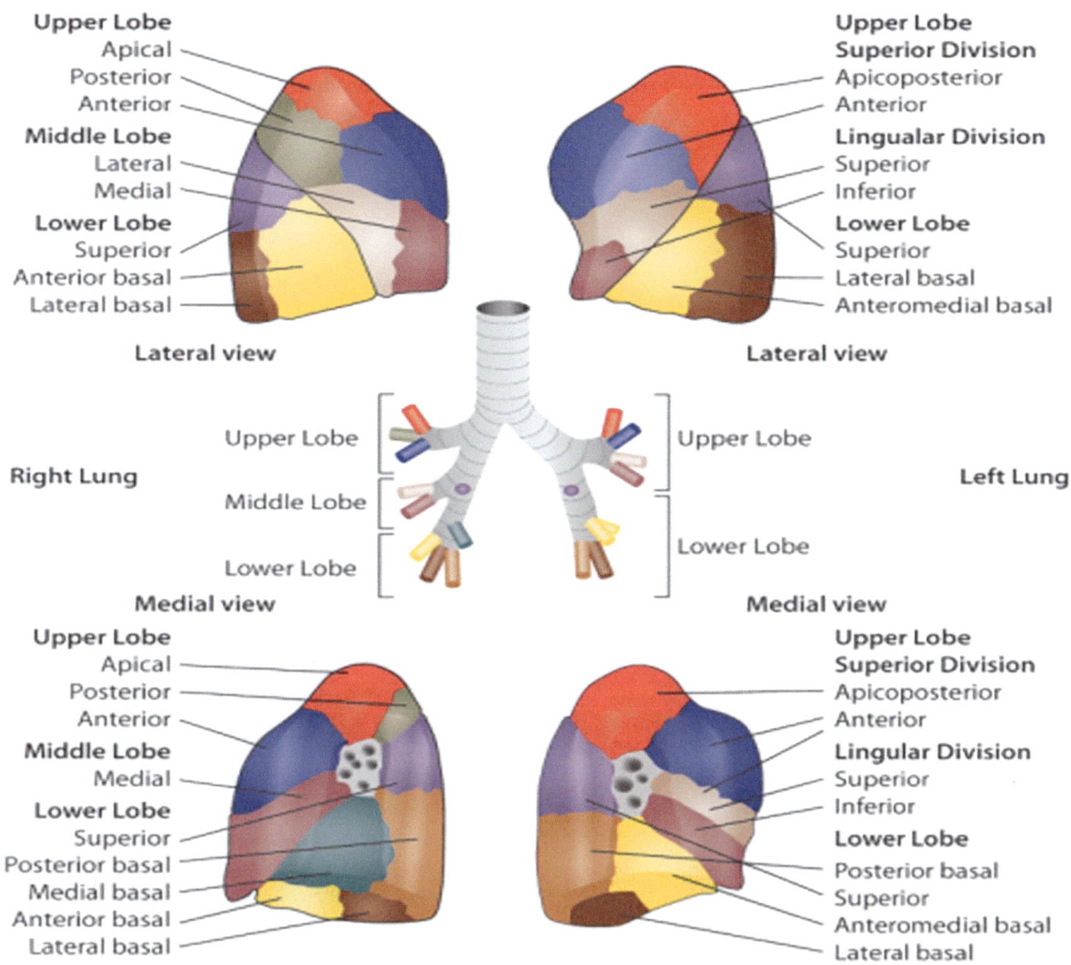

Fig. 1 Lung anatomy. (Adapted from SEER https://training.seer.cancer.gov/lung/anatomy/)

Smoke from cigarettes is a complex aerosol on its own, with nicotine serving as the main addictive component and tar serving as the particle residue left behind after nicotine and water have been eliminated. There are more than 50 known carcinogens in tobacco smoke, including polycyclic aromatic hydrocarbons (PAHs) and tobacco-specific N-nitrosamines (TSNAs), which are created when nicotine is nitro-sized during smoking. These carcinogens frequently causes DNA adducts that result in DNA mutations, increasing the risk of cancer development. The chance of developing lung cancer rises by over 30% among nonsmokers who are exposed to passive smoking, which appears to be another source of carcinogens [8].

Radon gas is the nuclear decay byproduct of radioactive Radium, which in turn is the decay product of uranium. Cancer-causing genetic mutations are brought on by the ionizing radiation created by radioactive decay. Lung cancer is also known to be caused by occupational exposure to various substances. Asbestos, Beryllium, Arsenic, Cadmium, Nickel, Silica, Solvents, Paints and Solvents, Chromium, Chloromethyl Ether, etc., are a few significant occupational agents [9].

The inhalation of particulate matter and other air contaminants is particularly pertinent to the post-industrial environment. Large cohort research revealed a link between persistent

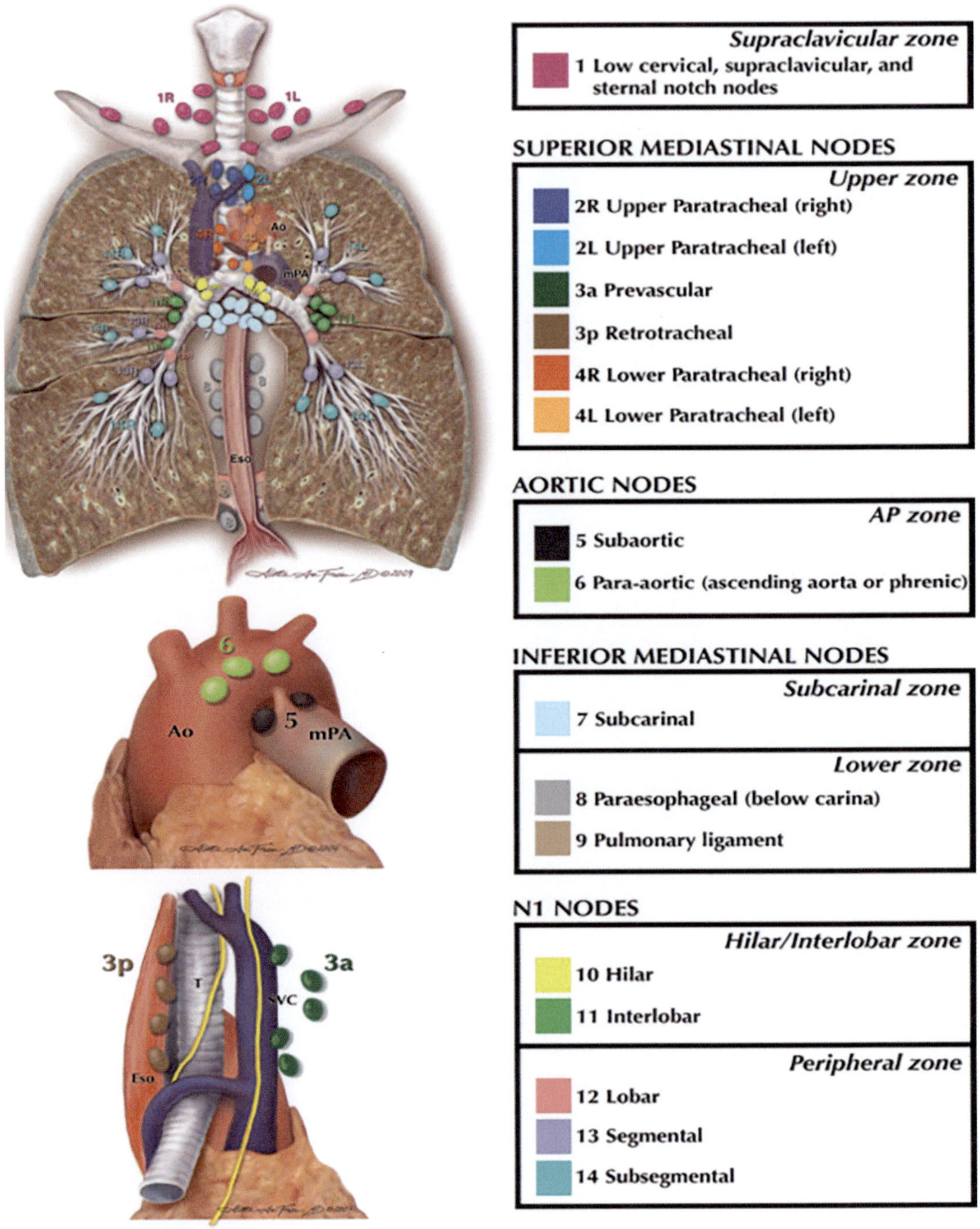

Fig. 2 The International Association for the Study of Lung Cancer (IASLC) lymph node map, including the proposed grouping of lymph node stations into "zones" for prognostic analyses [3]

exposure to fine particulate matter and lung cancer incidence and mortality.

2.2 Clinical Presentation

The clinical presentation of lung cancer depends on the stage at diagnosis. Often patients with early stage tumors are symptom-free, in which case the detection of cancer tends to be incidental. But this kind of presentation tends to be less common. More commonly, patients with lung cancer are diagnosed at an advanced stage where symptoms manifest due to primary tumors, metastatic sites, or paraneoplastic syndromes.

The most common symptoms caused by primary tumors are cough, hemoptysis, and dyspnea. Cough occurs in 70–90% of lung cancer patients, and it might be caused by a tumor interfering with bronchial peristalsis or by an ulceration of the bronchial mucosa. Since cigarette smoking also causes bronchorrhea and profuse mucus, the cough and sputum that are produced are nonspecific. Peripheral tumors can continue growing without manifestation of cough. In addition to fainting (cough syncope), rib fracture, or rupture of an emphysematous bleb, severe coughing episodes can also cause pneumothorax. Hemoptysis is a typical symptom affecting 25–40% of individuals. It might be caused by a tumor ulcerating the bronchial mucosa or by bronchial veins or venules rupturing, which would cause significant blood loss.

Another early symptom that affects roughly 60% of individuals is breathlessness. It might be out of proportion to radiological findings because of underlying lung abnormalities caused by smoking. A partial bronchial blockage strongly suggests wheezing, stridor, or an abrupt rise in dyspnea. These symptoms might be brought on by pressure and narrowing of the trachea or big bronchus. Dyspnea mainly arises from mechanical effects on the airways, lymphangitic spread, pleural effusion, hypercoagulability with pulmonary thromboembolism, and pericardial effusion. Chest pain is a frequent manifestation of lung cancer, which may exist even without obvious signs of the pleural, chest wall, or mediastinum invasion. The cause of this kind of pain can occasionally be unclear since the lung parenchyma lacks pain fibers. Pleural metastases can cause excruciating chest discomfort that requires narcotic medication. Squamous cell carcinoma frequently results in chronic chest discomfort with the invasion of the bony thorax. Due to the brachial plexus invasion (Pancoast syndrome), superior sulcus tumors often induce shoulder and arm pain. Brachial plexopathy, reflex sympathetic dystrophy, and Horner's syndrome are possible companion conditions. Pleural effusion is seen in 15–25% of patients with lung cancer. Pericardial effusion appears in 5–10% of patients and is often associated with a locally advanced progressive illness.

In addition to primary symptoms, organ-related symptoms result from metastatic disease. The brain, bone, liver, adrenals, and lungs are the most typical locations for lung cancer metastases. Headaches, skeletal pain, inexplicable loss of appetite and weight loss, and fatigue are common manifestations of metastatic symptoms. Lab abnormalities such as anemia, altered LFTs, or hypercalcemia should also highlight the possibility of metastatic dissemination. Liver enzyme abnormalities or staging workup imaging may be used to identify asymptomatic liver metastases during the presentation. Bony pain in the lower back, legs, and chest that is linked to high alkaline phosphate levels is typically seen in patients with bone metastases. Headache, nausea, loss of vision, hemiparesis, cranial nerve deficiency, and convulsions are all signs of brain metastases.

Lung cancer and paraneoplastic disorders frequently coexist. SCLC patients often experience hyponatremia caused by Syndrome of inappropriate antidiuretic hormone secretion syndrome (SIADH). The most frequent association with hypercalcemia owing to the ectopic synthesis of the parathyroid hormone-related peptide is squamous cell carcinomas. The Cushing syndrome, which results from ectopic corticotrophin production, is frequently linked to SCLC or, rarely, early stage carcinoid tumors. The most common symptoms of hypertrophic pulmonary osteoarthropathy are symmetrical, painful arthropathy of the limbs and characteristic findings of new periosteal bone growth of the long bones. Less frequent neurological syndromes include Lambert-Eaton myasthenic syndrome and encephalomyelitis-subacute sensory neuropathy, which are frequently linked to SCLC.

2.3 Diagnostic Investigations

Patients with complaints related to lung cancer need to undergo diagnostic tests for confirmation of diagnosis. The histological type of disease and staging are essential to guide the disease's management. A comprehensive history and physical examination of the patient is the first step in diagnosing the illness to find any signs and symptoms of lung cancer, whether they are local or metastatic, as well as any other coexisting conditions and the patient's overall health. It's also critical to have a thorough history of exposure to environmental toxins and tobacco usage. A physical examination of the chest can rule out pneumonia, pleural effusion, and airway blockage. Supraclavicular lymphadenopathy's involvement is ruled out through a proper neck examination.

2.3.1 Radiologic Examinations

X-ray of the chest (Fig. 3) is often the first investigation in a person with suspicious symptoms. It can demonstrate an opacity in the lung, widening of the mediastinum, pleural effusion, and post-obstructive consolidation, which can further guide a more detailed investigation.

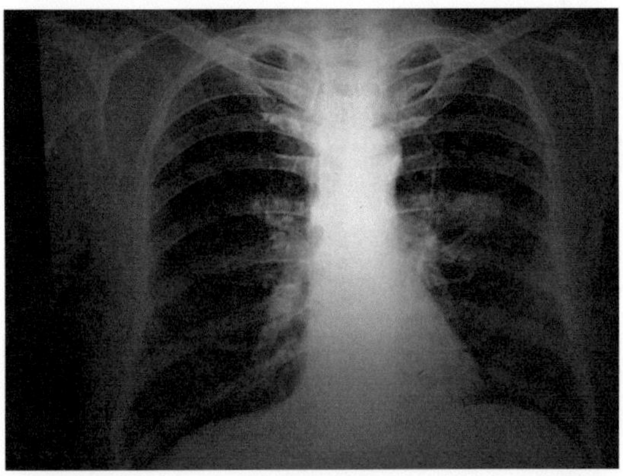

Fig. 3 Chest X-ray. Eighty years male, chronic smoker with cough and dyspnea for 15 days. Chest X-Ray suggestive of a lesion in the left upper lobe

All patients with a high suspicion of lung cancer should get a contrast-enhanced CT scan of their chest and upper abdomen unless contraindicated so that the entire liver and adrenal glands are visualized. Intravenous contrast helps distinguish mediastinal structures from vascular structures, making it easier to identify suspicious lymph nodes in the mediastinum. The size and other characteristics of the tumor are determined via a contrast enhanced CT (CECT) scan, which helps determine the T stage. Enlarged lymph nodes on a CT scan typically indicate lymphatic spread. When a lymph node's short axis diameter measures more than 1 cm, lymph nodal involvement is suspected in a confirmed lung cancer case. The other option is to get a PET CT scan (Fig. 4). This is increasingly becoming the investigation of choice, replacing a routine CT scan for several reasons. (1) It could avoid futile thoracotomy in approximately 20–30%. (2) It can aid in radiation planning, especially in differentiating tumors from atelectasis. (3) Ability to detect malignant disease in nodes and remote areas typically invisible on a CT scan. (4) PET CT scan can either upstage or downstage lung cancer by providing additional information than CECT.

Further, PET CT is also used for response assessment after chemoradiotherapy in locally advanced NSCLC. Maximum standardized uptake value is also shown to predict response in surgically and non-surgically managed patients.

MRI

MRI of the brain is routinely recommended to rule out brain metastases, which are seen in approximately 15–20% of patients at diagnosis. MRI has better sensitivity and specificity than CECT brain for detecting brain metastases. The incidence of brain metastases is higher in positive oncogene mutation status. MRI also provides information about leptomeningeal involvement in the brain, which is now more commonly seen in oncogene-mutated patients, especially in epidermal growth factor receptor mutations.

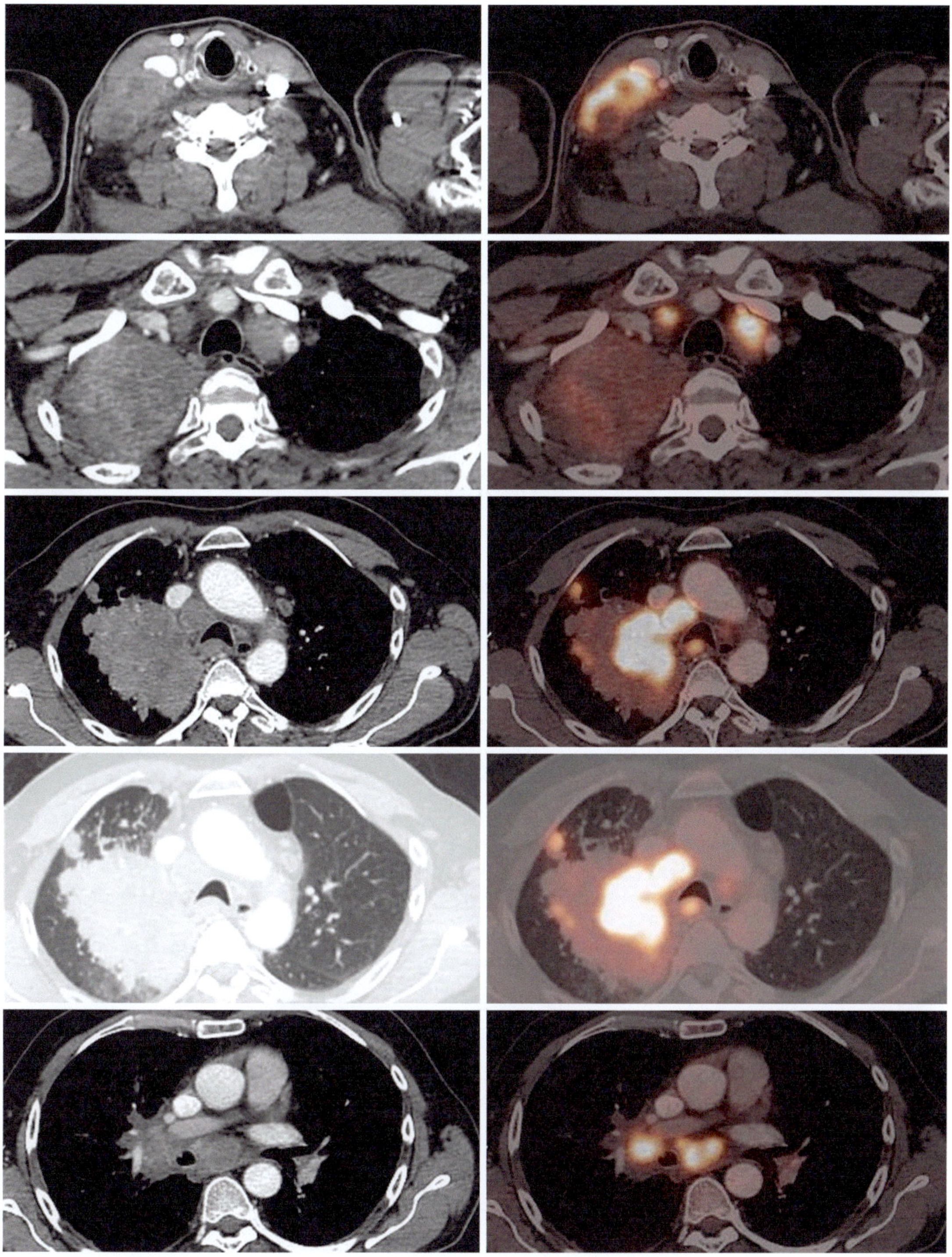

Fig. 4 PET CT showing a lesion in the right lung (PET avid) with associated atelectasis

2.3.2 Cytological and Histopathological Diagnosis

Sputum cytology or fiber-optic bronchoalveolar lavage or brushing cytology can be used for the initial cytological diagnosis of lung cancer. Fiber-optic bronchoscopy (FOB) makes it possible to see the tracheobronchial tree and obstructive growth, if any. If needed, lavage or cytologic brushings or transbronchial needle aspiration (TBNA) from visible lesions can be taken for cytological investigation. Pleural fluid cytology or cell block can also be done in patients presenting with pleural effusion to ease the diagnosis process.

Biopsy from the easily accessible lesion, either primary, supraclavicular nodes, or any metastatic lesions, is recommended for histopathological diagnosis. CT-guided percutaneous biopsy is crucial for making a diagnosis of a peripheral lung lesion. A biopsy is always preferable for pathological diagnosis and for making tissue available for molecular pathology in the precision oncology era (Table 1).

2.3.3 Histological Classification

Adenocarcinoma (35–40%) and squamous cell carcinomas (25–30%) are the two most common non-small cell lung cancer histologies. The table gives a comparison of salient features of predominant NSCLC histologies (Table 2).

Adenosquamous carcinoma and lung cancer, not otherwise specified (NOS), are some of the other histologies seen in NSCLC. Adenocarcinoma subtypes include lepidic, acinar, papillary, micropapillary, colloid, and fetal adenocarcinoma. Adenocarcinoma histology has been associated with various oncogene mutations like epidermal growth factor receptor and anaplastic lymphoma kinase, among various others (Fig. 5). Tyrosine kinase inhibitors directed against these oncogene mutations are FDA-approved and available for routine clinical use. WHO pathologic classification of lung tumors is being modified to incorporate all these recent advancements in NSCLC.

Table 1 Staging workup for lung cancer

Recommended imaging	*Invasive Procedures*	*Other Tests*
Chest X-ray, CT of Thorax and upper abdomen FDG-PET-CT MRI Brain Bone scan if FDG-PET-CT is not available	CT-guided biopsy Thoracocentesis Bronchoscopic/EUS/EBUS/ Robotic/navigational directed biopsy Bronchial lavage Mediastinoscopy	Pulmonary function tests Molecular marker testing Nutritional evaluation and malnutrition management
Laboratory examinations		
Complete blood count, renal function test, liver function test, alkaline phosphatase		

Table 2 Common pathological variants in NSCLC

Histological type	Squamous cell carcinoma	Adenocarcinoma	Large cell carcinoma
Frequency	Second most common	Most common	Lesser common
Predilection	Occurs in smokers	Occurs in nonsmokers and smokers, young adults, and women	Linked to smoking
Location	Central zone	Peripheral zone	Peripheral zone
Aggressiveness	Moderate growth	Slow growing	Fast growing
Other features	Seen more commonly in men, endobronchial pattern, cavitation frequent		Usually, poorly differentiated tumors

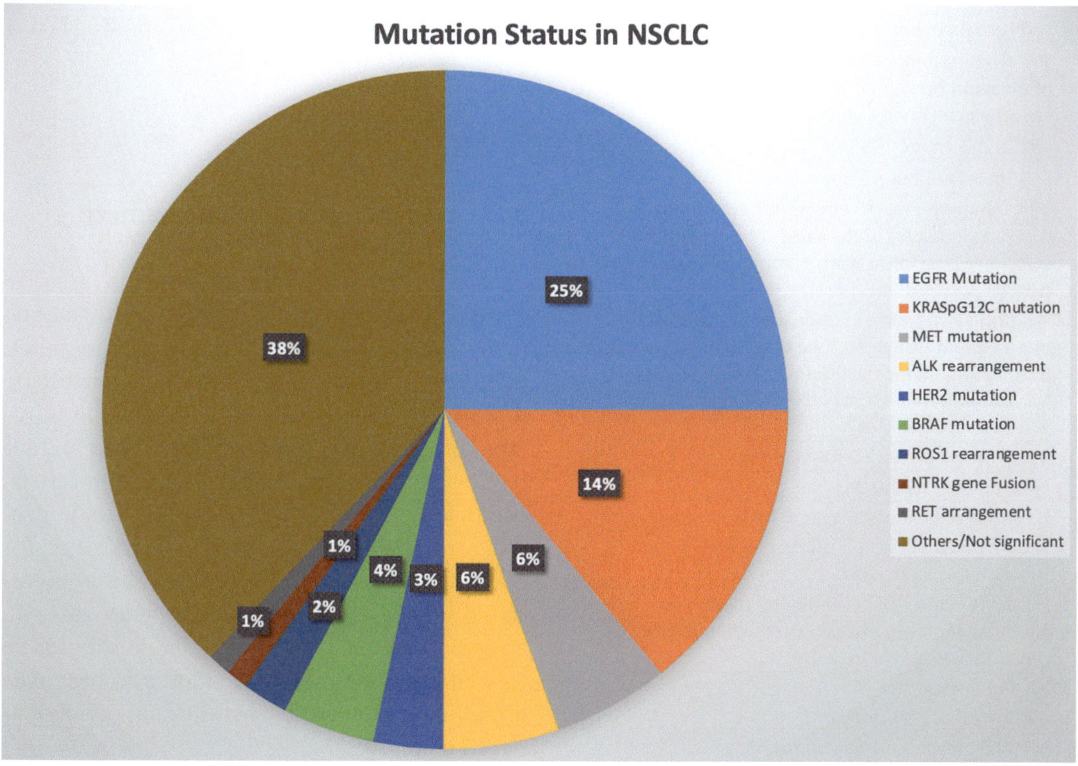

Fig. 5 Mutation status in NSCLC

Table 3 TNM staging of NSCLC

TNM staging—adapted from AJCC 8th edition
T: primary tumor
T0: no evidence of primary
Tis: Carcinoma in situ (CIS): Squamous cell CIS (SCIS) and adenocarcinoma with pure lepidic pattern ≤3 cm (AIS)
T1: primary tumor <3 cm surrounded by lung or visceral pleura, without main bronchus invasion
T1m1: minimally invasive adenocarcinoma (≤3 cm) with predominantly lepidic pattern (≤5 mm invasion)
T1a: ≤1 cm
T1b: >1 cm but ≤2 cm
T1c: >2 cm but ≤3 cm
T2: primary tumor>3 cm but ≤5 cm or involvement of the main bronchus, visceral pleura, or presence of atelectasis involving part or all of the lung
T2a: >3 cm but ≤4 cm
T2b: >4 cm but ≤5 cm
T3: primary tumor >5 cm but ≤7 cm or with separate nodule(s) in the same lobe or with the invasion of the chest wall, phrenic nerve, the parietal pericardium
T4: primary tumor >7 cm or with separate nodule(s) in a different ipsilateral lobe or with the invasion of the diaphragm, mediastinum, heart, great vessels, trachea, recurrent laryngeal nerve, esophagus, vertebral body, carina
N: regional lymph node involvement
N0: no nodal metastasis
N1: involvement of ipsilateral hilar lymph nodes
N2: involvement of ipsilateral mediastinal and/or subcarinal lymph nodes
N3: involvement of contralateral mediastinal, contralateral hilar, ipsilateral, or contralateral supraclavicular lymph nodes
M: distant metastasis
M0: no distant metastasis
M1: the presence of distant metastasis
M1a: separate nodule in a contralateral lobe; the presence of a pleural or pericardial nodule or pleural or pericardial effusions
M1b: solitary extra-thoracic metastasis
M1c: multiple extra-thoracic metastases in one or more organs

2.3.4 Staging of Non-small Cell Lung Cancer (Table 3)

The AJCC 9th edition staging classification for NSCLC is outlined in Tables 3 and 4.

2.3.5 Stage Grouping (Table 4)

Table 4 Group staging of NSCLC

T/M	Sub-category	N0	N1	N2	N3
T1	T1a	IA1	IIB	IIIA	IIIB
	T1b	IA2	IIB	IIIA	IIIB
	T1c	IA3	IIB	IIIA	IIIB
T2	T2a	IB	IIB	IIIA	IIIB
	T2b	IIA	IIB	IIIA	IIIB
T3	T3	IIB	IIIA	IIIB	IIIC
T4	T4	IIIA	IIIA	IIIB	IIIC
M1	M1a	IVA	IVA	IVA	IVA
	M1b	IVA	IVA	IVA	IVA
	M1c	IVB	IVB	IVB	IVB

3 Principles of Management (Fig. 6)

All patients should preferably be discussed in a multidisciplinary tumor board meeting, including specialists from surgical oncology, radiation oncology, medical oncology, radiology, bioimaging, pulmonologist, and palliative care departments. Psychiatrists, occupational and physiotherapists may provide ancillary support care. Treatment for NSCLC is planned according to the clinical-radiological stage, cardio-pulmonary reserve, and performance status. Patients should be treated concordantly with standard consensus guidelines, including institutional evidence-based medicine.

3.1 Localized (T1–3, N0–1) Non-small Cell Lung Cancer (NSCLC)

The cornerstone of treating early stage NSCLC is surgical resection. All patients who are planned for surgical excision should undergo invasive mediastinal staging before the surgical procedure.

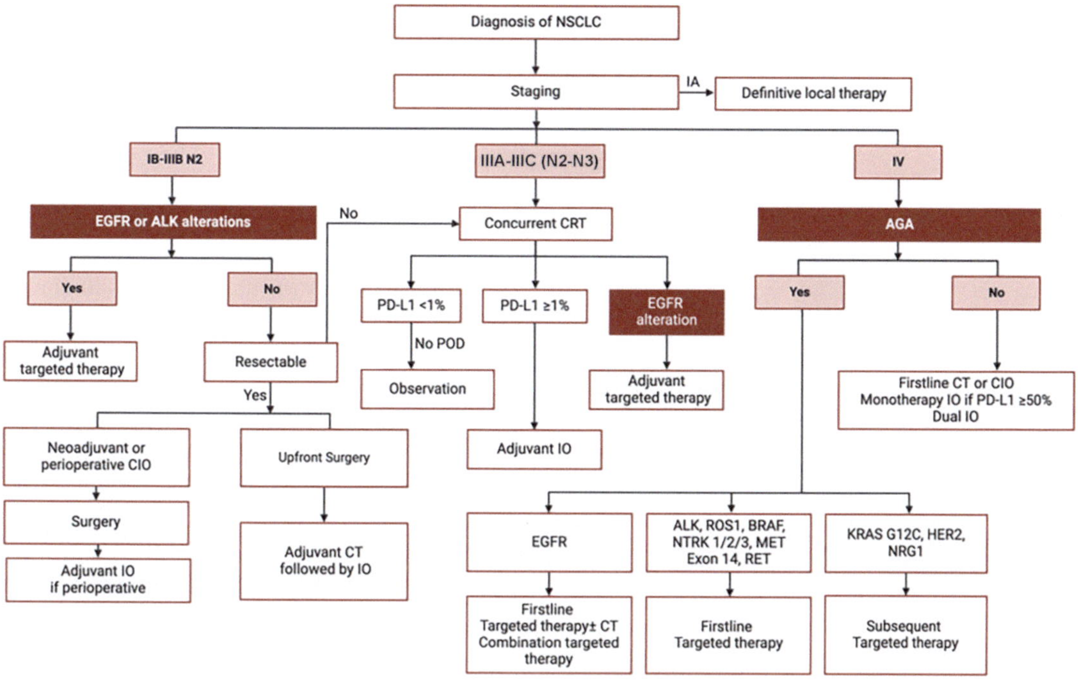

Fig. 6 Schematic initial management of NSCL (Note: AGA actionable genomic alterations; ALK anaplastic lymphoma kinase; CIO chemo-immunotherapy; CT chemotherapy; EGFR epidermal growth factor receptor; IO immunotherapy) [10]

3.2 Mediastinal Staging

Invasive mediastinal staging can be done either with endobronchial ultrasound (EBUS)/esophageal ultrasound (EUS)—fine needle aspiration from the hilar/mediastinal lymph nodes to rule out mediastinal nodal involvement, especially N3 disease or with mediastinoscopy. ESTS guidelines recommend doing EBUS/EUS guided needle aspiration before all the surgical procedures. If negative, mediastinoscopy is recommended to confirm negative mediastinal status (Fig. 7).

Invasive mediastinal staging could be avoided in imaging negative mediastinal nodes where the primary is ≤3 cm and located in peripheral one-third of the lung (Table 5).

Removal of 6 or more lymph nodes from hilar and mediastinal stations or sampling at least 3 lymph node stations including station 7 is recommended for intra-operative nodal assessment. Systematic mediastinal lymph node dissection is recommended while performing lobectomy. It typically involves removal of station 10, 11 and mediastinal stations like 2, 4, 7, 8, and 9. In left sided lung tumors, additional removal of stations 3, 5, and 6 are done preserving left recurrent laryngeal nerve. ACOSOG Z0030, a phase III RCT compared systematic sampling of mediastinal nodes with lymph nodal clearance and demonstarted no additional benefit with mediastinal lymph nodal clearance [11]. However, a very meticulous preoperative invasive mediastinal staging was done in this RCT. Further, a meta-analysis of five RCT concluded that in early NSCLC, a SMLND was associated with improved long-term survival but at the expense of slightly increased risk of postoperative morbidity including recurrent nerve palsy, chylothorax, and bleeding [12] (Table 6).

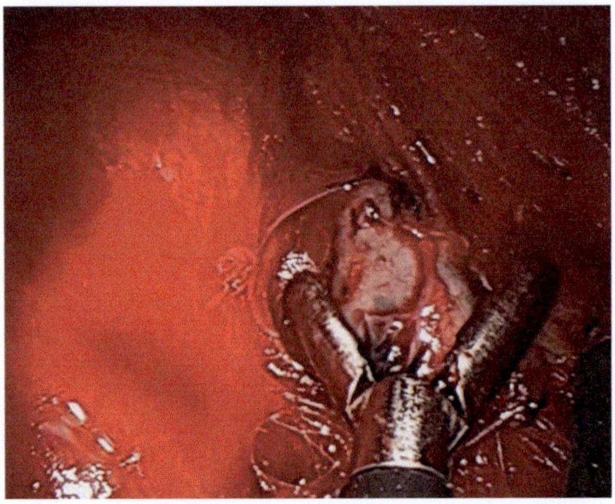

Fig. 7 Right lower paratracheal (Station 4R) node dissection during video- assisted mediastinoscopy (VAM)

Table 5 Lymph node accessibility for various mediastinal techniques

Lymph nodal basin (level)	EBUS	EUS	CM/ VAM	VATS
Highest mediastinal (1)	Yes	–	–	–
Upper paratracheal (2R, 2L)	Yes	Yes	Yes	Yes
Pre-vascular retrotracheal (3P)	Yes	Yes	–	Yes
Lower paratracheal (4R, 4L)	Yes	Yes	Yes	Yes
Subaortic (AP window) (5)	–	Yes	–	Yes
Para-aortic (6)	–	Yes	–	Yes
Subcarinal (7)	Yes	Yes	Yes	Yes
Paraoesophageal (8)	–	Yes	–	Yes
Pulmonary ligament (9)	–	Yes	–	Yes
Hilar(10)	Yes	–	Yes	Yes
Interlobar (11)	Yes	–	–	Yes

EBUS endobronchial ultrasound, *EUS* endoscopic ultrasound, *CM* cervical mediastinoscopy, *VAM* video assisted mediastinoscopy, *VATS* video assisted thoracoscopy surgery

Table 6 Factors affecting clinical outcomes in NSCLC

Patient related	Tumor related	Treatment related
Performance status	Stage	Completeness of resection
Weight loss	Tumor location	Addition of chemotherapy
Age	Histology subtype	Radiotherapy
Sex		
PFT		

4 Surgical Aspects

For patients with lung cancer, a number of surgical options are available, including wedge resection, segmentectomy, lobectomy, and pneumonectomy.

The recommended course of treatment for stage I or stage II lung cancer is surgical resection using a lobectomy or pneumonectomy along with systematic mediastinal lymph node dissection. The development of minimally invasive resection procedures (such VATS or RATS), which are linked to a decline in perioperative morbidity and a shorter hospital stay, has been surgery's most significant development in recent years.

4.1 Minimally Invasive Surgery Versus Open Surgery

CALGB 39802 trial [13] established the most authoritative and accepted definition of Video Assisted Thoracoscopic Surgery (VATS) lobectomy technique:

- No use of rib-spreading;
- Utility incision with a maximum length of upto 8 cm to deliver the specimen;
- Individual dissection of the vein, arteries and airway for the lobe;
- Standard lymph node sampling or dissection

Use of a small retractor may be acceptable in selected circumstances, such as complex procedures, like sleeve resections (Fig. 8)

The VATS approaches generally are performed using one to four thoracoscopic ports. The tumor-containing lung lobe must be removed together with the hilar and mediastinal lymph nodes, and all broncho-vascular systems must be tied off.

Minimally invasive techniques are now the current standard of care for NSCLC in its early stages. Recently, published randomized controlled trial comparing Open versus VATS lobectomy demonstrated better physical functioning at

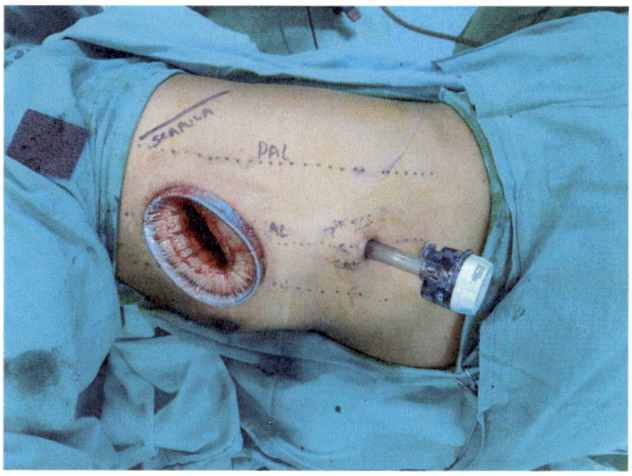

Fig. 8 Video-assisted thoracoscopic surgery (VATS)

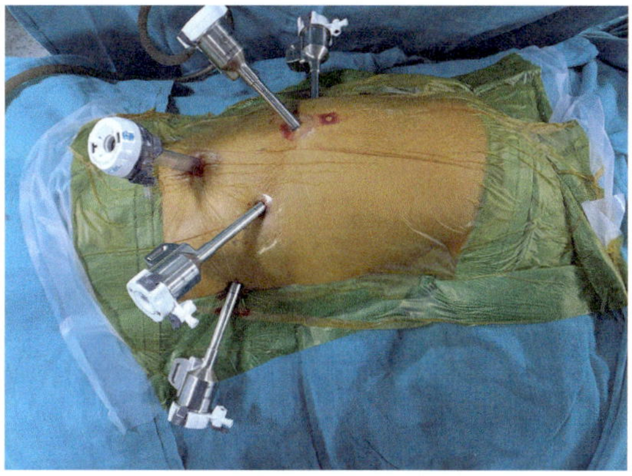

Fig. 9 Completely Portal Robotic Lobectomy (CPRL)/Robot-assisted thoracic surgery (RATS)

5-weeks after VATS. Serious adverse events were also less with VATS (31%) compared to open (38%). No difference in PFS and OS was seen between both the techniques. Hence, minimally invasive surgery like VATS is the practical standard of care and has advantages like reduced postoperative pain, in hospital complications, shorter hospital stays better quality of life with equivalent oncological outcomes. According to the multicenter VIOLET study [14], patients who had VATS lobectomies experienced better postoperative outcomes than those who had open lobectomies, including less pain, fewer acute complications, shorter hospital stays, better physical functioning after discharge, lower rehospitalization rates, and no difference in DFS or OS. Similar to thoracoscopic surgery, lobectomy performed using RATS has shown to produce better results, in comparison to open surgery. Based on the availability and training of robotic aided procedures, this might be a viable substitute for VATS at educational institutions (Fig. 9; Tables 7 and 8).

Table 7 Indications for VATS lobectomy (TO CHECK)

≤7 cm (T1, T2a, and T2b)	Recommended
N0 or N1 status	Recommended

Table 8 Contraindications for VATS lobectomy

Chest wall involvement including rib(s)	Recommended
Centrality of tumor if invading hilar structure(s)	Recommended
Previous thoracic surgery or pleurisy is not a contraindication	Highly recommended
FEV1 <30%	Recommended
DLCO <30%	Recommended

4.2 Extent of Lung Parenchyma Resection

Wedge resection, segmentectomy, or lobectomy (Figs. 10 and 11) are suitable for resection of early stage lung cancer, but the choice of resection depends on the patients' age, cardiopulmonary reserve, tumor size, and histology. All tumors resections, regardless of type, must have adequate disease free margins and adequate systematic lymphadenectomy.

The Lung Cancer Study Group established that limited pulmonary resections were associated with higher locoregional recurrence and higher death rate in comparison to lobectomy, thereby establishing the latter as the standard of care [15].

Lobectomy with systematic mediastinal lymph node dissection either open or video-assisted thoracoscopic surgery is the standard treatment of early stage NSCLC. Pneumonectomy could also be performed if indicated and in patients with good pulmonary reserve, however, it is not recommended in N2 positive nodes. For node negative early stage NSCLC, if pulmonary reserves are insufficient for lobectomy, wedge resections/segmentectomy could also be performed, however, it was shown to have inferior loco-regional control and overall survival (OS) in a randomized studies published in late 1990s.

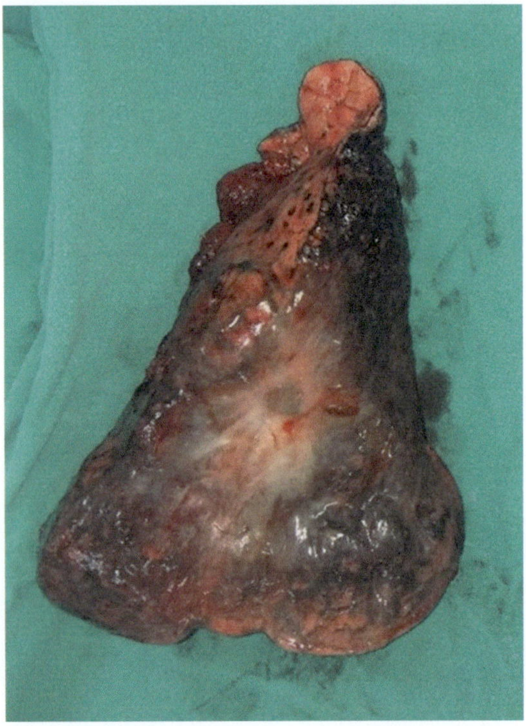

Fig. 10 A lobectomy specimen

However, a meta-analysis [16], reviewing survival data following limited resections for stage I lung cancer, published in 2005, noted that the survival differences may not be significant.

As a result, in a recent RCT [17], patients with clinical stage IA NSCLC were randomly assigned 1:1 to receive either lobectomy or segmentectomy.

The proportions of patients with local relapse were 10.5% for segmentectomy and 5.4% for lobectomy (p = 0.0018) However, improved overall survival was observed consistently across all predefined subgroups in the segmentectomy group. At 1 year follow-up, the significant difference in the reduction of median forced expiratory volume in 1 s between the two groups was 3·5% ($p < 0.0001$), which did not reach the predefined threshold for clinical significance of 10%. The 5-year relapse-free survival was 88·0% (95% CI 85.0–90.4) for segmentectomy and 87·9% (84.8–90.3) for lobectomy (HR 0.998; 95% CI 0.753–1.323; $p = 0.9889$).

Another trial, CALGB 140503 [18] conducted in the West to evaluate sublobar resections (anatomical segmentectomy and wedge resections) for clinically staged peripheral T1a N0 NSCLC, demonstrated non-inferiority to lobectomy with respect to disease-free survival and similar overall survival with the two procedures. The investigators did not observe any substantial difference between the two groups in the incidence of loco regional or distant recurrence.

Complications of surgical resections include bronchopulmonary leak, postoperative infec-

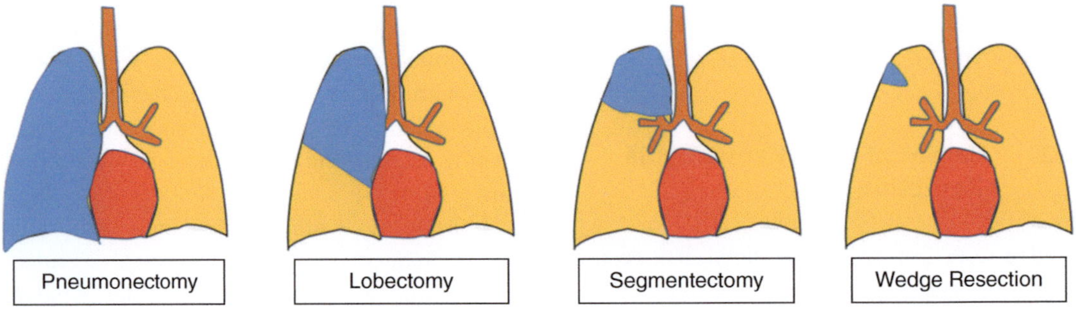

Fig. 11 Types of resection in the lung parenchyma (marked in blue). (Courtesy: Dr Anusheel Munshi, Principal Director and Head, Radiation Oncology, BLK Max, New Delhi)

tions, haemothorax, broncho-pleural fistula, cardio-pulmonary disorders, including supraventricular arrhythmias, respiratory failure and postoperative mortality. However, the incidences of all these complications are less than <10%. With improved and minimal surgical technique like VATS, anesthesia procedures, adoption of enhanced recovery after surgery (ERAS), improve peri-operative care, the complications and postoperative mortality rates have considerably reduced n the last few decades.

4.3 Functional Evaluation Before Treatment

Complete evaluation of all co-morbidities including ischemic heart disease, diabetes mellitus, and COPD is required. Pulmonologist should evaluate the patient before any surgical resections and chest physiotherapy including Incentive Spirometry needs to be started at least 2 weeks before surgery. Functional evaluation test like 6-minute walk test, shuttle walk test, stair-climbing test for evaluation of effort tolerance. Pulmonary function tests, forced expiratory volume in 1 second (FEV1) and diffusing capacity of the lungs for carbon monoxide (DLCO) are the most important components. Predicted postoperative values are calculated using the formula PPO value = [(total number of segments − segments being resected)/total no of segments] × observed value. A postoperative value of FEV1 and DLCO more than 60% are fit for anatomical lung resection. Values between 30% and 60% merit further evaluation. Values less than 30% are unfit for lung resection. 2D Echocardiography: Ejection fraction, pulmonary artery pressure. Regional wall motion abnormalities merit further cardiac evaluation in the form of a stress echocardiography. Cardiopulmonary exercise testing in patients with borderline pulmonary and cardiac function. Ventilation/Perfusion scan is recommended in patients with borderline pulmonary function in lesions where a ventilation perfusion mismatch is expected. For example, large tumors compressing a major proportion of lung, tumors with a central endo-bronchial component.

4.4 Systemic Therapy in Early Stage NSCLC

The choice of systemic therapy is usually different based on the histologies of NSCLC with pemetrexed-based chemotherapy and a Anti-VEGF therapy is preferred in adenocarcinoma than squamous cell carcinomas. The role of systemic therapy in early stage NSCLC is well established. Various published RCTs have evaluated the role of adjuvant chemotherapy in ES-NSCLC. In the ANITA trial [19], 840 NSCLC patients with stage I.B. (T2a, N0), stage II, or stage IIIA were randomly assigned to receive either postoperative vinorelbine/cisplatin or no intervention. Seven toxic deaths were reported in the chemotherapy group. However, grade 3/4 toxicities could be managed. In the chemotherapy group, the median survival was 66 months, compared to 44 months in the observation group, following a median follow-up of 76 months. Postoperative chemotherapy significantly increased (8.6%) the 5-year overall survival in patients with completely resected stage II and stage IIIA disease, despite the fact that there was no benefit in stage I.

The International Adjuvant Lung Cancer Trial [20] assessed patients with fully resected stage I, stage II, or stage III NSCLC for postoperative cisplatin-based Therapy (IALT). The study included 1867 patients with surgically removed lung cancer. With a median follow-up of 56 months, they were randomly assigned to undergo either cisplatin-based postoperative chemotherapy or observation. The 5-year survival rate for observation was 40% versus 45% for cisplatin-based Therapy.

The CALGB 9633 study [21] examined paclitaxel/carboplatin in patients with stage IB lung cancer (T2a, N0, M0). In this study, 344 patients with a median follow-up of 74 months either got paclitaxel/carboplatin or were left untreated (within 4–8 weeks following resection). Chemotherapy given after surgery was well tolerated; no adverse chemotherapy-related fatalities happened. A subset trial did, however, find a benefit for tumors smaller than 4 cm. Overall survival at 6 years did not change significantly from 3-year survival (80% vs. 73%, $p = 0.02$). Additionally, the LACE meta-analysis [22], which included 4584 patients from five of the major trials, revealed that giving cisplatin-based doublet chemotherapy postoperatively increased 5-year OS by 5.4%. This benefit was more pronounced in the higher stage compared to stage IB. Hence, adjuvant chemotherapy with a platinum doublet regimen is the standard treatment based on various randomized controlled trials and LACE meta-analysis. Overall, the general indications for adjuvant chemotherapy are tumor size >4 cm and pathological node-positive disease.

4.5 Neo-adjuvant Immunotherapies in Resectable NSCLC

Checkmate-816 [23], a phase III RCT compared Nivolumab plus chemotherapy with chemotherapy alone in resected stage IB to IIIA NSCLC with a primary endpoint of event-free survival and pathological complete response (CR) rates. The results showed a significant benefit in EFS of 31.6 versus 20.8 months, $p = 0.005$ in favor of combination therapy with pathological CR rates of 24% and 2.2%, $p < 0.001$. This benefit was seen across most subgroups with no increase in the incidence of adverse events. In an updated analysis, 5-yr overall survival was 65% and 55.4%, respectively. NADIM, a phase II RCT also showed a significant benefit in pathological CR rates of 36.2% vs 6.8% in favor of chemo-immunotherapy. PFS at 2 years was 67.3% vs 52.6% in the overall cohort, but in PD-L1 >1%, it was significant with a p-value of 0.015. There are various other RCTs which have demonstrated the benefit of peri-op or neo-adjuvant chemo-immunotherapy compared to chemotherapy alone in resectable NSCLC.

4.6 Adjuvant Targeted Therapy in Resected NSCLC

There have been numerous RCTs performed with the adjuvant TKI, especially in EGFR-positive NSCLC, with mixed results until the recently published ADAURA trial [24]. In the phase III randomized controlled ADAURA trial, adjuvant Osimertinib was administered for 36 months in stage IB to stage IIIA (AJCC 7th edition) non-squamous NSCLC patients with sensitizing EGFR mutation (exon19 or exon21). This led to a 37% absolute improvement in DFS at 24 months and translated into an 80% reduction in the risk of disease recurrence or death. The benefit was observed in all subgroups of patients, including 40% of patients who did not receive adjuvant chemotherapy. The magnitude of benefit was higher in Stage II–III patients (H.R.—0.17; 99.06% CI, 0.11 to 0.26; $p < 0.001$). The overall survival results are still awaited to make it a standard treatment option after surgical resection.

Similarly, data on EGFR TKIs as neo-adjuvant treatment is limited, although EGFR TKIs have been found to be a reasonable alternative to platinum-based chemotherapy in small trials. Neo-adjuvant EGFR-TKIs are also being tried in various RCTs like NeoADAURA [25].

4.7 Adjuvant Immunotherapy in Resected NSCLC

In a recently published phase III RCT [26] of adjuvant Atezolizumab versus best supportive care after completion of adjuvant chemotheraoy in surgically resected stages II to IIIA NSCLC, adjuvant atezolizumab for 1-year demonstrated significant disease-free survival advantage in patients with PD-L1 score of >1%. FDA, NCCN and EMA now approve this for eligible patients based on this study. There are ongoing studies of adjuvant immunotherapies with pembrolizumab and Nivoliumab in this cohort of patients.

4.8 Medically Inoperable Early Stage NSCLC

Due to poor pulmonary and cardiac function, if the patient is medically inoperable or not willing to surgery, stereotactic body radiotherapy (SBRT) is the treatment of choice in node-negative early stage NSCLC. With SBRT, one to eight sessions are routinely administered depending on the tumor location. Further details about SBRT lung are given in the chapter of Special Techniques—II (in Volume I, Chap. 19 of this book). In patients who are physically or technically unable to undergo SBRT, early stage tumor should be treated by moderately hypofractionated radiotherapy course.

4.9 Loco-regionally Advanced (T3–4 and N2–N3) NSCLC

Locally advanced NSCLC (LA-NSCLC) represents a heterogeneous group and requires multimodality management. Concurrent chemoradiotherapy, followed by Durvalumab, is the recommended treatment option according to the NCCN guidelines. However, controversies exist in single-station non-bulky mediastinal lymph nodes, as several institutions and guidelines do recommend neo-adjuvant treatment followed by surgery as one of the treatment options.

Radiotherapy alone has been used in the literature in patients for LA-NSCLC. Various RCTs compared radiation alone with the combination of chemotherapy and radiotherapy and demonstrated that combination therapy is superior to radiation alone in terms of 2-year OS. Auperin meta-analysis of RCTs [27] comparing sequencing of chemotherapy and radiotherapy demonstrated an absolute benefit of 4.5% in favor of concurrent chemoradiation therapy over sequential therapy with a H.R. of 0.84. Concomitant radiochemotherapy increased acute esophageal toxicity (grade 3–4) from 4% to 18% with a relative risk of 4.9 (95% CI, 3.1 to 7.8; $p < 0.001$). There was no significant difference regarding acute pulmonary toxicity.

Tri-modality treatment with neoadjuvant chemoradiation therapy followed by surgery is the standard treatment in Pancoast tumors or superior sulcus tumors with invasion of the chest wall or spine [28]. SWOG 9416 [29] demonstrated that induction chemoradiation therapy consisting of 2 cycles of cisplatin etoposide and 45 Gy of radiation followed by surgical resection provided a 5-year OS of 44% for all patients and 54% with complete surgical resection.

The effects of neoadjuvant chemoradiation followed by surgery have been examined in several studies on stage III (N2) NSCLC. Patients in the Intergroup 0139 [30] received induction chemo-irradiation treatment before being randomly assigned to receive additional radiotherapy or surgery. The results showed a similar median OS of 22.2 months versus 23.6 months and a 5-year OS of 20% vs. 27% ($p = 0.1$), respectively. In the surgery cohort, patients with pN0 status and who underwent lobectomy have improved survival compared to pN+ and pneumonectomy. ESPATUE [31], a phase III trial, also delivered induction chemoradiation therapy followed by randomization to either further radiotherapy boost or surgery. Patients received 45 Gy twice daily in the induction regimen. Approximately 65% (161/246) patients underwent randomization, and the results demonstrated no significant difference in the 5-year PFS of 35% vs. 32% and 5-year OS of 44% and 40%, respectively.

A German trial [32] compared neoadjuvant chemoradiation followed by surgery versus neoadjuvant chemotherapy followed by surgery and adjuvant radiation therapy. From a toxicity perspective, patients receiving CRT experienced significantly increased grade 3 or higher hematologic toxicity (10 vs. 1%) and esophagitis (19 vs. 4%). Essentially every surrogate endpoint favored preoperative CRT, with more patients undergoing complete resection (75 vs. 60%, $p = 0.0008$), nodal downstaging to N0–1 (46 vs. 29%, $p = 0.02$), and histopathologic response greater than 90% (60 vs. 20%, $p < 0.0001$). Despite these results, there were no differences in progression-free or overall survival or patterns of failure.

An important question is why such apparent pathologic differences did not translate into improved overall survival with CRT. Possible reasons could be (1) Increased time between the start of induction therapy and pathologic evaluation (the chemotherapy cohort would have had an increased pCR rate if more time had transpired) (2) Although radiation therapy increases the local pathologic response by adding cytotoxic therapy, it cannot influence the overall systemic therapy response to micrometastatic disease.

Most trials suggest avoiding pneumonectomy if neoadjuvant chemoradiation is used since this leads to increased adverse effects, including possibly higher postoperative mortality.

Direct comparison between neoadjuvant chemotherapy followed by surgery versus definitive chemoradiation has not been made in a properly conducted randomized setting. Hence, the question of whether definitive chemoradiation therapy is better or neoadjuvant therapy followed by surgery remains unanswered to date.

4.10 Postoperative Radiotherapy

In completely resected NSCLC patients, postoperative radiotherapy (PORT) has been a subject of considerable debate. The PORT meta-analysis [33] revealed adjuvant PORT is detrimental in stage I and II NSCLC with no detrimental effect seen in stage III NSCLC. A subset analysis of the ANITA trial [19] showed that in patients with pN2 disease, PORT improved 5-year OS after completion of adjuvant chemotherapy. Based on these, PORT was usually recommended based on individual practice for pN2 disease.

The long-awaited lung ART study [34], which began in 2010 and enrolled 501 patients, was published recently. Results showed a 3-year DFS of 47.1% in the PORT arm and 43.8% in the control arm (HR 0.85, 95% CI [0.67–1.07]; $p = 0.16$). Three-year OS was 66.5% in the PORT arm, compared with 68.5% in the control arm. Though mediastinal relapse was reduced by nearly 50% in patients receiving PORT, these patients experienced high rates of death secondary to cardiopulmonary toxicity. The authors therefore concluded that PORT should not be routinely administered in patients with pN2-resected NSCLC. In the Chinese PORT-C randomized trial [35], in patients with pIIIA-N2 NSCLC undergoing complete resection and adjuvant chemotherapy, PORT did not improve DFS as anticipated. However, the study did not elucidate the invasive nodal staging used pre-therapy and did not use neoadjuvant chemotherapy.

The PORT-C trial evaluated the effect of PORT using modern techniques on survival and safety in patients with pIIIA-N2 NSCLC after complete resection and adjuvant chemotherapy. The PORT-C randomized clinical trial was conducted in 394 patients with pIIIA-N2 NSCLC treated with complete resection and four cycles of platinum-based chemotherapy between January 2009 and December 2017. The 3-year DFS rates were 40.5% with PORT vs. 32.7% with observation (median, 22.1 vs. 18.6 months), and the difference in DFS was not statistically significant without adjustment (hazard ratio [H.R.], 0.84; 95% CI, 0.65–1.09; $p = 0.20$), In this phase 3 randomized clinical trial of patients with pIIIA-N2 NSCLC after complete resection and adjuvant chemotherapy, PORT did not improve DFS. Further studies exploring patients who might best benefit from PORT are needed. As of today, the use of PORT could be considered in a very select patient population as the involvement of multiple nodes, multiple stations involvement, or with extranodal extension after discussion in a multidisciplinary tumor board.

4.11 Systemic Therapy in Locally Advanced NSCLC

Neo-adjuvant chemotherapy in upfront resectable NSCLC with N0-N1 status is debated except for superior sulcus tumors, where neoadjuvant chemotherapy and radiation therapy before surgery is the standard of care. The results of adjuvant chemotherapy are very well established after the LACE meta-analysis [22] showed absolute benefit in overall survival. Various trials have assessed the efficacy of neoadjuvant chemotherapy with conflicting results. SWOG 9900 compared neoadjuvant chemotherapy versus surgery alone and demonstrated a non-significant increase in both median PFS and OS although this trial included patients who were upfront operable and N2 was excluded. Another phase II study of NACT with Cisplatin/Gemcitabine and a meta-analysis by Song et al. suggested overall survival (OS) benefit in the preoperative chemotherapy arm, which is similar to that attained with postoperative chemotherapy. The only published phase III RCT comparing surgery alone, NACT-Sx, with surgery-adjuvant CT is the NATCH trial [36] with DFS as the primary endpoint. The chemotherapy regimen used was three cycles of Paclitaxel and carboplatin. The results showed a non-significant increase in DFS in the preoperative chemotherapy arm compared to surgery alone, and more patients were able to receive preoperative CT than adjuvant CT.

Potential advantages of delivering neoadjuvant chemotherapy are downstaging of the primary tumor, treatment of micrometastases, better tolerability, and compliance rates, and assessing the disease biology. Response to neoadjuvant Therapy is a prognostic factor, and significant pathological response (MPR) [defined as <10% residual viable tumor in primary tumor and nodes] has been proposed to be a predictor of overall survival in patients treated with neoadjuvant therapy and is the primary endpoint of many ongoing neoadjuvant trials. Various chemotherapeutic regimens used in neoadjuvant regimens are platinum doublets like Cisplatin and Pemetrexed (nonsquamous), Paclitaxel, Gemcitabine, Vinorelbine, and Etoposide. If a patient is not eligible for Cisplatin-based chemotherapy, carboplatin is also used with similar efficacy.

The role of neoadjuvant chemotherapy is well established in patients with stage IIIA (N2) disease as mentioned above. A randomized study [37] compared surgery alone with neoadjuvant chemotherapy followed by surgery in 60 patients demonstrated a significant increase in DFS and OS in favor of neoadjuvant Therapy. Another RCT [38] compared perioperative chemotherapy with surgery alone in stage IIIA NSCLC showed a significant increase in overall survival with perioperative chemotherapy.

Postoperative chemotherapy should be administered to patients who did not receive preoperative chemotherapy. In completely resected N2 NSCLC, adjuvant radiation may or may not be necessary. The PORT meta-subset analysis's analysis revealed no differences in survival, however, a thorough review of the SEER database revealed that postoperative radiation improved survival for patients with N2 illness.

4.12 Radiation Therapy in LA-NSCLC

Concurrent chemoradiation therapy (CTRT) is the standard treatment for stage III NSCLC [27]. The standard dose of radiation therapy is 60–66 Gy in 30–33 fractions at 2 Gy per fraction over a period of six to six and a half weeks. With definitive CTRT, the expected median PFS ranges from 10 to 12 months and overall survival from 24 to 30 months. The survival has improved consistently in the RCTs of CTRT for stage III NSCLC. Despite this, approximately 30–40% of patients experience loco-regional relapse and 50% distal relapse.

Various strategies have been used to improve loco-regional control and OS for stage III NSCLC.

4.12.1 Dose Escalation

Radiotherapy dose: A dose of 60–66 Gy in 30–33 fractions is generally recommended for concurrent CTRT. Concomitant CTRT has shown to have better OS than sequential chemoradiation based on Auperin meta-analysis. Higher doses of R.T., like 74 Gy in 37 fractions, has shown to be inferior when compared to 60 Gy in 30 fractions in a landmark RTOG 0617 study [39]. The results showed inferior OS with a high dose (74 Gy) as compared to the standard dose (60 Gy). The median and 5-year OS was, 20.3 months vs. 28.7 months (p = 0.007) and 23% vs 32%

($p = 0.004$). There were various criticisms of this trial; a full high dose was given to the entire PTV rather than to subvolume like GTV, prolonged overall treatment time, and non-isotoxic dose escalation resulted in higher OAR doses like heart, lung, and esophagus. On multivariate analysis, heart dose, and maximum esophagitis grade were significant predictors of overall survival. Cetuximab therapy did not result in any improvement in survival outcomes. There are ongoing dose escalation studies evaluating the role of timing, type, and biological sub-volume dose escalation.

Other forms of dose escalation such as, (a) to resistant hypoxic sub volume or (b) mid-treatment boost to the residual or (c) post-treatment boost to the improve loco-regional control rates have also been investigated. PET-based dose escalation to FDG avid areas of primary tumor and nodes was tried in the NARLA 2 trial. Mid-treatment PET boost or SBRT boost to residual FDG avid areas are options for dose escalation. "Iso-toxic" individualized, tailored dose escalation (increasing radiation dose to pre-specified normal tissue dose constraints) can lead to increased tumor control probability with the same normal tissue complication probability. Sana et al. have tried dose escalation in a small cohort of patients, in the form of SBRT to residual disease after the end of conventional chemoradiation [40]. They found that such escalation was possible and well tolerated. However, to date, no study has found any significant benefit of dose escalation, and this technique remains investigational.

4.12.2 Altered Fractionation

Altered fractionation schedules like hyper fractionation, accelerated fractionation, and hypofractionation have also been tried in non-small cell lung cancer with limited success in improving survival outcomes. The U.K. trial of continuous hyper-fractionated accelerated radiotherapy (CHART) [41], to a dose of 54 Gy in 36 fractions of 1.5 Gy over 12 consecutive days compared with conventional radiotherapy dose of 60 Gy in 30 fractions, demonstrated a 2-year improved OS from 20% to 29% for CHART. No concurrent chemotherapy was given in this trial, and this trial showed the importance of tackling repopulation in NSCLC. Another study on altered fractionation with weekend less continuous hyper-fractionated accelerated radiotherapy (CHARTWEL) [42] delivering 60 Gy/40# over 2.5 weeks vs 66 Gy/33# over 6.5 weeks showed no difference in overall survival or local control rates.

Individual patient data meta-analysis of altered radiotherapy schedules showed an absolute benefit in OS of 2.5% at 5 years with an increased risk of acute esophageal toxicity. Concurrent chemoradiation using hypofractionated radiotherapy in a phase II SOCCAR study [43] was found to be safe and feasible using 50 Gy in 20 fractions over 4 weeks compared to sequential chemotherapy with cisplatin and vinorelbine. However, major concerns with hypo fractionation and concurrent CT use are the increased risk of late toxicities like radiation pneumonitis and esophagitis.

4.12.3 Technique of Radiotherapy

There are no RCT's comparing three-dimensional conformal radiotherapy versus intensity-modulated radiation therapy. However, a secondary analysis of RTOG 0617 between IMRT and 3D-CRT showed no significant difference in PFS, OS, L.F., and DMFS. IMRT plans did show a significant reduction in ≥grade 3 pneumonitis rate compared with 3D-CRT (7.9% vs. 3.5%, $p = 0.039$) and heart doses ($p < 0.05$). On multivariate analysis, heart doses like V40 Gy have significantly associated with OS A meta-analysis of ten retrospective studies also showed a significant reduction in the risk of pneumonitis, however with increased risk of esophagitis with no difference in OS

5 Radiation Therapy: Indications and Selection

5.1 Patient Selection

The majority of people with NSCLC benefit from radiotherapy. Overall, treatment options rely on the stage of the tumor as well as the patient's lung function, the extent of the disease, and performance status. Patients must have good P.S., adequate lung function (forced expiratory volume in 1 s [FEV1] >1 l or 40% predicted; transfer factor 40%), and disease that can be encompassed in a radiotherapy volume without undue risk of damaging normal tissue in order to be eligible for radical radiotherapy. Interstitial lung disease (ILD) patients are infrequently eligible. Such patients may need GAP scoring https://www.mdcalc.com/calc/2157/gap-index-idiopathic-pulmonary-fibrosis-ipf-mortality before the start of radiotherapy. If patients with impaired lung function have received enough counseling regarding the long-term dangers of breathlessness, they may still be eligible.

5.2 Radiation Indications and Uses in NSCLC (Table 9)

The principal objective of RT is maximizing tumor control with minimal side effects (Table 9). In nonrandomized trials, advanced technologies have been demonstrated to decrease toxicity and boost survival, including intensity-modulated R.T./volumetric modulated arc treatment (IMRT/VMAT), image-guided RT (IGRT), motion management techniques, and proton therapy.

Table 9 Indications of RT in NSCLC

1	Definitive Therapy for early stage NSCLC in patients with surgical contraindications
2	Definitive Therapy for locally advanced NSCLC, typically combined with chemotherapy.
3	Neoadjuvant or adjuvant Therapy (also known as preoperative or postoperative Therapy)
4	Salvage radiation therapy post definitive treatment, either surgery or chemoradiation therapy.
5	Palliative RT for bone, brain, liver, and adrenal metastases
6	Local ablative Therapy for oligo recurrent/oligoprogressive disease
7	Local consolidation radiation therapy for oligometastases

5.3 Simulation and Contouring

The planning of radiotherapy in lung cancer requires very careful attention as both the target volume and organs at risk are constantly moving with respiration. The planning CT scans should always be performed in the exact treatment position. For better target delineation whenever possible, intravenous contrast, with or without oral contrast, is advised, particularly in patients with central tumors or nodal involvement.

Simulation All lung cancer patients must be simulated with CT-based treatment planning. Usually, slice thickness should be less than 5 mm; the preferred is 2.5 mm, which can provide higher resolution digitally reconstructed radiographs for better localization during treatment delivery. The planning CT scan should cover the areas of interest as well as all the organs at risk with the lung from apex to their bases. Immobilization of the patient should be performed depending on the areas of interest and treatment plan, for example, if SBRT is to be performed, immobilization devices like customized vacuum cushion, which molds to the patients surface, or if the neck node is to be irradiated, a four clamp thermoplastic mask to be used (Fig. 12).

Immobilization devices help the patients' daily reproducibility on the treatment couch. Hence, the patient's position needs to be comfortable and simple.

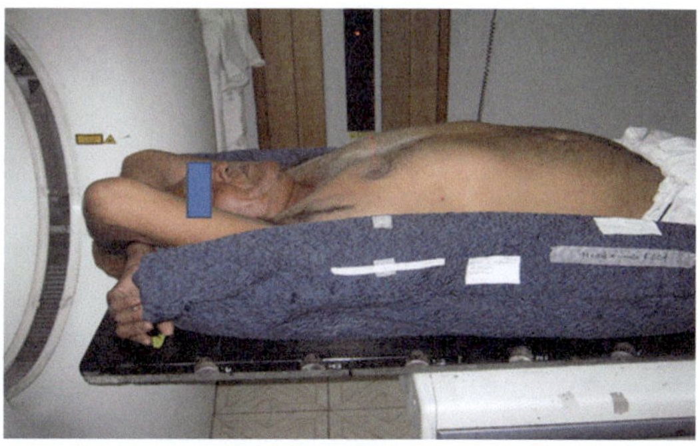

Fig. 12 Lung cancer patient simulation. Patient has been immobilized in a vacuum cushion bag

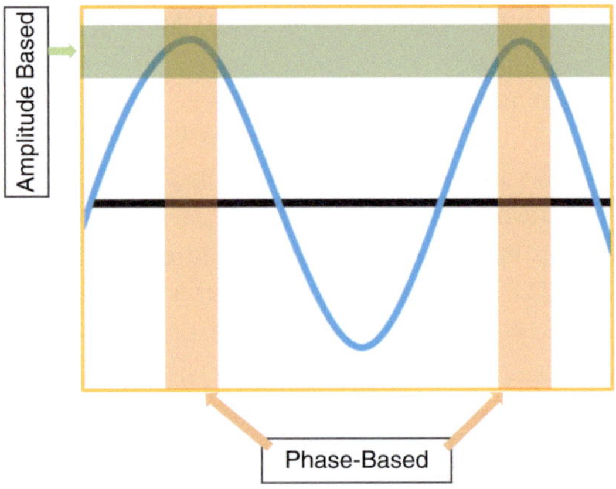

Fig. 13 Concept of phase-based and amplitude-based breath assessment and treating strategies. The solid blue line represents the respiratory cycle

Complex devices and patient positions need to be avoided. For SBRT, AAPM TG 101 recommends CT slice thickness to be between 1 and 3 mm.

5.4 Management of Tumor Motion

Respiratory motion can result in significant distortion of the target and organs at risk. These result in various types of artifacts like blurring, duplication, incomplete, and overlapping of images. Lung motion can extend significantly in all three orthogonal directions, maximum in craniocaudal directions, especially in the lower lobe (Fig. 13).

The location, size, lung function, and whether or not the tumor is attached to any mediastinal or chest wall affect how a lung tumor moves. Radiotherapy treatment planning for lung cancer requires taking into account the tumor motion either as tumor-encompassing methods like Internal Target Volume (ITV) or motion mitigation strategies. The AAPM Task Group Report 76 [44] recommends using motion management techniques when the range of motion is >5 mm in any direction.

However, one needs to use this technology with prudence, taking into account the patients age, disease stage and likely survival of the patient (Table 10).

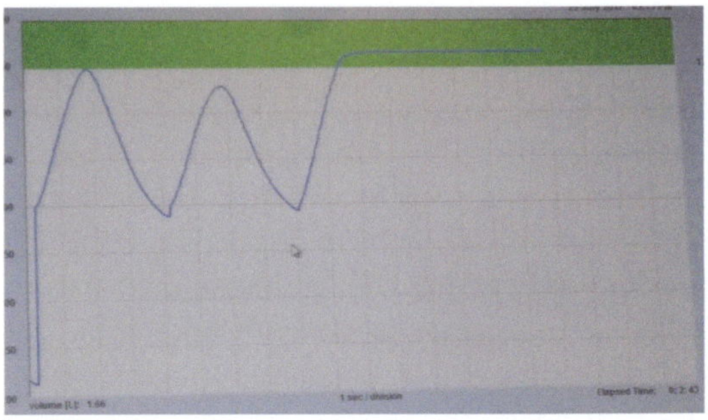

Fig. 14 DIBH in the lung cancer patient. The scan is done when the breath reaches the green band. Similarly, the treatment beam becomes on only when the patient's breath is in the green band

Table 10 Techniques available to assess lung motion

Technology	Advantages	Disadvantages
Fluoroscopy	Easily available and could provide a rough estimate of craniocaudal movement	Lacks the volumetric information of tumor and accurate assessment of motion
Slow CT scans(4 s per slice acquisition)	Provides a rough estimate of tumor motion and generates a motion envelope of all possible tumor excursions.	Require special scanners
Four-dimensional CT scans (4DCT).	Includes the spatial as well as temporal information of the tumor during the CT acquisition process, the most modern way of assessing motion	Require special add-on features in scanners

4DCT scanners acquire multiple CT slices throughout multiple respiratory cycles and subsequently generate multiple datasets for different respiratory cycle phases, which can be used to create a tumor envelope of the moving tumor called internal target volume (ITV) (Fig. 14; Table 11).

Table 11 Techniques for execution of 4 D treatments

Technology	Description	Advantages	Disadvantages
Abdominal compression methods	Examples include physical compressors to induce shallow breathing	Cost-effective technique	Uncomfortable for many patients Can displace tissues erratically
Deep Inspiratory Breath Hold (DIBH) (Fig. 14)	Treating the patient when a deep breath has been taken	Stable, reproducible method	Uncomfortable for some patients
Respiratory gating	Irradiating target while it is within a specific, predefined window of the breathing trajectory	It can be used in many patients unable to do breath hold	Some challenges in Q.A. and accurate delivery
Tracking techniques	The beam continuously tracks the tumor in all phases of respiration	The best way to account for target motion during treatment is to continually and dynamically direct the therapy beam at the moving target	This is the most difficult solution; both quality assurance and delivery can be very challenging
Maximum intensity projection (MIP)	Summation of the maximum intensities gives the iGTV for radiation planning	Simple, effective tool	Needs a lung parenchymal rim around the tumor. Issues with tumors abutting the chest wall and mediastinum

Table 12 Contouring for Ca lung

S No	Link	Comments
1	NRG oncology https://www.nrgoncology.org/ciro-lung	The RTOG consensus lung-contouring atlas
2	ICRU report 62 https://www.icru.org	Recommendations on the volumes and absorbed doses that are important in prescribing, recording and reporting photon beam therapy
3	ICRU report 83 https://www.icru.org	Provides information necessary to standardize techniques and procedures and to harmonize the prescribing, recording, and reporting IMRT
4	ESTRO ACROP guidelines [54]	ESTRO ACROP guidelines for contouring in Carcinoma Lung

6 Contouring Guidelines (Table 12)

Guidelines from the International Commission on Radiation Units Report No. 50 for defining targets have been applied to treating lung cancer. The gross tumor volume (GTV) is defined as a tumor visible by any imaging modality and grossly involved lymph nodes. The clinical target volume (CTV) is the anatomically defined area (e.g., the hilar or mediastinal lymph nodes or a margin around the grossly visible disease) believed to harbor microscopic disease. The planning target volume (PTV) includes a margin around the CTV to account for physiologic organ motion during treatment and day-to-day setup errors in fractionated Therapy and provide details of the current definitions of target volumes for 3D-RT and IMRT.

6.1 Gross Tumor Volume

The tumor visible on any imaging modality is defined as gross tumor volume. GTV demarcation on the planning-CT is required. If anatomically feasible, the GTV of the primary tumor and the GTV of the lymph node(s) should be delineated separately. The pre-set mediastinum window setting ($W = 400$ and $L = 20$) should be used to delineate lymph nodes and primary tumors invading the mediastinum or chest wall, whereas the pre-set lung window setting ($W = 1600$ and $L = 600$) should be used to delineate primary tumors surrounded by lung tissue. It is advised to define the GTV based on current CT and FDG-PET data. The GTV should not include the atelectasis/collapse regions that are apparent on the CT picture past the margin of the elevated FDG uptake.

Following induction chemotherapy, the GTV of the main tumor should be determined using the most recent CT scans. Still, pre-chemotherapy imaging, such as PET-CT, should also be considered. Based on pre-chemotherapy clinical, pathological, and imaging data, the GTV of the lymph nodes should encompass all implicated lymph nodes or lymph node stations, even if a node has entirely disappeared in recent imaging.

GTV lymph nodes are defined as lymph nodes that have had biopsy confirmation of malignancy or have been identified on FDG-PET as abnormal or suspicious. Suppose there is any doubt about the diagnosis. In that case, a node should be included in the GTV rather than excluded due to the inter-observer variability of reporting FDG-positive mediastinal nodes. Since the false negative rates of EBUS/EUS are high, lymph nodes that are FDG-PET positive but negative for EBUS/EUS should be included in the GTV.

6.2 Clinical Tumor Volume

The GTV-to-CTV expansions of 6 mm for squamous malignancies and 8 mm for adenocarcinomas are needed to cover the gross tumor and microscopic disease with 95% accuracy, according to a radiographic-histopathologic analysis of lung parenchymal illness [45]. However, these expansions should always be customized based on the location of the primary tumor and associated lymph nodes. The primary lesion's CTV need not enter the chest wall/ribs/mediastinum without radiographic evidence of invasion. The CTV should be edited from the anatomical barriers like bone, vessel, and air if there is no invasion into these. There are two ways to generate a CTV for the lymph nodes: using lymph node stations or expanding the GTV geometrically, analogous to the original tumor. The former method incorporates the entire pathologically involved lymph node station with at least a 5–8 mm margin around it (5–8 mm).

6.3 Planning Target Volume

The PTV is generated around the CTV by adding a margin to account for target motion and daily setup errors. Daily setup uncertainty varies according to the immobilization technique used and varies according to institutional practice.

Each institution should calculate the setup margin based on random and systematic errors, and accordingly, the PTV margin should be given. If an ITV is used for motion compensation and daily image-guided radiotherapy (IGRT) is used during treatment, typical margins for the PTV are usually 5–7 mm. If motion management is not used, margins are usually of greater magnitude due to the chances of missing the target due to motion. It has been demonstrated that daily IGRT-based setup considerably reduces residual errors and, as a result, planning margins (Fig. 15).

6.4 Radiotherapy Treatment Planning

The goal of treatment planning is to optimize the therapeutic ratio. The aim is to maximize the dose to the target while simultaneously minimizing the dose to surrounding normal organs. Radiation planning should use at least three-dimensional conformal radiation therapy

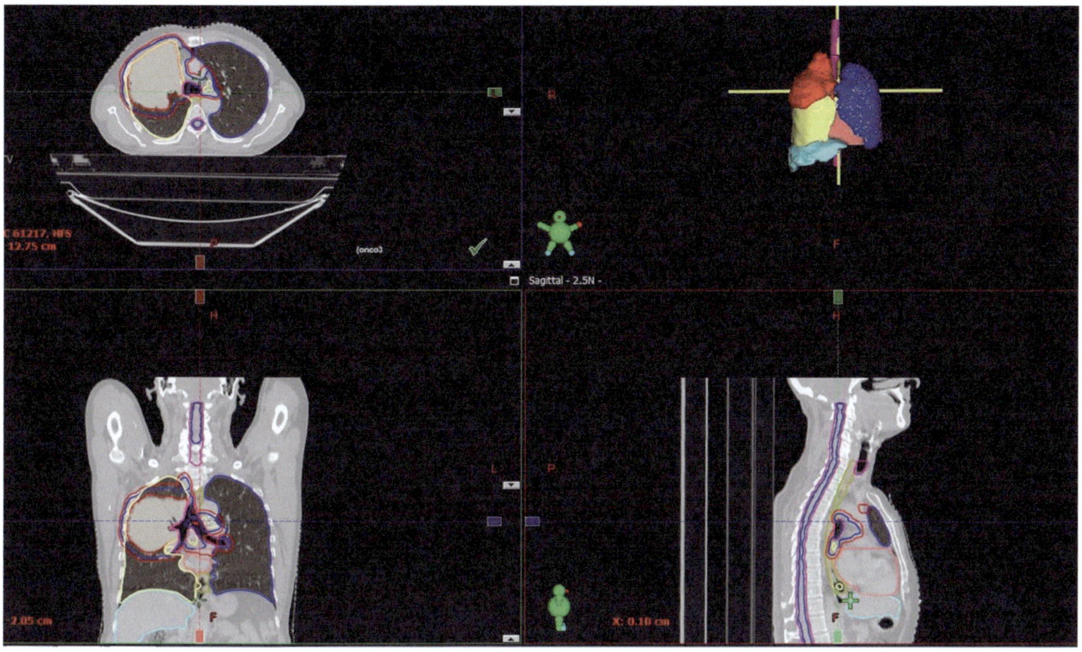

Fig. 15 GTV, CTV, and PTV contouring in a case of Ca Lung

(3DCRT) or intensity-modulated radiation therapy (IMRT) techniques for curative lung cancer treatment. A prospective trial (RTOG 0617) used definitive chemo/RT for patients with stage III NSCLC. IMRT was associated with a nearly 60% relative decrease in high-grade radiation pneumonitis (from 7.9% to 3.5%). Despite a higher proportion of stage IIIB and larger treatment volumes compared to 3D-CRT, there were similar survival and tumor control outcomes. As such, IMRT is preferred over 3D-CRT for radical chemoradiation in lung cancer [46]. Photon beam energy should be individualized based on the anatomic location of the tumors and beam paths. Generally, photon energies between 4 and 10 MV are recommended for beams passing through low-density lung tissue before entering the tumor. When there is no air gap before the beam enters the tumor, higher energies may improve the dose distribution, especially when using a smaller number of fixed beam angles. Examples include some large mediastinal tumors or those attached to the chest wall. Tissue heterogeneity correction and accurate dose calculation algorithms are recommended that account for buildup and lateral electron scatter effects in heterogeneous density tissues. Heterogeneity correction with simple pencil beam algorithms is not recommended. The respiratory motion should be managed when the motion is excessive. This includes (but is not limited to) forced shallow breathing with abdominal compression, accelerator beam gating with the respiratory cycle, dynamic tumor tracking, active breathing control (ABC), or coaching/biofeedback techniques. Motion-encompassing targeting is appropriate if the motion is minimal or the ITV is small. A useful resource for implementing respiratory motion management is the report of AAPM Task Group 76 [44] (Fig. 16).

6.5 B/L-Bilateral

For SBRT treatment, IMRT/VMAT treatment planning is preferable as the tumors are small and may be adjacent to critical structures to give bet-

Fig. 16 V 20 and V 5 in the context of lung radiotherapy planning

$$V\,20 = \frac{\text{Volume of B/L lung – PTV receiving 20 Gray OR MORE}}{\text{Total volume of B/L Lung – PTV}}$$

(represents intermediate dose area)

$$V\,5 = \frac{\text{Volume of B/L lung – PTV receiving 5 Gray OR MORE}}{\text{Total volume of B/L Lung – PTV}}$$

(represents low dose area)

Table 13 Commonly used doses for conventionally fractionated RT

Treatment type	Total dose	Fraction size	Treatment duration
Definitive RT with or without Chemotherapy	60–66 Gy	2 Gy	6–7 weeks
Preoperative RT	45–54 Gy	1.8–2 Gy	5 weeks
Postoperative RT			
Negative margins	50–54 Gy	1.8–2 Gy	5–6 weeks
Extracapsular nodal extension or positive microscopic margins	54–60 Gy	1.8–2 Gy	6 weeks
Gross residual tumor	60–66 Gy	2 Gy	6–7 weeks

ter conformality and minimize the dose to OAR. VMAT planning is generally preferred nowadays due to similar or better target coverage and shorter treatment time than conventional IMRT. In one such study, VMAT plans of SBRT were compared with traditional IMRT plans using the same optimization objective function and dose constraints, and the result demonstrated that the VMAT plan yielded improved target coverage and comparable normal tissue doses while reducing treatment time by approximately 60%. The faster radiation delivery with VMAT is also likely to substantially mitigate patient movement on the treatment table during a lengthy treatment procedure, thereby improving delivery quality. However, as with conventional IMRT, VMAT-based plans are also subject to the interplay effect, which must be considered depending on the mobility of the tumor and the degree of modulation of the MLC fields.

The prescription point in SBRT can differ based on institutional practices; For example, RTOG used isodose-based prescription (60–90% of isodose lines) to have inhomogeneous dose distribution inside the PTV and rapid dose fall-off outside the PTV. In contrast, some institutions use isocenter-based dose prescription where the prescribed to a point inside the PTV, usually the center of mass of the PTV. The studies have demonstrated no difference in local control between the two techniques.

For palliative treatment, beams can be arranged as either parallel-opposed anterior-posterior beams or using a three-dimensional technique. Target volume should be confirmed with the help of multileaf collimators for better conformality and to minimize the doses to nearby organs at risk (Tables 13 and 14).

RTOG 1306 https://clinicaltrials.gov/ProvidedDocs/96/NCT01822496/Prot_SAP_000.pdf last accessed on 6th Feb 2023

6.6 Plan Evaluation and Quality Assurance

Careful analysis of the dose volume histograms and the slice-by-slice dose distribution evaluation

Table 14 DVH dose constraints for radiation treatment planning

LUNG—3DCRT/IMRT for a prescription of 60 Gy in 30 fractions				
Structure	Metric	Ideal	Acceptable	Unacceptable
PTV	V60 Gy	≥95%	≥90%	<90%
	Min dose (0.03 cc)	≥55.8 Gy (93%)	≥54 Gy (90%)	<54 Gy
	Max dose (0.03 cc)	≤72 Gy (120%)	≤75 Gy (125%)	>75 Gy
	The minimum dose can fall below 93% of the prescribed dose provided it is at least 90% of the prescription dose if the areas of under-dosing are confined to regions of overlap with critical structures.			
Spinal cord	Max dose (0.03 cc)	≤50.5 Gy	≤52 Gy	>52 Gy
Lung (minus PTV)	V20 Gy	≤20%	≤30%	>35%
	Mean dose	≤20 Gy	≤22 Gy	>22 Gy
Heart		V60 < 1/3rd V45 < 2/3rd V40 < 100%		
Esophagus	Max dose (0.03 cc)	≤63 Gy	≤66 Gy	>66 Gy
	Mean dose	≤34 Gy	≤35 Gy	>35 Gy
Brachial plexus	Max dose (0.03 cc)	≤63 Gy	≤66 Gy	>66 Gy

Modified from RTOG 1306 protocol. https://clinicaltrials.gov/ProvidedDocs/96/NCT01822496/Prot_SAP_000.pdf

is essential for IMRT/VMAT plan evaluation. Organ contours and dose-volume-based organ constraints, planning margins for targets and OARs, intrafraction motion and impact on margins, inhomogeneity corrections, dose uniformity and "hot" or "cold" spots in the target region, normal tissue tolerance doses, and plan deliverability—that is, the presence of many low-intensity segments that could potentially be delivered—are just a few of the factors that need to be taken into account before radiation delivery.

6.7 Treatment Verification

Radiation delivery for lung cancer treatment is generally performed using IGRT-based systems, which can be acquired using megavoltage (MV) or kilovoltage (kV) based planar imaging, as well as volumetric cone beam CT to verify the target positioning prior to treatment (Fig. 17).

Daily verification or twice-weekly verification of the planning target volume can be done to ensure adequate coverage of PTV. Image-based verification also helps in adapting the treatment plan, especially in cases where lung collapse has resolved, a significant reduction in tumor volume thereby causing the anatomical shift, or new onset lung collapse or pleural effusion. The gating technique, which delivers radiation during a given phase of the breathing cycle or a tracking technique which tracks the tumor in real-time can be used for treatment delivery if tumor motion is larger, depending upon the availability and institutional expertise in using these complex delivery techniques. Image-guidance protocols, including type and frequency of imaging, as well as the need for gating or tracking, should be decided by the treatment planning team after consideration of factors such as stage of the disease, location of the tumor, degree of tumor mobility, and quality of the IMRT or SBRT treatment plan.

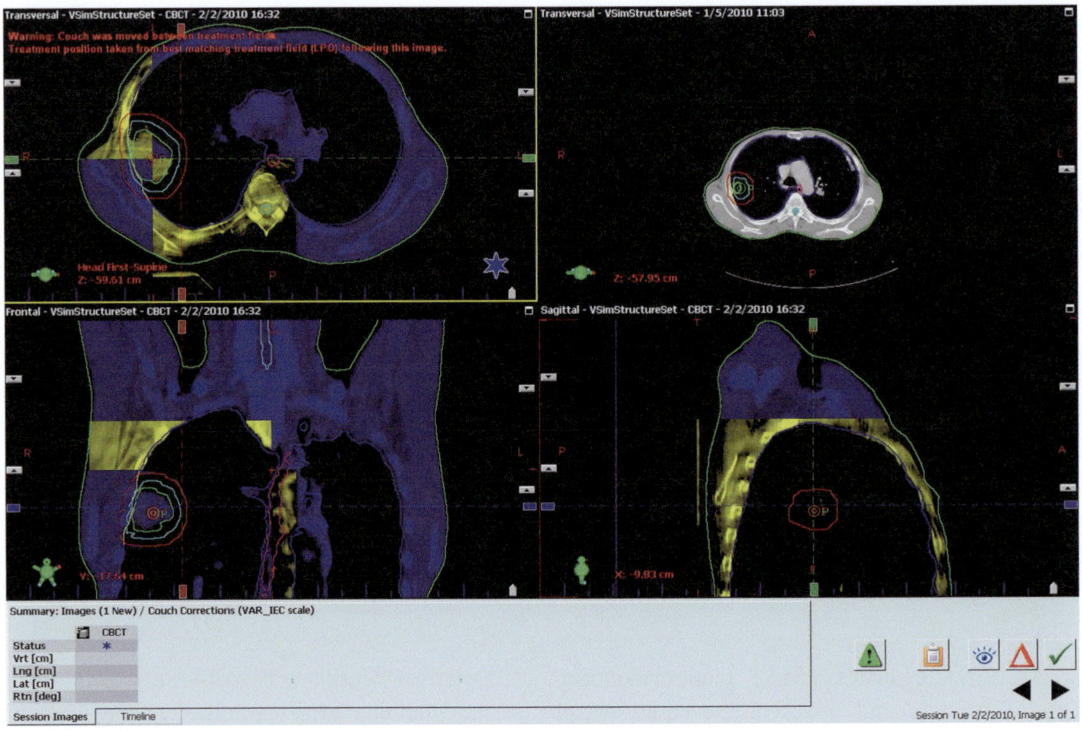

Fig. 17 On board cone beam CT (CBCT) in a case of carcinoma lung (just before treatment delivery)

7 Radiotherapy Sequelae

7.1 Radiation-Induced Toxicity

Radiation-induced toxicity is broadly divided as acute within (3 months) and chronic (beyond 3 months) (Table 15).

The reported incidence of brachial plexopathy in apical cancers treated with high-dose radiation may be as high as 16–20%. Usually, doses between 60 and 66 Gy are considered safe for the plexus—incidence rates for vertebral body fractures associated with thoracic radiation range from 8% to 17%.

The risk of radiation-induced toxicity is frequently impacted by the use of concomitant chemotherapy and radiation-related parameters such as total dose, dose per fraction, and organ at risk tolerances like lung minus PTV mean dose and volume receiving 20 Gy and 5 Gy. According to RTOG 0617, using IMRT was linked to a lower risk of pneumonitis of grade 3 or higher (8% vs. 20%; $p = 0.03$) but not esophagitis (30% vs. 39%; p = NS) or cardiovascular toxicity (11% vs. 21%; p = NS). Between IMRT and VMAT, no notable differences have been found.

Table 15 Toxicities related to thoracic radiation therapy

Acute toxicity	Late toxicities
Esophagitis	Radiation pneumonitis
Skin erythema	Lung fibrosis
Nausea	Esophageal/tracheobronchial stricture
Vomiting	Fistula
Decreased appetite	Cardiomyopathy
Lethargy	Brachial plexopathy
Dry cough	Myelopathy
Acute pericarditis	Second malignancies

7.2 Special Consideration on Pulmonary Toxicity

Thoracic radiation has a particularly well-documented history of causing lung damage. A 15–40% chance of radiation-induced pneumonitis (RP) and, in rare instances, lung fibrosis, are part of the pulmonary toxicity. Dry cough, dyspnea with exertion, and decreased effort tolerance are the typical symptoms of acute RP, which commonly appear within 6 weeks to 3 months. Late RP usually presents as chronic progressive dyspnea and can appear anywhere between 6 months and many years after radiation treatment. CT chest imaging studies are ideal because they are sensitive to subtleties of radiographic appearance. Acute RP frequently exhibits ground glass opacity, consolidation, or collapse, particularly in radiation environments. Radiographic evidence of bronchiectasis, fibrosis, chronic collapse, or loss of lung capacity are all associated with late RP.

Since RP is a clinical diagnosis, it's crucial to rule out any underlying infections or COPD flare-ups. RP is often graded using the Common Terminology Criteria for Adverse Events (CTCAE) (Grade—I Asymptomatic, only radiological or tomographic findings; II—Symptomatic, does not interfere with daily activities; III—Symptomatic, interferes with daily activities, requires supplemental O2; IV—Threatens life, requires mechanical ventilation support; and V—death).

The main course of treatment for RP consists of symptomatic interventions, such as steroids tapered off gradually. Supportive care is also provided with antibiotics, supplementary oxygen, and cough suppressants when necessary.

7.3 Response Assessment and Associated Challenges

The most used imaging technique for monitoring and assessing response is the CT chest. Contrary to post-surgery situations, it can frequently be difficult to interpret the results of a CT chest scan after radiation treatment. The evaluation is further complicated by early CT findings of diffuse consolidation, diffuse ground-glass opacity, patchy consolidation, and ground-glass opacity, as well as late CT findings of consolidation, volume loss, bronchiectasis, and scarring. Some of these difficulties may be resolved by a response evaluation review by a radiologist with experience in Lung cancer imaging and linkage with a treatment plan. PET avidity (6 months after therapy) or serial CT monitoring could be of considerable help in evaluating complex circumstances with aberrant CT characteristics.

7.4 Toxicities Associated with SBRT

Grades I–II radiation pneumonitis may occur in 25–30% of patients with grade III and above but occurs in less than 5% of patients. The incidence of RIP is usually higher in patients with interstitial lung disease. The decrease in pulmonary function parameters is also one of the toxicities associated with SBRT. Central and ultra-central tumors are more prone to toxicities like bronchial stenosis, esophagitis and subsequent stricture, bronco-pulmonary hemorrhage, and cartilage necrosis. Lesions adjacent to the chest wall can have chest wall pain, rib fractures, and chest wall fibrosis. If treated with a high dose per fraction, apical tumors can lead to brachial plexopathy.

7.5 Follow-Up

Most lung cancer follow-up policies are based on expert consensus and compelling data. Overall, there is not enough data to support a distinct follow-up strategy based on the cancer stage. There is no proof that more frequent testing may lead to the detection of more recurrences, which would be beneficial for survival.

The National Comprehensive Cancer Network (NCCN) advises performing CT chest +/− contrast scans every 3–6 months for the first 3 years, once every 6 months for the next 4–5 years, and once every year after that. The European Society of Medical Oncology (ESMO) suggests performing upper abdominal and thoracic CT scans every 6 months for the first 2 years and then once a year for the following 3 years. In the first 2 years following therapy, the most recent American society of clinical oncology (ASCO) guideline 2020 recommends a 6-monthly CT scan of the chest, including the adrenals, with or without contrast. According to ASCO guidelines, adding CT scans of the belly and pelvis is not beneficial; most patients just need a CT scan of the chest through the adrenals.

While there are some variations in frequency and timing, all the recommendations advise against using a routine MRI or PET scan to monitor NSCLC.

7.6 Quality of Life Issues

Improving the quality of life (QoL) is crucial for patients' treatment outcomes and is being increasingly acknowledged in practice. The prevalence of loco-regional diseases is high in this population, and the resulting intrathoracic symptoms are distressing until the final stage. When determining the scope and severity of these patient-reported symptomatic problems, QoL assessments are crucial. QoL tools could aid personalized therapy, palliative care, and rehabilitation strategies for cancer patients and survivors.

The European Organization for Research and Treatment of Cancer (EORTC) Quality of Life Questionnaire Core 30 (QLQ-C30) with a lung-specific module (LC 13) remains the most popular tool despite the availability of several standardized QoL instruments, such as Functional Assessment of Cancer Therapy-General (FACT-G), FACT-Lung cancer, and Lung Cancer Symptom Scale (LCSS). Assessment of longitudinal data, for example at pre-treatment, post-treatment, at follow-ups of 3 monthly intervals, provides a critical understanding of treatment-related toxicity and realized functional benefits. Data attrition is a significant problem in QoL studies, particularly in stage IV settings with constrained life expectancy. However, QoL evaluation provides accurate insight into patient-reported subjective concerns that may be important both during and after treatment.

7.7 Systemic Therapy in LA-NSCLC (Special Considerations)

Adopting different chemotherapy regimens for other histologies have also been tried, like Pemetrexed in nonsquamous histology. PROCLAIM, a phase III RCT compared Cisplatin –Pemetrexed combination with Cisplatin-Etoposide along with concurrent thoracic RT in nonsquamous histology patients, and the results showed no significant difference in PFS and OS Consolidation chemotherapy has also been tried to reduce the distant relapse rates. However, a pooled analysis of all studies did not reveal any benefit of consolidation chemotherapy. A meta-analysis of five studies showed an improvement in OS. However, no difference in PFS. Despite this, physicians and institutes differ in their practice of using consolidation chemotherapy after the completion of chemoradiation. The PACIFIC study [47] incorporated a programmed death-ligand 1 (PDL-1) inhibitor called Durvalumab after completion of CTRT in stage III inoperable elderly patients and non-elderly patients. It was a phase 3, double-blind, placebo-controlled, multicenter study in which patients who had not progressed following platinum-based cCRT were randomized to either Durvalumab or placebo for 12 months starting 1–42 days after cCRT. The results demonstrated a significant improvement in the median PFS of 16.8 vs 5.6 months with Durvalumab as compared to placebo ($p > 0.0001$). Patients who received Durvalumab had higher response rates (28.4% vs. 16.0%; $p < 0.001$), longer duration of response (72.8% vs. 46.8% of the patients had an ongoing response at 18 months), lower incidence of new lesions, (including new brain metastases) compared with placebo. There was significant improvement in 2-year OS of 66.3% vs 55.6% ($p = 0.002$). The improvement in PFS and OS was seen in all the pre-specified subgroups. The recent 4-year update reported a median OS of 47.5 months vs 29.1 months and 4-year PFS of

35.3% vs. 19.5%, respectively. In patients with EGFR mutated NSCLC without progression after CTRT, adjuvant Osimertinib improves progression free survival compared to placebo with median PFS of 39.1 months vs 5.6 months, respectively (p<0.001) [24].

The questions that remain are

- Should we dose escalate with CTRT
- Can we combine altered fractionation schedules with chemoradiation
- Can SBRT be given after NACT/NACTRT
- How can we further reduce the side effects of chemo RT
- What about chemoradiation in elderly/Low PS patients

7.8 Recurrent or Metastatic NSCLC

The treatment of recurrent NSCLC depends on the site of recurrence, number, and disease-free interval (Figs. 6 and 18).

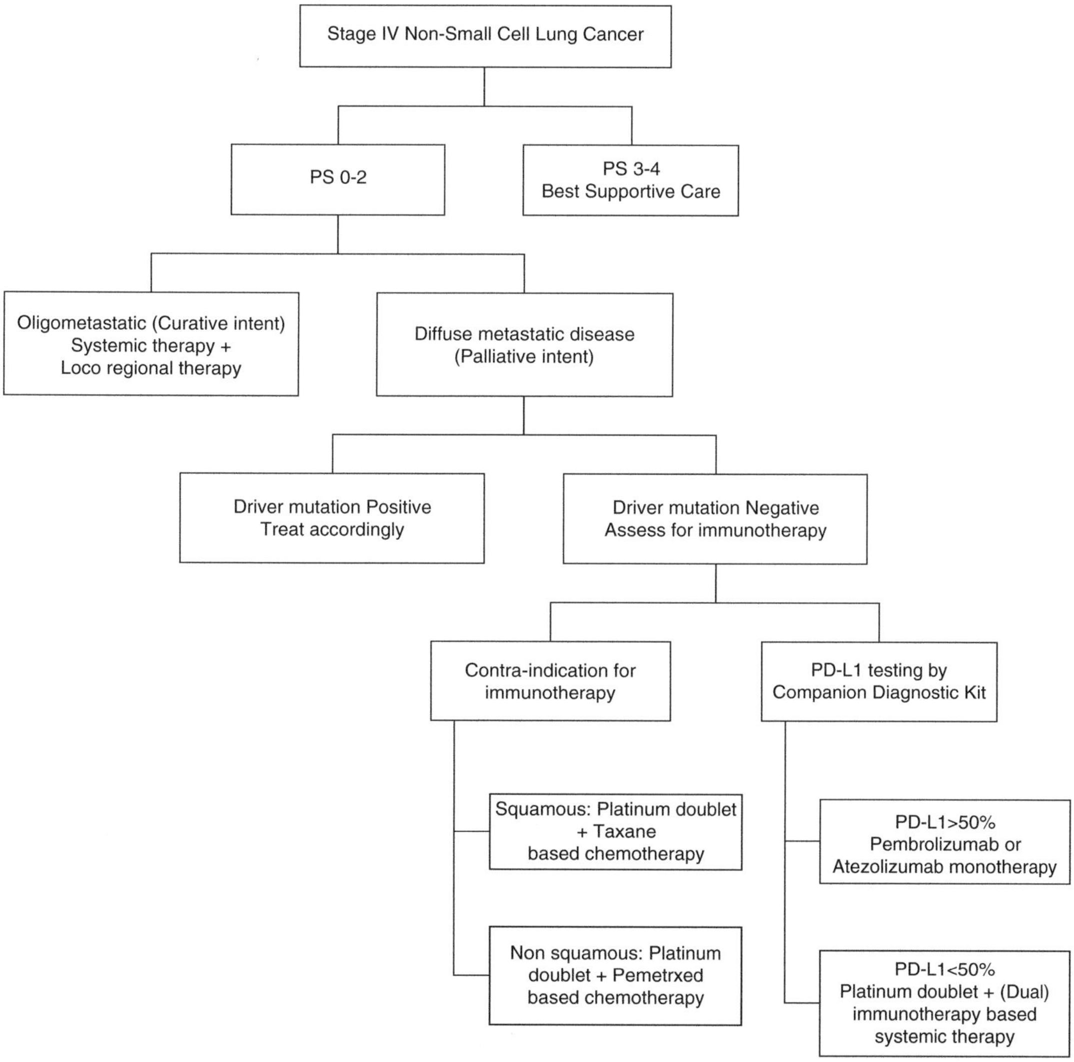

Fig. 18 Flowchart for management of metastatic NSCLC

In recurrent tumor, if surgically resectable, resections followed by systemic therapy should be considered. If radical radiation therapy is feasible for localized recurrent disease, RT should be used. The treatment of metastatic NSCLC is generally guided by the patient's performance status, comorbidities, oncogene mutation status, and PD-L1 status. During the last two decades, the treatment of metastatic NSCLC has evolved tremendously with molecular oncology-driven targeted therapy and immune checkpoint inhibitors. A detailed treatment of metastatic NSCLC is beyond the scope of this chapter, and only the salient points shall be presented.

In patients who have positive oncogene mutation status like Epidermal growth factor receptor (EGFR), Anaplastic lymphoma kinase (ALK), or ROS mutation, targeted therapy has become the standard of care. EGFR mutations are commonly seen in young females, non-smokers, and the Asian origin population. The most common and sensitizing mutation of EGFR is seen in exons 19 and 21. As given in the Table (Table 16) below, various tyrosine kinase inhibitors are approved for use in EGFR-positive mutation. The superiority of each of the first-line EGFR TKI in comparison with conventional platinum-based doublets was proven over the last decade through numerous trials (NEJ002, WJTOG 3405—Gefitinib, OPTIMAL, EURTAC—Erlotinib, LUX-Lung3, LUX-Lung 6—Afatinib). All the trials consistently showed improved ORR and PFS in comparison to the chemotherapy arm. The benefit of improvement in ORR and PFS was consistently seen across all age groups, genders, smoking status, and PS. However, none of the above studies could show an OS benefit, possibly due to the high level of crossover. The ARCHER 1050 (phase III) trial [48] compared dacomitinib with Gefitinib in the first-line setting and showed improved PFS (14.7 vs. 9.2 months; HR 0.59, $p < 0.0001$) and improved OS (34.1 vs. 26.8 months; HR 0.76; $p = 0.044$) in the dacomitinib arm. This was the first trial in which there was a significant improvement in OS with the use of a TKI. However, the ARCHER trial excluded patients with CNS metastasis at baseline, and hence its efficacy in CNS metastases is not known. The second instance where a TKI resulted in an overall survival advantage was in the FLAURA trial, where Osimertinib was compared with Gefitinib/Erlotinib in the first-line setting and showed a significant improvement in the PFS (18.9 vs. 10.2 months; HR 0.46; $p < 0.0001$) and OS (38.6 versus 31.8 months; HR 0.80, p 0.046). The FLAURA trial included patients with CNS metastasis (25%). Amongst patients with CNS metastasis, the PFS at 18 months was 58% (Osimertinib arm) versus 48% (Gefitinib/Erlotinib arm) (HR 0.48). Osimertinib is superior to 1st generation TKIs and has CNS activity. Hence, it is considered a preferred option in first-line treatment for NSCLC with sensitizing EGFR mutation. However, its cost is a major hindrance to its universal usage.

Table 16 Tyrosine kinase inhibitors in lung cancer

EGFR TKI	Type of inhibition	Indication
First generation TKI Gefitinib Erlotinib	Reversible	First-line therapy
Second generation TKI Afatinib Dacomitinib	Irreversible	First-line therapy
Third generation TKI Osimertinib	Irreversible	First-line therapy Second-line therapy for T790M mutation

7.8.1 TKI with Chemotherapy in the First Line

The concurrent administration of chemotherapy with EGFR TKI acts synergistically by inducing apoptosis and suppressing AKT and extracellular signal-regulated kinase phosphorylation, which may delay resistance. Oral TKI decreases the thymidylate synthase level, enhancing Pemetrexed's efficacy. The NEJ 009 study compared Gefitinib with Gefitinib + Pemetrexed + Carboplatin; there was a significant improvement in the ORR (67% vs. 84%), PFS (11.9 months vs. 20.9 months (HR 0.49; $p < 0.001$)) and OS (38.8 months vs. 50.9 months (HR 0.722)) in the combination arm. A study from Tata Memorial Hospital by Noronha et al. [5] showed an improved ORR (63% vs. 75%), PFS (8 months vs. 16 months (HR 0.51)) and OS (17 months vs. not reached; HR 0.45) with the combination of Gefitinib and chemotherapy. Based on the evidence from these two trials, Gefitinib plus chemotherapy is an alternative in patients who do not have access to osimertinib in the first-line setting.

7.8.2 ALK Rearranged NSCLC

Crizotinib in a first-generation ALK inhibitor that has activity in ALK-rearranged NSCLC. The phase III study, PROFILE 1014, compared Crizotinib with platinum–pemetrexed (without maintenance pemetrexed) as first-line treatment in ALK-rearranged advanced NSCLC. It demonstrated a significantly longer PFS (mPFS 10.9 vs. 7.0 months; HR 0.45; 95% CI 0.35–0.60; $p < 0.001$) and higher ORR with crizotinib compared with chemotherapy (ChT). Ceritinib are second-generation ALK inhibitors with good efficacy and intracranial activity in patients with ALK-rearranged NSCLC. Ceritinib improved ORR (72.5% vs. 26%), and PFS (16.6 vs. 8.1 months; HR 0.55, $p < 0.01$) when compared to chemotherapy in the ASCEND trial. Ceritinib had higher intracranial ORR (72.7% vs. 27.3%) as compared to chemotherapy in patients with CNS metastases. Alectinib (600 mg b.i.d.) was compared with crizotinib (250 mg b.i.d.) in the ALEX trial and demonstrated that Alectinib significantly improved the median PFS (34.8 vs. 10.9 months), and time to CNS progression (baseline CNS metastases mPFS 27.7 months vs. 7.4 months) compared to crizotinib. The updated result showed a 5-year OS of 62.5% vs. 46%, respectively. Alectinib is now recommended as the first-line treatment option for ALK-positive NSCLC. Brigatinib and Lorlatinib are the other two ALK-directed TKI compared against crizotinib, with better response rates.

7.8.3 Immunotherapy in Metastatic NSCLC

Compared to chemotherapy, immunotherapy (Table 17) for advanced NSCLC has produced a safer yet distinctive toxicity profile, better response rates, and higher overall survival. Without actionable driver mutations, immune checkpoint inhibitors have become the first line of treatment. Highly targeted humanized monoclonal antibodies are used in immunotherapy to target checkpoint signals like the programmed cell death receptor (PD-1) and programmed cell death ligand (PD-L1). Reactivating the immune system to attack the tumor is possible by inhibiting these receptors. Several regulatory bodies have approved the use of PD-1 inhibitors nivolumab and pembrolizumab, as well as PD-L1 inhibitors like atezolizumab for treating metastatic NSCLC.

Table 17 Immunotherapy agents

Type of ICI	Drugs
PD-1 inhibitors	Nivolumab, Pembrolizumab, Cemiplimab
PD-L1 inhibitors	Atezolizumab, Durvalumab, Avelumab
CTLA-4 inhibitors	Ipilimumab, Tremelimumab

The KEYNOTE-024 [49] & KEYNOTE-042 evaluated the role of Pembrolizumab monotherapy in advanced NSCLC. In the KEYNOTE-024 trial, patients with PD-L1 TPS ≥50% had a significantly higher PFS and OS when treated with Pembrolizumab as compared to a platinum-based chemotherapy doublet. The objective response rate was higher (Pembrolizumab 44.8% vs. chemotherapy 27.8%), with a longer duration of response in the pembrolizumab group. Similarly, in the KEYNOTE-042 study, the OS was significantly larger with pembrolizumab as compared to the chemotherapy group in all three TPS populations that is, ≥50% (HR 0·69, $p = 0.0003$), ≥20% (HR 0.77, $p = 0.0020$), and ≥1% (HR 0·81, $p = 0.0018$). Thus, based on the data from these two trials, Pembrolizumab monotherapy can be used as first-line therapy in patients with advanced NSCLC with PD-L1 TPS ≥1%.

The KEYNOTE-189 trial evaluated the role of adding Pembrolizumab to standard chemotherapy in patients with untreated metastatic non-squamous NSCLC without driver mutations. The KEYNOTE 407 assessed the same in squamous NSCLC. In both trials, the chemo-immunotherapy arm conferred superior PFS and OS compared with chemotherapy alone, regardless of the PD-L1 expression. The combination of

Pembrolizumab and chemotherapy is an approved standard first-line therapy option.

The IMpower110 phase 3 RCT compared atezolizumab with platinum-based chemotherapy for the first-line treatment of PD-L1-selected patients (n-205) with metastatic NSCLC. In the highest expression of the PD-L1 subgroup, the median OS was longer by 7.1 months in the atezolizumab group than in the chemotherapy group (20.2 months vs. 13.1 months; HR for death, 0.59; $p = 0.01$). Overall, PFS favored atezolizumab in the subgroups with a high blood-based TMB. In IMPower 130, treatment-naive patients with non-squamous metastatic NSCLC, combination of Atezolizumab + chemotherapy followed by atezolizumab maintenance was compared with chemotherapy alone (nab-paclitaxel and Carboplatin alone for 4–6 cycles) followed by supportive care or pemetrexed maintenance. The results showed a significant improvement in median OS and PFS in Atezolizumab + chemotherapy arm compared to the chemotherapy alone arm.

In the second line setting, CheckMate 017 (squamous histology) and CheckMate 057 [50] (non-squamous) showed a significant improvement in OS with Nivolumab compared to Docetaxel in a patient who had progressed on prior platinum-based chemotherapy. IN KEYNOTE-010 phase III RCT comparing Pembrolizumab with docetaxel chemotherapy, OS was significantly prolonged with Pembrolizumab [51]. Atezolizumab also showed improved OS when compared to chemotherapy. ICIs are approved for a second-line treatment options, and the choice of ICIs should be based on PD-L1 levels and affordability.

7.8.4 Chemotherapy in Negative Oncogene Mutation

For patients with PS of 0–2 who are not affordable or are ineligible for ICI's, histology-appropriate platinum-based doublet chemotherapy should be offered, with or without the addition of bevacizumab for those with non-squamous histology. Individual patient data (IPD) meta-analysis (MA) of supportive care and chemotherapy for non-small-cell lung cancer (NSCLC) of three studies showed the addition of chemotherapy resulted in a reduction in risk of death of 27% equivalent to an absolute improvement in survival of 10% at 1 year. Hence, systemic chemotherapy should be offered to all patients with stage IV NSCLC with PS 0–2.

7.9 First-Line Treatment for Non-squamous Lung Cancer

Compared with other platinum-based regimens, Pemetrexed platinum compounds showed a significant survival advantage in advanced non-small cell lung cancer, especially in non-squamous histology. Two studies have confirmed the differential efficacy of Pemetrexed with respect to histology in advanced NSCLC. Non-squamous patients treated with pemetrexed-based therapy experienced longer survival than the comparators (HR, 0.78 and 0.84, respectively), whereas squamous patients had shorter survival. (HR- 1.56 and 1.23, respectively). Therefore, pemetrexed platinum-based doublet should be the first-line treatment in advanced adenocarcinoma of the lung.

7.10 First-Line Treatment for Squamous Lung Cancer

Several chemotherapy agents (Gemcitabine/paclitaxel/vinorelbine) have been combined with platinum compounds, and all showed similar efficacy. The choice of doublets should be judged based on toxicity profile. Hence, platinum in combination with any third-generation cytotoxic agent (gemcitabine/paclitaxel/vinorelbine) should be considered in squamous lung cancer in the absence of contraindications.

7.11 Role of Radiation Therapy in Metastatic NSCLC

7.11.1 Brain Metastases

Approximately 10–20% of newly diagnosed patients with NSCLC have brain metastases (Fig. 19).

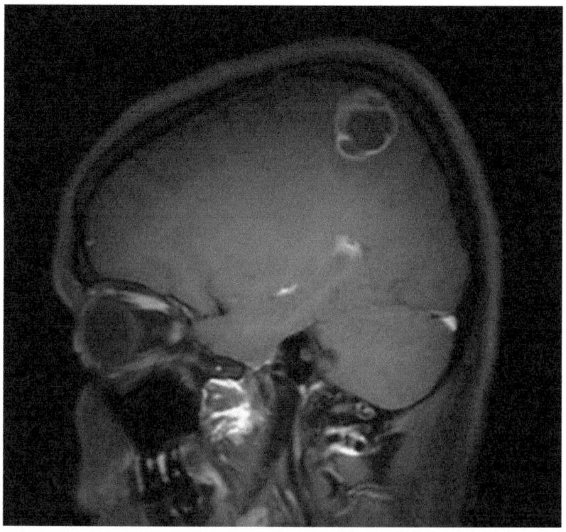

Fig. 19 High parietal metastasis shown on MRI brain in a case of NSCLC lung

In patients with brain metastases (BM), lung cancer is the most common primary seen in approximately 40–50% of cases. The incidence of BM is higher in patients with EGFR mutation and ALK rearrangement, approximately seen in 20–40% at presentation. Approximately 60–80% of NSCLC patients develop BM during the course of their disease. Brain metastases have a huge impact on OS and the quality of life of the patients. Steroids (oral/IV dexamethasone) are used to relieve vasogenic edema in patients with symptomatic brain metastases. For mildly symptomatic patients, dose of 4–8 mg/day, and for moderate to severe symptomatic patients, a dose of 16 mg/day in divided doses is recommended, to be gradually tapered over 2–4 weeks. In newly diagnosed patients who have not had a seizure, the use of prophylactic antiepileptic drugs (AEDs) is not recommended. When indicated, physicians may consider the use of levetiracetam over older AEDs to reduce the side effects. Brain metastases patients portend a very dismal prognosis with median OS ranging from 4 to 7 months. However, over the last decade or so, improvements in surgical resection techniques, advancement in radiation oncology techniques, and development of molecular driven therapies and immunotherapy have remarkably changed the management of brain metastases in NSCLC. The management of BM generally depends on the performance status of the patients, number of BM, age, and extracranial metastases status. There are various prognostic scoring systems to help in decision-making for treating BM like lung-specific graded prognostic assessment score, recursive partitioning analysis, and lung-molecular GPA with the incorporation of EGFR/ALK status. Further discussion of the management of brain metastasis is given in the chapter related to CNS.

7.11.2 Asymptomatic Brain Metastases

Its incidence ranges from 10% to 20% of all detected brain metastases done for standard staging investigations. The incidence is increasing gradually as MRI brain is being done frequently for driver mutation-positive patients as they are more prone to BM. Traditionally, in symptomatic BM, radiation therapy is delivered upfront to relieve the symptoms caused by vasogenic edema of brain metastases. However, in asymptomatic BM, various phase II studies in unselected populations of metastatic lung cancer evaluated upfront WBRT/SRS vs. delayed WBRT/SRS and did not demonstrate any survival benefit of treating upfront. However, intracranial response and fewer intracranial relapse rates were in favor of upfront RT. Asymptomatic brain metastases management has gained tremendous interest lately due to various CNS penetrating targeted agents. Higher generation TKIs with higher CNS penetration, like Osimertinib, Alectinib, Lorlatinib, has shown to effectively control brain metastases. Meta-analyses of retrospective studies have shown significantly better intracranial relapse rates and overall survival in favor of upfront WBRT/SRS versus delayed WBRT/SRS. However, alopecia and neurocognitive side effects of RT, particularly WBRT, and keeping RT as a salvage treatment modality in patients on higher generation TKIs especially have opened up a new debate on the timing of RT in asymptomatic BM. There are ongoing phase III RCT comparing upfront cranial radiotherapy (WBRT/

SRS) versus delayed CRT in asymptomatic brain metastases with positive oncogene mutation status like EGFR/ALK.

7.11.3 Bone Metastases

Bone is a frequent site of metastases in NSCLC, seen in approximately 30–40% at presentation. Bone metastases in NSCLC are predominantly lytic, with sclerotic lesions also commonly seen. Bone metastases exert a negative impact on quality of life (Fig. 20).

Bony destruction typically causes pain, mechanical instability, pathological fractures, hypercalcemia, and even paralysis from spinal cord compression. These skeletal-related events (SREs) occur in approximately 30% of patients with BM of NSCLC. Management of bone metastasis typically involves analgesics, bisphosphonates, radiotherapy, and surgery in some instances. Analgesia is based on the 3-step analgesic ladder developed by WHO with prompt oral administration of drugs in the following order: non-opioids (aspirin and paracetamol), then, as necessary, mild opioids, then strong opioids such as morphine, until the patient is free of pain. Surgical stabilization followed by palliative radiation therapy should be offered for unstable axial and appendicular lytic metastases. In patients who are unfit for surgical stabilization, palliative radiotherapy should be offered. Bisphosphonates (BPs) are a part of the standard of care for the treatment of bone metastases and the prevention of SREs. These include zoledronic acid, alendronate, pamidronate, and other pyrophosphate analogs. They concentrate in the skeleton and act by blocking the enzyme farsenyl diphosphate synthase in the HMG CoA reductase pathway.

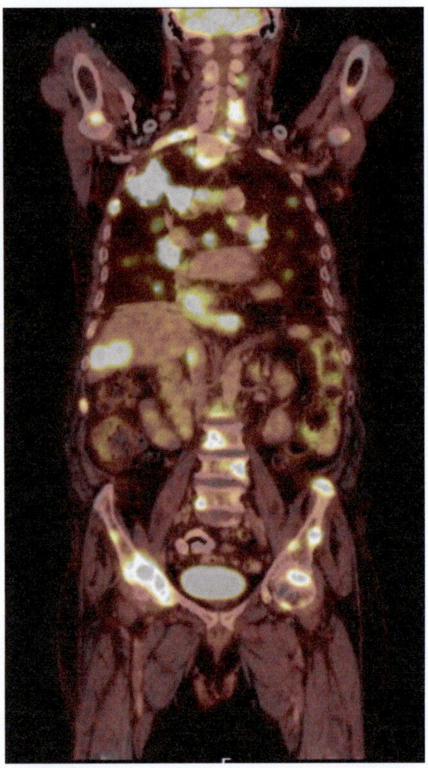

Fig. 20 PET CT of a lung cancer patient (NSCLC, adenocarcinoma) with diffuse metastatic disease (lymph nodes, lung nodules, bone metastasis, liver metastasis)

Further discussion of the role of radiotherapy in bone metastasis is given in related chapters.

With the increasing OS of NSCLC patients and advanced radiation technologies, SRS/SBRT for bone metastases for better pain and local control has been increasingly used, especially in patients with oligometastases. Various single-institution prospective and retrospective studies have shown the feasibility and toxicity profile of SRS/SBRT of spinal metastases. SRS/SBRT of spinal metastases resulted in good and faster pain control and local control of treated metastases with vertebral compression fracture rates of less than 10%. A phase II RCT comparing SRS of 24 Gy single fraction vs. 3D-CRT of 30 Gy in 10 fractions in painful spinal metastases did not show a significant difference in pain response at 3 months. However, pain relief was faster and more durable in the SRS arm compared to SBRT. In a prespecified secondary analysis, SBRT has shown a significant increase in bone density as compared to baseline, especially in lytic metastases. A phase III RCT of SBRT of 24 Gy in 2 fractions versus 3D-CRT of 30 Gy in 10 fractions have shown significantly better complete response rates (34% vs. 14%, $p = 0.0002$) with minimal grade 3–4 toxicity. In patients with non-spine bone metastases, a phase II RCT has demonstrated that SBRT is non-inferior to multi-fractionated radiotherapy (MFRT) in terms of pain response at various time points and should be considered in patients with reasonable chances of survival.

7.11.4 Spinal Cord Compression

Metastatic epidural spinal cord compression (MESCC) is an oncological emergency and is seen in approximately 15–20% of patients with lung cancer. Intravenous administration of steroids is recommended in neurologically symptomatic cord compression. In metastatic epidural spinal cord compression, surgical decompression followed by stabilization is recommended as the modality of choice. However, due to limited survival, rates of surgical decompression are very limited. Postoperative palliative radiotherapy to a dose of 20 Gy in 5 fractions or 30 Gy in 10 fractions should be offered. Further details have been given in relevant sections of the book (Fig. 21; Table 18).

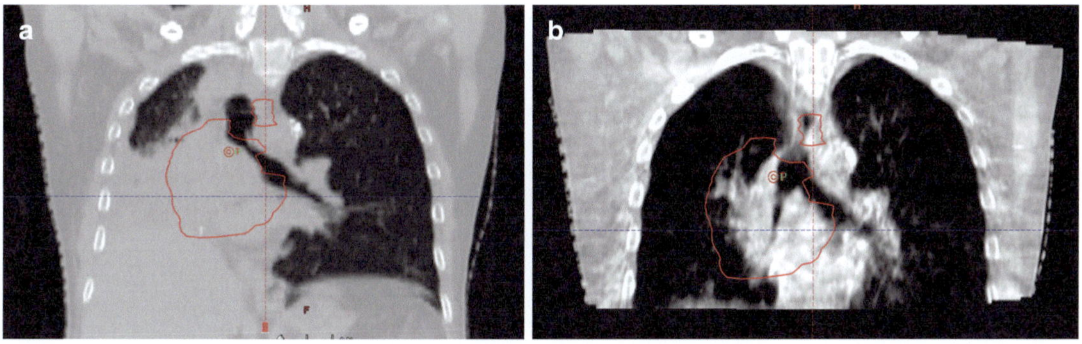

Fig. 21 Two coronal CT chest of a patient of locally advanced NSCLC who presented with obstructive atelectasis. Palliative radiotherapy can often prove beneficial if started early. Panel **a**: Pre radiotherapy. Panel **b**: Post 30 Gy/10 fractions of palliative radiotherapy with good re-expansion of the lung

Table 18 Palliative radiotherapy schedules in lung cancer

Clinical condition	Dose	Dose per fraction	Duration
SVC syndrome or obstruction-induced pneumonia	30 Gy	3 Gy	Two weeks
Bone metastases with a soft tissue mass	20 Gy–30 Gy	4 Gy to 3 Gy	1–2 weeks
Bone metastases without soft tissue mass	8 Gy	Single fraction	1 day
Bone metastases without soft tissue mass	20 Gy	4 Gy	One week
Brain metastases	*20–30 Gy (whole brain) and 18–30 Gy (SRS)*	*5–10 fraction (whole brain) and 1–5 fraction (SRS)*	*1–2 weeks (whole brain) and 1–5 days (SRS)*
Symptomatic chest disease in patients with poor PS	17 Gy	8.5 Gy	One week (2 # 1 week apart)
Recurrent/ unresolving hemoptysis	8 Gy to 20 Gy	8 Gy to 4 Gy	1 day to 1 week
Any metastasis in patients with poor performance status	8 Gy	8 Gy	1 day

7.12 Oligometastatic NSCLC

The concept of oligometastases in NSCLC has gained popularity in recent times owing to improvement in systemic therapy options, better staging modalities, and improved radiation delivery techniques especially SBRT and SRS with minimal toxicity. Approximately 10–15% of patients with NSCLC present with oligometastases during the course of their disease. This issue has been further discussed in the chapter related to metastatic/oligometastatic disease.

Prophylactic cranial irradiation may reduce the incidence of brain metastases, but there is no evidence of a survival benefit and the effect of prophylactic cranial irradiation on quality of life is not known [52, 53].

8 Prognosis, Results, Outcome, and Survival—Summary

Lung cancer has a dismal prognosis. Based on the stage, early lung cancer has a 5-year overall survival (OS) of 60–70% and locally advanced NSCLC of 40–45%. Metastatic NSCLC, depending on the oncogene mutation status, could have a 5-year OS rate of 20–30%, and non-oncogene mutation patients will have <10–15%. Progress in combined modalities and improved diagnostic staging show the increase in median survival: around 60 months for early stage (I, II); 24 months for locally advanced stage (III), and 6 to 12 months for metastatic stage. In the last decade or so, due to advancements in molecular targeted therapy, immune checkpoint inhibitors, and radiation delivery techniques, the survival rate of NSCLC has increased consistently across all stages.

Percepts Box

1. Overall, NSCLC is an aggressive disease with poor outcomes. Most patients present with locally advanced or metastatic disease.
2. Treatment decision in NSCLC is based on some of the following factors histological type, tumor size and location, involvement of pleura, surgical margins, location of lymph nodes by station, tumor grade and lymphovascular invasion
3. Surgery is potentially the most curative therapeutic option for NSCLC
4. Postoperative chemotherapy may provide an additional benefit to patients with resected NSCLC.
5. Radiation therapy combined with chemotherapy is the treatment of choice for locally advanced NSCLC.
6. Radiation therapy has a critical role in early stage NSCLC (SBRT), locally advanced stage (chemoradiation), oligometastatic disease (SBRT to oligomets), and metastatic disease (palliative radiotherapy)
7. Role of PCI in NSCLC is not established
8. The identification of gene mutations in lung cancer has led to the development of molecularly targeted therapy and immune check-point inhibitor (ICI) drugs to improve the survival of subsets of patients with locally advanced and metastatic disease

Multiple Choice Questions

1. The most frequently seen paraneoplastic syndrome in NSCLC
   (a) Hypercalcemia/SIADH
   (b) Lambert-Eaton syndrome
   (c) Polycythemia
   (d) Cushing syndrome
2. A 63-year-old male presents with a 3.4 cm lesion in the right upper lobe on chest x-ray. Further PET scan revealed involvement of ipsilateral hilar lymph node and right sided moderate pleural effusion. What would be the TNM staging of this patient?

(a) T2bN2M0
(b) T2aN1M0
(c) T2aN1M1a
(d) T3N2M1b

3. For an adequate mediastinal staging, how many lymph node stations should be sampled minimally?
(a) 1
(b) 2
(c) 3
(d) 4
4. For a medically inoperable Stage IB NSCLC patient, what mode of treatment would be considered the most appropriate?
(a) SBRT
(b) CTRT
(c) CT alone
(d) None
5. Most common histological variant of NSCLC
(a) Squamous cell carcinoma
(b) Adenocarcinoma
(c) Large cell carcinoma
(d) Adenosquamous carcinoma
6. Most common EGFR mutation in Adenocarcinoma of the lung is?
(a) Exon 19
(b) Exon 20
(c) Exon 21
(d) Both (a) and (c)
7. A 55-year patient presents with a T3N0M0 superior sulcus tumor. What would the preferred mode of treatment?
(a) CRT
(b) NACT followed by surgery
(c) Surgery followed by adjuvant CRT
(d) CRT followed by surgery
8. What is the standard treatment for Stage III NSCLC
(a) Concurrent CRT
(b) NACT followed by surgery followed by adjuvant RT
(c) RT alone
(d) Surgery followed by adjuvant CTRT
9. The AAPM task group report 76 recommends using a motion management technique beyond what range of motion?
(a) 5 mm
(b) 1 cm
(c) 2 mm
(d) 8 mm
10. For adenocarcinoma of the lung, how much is the recommended GTV to CTV expansion"
(a) 3 mm
(b) 5 mm
(c) 8 mm
(d) 6 mm
11. IMRT is preferred over 3DCRT to irradiate lungs. Which parameter among these can best explain this preference?
(a) Improved PFS with IMRT
(b) Improved OS with IMRT
(c) Improved DMFS with IMRT
(d) Decreased incidence of Grade 3 pneumonitis
12. What values of FEV1 and DLCO is needed for the patient to be considered for surgery?
(a) >90%
(b) >60%
(c) >40%
(d) Any value is fine.
13. Most common dose regimen in conventionally fractionated RT
(a) 45–50 Gy
(b) 50–54 Gy
(c) 55–60 Gy
(d) 60–70 Gy
14. All of the following are TKI inhibitors except
(a) Erlotinib
(b) Osimertinib
(c) Crizotinib
(d) Afatinib
15. What is the dose of Durvalumab?
(a) 5 mg/kg
(b) 50 mg/kg
(c) 10 mg/kg
(d) 1 mg/kg

Answer Key

1. (a)
2. (c)
3. (c)
4. (a)
5. (b)

6. (d)
7. (d)
8. (a)
9. (a)
10. (c)
11. (d)
12. (b)
13. (d)
14. (c)
15. (c)

References

1. https://gco.iarc.fr/today/data/factsheets/populations/900-world-fact-sheets.pdf.
2. https://www.who.int/news-room/fact-sheets/detail/cancer.
3. https://pubs.rsna.org/doi/10.1148/rg.346130097.
4. https://gco.iarc.fr/. Last accessed 6 Feb 2023.
5. Noronha V, Pinninti R, Patil VM, Joshi A, Prabhash K. Lung cancer in the Indian subcontinent. South Asian J Cancer. 2016;5(3):95–103.
6. Zhou W, Liu G, Hung RJ, Haycock PC, Aldrich MC, Andrew AS, Arnold SM, Bickeböller H, Bojesen SE, Brennan P, Brunnström H, Melander O, Caporaso NE, Landi MT, Chen C, Goodman GE, Christiani DC, Cox A, Field JK, Johansson M, Kiemeney LA, Lam S, Lazarus P, Le Marchand L, Rennert G, Risch A, Schabath MB, Shete SS, Tardón A, Zienolddiny S, Shen H, Amos CI. Causal relationships between body mass index, smoking, and lung cancer: univariable and multivariable Mendelian randomization. Int J Cancer. 2021;148(5):1077–86.
7. Smoking and health: report of the Advisory Committee to the Public Health Service Surgeon General. Washington: U.S. Department of Health, Education, and Welfare, Public Health Service, Center for Disease Control; 1964. PHS Publication No. 1103.
8. Kurmi OP. Household air pollution, passive smoking, and lung cancer: do we know enough about this conundrum? Am J Respir Crit Care Med. 2022;206(9):1065–7.
9. Hecht SS. Tobacco smoke carcinogens and lung cancer. J Natl Cancer Inst. 1999;91(14):1194–210.
10. Jeon H, Wang S, Song J, Gill H, Cheng H. Update 2025: Management of non-small-cell lung cancer. Lung. 2025;203:53. https://doi.org/10.1007/s00408-025-00801-x.
11. Darling GE, Allen MS, Decker PA, Ballman K, Malthaner RA, Inculet RI. Randomized trial of mediastinal lymph node sampling versus complete lymphadenectomy during pulmonary resection in the patient with N0 or N1 (less than hilar) non-small cell carcinoma: results of the American College of Surgery Oncology Group Z0030 Trial. J Thorac Cardiovasc Surg. 2011;141(3):662–70.
12. Mokhles S, Macbeth F, Treasure T, Younes RN, Rintoul RC, Fiorentino F. Systematic lymphadenectomy versus sampling of ipsilateral mediastinal lymph-nodes during lobectomy for non-small-cell lung cancer: a systematic review of randomized trials and a meta-analysis. Eur J Cardiothorac Surg. 2017;51(6):1149–56. https://doi.org/10.1093/ejcts/ezw439. Erratum in: Eur J Cardiothorac Surg. 2018 Oct 1;54(4):795. PMID: 28158453; PMCID: PMC6095012.
13. Swanson SJ, Herndon JE II, D'Amico TA, Demmy TL, Mc Kenna RJ Jr, Green MR, et al. Video-assisted thoracic surgery lobectomy: report of CALGB 39802—a prospective, multi-institution feasibility study. J Clin Oncol. 2007;25:4993–7.
14. Yan TD, et al. Video-assisted thoracoscopic surgery lobectomy at 20 years: a consensus statement. Eur J Cardiothorac Surg. 2014;45:633–9.
15. Lung Cancer Study Group, Ginsberg RJ, Rubintein LV, et al. Randomized trial of lobectomy versus limited resection for T1N0 non-small-cell lung cancer. Ann Thorac Surg. 1995;60:615–23.
16. Nakamura H, Kawasaki N, Taguchi M, Kabasawa K. Survival following lobectomy vs limited resection for stage I lung cancer: a meta-analysis. Br J Cancer. 2005;92:1033–7.
17. Saji H, Okada M, Tsuboi M, Nakajima R, Suzuki K, Aokage K, Aoki T, Okami J, Yoshino I, Ito H, Okumura N, Yamaguchi M, Ikeda N, Wakabayashi M, Nakamura K, Fukuda H, Nakamura S, Mitsudomi T, Watanabe SI, Asamura H, West Japan Oncology Group and Japan Clinical Oncology Group. Segmentectomy versus lobectomy in small-sized peripheral non-small-cell lung cancer (JCOG0802/WJOG4607L): a multicentre, open-label, phase 3, randomised, controlled, non-inferiority trial. Lancet. 2022;399(10335):1607–17.
18. Nasser A, Xiaofei W, David K, Colleen W, Rodney L, Dennis W, Jeffrey P, Jones David R, Massimo C, Ashrafi Ahmad S, Moishe L, Kazuhiro Y, Stephen Y, Mitchell John D, Harvey P, Robert K, Thomas B, Daniel M, Kohman Leslie J, Stinchcombe Thomas E, Everett V. Lobar or sublobar resection for peripheral stage IA non-small-cell lung cancer. N Engl J Med. 2023;388:489–98.
19. Douillard JY, Rosell R, De Lena M, Carpagnano F, Ramlau R, Gonzáles-Larriba JL, Grodzki T, Pereira JR, Le Groumellec A, Lorusso V, Clary C, Torres AJ, Dahabreh J, Souquet PJ, Astudillo J, Fournel P, Artal-Cortes A, Jassem J, Koubkova L, His P, Riggi M, Hurteloup P. Adjuvant vinorelbine plus cisplatin versus observation in patients with completely resected stage IB-IIIA non-small-cell lung cancer (Adjuvant Navelbine International Trialist Association [ANITA]): a randomized controlled trial. Lancet Oncol. 2006;7(9):719–27.

20. Arriagada R, Dunant A, Pignon JP, Bergman B, Chabowski M, Grunenwald D, Kozlowski M, Le Péchoux C, Pirker R, Pinel MI, Tarayre M, Le Chevalier T. Long-term results of the international adjuvant lung cancer trial evaluating adjuvant Cisplatin-based chemotherapy in resected lung cancer. J Clin Oncol. 2010;28(1):35–42.
21. Strauss GM, Herndon JE 2nd, Maddaus MA, Johnstone DW, Johnson EA, Harpole DH, Gillenwater HH, Watson DM, Sugarbaker DJ, Schilsky RL, Vokes EE, Green MR. Adjuvant Paclitaxel plus carboplatin compared with observation in stage I.B. non-small-cell lung cancer: CALGB 9633 with the Cancer and Leukemia Group B, Radiation Therapy Oncology Group, and North Central Cancer Treatment Group Study Groups. J Clin Oncol. 2008;26(31):5043–51.
22. Pignon JP, Tribodet H, Scagliotti GV, Douillard JY, Shepherd FA, Stephens RJ, Dunant A, Torri V, Rosell R, Seymour L, Spiro SG, Rolland E, Fossati R, Aubert D, Ding K, Waller D, Le Chevalier T, LACE Collaborative Group. Lung adjuvant cisplatin evaluation: a pooled analysis by the LACE Collaborative Group. J Clin Oncol. 2008;26(21):3552–9.
23. Forde PM, Spicer J, Lu S, Provencio M, Mitsudomi T, Awad MM, Felip E, Broderick SR, Brahmer JR, Swanson SJ, Kerr K, Wang C, Ciuleanu TE, Saylors GB, Tanaka F, Ito H, Chen KN, Liberman M, Vokes EE, Taube JM, Dorange C, Cai J, Fiore J, Jarkowski A, Balli D, Sausen M, Pandya D, Calvet CY, Girard N, CheckMate 816 Investigators. Neoadjuvant nivolumab plus chemotherapy in resectable lung cancer. N Engl J Med. 2022;386(21):1973–85.
24. Wu YL, Tsuboi M, He J, John T, Grohe C, Majem M, Goldman JW, ADAURA Investigators, et al. Osimertinib in resected *EGFR*-mutated non-small-cell lung cancer. N Engl J Med. 2020;383(18):1711–23.
25. Tsuboi M, Weder W, Escriu C, Blakely C, He J, Dacic S, Yatabe Y, Zeng L, Walding A, Chaft JE. Neoadjuvant osimertinib with/without chemotherapy versus chemotherapy alone for *EGFR*-mutated resectable non-small-cell lung cancer: NeoADAURA. Future Oncol. 2021;17(31):4045–55.
26. Felip E, Altorki N, Zhou C, Csőszi T, Vynnychenko I, Goloborodko O, Luft A, Akopov A, Martinez-Marti A, Kenmotsu H, Chen YM, Chella A, Sugawara S, Voong D, Wu F, Yi J, Deng Y, McCleland M, Bennett E, Gitlitz B, Wakelee H, IMpower010 Investigators. Adjuvant atezolizumab after adjuvant chemotherapy in resected stage IB-IIIA non-small-cell lung cancer (IMpower010): a randomized, multicentre, open-label, phase 3 trial. Lancet. 2021;398(10308):1344–57.
27. Aupérin A, Le Péchoux C, Rolland E, Curran WJ, Furuse K, Fournel P, Belderbos J, Clamon G, Ulutin HC, Paulus R, Yamanaka T, Bozonnat MC, Uitterhoeve A, Wang X, Stewart L, Arriagada R, Burdett S, Pignon JP. Meta-analysis of concomitant versus sequential radiochemotherapy in locally advanced non-small-cell lung cancer. J Clin Oncol. 2010;28(13):2181–90.
28. Lin TY, Atrchian S, Humer M, Siever J, Lin A. Clinical outcomes of Pancoast tumors treated with trimodality therapy. J Thorac Dis. 2021;13(6):3529–38.
29. Barnes JB, Johnson SB, Dahiya RS, Temes RT, Herman TS, Thomas CR Jr. Concomitant weekly cisplatin and thoracic radiotherapy for Pancoast lung tumors: pilot experience of the San Antonio Cancer Institute. Am J Clin Oncol. 2002;25(1):90–2.
30. Albain KS, Swann RS, Rusch VW, Turrisi AT 3rd, Shepherd FA, Smith C, Chen Y, Livingston RB, Feins RH, Gandara DR, Fry WA, Darling G, Johnson DH, Green MR, Miller RC, Ley J, Sause WT, Cox JD. Radiotherapy plus chemotherapy with or without surgical resection for stage III non-small-cell lung cancer: phase III randomized controlled trial. Lancet. 2009;374(9687):379–86.
31. Eberhardt WE, Pöttgen C, Gauler TC, Friedel G, Veit S, Heinrich V, Welter S, Budach W, Spengler W, Kimmich M, Fischer B, Schmidberger H, De Ruysscher D, Belka C, Cordes S, Hepp R, Lütke-Brintrup D, Lehmann N, Schuler M, Jöckel KH, Stamatis G, Stuschke M. Phase III study of surgery versus definitive concurrent chemoradiotherapy boost in patients with resectable stage IIIA(N2) and selected IIIB non-small-cell lung cancer after induction chemotherapy and concurrent chemoradiotherapy (ESPATUE). J Clin Oncol. 2015;33(35):4194–201.
32. Thomas M, Rube C, Hoffknecht P, Macha HN, Freitag L, Linder A, et al. Effect of preoperative chemoradiation in addition to preoperative chemotherapy: a randomized trial in stage III non-small-cell lung cancer. Lancet Oncol. 2008;9:636–48.
33. Postoperative radiotherapy in non-small-cell lung cancer: systematic review and meta-analysis of individual patient data from nine randomised controlled trials. PORT Meta-analysis Trialists Group. Lancet. 1998;352(9124):257–63.
34. Le Pechoux C, Pourel N, Barlesi F, Lerouge D, Antoni D, Lamezec B, et al. Postoperative radiotherapy versus no postoperative radiotherapy in patients with completely resected non-small-cell lung cancer and proven mediastinal N2 involvement (Lung ART): an open-label, randomized, phase 3 trial. Lancet Oncol. 2022;23(1):104–14.
35. Hui Z, Men Y, Hu C, Kang J, Sun X, Bi N, Zhou Z, et al. Effect of postoperative radiotherapy for patients with pIIIA-N2 non-small cell lung cancer after complete resection and adjuvant chemotherapy: the phase 3 PORT-C randomized clinical trial. JAMA Oncol. 2021;7(8):1178–85.
36. Felip E, Rosell R, Maestre JA, Rodríguez-Paniagua JM, Morán T, Astudillo J, Spanish Lung Cancer Group, et al. Preoperative chemotherapy plus surgery versus surgery plus adjuvant chemotherapy versus surgery alone in early-stage non-small-cell lung cancer. J Clin Oncol. 2010;28:3138–45.
37. Rosell R, Gómez-Codina J, Camps C, Maestre J, Padille J, Cantó A, et al. A randomized trial comparing preoperative chemotherapy plus surgery with sur-

gery alone in patients with non-small-cell lung cancer. N Engl J Med. 1994;330:153–8.
38. Roth JA, Fossella F, Komaki R, Ryan MB, Putnam JB Jr, Lee JS, et al. A randomized trial comparing perioperative chemotherapy and surgery with surgery alone in resectable stage IIIA non-small-cell lung cancer. J Natl Cancer Inst. 1994;86:673–80.
39. Bradley JD, Paulus R, Komaki R, Masters G, Blumenschein G, Schild S, Bogart J, Hu C, Forster K, Magliocco A, Kavadi V, Garces YI, Narayan S, Iyengar P, Robinson C, Wynn RB, Koprowski C, Meng J, Beitler J, Gaur R, Curran W Jr, Choy H. Standard-dose versus high-dose conformal radiotherapy with concurrent and consolidation carboplatin plus Paclitaxel with or without cetuximab for patients with stage IIIA or IIIB non-small-cell lung cancer (RTOG 0617): a randomized, two-by-two factorial phase 3 study. Lancet Oncol. 2015;16(2):187–99.
40. Karam SD, Horne ZD, Hong RL, McRae D, Duhamel D, Nasr NM. Dose escalation with stereotactic body radiation therapy boost for locally advanced non-small cell lung cancer. Radiat Oncol. 2013;8:179.
41. Saunders M, Dische S, Barrett A, Harvey A, Gibson D, Parmar M. Continuous hyperfractionated accelerated radiotherapy (CHART) versus conventional radiotherapy in non-small-cell lung cancer: a randomized multicentre trial. CHART Steering Committee. Lancet. 1997;350(9072):161–5.
42. Baumann M, Herrmann T, Koch R, Matthiessen W, Appold S, Wahlers B, CHARTWEL-Bronchus Study Group. Final results of the randomized phase III CHARTWEL-trial (ARO 97-1) comparing hyper fractionated-accelerated versus conventionally fractionated radiotherapy in non-small cell lung cancer (NSCLC). Radiother Oncol. 2011;100(1):76–85.
43. Maguire J, Khan I, McMenemin R, O'Rourke N, McNee S, Kelly V, Peedell C, Snee M. SOCCAR: a randomised phase II trial comparing sequential versus concurrent chemotherapy and radical hypofractionated radiotherapy in patients with inoperable stage III non-small cell lung cancer and good performance status. Eur J Cancer. 2014;50(17):2939–49.
44. Keall PJ, et al. The management of respiratory motion in radiation oncology report of AAPM Task Group 76. Med Phys. 2006;33:3874–900.
45. Giraud P, Antoine M, Larrouy A, Milleron B, Callard P, De Rycke Y, et al. Evaluation of microscopic tumor extension in non-small-cell lung cancer for three-dimensional conformal radiotherapy planning. Int J Radiat Oncol Biol Phys. 2000;48:1015–24.
46. Liu MB, et al. Clinical impact of dose overestimation by effective path length calculation in stereotactic ablative radiation therapy of lung tumors. Pract Radiat Oncol. 2013;3:294–300.
47. Socinski MA, Özgüroğlu M, Villegas A, Daniel D, Vicente D, Murakami S, Hui R, Gray JE, Park K, Vincent M, Mann H, Newton M, Dennis PA, Antonia SJ. Durvalumab after concurrent chemoradiotherapy in elderly patients with unresectable stage III non-small-cell lung cancer (PACIFIC). Clin Lung Cancer. 2021;22(6):549–61.
48. Wu YL, Cheng Y, Zhou X, Lee KH, Nakagawa K, Niho S, Tsuji F, Linke R, Rosell R, Corral J, Migliorino MR, Pluzanski A, Sbar EI, Wang T, White JL, Nadanaciva S, Sandin R, Mok TS. Dacomitinib versus Gefitinib as first-line treatment for patients with EGFR-mutation-positive non-small-cell lung cancer (ARCHER 1050): a randomized, open-label, phase 3 trial. Lancet Oncol. 2017;18(11):1454–66. https://doi.org/10.1016/S1470-2045(17)30608-3.
49. Reck M, Rodríguez-Abreu D, Robinson AG, Hui R, Csőszi T, Fülöp A, Gottfried M, Peled N, Tafreshi A, Cuffe S, O'Brien M, Rao S, Hotta K, Leiby MA, Lubiniecki GM, Shentu Y, Rangwala R, Brahmer JR, KEYNOTE-024 Investigators. Pembrolizumab versus chemotherapy for PD-L1-positive non-small-cell lung cancer. N Engl J Med. 2016;375(19):1823–33.
50. Borghaei H, Gettinger S, Vokes EE, Chow LQM, Burgio MA, de Castro CJ, Pluzanski A, Arrieta O, Frontera OA, Chiari R, Butts C, Wójcik-Tomaszewska J, Coudert B, Garassino MC, Ready N, Felip E, García MA, Waterhouse D, Domine M, Barlesi F, Antonia S, Wohlleber M, Gerber DE, Czyzewicz G, Spigel DR, Crino L, Eberhardt WEE, Li A, Marimuthu S, Brahmer J. Five-year outcomes from the randomized, phase III trials checkmate 017 and 057: nivolumab versus docetaxel in previously treated non-small-cell lung cancer. J Clin Oncol. 2021;39(7):723–33.
51. Herbst RS, Garon EB, Kim DW, Cho BC, Gervais R, Perez-Gracia JL, Han JY, Majem M, Forster MD, Monnet I, Novello S, Gubens MA, Boyer M, Su WC, Samkari A, Jensen EH, Kobie J, Piperdi B, Baas P. Five year survival update from KEYNOTE-010: pembrolizumab versus docetaxel for previously treated, programmed death-ligand 1-positive advanced NSCLC. J Thorac Oncol. 2021;16(10):1718–32.
52. Lester JF, MacBeth FR, Coles B. Prophylactic cranial irradiation for preventing brain metastases in patients undergoing radical treatment for non-small-cell lung cancer: a Cochrane Review. Int J Radiat Oncol Biol Phys. 2005;63(3):690–4.
53. Pöttgen C, Eberhardt W, Grannass A, et al. Prophylactic cranial irradiation in operable stage IIIA non small-cell lung cancer treated with neoadjuvant chemoradiotherapy: results from a German multicenter randomized trial. J Clin Oncol. 2007;25(31):4987–92.
54. Nestle U, De Ruysscher D, Ricardi U, Geets X, Belderbos J, Pöttgen C. ESTRO ACROP guidelines for target volume definition in the treatment of locally advanced non-small cell lung cancer. Radiother Oncol. 2018;127(1):1–5.

Online Links

https://econtour.org/references (Contouring guidelines for various body sites)

http://eqd2.com/ (EQD2 calculator)

https://www.mdcalc.com/calc/2157/gap-index-idiopathic-pulmonary-fibrosis-ipf-mortality (Calculating mortality in idiopathic pulmonary fibrosis)

https://www.youtube.com/watch?v=6TXUYm-OQhTk&t=137s (SBRT lung)

https://www.youtube.com/watch?v=6TXUYm-OQhTk&t=137s (Panel discussion early lung cancer)

Small Cell Lung Cancer

Prabhat Singh Malik, Sindhura Chitikela,
and Soumyajit Roy

1 Introduction

Small cell lung cancer (SCLC) is a highly aggressive malignancy with dismal outcomes, representing around 15% of all lung cancers. It occurs almost exclusively in smokers and is characterized by rapid cellular proliferation, genomic instability, high tumor mutation burden, and a higher propensity for distant metastasis. It originates from neuroendocrine cells in the bronchial epithelium and almost always shows functional loss of tumor suppressor genes TP53 and RB1. Patients present with a short duration of illness and rapidly progressing symptoms. Up to 70% of patients present with distant metastasis at diagnosis, with common sites being the lung, brain, liver, adrenal, and bone. SCLC is characterized by high platinum sensitivity; however, responses are short-lived. The addition of immune checkpoint inhibitors to platinum-based chemotherapy has improved survival, though modestly. With recent advances in gene expression profiling and transcriptomics, various molecular subtypes of SCLC have been identified, which are opening up newer therapeutic avenues.

P. S. Malik (✉) · S. Chitikela
Department of Medical Oncology, Dr B.R.A. Institute Rotary Cancer Hospital, All India Institute of Medical Sciences, New Delhi, India

S. Roy
Radiation Oncology, UH Seidman Cancer Center, Case Western Reserve University, Cleveland, OH, USA

2 Epidemiological Aspects and Risk Factors

Lung cancer is the second most common cancer and the most common cause of cancer mortality worldwide, according to the GLOBOCAN 2020. SCLC constitutes around 15% of all lung cancers. The incidence of SCLC has been decreasing over 3 decades [1]. SCLC was predominant in males; however, narrowing of the gap between males and females has been observed with an increase in females with SCLC, possibly attributable to smoking in females.

Cigarette smoking is one strong risk factor for the occurrence of SCLC. More than 90% of cases of SCLC occur in current or former smokers who are commonly heavy smokers. Two percent of cases of SCLC arise in never smokers. It was previously reported that current smokers had a higher risk of SCLC compared to that of former smokers [2]. A meta-analysis reported the highest association of smoking with SCLC compared to other histological types of lung cancer, with an odds ratio (OR) of 72.5 for current smokers [3].

Other possible risk factors of SCLC in never smokers explored were air pollution, radon exposure, and prior chronic pulmonary diseases like chronic obstructive pulmonary disease [4, 5]. Genetic susceptibility is also known to contribute to the occurrence of SCLC [6]. A proportion of SCLC occurs secondary to the histological transformation of EGFR-mutated non-small cell lung cancer to SCLC.

B. K. Mohanti et al. (eds.), *Radiation Oncology – Principles, Precepts and Practice*,
https://doi.org/10.1007/978-981-95-5171-2_7

3 Clinical Symptoms and Signs

The most common presentation includes a hilar mass with bulky mediastinal lymphadenopathy with or without distant metastasis. Patients present with a short duration of illness, usually less than 3 months, with rapidly progressing symptoms. Approximately 70% of patients present with metastases at diagnosis [7]. Symptoms can either be due to intrathoracic disease or as a result of metastases to the brain, liver, bone, and paraneoplastic syndromes. Usual symptoms include cough, dyspnea, chest pain, weight loss, swelling of the face, neck, and upper limbs as a result of compression of the superior vena cava, dysphagia, and hoarseness of voice. Patients with metastases can present with bone pain, jaundice, altered sensorium, neurological deficits, seizures, and other systemic symptoms. SCLC is frequently associated with paraneoplastic syndromes as a result of aberrant immune upregulation, causing remote effects associated with he malignancy. Endocrine paraneoplastic syndromes include the syndrome of inappropriate anti-diuretic hormone (SIADH), Cushing syndrome, hypoglycemia, hyperglycemia, and hypercalcemia. Paraneoplastic neurological syndromes (PNSs) include sensory neuropathy, Lambert-Eaton syndrome, encephalomyelitis, dermatomyositis, opsoclonus myoclonus, etc. Some of the causative onconeural antibodies for PNSs are identified, such as Anti-Hu, Anti-Ri, Anti-CAR, Anti-amphiphysin, Anti-CV2. Table 1 summarizes various paraneoplastic syndromes associated with SCLC.

Mohan et al. have reported that more than half of the patients (57%) have a high symptom burden (>5 symptoms) at the time of presentation. Symptom burden generally correlates with overall survival in SCLC [8].

Table 1 Paraneoplastic syndromes associated with SCLC

Type	Mediator	Incidence	Clinical features	Laboratory features and diagnosis
Endocrine				
SIADH (syndrome of inappropriate ADH secretion)	ADH (anti-diuretic hormone)	15%	Falls, lethargy, altered sensorium, seizures	Hyponatremia Increased urine osmolality
Cushing syndrome	ACTH	5%	Edema, abdominal striae, central obesity, edema	Hypokalemia, hypertension, elevated ACTH on dexamethasone suppression test
Neurological				
Lambert-Eaton myasthenic syndrome	Anti-voltage-gated calcium channels	1–3%	Weakness, fatigue that improves with activity	
Encephalitis	Anti-Hu	<1%	Seizures, mood changes, hallucinations	Antibodies in serum
Sensory neuronopathy	Anti-Hu	<1%	Subacute, asymmetric paresthesias, more in upper limbs	CSF pleocytosis, increased protein, and antibodies in serum
Cerebellar degeneration	Anti-Hu Anti-Yo Anti-Ri Anti-CAR	<1%	Limb and gait ataxia, dysarthria, nystagmus, and mental status changes	Antibodies in serum
Opsoclonus-myoclonus	Anti-Hu Anti-Ri	<1%	Involuntary rapid eye movements Multifocal myoclonus	Antibodies in serum
Stiff person syndrome	Anti-amphiphysin	<1%	Mood changes, increased tone	Antibodies in serum

4 Pathology

SCLC is a high-grade neuroendocrine carcinoma. Various neuroendocrine tumors of the lung, as per the WHO classification 2021, include (also summarized in Table 2)

1. Diffuse idiopathic neuroendocrine cell hyperplasia
2. Typical carcinoid
3. Atypical carcinoid
4. Large cell neuroendocrine carcinoma
5. Small cell neuroendocrine carcinoma

Small cell neuroendocrine carcinoma includes two subtypes, pure SCLC (80%) and combined SCLC (20%). Diagnosis of SCLC is primarily based upon light microscopy findings of small round blue cell tumors with sparse cytoplasm and finely dispersed chromatin without distinct nucleoli. SCLC can coexist with other non-small cell histologies like squamous cell carcinoma, adenocarcinoma, and large cell carcinoma, and is considered a combined SCLC irrespective of the percentage of the non-small cell component. Large cell neuroendocrine carcinoma may co-exist with SCLC in approximately 4–16% of all SCLCs, and due to overlapping morphological features, large cell component should constitute at least 10% of tumor tissue to be considered a combined type SCLC. Small cell transformation may also be observed in EGFR mutation-positive adenocarcinoma after treatment with tyrosine kinase inhibitors.

Table 2 Pathological classification of neuroendocrine tumors of lung

Tumor histology	Histopathology criteria
Diffuse idiopathic neuroendocrine cell hyperplasia	Multifocal hyperplasia of neuroendocrine cells in the bronchiolar epithelium, associated with multiple carcinoid tumorlets <5 mm
Typical carcinoid	Carcinoid morphology with <2 mitoses/10 hpf No necrosis and >0.5 cm
Atypical carcinoid	Carcinoid morphology with 2–10 mitoses/10 hpf or necrosis (punctuate)
Large cell neuroendocrine carcinoma	Neuroendocrine morphology High mitotic rate >10/10 hpf Necrosis Large cell size, abundant cytoplasm, low NC ration, vesicular fine chromatin
Small cell neuroendocrine carcinoma	Small-sized cells with scant cytoplasm and finely granular chromatin, absent or faint nucleoli High mitotic rate >11 mitoses/10 hpf Frequent necrosis

On immunohistochemistry, tumor cells are usually immune-positive for cytokeratin, thyroid transcription factor 1 (TTF1), and other markers of neuroendocrine and neural differentiation, which include synaptophysin, chromogranin, CD56 or neural cell adhesion molecule, and neuron-specific enolase (NSE).

5 Pathogenesis and Genomic Abnormalities

Mutation profiling reveals that SCLC exhibits a characteristic smoking signature, suggesting tobacco-related carcinogenesis for the development of SCLC. SCLC arises from pulmonary neuroendocrine cells. The neuroendocrine or non-neuroendocrine fate of pluripotent progenitor cells is primarily regulated by ASCL1 and NOTCH. NOTCH is inhibited by smoking and eventually leads to upregulation of ASCL1, which directs the neuroendocrine differentiation.

SCLC genome exhibits a high mutational burden. It is characterized by near-universal loss of dual tumor suppressor genes TP53 and RB1 in almost 90% of cases. A subset of tumors is characterized by MYC gene alterations in up to 20%. Other genetic alterations found in SCLC involve PTEN, NOTCH, CREBBP, and KMT2D.

The genomic landscape doesn't define a specific classification in SCLC. However, more recently, based on the predominant expression of transcription factors, 4 different biologically distinct transcriptomic subtypes of SCLC have been identified, namely SCLC A (high ASCL1 expression), SCLC N (high NEUROD1 expression), SCLC P (high POU2F3 expression) and SCLC I (inflamed subtype) that lacks expression of ASCL1, NEUROD1, and POU2F3 transcription factors. SCLC I tumors are characterized by epithelial-mesenchymal transition, higher immune cell infiltration, immune checkpoints, and thereby their sensitivity to immunotherapy [9]. Further, based on this transcriptomic classification, various therapeutic vulnerabilities of individual subtypes are being proposed. Based on preclinical studies, SCLC A tumors were identified to be sensitive to BLC2 inhibitors, SCLC N to Aurora kinase inhibitors, and SCLC P to PARP inhibitors [10]. This classification might open up new avenues of targeted therapy in SCLC.

6 Integrated Management Plan, Including Diagnostic Tests, Staging

Since SCLC is a high-grade, aggressive malignancy, a timely diagnostic and staging workup is crucial and has to be done as soon as possible. Diagnosis relies on biopsy (preferred) or cytology from the lung mass showing characteristic light microscopy findings and confirmation by immunohistochemistry (Table 3).

Given the common presentation of SCLC with central tumors and bulky mediastinal lymph nodes, biopsies are often obtained by bronchoscopy. Alternatively, a transthoracic biopsy from the mediastinal mass can be attempted. Biopsy from a metastatic lesion can also be considered in case of poor accessibility to the primary lesion.

Table 3 Diagnosis and staging workup

Clinical assessment
History and physical examination
Smoking history
History of comorbidities
Assessment for paraneoplastic syndromes
Laboratory investigations
Hemogram with peripheral smear
Liver and kidney function tests
Serum LDH
Serum electrolytes
Blood glucose
Staging
Contrast-enhanced CT chest abdomen with bone scintigraphy or PET/CT
Contrast-enhanced MRI brain
Bone marrow aspirate and biopsy if abnormal blood counts or leucoerythroblastic picture or presence of nucleated RBCs on peripheral smear
Tumor biopsy
Bronchoscopy or transthoracic
Pulmonary function tests
FEV1, FVC, DLCO in patients who are candidates for radiation or surgery

In addition to clinical assessment, routine laboratory investigations and workup should include imaging of the chest and systemic imaging with contrast-enhanced CT and bone scintigraphy or a whole-body FDG PET/CT. Contrast-enhanced MRI brain is recommended for the assessment of brain metastases. In case of abnormal blood counts or presence of nucleated RBCs or leukoerythroblastic picture, bone marrow aspiration and biopsy are to be performed to rule out involvement by metastasis.

The role of PET CT in SCLC is controversial. In a systematic review and meta-analysis of 9 studies, a change in staging was observed in 15% of patients, and it did not reflect in the survival of patients irrespective of the modality used [10]. The same holds true as per the data on the role of PET CT from the recently reported CONVERT trial [11]. However, FDG PET CT had a higher sensitivity for detecting bone metastases of 87% compared to 37% with bone scintigraphy. FDG PET CT has no role in the detection of brain metastases [10, 11].

Assessment of circulating tumor cells and/or circulating tumor DNA (ctDNA) in SCLC is still investigational. They might have a prognostic value and also would be useful in understanding the genomic evolution and intratumoral heterogeneity [12].

7 Staging

Two systems are used in clinical practice for the staging of SCLC [13].

1. AJCC 8th edition Tumor node metastasis (TNM) staging for lung cancer
2. Veterans Administration Lung Study Group (VALSG) divides SCLC into limited and extensive-stage SCLC
   2.1. Limited stage SCLC constitutes a tumor confined to one hemithorax and can be encompassed in a single radiation port, without malignant pleural and pericardial effusion

2.2. Extensive stage SCLC constitutes a disease not meeting the criteria for limited-stage. This includes distant metastases, malignant pleural or pericardial effusion, contralateral supraclavicular and contralateral hilar lymph node

TNM staging provides precise anatomical characteristics and nodal involvement, thereby being useful in formulating prognostic information. Though the TNM system is the preferred staging system, VALSG staging is still the most widely used staging system in routine clinical practice and clinical trials, as it primarily decides the patient's candidacy for definitive chemoradiation or systemic therapy.

8 Integrated Treatment Plan

Treatment of SCLC mainly involves a multidisciplinary approach, with assessment by a pulmonologist, radiation oncologist, medical oncologist, and palliative medicine physician. Once the diagnosis of SCLC is made and staging ascertained, treatment depends on the performance status of the patients and fitness for therapy. The algorithm detailed below depicts the flow of treatment of SCLC as per the stage (Figs. 1 and 2).

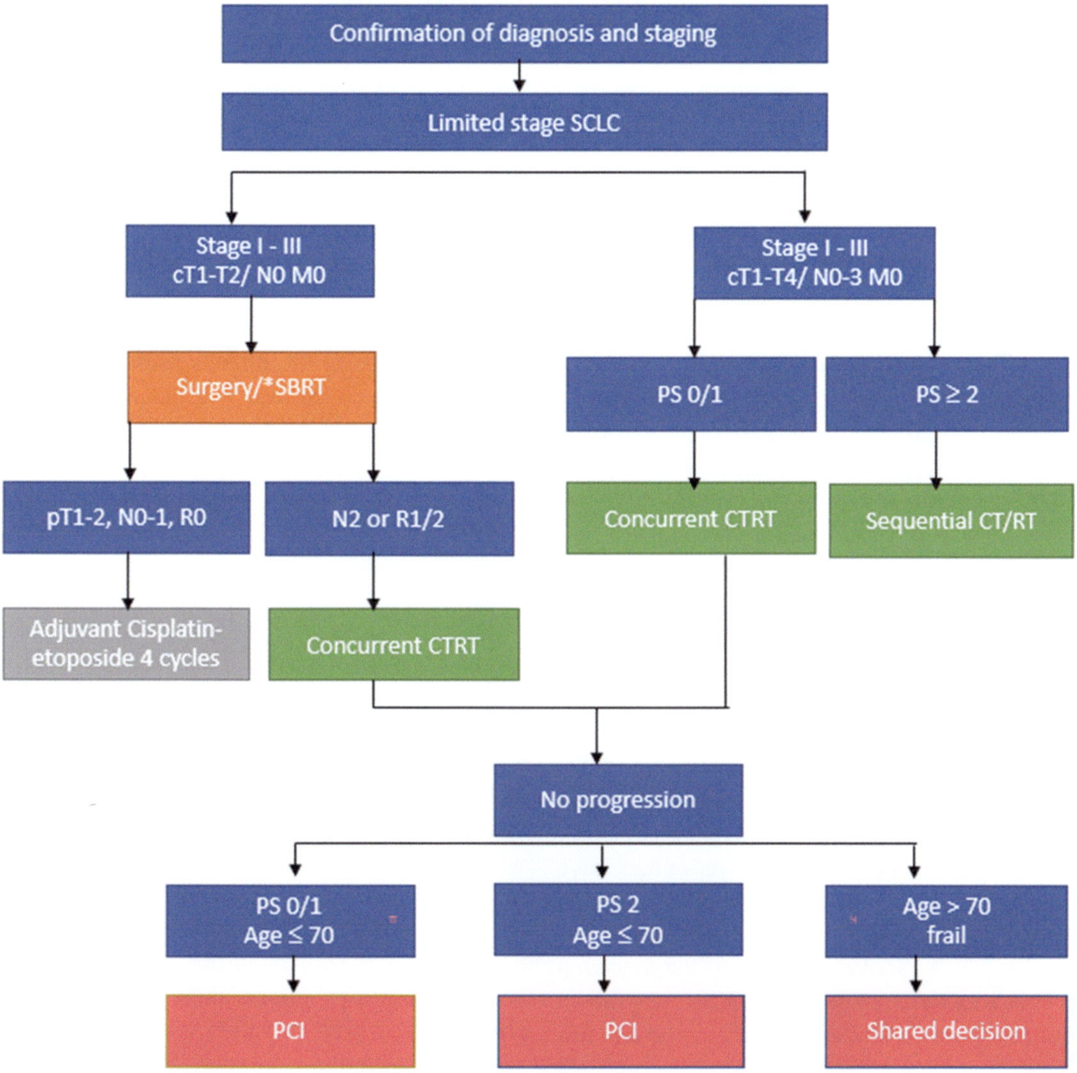

Fig. 1 Limited stage SCLC—management workflow

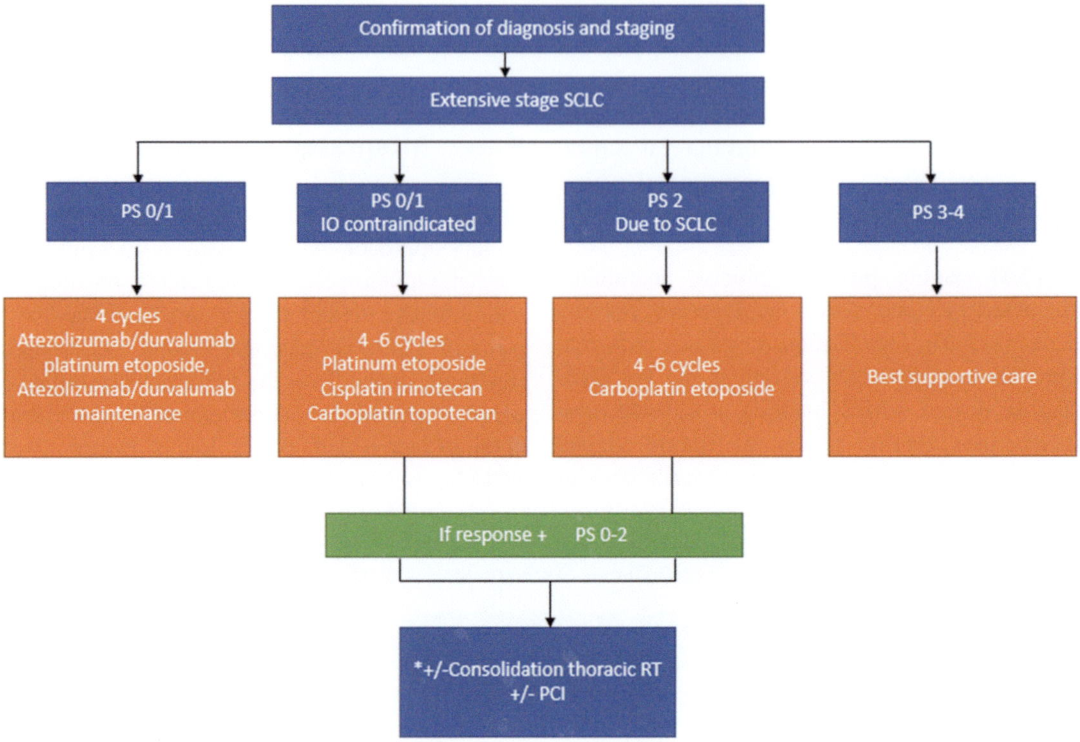

Fig. 2 Extensive stage SCLC—management workflow

9 Surgical Aspects

The role of surgery in SCLC is limited to patients with smaller tumors, stage I disease with T1–T2, node-negative tumors, with no evidence of distant metastases. These patients account for less than 5% of SCLC. Treatment mainly involves resection of the primary by lobectomy with mediastinal lymph node dissection, followed by adjuvant chemotherapy. Adjuvant RT can be considered in cases of N2 disease or margin-positive disease.

Surgery and chemoradiation have been evaluated as treatment modalities for treating stage I SCLC. However, no prospective trials are comparing the two. Few retrospective studies have shown that outcomes were better in patients treated with a surgical approach over chemoradiotherapy. A study comparing surgery and chemoradiation in stage I–IIIA SCLC has shown that lobectomy with adjuvant chemotherapy has resulted in significantly longer survival of 48 months versus 28 months with concurrent chemoradiation in patients with stage I, II SCLC, with higher benefit in stage I tumors [14]. In a report from the IASLC project, 5-year overall survival with surgery in stage I SCLC was reported to be around 48% while other studies reported 5-year survival of around 25–36% with chemoradiation [15].

Surgery alone in early-stage SCLC had resulted in poor outcomes. There are no randomized controlled trials that evaluated the role of adjuvant chemotherapy. A retrospective study of a population-based cohort of 1574 patients, with pT1-T2 N0 SCLC, revealed that adjuvant chemotherapy with or without radiation was associated with improved 5-year survival compared to that of surgery alone (53% versus 40%) and a median overall survival of 66 versus 42 months. On further analysis, it was found that the use of adjuvant chemotherapy alone and the use of adjuvant chemotherapy with radiation to the brain were associated with improved survival, and no difference was observed in patients with adjuvant chemotherapy with thoracic radiation [16].

Adjuvant thoracic radiation was associated with better 5-year overall survival in patients with pathologic N2 disease (29% versus 19%), but not in patients with node-negative or N1 disease [17]. Hence, adjuvant RT is recommended in patients with either N2 disease or margin-positive post-resection.

10 Systemic Therapy Aspects

10.1 Chemotherapy

Chemotherapy is an important aspect of treatment in all stages of SCLC. Various chemotherapeutic agents active in SCLC include platinum compounds (cisplatin, carboplatin), camptothecins (irinotecan, topotecan), podophyllotoxins (etoposide), taxanes (paclitaxel, docetaxel), vinca alkaloids (vinorelbine), alkylating agents (cyclophosphamide, ifosfamide, temozolomide), and anthracyclines (doxorubicin, epirubicin, amrubicin). Etoposide-cisplatin (EP) is the regimen of choice for the treatment of SCLC. In patients who are not candidates for cisplatin, carboplatin etoposide can be considered. Other chemotherapy regimens evaluated in limited-stage SCLC include cyclophosphamide, doxorubicin/epirubicin, vincristine (CAV/CEV), EP alternating CAV, and cisplatin irinotecan. However, EP remained the regimen of choice over decades because of high response rates of up to 80%, ease of combining with concurrent radiation, and better tolerability with less myelotoxicity and mucositis compared to CAV [18]. EP, when compared to CEV in a phase 3 randomized controlled trial, showed that EP resulted in better survival of 14.5 months versus 9.7 months in the CEV arm in limited-stage SCLC. There was no significant difference in survival between the two arms in extensive-stage SCLC [19]. A survival benefit with cisplatin-based regimens over other alkylator-based regimens was also reported in a meta-analysis [20].

Carboplatin can be substituted in place of cisplatin in cisplatin-ineligible patients. Overall response rates, progression-free survival, and overall survival were reported to be similar with cisplatin or carboplatin-containing regimens, with higher hematological toxicity with carboplatin and non-hematological toxicities like nephrotoxicity, metabolic abnormalities with cisplatin. A meta-analysis comparing cisplatin-based versus carboplatin-based regimens in SCLC has reported that there is no difference in efficacy between cisplatin and carboplatin, but there are differences in the toxicity profile [21].

The combination of irinotecan with cisplatin was extensively studied in both limited-stage and extensive-stage SCLC. Irinotecan cisplatin was compared to cisplatin etoposide in limited-stage SCLC in two randomized controlled trials. JCOG02020 was a phase 3 trial that evaluated the role of consolidation with either irinotecan plus cisplatin or etoposide plus cisplatin in patients treated with induction cisplatin etoposide and accelerated hyperfractionated RT and reported no difference in overall survival between the two regimens [22]. Another trial JCOG1205/1206, evaluated irinotecan-cisplatin combination in completely resected stage I–III high-grade neuroendocrine carcinoma of the lung. This trial reported similar 3-year recurrence-free survival as that of cisplatin etoposide of up to 65%. Overall, grade 3/4 adverse events were common in the cisplatin etoposide arm, with febrile neutropenia in 20% versus 4% in the irinotecan cisplatin arm; however, grade 3/4 diarrhea was common in the irinotecan cisplatin arm (8% versus 1%) [23].

Several trials have evaluated the role of platinum irinotecan combination in extensive stage SCLC. JCOG9511 was a randomized controlled trial that evaluated cisplatin etoposide versus cisplatin irinotecan. Higher response rates of 84% versus 68%, with longer median survival (12.8 months versus 9.4 months) were reported in irinotecan-based arm compared to cisplatin etoposide. Irinotecan platinum resulted in higher grade 3 /4 diarrhea (17% versus 0%) and lesser neutropenia (65% versus 92%) compared to cisplatin etoposide arm [24]. However, other trials did replicate these results and showed similar response rates and survival with irinotecan-based regimens [25–27]. In SWOGS0124, which randomized 671 patients with extensive stage SCLC, median progression-free survival, overall survival as well as response rates were all similar in the irinotecan and etoposide arms, with similar toxicity profiles [27].

10.2 Systemic Therapy in Limited-Stage SCLC (LS-SCLC)

Cisplatin-based chemotherapy with concurrent thoracic radiation is the standard of care for limited-stage SCLC. Concurrent chemoradiation resulted in better overall survival and intrathoracic tumor control when compared to chemotherapy alone. In a meta-analysis of trials, concurrent chemoradiation resulted in a 3-year overall survival of 14.3% vs 8.9% with chemotherapy alone [28]. Cisplatin etoposide is the preferred chemotherapy regimen of choice.

The addition of paclitaxel to cisplatin etoposide in limited stage SCLC either sequentially or concurrently with RT has been evaluated; however, it did not consistently result in improved outcomes at the cost of increased mucositis, esophagitis, and neutropenia [29–32]. The use of bevacizumab with concurrent chemoradiation had increased the formation of tracheoesophageal fistulae, resulting in early termination of clinical trials [33].

10.3 Systemic Therapy in Extensive Stage SCLC (ES-SCLC)

Chemotherapy with cisplatin/carboplatin etoposide is the mainstay treatment of extensive stage SCLC. Four to six cycles of chemotherapy are usually administered. Immunotherapy (atezolizumab or durvalumab), when added to chemotherapy, had resulted in an additional benefit. Thoracic radiation and prophylactic cranial irradiation may be considered in patients who respond to chemotherapy, as discussed in the earlier section.

Objective response rates with systemic chemotherapy are around 40–70% including complete response rates of 10%. Unfortunately, the responses to chemotherapy are short-lived, leading to early relapses. Various other intensification approaches, like the addition of bevacizumab, ifosfamide, and palifosfamide, have been tried to improve outcomes in extensive stage SCLC; however, none of the approaches have superseded the platinum etoposide combination, which has remained the standard of care chemotherapy over the last 4 decades.

The role of bevacizumab was evaluated in two randomized controlled trials IFCT 0802 and SALUTE. None of them reported an increase in overall survival with the addition of bevacizumab to chemotherapy [34, 35].

Recent studies have shown benefit in outcomes of extensive stage SCLC with the use of immune checkpoint inhibitors. Atezolizumab and durvalumab, anti-PDL1 antibodies, when combined with platinum etoposide combination chemotherapy during induction and continued as maintenance till progression, have resulted in improved progression-free survival and overall survival over chemotherapy alone in extensive stage SCLC in recent phase 3 trials.

IMPOWER133 was a phase 3 randomized controlled trial, which evaluated atezolizumab plus carboplatin and etoposide in patients with treatment naïve extensive stage SCLC against carboplatin etoposide and placebo. Overall response rates were similar in both groups with longer progression-free survival in atezolizumab arm of 5.2 months vs 4.3 months in the placebo arm (HR 0.77) and longer overall survival of 12.3 months in the atezolizumab arm of 12.3 months compared to 10.3 months (HR 0.70), 18-month overall survival of 34% vs 21%, irrespective of PDL1 status. Similar rates of toxicities were observed in both groups with grade 3 toxicities observed up to 58% in each arm [36].

Similarly, CASPIAN, a phase 3 randomized controlled trial evaluated the role of durvalumab plus platinum etoposide chemotherapy in the treatment-naive extensive stage SCLC. Patients were randomly assigned to one of the 3 study groups, durvalumab plus chemotherapy, durvalumab plus chemotherapy, and tremelimumab and chemotherapy. Durvalumab was continued as maintenance till progression. Patients in the durvalumab plus platinum etoposide arm had better overall response rates of 68% vs 58%, better progression-free survival, 2 yr progression-free survival of 11% vs 2.9% with chemotherapy alone (HR 0.80), and also a better overall survival of 12.9 months vs 10.5 months with chemotherapy [37]. The addition of tremelimumab, an anti-CTLA4 inhibitor, did not result in any additional benefit in response rates or survival, but rather had increased toxicity [38].

Pembrolizumab with platinum etoposide in treatment naïve extensive stage SCLC was evaluated in a phase 2 trial and resulted in improved progression-free survival 12 month progression-free survival of 13.6% versus 3.1% in comparison with chemotherapy, however, did not result in significant improvement in overall survival [39].

10.4 Systemic Therapy for Refractory and Relapsed Disease

Relapse SCLC is generally considered a chemo-refractory disease, unlike treatment naïve SCLC. It is postulated that the Wnt signaling pathway confers chemoresistance in relapse SCLC [40].

Patients who relapse more than 6 months after completion of chemotherapy are still considered to be platinum sensitive, and rechallenging with the same platinum combination may be considered. Most of the data of reinduction with primary platinum-based regimen comes from retrospective series, which showed an improvement in progression-free survival over non-rechallenge group [41]. A phase 3 randomized controlled trial evaluated the superiority of carboplatin etoposide over single-agent topotecan in patients with SCLC who relapsed after 90 days of completion of chemotherapy. Patients who received platinum combination chemotherapy had a longer median progression-free survival of 4.7 months versus 2.7 months with topotecan (HR 0.57). There was a higher risk of neutropenia, febrile neutropenia, and thrombocytopenia with topotecan compared to carboplatin etoposide combination [42].

If patients relapse within 6 months of completion of chemotherapy or progress on first-line therapy, it is considered to be resistant or refractory disease and requires further lines of chemotherapy. Response rates to various second-line regimens are modest (around 10%).

Lurbinectedin, an alkylating agent and a selective inhibitor of oncogenic transcription, is approved for the treatment of relapsed or refractory SCLC. It was evaluated in a single-arm phase 2 study in which patients with SCLC after the failure of platinum-based chemotherapy were recruited. It resulted in an overall response rate of 35%, with a median duration of response of 5 months. Responses and survival outcomes were better in platinum-sensitive relapse compared to resistant relapse (44 vs 22% and 4.5 months vs 2.6 months, respectively) [43]. The role of lurbinectedin in patients with brain metastases remains questionable.

Single agent topotecan was evaluated in comparison to best supportive care or cyclophosphamide doxorubicin vincristine (CAV) chemotherapy and has shown to result in response rates of 10–20% and a median overall survival of 25 weeks [44, 45]. Both intravenous and oral forms are approved for the second-line treatment of SCLC.

Single-agent irinotecan is another option in relapsed SCLC. In single arm phase 2 studies, response rates of around 16% were observed in overall cohort patients, 4% in resistant relapse compared to 35% in platinum-sensitive disease. Cardinal toxicities of irinotecan include diarrhea and neutropenia.

Other options include single agent paclitaxel, which resulted in response rates of up to 20–30% when used as third line therapy, however, with short-lasting responses [46]. Paclitaxel carboplatin combination was also evaluated in patients with relapsed SCLC, which resulted in a response rate of 33% and a disease control rate of 65%, with a median progression-free survival of 4 months and a median overall survival of 8.7 months [47].

Response rates with single agent vinorelbine, temozolomide, gemcitabine have been reported to be around 10–20% [48–50]. Temozolomide showed better intracranial response rates of 38% in patients with brain metastases [48].

Rovalpituzumab tesirine (Rova T), an antibody drug conjugate, that binds to delta-like protein (DLL3), a NOTCH ligand, that is highly expressed in SCLC tumor cells was evaluated in a phase 1 study and showed an overall response rate of 18% which rose to 39% in tumors with DLL3 expression of ≥50% [51]. TRINITY is a phase 2 study that evaluated the role of Rova T in relapsed SCLC, post at least 2 lines of therapy which showed an overall response rate of 12.4% and a median overall survival of 5.7 months [52].

With progress in molecular subtyping of SCLC, the current focus is on targetable genomic alterations which are so far been lacking. The role of PARP inhibitors and aurora kinase inhibitors is being explored (NCT04728230).

In patients with poor performance status, management should focus primarily on symptoms palliation and supportive care. Patients with poor performance due to a high disease burden may still be treated with chemotherapy along with supportive care.

11 Radiation Therapy for Limited-Stage SCLC

11.1 Stereotactic Body Radiation Therapy in SCLC

With the advent of low dose computed tomographic technology, there has been a significant rise in the screening-detected early-stage lung cancer of whom about 10% belong to the small cell category [53]. Currently, surgery has a limited role in the management of early-stage small cell lung cancer (SCLC). Stereotactic body radiation therapy (SBRT) is an effective modality of definitive management for these patients, especially those who are inoperable. In a multi-institutional study of SBRT in early SCLC, 3-year local control, disease-specific survival, and overall survival rates were 96.1%, 64.4%, and 34%, respectively with about 5% incidence of grade 2 or higher pneumonitis [54]. A majority (45.8% of the recurrences) of the patients had a distant failure which was also one of the important findings from a systematic review by Rathod et al. [55]. Based on such patterns of failure, SBRT followed by adjuvant systemic therapy could be a viable treatment option for early (T1-T2bN0) SCLC. However, the use of SBRT should be practiced with caution for patients with "ultra central" tumors, which includes tumors whose planning target volume directly contacts or overlaps the proximal bronchial tree, trachea, and mainstem bronchus, esophagus, pulmonary vein, or pulmonary artery. The propensity for lymph node metastases is higher with central versus peripheral lesions, and ultra central tumors that often encroach on mediastinal structures, which increases the risk of toxicity with SBRT [56].

11.2 Evidence for Combining Radiation Therapy with Chemotherapy in Limited-Stage Small Cell Lung Cancer

The combination of radiation therapy with chemotherapy remains the standard of care for limited stage SCLC. In a meta-analysis of 11 randomized controlled trials, Warde et al. showed a significant improvement in local control (47% vs. 24%) with the combination of chemotherapy and radiation therapy in limited-stage SCLC [57]. Combined modality treatment conferred a 5.4% improvement in 2-yr overall survival (20% vs. 15%). Patients with age less than 60 years had maximum benefit from combined modality therapy. There was no significant difference in treatment-related death. In another meta-analysis of 2140 patients with limited stage SCLC there was a 14% relative reduction in the risk of mortality with the addition of radiation therapy to chemotherapy [28]. Absolute overall survival benefit was 5.4% (14.3% vs. 8.9%) at 3 years with younger patients (age <55 years) deriving higher benefit from the combined modality therapy compared to patients with age more than 70 years.

11.3 Relative Sequencing of Chemotherapy and Radiation Therapy in Limited Stage Small Cell Lung Cancer

Concurrent chemoradiation therapy is the standard of care management for medically fit patients with limited-stage SCLC. Historically, there were some controversies concerning the sequencing of chemotherapy and thoracic radiation therapy (TRT) in these patients. Three randomized trials demonstrated a benefit of early initiation of radiation therapy [58–60] while three other trials failed to show any benefit of early radiation therapy [61–63] (Table 4). Subsequently, two meta-analyses from De Ruysscher et al. provided robust evidence in favor of concurrent chemoradiation therapy in limited stage SCLC. According to a meta-analysis published in 2006, the time between the first day of systemic therapy to the end of TRT (SER) should be <30 days. In this meta-analysis of 4 randomized controlled trials, 5-year overall survival was superior in shorter (<30 days) vs. longer SER arms (relative risk [RR]: 0.62, 95% confidence intervals [CI]: 0.49–0.80, $p = 0.0003$). Each week's extension of SER beyond that of the study arm with the shortest SER resulted in a 1.83% absolute decrease in the 5-year overall survival rate. Shorter SER portended a higher incidence of severe esophagitis (RR: 0.55, 95% CI: 0.42–0.73, $p < 0.0001$) [64]. In a second meta-analysis of 7 randomized controlled trials from 2006, 5-year overall survival was superior with early addition of TRT (odds ratio [OR] for 5-year overall survival: 0.64; 95% CI: 0.44–0.92, $p = 0.02$) in patients who received platinum-based chemotherapy [65]. Considering studies with an overall treatment time of TRT of less than 30 days, the 5-year survival (OR: 0.56, 95% CI: 0.37–0.85; $p = 0.006$) was significantly higher with the early addition of TRT. However, this effect was not evident for 2-year overall survival (OR: 0.70, 95% CI: 0.46–1.06), and neither was any favorable effect of early TRT on local control (OR: 0.68; 95% CI: 0.40–1.17). Early TRT was associated with a 50% relative increase in the odds of severe esophagitis (OR: 1.50; 95% CI: 1.03–2.20) and 95% relative increase in the odds of severe pneumonitis (OR: 1.95; 95% CI: 0.96–3.94).

Subsequently, in a more contemporary meta-analysis published in 2016 by De Ruysscher, individual patient data of 2668 patients from 12 randomized controlled trials were included [66]. However, 2305 patients from 9 randomized controlled trials were evaluable. Earlier or shorter radiation therapy was associated with a 21% relative reduction in the risk of mortality (HR: 0.79; 95% CI: 0.69–0.91) when compliance with chemotherapy regimens was similar in both arms. In contrast, shorter or earlier TRT was associated with a 19% relative increase in the risk of mortality (HR: 1.19, 95% CI: 1.05–1.34) when there was a difference in compliance with chemotherapy between the two regimens. The interaction of treatment effect on overall survival and compliance to chemotherapy was highly significant ($p < 0.0001$). Earlier or shorter TRT extended the 5-year mean survival time by 4.2 months (95% CI: 1.8–6.7, absolute measures: 28.9 vs. 24.7 months) for trials with similar compliance while reducing the 5-year mean survival time by 3.1 months (95% CI: 1.3–4.9, absolute measures: 17.5 vs. 20.6 months) in trials with differing compliance to chemotherapy between the two sequencing regimens. Earlier or shorter TRT resulted in a significantly higher risk of severe neutropenia (OR: 1.54, 95% CI: 1.19–2.00), esophagitis (OR: 1.93; 95% CI: 1.45–2.56), and cardiac toxicities (OR: 3.12; 95% CI: 1.46–6.68), respectively. Although there was evidence of a higher risk of pneumonitis with earlier or shorter TRT (OR: 1.50, 95% CI: 0.86–2.62), this did not reach the conventional level of statistical significance ($p = 0.16$).

Early use of both modalities leads to more accurate radiation therapy planning and shorter overall treatment time, however, at the cost of

Table 4 Studies that investigated the timing of radiation therapy and chemotherapy in limited-stage SCLC

Author	Treatment arms	Progression-free survival	Overall survival	Toxicity
Murray [58]	TRT (40 Gy in 15 fractions) with C1 of chemotherapy (wk 3) Vs. TRT after 3 cycles of CAV and 3 cycles of EP (wk 15)	Median: 15.4 mo vs. 11.8 mo ($p = 0.036$)	Median: 21.2 mo vs. 16.0 mo ($p = 0.008$)	Early TRT was associated with higher and more severe anemia, esophagitis, and dermatitis
Jeremic [59]	EP + TRT (54 Gy in 36 fractions over 18 days) f/b 4 cycles of EP Vs. 2 cycles of EP f/b TRT followed by 2 cycles of EP[a]	3-year LRFS: 73% vs. 61% ($p = 0.011$) 3-year DMFS: 56% vs. 57% ($p = 0.48$)	Median: 34 vs. 26 mo ($p = 0.052$)	Acute grade ≥3 esophagitis rate 29% vs. 25% Late grade ≥3 esophagitis in one patient in each arm Late grade ≥3 bronchopulmonary toxicity in 1 patient of early TRT arm
Takada [60]	TRT (45 Gy in 30 fractions over 15 days) with concurrent EP (day 2 of C1) Vs. Induction EP × 4 f/b TRT[a]	Superior progression-free survival rate in the concurrent arm ($p = 0.08$)	Median: 27.2 mo vs. 19.7 mo ($p = 0.097$)	More severe myelosuppression in the concurrent arm (grade ≥3; 88% vs. 54%, $p < 0.001$) Grade ≥3 esophagitis in 9% vs. 4% patients ($p = 0.17$) Overall, 3 and 4 treatment related deaths in the concurrent and sequential arm, respectively.
Perry [61]	TRT (50 Gy in 25 fractions/5 wks) on day 1 of C1 Vs. TRT on day 64 (C4) Vs. Chemotherapy alone[a, b]	Median time to failure: 11 vs. 11.2 vs. 8.7 mo ($p = 0.0004$)[c]	13.0 vs. 14.5 vs. 13.6 mo ($p = 0.007$)[c]	
Spiro [62]	TRT (40 Gy in 15 fractions) with C2 (CAV alternating with EP) Vs. TRT with C6 (CAV alternating with EP)[a]	10.6 vs. 11.3 mo ($p = 0.17$)	Median: 13.7 vs. 15.1 mo ($p = 0.23$)	Higher rates of nonhematological toxicities in the concurrent arm (39% vs. 23%, $p = 0.001$) Grade ≥3 esophagitis in 8% vs. 3% patients No difference in hematological toxicities
Sun [63]	TRT (52.5 Gy over 25 fractions over 5 weeks) with C1 of EP Vs. TRT with C3 of EP	Median: 12.4 vs. 11.2 mo ($p = 0.60$)	Median 24.1 vs. 26.8 mo ($p = 0.69$)	Grade ≥3 esophagitis in 3.6% ($n = 4$) vs. 0.9% ($n = 1$) patients Grade ≥3 pneumonitis in 4.5% ($n = 5$) vs. 2.8% ($n = 3$) patients Febrile neutropenia was higher in the early TRT arm (21.6% vs. 10.2%, $p = 0.02$)

TRT Thoracic radiation therapy, *C* Cycle, *CAV* Cyclophosphamide + Adriamycin + Vincristine, *EP* Etoposide + Cisplatin, *wk* week, *mo* months, *EP* Etoposide + Cisplatin, *LRFS* Local recurrence-free survival, *DMFS* Distant metastasis-free survival

[a]All responders received PCI

[b]Chemotherapy regimen included Cyclophosphamide + Vincristine + Etoposide, which was later replaced by Adriamycin

[c]Both median overall survival and time to clinical failure were worse in arm III than I + II (SS) but could not demonstrate whether arm I or II was superior

higher treatment complications such as higher risk of esophagitis, pneumonitis, and myelosuppression. It is recommended to start the radiation therapy with the first or second cycle of chemotherapy in patients who are fit enough to tolerate TRT concurrently with systemic therapy. However, in patients with poor performance status or those who are at a higher risk of treatment-induced toxicities, sequential chemoradiation therapy could be offered instead of concomitant chemoradiation therapy.

11.4 Time-Dose-Fraction Schedule for Thoracic Radiation Therapy in Limited Stage Small Cell Lung Cancer

The standard dose of TRT for small cell lung cancer is 45 Gy in 30 fractions over 3 weeks at 1.5 Gy per fraction twice daily (at least 6 hours apart). This is based on results from the landmark phase III randomized controlled study by Turrisi et al. [67]. In this study, 417 patients were treated with concurrent chemoradiation therapy using one of the following two regimens—45 Gy in 25 fractions over 5 weeks vs. 45 Gy in 30 fractions over 3 weeks at 1.5 Gy twice daily. Fields were taken off the spinal cord at 36 Gy. Patients with complete response (CR) received PCI 25 Gy/10 fractions. At a median follow-up of 8 years, there was a 10% improvement (26% vs. 16%) in the 5-year overall survival, 16% (36% vs. 52%) improvement in rates of local failure, and 5% improvement (29% vs. 24%) in the 2-year failure-free survival with twice-daily regimen. Although the twice-daily TRT regimen resulted in a more than two-fold increase in grade 3 or higher esophagitis rates (27% vs. 11%), there was no difference between the groups concerning the incidence of grade 4 esophagitis, and there were no reports of permanent stricture due to the acute esophagitis. It is noteworthy that there was a 60–70% risk of esophagitis with twice-daily regimen in the subgroup of patients aged >70. Therefore, the twice-daily regimen should be used with caution in these patients.

In another phase III randomized controlled study (CONVERT) with a superiority design, the authors randomized patients to 66 Gy of TRT in 33 fractions over 6.5 weeks or 45 Gy in 30 fractions over 3 weeks at 1.5 Gy per fraction twice daily [68]. Radiotherapy commenced on day 1 of cycle 2 of chemotherapy. The authors designed this study with the hypothesis that once-daily regimen would result in a 12% higher overall survival at 2 years compared to the twice-daily regimen. Compliance rates with chemotherapy were 91% in the twice-daily group and 88% in the once-daily group. More patients received the full dose of radiotherapy in the twice-daily group (98% twice-daily vs 83% once-daily; $p < 0.0001$). Overall survival at 2 years was 56% in the twice-daily group and 51% in the once-daily group (absolute difference between the treatment groups 5.3% [95% CI: −3.2–13.7%]). Overall survival at 5 years was 34% in the twice-daily group and 31% in the once-daily group (absolute difference 2.8% [95% CI: −6.4–12.0%]). Significantly more grade 4 neutropenia was noted in the twice-daily group than in the once-daily group (49% vs 38%; $p = 0.05$), although there was no difference in the rates of grade 3 or higher febrile neutropenia. Acute grade 3 or higher esophagitis rates were 18% and 19% in the two arms, respectively. Overall, 4 patients in the once-daily group developed grade 3 esophagitis. Six patients in each group developed grade 3–4 pneumonitis, while 3 and 2 patients in the twice-daily group and once-daily group developed grade 3 pulmonary fibrosis. Due to the superiority study design, it is impossible to conclude if the 66 Gy once-daily regimen is non-inferior to 45 Gy.

Another phase III randomized controlled trial, CALGB 30610/RTOG 0538 trial compared 45 Gy in 30 fractions (twice-daily) with 70 Gy in 35 fractions (once-daily) and 61.2 Gy (28.8 Gy in 16 fractions [one fraction per day] followed by 32.4 Gy in 18 fractions [two fractions per day]). The results have only been presented as abstract forms [69]. Planned discontinuation of the 61.2 Gy arm was done based on interim toxicity analysis, with patients then randomized 1:1 in the two remaining arms. TRT was given starting with either the 1st or 2nd (of 4 total) chemotherapy cycles. After an approximate median follow-up of 3 years, there was no significant between-arm difference in overall survival (median for once-daily vs. twice-daily: 30.5 vs. 28.7 months, HR: 0.94; 95% CI: 0.76–1.20) or progression-free survival (HR: 0.96; 95% CI: 0.78–1.18), respectively. Most grade 3+ hematologic and non-hematologic adverse events (AEs) were similar between cohorts.

Based on these studies and based on the recent American Society of Radiation Oncology (ASTRO guideline), once-daily regimen could be used in patients for whom twice-daily regimen is not feasible for logistical reasons, or in whom there is an increased risk of grade 4 neutropenia [70]. Based on this evidence, the current NRG RTOG phase II/III trial (LU005; NCT03811002) allows both the TRT regimens as the standard of care as part of their trial investigating the role of atezolizumab in conjunction with chemoradiation therapy.

In a recent phase II randomized controlled trial, 45 Gy in 30 fractions at 1.5 Gy per fraction twice-daily regimen was tested against a higher dose regimen of 60 Gy in 40 fractions at 1.5 Gy per fraction twice daily [71]. TRT is started approximately 3–4 weeks after the first day of the first cycle of platinum and etoposide. The target volume included primary tumor and PET-avid nodes. Responders were offered prophylactic cranial irradiation of 25–30 Gy. At a median follow-up of 4 years, there was a substantial improvement in 2-year overall survival (74.2% vs. 48.1%, OR: 3.09 [95% CI: 1.62–5.89]). Common grade 3 or higher adverse events were mainly related to myelosuppression and esophagitis (21% in the high-dose group vs. 18% in the low-dose group). Both treatment regimens had similar numbers of serious adverse events (55 vs. 56) and treatment-related deaths (3 vs. 3). However, this regimen needs further investigation before integration into routine clinical practice.

11.5 Target Volume of Thoracic Radiation Therapy in Limited-Stage Small-Cell Lung Cancer

When sequential chemoradiation therapy is used, the inclusion of post-chemotherapy residual tumor as the target volume does not lead to any compromise in local control or survival. This was initially shown in the SWOG study [72]. In this study, 191 patients with partial response or stable disease after induction chemotherapy were randomly assigned to pre-chemotherapy large field vs. post-chemotherapy small field TRT. There was no difference in the median survival (51 weeks vs. 46 weeks from registration for maintenance) and duration of remission (31 vs. 30 weeks). Myelosuppression was higher in patients treated with a larger field, but no difference was noted in the incidence of radiation pneumonitis. This has been confirmed in the contemporary Chinese study by Hu et al., which randomized 309 patients to pre-chemotherapy vs. post-chemotherapy target volume after 2 cycles of induction chemotherapy using cisplatin and etoposide [73]. Lymph node regions originally involved before induction chemotherapy were included as a nodal CTV for both arms, even if there was complete resolution of the nodes after induction chemotherapy. After a median follow-up of 54 months for the surviving patients, 5-year overall survival was 22.8% vs. 28.1% for patients treated with post-chemotherapy vs. pre-chemotherapy target volumes, respectively. Similarly, there was no difference in the 3-year local or regional progression-free survival between the two regimens. Based on these trials, for patients undergoing TRT after cycle 1 of chemotherapy, it is often recommended to include the craniocaudal extent of the pre-chemotherapy target volume, but the target can be reduced in all other directions based on the response to chemotherapy. PET-avid lymph nodes at baseline should be included in the target volume. However, there is no additional benefit of elective nodal radiation in SCLC if PET/CT has been used as part of the initial staging evaluation [74]. A four-dimensional computed tomography scan with respiratory gating is preferable for radiation therapy simulation purposes. If free breathing is used, additional motion management techniques should be considered. Intravenous contrast is preferred, and a pre-chemotherapy PET scan should be registered with the planning CT scan to guide target delineation. Approximately 5 mm expansion around the internal target volume is provided to generate the clinical target volume. The clinical target volume to planning target volume expansion is usually guided by the institutional policy. However, at least 4 mm radial and 5–7 mm craniocaudal margin should be used.

11.6 Evidence for Combining Thoracic Radiation Therapy with Chemotherapy in Extensive-Stage Small-Cell Lung Cancer

Patients with extensive stage SCLC (ES-SCLC) have a poor prognosis with a median overall survival of 8–13 months [24, 75]. Palliative chemotherapy for four to six cycles was the standard treatment for this group of patients until the recent studies (IMPower133 and CASPIAN) showed an almost 30% reduction in the hazard of death with the addition of atezolizumab or durvalumab [19, 36, 38, 76].

Several trials have assessed whether the addition of thoracic radiotherapy (TRT) might improve outcomes. One of them was a small single-arm study with 33 patients who received chest radiation therapy (40 Gy in 15 fractions) with PCI (25 Gy in 10 fractions) simultaneously 4–8 weeks after completion of chemotherapy. Target volume included the post-chemotherapy residual chest disease plus a margin. Chest recurrence took place in 16 patients, of whom seven were in-field and five were symptomatic [77]. Jeremic et al. found a small but statistically significant benefit in terms of overall survival by adding TRT to complete responders after chemotherapy [78], and these results were later confirmed by Giuliani et al. [79] and Palma et al. in a meta-analysis [80]. Another recent randomized controlled study (CREST) by Slotman et al. showed that the addition of TRT (30 Gy in 10 fractions) in patients with any response after 4–6 cycles of chemotherapy improves overall survival by 10% (13% [95% CI: 9–19] vs. 3% [95% CI: 2–8]) at 2 years. Of note, the primary endpoint of this study was 1-year overall survival, which was not significantly different between the two groups (33% [95% CI: 27–39] vs. 28% [95% CI: 22–34]) [81]. RTOG 0937 randomized patients with extensive stage SCLC with 4 or fewer sites of metastases to consolidative TRT and PCI after complete or partial response to chemotherapy vs. PCI alone after chemotherapy. PCI consisted of 25 Gy in 10 fractions. TRT consisted of 45 Gy in 15 fractions to the post-chemotherapy volumes, including the site of the primary and involved nodal regions at diagnosis. Metastases were treated if they did not have a complete response to chemotherapy. If normal tissue dose constraints were unable to be met with this dose, dose reduction to 30–40 Gy was allowed. Although the trial showed some benefit in terms of time to progression (53.3% vs. 14.5% at 3 months and 79.6% vs. 75% at 12 months); there was no difference in the 1-year overall survival (60.1% for PCI vs. 50.8% for PCI + TRT, HR: 1.44; 95% CI: 0.82–2.53) between the two groups. Of note, the absolute rates of 1-year overall survival were significantly high in the two groups and exceeded what was predicted at the time of designing the study. There were numerically higher rates of grade 3 or higher toxicity in the PCI + TRT arm (36% vs. 23%, $p = 0.24$). There was one death attributed to protocol therapy, and the patient had radiation-induced pneumonitis. One could hypothesize that the TRT arm suffered from non-cancer-specific deaths secondary to cardiopulmonary toxicities from high-dose TRT, which abrogated the difference in overall survival between the two groups.

Although the IMpower 133 trial did not allow TRT, approximately 80–85% of patients had locoregional disease burden and only 2.5% of patients on the atezolizumab arm experienced a complete response [36]. Therefore, there is a scope for maximizing the response by adding TRT in these patients. Additionally, TRT might enhance the effect of immunotherapy in these patients. Although the immunogenic action of radiation therapy has been shown in preclinical models, this needs to be proven under specific clinical scenarios [82–84]. To conclude, TRT to a total dose of 30–40 Gy in 10–15 fractions has been proven to be beneficial in patients with extensive stage SCLC and should be considered in patients with a high burden of loco-regional disease despite being treated with immunotherapy. However, the sequencing and dose of TRT in the era of chemo-immunotherapy remain to be answered from ongoing and future clinical trials (NCT03043599; NCT04462276; NCT04402788; NCT04636762; NCT04951115).

11.7 Role of Prophylactic Cranial Radiation Therapy in Small Cell Lung Cancer

SCLC has a propensity to develop early metastasis, and the brain is the most common site of metastasis with a cumulative incidence of 50% at 2 years. Extrapolating outcomes from pediatric acute lymphoblastic leukemia, investigators encouraged the use of prophylactic cranial irradiation (PCI), intending to attain sterilization within the CNS, a sanctuary site for SCLC. The overarching goal was to improve overall survival and quality of life metrics.

No randomized trial has ever demonstrated any benefit of PCI in limited-stage SCLC. A meta-analysis of seven randomized controlled trials (n = 987) by Auperin et al. showed a 16% reduction in the risk of mortality (RR: 0.84, 95% CI: 0.73–0.97) by use of PCI. Absolute reduction in the mortality was 5.4% at 3 years. A higher dose of PCI was associated with a greater decrease in the risk of brain metastasis (8 Gy, 24–5 Gy, 30 Gy, and 36–40 Gy; p-value for trend = 0.02). However, there was no difference in overall survival among the various time-dose-fraction schedules. The interpretation of the findings merits caution in light of high variability in the criteria for entry, treatment, and assessment of patients enrolled in these studies. Furthermore, in the era when these trials were conducted, no patient had a CNS evaluation by MRI. A proportion of patients in the meta-analysis were from the pre-CT era, when the only method of CNS evaluation was pneumoencephalography. In a single institutional study of 481 patients, the prevalence of brain metastases in the CT era was 10% versus 24% in the MRI era. All of those in the CT era were symptomatic, whereas approximately one-half of those detected by MRI were asymptomatic [85]. Therefore, the benefit of PCI potentially originated from the treatment of disease that would now clearly be recognized and treated with whole brain radiotherapy or stereotactic radiosurgery, whereas patients without evidence of disease could be spared PCI [86]. Overall stage migration with the use of PET/CT is also an important consideration that questions the results of the Auperin meta-analysis in the present era. For example, in a Korean study, there was a significant reduction in the risk of intracranial metastasis (13.3% vs. 37.0%, p = 0.020) in the subgroup of patients who were not staged using PET/CT while there was no evidence of benefit (34.3% vs. 41.1%, p = 0.24) in patients who were staged initially using PET/CT [87]. Finally, with the advent of low-dose CT screening, more patients are being diagnosed with stage I or II SCLC who are at less risk of CNS metastasis [88, 89]. Therefore, the relative benefit of PCI in this patient population remains questionable.

Two randomized trials investigated the role of PCI in extensive-stage SCLC [90, 91]. The contrasting findings between the two trials could be attributed to several factors. In contradistinction to the EORTC study, all patients in the Japanese study underwent MRI brain as part of baseline staging and had regular follow-up CNS imaging with MRI, while brain imaging was not part of standard staging and follow-up procedures in the EORTC study unless there were symptoms indicative of intracranial metastasis [90, 91]. An additional important factor that could explain the conflicting results is the use of second-line chemotherapy in more than 4/5th of patients in both treatment groups in the Japanese study, which could have stretched the overall survival in both groups and potentially narrowed any difference in overall survival between the control and study groups, respectively. In a nutshell, both studies provide important information on two different study populations within the overall domain of extensive-stage SCLC. One additional concern of PCI is radiation-induced toxicities, although none of the studies showed any significant change in cognitive functioning. In the Japanese study, PCI was not associated with any change in the mini-mental status examinations. In the EORTC study, PCI was associated with increased severity of fatigue, anorexia, and nausea for up to 3 months. However, there was no substantial difference in the global health status, emotional, and cognitive functioning. With the advent of hippocampal sparing techniques and concurrent use of memantine, there has been a significant improvement in the therapeutic index of PCI [92, 93].

In the NRG CC001 trial, 518 patients with brain metastasis were randomized to whole brain radiation therapy (WBRT) with memantine versus whole brain radiation therapy with hippocampal avoidance (HA-WBRT) using intensity modulation in conjunction with memantine. HA-WBRT resulted in a 26% relative reduction in the risk of cognitive failure (adjusted HR: 0.74; 95% CI: 0.58–0.95, $p = 0.02$). This difference could be attributed to less deterioration in executive function at 4 months (23.3% v 40.4%; $p = 0.01$) and learning and memory at 6 months (11.5% v 24.7% [$p = 0.049$] and 16.4% v 33.3% [$p = 0.02$], respectively). Additionally, HA-WBRT with memantine resulted in less fatigue, less difficulty with remembering things, and less difficulty with speaking at 6 months relative to WBRT with memantine [92].

In the PREMER study, 150 patients with SCLC were randomized to PCI vs. HA-PCI (dose: 25 Gy in 10 fractions over 2 weeks). Overall, 71.3% of patients had limited-stage SCLC. The primary objective was the delayed free recall using the Free and Cued Selective Reminding Test (FCSRT) at 3 months. A decrease of 3 points or greater from baseline was considered a decline in this study. After a median follow-up of 40.4 months, the decline in delayed free recall from baseline to 3 months was substantially lower in the HA-PCI arm (5.8% vs. 23.5%, OR: 5.00, 95% CI: 1.57–15.86). There was no significant difference in cumulative incidence of brain metastases at 2 years between the HA-PCI vs. PCI groups (22.8% [95% CI: 14.1–32.9] vs. 17.7% [95% CI, 10.0–27.3]), respectively. Only one patient with extensive SCLC in the HA-PCI arm had an isolated brain metastasis in the dentate gyrus, which was salvaged using SRS. Acknowledging the limitation of missing data over long term, HA-PCI was associated with less decline in total recall at 24 months (relative to baseline) compared to PCI (47.6% vs. 14.2%, $p = 0.019$) [93].

Based on these results from various randomized controlled trials, it is undeniable that PCI (especially with use of hippocampal avoidance) might be beneficial in a select group of SCLC patients who obtain excellent overall control of disease with first-line treatment and might develop recurrences in the CNS, which could lead to death. However, serial MRI surveillance in these patients might catch these recurrences at the earlies, which might enable the physicians to treat them with SRS and/or whole brain radiation therapy. The ongoing MAVERICK (SWOG1827) trial will provide a clear idea of which approach is superior in patients with SCLC. Till then, PCI should be discussed and offered to patients with SCLC who have at least some responses to first-line systemic therapy, regardless of their disease burden, and whenever possible, should be used with hippocampal avoidance technique in conjunction with memantine.

12 Palliative Care, Follow-Up, and Quality of Life Issues

Considering the aggressive nature and poor prognosis associated with SCLC, addressing palliative needs and quality of life issues are equally important. An open discussion involving patients and caregivers, about the prognosis, goals of treatment and supportive care should be done early in the course of the disease. Involvement of palliative care physicians and psychologists/counselors should be encouraged. Counselling regarding smoking cessation should be carried out from the beginning. Good management of thoracic symptom burden and improvement in breathing status would increase the tolerance for systemic chemotherapy, immunotherapy, and thoracic irradiation.

Since SCLC at diagnosis is a chemoresponsive disease, patients with a high disease burden show improvement in quality of life with chemotherapy. However, considering the limited life expectancy, particularly in extensive stage SCLC, the risk of toxicities should not outweigh the symptomatic benefit. Long-term toxicities become more relevant in the context of limited-stage SCLC treated with curative intent and also to some of the exceptional responders, even in extensive-stage SCLC in the current chemo-immunotherapy era. More recent radiation techniques minimize long-term toxicities like pneumonitis. Hippocampal sparing PCI in SCLC results in a lower risk of neurocognitive decline without affecting overall survival [93].

13 Follow-Up

Small cell lung cancer is associated with a high risk of relapse, almost 75% of limited stage SCLC and around 90% of extensive stage SCLC relapsing in the first 2 years of diagnosis. After completion of treatment, follow-up is recommended every 3 months in the first 2 years, 6 monthly in the 3rd year, then annually. More frequent follow-up may be done for extensive stage SCLC [13]. Surveillance imaging may be done particularly in the first 2 years; however, there is a paucity of data regarding the frequency of imaging and its impact on survival. Smoking cessation counselling and addressing survivorship issues should be part of every follow-up visit.

14 Future Direction

Recently proposed transcriptomic classification has renewed hopes for opening up therapeutic avenues for personalized targeted therapy in SCLC. This has been possible due to better understanding of the molecular characteristics of small cell lung cancer using genetically engineered mouse models, SCLC cell lines, patient-derived in-vivo models and primary human tumors. Elucidation of therapeutic resistance mechanisms is required to expand the treatment landscape of relapse SCLC. Liquid biopsy-based approaches might be useful to understand the tumor dynamics over the period of time and during treatment.

Most patients of SCLC are diagnosed in the advanced stage, further highlighting need of prevention and early detection. Annual low-dose CT-based screening fails to detect early-stage SCLC due to the aggressive behavior of disease [53]. However, blood-based detection by mutational, proteomic, or multiparameter approaches has potential. Detection of neuroendocrine markers using mass spectrometry is one such potential strategy [94].

The advent of chemo-immunotherapy has led to an improvement in survival though modestly in patients with extensive SCLC. Recent study has shown, Even in limited stage SCLC adjuvant Durvalumab after definitive chemoradiation has shown to improve overall survival and progression free survival [95]. However, identification of a predictive biomarker for selecting patients for immune checkpoint inhibitors is an unmet need. Current focus of research is also to identify complementary immune activation pathways and evaluation of various combination approaches like bi-specific T cell engagers, NK cell activators, DNA damage response inhibitors, and epigenetic targeted agents to further enhance immune responsiveness of SCLC. Compared to the past, in current scenario, the role of radiotherapy, in combination with chemoimmunotherapy requires greater integration. The biological, technological and clinical skills in radiation oncology can be utilized for improved dose, fractionation regimes in thoracic, PCI, and metastatic sites encompassing the management trajectory of SCLC [96].

Percepts Box

1. Small cell lung cancer is aggressive cancer associated with smoking and is associated with a high symptom burden.
2. Unlike NSCLC, SCLC lacks mutation in the RAS-RAF-RTK pathway, rather characterised by tumor suppressor loss mainly TP53 and Rb which are not therapeutically targetable.
3. Recently proposed transcriptomic classification might uncover therapeutic vulnerabilities to novel agents and the development of precision-targeted therapy for SCLC.
4. Veterans Administration Lung Study Group (VALSG) staging system, dividing SCLC into limited stage or extensive stage based on the feasibility of thoracic radiation still remains the most commonly used staging system. However, it is encouraged to use the TNM system proposed by AJCC 8th edition for a better description.
5. Surgery or SBRT followed by adjuvant chemotherapy could be considered for early-stage non-metastatic SCLC (T1/T2N0).
6. Concomitant chemoradiation therapy is the standard of care for limited-stage SCLC. Thoracic radiation therapy with 45 Gy in 30 fractions at 1.5 Gy per fraction twice daily or 66 Gy in 33 fractions over 6.5 weeks is the current standard. However, dose-escalated BID regimens (60 Gy in 40 fractions at 1.5 Gy per fraction twice daily) have shown superior results compared to 45 Gy in 30 fractions at 1.5 Gy per fraction twice daily.
7. Platinum-based combination chemotherapy with atezolizumab or durvalumab is the new standard of care for extensive SCLC. However, in LMIC (low and middle income countries) setting platinum-based doublet chemotherapy remains the standard.
8. Carboplatin may be replaced for cisplatin in unfit patients.
9. Patients with extensive stage SCLC, not suitable for immunotherapy, may be treated with consolidative thoracic radiation therapy after initial chemotherapy.
10. The role of radiation therapy is controversial in patients with extensive stage SCLC who are treated with chemotherapy and immunotherapy combination. However, thoracic radiation therapy should be discussed in such patients with a high loco-regional disease burden.
11. PCI should be discussed and offered as a part of the multidisciplinary treatment in patients with SCLC who had some response to initial systemic therapy.
12. A total dose of 25 Gy in 10 fractions over 2 weeks with hippocampal avoidance (with/without memantine) is the standard of care for PCI.

15 Conclusion/Overview

SCLC is an aggressive malignancy, more common in smokers. It is extremely chemo-sensitive, though associated with higher rates of relapse following treatment. Platinum based chemotherapy, thoracic radiation form major components of therapy for SCLC. Prophylactic cranial irradiation can be considered in patients with response to initial systemic therapy.

Multiple Choice Questions

1. Which of the following are the hallmark genomic features of SCLC?
   (a) EGFR and BRAF alterations

   (b) EGFR and ALK alterations
   (c) TP53 and RB alterations
   (d) KRAS and BRAF alterations
2. Indication of bone marrow evaluation in patients with SCLC are all except:
   (a) Pancytopenia
   (b) Leukoerythroblastic picture
   (c) Presence of nucleated RBCs on peripheral smear
   (d) Neutrophilia
3. A 50 year old man, chronic smoker, recently diagnosed case of small cell carcinoma lung with liver metastases was brought to the emergency department with drowsiness. On admission patient had no distress, pulse rate was 104/min, blood pressure of 110/70 mmHg, respiratory rate of 24/min, SpO_2 98% on room air. There were no focal neurologic deficits. Laboratory evaluation revealed serum Na 124 mmol/L, K 3.5 mEq/L, glucose 120 mg/dL. What is the suspected diagnosis?
   (a) Cushing syndrome
   (b) Lambert Eaton myasthenic syndrome
   (c) Syndrome of inappropriate antidiuretic hormone secretion
   (d) Encephalitis
4. A 65 year old male had a right upper lobe mass and bronchoscopy biopsy revealed small cell carcinoma. Patient now complains of headache, dizziness on leaning forward. Examination revealed dilated engorged veins over chest, neck, right upper limb with facial plethora. What is the appropriate treatment modality for this patient?
   (a) Chemotherapy
   (b) Radiation
   (c) Corticosteroids
   (d) Endovascular stenting
5. Usual features of SCLC include all except
   (a) Common in smokers
   (b) Presents with peripheral seated mass
   (c) Bulky mediastinal nodes
   (d) SVC more common than non-small cell lung cancer
6. The most common paraneoplastic syndrome associated with SCLC?
   (a) SIADH
   (b) Lambert-Eaton syndrome
   (c) Opsoclonus-Myoclonus
   (d) Cerebellar degeneration
7. 55 year old male smoker presented with a history of cough over the last 3 months. CECT Thorax revealed a 5.5 cm lesion is the left upper lobe and a 2 cm right hilar lymph node. MRI brain was normal. A biopsy was done which showed a SCLC. Patient is an avid runner but complains that he isn't able to run as much as before. However, he has no problems working his job as a software engineer. What treatment mode would you recommend?
   (a) Immunotherapy + chemotherapy alone
   (b) Surgery followed by adjuvant radiation
   (c) Immunotherapy + chemotherapy followed by Thoracic RT
   (d) Best supportive care
8. Benefit of adding atezolizumab to chemotherapy in treatment naïve extensive stage SCLC was established by which trial?
   (a) IMpower 133
   (b) Mona Lisa
   (c) CASPIAN
   (d) RAPID-O
9. Most common site of metastasis in SCLC?
   (a) Bone
   (b) Liver
   (c) Brain
   (d) Adrenal
10. The CASPIAN trial established the role of which drug in the treatment of SCLC
   (a) Atezolizumab
   (b) Nivolumab
   (c) Ipulimumab
   (d) Durvalumab

Answer Key

1. (c)
2. (d)
3. (c)
4. (a)
5. (b)
6. (a)
7. (c)

8. (a)
9. (c)
10. (d)

References

1. Cittolin-Santos GF, Knapp B, Ganesh B, Gao F, Waqar S, Stinchcombe TE, Govindan R, Morgensztern D. The changing landscape of small cell lung cancer. Cancer. 2024;130:2453–61. https://doi.org/10.1002/cncr.35281.
2. Barbone F, Bovenzi M, Cavallieri F, Stanta G. Cigarette smoking and histologic type of lung cancer in men. Chest. 1997;112(6):1474–9. https://doi.org/10.1378/chest.112.6.1474.
3. Khuder SA. Effect of cigarette smoking on major histological types of lung cancer: a meta-analysis. Lung Cancer. 2001;31(2):139–48. https://doi.org/10.1016/S0169-5002(00)00181-1.
4. Lamichhane DK, et al. Lung cancer risk and residential exposure to air pollution: a Korean population-based case-control study. Yonsei Med J. 2017;58(6):1111–8. https://doi.org/10.3349/ymj.2017.58.6.1111.
5. Torres-Durán M, et al. Small-cell lung cancer in never-smokers. ESMO Open. 2021;6(2):100059. https://doi.org/10.1016/j.esmoop.2021.100059.
6. Wang J, et al. Genetic predisposition to lung cancer: comprehensive literature integration, meta-analysis, and multiple evidence assessment of candidate-gene association studies. Sci Rep. 2017;7(1):8371. https://doi.org/10.1038/s41598-017-07737-0.
7. Malik PS, Sharma MC, Mohanti BK, Shukla NK, Deo SV, Mohan A, Kumar G, Raina V. Clinicopathological profile of lung cancer at AIIMS: a changing paradigm in India. Asian Pac J Cancer Prev. 2013;14(1):489–94.
8. Mohan A, et al. Survival in small cell lung cancer in India: prognostic utility of clinical features, laboratory parameters and response to treatment. Indian J Cancer. 2006;43(2):67. https://doi.org/10.4103/0019-509X.25887.
9. Gay CM, et al. Patterns of transcription factor programs and immune pathway activation define four major subtypes of SCLC with distinct therapeutic vulnerabilities. Cancer Cell. 2021;39(3):346–60.e7. https://doi.org/10.1016/j.ccell.2020.12.014.**
10. Martucci F, et al. Impact of 18F-FDG PET/CT in staging patients with small cell lung cancer: a systematic review and meta-analysis. Front Med. 2020;6. [Online]. Available: https://www.frontiersin.org/article/10.3389/fmed.2019.00336. Accessed 19 Jan 2022.
11. Manoharan P, et al. 18F-Fludeoxyglucose PET/CT in SCLC: analysis of the CONVERT randomized controlled trial. J Thorac Oncol. 2019;14(7):1296–305. https://doi.org/10.1016/j.jtho.2019.03.023.
12. Nong J, et al. Circulating tumor DNA analysis depicts subclonal architecture and genomic evolution of small cell lung cancer. Nat Commun. 2018;9(1):1. https://doi.org/10.1038/s41467-018-05327-w.
13. Ganti AKP, et al. Small cell lung cancer, version 2.2022, NCCN clinical practice guidelines in oncology. J Natl Compr Canc Netw. 2021;19(12):1441–64. https://doi.org/10.6004/jnccn.2021.0058.**
14. Wakeam E, et al. Surgery versus chemotherapy and radiotherapy for early and locally advanced small cell lung cancer: a propensity-matched analysis of survival. Lung Cancer. 2017;109:78–88. https://doi.org/10.1016/j.lungcan.2017.04.021.*
15. Vallières E, et al. The IASLC lung cancer staging project: proposals regarding the relevance of TNM in the pathologic staging of small cell lung cancer in the forthcoming (seventh) edition of the TNM classification for lung cancer. J Thorac Oncol. 2009;4(9):1049–59. https://doi.org/10.1097/JTO.0b013e3181b27799.*
16. Yang C-FJ, et al. Role of adjuvant therapy in a population-based cohort of patients with early-stage small-cell lung cancer. J Clin Oncol. 2016;34(10):1057–64. https://doi.org/10.1200/JCO.2015.63.8171.*
17. Wong AT, Rineer J, Schwartz D, Schreiber D. Assessing the impact of postoperative radiation therapy for completely resected limited-stage small cell lung cancer using the National Cancer Database. J Thorac Oncol. 2016;11(2):242–8. https://doi.org/10.1016/j.jtho.2015.10.011.*
18. Fukuoka M, et al. Randomized trial of cyclophosphamide, doxorubicin, and vincristine versus cisplatin and etoposide versus alternation of these regimens in small-cell lung cancer. JNCI J Natl Cancer Inst. 1991;83(12):855–61. https://doi.org/10.1093/jnci/83.12.855.**
19. Sundstrøm S, et al. Cisplatin and etoposide regimen is superior to cyclophosphamide, epirubicin, and vincristine regimen in small-cell lung cancer: results from a randomized phase III trial with 5 years' follow-up. J Clin Oncol. 2002;20(24):4665–72. https://doi.org/10.1200/JCO.2002.12.111.**
20. Pujol J-L, Carestia, Daurès J-P. Is there a case for cisplatin in the treatment of small-cell lung cancer? A meta-analysis of randomized trials of a cisplatin-containing regimen versus a regimen without this alkylating agent. Br J Cancer. 2000;83(1):1. https://doi.org/10.1054/bjoc.2000.1164.
21. Rossi A, et al. Carboplatin- or cisplatin-based chemotherapy in first-line treatment of small-cell lung cancer: the COCIS meta-analysis of individual patient data. J Clin Oncol. 2012;30(14):1692–8. https://doi.org/10.1200/JCO.2011.40.4905.**
22. Kubota K, et al. Etoposide and cisplatin versus irinotecan and cisplatin in patients with limited-stage small-cell lung cancer treated with etoposide and cisplatin plus concurrent accelerated hyperfractionated thoracic radiotherapy (JCOG0202): a randomised phase 3 study. Lancet Oncol. 2014;15(1):106–13. https://doi.org/10.1016/S1470-2045(13)70511-4.**

23. Kenmotsu H, et al. Randomized phase III study of irinotecan plus cisplatin versus etoposide plus cisplatin for completely resected high-grade neuroendocrine carcinoma of the lung: JCOG1205/1206. J Clin Oncol. 2020;38(36):4292–301. https://doi.org/10.1200/JCO.20.01806.**
24. Noda K, et al. Irinotecan plus cisplatin compared with etoposide plus cisplatin for extensive small-cell lung cancer. N Engl J Med. 2002;346(2):85–91. https://doi.org/10.1056/NEJMoa003034.**
25. Hanna N, et al. Randomized phase III trial comparing irinotecan/cisplatin with etoposide/cisplatin in patients with previously untreated extensive-stage disease small-cell lung cancer. J Clin Oncol. 2006;24(13):2038–43. https://doi.org/10.1200/JCO.2005.04.8595.**
26. Zatloukal P, et al. A multicenter international randomized phase III study comparing cisplatin in combination with irinotecan or etoposide in previously untreated small-cell lung cancer patients with extensive disease. Ann Oncol. 2010;21(9):1810–6. https://doi.org/10.1093/annonc/mdq036.**
27. Lara PN, et al. Phase III trial of irinotecan/cisplatin compared with etoposide/cisplatin in extensive-stage small-cell lung cancer: clinical and pharmacogenomic results from SWOG S0124. J Clin Oncol. 2009;27(15):2530–5. https://doi.org/10.1200/JCO.2008.20.1061.**
28. Pignon J-P, et al. A meta-analysis of thoracic radiotherapy for small-cell lung cancer. N Engl J Med. 1992;327(23):1618–24. https://doi.org/10.1056/NEJM199212033272302.
29. Baas P, et al. Concurrent chemotherapy (carboplatin, paclitaxel, etoposide) and involved-field radiotherapy in limited stage small cell lung cancer: a Dutch multicenter phase II study. Br J Cancer. 2006;94(5):5. https://doi.org/10.1038/sj.bjc.6602979.**
30. Ettinger DS, et al. Study of paclitaxel, etoposide, and cisplatin chemotherapy combined with twice-daily thoracic radiotherapy for patients with limited-stage small-cell lung cancer: a Radiation Therapy Oncology Group 9609 Phase II Study. J Clin Oncol. 2005;23(22):4991–8. https://doi.org/10.1200/JCO.2005.00.414.**
31. Hainsworth JD, et al. Paclitaxel, carboplatin, and extended-schedule etoposide in the treatment of small-cell lung cancer: comparison of sequential phase II trials using different dose-intensities. J Clin Oncol. 1997;15(12):3464–70. https://doi.org/10.1200/JCO.1997.15.12.3464.*
32. Levitan N, et al. Multi-institutional phase I/II trial of paclitaxel, cisplatin, and etoposide with concurrent radiation for limited-stage small-cell lung carcinoma. J Clin Oncol. 2000;18(5):1102. https://doi.org/10.1200/JCO.2000.18.5.1102.
33. Spigel DR, et al. Tracheoesophageal fistula formation in patients with lung cancer treated with chemoradiation and bevacizumab. J Clin Oncol. 2010;28(1):43–8. https://doi.org/10.1200/JCO.2009.24.7353.
34. Pujol J-L, et al. Randomized phase II–III study of bevacizumab in combination with chemotherapy in previously untreated extensive small-cell lung cancer: results from the IFCT-0802 trial†. Ann Oncol. 2015;26(5):908–14. https://doi.org/10.1093/annonc/mdv065.
35. Spigel DR, et al. Randomized phase II study of bevacizumab in combination with chemotherapy in previously untreated extensive-stage small-cell lung cancer: results from the SALUTE trial. J Clin Oncol. 2011;29(16):2215–22. https://doi.org/10.1200/JCO.2010.29.3423.
36. Horn L, et al. First-line atezolizumab plus chemotherapy in extensive-stage small-cell lung cancer. N Engl J Med. 2018;379(23):2220–9. https://doi.org/10.1056/NEJMoa1809064.**
37. Paz-Ares L, et al. Durvalumab plus platinum–etoposide versus platinum–etoposide in first-line treatment of extensive-stage small-cell lung cancer (CASPIAN): a randomised, controlled, open-label, phase 3 trial. Lancet. 2019;394(10212):1929–39. https://doi.org/10.1016/S0140-6736(19)32222-6.**
38. Goldman JW, et al. Durvalumab, with or without tremelimumab, plus platinum–etoposide versus platinum–etoposide alone in first-line treatment of extensive-stage small-cell lung cancer (CASPIAN): updated results from a randomised, controlled, open-label, phase 3 trial. Lancet Oncol. 2021;22(1):51–65. https://doi.org/10.1016/S1470-2045(20)30539-8.**
39. Rudin CM, et al. Pembrolizumab or placebo plus etoposide and platinum as first-line therapy for extensive-stage small-cell lung cancer: randomized, double-blind, phase III KEYNOTE-604 study. J Clin Oncol. 2020;38(21):2369–79. https://doi.org/10.1200/JCO.20.00793.*
40. Wagner AH, et al. Recurrent WNT pathway alterations are frequent in relapsed small cell lung cancer. Nat Commun. 2018;9(1):1. https://doi.org/10.1038/s41467-018-06162-9.*
41. Genestreti G, et al. Outcomes of platinum-sensitive small-cell lung cancer patients treated with platinum/etoposide rechallenge: a multi-institutional retrospective analysis. Clin Lung Cancer. 2015;16(6):e223–8. https://doi.org/10.1016/j.cllc.2015.04.006.
42. Baize N, et al. Carboplatin plus etoposide versus topotecan as second-line treatment for patients with sensitive relapsed small-cell lung cancer: an open-label, multicentre, randomised, phase 3 trial. Lancet Oncol. 2020;21(9):1224–33. https://doi.org/10.1016/S1470-2045(20)30461-7.*
43. Lurbinectedin as second-line treatment for patients with small-cell lung cancer: a single-arm, open-label, phase 2 basket trial. Lancet Oncol. https://www.thelancet.com/journals/lanonc/article/PIIS1470-2045(20)30068-1/fulltext. Accessed 24 Apr 2022.
44. O'Brien MER, et al. Phase III trial comparing supportive care alone with supportive care with oral topotecan in patients with relapsed small-cell lung cancer. J Clin Oncol. 2006;24(34):5441–7. https://doi.org/10.1200/JCO.2006.06.5821.
45. von Pawel J, et al. Topotecan versus cyclophosphamide, doxorubicin, and vincristine for the treat-

ment of recurrent small-cell lung cancer. J Clin Oncol. 1999;17(2):658. https://doi.org/10.1200/JCO.1999.17.2.658.
46. Smit EF, Fokkema E, Biesma B, Groen HJM, Snoek W, Postmus PE. A phase II study of paclitaxel in heavily pretreated patients with small-cell lung cancer. Br J Cancer. 1998;77(2):2. https://doi.org/10.1038/bjc.1998.54.
47. Mouri A, et al. Combination therapy with carboplatin and paclitaxel for small cell lung cancer. Respir Investig. 2019;57(1):34–9. https://doi.org/10.1016/j.resinv.2018.09.004.
48. Pietanza MC, et al. Phase II trial of temozolomide in patients with relapsed sensitive or refractory small cell lung cancer, with assessment of methylguanine-DNA methyltransferase as a potential biomarker. Clin Cancer Res. 2012;18(4):1138–45. https://doi.org/10.1158/1078-0432.CCR-11-2059.
49. Furuse K, et al. Phase II study of vinorelbine in heavily previously treated small cell lung cancer. Oncology. 1996;53(2):169–72. https://doi.org/10.1159/000227555.
50. Masters GA, et al. Phase II trial of gemcitabine in refractory or relapsed small-cell lung cancer: Eastern Cooperative Oncology Group Trial 1597. J Clin Oncol. 2003;21(8):1550–5. https://doi.org/10.1200/JCO.2003.09.130.
51. Rudin CM, et al. Rovalpituzumab tesirine, a DLL3-targeted antibody-drug conjugate, in recurrent small-cell lung cancer: a first-in-human, first-in-class, open-label, phase 1 study. Lancet Oncol. 2017;18(1):42–51. https://doi.org/10.1016/S1470-2045(16)30565-4.
52. Morgensztern D, et al. Efficacy and safety of rovalpituzumab tesirine in third-line and beyond patients with DLL3-expressing, relapsed/refractory small-cell lung cancer: results from the phase II TRINITY study. Clin Cancer Res. 2019;25(23):6958–66. https://doi.org/10.1158/1078-0432.CCR-19-1133.
53. Reduced lung-cancer mortality with low-dose computed tomographic screening. NEJM. https://www.nejm.org/doi/10.1056/NEJMoa1102873?url_ver=Z39.88-2003&rfr_id=ori:rid:crossref.org&rfr_dat=cr_pub%20%200www.ncbi.nlm.nih.gov. Accessed 24 Apr 2022.
54. Verma V, et al. Multi-institutional experience of stereotactic ablative radiation therapy for stage I small cell lung cancer. Int J Radiat Oncol Biol Phys. 2017;97(2):362–71. https://doi.org/10.1016/j.ijrobp.2016.10.041.*
55. Rathod S, Koul R, Bashir B, Chowdhury A, Dubey A. Role of stereotactic body radiation therapy in early stage small cell lung cancer in the era of lung cancer screening: a systematic review. Am J Clin Oncol. 2019;42(2):123–30. https://doi.org/10.1097/COC.0000000000000489.*
56. Tekatli H, et al. Outcomes of hypofractionated high-dose radiotherapy in poor-risk patients with "ultracentral" non–small cell lung cancer. J Thorac Oncol. 2016;11(7):1081–9. https://doi.org/10.1016/j.jtho.2016.03.008.**
57. Warde P, Payne D. Does thoracic irradiation improve survival and local control in limited-stage small-cell carcinoma of the lung? A meta-analysis. J Clin Oncol. 2016. https://doi.org/10.1200/JCO.1992.10.6.890.*
58. Murray N, et al. Importance of timing for thoracic irradiation in the combined modality treatment of limited-stage small-cell lung cancer. The National Cancer Institute of Canada Clinical Trials Group. J Clin Oncol. 1993;11(2):336–44. https://doi.org/10.1200/JCO.1993.11.2.336.**
59. Jeremic B, Shibamoto Y, Acimovic L, Milisavljevic S. Initial versus delayed accelerated hyperfractionated radiation therapy and concurrent chemotherapy in limited small-cell lung cancer: a randomized study. J Clin Oncol. 1997;15(3):893–900. https://doi.org/10.1200/JCO.1997.15.3.893.**
60. Takada M, et al. Phase III study of concurrent versus sequential thoracic radiotherapy in combination with cisplatin and etoposide for limited-stage small-cell lung cancer: results of the Japan Clinical Oncology Group Study 9104. J Clin Oncol. 2002;20(14):3054–60. https://doi.org/10.1200/JCO.2002.12.071.**
61. Perry MC, Herndon JE, Eaton WL, Green MR. Thoracic radiation therapy added to chemotherapy for small-cell lung cancer: an update of Cancer and Leukemia Group B Study 8083. J Clin Oncol. 1998;16(7):2466–7. https://doi.org/10.1200/JCO.1998.16.7.2466.**
62. Spiro SG, et al. Early compared with late radiotherapy in combined modality treatment for limited disease small-cell lung cancer: a London lung cancer group multicenter randomized clinical trial and meta-analysis. J Clin Oncol. 2006;24(24):3823–30. https://doi.org/10.1200/JCO.2005.05.3181.**
63. Phase III trial of concurrent thoracic radiotherapy with either first- or third-cycle chemotherapy for limited-disease small-cell lung cancer. ScienceDirect. https://www.sciencedirect.com/science/article/pii/S0923753419368115?via%3Dihub. Accessed 24 Apr 2022.**
64. De Ruysscher D, et al. Time between the first day of chemotherapy and the last day of chest radiation is the Most important predictor of survival in limited-disease small-cell lung cancer. J Clin Oncol. 2006;24(7):1057–63. https://doi.org/10.1200/JCO.2005.02.9793.*
65. Systematic review and meta-analysis of randomised, controlled trials of the timing of chest radiotherapy in patients with limited-stage, small-cell lung cancer. ScienceDirect. https://www.sciencedirect.com/science/article/pii/S0923753419575548?via%3Dihub. Accessed 24 Apr 2022.
66. Impact of thoracic radiotherapy timing in limited-stage small-cell lung cancer: usefulness of the individual patient data meta-analysis. ScienceDirect. https://www.sciencedirect.com/science/article/pii/S0923753419358971?via%3Dihub. Accessed 24 Apr 2022.*

67. Turrisi AT, et al. Twice-daily compared with once-daily thoracic radiotherapy in limited small-cell lung cancer treated concurrently with cisplatin and etoposide. N Engl J Med. 1999;340(4):265–71. https://doi.org/10.1056/NEJM199901283400403.**
68. Faivre-Finn C, et al. Concurrent once-daily versus twice-daily chemoradiotherapy in patients with limited-stage small-cell lung cancer (CONVERT): an open-label, phase 3, randomised, superiority trial. Lancet Oncol. 2017;18(8):1116–25. https://doi.org/10.1016/S1470-2045(17)30318-2.**
69. Bogart JA, et al. Phase 3 comparison of high-dose once-daily (QD) thoracic radiotherapy (TRT) with standard twice-daily (BID) TRT in limited stage small cell lung cancer (LSCLC): CALGB 30610 (Alliance)/RTOG 0538. J Clin Oncol. 2021;39(15_suppl):8505. https://doi.org/10.1200/JCO.2021.39.15_suppl.8505.**
70. Simone CB, et al. Radiation therapy for small cell lung cancer: an ASTRO clinical practice guideline. Pract Radiat Oncol. 2020;10(3):158–73. https://doi.org/10.1016/j.prro.2020.02.009.**
71. Grønberg BH, et al. High-dose versus standard-dose twice-daily thoracic radiotherapy for patients with limited stage small-cell lung cancer: an open-label, randomised, phase 2 trial. Lancet Oncol. 2021;22(3):321–31. https://doi.org/10.1016/S1470-2045(20)30742-7.**
72. Kies MS, et al. Multimodal therapy for limited small-cell lung cancer: a randomized study of induction combination chemotherapy with or without thoracic radiation in complete responders; and with wide-field versus reduced-field radiation in partial responders: a Southwest Oncology Group Study. J Clin Oncol. 1987;5(4):592–600. https://doi.org/10.1200/JCO.1987.5.4.592.**
73. Hu X, et al. Final report of a prospective randomized study on thoracic radiotherapy target volume for limited-stage small cell lung cancer with radiation dosimetric analyses. Cancer. 2020. Wiley Online Library. https://acsjournals.onlinelibrary.wiley.com/doi/10.1002/cncr.32586. Accessed 24 Apr 2022.*
74. van Loon J, et al. Selective nodal irradiation on basis of (18)FDG-PET scans in limited-disease small-cell lung cancer: a prospective study. Int J Radiat Oncol Biol Phys. 2010;77(2):329–36. https://doi.org/10.1016/j.ijrobp.2009.04.075.
75. Lally BE, et al. Trends in the outcomes for patients with limited stage small cell lung cancer: an analysis of the surveillance, epidemiology, and end results database. Lung Cancer. 2009;64(2):226–31. https://doi.org/10.1016/j.lungcan.2008.08.010.
76. Allen J, Jahanzeb M. Extensive-stage small-cell lung cancer: evolution of systemic therapy and future directions. Clin Lung Cancer. 2008;9(5):262–70. https://doi.org/10.3816/CLC.2008.n.041.
77. Yee D, et al. Clinical trial of post-chemotherapy consolidation thoracic radiotherapy for extensive-stage small cell lung cancer. Radiother Oncol. 2012;102(2):234–8. https://doi.org/10.1016/j.radonc.2011.08.042.**
78. Jeremic B, et al. Role of radiation therapy in the combined-modality treatment of patients with extensive disease small-cell lung cancer: a randomized study. J Clin Oncol. 1999;17(7):2092–9. https://doi.org/10.1200/JCO.1999.17.7.2092.**
79. Giuliani ME, et al. Clinical outcomes of extensive stage small cell lung carcinoma patients treated with consolidative thoracic radiotherapy. Clin Lung Cancer. 2011;12(6):375–9. https://doi.org/10.1016/j.cllc.2011.03.028.*
80. Palma DA, Warner A, Louie AV, Senan S, Slotman B, Rodrigues GB. Thoracic radiotherapy for extensive stage small-cell lung cancer: a meta-analysis. Clin Lung Cancer. 2016;17(4):239–44. https://doi.org/10.1016/j.cllc.2015.09.007.
81. Slotman BJ, et al. Use of thoracic radiotherapy for extensive stage small-cell lung cancer: a phase 3 randomised controlled trial. Lancet. 2015;385(9962):36–42. https://doi.org/10.1016/S0140-6736(14)61085-0.*
82. Deng L, et al. Irradiation and anti-PD-L1 treatment synergistically promote antitumor immunity in mice. J Clin Invest. 2014;124(2):687–95. https://doi.org/10.1172/JCI67313.
83. Dovedi SJ, et al. Fractionated radiation therapy stimulates antitumor immunity mediated by both resident and infiltrating polyclonal T-cell populations when combined with PD-1 blockade. Clin Cancer Res. 2017;23(18):5514–26. https://doi.org/10.1158/1078-0432.CCR-16-1673.
84. Formenti SC, et al. Radiotherapy induces responses of lung cancer to CTLA-4 blockade. Nat Med. 2018;24(12):1845–51. https://doi.org/10.1038/s41591-018-0232-2.
85. Seute T, Leffers P, ten Velde GPM, Twijnstra A. Detection of brain metastases from small cell lung cancer: consequences of changing imaging techniques (CT versus MRI). Cancer. 2008;112(8):1827–34. https://doi.org/10.1002/cncr.23361.
86. Rusthoven CG, et al. Evaluation of first-line radiosurgery vs whole-brain radiotherapy for small cell lung cancer brain metastases: the FIRE-SCLC cohort study. JAMA Oncol. 2020;6(7):1028–37. https://doi.org/10.1001/jamaoncol.2020.1271.*
87. Choi M, Lee Y, Moon SH, Han J-Y, Kim HT, Lee JS. Effect of accurate staging using positron emission tomography on the outcomes of prophylactic cranial irradiation in patients with limited stage small-cell lung cancer. Clin Lung Cancer. 2017;18(1):77–84. https://doi.org/10.1016/j.cllc.2016.06.012.
88. Xu J, et al. Prophylactic cranial irradiation for patients with surgically resected small cell lung cancer. J Thorac Oncol. 2017;12(2):347–53. https://doi.org/10.1016/j.jtho.2016.09.133.*
89. Wu AJ, et al. Patterns of failure in limited-stage small cell lung cancer: implications of TNM stage for prophylactic cranial irradiation. Radiother Oncol. 2017;125(1):130–5. https://doi.org/10.1016/j.radonc.2017.07.019.

90. Slotman B, et al. Prophylactic cranial irradiation in extensive small-cell lung cancer. N Engl J Med. 2007;357(7):664–72. https://doi.org/10.1056/NEJMoa071780.*
91. Takahashi T, et al. Prophylactic cranial irradiation versus observation in patients with extensive-disease small-cell lung cancer: a multicentre, randomised, open-label, phase 3 trial. Lancet Oncol. 2017;18(5):663–71. https://doi.org/10.1016/S1470-2045(17)30230-9.*
92. Brown PD, et al. Hippocampal avoidance during whole-brain radiotherapy plus memantine for patients with brain metastases: phase III trial NRG oncology CC001. J Clin Oncol. 2020;38(10):1019–29. https://doi.org/10.1200/JCO.19.02767.**
93. Rodríguez de Dios N, et al. Randomized phase III trial of prophylactic cranial irradiation with or without hippocampal avoidance for small-cell lung cancer (PREMER): a GICOR-GOECP-SEOR study. J Clin Oncol. 2021;39(28):3118–27. https://doi.org/10.1200/JCO.21.00639.**
94. Taguchi A, et al. Lung cancer signatures in plasma based on proteome profiling of mouse tumor models. Cancer Cell. 2011;20(3):289–99. https://doi.org/10.1016/j.ccr.2011.08.007.
95. Cheng Y, Spigel DR, Cho BC, Laktionov KK, et al. ADRIATIC Investigators. Durvalumab after Chemoradiotherapy in Limited-Stage Small-Cell Lung Cancer. N Engl J Med. 2024;391:1313–27 https://doi.org/10.1056/NEJMoa2404873
96. Borghetti P, Ramella S, Ricardi U. The role of radiotherapy in small cell lung cancer: a new paradigm for the radiation oncologist. Front Oncol. 2025;14:1541527. https://doi.org/10.3389/fonc.2024.1541527

Online Links

https://www.youtube.com/watch?v=2dWURnkuoJ8
https://www.youtube.com/watch?v=9anrSXFMEeM
https://www.youtube.com/shorts/nZ044EicYO4
https://www.youtube.com/watch?v=lMFIkBMlF_M
https://www.esmo.org/guidelines/guidelines-by-topic/lung-and-chest-tumours/small-cell-lung-cancer
https://jnccn.org/view/journals/jnccn/19/12/article-p1441.xml
https://www.sciencedirect.com/science/article/pii/S1879850020300539

Mediastinal Tumours

Ahitagni Biswas, Rakesh Kapoor, Kannan Periasamy, Namrata Das, Prabhat Singh Malik, and Sunil Kumar

1 Introduction

The mediastinum is the midline compartment of the thoracic cavity that separates the two pleural cavities. It contains vital organs like the heart and serves as a conduit for structures to pass in and out of the thoracic cavity [1, 2].

Mediastinal tumours are rare and heterogeneous since they can arise from any of the mediastinal structures. They are commonly asymptomatic, with the location and type of tumour varying by demography. In adults, anterior mediastinal tumours like thymic epithelial neoplasms, lymphomas and germ cell tumours are commonest. In children, more than half of the tumours are neurogenic in origin arising in the posterior mediastinum [3].

Disease management strategies and outcomes vary with the histologic type of tumour, its location, aggressiveness and the symptom burden. Surgery is the main modality when the disease is accessible and operable. In most of the malignant tumors showing aggressiveness, systemic chemotherapy is considered in different settings, preoperative, adjuvant, or, as sole modality with curative or palliative intent. For example, in an International Thymic Malignancy Interest Group (ITMIG)/International Association for the Study of Lung Cancer (IASLC) retrospective analysis, surgery (40%) alone was the commonest treatment modality for thymic tumours followed by surgery with radiotherapy (19%). The ITMIG is an international organisation that is spearheading data collection and research in thymic and other mediastinal malignancies [4, 5].

2 Anatomy

The mediastinum is the central portion of the thoracic cavity extending superoinferiorly from the thoracic inlet to the diaphragm, antero-posteriorly from sternum to vertebral bodies, and enclosed laterally on each side by mediastinal pleura. Models for classifying mediastinal compartments have evolved from X-ray-based systems to CT-based divisions as given by the Japanese Association for Research on Thymus (JART) and ITMIG models [1, 6].

A. Biswas (✉) · N. Das
Department of Radiation Oncology, All India Institute of Medical Sciences, New Delhi, Delhi, India

R. Kapoor · K. Periasamy
Department of Radiotherapy & Oncology, Postgraduate Institute of Medical Education and Research, Chandigarh, India

P. S. Malik
Department of Medical Oncology, All India Institute of Medical Sciences, New Delhi, India

S. Kumar
Department of Surgical Oncology, All India Institute of Medical Sciences, New Delhi, India

B. K. Mohanti et al. (eds.), *Radiation Oncology – Principles, Precepts and Practice*,
https://doi.org/10.1007/978-981-95-5171-2_8

Four-Compartment Model Traditional anatomical division of the mediastinum is into superior and inferior mediastinum by the transverse thoracic plane that passes anteriorly from the sternal angle to the T4–T5 junction posteriorly. The superior mediastinum contains the trachea and upper portion of the great vessels and thymus. The inferior mediastinum is further split into three parts—anterior, middle and posterior by the pericardium. The anterior mediastinum mainly includes thymus, lymph nodes and fat. The middle mediastinum contains the heart and pericardium, origin of the great vessels, main bronchi and nerves like the vagus and the recurrent laryngeal. The oesophagus, thoracic aorta, thoracic duct, sympathetic trunk and thoracic splanchnic nerves are present in the posterior compartment. The JART is a modern CT-based four-compartment classification where the superior and the anterior mediastinum are separated by the anatomical line defined by the intersection of the caudal margin of the left innominate vein with the trachea. This falls in line with the IASLC nodal level borders. Another difference is that the oesophagus is included in the middle mediastinum [2, 7].

Three-Compartment Model The three-compartment models are popular since they follow natural anatomical borders. There is no division between the superior and anterior mediastinum. The popular Shield's classification is slowly being superseded by the CT-based ITMIG classification, where the mediastinum is divided into prevascular, visceral and paravertebral compartments based on the cross-sectional imaging (Fig. 1) [8]. The clinical significance of the 3 compartments is attached to the compartment--based tumor types of primary mediastinal tumors: A. anterior compartment-thymic tumors (thymoma, thymic carcinoma, neuroendocrine thymic tumor), lymphomas (HD, NHL), germ cell tumors, thyroid/parathyroid tumors, metastases; B. medial/visceral compartment-lung (bronchogenic, benign and malignant), lymphomas, metastases; C. posterior compartment-neurogenic tumors (schwannoma, malignant peripheral nerve sheath tumor, paraganglioma, pheochromocytoma, neuroblastoma, ganglio-neuroblastoma), non-neurogenic tumors (chordoma, chondrosarcoma, Ewing's sarcoma).

3 Epidemiology and Risk Factors

Mediastinal tumours are rare and encompass a spectrum of clinical and pathological entities. In surgical series, around 60% of resected tumours were thymomas, neurogenic tumours and benign cysts. The other 30% consisted of lymphomas, teratomas and granulomatous diseases. A similar distribution was reported in an Indian series of 91 patients with thymomas (39%), lymphomas (30%) and germ cell tumours (15%) being the top three aetiologies in adults [9]. The anterior mediastinum is the commonest site of origin and includes the following in descending order of incidence across multiple series: thymic epithelial neoplasm (35%), lymphoma (25%), thyroid mass (15%) and germ cell tumour (benign teratoma:15%, malignant: 10%). Middle and posterior mediastinal masses form 50% of the total, with lymphomas and neurogenic tumours being the commonest types (Table 1) [9–12].

The age and sex of the patient are the key demographics that influence the distribution of tumours. In adults more than 40 years of age, regardless of sex, thymic neoplasms and substernal goitres make up two-thirds of all anterior mediastinal tumours. In women between 10 and 39 years, lymphomas (Hodgkin's disease/HD or Mediastinal Large Cell Non-Hodgkin's Lymphoma/MLC-NHL), thymic neoplasms (>20 years) and benign teratomas (<25 years) are commonest. In males between 10–39 years, there is no predominant subtype with germ cell tumours, lymphomas and thymic neoplasms being equally present. For children less than 10 years, the posterior mediastinum is the commonest site of origin of neurogenic tumours, followed by rare anterior mediastinal lymphomas (Table 2) [12, 13].

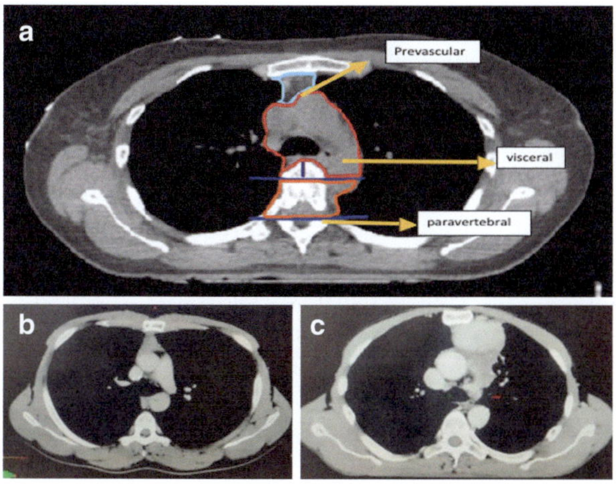

d ITMIG Mediastinal Compartments (summarized)

Compartment	Boundaries	Major Contents
Prevascular	Superior: Thoracic inlet Inferior: Diaphragm Anterior: Sternum Lateral: Mediastinal pleural reflection Posterior: Anterior aspect of pericardium	Thymus, fat, lymph nodes, left brachiocephalic vein
Visceral	Superior: Thoracic inlet Inferior: Diaphragm Anterior: Posterior boundary of prevascular compartment Posterior: Vertical line connecting a point on each thoracic vertebral body at 1 cm posterior to its anterior margin	Nonvascular: trachea, carina, esophagus, lymph nodes Vascular: Heart, aortic arch, thoracic duct
Paravertebral	Superior: Thoracic inlet Inferior: Diaphragm Anterior: Posterior boundary of visceral compartment Posterior: Vertical line against posterior margin of chest wall at the lateral margin of transverse process of thoracic spine	Paravertebral soft tissue

Fig. 1 (**a**) Axial CT slice showing ITMIG's 3 compartment model, (**b**) mass in prevascular compartment, (**c**) mass in visceral compartment, (**d**) ITMIG compartment boundaries

Table 1 Distribution of mediastinal lesions by anatomical location

Superior mediastinum	Anterior mediastinum	Middle mediastinum	Posterior mediastinum
Thymic epithelial tumour	Teratoma	Pericardial-bronchogenic-mediastinal cyst	Neurogenic tumours
Ectopic thyroid tissue	Mediastinal lymphoma	Mediastinal lymphoma	Oesophageal disease
	Mediastinal germ cell tumour		
	Thymic epithelial tumour		

Table 2 Distribution of mediastinal lesions by age

Children	Adults
Neurogenic tumours (40%)	Thymic epithelial tumour (TET) (30%)
Neuroblastoma (27%)	Germ cell tumours (GCTs)
Teratoma and lymphoma	Lymphoma
Enteric cyst, ganglioneuroma (<1%)	

4 Clinical Symptoms and Signs, Pathology

4.1 Clinical Symptoms

Asymptomatic presentation with an incidentally detected mediastinal mass detected on chest x-ray or computed tomography for unrelated reasons is common. In symptomatic patients, the presenting symptoms are varied.

1. Compressive symptoms: Cough, dyspnoea, stridor (airway); dysphagia (oesophagus)
2. Superior vena cava obstruction features: puffiness of face, neck, distended neck and chest veins
3. Hoarseness of voice (Xth cranial nerve/recurrent laryngeal nerve involvement), Horner's syndrome (brachial plexus involvement)
4. Systemic symptoms: fever, night sweats, weight loss (lymphoma); features of myasthenia gravis (thymoma)

4.2 Signs

1. General physical examination:
   (a) Thyroid swelling: to rule out retrosternal extension to mediastinum.
   (b) All lymph node sites have to be examined if a lymphoma is suspected.
   (c) Bilateral testes should be examined to rule out germ cell tumours.

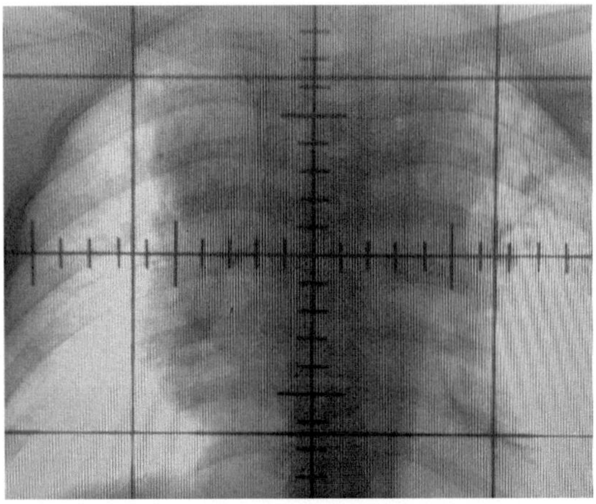

Fig. 2 A mediastinal mass on simulation chest X-ray for radiation planning

2. Paraneoplastic syndromes: Myasthenia gravis, pure red cell aplasia, agammaglobulinemia, and hypogammaglobulinemia may be associated with thymic epithelial neoplasms.
3. Imaging features:
   (a) Chest X-Ray: both PA and lateral views required
      (i) Mediastinal masses make obtuse margins with lung and do not have air bronchograms (Fig. 2)
   (b) CT chest: Mediastinal masses
   (c) 18-F FDG PET/CT scan: In mediastinal lymphomas helps identify biopsy site, monitor treatment response
   (d) MRI chest: It can rule out thymic cyst and hyperplasia and avoid unnecessary thymectomy in equivocal cases
   (e) MRI spine: required for posterior mediastinal masses
   (f) Scrotal ultrasound: to rule out a testicular swelling (in case of mediastinal germ cell tumor)
   (g) Scans in special situations: ^{131}I-MIBG scan: thoracic neuroblastoma, phaeochromocytoma; ^{68}Ga-DOTATATE PET/CT scan: thymic neuroendocrine tumours; ^{99m}Tc- pertechnetate scan (or 123-Iodine/131-Iodine scan): suspected ectopic thyroid masses
4. Serum tumour markers:
   (a) Alpha-fetoprotein (α-FP): may be raised in patients with mediastinal yolk sac tumour/endodermal sinus tumours.
   (b) Beta-human chorionic gonadotropin (β-HCG): may be raised in patients with mediastinal choriocarcinoma, embryonal carcinoma and to a lesser extent in seminoma.
   (c) Lactate dehydrogenase: may be raised in patients with mediastinal lymphoma as well as germ cell tumour. It reflects the tumour burden and may serve as a prognostic marker in patients with mediastinal lymphoma.

4.3 Pathology

In the 2015 WHO classification (4th edition), mediastinal tumours have been described under tumours of the thymus and heart. The tumours of the thymus contain epithelial neoplasms which include the spectrum from thymomas to thymic carcinoma, mediastinal germ cell tumours, lymphomas, etc. (Table 3).

Integrated Management Plan Fig. 3

5 Thymic Epithelial Tumours

Thymic epithelial tumours arise in the anterior mediastinum from thymic remnants. They include thymomas and thymic carcinomas. These are rare tumours, and western registries estimate a prevalence of around 1.5 cases per million [14, 15]. They occur in the age group of 40–60 years with no gender predisposition. Patients with thymomas are generally asymptomatic and are usually identified either with mediastinal widening or an anterior mediastinal mass on chest X-ray or CT performed for a different purpose. Metastases are uncommon with thymomas, but they are locally invasive to pericardium, heart, great vessels, lungs and sternum. Paraneoplastic syndromes commonly associated with thymomas include myasthenia gravis, pure red cell aplasia (PRCA) and acquired hypogammaglobulinemia.

Table 3 Summary of 2015 WHO classification of mediastinal tumours

Epithelial tumours	Thymoma (A, AB, B1–3) Thymic carcinoma NUT carcinoma Thymic endocrine tumours
Lymphomas of the mediastinum	Primary mediastinal B-cell lymphoma (PMBCL) Extranodal marginal zone lymphoma (MALT lymphoma) Hodgkin lymphoma T-cell lymphoblastic lymphoma/leukaemia B-cell lymphoma, unclassifiable, with features intermediate between diffuse large B cell and classical Hodgkin lymphoma (synonymous with mediastinal grey zone lymphoma, MGZL)
Germ cell tumour of the mediastinum	Seminoma Embryonal carcinoma Choriocarcinoma Yolk sac tumour Mixed germ cell tumour
Histiocytic and dendritic cell neoplasms of the mediastinum	
Myeloid sarcoma and extramedullary acute myeloid leukaemia	
Soft tissue tumours of the mediastinum	
Ectopic tumours of the thymus	
Metastasis to the mediastinum or thymus	

Approximately 10–15% of myasthenia gravis patients have thymoma, and almost half of the patients with thymoma have myasthenia gravis as paraneoplastic syndrome [16].

5.1 Staging and Risk Assessment

The staging of thymic cancers was usually done using the Masaoka staging system which guides treatment decisions (Table 4) [17]. The WHO histologic classification has prognostic value and is incorporated in decision-making algorithms [18]. The first TNM staging system for these cancers was published in the eighth edition by the American Joint Committee on Cancer (AJCC).

5.2 Management

For operable cases, characteristic CT chest supplemented by clinical signs are diagnostic. A core needle biopsy is required if neoadjuvant treatment is planned for locally advanced disease.

5.3 Treatment

5.3.1 Surgery

Total or extended thymectomy is the main treatment for thymic tumours, as complete clearance is associated with improved progression-free survival and overall survival. Patients with myasthenia gravis must undergo treatment for the same before undergoing surgical resection, as there is high risk of respiratory failure.

5.3.2 Systemic Therapy

For patients with borderline or potentially resectable disease, neoadjuvant treatment in the form of chemotherapy or chemoradiation may be considered to facilitate complete resection with negative margins. The three most commonly used neoadjuvant chemotherapy regimens include CAP [Cyclophosphamide, Adriamycin and Cisplatin], EP [Etoposide and Cisplatin] and TP [Paclitaxel and Carboplatin]. Preoperative chemoradiotherapy generally involves delivery of radiation to a dose of 45 Gy in 25 fractions over 5 weeks in combination with EP or TP. Studies have reported response rates of 70%

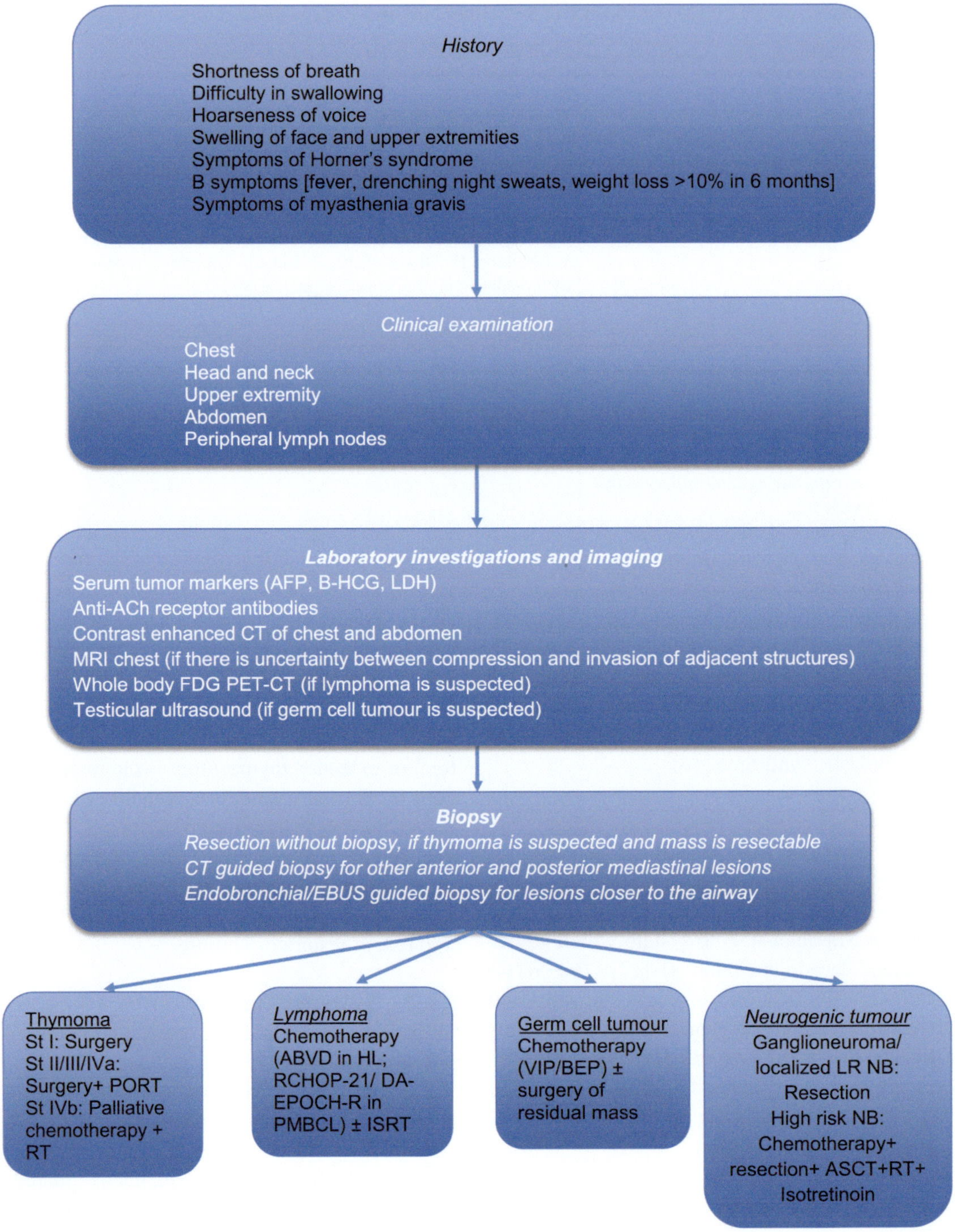

Fig. 3 Diagnostic and therapeutic approach to a patient with mediastinal tumour

Table 4 Masaoka staging system of thymic epithelial neoplasms [17]

Stage	Description
I	Macroscopically completely encapsulated tumour No microscopic capsular invasion
IIa	Macroscopic invasion into surrounding mediastinal fat and/or pleura
IIb	Microscopic capsular invasion
III	Macroscopic invasion into surrounding organs
IVa	Pleural or pericardial implants/dissemination
IVb	Haematogenous or lymphatic metastases

and resectability rates of 36–69% with neoadjuvant therapy [19–21]. Patients with distant metastatic disease are usually managed with palliative chemotherapy with reservation of palliative radiotherapy for local symptoms. Pembrolizumab or targeted therapies such as EGFR or VEGF inhibitors may be explored in patients who have progressed on chemotherapy [22, 23].

Chemotherapy Regimens

CAP

Injection Cyclophosphamide 500 mg/m^2 intravenous Day 1
Injection Adriamycin 50 mg/m^2 intravenous Day 1
Injection Cisplatin 50 mg/m^2 intravenous Day 1
Given every 3 weeks

EP

Injection Cisplatin 60 mg/m^2 intravenous Day 1
Injection Etoposide 120 mg/m^2 intravenous Day1–D3
Given every 3 weeks

5.4 Radiotherapy

Indications and Selection

1. Post-operative RT: Adjuvant radiation is recommended in patients with positive margins, gross residual disease and stage III–IV disease due to overall survival benefit. The evidence for the same in stage II disease is variable but should be considered for B2 histology onwards [24–26].
2. Definitive radiation with or without chemotherapy: Medically inoperable patients and those with unresectable tumours.
3. Neoadjuvant chemoradiotherapy: In borderline resectable cases, radiotherapy may be combined with concurrent chemotherapy.
4. Hemi thoracic radiation: In select cases (stage IVA thymoma) to treat ipsilateral pleura.

Radiotherapy Planning

Pre-treatment checklist should include operative notes, preoperative images, baseline tests including a pulmonary function test (PFT) and ECHO if high heart doses are unavoidable. Immobilisation with hands above head with a vac-lock or thermoplastic cast can be used. A 4D-CT scan should be used whenever available. The planning CT scan should have ≤3 mm slice thickness with the addition of IV contrast to better visualise mediastinal structures. For adjuvant RT, the baseline diagnostic images should be fused to the planning CT for better target delineation [27].

Target Delineation

1. Gross Tumour Volume: the residual disease in R2 resection or gross disease in definitive or neoadjuvant setting.
2. Clinical Target Volume: For adjuvant cases, it encompasses the post-operative tumour bed at risk guided by intraoperative findings, surgical clips and preoperative tumour extent. Guidance from the operating surgeon has shown to improve volume delineation accuracy [28]. In cases with gross disease, a margin of 0.5–1 cm for CTV is acceptable.
3. Planning Target Volume: CTV plus 1–1.5 cm without 4D-CT and daily kV verification, maybe reduced to 0.5 cm if both are present [27].

Treatment planning should be by conformal techniques to minimise doses to lung and mediastinal structures like the heart and the oesophagus (Fig. 4). Though direct head-to-head trials have not been done, intensity-modulated radiotherapy (IMRT) is expected to provide better conformality over three-dimensional conformal

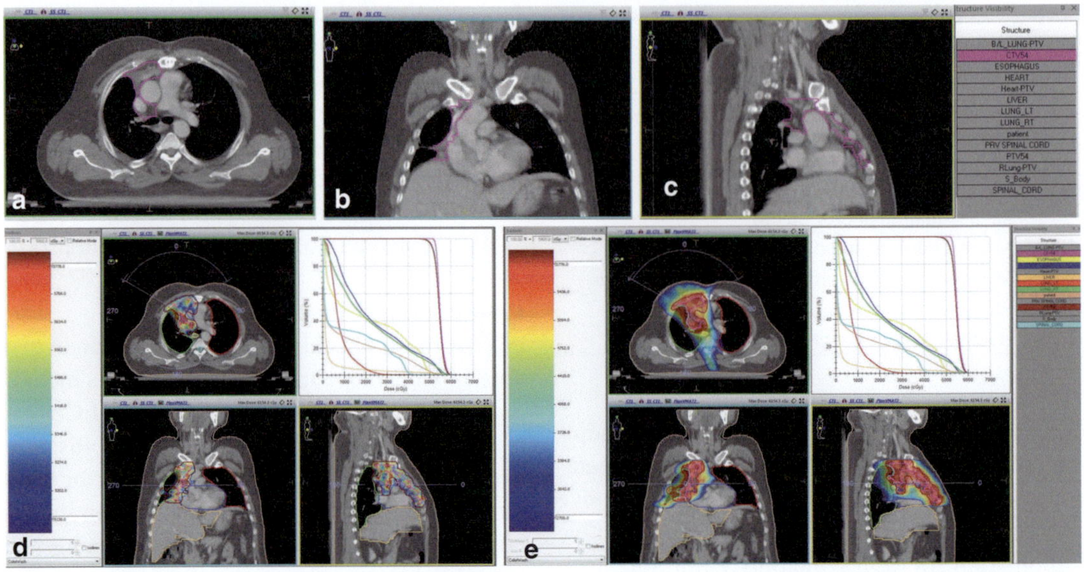

Fig. 4 In a 47-year-old male patient with Masaoka stage III thymoma (WHO type A) undergoing postoperative radiotherapy to a dose of 54 Gray in 30 fractions over 6 weeks after R1 resection, the clinical target volume (CTV) comprised the tumour bed, as seen on axial (**a**), coronal (**b**) and sagittal (**c**) sections of the contrast enhanced planning CT scan. A 1 cm isotropic expansion was given to the CTV to generate the planning target volume (PTV), to which the dose was prescribed. Postoperative adjuvant RT delivered by coplanar partial arc volumetric modulated arc therapy (VMAT) technique with 6 MV X-rays on Elekta Versa HD linear accelerator. 95–107% of the prescribed dose (54 Gray) colourwash demonstrates dose sculpting around the target volumes and the cumulative dose volume histogram (DVH) shows adequate coverage of the target volumes with simultaneous sparing of the critical organs at risk (**d**). 50–107% of the prescribed dose colourwash demonstrates the irradiated volume (**e**)

radiotherapy (3D-CRT) by extrapolating from lung cancer. The normal tissue organs at risk constraints are similar to that of lung cancer. A recent meta-analysis [25] has shown that 3-D image based modern radiotherapy techniques achieve statistically higher disease control and improved survival from 2015 onward, compared to the previous years' outcomes.

Radiotherapy Dose

1. Adjuvant: Adjuvant radiotherapy should be started within 3 months of surgery, preferably as soon as the surgical wound heals. The dose recommended in the adjuvant setting is usually 45 Gy in 25 fractions over 5 weeks.
2. Areas of positive margins should be given a minimum of 54 Gy.
3. For definitive RT or gross residual disease, doses of up to 60 Gy should be used.

Results and outcome: The five- and ten-year overall survival (OS) in patients with thymomas is 90% whereas the five-year rate varies from 30 to 50% for thymic carcinomas [25, 29, 30]. Completeness of resection and 3-D image based modern radiotherapy delivery are the most important indicators of survival [25, 31].

5.5 Indian Experience

In a retrospective study of 62 patients with thymoma treated at Tata Memorial Hospital, Mumbai with multimodality approach from 2006 to 11, 57% of the patients had early (stage I–II) tumours [32]. The most common histopathological subtype was WHO subtype B (49%). The mean tumour size was 5.3 cm in patients with myasthenia and 7.6 cm in the entire cohort. The median OS was 60 months and the 3-year OS rate was 90% (94% in resectable tumours versus 81% in unresectable tumours). Masaoka stage was the only significant prognostic factor on multivariate analysis (MVA) of OS.

In another retrospective study of 7I patients with thymoma treated at All India Institute of Medical Sciences, New Delhi with multimodality approach from 1999 to 2013, 91.5% of the patients had advanced (stage III–IV) tumours [33]. Association with myasthenia was noted in 44% patients. Three patients had pure red cell aplasia (PRCA) documented. A majority of the patients (80.3%) were treated with surgery (radical thymectomy) followed by post-operative RT. The median follow-up was 19.3 months. The 2-year and 3-year PFS rates were 78.3% and 57.1%, respectively. On univariate analysis of PFS, surgery and Masaoka stage were significant prognostic factors. Masaoka stage retained prognostic significance on MVA of PFS.

6 Germ Cell Tumour

Primary extragonadal germ cell tumours are solid tumours arising from midline sites of the body with no evidence of gonadal disease. These are rare tumours comprising less than 5% of all germ cell tumours with the mediastinum being the commonest site [34]. They are usually divided into seminomas and non-seminomatous germ cell tumours. Mediastinal seminomas, often diagnosed between the ages of 20 and 40, account for 2–4% of mediastinal tumours and approximately one third of mediastinal GCTs [35]. Approximately three-fourths of patients are symptomatic at diagnosis. Mediastinal non-seminomatous germ cell tumours, often associated with marked elevation of α-FP and/or β-HCG, include yolk sac tumours, embryonal carcinoma, teratomas and mixed tumours (Table 5).

Table 5 Germ cell tumours of the mediastinum

Seminoma
Embryonal carcinoma
Yolk sac tumour
Choriocarcinoma
Teratoma
Teratoma, mature
Teratoma, immature
Mixed germ cell tumour
Germ cell tumours with somatic-type solid malignancy
Germ cell tumours with associated haematological malignancy

6.1 Treatment

Surgery is the curative treatment for mature teratomas as these tumours are relatively insensitive to both radiation and chemotherapy. Subtotal resection can be attempted in symptomatic patients if complete resection is not possible. VIP [Etoposide, Ifosfamide, Cisplatin] chemotherapy followed by surgical resection is recommended in patients with immature teratomas [36, 37]. As these patients often require surgery after completion of chemotherapy, BEP chemotherapy is generally not preferred due to associated high risk of postoperative pulmonary complications [38]. Other non-seminomatous GCTs are treated with four cycles of VIP, and surgical resection is usually reserved for patients with post-chemotherapy residual mass [39]. For patients with mediastinal seminomas, surgery is usually not performed upfront as they are highly sensitive to chemotherapy and radiation therapy. Three cycles of BEP [Bleomycin, Etoposide, Cisplatin] regimen or four cycles of EP regimen are recommended for good risk [mediastinal seminoma with no extrapulmonary metastases] tumours, and four cycles of BEP are recommended for intermediate risk [mediastinal seminoma with extrapulmonary metastases] tumours, as chemotherapy provides longer disease-free survival in 90% of treated patients. Surgical resection may be considered in patients with a PET-positive post-chemotherapy residual mass of $\geq$3 cm [40, 41]. Radiation therapy, including mediastinum and bilateral supraclavicular fossae, is generally not preferred as first-line treatment as there is risk of late toxicities and usually considered in patients with contraindications to chemotherapy. Radiotherapy, given selectively, combined with systemic chemotherapy or targeted drug is a viable option for inoperable mediastinal germ cell tumors [35].

6.2 Chemotherapy Regimens

BEP

Injection Bleomycin 30 units IV on Day 1, 8, 15 or Day 2, 9, 16

Injection Etoposide 100 mg/m^2 IV on Days 1–5

Injection Cisplatin 20 mg/m^2 IV on Days 1–5

Given every 3 weeks

EP

Injection Etoposide 100 mg/m^2 IV on Days 1–5

Injection Cisplatin 20 mg/m^2 IV on Days 1–5

Given every 3 weeks

VIP

Injection Etoposide 75 mg/m^2 IV on Days 1–5

Injection Ifosfamide 1200 mg/m^2 on Days 1–5 (with MESNA uroprotection)

Injection Cisplatin 20 mg/m^2 IV on Days 1–5

Given every 3 weeks

7 Lymphoma

Lymphomas involving the mediastinum may be either primary mediastinal lymphoma or could be part of the involvement of systemic lymphoma. Primary mediastinal B-cell lymphomas (PMBCL) and Hodgkin lymphomas (HL) are the most common primary mediastinal lymphomas, usually involving the anterior mediastinum. Primary mediastinal B-cell lymphoma is an aggressive malignancy predominantly seen between the ages of 30 and 40 with a female preponderance. Patients generally present with bulky mediastinal mass (>10 cm) with stage I or II disease. Distant spread at initial presentation is less common. Vascular encasement on imaging is seen in approximately two-thirds of cases. The diagnostic and staging workup is similar to other high-grade lymphomas. Unlike Hodgkin lymphomas that typically express CD15 and 30, patients with primary mediastinal B-cell lymphomas express pan B-cell markers [CD20 and CD79a] and MAL-1 and CD200. In addition, PMBCL may show variable expression of CD30. Patients are classified as having limited-stage or advanced-stage disease. For patients with limited stage PMBCL, R-CHOP [Rituximab, Cyclophosphamide, Doxorubicin, Vincristine and Prednisolone] for 6 cycles followed by involved site radiation therapy (ISRT) to the mediastinum to a dose of 30 Gy in 15 fractions over 3 weeks is recommended. Dose-adjusted EPOCH-R [Etoposide, Prednisolone, Vincristine, Cyclophosphamide, Doxorubicin and Rituximab] for 6–8 cycles may be considered in patients not willing for mediastinal radiotherapy and in young females [42–44]. In Hodgkins lymphoma, ABVD [Adriamycin, Bleomycin, Vinblastine and Dacarbazine] for 4–6 cycles is given, followed by mediastinal radiotherapy to a dose of 20–30 Gy in 10–15 fractions over 2–3 weeks. In early-stage HL, all initially involved lymph nodes or extranodal sites are encompassed in the RT portal, whereas only the site of prechemotherapy bulk or post-chemotherapy metabolically active residual disease is addressed in advanced HL.

Involved field radiotherapy [IFRT], ISRT, and involved node radiotherapy [INRT] are three different contemporary radiation therapy techniques in lymphomas. In IFRT, the entire initially involved lymph node regions, based on traditional bony anatomical landmarks, are irradiated. In ISRT and INRT, only the initially involved lymph nodes are irradiated (Fig. 5). In this context, prechemotherapy whole body 18F-FDG-PET/CT scan should be done, preferably in the radiotherapy treatment position and should be subsequently electronically fused with the planning CT scan. The GTV is delineated on the baseline PET/CT scan and adapted on the planning CT scan. Notably, ISRT differs from INRT by including a safety margin (craniocaudal expansion of 1.5 cm along the lymphatic chain) to the GTV to generate the CTV. A further expansion of 5–10 mm (depending upon respiratory motion management strategy) is given to the CTV to generate the PTV. The basic prerequisite for both ISRT and INRT is to have an accurate prechemotherapy extent of disease. If the initial extent of disease is uncertain, IFRT is recommended rather than ISRT or INRT.

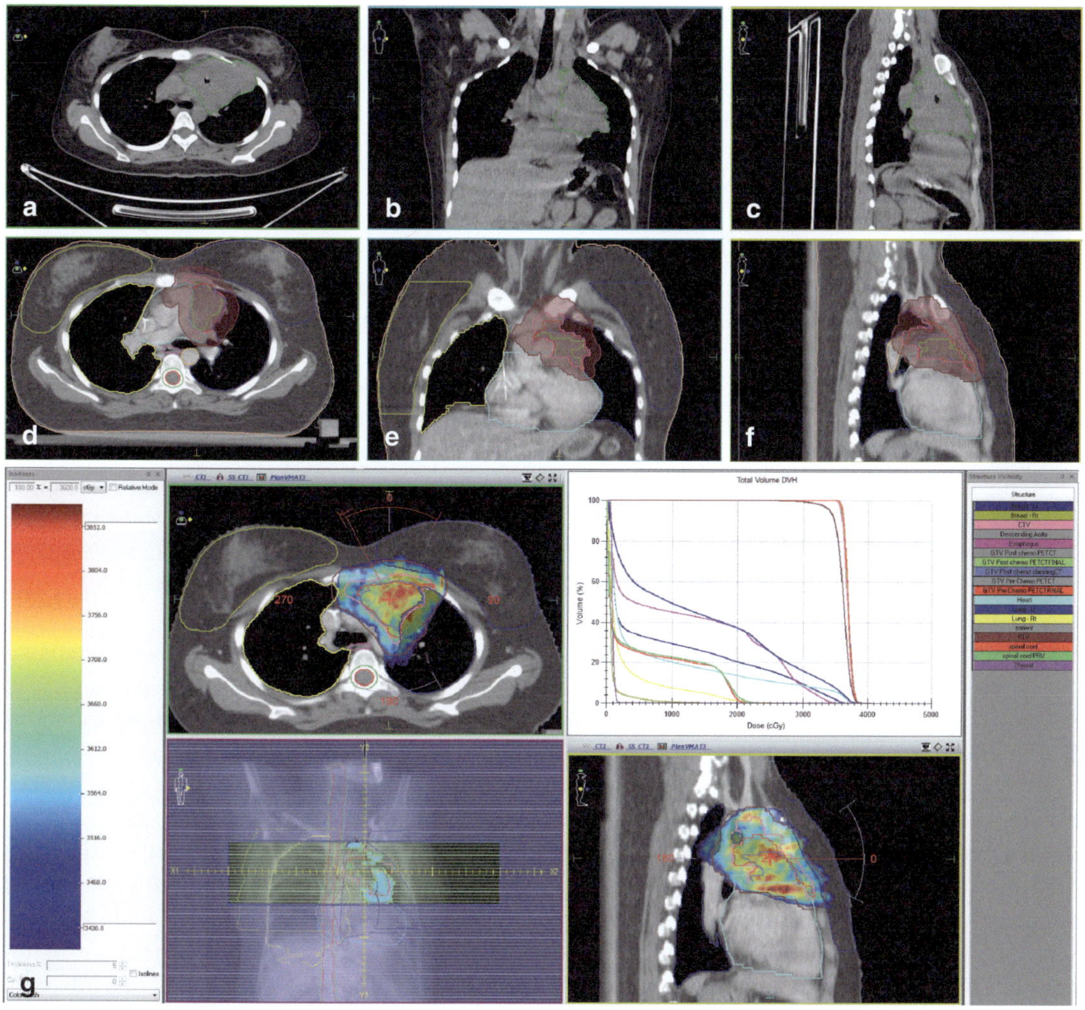

Fig. 5 A 24-year-old female patient with primary mediastinal B-cell lymphoma (thymic type) stage I underwent consolidative involved site radiotherapy (ISRT) to a dose of 36 Gray in 20 fractions over 4 weeks after obtaining partial metabolic response (Deauville score 4) to 6 cycles of dose adjusted R-EPOCH regimen. The gross tumour volume (GTV) was initially contoured on the baseline whole body PET-CT scan and the same may be appreciated on the axial (**a**), coronal (**b**) and sagittal (**c**) sections of the baseline CT. The adapted and residual GTVs, the clinical target volume (GTV+ 1.5 cm anatomically constrained craniocaudal expansion along the lymphatic chain), the planning target volume (CTV+ 1 cm isotropic expansion) and the critical organs at risk (OARs), subsequently delineated on the contrast enhancing planning CT scan, may be seen on the axial (**d**), coronal (**e**) and sagittal (**f**) sections. She underwent ISRT by non-coplanar partial arc volumetric modulated arc therapy (VMAT) technique with 6 MV X-rays on Elekta Versa HD linear accelerator. 95–107% of the prescribed dose (36 Gray) colourwash demonstrates dose sculpting around the target volumes and the cumulative dose volume histogram (DVH) shows adequate coverage of the target volumes with simultaneous sparing of the OARs (the mean radiation dose to heart- 6.6 Gray, right lung- 2.5 Gray, left lung- 13.87 Gray, right breast- 0.86 Gray, left breast- 8.36 Gray) (g). The end-of-treatment whole body PET-CT scan revealed a complete metabolic response

7.1 Chemotherapy Regimens

ABVD

Injection Adriamycin 25 mg/m^2 IV Day 1 and 15
Injection Bleomycin 10 U/m^2 IV Day 1 and 15
Injection Vinblastine 6 mg/m^2 IV Day 1 and 15
Injection Dacarbazine 375 mg/m^2 IV Day 1 and 15
Given every 4 weeks

R-CHOP

Injection Rituximab 375 mg/m^2 IV Day 1
Injection Cyclophosphamide 750 mg/m^2 IV Day 1
Injection Doxorubicin 50 mg/m^2 IV Day 1
Injection Vincristine 1.4 mg/m^2 (capped at 2 mg) IV Day 1
Tab Prednisolone 100 mg OD Day 1–5

8 Neurogenic Tumour

Neurogenic tumours, though rare, form the majority of posterior mediastinal masses. In children, they are the commonest site of mediastinal tumours overall. The majority are benign (15% in adults, 50% in children) and are often asymptomatic, thus reaching large sizes. Dumbbell tumours are those that extend into the spinal foramina. In such cases, paraparesis may occur due to spinal cord compression. During workup, CEMRI of the spine is required to determine the extent of disease because surgery in these cases is often a collaborative thoracic surgery-neurosurgery venture.

Broadly, neurogenic tumours can be grouped based on their neural cell of origin (Table 6):

8.1 Tumours Arising from Nerve Sheath

Schwannomas and neurofibromas are benign and the commonest of all neurogenic tumours. In 25–40% cases, these are associated with Neurofibromatosis Type 1. Surgical resection is the standard approach in these cases. The malignant counterparts of these tumours are malignant peripheral nerve sheath tumors (MPNSTs) are aggressive in nature and constitute 10% of soft tissue sarcomas. The treatment for MPNSTs of mediastinum is individualised on the principles of management of soft tissue sarcomas in general. Radiation has been identified as a causative factor for a few reported cases of radiation-induced MPNSTs. MPNSTs associated with NF1 tend to have a worse prognosis.

In a case series of six patients with mediastinal MPNST from Japan, three patients who could undergo R0 resection had long-term survival. Adjuvant radiation and chemotherapy were given to three patients each [45]. The benefits of adjuvant radiotherapy can only be extrapolated from MPNSTs of other sites. An Indian series of MPNSTs across all sites showed both a disease-free survival (DFS) and OS benefit with the addition of post-operative radiotherapy [46]. Though an OS benefit with adjuvant radiotherapy has not been consistently established, a locoregional failure-free survival has been observed across multiple studies [47–49]. In locally advanced and metastatic cases, a DFS benefit has been seen with palliative radiotherapy [50]. Resection is the most important predictor for survival in MPNSTs [48].

Table 6 Neurogenic tumours of the mediastinum

Nerve tumours	Sympathetic ganglia tumour	Paraganglia cell tumour
Neurofibroma	Ganglioneuroma	Paraganglioma (Phaeochromocytoma)
Schwannoma	Ganglioneuroblastoma	
Malignant peripheral nerve sheath tumour (MPNST)	Neuroblastoma	

8.2 Tumour Arising from Sympathetic Ganglia

A posterior mediastinal mass with calcification in childhood is suggestive of a neurogenic tumour, probably originating from the sympathetic ganglion. These tumours may be benign, e.g. ganglioneuroma (more common in older children), or malignant, e.g. ganglioneuroblastoma and neuroblastoma (more common in children younger than 3 years) [51]. The most common neurogenic tumour in this location is neuroblastoma. Mediastinal neuroblastoma constitutes 11–26% of all neuroblastoma. Compared to abdominal neuroblastoma, mediastinal neuroblastoma presents more frequently in early stage and is associated with relatively better prognosis [52]. The management of mediastinal neuroblastoma depends upon tumour stage, biology and the risk-stratum. Early-stage low-risk tumours may be managed by surgical resection alone. Advanced stage high-risk tumours usually require multimodality treatment in the form of multi-agent chemotherapy [Cyclophosphamide, Doxorubicin, Cisplatin/Carboplatin, Etoposide], surgery, high dose chemotherapy [Busulfan and Melphalan] and autologous stem cell transplant followed by post-transplant radiation therapy, differentiation therapy [13-cis retinoic acid] and immunotherapy [anti-ganglioside 2 (GD2) antibody]. Post-transplant radiation therapy to the tumour bed and post-induction MIBG-avid metastatic sites 21 Gy in 14 fractions over 14 working days is usually given on Day 60 of transplant by 3D-CRT or IMRT (Fig. 6). A large majority of the young children (<3 years) require sedation or general anaesthesia to aid immobilisation before radiation therapy. Compared to 3D-CRT, IMRT plans result in better conformity and sparing of the critical organs at risk, but may be associated with higher integral dose and low dose bath. In this context, proton beam therapy may lead to comparable target coverage with even lower collateral dose to surrounding organs at risk (due to Bragg peak) and hence is being explored in clinical trials [53]. Higher expenditure and limited availability are some of the obstacles to widespread adoption of this technology.

9 Endocrine Tumours

9.1 Thyroid Tumours

Direct extension of thyroid tumours to the superior and anterior mediastinum is common. Benign goitres are slow-growing and surgical resection is sufficient. Thyroid carcinomas have a more rapid course. Surgical resection followed by radioiodine remnant ablation and supraphysiological doses of levothyroxine is the treatment in differentiated thyroid cancers. Radiotherapy can be used for palliation of symptomatic metastatic sites or in inoperable cases [54].

Ectopic mediastinal thyroid tumours without connection to the cervical thyroid gland are rare. Both follicular and papillary carcinomas have been reported to arise from ectopic thyroid tissue. The treatment is surgical resection followed by radio-iodine therapy, similar to that of primary thyroid cancer [55, 56].

10 Tracheal Tumours

Primary tumours of the trachea are almost always malignant in adults (90%), with squamous cell carcinoma and adenoid cystic carcinoma being the commonest subtypes. In children, however, only 10–30% are malignant. Endoscopic resection or laser/electrocautery fulguration may suffice for benign tumours in children [57].

Upfront surgery has been associated with improved survival—180 months versus 48 months with non-surgical management in an individual patient data meta-analysis. Radiotherapy plays a key role in the adjuvant, definitive and palliative setting. In unresectable tumours, a dose of more than 60 Gy is associated with improved survival [58]. After surgery, adjuvant radiotherapy is routinely advocated for all patients with factors such as type of resection, lymphatic invasion and thyroid gland involvement providing prognostic value [59]. In a French study, the 5-year survival improved with adjuvant radiotherapy in patients after both complete resection (74% vs. 53%) and incomplete resection (45% vs. 0%) [60]. Endoluminal brachyther-

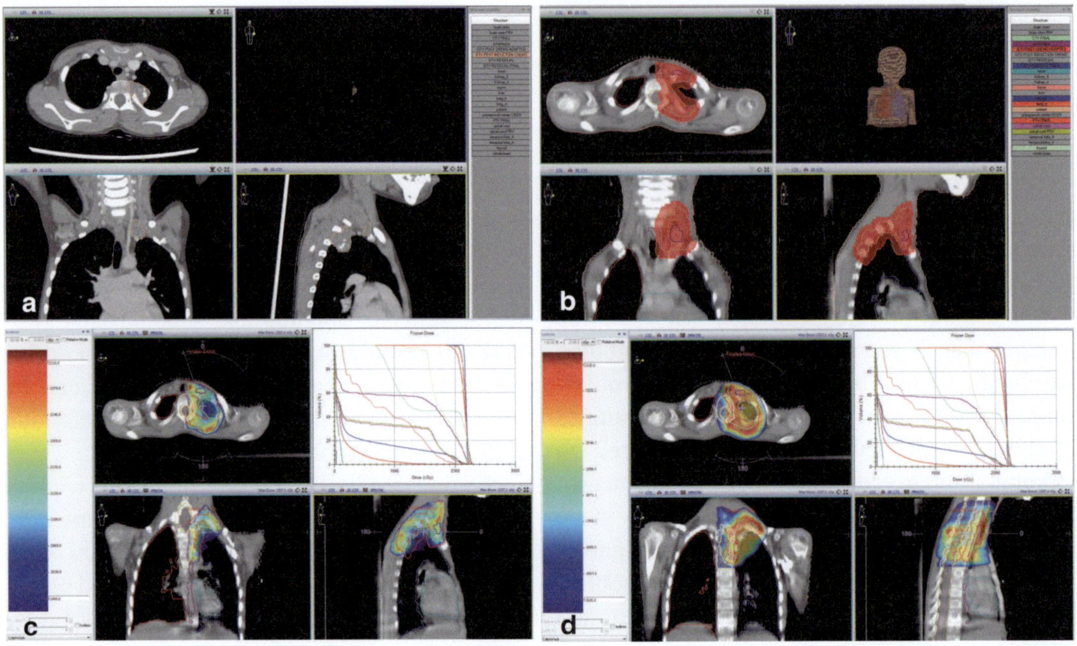

Fig. 6 A 6-year-old male child with high risk, *MYCN* non-amplified neuroblastoma of the left paraspinal region (D1–D4) with metastasis to the left supraclavicular fossa underwent post-transplant radiotherapy to a dose of 21 Gray in 14 fractions over 3 weeks on day-60. The residual gross tumour volume (GTV) was initially contoured on the post-induction chemotherapy CT scan (**a**). The adapted post-induction and post-transplant residual GTVs, the clinical target volume (GTV+ 1 cm anatomically constrained expansion), the planning target volume (CTV+ 0.5 cm isotropic expansion) and the critical organs at risk (OARs) were subsequently delineated on the contrast enhancing planning CT scan (**b**). He underwent post-transplant RT by coplanar partial arc volumetric modulated arc therapy (VMAT) technique with 6 MV X-rays on Elekta Synergy S linear accelerator. 95–110% of the prescribed dose (21 Gray) colourwash demonstrates dose sculpting around the target volumes and the cumulative dose volume histogram (DVH) shows adequate coverage of the target volumes with simultaneous sparing of the OARs (the mean radiation dose to heart- 0.42 Gray, right lung- 1.3 Gray, left lung- 2.84 Gray, thyroid gland- 15.18 Gray, larynx- 8.23 Gray) (**c**). The primary ossification centres (C6–D5) were symmetrically irradiated ($D95 \geq 15.2$ Gy) to limit the lateral (left to right) radiation dose gradient below 5 Gray to prevent late scoliosis (**d**)

apy has been used in a few specialised centres, both as a boost post-external beam radiotherapy in radical patients and for symptom palliation in advanced cases [61].

In view of the rarity and poor prognosis of tracheal tumours, a combined modality approach is essential for the management of malignant tracheal tumours. Surgical management of tumours in centres of expertise should be encouraged. Radiotherapy with modern techniques should be offered to almost all patients in the adjuvant setting. It also provides durable local control rates in inoperable patients provided high doses are delivered.

11 Cardiac Tumours

Primary cardiac tumours are rare and often diagnosed after death. Metastasis from lung cancer is the commonest presentation and needs to be ruled out. The symptoms mimic those of heart failure and thus, presentation of primary tumours is often in an advanced stage.

Nearly 75% of all cardiac tumours are benign, with atrial myxomas arising from the interatrial septum forming the majority. Surgical resection is curative for these lesions.

The remaining one-fourth of malignant tumours comprises primarily of sarcomas that originate from the myocardium with angiosarcoma, rhabdomyosarcoma and undifferentiated/NOS being the three commonest histologies in decreasing order of frequency. Primary mesothelioma arising from the pericardium is another rare, malignant primary tumour that almost always presents with metastasis [62].

Surgical resection, whenever possible, should be attempted in malignant primary tumours. However, this often is the exception rather than the norm because the majority of patients present with metastatic disease. Surgery for a sarcoma should be followed by adjuvant radiotherapy to reduce local recurrence. There is also a potential role of heart transplantation for unresectable, non-metastatic tumours [63]. Primary pericardial tumours often are symptomatic on presentation, requiring pericardiocentesis or pericardiectomy. Treatment for pericardial mesothelioma can be extrapolated from pleural mesothelioma. Following primary surgical resection, adjuvant chemotherapy with pemetrexed and cisplatin should be considered [64].

12 Miscellaneous and Rare Tumours

12.1 NUT Carcinoma

NUT Carcinoma [synonyms: NUT midline carcinoma; thymic carcinoma with t(15;19)] is a rare, aggressive, poorly differentiated carcinoma with a median survival of 5–6 months. Presentation can be across all age groups. Due to its rapid clinical course, disease is usually locally advanced with pleural and lung invasion on presentation. Metastasis is common, commonly to bones. The anterior mediastinum is the commonest location with infiltration of local structures on imaging. Whole body PET/CT is the imaging modality of choice to assess baseline disease status, metastatic burden and monitor response. Tissue diagnosis is established with diffuse positivity of Nuclear protein in Testis (NUT) on IHC and the characteristic translocation [t(15;19)] and fusion of the *NUT* gene to *BRD4* (70%), *BRD3* (6%), etc.

Complete resection and radiotherapy are associated with improved survival. However, resectability is often not possible in view of advanced stage at presentation, and treatment has to be individualised. In a review of 119 patients with NUT carcinomas from all sites, 26% arose from the mediastinum. Radiotherapy was used radically in 17 (median dose = 64.5 Gy), post-operatively in 9 (median dose = 63 Gy), pre-operatively in 1 (dose = 66 Gy) and with palliative intent (dose of 20–30 Gy) in 10 patients, respectively [65]. There are ongoing clinical trials of Bromodomain Extra-Terminal (BET) inhibitors targeting BRD4 protein, which plays a significant role in NUT carcinoma as mentioned above.

12.2 Thymic Neuroendocrine Tumour

Thymic neuroendocrine tumours (NETs), commonly known as thymic carcinoids, are the rarest of primary thymic epithelial neoplasms, comprising less than 5% of the total. These are often associated with endocrinopathies like Cushing's syndrome, acromegaly, MEN-1 syndrome, etc. Nearly 25% patients of thymic NETs are diagnosed with MEN-1 syndrome, underlying the consideration of prophylactic thymectomy in MEN-1 patients [66].

These are aggressive tumours with a high propensity to recur locally and metastasise. Adequate surgery is the primary prognostic factor. For adjuvant treatment, lung neuroendocrine tumour principles can be extrapolated. Adjuvant local radiotherapy may be provided to incompletely resected, well-differentiated (typical) and moderately differentiated (atypical) NETs. However, for poorly differentiated histologies, adjuvant radiotherapy should be provided to all, regardless of resection status. Adjuvant chemotherapy with platinum and etoposide is given for all poorly differentiated tumours, whereas evidence is unclear for atypical tumours [67].

13 Mediastinal Lymphadenopathy

Mediastinal lymphadenopathy as such is not considered as a primary tumour of mediastinum. But in India and in few developing countries where tuberculosis is common, there is high propensity of only mediastinal lymphadenopathy at presentation. Therefore, it is imperative to discuss this as an individual entity for reasons related to various differentials of malignant tumour. Mediastinal lymph nodes are said to be significant if short axis diameter is >1 cm on cross-sectional imaging. Though they can occur at any part of mediastinum secondary to inflammatory or neoplastic lesions, the most common location is the middle mediastinum. Malignancies such as lung cancer, breast cancer and oesophageal carcinomas have high risk of spread to mediastinal lymph nodes. Apart from cancerous lesions, non-neoplastic conditions such as tuberculosis, histoplasmosis, sarcoidosis and pneumoconiosis frequently result in mediastinal lymphadenopathies.

14 Surgical Aspects of Mediastinal Tumours

14.1 Approach and Techniques

The approaches to surgery depend upon various conditions like disease factors (location, extent of the tumour, relation to important anatomical structures like major vessels, airways, lungs, pericardium and heart, neural structures, requirement for mobilisation and reconstruction), patient factors (body structure, ability to withstand long duration anaesthesia, haemodynamics) and institutional factors (available infrastructure and expertise of the surgical team). Broadly the surgical approaches can be divided into two groups: the open approach and the minimally invasive approach. Minimally invasive approaches can be either video-assisted thoracoscopic surgery (VATS) or robotic-assisted approach and have perioperative advantages of being less painful with shorter hospital stay and fewer chances of wound infection and are considered to be the first choice. It also allows the surgical treatment to be offered to patients with borderline respiratory function who may not tolerate an open surgical approach. Judicious selection of cases (tumours less than 5 cm, non-invasive tumours and availability of technical expertise and an experienced team) is of paramount importance.

The use of minimally invasive techniques like VATS and robotics has recently been taken up in most centres. The approach for right-sided tumours is a right-sided VATS using a 4–5 cm traditional utility incision in the 5th intercostal space (ICS) and additional ports for camera and assistant as necessary. If tumours are smaller, VATS is an option using a 2–3 cm utility incision in the 5th ICS. Similarly, a left-sided approach can be used for tumour located towards the left side. In centrally placed tumours, subxiphoid approach is a well-known procedure. VATS causes less muscle traction and injury resulting in better postoperative pain-free periods and faster recovery. Currently, uniportal techniques have been found to be equally safe and promising with respect to perioperative outcomes like hospital stay and 30-day morbidity rates [68]. In this technique, 5 or 10 mm 30° video camera is used along with other instruments through the single port placed in 4th or 5th ICS.

With the launch of da Vinci surgical systems, robotic surgery has paved its way into the current era of thoracic surgery. The advantages of robotics over VATS are seven degrees of freedom of movement and control, thereby allowing to handle even complicated cases in deep cavities using the minimally invasive technique. Investigators comparing robot-assisted thoracoscopic surgery (RATS) with multi-portal VATS have reported shorter chest tube placement time (2.21 ± 1.11 vs. 2.43 ± 0.88 days, $p = 0.001$) and hospital stay (3.62 ± 1.21 vs. 4.07 ± 1.75 days, $p = 0.001$), without any rise in complication rates [69].

The open approach is preferred for large and invasive tumours. Patients who present with mediastinal tumours invading resectable structures like the mediastinal pleura, pericardium or adjacent lung should undergo primary curative surgical treatment with the aim of achieving an R0 resection. The usual approach to mediastinal tumours is median sternotomy for open surgery. For tumours located more towards either side of the mediastinum, a unilateral thoracotomy can also provide adequate exposure. Combining the partial sternotomy and limited thoracotomy (the hemiclamshell approach) becomes useful in cases with a larger tumour extending on either side, i.e. towards left or right hemithorax, with possible invasion of the surrounding structures or invasion of the lung. Frequently, these tumours invade the surrounding structures like the SVC, brachiocephalic vein, subclavian, carotid and innominate vessels necessitating extensive resection and reconstruction. An anterior open approach can provide adequate exposure in these scenarios with a central invasive focus. A situation like the involvement of the tumour with the right main bronchus requiring mobilisation and sleeve resection can be better approached from the right lateral side. Occasionally, neurogenic tumours extend to the spinal foramen and require cooperation between a thoracic surgeon and neurosurgeon. In general, a proper preoperative evaluation is key to a safe and successful strategy involving a multidisciplinary team.

14.2 Surgery for Invasive Mediastinal Tumours with Reconstruction or Bypass

Mediastinal tumours invading the adjacent major vasculature may need resection and reconstruction of vessels for complete removal of the tumour. Arterial resection almost always requires reconstruction, whereas in tumours invading veins (e.g. brachiocephalic or subclavian veins) decision to do reconstruction depends on the development of collateral veins. Veinous reconstruction may not be required in patients with prolonged obstruction of the veins where collaterals have developed. For instance, the removal of a segment of the left brachiocephalic vein in a patient with long-duration venous obstruction/thrombosis may not require reconstruction and the vein may be simply ligated. Resection of superior vena cava almost always requires reconstruction.

Situations where arterial resection is done (e.g. brachiocephalic, subclavian or axillary artery) necessitate reconstruction. Such surgeries may require a cardiopulmonary bypass, not just for reconstruction but also to assess and complete primary resection of the tumour with tumour-free margins. The conduit for reconstruction can be biological graft, including an autograft (like internal jugular vein) or an allograft, which is preferred if available. Alternatives are prosthetic grafts like polytetrafluoroethylene (PTFE). In cases where only a part of the circumference of the vessel has been resected, a venous patch from an opened segment of saphenous vein or a part of any resected vein may be used for reconstruction.

Dense adhesions or frank tumour infiltration of the pericardium requires the removal of a part of it. Pericardial defects thus formed require patch cover (using a bovine pericardium or a prosthetic graft), especially if the defect is large (more than 5 cm) or around the ventricles.

14.3 Hyperthermic Intrathoracic Chemotherapy

Recently, hyperthermic intrathoracic chemotherapy (HITHOC) has emerged as a new modality of treatment [70]. In this process, chemotherapy is circulated through a perfusion pump after adequate dilution, and the drug is instilled into the thoracic cavity for a variable time (60–120 min) at a set temperature of 40–45 °C [71]. Drugs commonly used are Cisplatin in isolation or in combination with other cytotoxics like Doxorubicin, Epirubicin, Oxaliplatin, and Mitomycin [72]. This procedure is indicated in tumours (especially thymomas) presenting with pleural nodules. Studies have found varying response rates to the HITHOC treatment with some authors reporting manageable toxicities, lower recurrence rates, longer overall and disease-free survival [73].

15 Conclusion

Mediastinal tumours are very heterogeneous and differential diagnoses are formulated based on information such as age, sex, clinical presentation and imaging findings. In clinical care for patients with mediastinal tumours, the entity of mediastinal mass syndrome (MMS) is a complex life-threatening situation. Giant anterior mediastinal mass, ≥10 cm., may cause MMS, often characterised by sudden and severe haemodynamic and respiratory decompensation. The patho-physiology involves the tumour often growing unnoticed, heart/great vessel (superior vena cava, pulmonary artery) compression, and/or central tracheo-bronchial compression. Airway management, cardiac support and decompression of the giant tumor (by surgery, chemotherapy or radiotherapy) become emergency therapeutic measures. Surgery of the mediastinum requires caution for anesthesia and surgical procedure. The MMS classification (safe, uncertain, and unsafe) requires careful consideration before surgery, chemotherapy or thoracic radiotherapy (depending upon tumor type- thymoma, germ cell tumor, lymphoma, teratoma etc.) [74]. With the increasing incidence of precise diagnosis for most of the mediastinal tumours in the present era of sophisticated radiological imaging, and molecular pathology, the management of mediastinal tumours has significantly improved, and has become tailored leading to increased overall and disease-free survival. Recent advances in surgical techniques (VATS, RATS), radiotherapy techniques (IMRT, IMPT, respiratory motion management) and systemic therapy (novel targeted biological agents and immune checkpoint inhibitors) have the potential to further improve treatment outcome, simultaneously mitigate treatment-related acute and late morbidities and optimise health-related quality of life.

Percepts Box

1. The anterior mediastinum is the most common site of mediastinal tumours with thymic epithelial neoplasms being the most common tumour.
2. In adult males over 40 years, substernal goitres are the most common tumours, while in women between 10 and 39 years, lymphomas are the most common mediastinal tumours.
3. Patients with mediastinal tumour may be asymptomatic at presentation with the tumour being detected incidentally. When symptomatic, they could present with compressive symptoms or features of SVCO, Horner's syndrome or general systemic features. Mediastinal mass syndrome should be diagnosed early.
4. Certain tumours, like thymic epithelial tumours, could be associated with paraneoplastic syndromes like Myasthenia gravis, red cell aplasias, etc.
5. Tumours like nonseminomatous germ cell tumours (GCT) or seminomas may be associated with raised serum tumour marker levels.
6. Thymic epithelial tumours comprise thymomas or thymic carcinomas. These are staged according to the Masoaka-Koga staging system. They are most commonly seen in 40–60--year age group.
7. The mainstay of treatment in thymic epithelial tumours is surgery, usually a total or extended thymectomy. In potentially resectable cases, they could be treated by NACT or NACTRT.
8. Post-operative RT is indicated in positive margins, gross residual disease and stage III-IV disease to improve OS in patients with thymoma. Recommended dose is 45 Gy in 25

(continued)

fractions, dose should be increased to 54 Gy in R1 resection.

9. Primary extragonadal GCTs are rare tumours but are most commonly found in the mediastinum. Mature teratomas are relatively resistant to both chemo and radiotherapy and are commonly treated with excision. Immature teratomas are treated with NACT followed by surgery. RT is generally not considered as a part of 1st line therapy and is reserved for patients who cannot receive chemotherapy.
10. Primary mediastinal lymphomas are usually Hodgkin's lymphoma (HL) or primary mediastinal B-cell lymphomas (PMBCL). The latter is further classified as limited stage or advanced stage disease, is more aggressive and expresses CD20, CD79a and MAL-1 and CD200.
11. Limited-stage PMBCL is usually treated with chemoimmunotherapy (R-CHOP) followed by ISRT (30 Gy/15 fractions). There is an attempt to avoid the late effects of mediastinal radiotherapy by using more intensive chemotherapy (dose adjusted EPOCH-R) particularly in young females.
12. HL is treated with ABVD chemotherapy (4–6 cycles) followed by mediastinal RT (20–30 Gy in 10–15 fractions).
13. Neurogenic tumours are rare, although mostly benign tumours and are the most common type of posterior mediastinal tumours. They are grouped based on their neural cell of origin- nerve sheath tumours, sympathetic or parasympathetic ganglia tumours.
14. Schwannomas and neurofibromas are benign and are the most common type of nerve sheath tumours. In up to 40%, they are associated with NF-I. When associated with NF-1, the malignant counterpart, MPNST, has a poorer prognosis. Treatment is highly individualised.
15. Sympathetic ganglia tumours can either be benign (ganglioneuroma) or malignant (ganglioneuroblastoma or neuroblastoma). Early-stage tumours can be managed with surgery alone, whereas advanced stages usually need some form of adjuvant therapy. Radiotherapy is an important component of multimodality management of high-risk neuroblastoma.
16. Endocrine tumours like thyroid carcinoma have a rapid course. These are treated by surgical removal followed by radio-iodine ablation in case of any remnants and Levothyroxine. RT is usually given for palliation or in inoperable cases.
17. Primary tracheal tumours are almost always malignant in adults but are benign in up to 70% in children. Surgery and adjuvant RT are the mainstay of treatment in malignant cases. In benign tumours, however, endoscopic resection or laser/electrocautery fulguration could suffice.
18. Cardiac tumours are rare and are often diagnosed only after death. However, 75% of the tumours are benign, with atrial myxoma being the most common type cured by surgery. Malignant forms include tumours like angiosarcoma and rhabdomyosarcoma. These are treated with surgery when possible and adjuvant RT.
19. Surgery in mediastinal tumours is divided into open approach and minimally invasive (VATS and RATS). The latter is used in small, less invasive tumours and needs technical and surgical expertise. The former is preferred for larger, invasive tumours and is usually performed using a median sternotomy approach.

(continued)

20. When tumours invade vasculature, surgery is always associated with reconstruction using either an autograft or an allograft (preferred). In some cases, a cardiopulmonary bypass may also be needed.
21. Recent advances in radiotherapy techniques (IMRT, IMPT, respiratory motion management) and systemic therapy (novel targeted biological agents and immune checkpoint inhibitors) may improve treatment outcomes, simultaneously mitigate treatment-related acute and late morbidities and optimise health-related quality of life.

Multiple Choice Questions

1. The most common site of mediastinal tumours is
   (a) Superior mediastinum
   (b) Anterior mediastinum
   (c) Posterior mediastinum
   (d) Middle mediastinum
2. The most common mediastinal tumour is
   (a) Lymphoma
   (b) Germ cell tumour
   (c) Thymoma
   (d) None of the above
3. The most common mediastinal lesion in children is
   (a) Neuroblastoma
   (b) Lymphoma
   (c) Ganglioneuroma
   (d) Neurogenic tumours
4. ^{68}Ga-DOTATATE PET/CT scan is used to detect
   (a) Thoracic neuroblastoma
   (b) Phaeochromocytoma
   (c) Ectopic thyroid masses
   (d) Thymic neuroendocrine tumours
5. Masoaka staging system is used to classify
   (a) Thymic epithelial neoplasm
   (b) Thoracic neuroblastoma
   (c) Hodgkin's disease
   (d) Germ cell tumour
6. The most common chemotherapy regimen(s) used to treat thymic neoplasms is/are
   (a) CAP
   (b) EP
   (c) Both A and B
   (d) None of the above
7. All of the following are indications for adjuvant RT in thymoma except
   (a) Stage III disease
   (b) Positive margins
   (c) Stage II with B1 histology
   (d) Gross residual disease
8. Recommended RT dose in a definitive setting of thymic carcinoma is
   (a) 45 Gy
   (b) 54 Gy
   (c) 60 Gy
   (d) 70 Gy
9. Treatment of immature teratoma is
   (a) Upfront surgery
   (b) NACT followed by surgery
   (c) RT alone
   (d) Observation
10. The most common mediastinal lymphoma is
    (a) Hodgkin lymphoma
    (b) DLBCL
    (c) Follicular lymphoma
    (d) MALToma
11. The classical dumbbell-shaped tumours are seen in
    (a) Neurogenic tumours
    (b) Lymphoma
    (c) Germ cell tumour
    (d) Thymic carcinoma
12. The most common tumour in the posterior mediastinum is
    (a) Lymphoma
    (b) Neurogenic tumours
    (c) Germ cell tumour
    (d) Tracheal tumours
13. The recommended RT dose in PMBCL is
    (a) 60 Gy/30 fractions
    (b) 20 Gy/10 fractions
    (c) 45 Gy/25 fractions
    (d) 30 Gy/15 fractions

14. Treatment of choice in limited-stage PMBCL is
    (a) Induction chemotherapy followed by surgery
    (b) Chemotherapy alone
    (c) Induction chemotherapy followed by RT in case of partial metabolic response
    (d) RT alone
15. The most common cardiac tumour is
    (a) Angiosarcoma
    (b) Rhabdomyosarcoma
    (c) Primary mesothelioma
    (d) Atrial myxoma
16. The most common site of metastasis in NUT carcinoma is
    (a) Heart
    (b) Bone
    (c) Liver
    (d) Brain
17. MEN-1 syndrome is most commonly associated with
    (a) Thymic carcinoids
    (b) Neuroblastoma
    (c) Ganglioneuroma
    (d) Ganglioneuroblastoma
18. Which of the following is not a safe indication for minimally invasive surgery?
    (a) Tumours >10 cm
    (b) Tumours <5 cm
    (c) Non-invasive tumours
    (d) Availability of experienced team

Answer Key

1. (b)
2. (c)
3. (d)
4. (d)
5. (a)
6. (c)
7. (c)
8. (c)
9. (b)
10. (a)
11. (a)
12. (b)
13. (d)
14. (c)
15. (d)
16. (b)
17. (a)
18. (a)

References

1. Asamura HYM. Shields' general thoracic surgery. Wolters Kluwer Health; 2018. p. 3776–91.
2. Gray's Anatomy for Students. 124–233. Elsevier; 2019.
3. Su SCY. Adult chest surgery. 2nd ed. McGraw Hill Professional; 2014. p. 1234–40.
4. International Thymic Malignancy Interest Group. ITMIG. https://itmig.org/
5. Nicholson AG, et al. The IASLC/ITMIG Thymic Epithelial Tumors Staging Project: proposals for the T component for the Forthcoming (8th) Edition of the TNM Classification of Malignant Tumors. J Thorac Oncol. 2014;9:S73–80. https://doi.org/10.1097/jto.0000000000000303.
6. Moore KL, Dalley AF, Agur AMR. Clinically oriented anatomy. Lippincott Williams & Wilkins; 2013. p. 1171.
7. Fujimoto K, et al. Proposal for a new mediastinal compartment classification of transverse plane images according to the Japanese Association for Research on the Thymus (JART) General Rules for the Study of Mediastinal Tumors. Oncol Rep. 2014;31:565–72. https://doi.org/10.3892/or.2013.2904.
8. Carter BW, et al. A modern definition of mediastinal compartments. J Thorac Oncol. 2014;9:S97–101.
9. Dubashi B, Cyriac S, Tenali SG. Clinicopathological analysis and outcome of primary mediastinal malignancies – a report of 91 cases from a single institute. Ann Thorac Med. 2009;4:140–2.
10. Strollo DC, Rosado de Christenson ML, Jett JR. Primary mediastinal tumors. Part 1: Tumors of the anterior mediastinum. Chest. 1997;112:511–22.
11. Strollo DC, Rosado-de-Christenson ML, Jett JR. Primary mediastinal tumors: Part II. Tumors of the middle and posterior mediastinum. Chest. 1997;112:1344–57.
12. Carter BW, Marom EM, Detterbeck FC. Approaching the patient with an anterior mediastinal mass: a guide for clinicians. J Thorac Oncol. 2014;9:S102–9. https://doi.org/10.1097/jto.0000000000000294.
13. Detterbeck F. ESTS textbook of thoracic surgery. Exeter: European Society of Thoracic Surgeons; 2014.
14. Marx A, et al. The 2015 World Health Organization classification of tumors of the thymus: continuity and changes. J Thorac Oncol. 2015;10:1383–95.
15. Engels EA. Epidemiology of thymoma and associated malignancies. J Thorac Oncol. 2010;5:S260–5.

16. Safieddine N, et al. Prognostic factors for cure, recurrence and long-term survival after surgical resection of thymoma. J Thorac Oncol. 2014;9:1018–22.
17. Masaoka A, Monden Y, Nakahara K, Tanioka T. Follow-up study of thymomas with special reference to their clinical stages. Cancer. 1981;48:2485–92.
18. Weis C-A, et al. The impact of thymoma histotype on prognosis in a worldwide database. J Thorac Oncol. 2015;10:367–72.
19. Kim ES, et al. Phase II study of a multidisciplinary approach with induction chemotherapy, followed by surgical resection, radiation therapy, and consolidation chemotherapy for unresectable malignant thymomas: final report. Lung Cancer. 2004;44:369–79.
20. Huang J, et al. Feasibility of multimodality therapy including extended resections in stage IVA thymoma. J Thorac Cardiovasc Surg. 2007;134:1477–83.; discussion 1483–4.
21. Korst RJ, et al. Neoadjuvant chemoradiotherapy for locally advanced thymic tumors: a phase II, multi-institutional clinical trial. J Thorac Cardiovasc Surg. 2014;147:36–44, 46.e1.
22. Cho J, Kim HS, Ku BM, Choi YL, et al. Pembrolizumab for patients with refractory or relapsed thymic epithelial tumor: an open-label Phase II Trial. J Clin Orthod. 2019;37(24):2162–70. https://doi.org/10.1200/JCO.2017.77.3184.
23. Rajan A, Giaccone G. Targeted therapy for advanced thymic tumors. J Thorac Oncol. 2010;5:S361–4.
24. Lim YJ, et al. Survival impact of adjuvant radiation therapy in masaoka stage II to IV thymomas: a systematic review and meta-analysis. Int J Radiat Oncol Biol Phys. 2016;94:1129–36.
25. He T, Yao J, Chen J, Liu T, Dang J. Postoperative radiotherapy for completely resected thymoma and thymic carcinoma: a systematic review and meta-analysis. PLoS One. 2024;19:e0308111. https://doi.org/10.1371/journal.pone.0308111
26. Girard N, et al. Thymic epithelial tumours: ESMO Clinical Practice Guidelines for diagnosis, treatment and follow-up. Ann Oncol. 2015;26(Suppl 5):v40–55.
27. Gomez D, Komaki R, Yu J, Ikushima H, Bezjak A. Radiation therapy definitions and reporting guidelines for thymic malignancies. J Thorac Oncol. 2011;6:S1743–8.
28. Marcuse F, et al. Optimal delineation of the clinical target volume for thymomas in the post-resection setting: a multi-center study. Radiother Oncol. 2021;165:8–13.
29. Eng TY, Fuller CD, Jagirdar J, Bains Y, Thomas CR Jr. Thymic carcinoma: state of the art review. Int J Radiat Oncol Biol Phys. 2004;59:654–64.
30. Zhao Y, et al. Surgical treatment of thymoma: an 11-year experience with 761 patients. Eur J Cardiothorac Surg. 2016;49:1144–9.
31. Huang J, et al. Comparison of patterns of relapse in thymic carcinoma and thymoma. J Thorac Cardiovas Surg. 2009;138:26–31. https://doi.org/10.1016/j.jtcvs.2009.03.033.
32. Rathod S, et al. Thymoma: first large Indian experience. Indian J Cancer. 2014;51:109–12.
33. Julka PK, et al. Outcomes of thymoma treated with multimodality approach: a tertiary cancer center experience of 71 patients. Tumori. 2017;103:572–6.
34. Bokemeyer C, et al. Extragonadal germ cell tumors of the mediastinum and retroperitoneum: results from an international analysis. J Clin Oncol. 2002;20:1864–73.
35. Kang J, Mashaal H, Anjum F. Mediastinal Germ Cell Tumors. 2023. In: StatPearls [Internet]. Treasure Island (FL): StatPearls Publishing; 2025. PMID: 33085379.
36. Lewis BD, et al. Benign teratomas of the mediastinum. J Thorac Cardiovasc Surg. 1983;86:727–31.
37. Takeda S-I, et al. Primary germ cell tumors in the mediastinum: a 50-year experience at a single Japanese institution. Cancer. 2003;97:367–76.
38. Ranganath P, Kesler KA, Einhorn LH. Perioperative morbidity and mortality associated with bleomycin in primary mediastinal nonseminomatous germ cell tumor. J Clin Oncol. 2016;34:4445–6. https://doi.org/10.1200/jco.2016.69.8910.
39. Vuky J, et al. Role of postchemotherapy adjunctive surgery in the management of patients with nonseminoma arising from the mediastinum. J Clin Oncol. 2001;19:682–8.
40. Schultz SM, Einhorn LH, Conces DJ Jr, Williams SD, Loehrer PJ. Management of postchemotherapy residual mass in patients with advanced seminoma: Indiana University experience. J Clin Oncol. 1989;7:1497–503.
41. Puc HS, et al. Management of residual mass in advanced seminoma: results and recommendations from the Memorial Sloan-Kettering Cancer Center. J Clin Oncol. 1996;14:454–60.
42. Dunleavy K, et al. Dose-adjusted EPOCH-rituximab therapy in primary mediastinal B-cell lymphoma. N Engl J Med. 2013;368:1408–16.
43. Rieger M, et al. Primary mediastinal B-cell lymphoma treated with CHOP-like chemotherapy with or without rituximab: results of the Mabthera International Trial Group study. Ann Oncol. 2011;22:664–70.
44. Hamlin PA, et al. Primary mediastinal large B-cell lymphoma: optimal therapy and prognostic factor analysis in 141 consecutive patients treated at Memorial Sloan Kettering from 1980 to 1999. Br J Haematol. 2005;130:691–9.
45. Nakajima Y, et al. Long-term progress of six cases of malignant peripheral nerve sheath tumors of the mediastinum that underwent surgical treatment: case report series. Int J Surg Case Rep. 2016;24:185–7.
46. Kar M, Deo SV, Shukla NK, Malik A, DattaGupta S, Mohanti BK, Thulkar S. Malignant peripheral nerve sheath tumors (MPNST)–clinicopathological study and treatment outcome of twenty-four cases. World J Surg Oncol. 2006;455. https://doi.org/10.1186/1477-7819-4-55.
47. Lucas C-HG, et al. Histopathologic findings in malignant peripheral nerve sheath tumor predict response

to radiotherapy and overall survival. Neurooncol Adv. 2020;2:vdaa131.
48. Martin E, et al. A nationwide cohort study on treatment and survival in patients with malignant peripheral nerve sheath tumours. Eur J Cancer. 2020;124:77–87.
49. Yuan ZN, et al. Clinicopathological features and prognosis of malignant peripheral nerve sheath tumor: a retrospective study of 140 cases. Zhonghua Zhong Liu Za Zhi. 2017;39:439–44.
50. Sobczuk P, et al. Systemic treatment for advanced and metastatic malignant peripheral nerve sheath tumors – a sarcoma reference center experience. J Clin Med Res. 2020;9:3157.
51. Verma S, Kalra K, Rastogi S, Sidhu HS. Clinical approach to childhood mediastinal tumors and management. Mediastinum. 2020;4:21.
52. Suita S, et al. The characteristics of mediastinal neuroblastoma. Eur J Pediatr Surg. 2000;10:353–9.
53. Bagley AF, et al. Efficacy of proton therapy in children with high-risk and locally recurrent neuroblastoma. Pediatr Blood Cancer. 2019;66:e27786.
54. Ferreira M, de Leal CTS, Ferreira LV, Ezequiel DGA, Costa MB. Atypical presentation of a medullary thyroid carcinoma producing Acth and serotonin. Case Rep Oncol. 2019;12:742–8.
55. Shah BC, et al. Ectopic thyroid cancer. Ann Thorac Cardiovasc Surg. 2007;13:122–4.
56. Karim F, Inam H, Choudry UK, Hasnain Fatimi S. Ectopic follicular variant of papillary thyroid carcinoma in anterior mediastinum with a normal thyroid gland. A case report. Int J Surg Case Rep. 2018;51:213–7.
57. Macchiarini P. Primary tracheal tumours. Lancet Oncol. 2006;7:83–91.
58. Mallick S, Benson R, Giridhar P, Rajan Singh A, Rath GK. Demography, patterns of care and survival outcomes in patients with malignant tumors of trachea: a systematic review and individual patient data analysis of 733 patients. Lung Cancer. 2019;132:87–93.
59. Honings J, et al. Pathologic characteristics of resected squamous cell carcinoma of the trachea: prognostic factors based on an analysis of 59 cases. Virchows Arch. 2009;455:423–9.
60. Regnard JF, Fourquier P, Levasseur P. Results and prognostic factors in resections of primary tracheal tumors: a multicenter retrospective study. The French Society of Cardiovascular Surgery. J Thorac Cardiovasc Surg. 1996;111:808–13.; discussion 813–4.
61. Harms W, et al. Treatment of primary tracheal carcinoma. The role of external and endoluminal radiotherapy. Strahlenther Onkol. 2000;176:22–7.
62. Leja MJ, Shah DJ, Reardon MJ. Primary cardiac tumors. Tex Heart Inst J. 2011;38:261–2.
63. Goldstein DJ, Oz MC, Rose EA, Fisher P, Michler RE. Experience with heart transplantation for cardiac tumors. J Heart Lung Transpl. 1995;14:382–6.
64. Godar M, Liu J, Zhang P, Xia Y, Yuan Q. Primary pericardial mesothelioma: a rare entity. Case Rep Oncol Med. 2013;2013:283601.
65. Giridhar P, Mallick S, Kashyap L, Rath GK. Patterns of care and impact of prognostic factors in the outcome of NUT midline carcinoma: a systematic review and individual patient data analysis of 119 cases. Eur Arch Otorhinolaryngol. 2018;275:815–21.
66. Filosso PL, et al. Neuroendocrine tumors of the thymus. J Thorac Dis. 2017;9:S1484–90.
67. Baudin E, et al. Lung and thymic carcinoids: ESMO Clinical Practice Guidelines for diagnosis, treatment and follow-up☆. Ann Oncol. 2021;32:439–51.
68. Wu C-F, et al. Single-port video-assisted thoracoscopic mediastinal tumour resection. Interact Cardiovasc Thorac Surg. 2015;21:644–9.
69. Zeng L, et al. Uniportal video-assisted thoracoscopic surgery and robot-assisted thoracoscopic surgery are feasible approaches with potential advantages in minimally invasive mediastinal lesions resection. Gland Surg. 2021;10:101–11.
70. Patel MD, et al. Hyperthermic Intrathoracic Chemotherapy (HITHOC) for Pleural Malignancies-Experience from Indian Centers. Indian J Surg Oncol. 2019;10:91–8.
71. Ried M, et al. State of the art: diagnostic tools and innovative therapies for treatment of advanced thymoma and thymic carcinoma. Eur J Cardiothorac Surg. 2016;49:1545–52.
72. Aprile V, et al. Hypertermic Intrathoracic Chemotherapy (HITHOC) for thymoma: a narrative review on indications and results. Ann Transl Med. 2021;9:957.
73. Mendogni P, Orlandi R, Ambrogi M, Lucchi M, et al. Hyperthermic intrathoracic chemotherapy (HITHOC) in stage IVA thymomas: a narrative review. Mediastinum. 2025;9:16. https://doi.org/10.21037/med-25-8
74. Tani K, Kimura D, Matsuo T, Sasaki T, Kimura S, Muto C, Minakawa M. Perioperative strategies and management of giant anterior mediastinal tumors: a narrative review. Mediastinum. 2024;8:34. https://doi.org/10.21037/med-23-40.

Online Links

https://www.youtube.com/watch?v=MKRGFL7RjRI
https://www.youtube.com/watch?v=MD0C9-CLhew
https://www.youtube.com/watch?v=GrPcP0FVUto

Esophageal Cancer

Sunil Kumar, Supriya Mallick, Adrija Ghosh,
Naveen Kumar, Sandeep K. Bhoriwal,
Atul Sharma, and S. V. S. Deo

1 Introduction and Epidemiology

Esophageal cancer is one of the most common and lethal gastrointestinal cancer traditionally associated with poor long-term survival. As per Globocan 2020 data, esophageal cancer ranks seventh in terms of incidence, with the overall incidence of carcinoma esophagus just above 6,00,000 cases accounting for 3.1% of the total cancer cases. It is the sixth leading cause of cancer-related mortality [1]. The incidence and cancer-related mortality are very high in Asian countries. In India, the incidence of esophageal cancer has been increasing remarkably over the last three decades, and as per projections of NCRP for 2020, more than 50,000 cases were expected with a cumulative risk of one in 270 and the risk of one in 201 in 370 in males and females, respectively [2]. At present, esophageal cancer is the most common gastrointestinal malignancy overall in India. Over half of the patients diagnosed with esophageal cancer present with a locoregionally advanced stage, while 40% of patients present with upfront metastatic disease. Up to 50% of patients presenting with localized esophageal cancer are inoperable, and of the remaining patients, 20% patients will have unresectable disease and only one-third of newly diagnosed patients will undergo potentially curative surgery. In the recent past, the landscape of esophageal cancer management has undergone a major evolution. Multidisciplinary collaboration now forms the backbone of therapy for esophageal cancer.

S. Kumar (✉) · S. K. Bhoriwal
Department of Surgical Oncology, IRCH, AIIMS, New Delhi, India

S. Mallick · A. Ghosh
Department of Radiation Oncology, National Cancer Institute (Jhajjar), AIIMS, New Delhi, India

N. Kumar
Department of Surgical Oncology, National Cancer Institute (Jhajjar), AIIMS, New Delhi, India

A. Sharma
Department of Medical Oncology, MAX Hospital, New Delhi, India

S. V. S. Deo
Department of Surgical Oncology, MAX Hospital, Saket, New Delhi, Delhi, India

1.1 The Changing Pattern

The two most common histological variants of esophageal cancer are squamous cell carcinoma and adenocarcinoma. In recent years, the western world has observed an increasing ratio of adenocarcinoma to squamous cell carcinoma, with adenocarcinoma being the most common variant over the last three decades. The changing dietary patterns and obesity associated with increased chances of esophageal reflux are presumed to drive the sequence of metaplasia to display in the form of Barrett's esophagus, which is considered

B. K. Mohanti et al. (eds.), *Radiation Oncology – Principles, Precepts and Practice*,
https://doi.org/10.1007/978-981-95-5171-2_9

to be a precursor of adenocarcinoma. India has witnessed an increasing incidence of adenocarcinoma as well although squamous cell carcinoma is still the predominant variant. The typical esophageal cancer in India is a squamous cell carcinoma located in the middle third of the esophagus.

2 Anatomy

The esophagus is located in the posterior mediastinum. With respect to management implications, the esophagus can be divided into three parts: the upper esophagus extends from cricopharynx to the azygous vein, the middle third extends from the azygous vein to the level of the inferior pulmonary vein, and the lower third is considered to extend from inferior pulmonary vein to the gastroesophageal junction. Anatomy and histology of esophagus are depicted in Fig. 1a–d. Being a long tubular structure, esophagus is surrounded by some critical structures like the trachea, bronchi, aorta and vertebrae. The pericardium overlying the left atrium is in direct contact. As peri-esophageal fat may be, absent in nutritionally compromised patients, radiological interpretation of the circumferential extent of tumor becomes tricky and may alter the treatment planning. It also poses challenges in the circumferential clearance of tumor, essential for margin-free surgical resection.

3 Etiology

Hereditary Factors Increased incidence of esophageal cancer has been reported in patients with Peutz-Jeghers syndrome and in patients with germline PTEN mutation. Familial aggregation is associated with SCC and Barrett's esophageal cancers [3, 4].

Squamous Cell Carcinoma The incidence varies among geographical locations, with highest rates in Northern Iran, Central Asia, and North Central China, the so-called esophageal cancer belt [5]. Major risk factors are the use of tobacco (particularly smoking and chewing) and alcohol, which have been found to work synergistically. Insufficiency or marginal deficiency of micronutrients (vitamins A and E), which have antioxidant properties, contribute to the etiology. Table 1 shows risk factors for SCC and adenocarcinoma.

The contribution of endogenously formed nitrosamine (formed in the stomach under favourable conditions of acidic pH) has been postulated with a combination of high levels of nitrates and nitrites in drinking water and secondary amines in moldy foods [6]. However, clear evidence about the exact role of nitrosamine and polycyclic hydrocarbons is still lacking, and so is the role of HPV infection [7].

Genome-wide association studies (GWAS) in Japan have shown that functionally variant alcohol dehydrogenase 1B and aldehyde dehydrogenase 2, coupled with alcohol and smoking, synergistically increase the risk of esophageal squamous cell carcinoma [8]. Genetic factors leading to low activity of cell cycle regulation and Notch signalling have been implicated in the pathogenesis.

3.1 *Adenocarcinoma*

The most important etiological factor for esophageal adenocarcinoma is gastroesophageal reflux disease (GERD), which causes irritation and inflammation of lower esophageal mucosa, leading to Barrett's esophagus (metaplasia of the mucosa) and subsequently to esophageal adenocarcinoma.

Reflux caused by surgical procedures like esophago-gastro-duodenostomy has been shown to induce malignant changes in animal models. Oxidative stress in combination with aberrant arachidonic acid metabolism promotes inflammation and genetic mutations for the development of esophageal adenocarcinoma. These changes are particularly inhibited by antioxidants like vitamin E, and inhibitors of pro-inflammatory eicosenoids (like Celecoxib, Zileuton, and Bestatin) have been shown to inhibit the formation of esophageal adenocarcinoma in animal models and are being explored as preventive measures in human trials.

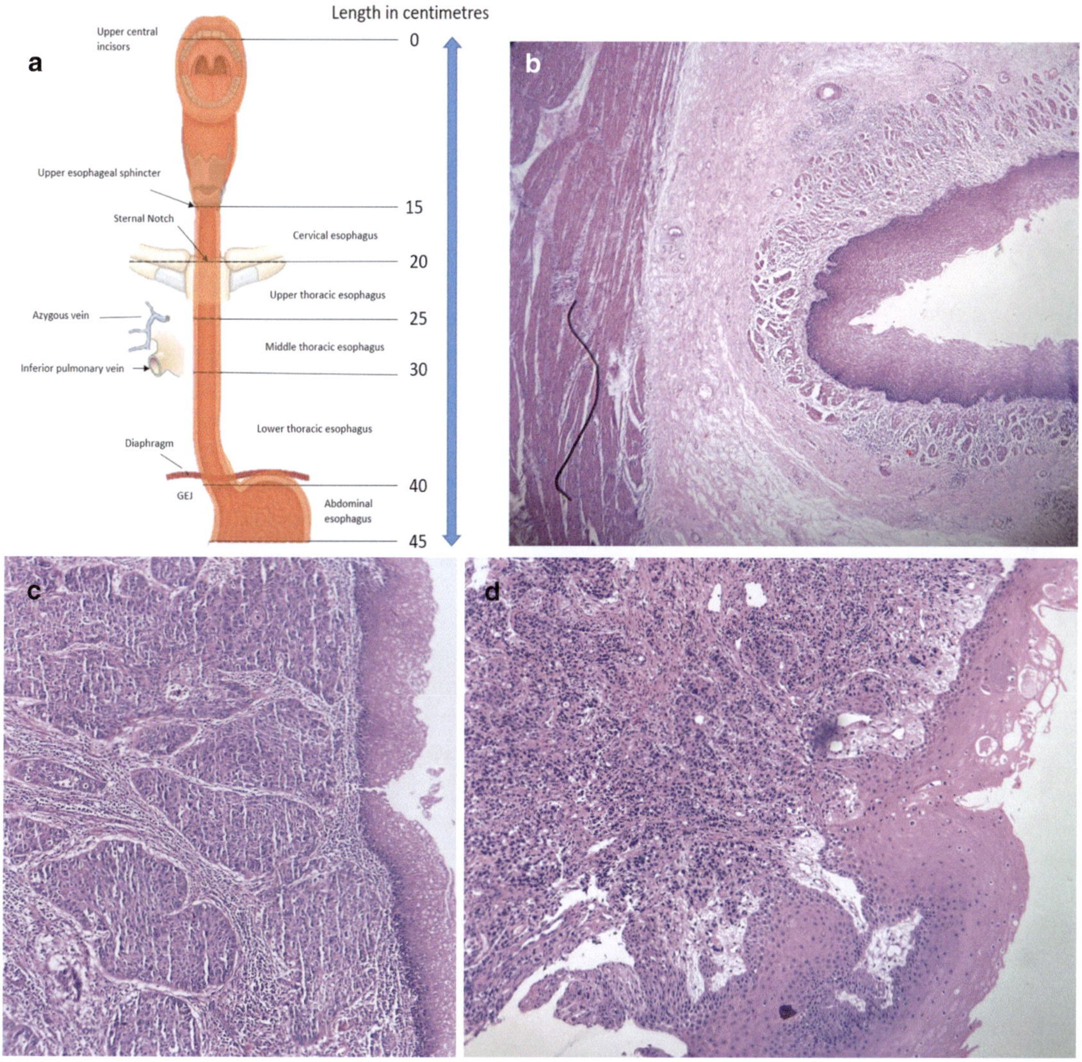

Fig. 1 (**a**) Normal esophageal anatomy. (**b**) Normal esophageal mucosa. (Courtesy: Dr. Priyanka Bhatia, DNB Pathology, Consultant histopathology and cytopathology, Department of Laboratory Sciences, Manipal Hospital Dwarka.) (**c**) Moderately differentiated squamous cell carcinoma esophagus. (Courtesy: Dr. Priyanka Bhatia, DNB Pathology, Consultant histopathology and cytopathology, Department of Laboratory Sciences, Manipal Hospital Dwarka.) (**d**) Adenocarcinoma esophagus. (Courtesy: Dr. Priyanka Bhatia, DNB Pathology, Consultant histopathology and cytopathology, Department of Laboratory Sciences, Manipal Hospital Dwarka.)

4 Clinical Presentation

Clinical presentation of esophageal carcinoma varies from minimal or no symptoms in very early stage disease to frank dysphagia, which varies as per the extent of luminal obstruction. The extent or grade of dysphagia is an important consideration in the management of the patient. It may lead to regurgitation and absolute dysphagia. There may be associated chest pain after swallowing.

Grades of dysphagia:

- Grade 1: Difficulty in swallowing solid food, but can swallow with some effort
- Grade 2: Can swallow semisolid food only
- Grade 3: Can swallow liquids only, but no solid or semisolid food

Table 1 Risk factors for esophageal SCC and adenocarcinoma

Squamous cell carcinoma (SCC)	Adenocarcinoma
Demographic and socio-economic factors	Gastro-esophageal Reflux Disease (GERD) and esophageal gas exposure
Smoking and alcohol	Smoking and alcohol
Dietary factors	Obesity and metabolic syndromes
Underlying esophageal disease	HPV
Prior gastrectomy	
Atrophic gastritis	
Human papilloma virus (HPV)	
Upper aerodigestive tract cancers	
Tylosis	
Bisphosphonates	
Poor oral hygiene	

Note: Protective factors for esophageal adenocarcinoma include Cereal fibres and NSAIDS

Grade 4: Absolute dysphagia (not able to swallow solids or liquids either)

Patients with significant reflux may present with cough and change in voice because of persistent microaspirations. Typically, patients complain of a sensation of obstruction of food bolus, which is of recent onset and progressing in severity. Patients with advanced tumors may present with associated hoarseness of voice and symptoms of fistulous connection between esophagus and airway, like the onset of cough immediately after swallowing food, which may be associated with copious foul-smelling sputum. Commonly, there is a history of significant loss of weight without loss of appetite. It is very common in Indian scenarios to come across patients who have had weight loss of more than 10–20% and a rapid fall in the general condition and performance of the patient, which is an important factor in deciding the treatment plan. There may be a history of hematemesis and melaena. On clinical examination, particular attention should be paid to the presence of supraclavicular and cervical lymphadenopathy.

4.1 Work-Up and Investigations

It is important to have a high index of suspicion for an early diagnosis, as the stage of the presentation plays an important role in the overall management and prognosis of the disease. Table 2 represents the diagnostic workup for esophageal cancer patients. The diagnostic investigation to confirm the presence and histological type of malignancy is upper gastro-intestinal (GI) endoscopy and a guided biopsy, which is generally the initial mode of investigation. After that, radiological imaging is required to ascertain the extent of the disease involvement. The most important investigation to stage the disease is CECT of the chest and abdomen (with oral and intravenous contrast) or PET-CT if accessible and affordable. PET-CT is preferred over CECT for its higher sensitivity and specificity for nodal involvement. Endoscopic ultrasound plays an important role in evaluating the local regional extent of the disease, specifically the T stage. Barium swallow study, which was commonly used in earlier times, is now more of historical importance, although, in patients with non-passable growth on endoscopy, it is sometimes used to know the track of the compromised lumen before any endoscopic intervention like Ryle's tube or stent placement.

5 Upper GI Endoscopy

Upper GI endoscopy is an important investigation to localize and characterize the lesion (Fig. 2). The early tumor appears as an ulcer,

Table 2 Diagnostic workup of esophageal carcinoma

History and physical examination
Routine blood investigations including spirometry and cardiac evaluation
Establishing diagnosis with upper GI endoscopy and biopsy
Metastatic work up—contrast-enhanced CT of chest, abdomen, and pelvis or whole body FDG PET-CT
Bronchoscopy to rule out tracheal infiltration, if necessary
Multidisciplinary evaluation by surgical, medical, and radiation oncologists

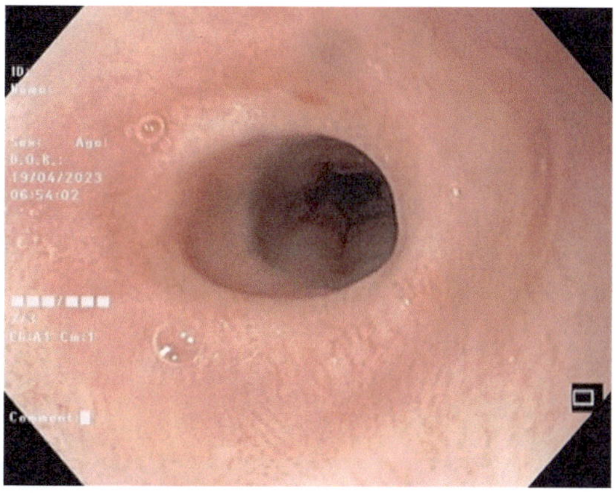

Fig. 2 Normal esophageal lumen on endoscopy

nodule or plaque with passable scope whereas

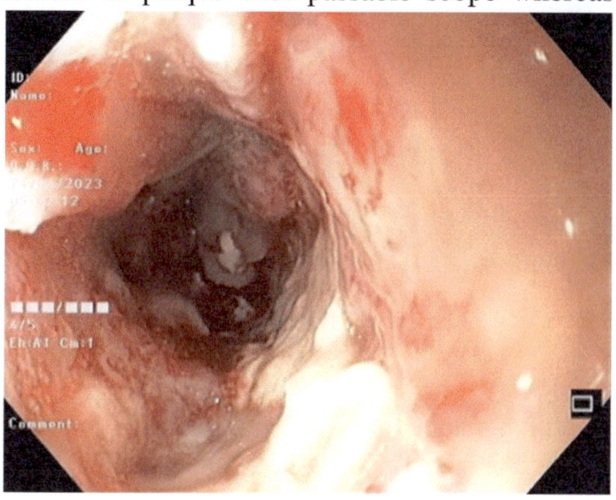

Fig. 3 A typical appearance of esophageal malignancy, causing obstruction in the lumen

advanced disease generally presents as a stricture or ulcerated mass obstructing the lumen where scope cannot pass across the growth or can be passed only with difficulty (Fig. 3). Appearance (proliferative vs infiltrative), the extent of longitudinal and circumferential involvement, the presence of skip lesions and changes in mucosa like Barrett's esophagus should be noted with the use of additional tools like chromoendoscopy and narrow band imaging (NBI). The tumors with primarily the proliferative and intraluminal components have a better prognosis than infiltrative tumors. The diagnostic accuracy depends on the number of biopsies taken, and a minimum of six random biopsies is recommended for better diagnostic yield. Graham et al. performed a prospective trial on the number of biopsies on 202 consecutive patients. This study found a total of seven biopsy specimens increased accuracy by more than 98% [9]. In cases with tight, stricturous, or infiltrative growth, a brush cytology may be an alternative if no clear growth is visible.

5.1 Pathological Features on Biopsy

A detailed biopsy report indicating the type of malignancy (Squamous or adenocarcinoma), the level of differentiation, presence of high-risk features like lymphovascular invasion (LVI) and perineural invasion (PNI), plays an important role in treatment decision-making.

5.2 CECT and PET-CT

Contrast-enhanced CT scan and the fluorine-18 (18F) fluorodeoxyglucose (FDG) positron emission tomography (PET) scan are the main investigations to stage the disease. CT scan is highly accurate for the involvement of extra-esophageal structures like aorta, trachea, bronchus, atrium, inferior pulmonary vein, diaphragm, and suspected trachea-esophageal or esophago-pleural fistula. In patients with suspected infiltration of trachea or bronchus, a fibreoptic bronchoscopy should be done, although it is more helpful only in cases with mucosal involvement of the airway or obvious compression. CT scan has a limited role in the assessment of depth of infiltration by tumor (T stage). Figure 4 shows PET-CT in a case of cancer esophagus-lower one-third.

FDG PET/CT scan has higher sensitivity for detecting esophageal cancer, but again, it has a limited role for the T stage and to look for surrounding organ invasion.

Both these investigations have suboptimal sensitivity for detecting the locoregional nodes (CT scan: 30–40%, PET scan: ~51%) compared to endoscopic ultrasound (having sensitivity

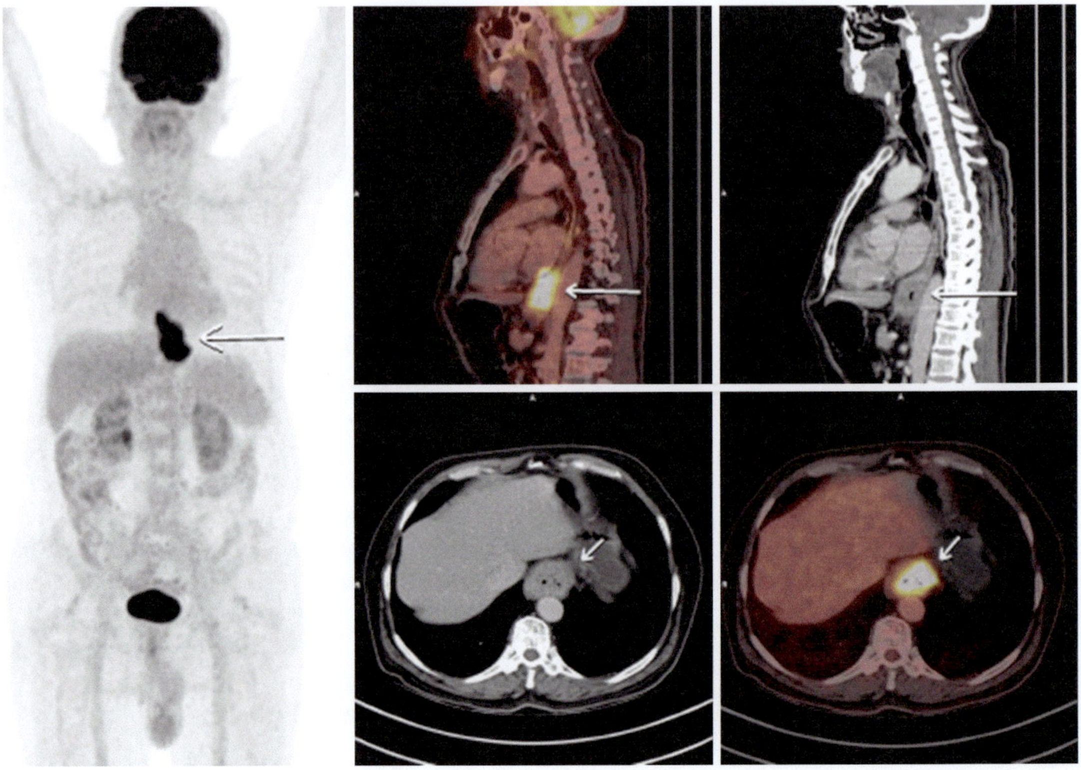

Fig. 4 PET-CT in a case of CA esophagus (lower 1/3). (Courtesy: Dr. Ankur Pruthi, Consultant and Head, Nuclear Medicine & PET CT, Manipal Hospital, Dwarka, New Delhi)

(~85%), but PET-CT plays an important role in the assessment of distant metastasis.

Apart from its diagnostic value, PET-CT plays an important role in the assessment of the response to neo-adjuvant therapy. It correlates well with pathological response, and the response as assessed by using the PET response criteria in solid tumors (PERSIST criteria) may be used for planning a surgical resection after neo-adjuvant treatment. Apart from SUVmax, which is commonly used for describing the tumor activity, other parameters like tumor-to-liver ratio (TLR) of the uptake and percentage change in activity after neo-adjuvant treatment correlate well with pathological response [10]. Assessment of response should be done 4–6 weeks after completion of neo-adjuvant treatment.

Given the prevalence of granulomatous diseases like tuberculosis in India, a cautious interpretation (particularly of nodal involvement) should be done to avoid overstaging, and the activity of the tumor vs node may be a helpful indicator.

5.3 Endoscopic Ultrasound (EUS)

Endoscopic ultrasound (EUS) is the preferred investigation for both depth of tumor infiltration (T stage) and nodal involvement (N stages) (Fig. 5). It uses a high-frequency (7.5–12 MHz) ultrasound that provides detailed images of the tumor and its infiltration into different esophageal layers. The sensitivity and specificity of EUS for evaluating the T stage range from 80% to 92% and 94% to 97%, respectively. The accuracy of EUS varies as per the T-stage, with lower sensitivity for T1 and T2 tumors than for T3 and T4 tumors. Luo et al. showed a sensitivity of 66–77% for T1, T2 tumors, whereas 84–87% for

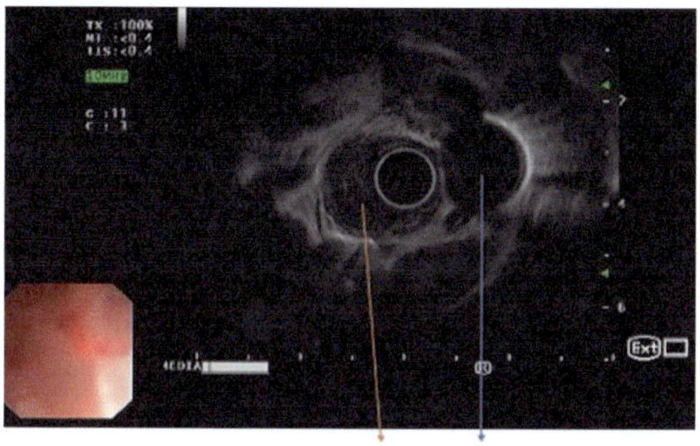

Fig. 5 Esophageal malignancy on endoscopic ultrasound (orange arrow) and aorta (blue arrow)

T3, T4 tumors [11]. In general, the EUS tends to overstage T2 and understage T3 tumors.

Note: Fig. 5: shows esophageal wall tumor (orange arrow) and nearby aorta lumen (blue arrow). EUS also helps in nodal staging. The EUS criteria for malignant involvement of nodes are a size of more than 10 mm in short-axis diameter, rounded shape, smooth border and an echo-poor pattern with loss of hilar delineation. The presence of all four features indicates an 80–100% chance of involvement by the tumor. The accuracy of EUS for nodes can also be improved by taking FNA. After neoadjuvant therapy, the accuracy of EUS is limited and is not reliable. The EUS leads to upstaging of the disease because of the treatment-induced fibrosis. A study comparing EUS-FNA, CT Scan, and EUS alone for the preoperative N stage in 125 patients found higher sensitivity (83% vs. 29%; $P < 0.001$) for the EUS-FNA [12].

One of the limitations of EUS is that the regular endoscope cannot be passed through the obstructing or stricturous tumors, which accounts for nearly 30% of cases in the Indian scenario. For these situations, miniature EUS probes are available that can be passed through the smaller lumen. However, these devices have a very limited depth of penetration (approximately 3 cm) and they do not provide detailed information. Availability of EUS facilities and expertise is still very limited in India, and staging through EUS is not routine at most of the centres.

5.4 Correlation Between T and N Stages

Anatomically esophagus is unique in having two lymphatic channels: the periesophageal lymphatic channel and a rich submucosal lymphatic channel, which are connected. Involvement of submucosa by the tumor (T1b) leads to a high probability of lymph nodal metastasis (varying from 20% to 50% in various studies). Compared to this, tumors localized up to mucosa or lamina propria (T1a) have much lower chances of lymph nodal metastasis (usually <5%). Because of the extensive submucosal channel, tumor extension along the submucosal route is common, and a higher surgical resection margin (ideally 5 cm) is required proximally.

For T2 tumors, the overstaging of N stage has been found in up to 63% of the patients [13], and for this category, upfront surgery remains the first treatment. The probability of nodal metastasis in T3 and T4 tumors has been described to be >60%. TNM staging for esophageal cancer is shown in Table 3 [14].

6 GEJ Tumor Classification

Gastro-esophageal junction has a unique anatomical location and is defined as the transition line between gastric columnar epithelium and esophageal squamous epithelium. As tumors in this area are primarily a result of chronic reflux and mostly adenocarcinoma, their lymphatic spread is both in lower mediastinum as well as in abdominal compartment. Siewert et al. [15] classified the GE junctional adenocarcinomas into three types based on the location of the epicenter of the tumor mass (Fig. 6):

Type I: Epicenter lying from 1 to 5 cm above the GE junction (lower esophageal tumors)

Type II: Epicenter within 1 cm above and 2 cm below the GE junction (true GE junction tumors)

Type III: Epicenter lying beyond 2 cm below the GE junction in stomach (gastric tumors)

Table 3 TNM staging of esophageal and gastroesophageal tumors

Primary tumor (T), squamous cell carcinoma, and adenocarcinoma	
T category	*T criteria*
Tx	Tumor cannot be assessed
T0	No evidence of primary tumor
T1	Tumor invades the lamina propria, muscularis mucosa, and submucosa
T1a	Tumor invades the lamina propria and muscularis propria
T1b	Tumor invades submucosa
T2	Tumor invades muscularis propria
T3	Tumor invades adventitia
T4	Tumor invades adjacent structures
T4a	Tumor invades pleura, pericardium, azygous vein, diaphragm, or peritoneum
T4b	Tumor invades other adjacent structures such as aorta, vertebral body, or airway

Regional nodes (N) squamous cell carcinoma and adenocarcinoma	
N category	*N criteria*
Nx	Regional lymph nodes cannot be assessed
N0	No regional lymph nodes
N1	Metastases to 1–2 regional lymph nodes
N2	Metastases to 3–6 regional lymph nodes
N3	Metastases to 7 or more regional lymph nodes

Distant metastases (M), squamous cell carcinoma, and adenocarcinoma	
M0	No distant metastases
M1	Distant metastases

Clinical staging			
When cT is	N is	M is	Then stage group is
Tis	N0	M0	0
T1	N0–1	M0	I
T2	N0–1	M0	II
T3	N0	M0	II
T3	N1	M0	III
T1–3	N2	M0	III
T4	N0–2	M0	IVA
Any T	N3	M0	IVA
Any T	Any N	M1	IVB

Pathological staging					
pT is	pN is	pM is	Grade	Location	Stage
Tis	N0	M0	N/A	Any	0
T1a	N0	M0	G1	Any	IA
T1a	N0	M0	G2–3	Any	IB
T1a	N0	M0	Gx	Any	IA
T1b	N0	M0	G1–3	Any	IB
T1b	N0	M0	Gx	Any	IB
T2	N0	M0	G1	Any	IB
T2	N0	M0	G2–3	Any	IIA
T2	N0	M0	Gx	Any	IIA
T3	N0	M0	Any	Lower	IIA
T3	N0	M0	G1	Upper/middle	IIA
T3	N0	M0	G2–3	Upper/middle	IIB

(continued)

Table 3 (continued)

T3	N0	M0	Gx	Any	IIB
T3	N0	M0	Any	Location X	IIB
T1	N1	M0	Any	Any	IIB
T1	N2	M0	Any	Any	IIIA
T2	N1	M0	Any	Any	IIIA
T2	N2	M0	Any	Any	IIIB
T3	N1–2	M0	Any	Any	IIIB
T4a	N0–1	M0	Any	Any	IIIB
T4a	N2	M0	Any	Any	IVA
T4b	N0–2	M0	Any	Any	IVA
Any T	N3	M0	Any	Any	IVA
Any T	Any N	M1	Any	Any	IVB

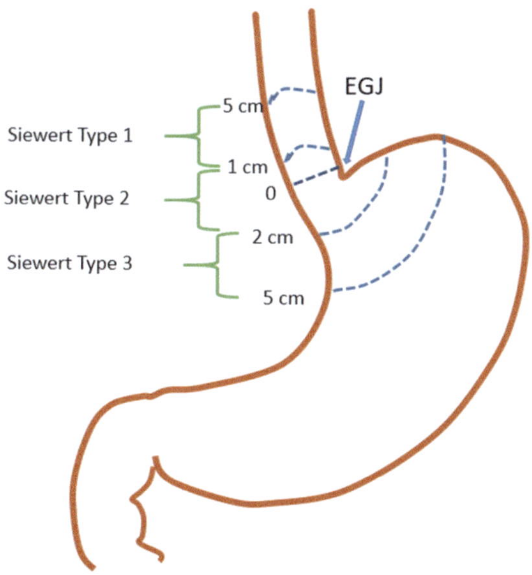

Fig. 6 Seiwert's classification. EGD = Esophgagogastric junction. (Courtesy: Anusheel Munshi, Head, Radiation Oncology, BLK MAX Hospital, Delhi)

In the eighth edition of TNM classification, types I and II and staged as esophageal adenocarcinoma and type III has been staged as per gastric cancer staging system. Similarly, their management has been on the respective lines.

6.1 Assessment of General Condition

As the management of esophageal cancer involves multimodality approach most of the time, it is important to assess the overall general condition and performance status (ECOG status) at the beginning of the treatment planning. It involves the assessment of nutritional, respiratory parameters, and comorbidity status. Assessment of the likely tolerance of the planned treatment is of paramount importance. Apart from a routine blood hemogram and biochemistry pulmonary function test should be done. Assessment of socio-economic status is equally important as the treatment for esophageal cancer is generally time taking and has significant economic implications, particularly for the patients in India, where the cost of the treatment is mostly borne by the patient.

6.2 Basic Principles of Management

In general, the management of esophageal malignancy involves a multi-disciplinary approach (including surgical, medical, radiation oncologists, anesthetist, radiologists, endoscopy expert, pathologist, nutritionist, physiotherapists and palliative care personnel) and should be a protocol-based treatment. Evidence suggests that high-volume centres have better treatment outcomes, both in peri-operative as well as long-term periods. The mainstay of curative treatment remains surgical resection irrespective of the histology.

The factors deciding the management are

- Location of the tumor (upper third or cervical vs middle and lower third)
- Stage of the tumor (early/low risk vs locally advanced/high risk vs metastatic)

- Performance status of the patient
- Comorbidities

It is now accepted that biologically squamous cell carcinoma and adenocarcinoma are totally different diseases, and their management also differs in approaches.

As per the stage, the treatment algorithm for squamous cell carcinoma can be classified as follows:

Mucosal disease (Tis and T1a): options of Endoscopic mucosal resection and esophagectomy

T1b to T2 disease with low-risk features: Upfront surgery as primary treatment option

Well differentiated
Less than 3 cm in size
No aggressive features like LVI and PNI
No evidence of nodal metastasis

Presence of high-risk features (Poorly differentiated tumor, size more than 3 cm, presence of LVI & PNI and nodal metastasis) or T3 and T4a disease: Neo-adjuvant treatment followed by surgical resection

T4b (surgically inoperable) disease: Definitive chemo-radiation

Distant metastatic (M1) disease: Palliative approaches for symptom management

6.3 Prehabilitation

Prehabilitation involves the management of factors that have a bearing on the successful completion of the planned treatment. Since most of the patients in India are nutritionally depleted at the time of presentation, reinstatement of enteral nutrition is the priority before starting any cancer-directed treatment. It can be achieved either by the placement of an endoscopy-guided nasogastric tube, which is simple and cost-effective. In cases where it is either not successful or not tolerated by the patient, options of image-guided or surgical feeding jejunostomy are there. Feeding gastrostomy should be avoided so that the stomach can be used as a conduit in case an esophagectomy is done. A nutritionist should be consulted to design a liquid-based diet rich in protein and calories to compensate for the catabolic effect of the tumor.

Apart from nutrition, cessation of smoking and alcohol intake, home spirometry exercises to improve respiratory function, and optimization of comorbidities like diabetes, hypertension, and chronic obstructive pulmonary disease are strongly recommended.

Management Figures 7 and 8 summarize the management of esophageal squamous cell carcinoma and adenocarcinoma.

6.4 Endoscopic Treatment

Endoscopic management for very early or screen-detected tumors (Tis and T1a, limited to mucosa only) involves endoscopic mucosal resection (EMR) with or without endoscopic radiofrequency ablation. Endoscopic resection is a good alternative and preferred option for superficial esophageal cancer if expertise is available. The ideal candidate for EUS-guided resection has solitary, small <2 cm in diameter, flat mucosal lesions without lymphovascular invasion. The prerequisites are the willingness for close follow-up and multiple biopsies during follow-up. The patients are also informed of the small chances of nodal metastasis and procedural risks.

The majority of the trials are observational or non-randomized. A meta-analysis of 21 studies has shown a 90% (95% CI 87–94%) complete R0 resection after endoscopic mucosal resection. The common complications were esophageal stenosis and perforation [16]. Another study of 349 patients with high-grade dysplasia or intramucosal adenocarcinoma has shown a complete response in 96.6% of the treated patients. Recurrence was noted in 21.5% and surgery was needed in 3.7% only [17].

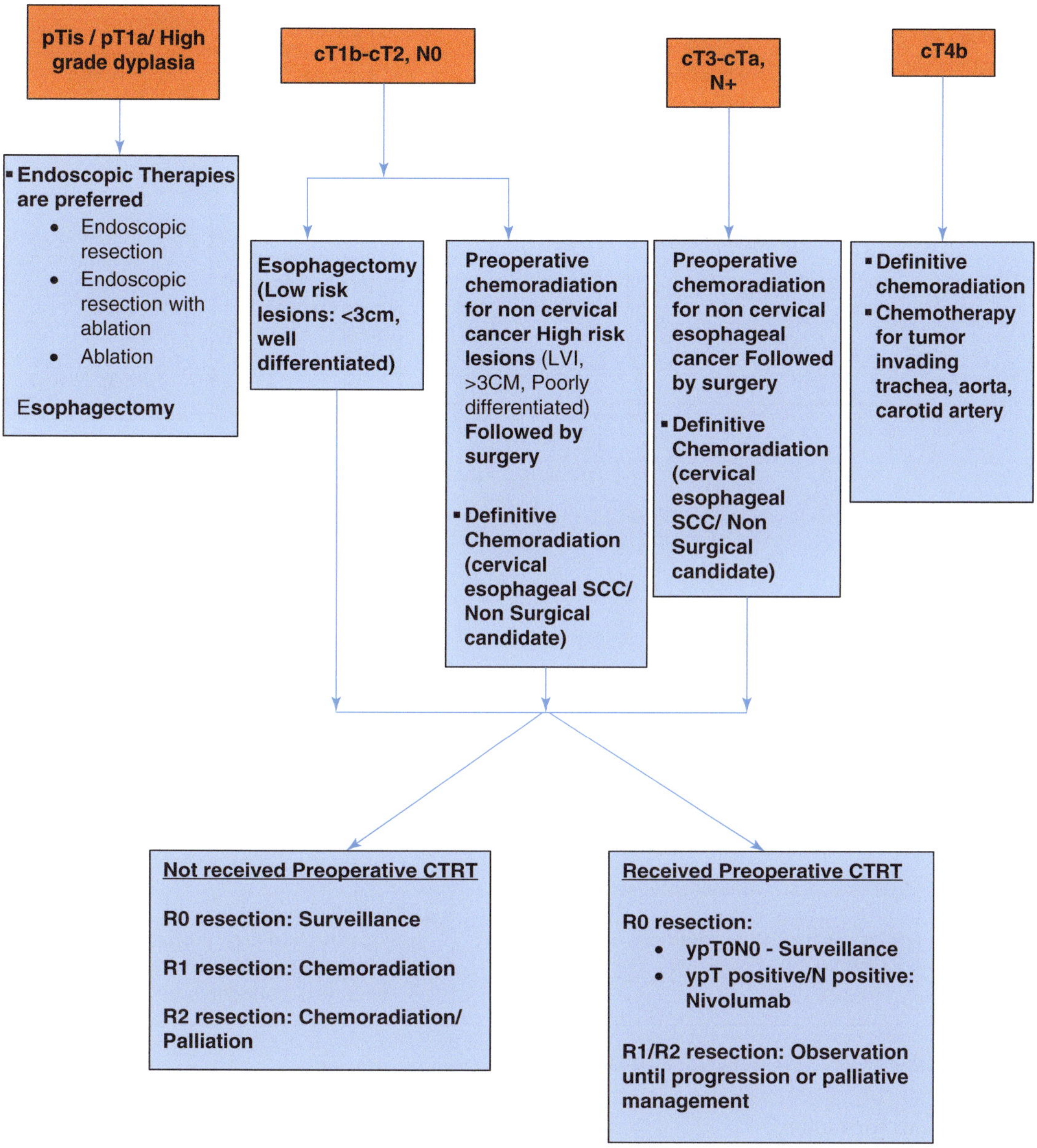

Fig. 7 Management algorithm for squamous cell carcinoma of esophagus

6.5 Principles of Surgical Treatment

Although the management of esophageal cancer is multimodal, surgery remains the most important curative modality. At the same time, because of the extensive and complicated nature of the surgical procedure, it is considered one of the most challenging undertakings in the entire oncological spectrum. The first and most important condition for successful outcome of esophageal resection is an appropriate selection of patient (in terms of resectability of the tumor and operability of the patient as determined by cardio-pulmonary reserve). The other important factors are good prehabilitation, meticulous surgical technique, availability of postoperative intensive care, and surgical expertise to manage surgical complications.

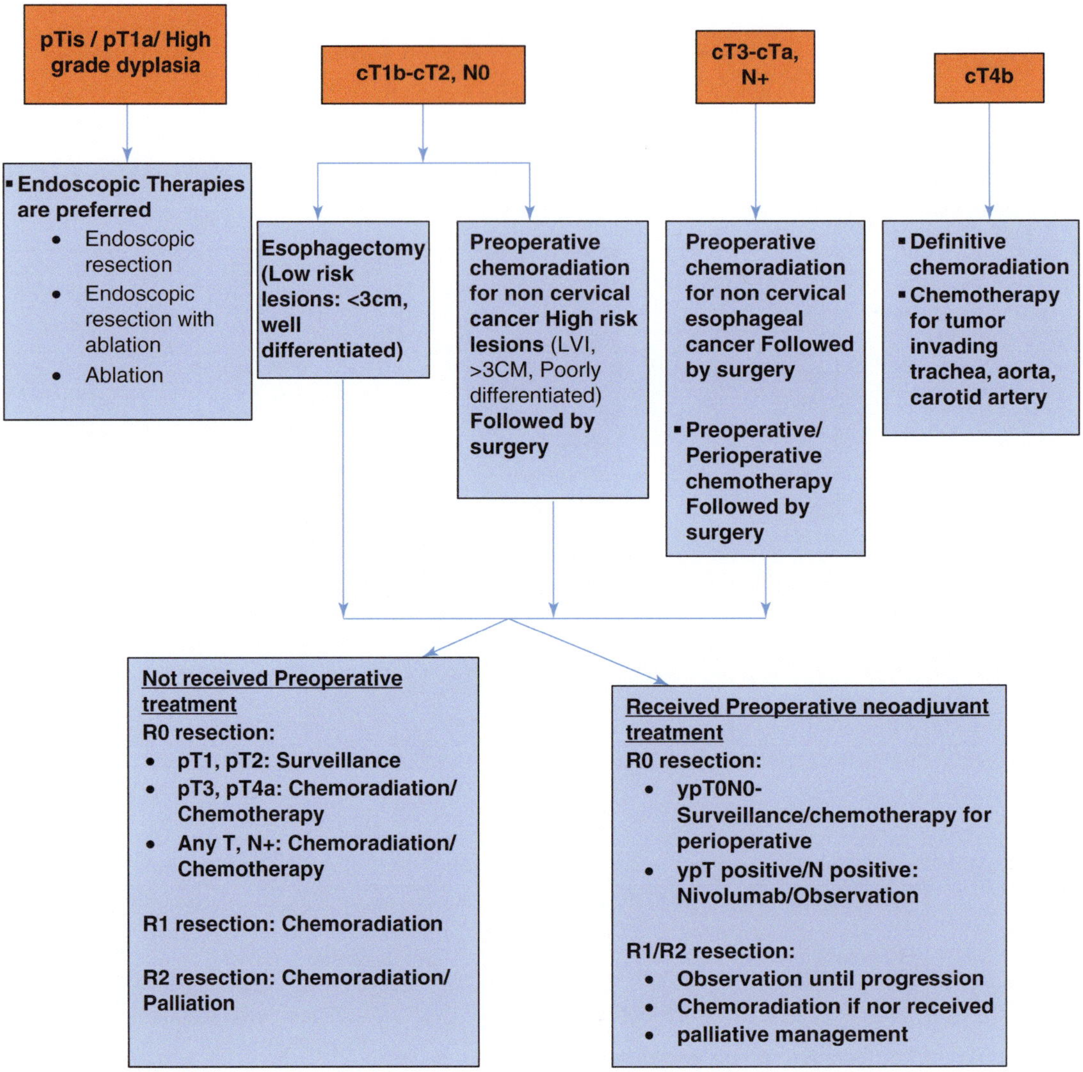

Fig. 8 Management of adenocarcinoma of esophagus or esophagogastric junction

Indications for surgery:

1. Early stage disease (upto T2 in the absence of high-risk features as mentioned previously) in an upfront setting
2. After neo-adjuvant treatment for locally advanced disease (T3/T4a)
3. Localized residual disease (incomplete response following definitive CT-RT) in carefully selected patients with good general condition
4. "Salvage esophagectomy" for cervical esophageal cancer after definitive CT-RT

6.6 Approaches for Surgical Resection

A number of approaches have been used for surgical resection of esophageal tumors. The most important factors influencing the approach are the location and extent of nodal involvement of the tumor and performance status of the patient (presence of compromised respiratory function). Broadly, the surgical approaches may be divided into transthoracic (Fig. 9) and transhiatal approaches.

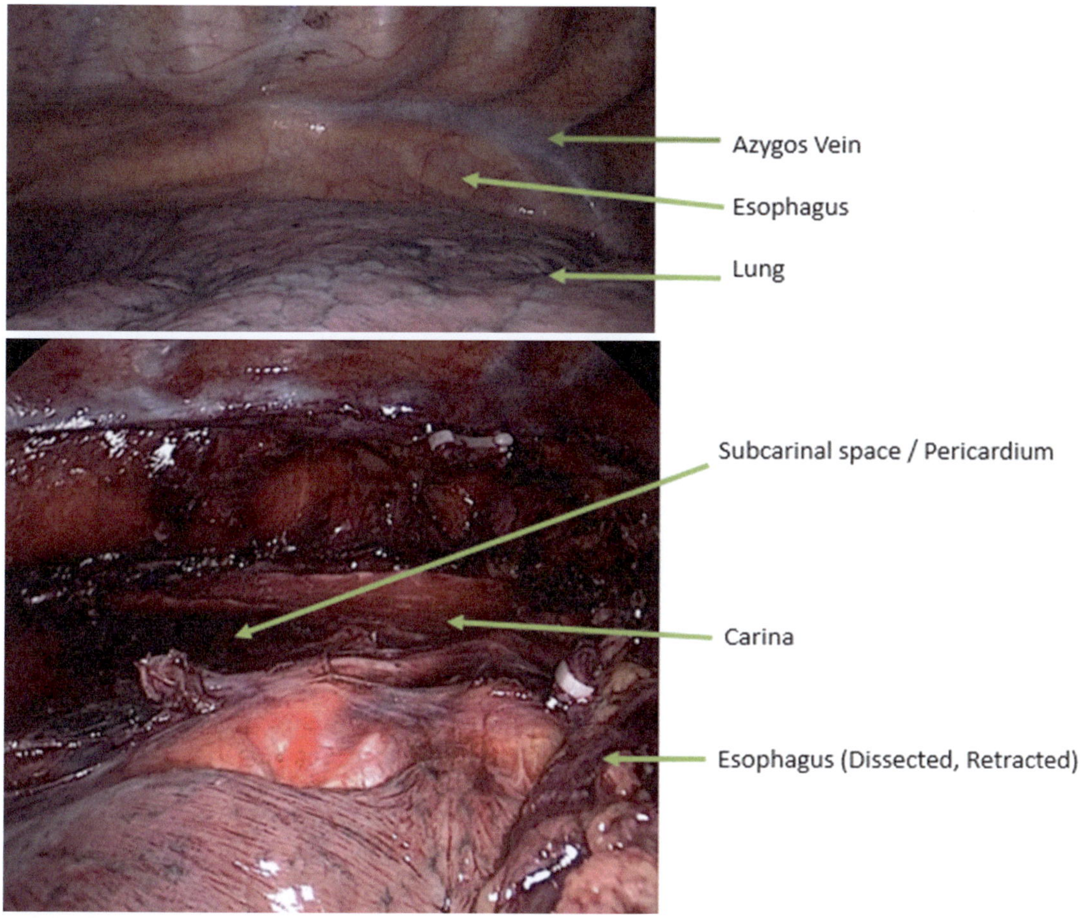

Fig. 9 Transthoracic surgery in carcinoma esophagus. (Courtesy: Dr. Shubham Jain, Senior Director, Surgical Oncology, Fortis Flt. Lt. Rajan Dhall Hospital, Vasant Kunj, Delhi)

Transthoracic approach is usually used for all the middle-third tumors and for lower-third tumors as per the experience and choice of the surgeon. A systematic mediastinal lyphadenectomy can be performed under the vision and surgery can be performed both through open and minimal access methods (thoracoscopic or robot-assisted).

Transhiatal approach does not require a thoracotomy and has been found to be associated with lesser chance of pulmonary complications. At the same time, essentially it is for lower third tumors with no evidence of mediastinal nodal metastasis as a systematic mediastinal nodal dissection is not feasible through this approach. Meta-analysis comparing these two approaches showed better long-term survival for the transthoracic approach, although it did not reach statistical significance. We reserve the transhiatal approach only for GE junction or lower esophageal adenocarcinomas with compromised respiratory function.

Various approaches used for esophagectomy are:

1. Transthoracic esophagectomy with removal of entire intra-thoracic esophagus with cervical anastomosis (McKeown's tri-incision method: open thoracotomy or minimal access approach: thoracoscopic or combination of open thoracotomy and laparoscopic or robotic)
2. Ivor Lewis esophagectomy (partial esophagectomy with partial gastrectomy) with intrathoracic anastomosis in right thorax (open or minimal access)

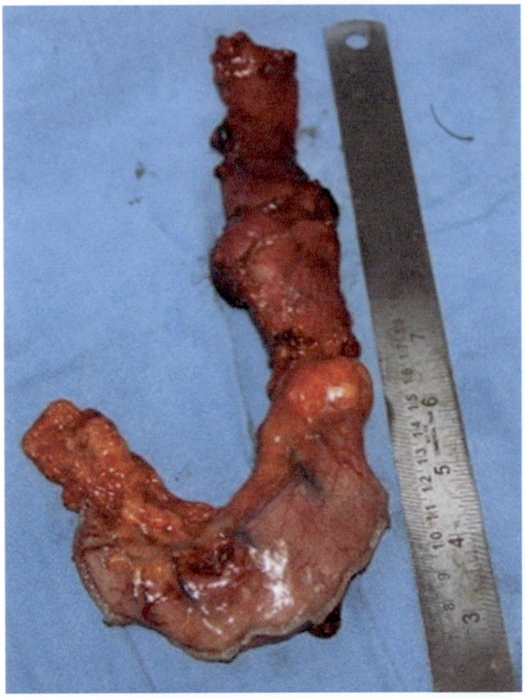

Fig. 10 A typical esophagectomy surgical specimen

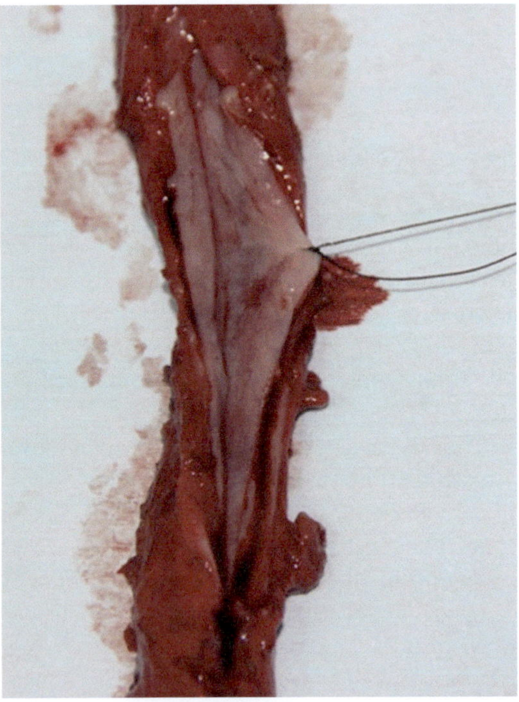

Fig. 11 Esophagectomy specimen showing good response to neoadjuvant therapy

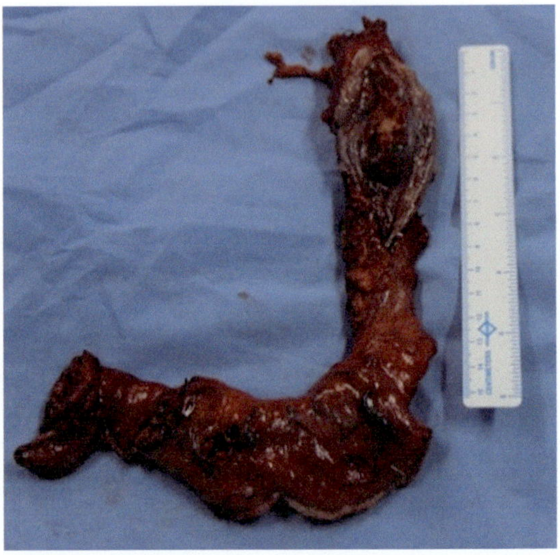

Fig. 12 Esophagectomy specimen with poor response to neoadjuvant therapy

3. Left thoraco-abdominal approach (partial esophagectomy with partial or total gastrectomy) with anastomosis in the left thorax
4. Transhiatal approach

All the methods may be through an open incision or minimal access approaches (Figs. 10, 11, and 12). Over the recent years, an increasing number of minimally access esophagectomies have been performed. The feasibility and safety of minimal access approaches have been established in various studies [18]. The long-term oncological outcomes have also been found to be equivalent to open approaches. Although there is no strong evidence to suggest one approach over the other, the choice depends on the experience and expertise of the surgical team. With the advantages of lesser post-operative pain, less blood loss, lower duration of ICU and hospital stay, and faster return to activity, minimal access esophagectomy is here to stay and will become the preferred method in future.

6.7 Surgical Margins

Surgical resection aims to achieve a tumor-free margin both longitudinally as well as circumferentially. Because of the possible submucosal spread, a longitudinal margin of 5 cm is preferred. Circumferentially, esophagectomy with the removal of peri-esophageal fat helps in getting a margin-free (R-0) resection.

6.8 Lymphadenectomy

Lymphadenectomy for esophageal cancer has been a matter of great debate for decades and conclusive evidence for the extent of nodal dissection is still lacking. It may be classified based on the removal of the lymph nodes in the following "fields" or nodal basins:

1. Abdominal
2. Mediastinal which may be infra azygous or supra-azygous, including removal of the lymph nodes along the recurrent laryngeal nerves.
3. Lower cervical lymph nodal dissection

Depending on the number of fields dissected, the lymphadenectomy can be classified either as two-field or three-field. A minimum of 15 nodes need to be dissected for adequate nodal staging. Apart from the number, the number of nodal stations dissected indicates the thoroughness of the nodal dissection. A complete mediastinal lymph nodal dissection involves the removal of the lymph nodes around the esophagus from the abdominal hiatus up to the thoracic inlet, including the removal of nodes along both the recurrent laryngeal nerves. In the absence of conclusive evidence from any large-scale study in favor of three-field lymphadenectomy, it's advantages in survival outcomes remain controversial, and it is not routinely practised. The high incidence (upto 30%) of recurrent laryngeal palsy associated with three-field lymphadenectomy has been a matter of apprehension [19]. At the most extensive lymphadenectomy helps in accurate pathological staging with a possible "stage migration" phenomenon. It remains a policy of the surgeon based on experience. We have a routine policy of two-field lymphadenectomy.

6.9 Reconstruction Rechnique

The first and the most common choice for replacement of the resected esophagus remains to be gastric conduit placed in the esophageal bed through the mediastinal route. Other options (generally exercised in cases of failure of gastric conduit) are colon interposition and pedicled or free jejunal segment. Anastomosis may be made either in neck or thorax (esophago-gastric anastomosis) using either the hand-sewn or stapled method, with no difference in outcomes of either method.

6.10 Multimodal Management for Loco-Regionally Advanced Disease

Historically, with surgery being the only therapy for stage I–III esophageal cancer, overall survival (OS) rates barely exceeded 1 year. The first cervical esophageal resection was performed by Czerny in 1897. Before 1978, 5 year OS stood dismally at 9.6% [20]. There has been an 11% improvement in survival over the past 30 years. The 5 year OS for patients with localized and regional disease, however, remains low at 33.7% and 16.7% respectively [21]. The poor long-term outcomes with single modality therapy provoked research into the multimodality approach to treat non-metastatic locoregionally advanced esophageal disease. For early T1–2N0 esophageal cancers amenable to surgery, single modality surgical management is still the treatment of choice, but survival rates drastically fall with progress in the T stage and nodal involvement. International guidelines recommend neoadjuvant treatment for all tumors with T3 or greater and N+ tumors. The combination of chemotherapy with radiotherapy provides a radio-sensitizing effect on the tumor, downstages the disease, and improves local control while potentially eradicating micrometastatic disease, thereby facilitating long-term survival. The improvement in toxicity management has given rise to include T2 with high-risk biopsy features to be considered for pre-operative chemo-radiotherapy.

Almost all the permutations and combinations of surgery, chemotherapy, and radiotherapy have been tried over the last four decades. Barring a few, all the studies clubbed adenocarcinoma and squamous cell carcinoma together, although the biological differences between the two histologies are now apparent. A vast majority of the studies from west have included adenocarcinoma predominantly, whereas most of the Japanese studies report on squamous cell carcinoma. A variety of chemotherapy and radiotherapy protocols have been tried and response pattern for different regimens for these two histologies is remarkably different. For example, squamous cell carcinoma has shown a better response to neo-adjuvant chemoradiation compared to adenocarcinoma.

Various common combinations of treatments are as follows:

- Preoperative radiotherapy
- Neo-adjuvant chemoradiotherapy followed by surgery
- Neo-adjuvant chemotherapy followed by surgery
- Adjuvant chemotherapy with or without radiotherapy
- Definitive chemoradiotherapy

7 Preoperative RT

Radiotherapy, when used as a monotherapy historically, provided similar LRC rates as did the surgery. Exner first described the treatment of oesophageal cancer with radium in 1904 [22].

The rationale for using preoperative RT is to:

1. Increase resectability
2. Increased tumor radio-responsiveness secondary to improved tumor oxygenation
3. Decreased likelihood of dissemination at the time of surgery
4. Avoidance of surgery in patients with rapidly progressive disease

Five randomized trials (Table 4) evaluated the role of preoperative RT in esophageal cancer: The Meta-Analysis by the Oesophageal Cancer Collaborative Group (Arnott et al.) in 2005 updated the data from five randomized trials of >1000 patients comparing preop RT alone vs surgery alone. The majority of patients had SCC. After a median follow-up of 9 years, the hazard ratio for death was 0.89, suggesting an 11% reduction in the overall risk of death, with an absolute survival benefit of 4% at 5 years with the use of preoperative radiotherapy ($p = 0.06$). There were no differences observed in the resectability rates, local failure, or survival in almost all reported individual studies [27].

8 Neo Adjuvant Chemoradiotherapy (NACTRT) Followed by Surgery

The role of preoperative CTRT was evaluated by U.S. Intergroup Trial (1990–1995) which showed a 57% failure to control local disease (including 41% failure to resect all local disease) and a 50% distant failure rate in patients who did have a complete resection [28]. Wayman et al. in 2007 reported that with preop CTRT, 34% of patients

Table 4 Trials evaluating the role of preoperative RT in esophageal cancer

Author	Patients	Dose	Fraction	Local failure		5 year survival	
				Surgery	RT + surgery	Surgery	RT + surgery
Launois et al. [23]	109	40 Gy	NA	NA	NA	12	10
Gignoux et al. [24]	229	33 Gy	3.3 Gy/#	67	46	8	10
Arnott et al. [25]	176	20 Gy	2 Gy/#	NA	NA	17	9
Wang et al. [26]	160	40 Gy	2 Gy/#	NA	NA	30	35

had distant failure; 19% had local failure; 14% had a locoregional nodal failure and 6% had peritoneal seeding [29]. Six randomized studies evaluated the 5-year results with preop CTRT and subsequently, two Meta-analyses confirmed improved OS, R0 resection rate, and local control rates with the addition of pre-operative CTRT in comparison to surgery alone [30, 31]. Mariette et al. [32] and Bosset et al. [33] reported no excess mortality for patients treated with preoperative CTRT followed by surgery compared to surgery alone. Subsequently, the FFCD 9102 trial [34] was undertaken to compare, in responders only, chemoradiation alone with chemoradiation followed by surgery in 444 patients with locally advanced T3N0–1M0 adenocarcinoma of the thoracic esophagus. Patients with tumors within 18 cm from the upper incisor/infiltrating the gastric cardia or tracheobronchial tree, M1, N3, weight loss >15%, or comorbidities, were excluded. The primary endpoint was OS. Patients received two cycles of fluorouracil (FU) and cisplatin (days 1–5 and 22–26) and either conventional (46 Gy in 4.5 weeks) or split-course (15 Gy, days 1–5 and 22–26) concomitant radiotherapy. Patients with a response and no contraindication to either treatment were randomly assigned to surgery (arm A) or continuation of chemoradiation (arm B; three cycles of FU/cisplatin and either conventional [20 Gy] or split-course [15 Gy] radiotherapy). Chemoradiation was considered equivalent to surgery if the difference in 2-year survival rate was less than 10%. Stahl et al. [35] randomized patients with locally advanced SCC to either induction chemotherapy followed by chemoradiotherapy (40 Gy) followed by surgery (arm A), or the same induction chemotherapy followed by chemoradiotherapy (at least 65 Gy) without surgery (arm B). Local disease control was significantly higher in the surgery arm (64% vs 41%, $p < 0.05$), but median survival remained quite similar in both arms (16.4 vs 14.9 months, p = NS). Long-term data from the POET trial reported favorable local progression-free survival when radiotherapy was added to preoperative chemotherapy [36]. The above discussion highlights that pre-operative CTRT plays an important role in the management of locally advanced carcinoma esophagus. Figure 13 shows treatment response for neoadjuvant chemoradiation in a case of Carcinoma esophagus (pre and post NACTRT).

Performing surgery after NACTRT is safe. The last two trials [35, 36] also pointed out that a group of patients may be managed with a non-surgical approach without compromising survival outcomes.

Neoadjuvant concurrent chemoradiotherapy thus has shown a significant survival advantage compared to upfront surgery alone, regardless of tumor location or histology. Three large PHASE III randomized trials published their results in favor of trimodally therapy for resectable esophageal cancers. These include the CALGB 9781 [37] and the Dutch CROSS trial [38] (where a majority of the patients had Adenocarcinoma histology); and the Chinese NEOCRTEC 5010 [39] trial, where only esophageal SCC was recruited. A persistent survival benefit was shown in all three trials with NACTRT in comparison to surgery alone. There were no differences in postop morbidity/mortality rates between the two groups in all three trials.

The CALGB 9781 trial was closed early due to poor accrual, but the results were significant. Patients were randomly assigned to either esophagectomy with node dissection alone or cisplatin 100 mg/m(2) and fluorouracil 1000 mg/m(2)/day for 4 days on weeks 1 and 5, concurrent with radiation therapy (50.4 Gy total: 1.8 Gy/fraction over 5.6 weeks), followed by esophagectomy with node dissection. The median follow-up was 6 years. An intent-to-treat analysis showed a median survival of 4.48 vs 1.79 years in favour of trimodality therapy (exact stratified log-rank, $p = 0.002$). Five-year survival was 39% (95% CI, 21–57%) vs 16% (95% CI, 5–33%) in favour of trimodality therapy.

The largest and practice-defining landmark trial was the Dutch CROSS trial. Patients with operable carcinoma esophagus or GE junction were randomly assigned to receive surgery alone or weekly administration of carboplatin (doses titrated to achieve an AUC of 2 mg/ml/min) and paclitaxel (50 mg/m^2 of TBSA) for 5 weeks and concurrent radiotherapy (41.4 Gy in 23 fractions, 5 days/week), followed by surgery. The R0 resection rates were significantly higher in the

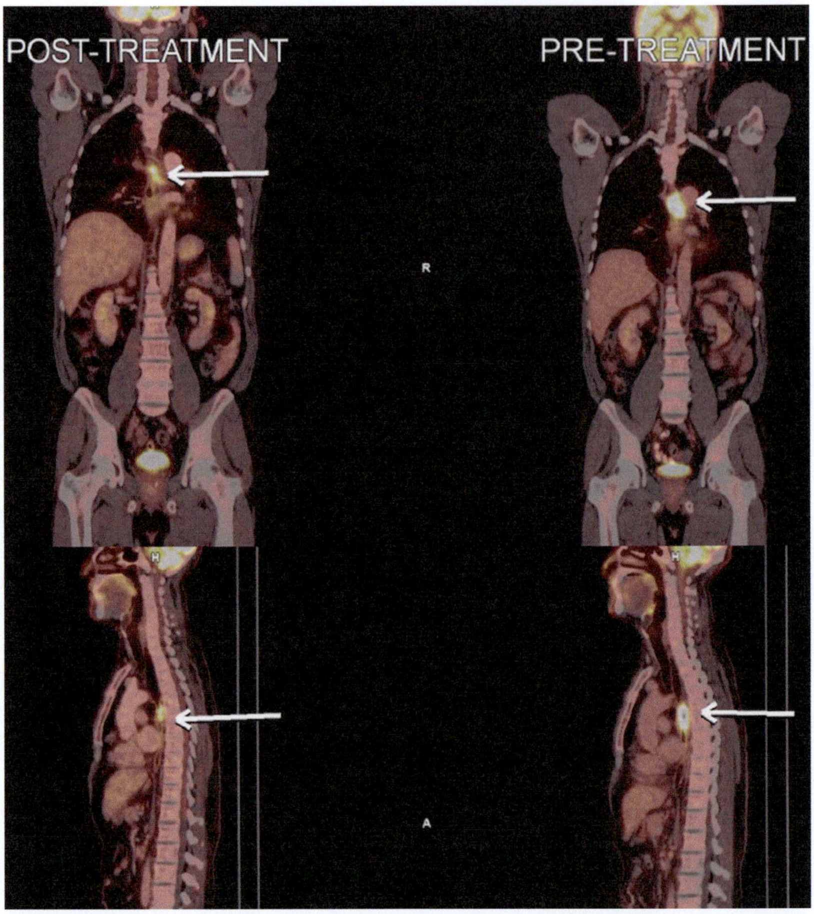

Fig. 13 Neo-adjuvant chemoradiation in a case of Carcinoma esophagus (post and pre treatment). (Courtesy: Dr. Ankur Pruthi, Consultant and Head, Nuclear Medicine & PET CT, Manipal Hospital, Dwarka, New Delhi)

NACTRT arm (92% vs 69%), and 29% of the NACTRT arm had pathological CR. The rate of path CR was 49% for the SCC cohort. The median F/U was 84 months. The median OS was 48.6 months vs 24 months, and a 5-year OS of 47% vs 33% in favour of the NACTRT arm. Updated analysis revealed a more profound benefit in patients with SCC, with median OS (81.6 months vs 21.1 months) favoring NACTRT. Patients with adenocarcinoma histology also had a significant survival advantage with NACTRT 43·2 months vs 27·1 months ($p = 0.038$). Overall recurrence rates were 35% vs 58% in favour of NACTRT, thus indicating that both LRR and peritoneal carcinomatosis were significantly reduced with the neoadjuvant treatment.

The NEOCRTEC 5010 trial evaluated the survival and safety of NACRT plus surgery with surgery alone in patients with locally advanced ESCC. In NACRT group, patients received vinorelbine 25 mg/m^2 intravenously (IV) on days 1 and 8 and cisplatin 75 mg/m^2 IV on days 1, or 25 mg/m^2 IV on days 1–4 every 3 weeks for two cycles, with a total concurrent radiation dose of 40.0 Gy administered in 20 fractions of 2.0 Gy on 5 days/week. In both groups, patients underwent McKeown or Ivor- Lewis esophagectomy. The pathological complete response rate was 43.2% in NACRT group. Compared with group S, group CRT had a higher R0 resection rate (98.4% vs 91.2%; $p = 0.002$), a better median overall survival (100.1 months vs 66.5 months; hazard ratio, 0.71; 95% CI, 0.53–0.96; $p = 0.025$), and a prolonged disease-free survival (100.1 months vs 41.7 months; hazard ratio, 0.58; 95% CI, 0.43–0.78; $P < 0.001$).

Several subsequent meta-analyses reconfirmed the impact of NACTRT on OS when compared to all other treatment approaches, including surgery alone; NACT, or NART [40, 41]. In the meta-analysis by Sjoquist et al. [42], the hazard ratio of 0.78 was noted with NACTRT, yielding an absolute survival benefit of 8.7% at 2 years, and NNT to prevent one death being 11. This was significant across histologies, and the advantage was not offset by perioperative mortality.

Newer trials viz. PROTECT 1402 [43] by Messager et al. and another phase II trial by Leichman et al. [44] have shown encouraging results for an alternative chemotherapy regimen of FOLFOX. However, data from the phase III trial is yet to confirm the findings.

8.1 Neoadjuvant Chemotherapy (NACT) Followed by Surgery

Neoadjuvant chemotherapy has been tried since the 1980s with different regimes and has been tested both in preoperative as well as in perioperative settings (Table 5). The primary objective of this strategy has been a combination of downstaging of tumor and treatment of micrometastatic disease. It also gives an idea about the biological behavior of the tumor. The trials involving perioperative strategy (e.g., MAGIC trial and FLOT 4 study) mostly included patients with adenocarcinoma and had a mixed population of the stomach, gastroesophageal junction, and lower esophageal tumors. The largest trial comparing preoperative chemotherapy plus surgery versus surgery alone (MRCOWG OE02) had a total of 802 patients, including 533 patients

Table 5 Trials evaluating the role of preoperative chemotherapy in esophageal cancer

Author	Patients	Preop chemo	RT	R0 resection (%)	pCR (%)	Median Survival (m)	5 year survival (%)
Forastiere et al. [45]	43	Cisplatin 20 mg/m²/day on D1–5; 17–21 Vinblastine 1 mg/m²/day on D1–4; 17–20 5FU 300 mg/m²/day on D1–21	3750 R/15# 4500 R/15#	84	24	29	34
Bedenne et al. [46]	94	Cisplatin 20 mg/m²/day 5FU 800 mg/m²/day D1–5; 22–26	30 Gy/10# split course D1–5; 22–26	82	20	17	23
Urba et al. [47]	50	Cisplatin 20 mg/m²/day on D1–5; 17–21 Vinblastine 1 mg/m²/day on D1–4; 17–20 5FU 300 mg/m²/day on D1–21	45 Gy/30#/BID	90	28	17	22
Posner et al. [48]	44	5FU, cisplatin, and interferon in various schedules	40 Gy/20# 45 Gy/30#/BID	81	24	28	32
Kleinberg et al. [49]	92	Cisplatin 20 or 26 mg/m²/day D1–5; 26–30 5FU 225 or 300 mg/m²/day D1–30	44 Gy/22#	87	37	35	40
Tepper et al. [50]	30	Cisplatin 100 mg/m² and 5FU 1000 mg/m²/day × 4 days, week 1 and 5	50.4 Gy/25#	NA	40	54	39

with adenocarcinoma of GE junction or lower esophagus, showed a significant overall survival difference favouring neoadjuvant chemotherapy for adenocarcinoma compared with surgery alone [51]. The FNCLCC ACCORD 07 [52] trial had shown a 14% benefit in OS at 5 years with perioperative cisplatin and 5FU. Neo-AEGIS (Neoadjuvant trial in Adenocarcinoma of the Esophagus and Esophago-Gastric Junction International Study) [53] compared the CROSS regimen with modified MAGIC or FLOT regimen for locally advanced adenocarcinoma esophagus or GE junction. The trial reported non-inferior outcomes with either of the treatment approaches and the 3-year estimated survival probability of 56–57%.

The strategy of neoadjuvant chemotherapy has increased the R-0 resection rate and has resulted in improvements in 5-year overall survival to the tune of 13–15%. Patients with adenocarcinoma of GE junction/lower esophagus with T3/T4 tumors or those with evidence of nodal metastasis should be considered for neoadjuvant chemotherapy. The choice of regimen may include Cisplatin + 5 FU, FLOT (Docetaxel, Oxaliplatin, 5-FU, and Leucovorin), or Paclitaxel + Carboplatin.

8.2 Preoperative Chemotherapy for Squamous Cell Carcinoma

A vast majority of trials conducted for the evaluation of neoadjuvant chemotherapy had a predominance of adenocarcinoma in the study population, and for squamous cell carcinoma, the results were either of subgroup analysis or an extrapolation of the statistics for adenocarcinoma. Because of the limited number (<100) of patients with squamous cell carcinoma, they lacked sufficient power for conclusive evidence.

The MRCOWG trial OE-02 compared preoperative chemotherapy (2 cycles of Cisplatin 80 mg/m^2 on day 1 and 5-FU 1000 mg/m^2/day from day 1 to 4 every 3 weeks) with surgery alone. The subgroup of squamous cell carcinoma had 269 patients, and the 5-year overall survival was better in the neoadjuvant chemotherapy arm (25.5% vs 17%). A pooled analysis of ten studies involving a total of 2061 patients comparing NACT followed by surgery with surgery alone showed a survival benefit of 5% for the NACT arm [42].

The most important evidence for preoperative chemotherapy in squamous cell carcinoma came from the JCOG 9907 trial, which showed a significant improvement in overall survival over adjuvant chemotherapy (55% vs 43%, HR 0.73, $p = 0.04$) [54].

The recently completed JCOG 1109 NExT study comparing two preoperative chemotherapy regimens and preoperative chemoradiotherapy has published its results, which has generated great interest. It included 601 patients with only squamous cell carcinoma histology up to stage III (excluding T4 tumors) randomized in 1:1:1 fashion to preoperative Cisplatin + 5 FU (NeoCF), Docetaxel + Cisplatin + 5 FU (NeoCF+D), and CF + concurrent radiation (NeoCF+RT, 41.4 Gy) in 3 arms. The 3-year overall survival (OS) in the 3 arms: NeoCF, NeoCF+D, and NeoCF+RT were 62.6%, 72.1% and 68.3% respectively. After a median survival of 4.2 years, the median OS in NeoCF and NeoCF+RT were 4.6 years and 6 years, respectively, while it was yet to be reached in the NeoCF+D arm. This study, after a median follow-up of 50+ Months has shown that NeoCF+D chemotherapy regimen had a higher incidence of treatment-related toxicities, and incomplete therapy course [55].

8.3 NACTRT Versus NACT

Before JCOG 1109, there were not enough randomized studies to compare these two modalities head-to-head separately for different histologies. NeoRes I, which was a phase II randomized study comparing NACTRT with NACT in T1N1 or T2-3N0-1 M0-1a tumors, included esophageal adenocarcinoma (131 patients) and squamous cell carcinoma (50 patients) using three cycles of Cisplatin and 5-FU at 3 weekly intervals with or without radiotherapy (40 Gy/20 fractions/4 weeks). Although the NACTRT arm had a higher

PCR rate (28% vs 9% in NACT), 5-year progression-free and overall survival were not significantly different. Postoperative complications appeared to be more severe in the NACTRT arm. Higher rates of treatment-related toxicity and postoperative mortality appeared to negate the advantages of higher PCR and R-0 resection [56]. Similar results were found in the meta-analysis, which included three eligible randomized trials comparing NACTRT with NACT in a total of 375 patients. Higher PCR and R-0 resection rates did not significantly affect overall survival [57].

Particularly, adenocarcinoma of the esophagus remains a challenge, and both preoperative CTRT and preoperative CT have similar long-term results and the value of adding radiation to the treatment plan is being questioned because of these similar outcomes.

In general, although NACTRT is associated with higher PCR and R-0 resection, it also has higher toxicity and no proven superior survival benefit compared to NACT. These outcomes are more relevant in the Indian scenario where a majority of the patients are nutritionally compromised and tolerance to concurrent CT-RT regime may not be optimal. Therefore, a cautious approach is often required to balance the advantages and post-treatment complications. NACT may have the theoretical advantage of acting as a triage method to see the response and tolerance to the regimen. Dense fibrotic response after NACTRT may obliterate the planes of circumferential dissection during surgery, which is more relevant in middle-third tumors. Even for NeoCF+D regime, the tolerance, compliance and toxicity profile need to be carefully weighed in India. We tried the weekly Paclitaxel and Carboplatin regime (instead of 3-weekly) and found it to be better tolerated.

Overall, loco-regional and distant failure remains a concern and more tailored treatment according to risk stratification using easily identifiable biomarkers such as postoperative lymph node status, R0 resection, and the presence or absence of mismatch repair deficiency should be looked into.

9 Definitive Chemoradiation (CTRT)

Concurrent chemoradiotherapy has consistently shown superior survival indices in comparison to RT alone, thereby making concurrent treatment the current standard of care for the inoperable disease. The landmark RTOG (Radiation Therapy Oncology Group) 85-01 [58] enrolled patients with both SCC and adenocarcinoma and was prematurely closed due to a significant survival advantage both locoregionally and distantly. 123 patients with non-metastatic carcinoma esophagus were enrolled (80% SCC and 20% AdenoCA). CTRT arm of 50 Gy/25 fractions/5 weeks with 4 cycles of 5FU (1000 mg/m^2 D1–4, week 1,5,8,11) + CDDP (75 mg/m^2 D1), was compared to RT alone with 64 Gy/32 fractions/6.4 weeks. Patients with gastric/supraclavicular LN/mediastinal LN were excluded. Median OS was reported to be 12.5 months in CTRT arm compared to 8.9 months in RT alone arm ($p = 0.001$). Estimated 2- and 3-year survival was 36% and 33% in the CTRT arm compared to 10% and 0% in RT alone arm. Long-term follow-up results of the RTOG 85-01 trial by Cooper et al. [59] showed that the persistence of disease was the predominant pattern of failure. Combined modality treatment in long term cured more patients than RT alone. 8-year survival with CTRT was 22%. No difference in late toxicities was noted between the two arms. The projected 10-year OS with CTRT was 20%. No deaths after 5 years occurred due to disease. The 5-year survival of SCC was 21% vs 13% for AdenoCA (p = 0.15), i.e., no difference in survival based on histology. The approach of CTRT with concurrent paclitaxel and carboplatin is safe and feasible in Indian patients [60].

However, a dismal locoregional failure rate of around 50% at 1 year led to further investigation in the RTOG 94-05 INT 0123 trial [61] that wanted to evaluate the role of dose escalation in CTRT for Esophageal Cancer. A standard dose regimen of 50.4 Gy/28#/5.5 weeks was compared to a dose-escalated RT schedule of 64.8 Gy/36#/7.1 weeks. The chemotherapy regimen was common between the two arms = 5FU

(1000 mg/m² D1–4 iv week 1,5,8,11) + CDDP (75 mg/m² D1). The trial was closed early as the interim analysis did not show a survival advantage with dose escalation, and the incidence of grade 3 or higher toxicity was higher in high-dose RT arm. Xu et al. in a phase III trial randomized 319 patients, deemed inoperable, to receive either 60 Gy with 50 Gy to the primary and regional lymph nodes along with concurrent Docetaxel followed by two additional cycles of chemotherapy. One, 3-year locoregional PFS and OS were similar in both arms but a higher dose was associated with significantly higher pneumonitis ($p = 0.03$) [62]. The ARTDECO trial randomized patients with inoperable or medically unresectable carcinoma esophagus to receive either 50.4 Gy or 61.6 Gy along with concurrent carboplatin and paclitaxel once a week for 6 weeks. The study reported no difference in terms of local or locoregional PFS or OS; similarly toxicity was not different in both arms [63].

9.1 Elective Nodal Radiation

Elective nodal irradiation has been debated for the management of carcinoma esophagus as it increases target volume and subsequent risk of radiation pneumonitis. Zhao et al. in a retrospective study, compared failure patterns and effects of elective nodal irradiation (ENI) or involved field irradiation (IFI) for cervical and upper thoracic esophageal squamous cell carcinoma (SCC) patients [64]. The authors reported in-field recurrence in 44% of patients, and 46% failed with distant mets with or without regional failure. Zhu et al. performed the pattern of failure analysis of the patients treated in the ESO-Shanghai 1 trial. Patients were treated to a dose of 61.2 Gy by the IMRT technique along with involved nodal irradiation. The authors reported 86% 3-year extensive elective nodal control and 94.3% extensive elective nodal control-only rates. These extensive elective nodes received an incidental dose of 23.2 Gy as they were located 2 cm away from the PTV [65].

9.2 Altered Fractionation

Several trials were undertaken to evaluate the role of altered fractionation radiotherapy in the treatment of esophageal cancer. It has been found that if the dose per fraction is reduced (i.e., in hyperfractionation) there is a sparing of late-reacting normal tissues relative to those, which respond early. Low α/β values (1.5–5 Gy) have been observed for late-reacting normal tissues and indicate that radiation damage should be greatly spared by the use of dose fractions smaller than the 2 Gy, as used in conventional radiotherapy. However, the high α/β values (6–14 Gy) observed for acutely responding normal tissues indicate that the response is relatively linear over the dose range of clinical interest. Hence late toxicities remain at par even if lower doses per fraction are administered. If tumors respond in the same way as acutely responding normal tissues then hyperfractionation might confer a therapeutic gain relative to late-responding normal tissues [66].

Accelerated repopulation is one of the main reasons for the local failure of tumors after radiotherapy, which allows the surviving stem cells to thrive and repopulate more aggressively than before the start of treatment. Marcu et al. showed that prolonging the treatment time may lead to a decrease in the effective dose by 0.59 Gy/day due to the accelerated repopulation that starts after 4 weeks in the tumor cells [67]. A phase II study by Choi N et al. evaluated the role of twice-daily radiotherapy of 58.4 Gy/34 fractions/5 weeks as a concurrent boost during two chemotherapy cycles in NACTRT for resectable esophageal cancer. The 5-year OS (56% vs 24%, $p = 0.0214$) and DFS (48% vs 6%) were significantly better for patients with a pathological CR and minimal residual disease [68].

Stuart et al. undertook a study to evaluate the outcomes and treatment-related mortality and morbidity patterns of patients treated with neoadjuvant hyperfractionated accelerated chemoradiation for resectable esophageal cancer [69]. Two hundred and fifty patients with resectable esophageal cancer treated with preoperative hyperfractionated accelerated chemoradiotherapy (45 Gy in 30 twice-daily fractions over 3 weeks) followed by planned transhiatal esophagectomy were analyzed. Median OS was 35.1 months for patients who underwent esophagectomy after the specified neoadjuvant therapy. Neoadjuvant twice-daily chemoradiation for esophageal cancer could thus be a safe and effective alternative to daily fractionation with low treatment-related mortality and long-term outcomes similar to standard fractionation courses.

Newer randomized studies have found utility in other chemotherapy regimens when used as radiosensitizers. Phase II/III PRODIGE 5/ ACCORD 17 trial [70] showed promising results with concurrent FOLFOX, although survival endpoints were not statistically superior.

10 Can Surgery Be Avoided in CA Esophagus

The prognosis and survival in esophageal cancer(EC) without undergoing surgery gained attention with incremental improvements in the chemotherapy regimens and simultaneous developments in technological and biological basis of radiotherapy in the last 30 years. A nonoperative approach is indicated for squamous cell carcinoma (SCC) of the cervical esophagus. Currently, other than cervical esophagus, esophageal cancer is always evaluated for surgery. In the esophageal SCC studies by Alexandrou A et al. [71] and Koppert LB et al. [72], surgery has shown improved disease control. However, neoadjuvant/preoperative NACT or NACRT is suitable for operable EC patients with good performance status and those below 70 years age. First, pathological CR rates would range 25% to 40% in SCC, and 5% to 30% in adenocarcinoma. Second, perioperative mortality was found to be higher for SCC than for adenocarcinoma, perhaps due to associated comorbidity and higher tumor location. In the Cochrane meta-analysis of randomized controlled studies comparing neoadjuvant versus definitive chemoradiation, mostly in SCC patients, there was no survival difference between the definitive chemoradiation group and the surgical group, while higher treatment-related mortality was shown in the surgical group [73]. In a long-term analysis of the FFCD 9102 trial by Vincent J et al., higher OS was shown for clinical non-responders who underwent surgery, than those who did not (17 vs. 5.5 months, respectively), suggesting efficacy for a non-operative approach in chemoradiation responders only [74].

In a multi-institutional cooperative group setting by RTOG 0113 [75], patients with localized unresectable/inoperable EC were randomly assigned to receive either induction with fluorouracil, cisplatin, and paclitaxel and then fluorouracil plus paclitaxel with 50.4 Gy of radiation (arm A) or induction with paclitaxel plus cisplatin and then the same chemotherapy concomitantly with 50.4 Gy of radiation (arm B). Though this was a phase II trial, 2-year survival rates were 56%(Arm-A) and 37%(Arm-B); however the toxicities were of clinical concern; Grade 3 and 4 encountered in more than 70% of patients in both groups. In our clinical practice, it is realised that one-third of EC patients receiving chemoradiotherapy would show complete response. This group of responders can be considered a special cohort for active surveillance by endoscopy, biopsy, and if necessary CT/PET-CT scan imaging. Proper counselling, timely follow-up tests, and a provision of surgery are integral to such a surveillance.

11 Intraluminal Radiotherapy (ILRT)

Intraluminal radiotherapy (ILRT) for oesophageal cancers provides high conformal dose to a small tumor volume while sparing the adjacent critical organs (like lung, heart). ILRT can be used in both curative and palliative settings. Figure 14 shows the schematic diagram of esophageal applicator.

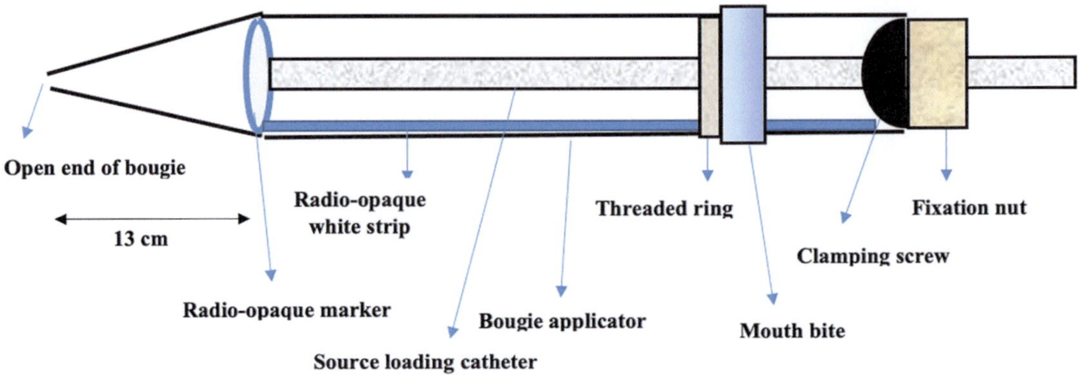

Fig. 14 Schematic representation of various parts of esophageal bougie (intraluminal applicator). (Courtesy: Dr Khushboo Rastogi, Department of Radiation Oncology, BLK Max, New Delhi)

11.1 Curative Setting

Indications:

1. Thoracic esophageal cancer (both SCC and adenocarcinoma)
2. Unifocal tumor
3. No e/o distant metastatic disease
4. Maximum length not more than 10 cm
5. Typically used as a boost after external beam radiotherapy (EBRT)

Contraindications:

1. Tracheal or bronchial involvement
2. Cervical esophagus and type II/III GE junction location
3. Stenosis that cannot be bypassed

Guiding principles:

1. Brachytherapy should follow EBRT
2. Avoid concurrent chemotherapy with ILRT
3. Applicator should have an external diameter of ≥10 mm

Dose recommendations (after 4–5 weeks of EBRT):

1. HDR 10–12 Gy in two fractions of 5–6 Gy each
2. Spaced at weekly intervals

Process of ILRT

1. Following completion of EBRT, a gap of 1–2 weeks is preferred before considering the patient for ILRT.
2. Pre-anaesthetic check-up and Gastroenterology opinion to be sought before planning ILRT.
3. Patient is admitted 1 day prior to procedure and advised overnight fasting.
4. Under sedation, endoscopy is performed (in endoscopy suite) to visualize the tumor, and the proximal and distal borders are noted (from the incisors).
5. Once tumor extent is documented, endoscope is removed leaving a guide wire in situ. The applicator (esophageal bougie—Fig. 14) is then inserted into the esophagus over the guide wire and placed in a way that the radio-opaque ring at its distal end comes to lie approx. 2 cm below the PTV (tumor + margin).
6. Gross tumor volume (GTV) is delineated on the planning CT scan, and a PTV margin of 2 cm is given in cranio-caudal directions.
7. Dose is prescribed at 5 mm from the surface (Fig. 15).
8. Once planning is done, the after-loading machine is connected by means of transfer tubes, and treatment is performed.
9. After treatment is completed, the applicator is removed.
10. Patient is kept under observation till fully conscious and stable.

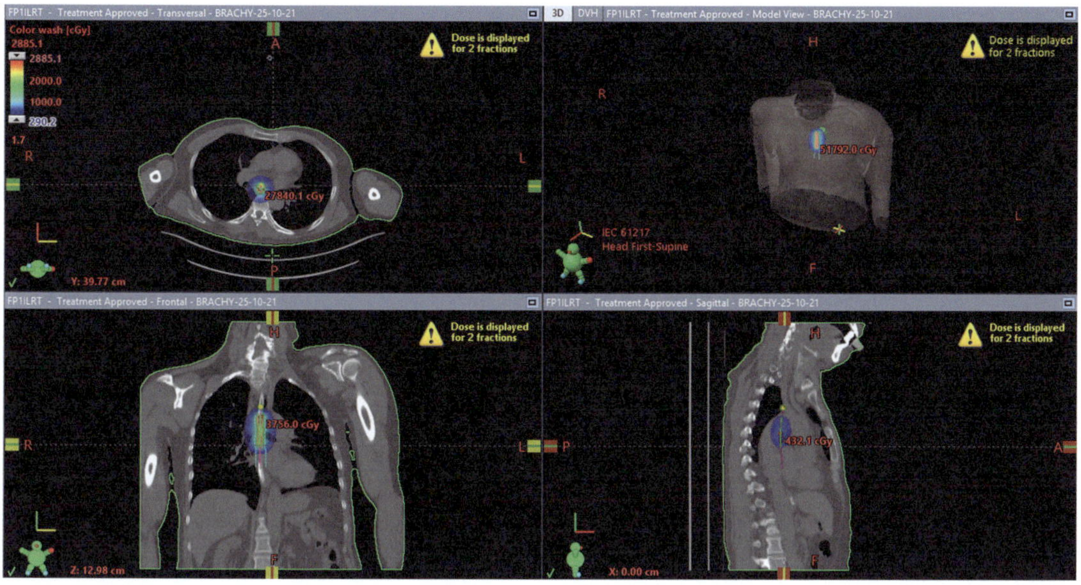

Fig. 15 ILRT planning in a patient of CA esophagus

11.2 Palliative Setting

Indications for palliative ILRT in carcinoma esophagus include (a) Unresectable local disease progression/recurrence after definitive radiation treatment (b) Adeno- or squamous cancers of the thoracic esophagus with or without distant metastasis (c) Dysphagia (d) Tumor haemorrhage.

Typically, a dose of HDR 6–24 Gy in 1–4 fractions is recommended.

Complete Kit for ILRT (GammaMedPlus)

1. Esophageal bougie (varying diameters—8, 10, 12, 14 mm) with bite protector and fixation (over the mouth)**
2. Strap for fixation mask and bite protector bougie
3. Cleaning set for esophageal bougie
4. Clamping screws for bougie
5. Seldinger guide wire, 2600 mm × 0.032″, sterile
6. Tube catheter, 3.2 mm diameter
7. Source guide tube support

**Esophageal ILRT Applicator should be CT scan imaging compatible, radio-opaque markers along entire length of bougie for easy identification, radio-opaque ring 13 cm above distal conical end of bougie.

12 Brachytherapy Boost

Gaspar et al. [76] in a multi-institutional, prospective study RTOG 9207 evaluated the feasibility of a brachytherapy boost in the form of HDR/LDR boost on week 8 post EBRT of 50 Gy/25#/5 weeks with concurrent 5-FU/cisplatin chemotherapy. HDR schedule of −15 Gy @5-Gy fractions at weeks 8, 9, and 10 or LDR brachytherapy one session 20 Gy dose during week 8 was followed. The HDR dose was decreased to 10 Gy in two 5-Gy fractions given in weeks 8 and 9. The local persistence/local recurrence rate was 63%. The 1-year actuarial fistula development rate was 18% and the overall treatment-related mortality rate was 8%. The incidence of fistulas made the authors urge caution in employing Esophageal Brachytherapy, particularly when used in conjunction with chemotherapy.

Intending to improve the results of the treatment of esophageal cancer, Okawa et al. [77] undertook a multi-institutional, randomized trial to evaluate external irradiation alone and in combination with intraluminal brachytherapy in esophageal SCC. The patients assigned to receive external irradiation alone received boost EBRT irradiation of 10 Gy/week on a schedule similar to the previous one and with the same or smaller irradiation field. Intraluminal brachytherapy was performed, as a rule, with the reference dose point set at a depth of 5 mm of the esophageal submucosa, and a total of 10 Gy was irradiated at a daily dose of 5 Gy, on a once-weekly schedule with low-dose-rate or high-dose-rate brachytherapy equipment. The cause-specific survival rate at 5 years was 27% in the external irradiation alone group and 38% in the intraluminal brachytherapy combined group ($p = 0.385$). However, in the patients with 5 cm or less tumor length, the cause-specific survival rate was 64% at 5 years in the intraluminal brachytherapy boost group, which showed a significant improvement over 31.5% in the external irradiation alone group ($p = 0.025$). The incidence of early and late complications did not differ according to whether intraluminal brachytherapy was used. They thus found intraluminal brachytherapy to be superior to external beam radiotherapy when used as a boost in a subgroup of patients with small tumors less than 5 cm in length. This improvement in survival was, however, not associated with an increase in treatment-related toxicity.

The American Brachytherapy Society (ABS) guidelines proposed Recommendations were made for brachytherapy in the definitive and palliative treatment of esophageal cancer [78].

(A) Definitive treatment: good candidates for brachytherapy include patients with unifocal thoracic adeno- or squamous cancers ≤10 cm in length, with no evidence of intra-abdominal or metastatic disease. Contraindications include tracheal or bronchial involvement, cervical esophagus location, or stenosis that cannot be bypassed. The esophageal brachytherapy applicator should have an external diameter of 6–10 mm. If 5FU-based chemotherapy and 45–50-Gy external beam are used, recommended brachytherapy is either: (i) HDR 10 Gy in 2 weekly fractions of 5 Gy each; or (ii) LDR 20 Gy in a single course at 0.4–1 Gy/h. All doses are specified 1 cm from the mid-source or mid-dwell position. (Fig. 15).

Brachytherapy should follow external beam radiation therapy and should not be given concurrently with chemotherapy.

(B) Palliative treatment: Patients with adeno- or squamous cancers of the thoracic esophagus with distant metastases or unresectable local disease progression/recurrence after definitive radiation treatment should be considered for brachytherapy with palliative intent. After a limited dose (30 Gy) EBRT, the recommended brachytherapy is either: (i) HDR 10–14 Gy in one or two fractions; or (ii) LDR 20–25 Gy in a single course at 0.4–1 Gy/h. The need for external beam radiation in newly diagnosed patients with a life expectancy of fewer than 3 months is controversial. In these cases, HDR of 15–20 Gy in two to four fractions or LDR of 25–40 Gy at 0.4–1 Gy/h may be of benefit.

13 Adjuvant RT

To date, there is no level I evidence regarding the practice of radiotherapy in the adjuvant setting in esophageal cancer. Some trials that tried to evaluate the same had inconsistent results.

Schreiber et al. in 2010 [79], undertook a retrospective analysis of the SEER database to assess the impact of radiotherapy after esophagectomy in locally advanced esophageal cancer. Adjuvant RT was shown to have a benefit in OS (absolute benefit of 6 months) and DSS (3.5% at 3 years). Subgroup analysis revealed the OS and DSS were limited to AJCC stage III disease only (T3N1 or T4N0–1), irrespective of histology. Thus, this large population-based review supported the use of postoperative radiation for stage III SCC and AC of the esophagus. But owing to the retrospective nature of this study, this was an underpowered study not suitable to establish a stand of care guidelines.

Wei Deng undertook a Prospective, Phase III, Randomized Controlled Trial (RCT) to evaluate the efficacy and safety of postoperative radiotherapy in patients with pathological T2–3N0M0 thoracic esophageal squamous cell carcinoma. Patients were randomly assigned to surgery alone or to receive postoperative radiotherapy of 50.4 Gy in the supraclavicular field and 56 Gy in the mediastinal field in 28 fractions over 6 weeks. The interim analysis was published in 2020 [80] that revealed a significant benefit in the 3-year disease-free survival rates with post-op radiotherapy (75.1% vs 58.7%; $p = 0.030$) and reduced Local-regional recurrence with radiotherapy (10.0% vs. 32.5%, $p = 0.001$). The overall survival and distant metastasis rates were not significantly different between the two groups. Grade 3 toxicity rate related to radiotherapy was 12.5%. Postoperative radiotherapy significantly increased disease-free survival and decreased local regional recurrence rate in patients with pathological T2–3N0M0 thoracic esophageal squamous cell carcinoma with acceptable toxicities in this interim analysis.

A recent phase III trial by Wenjie et al. [81] published in 2021, evaluated the role of adjuvant therapy (post-op RT: PORT/postop Chemo-RT: POCRT) in stage IIB—III Esophageal SCC undergoing R0 resection upfront. The trial was prematurely closed after 5 years of enrolment and a median F/U of 56.4 months. A Median OS benefit of 20.2 months and a median DFS benefit of 30.8 months were noted with adjuvant therapy. Locoregional failure was the predominant pattern of failure in the surgery-alone arm. POCRT showed lower distant failure than PORT alone. Radiation plays important role in the salvage of recurrent tumors after surgery. Patients with good PS, lower group stage, node negativity at index surgery, longer disease-free interval, nodal recurrence (as compared to anastomotic site recurrence), smaller disease volume, single site of recurrence, RT dose >50 Gy, conformal RT, use of concomitant chemotherapy and good radiological response after radiotherapy are a better candidate for salvage radiation [82]. Table 6 shows trials on adjuvant radiotherapy.

14 Palliative External RT

There are no big randomized studies evaluating the role of RT in palliation in esophageal cancer. A retrospective analysis by Murray et al. in 2012 [87] showed that short-course EBRT (most commonly 20 Gy/5#) might be an effective means to palliate dysphagia in patients with incurable EC while being non-invasive at the same time. Following radiotherapy, 75% of patients experienced an improvement in dysphagia and 25% of patients gained weight. The median stent (and retreatment)-free survival was 4.9 months. Median overall survival was 6.1 months. However, a median delay of 1–2 months was noted between RT completion and symptomatic relief.

Welsch et al. in 2016 [88] undertook a retrospective study to evaluate the survival and symptom relief after palliative RT in esophageal cancer. RT was given as EBRT alone, Brachytherapy alone, or a combination of EBRT and Brachytherapy. The 6-month Dysphagia free survival was 90% ± 4%; 37 ± 75; and 92% ± 5% respectively in the three arms with a median response duration of 5 months. The median period to dysphagia improvement was 26 weeks

Table 6 Trails on adjuvant RT

Reference	No of patients		5-year survival		*P* value	Treatment modality (%)
	R0	R1	R0	R1		
Zafirellis et al. [83]	82	57	45.3	14.4	<0.001	Op alone
Hofstetter et al. [84]	864	130	29	5	0.0001	Op alone—47 NACT—17 NART—14 NACTRT—22
Mulligan et al. [85]	163	49	16.0	6.0	<0.001	± NACTRT
Kelsen et al. [86]	270	43	39	13	<0.0001	NACT

for patients who were treated with EBRT ± BT and 16 weeks for patients who were treated with BT alone. Laskar et al. and Vivekanandam et al. reported significant improvement in dysphagia relief and symptom scores with the addition of external beam radiotherapy (EBRT) to intraluminal brachytherapy (ILBT) [89, 90].

A multicentre randomized trial by Homs et al. in 2004 [91] evaluated 209 patients with dysphagia from inoperable carcinoma of Esophagus/GEJn who underwent either metal stent placement or Single dose brachytherapy 12 Gy. Dysphagia improved more rapidly after stent placement than after brachytherapy, but long-term relief of dysphagia was better after brachytherapy. Stent placement had more complications than brachytherapy, which was mainly due to an increased incidence of late hemorrhage. Quality-of-life scores were in favor of brachytherapy compared with stent placement. Despite slow improvement, single-dose brachytherapy gave better long-term relief of dysphagia with fewer complications than metal stent placement.

Amdal et al. in 2013 [92] undertook a phase III randomized study to compare Palliative brachytherapy with and without self-expanding metallic stent (SEMS) in Stage IV esophageal cancer. Patients receiving SEMS followed by brachytherapy had significantly improved dysphagia at the first follow-up compared to patients receiving brachytherapy alone ($n = 35$). A difference in pain was not observed. At the second follow-up, however, patients in both arms ($n = 21$) had less dysphagia. For the relief of dysphagia, SEMS followed by brachytherapy is preferable and safe for patients in need of immediate alleviation.

Another retrospective analysis by Martin et al. in 2020 [93] was undertaken to evaluate in stage IV esophageal Ca, the outcomes and adverse effects of palliative RT (1593 patients) in comparison to esophageal stenting (364 patients). The cumulative incidence of adverse effects at 6 months was significantly higher in the stenting arm (12.45% vs 21.7%). Multivariate analysis showed that RT had more rapid and durable pain relief in comparison to stenting, with no difference in the dysphagia impact. Compared to esophageal stenting, radiotherapy was found to be associated with a decreased risk of adverse effects, greater pain relief, and equivalent relief of moderate to severe dysphagia over time. However, the disparity between the sample size of the two arms poses definite doubt regarding the generalizability of the analysis.

Palliation and best supportive care, thus, are of paramount importance in the treatment paradigm of stage IV esophageal cancer.

15 Radiation Techniques

Simulation The radiation oncologist should know the extent of disease based on endoscopy and imaging before simulation. Simulation can depend on site of tumor. For cervical oesophageal tumors, patient is simulated in supine position with arms by the side to cover the supraclavicular lymph nodes. For mid-thoracic, distal oesophageal, and GEJ tumors, patient is simulated in supine position with arms overhead. An immobilization device (thermoplastic mask, VacLoc with wing board) is used to minimize daily setup errors. For GEJ tumors with stomach involvement, it is preferable to advice

Table 7 Contouring guidelines for Esophageal and GEJ Tumors

GTV	Pre-chemotherapy extent of disease
CTV (include tumor bed and nodal regions at risk)	Superio-inferiorly—3–4 cm and radially—0.5–1 cm to GTV, involved nodes—0.3–0.5 cm circumferential margin For tumors above carina—include supraclavicular Lymph nodes For tumors of distal esophagus and GEJ the tumor should include celiac nodes
PTV	As per institutional protocol No IGRT—0.5–1 cm IGRT—0.3–0.5 cm

GTV gross tumor volume, *CTV* clinical target volume, *PTV* planning treatment volume, *IGRT* image guided radiotherapy, *GEJ* gastro-esophageal junction patient to come in empty stomach. Radiotherapy planning CT contrast/non-contrast is done with slice thickness of 3–5 mm. In NACT-RT or definitive CT-RT, radiotherapy planning PET-CT is preferred. 4DCT can be used for distal or GEJ tumors.

Contouring For designing radiotherapy fields, it is important to accurately delineate target volumes and organs at risk (OARs). Historically, two-dimensional fields were based on bony landmarks, but expert contouring guidelines are needed for more conformal radiotherapy techniques like intensity-modulated radiotherapy (IMRT). Wu et al., framed an expert consensus guidelines for IMRT in oesophageal and GEJ tumors [94]. Table 7 shows target volume delineation. Gross tumor margins (GTV) is determined based on endoscopy and imaging. GTV to Clinical target volume (CTV) expansion includes 3–5 cm superior-inferiorly to account for submucosal spread and 0.5–1 cm radially. CTV should be cropped from normal anatomical structures. There is no consensus on elective nodal radiation, however, for upper esophageal tumors periesophageal, mediastinal and supraclavicular lymph nodes should be included. For distal and GEJ tumors periesophageal, mediastinal, perigastric and celiac lymphatics should be considered (Figs. 16 and 17). Planning target volume (PTV) is based upon institutional protocol. Organs at risk includes: lungs, liver, kidneys, heart and spinal cord.

Radiotherapy prescription and dose to organs at risk (Tables 8 and 9):

3D-conformal RT via three or four fields is the standard technique for esophageal cancer, with NCCN suggesting IMRT in cases when OAR constraints cannot be met [95]. Retrospective data suggest IMRT benefit in reducing cardiac toxicity, but the selection and follow-up bias remains the issue and further study is necessary. Institutional protocol to reduce lung, heart and liver dose with IMRT planning are routinely done.

Lin et al. in 2012 [96] retrospectively assessed 676 patients treated at MDACC with CTRT (413 3D-CRT, 263 IMRT) with stage IB–IVA esophageal cancer. Compared with IMRT, 3D-CRT

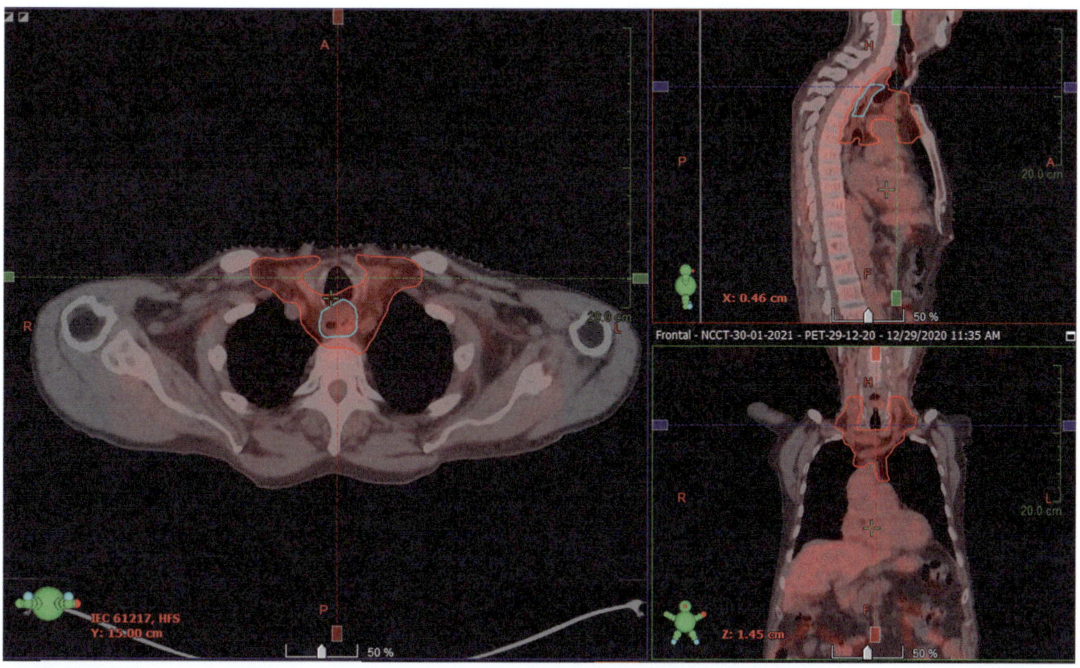

Fig. 16 Contouring of cervical esophageal tumor (Cyan = Gross tumor volume, Red = Planning tumor volume)

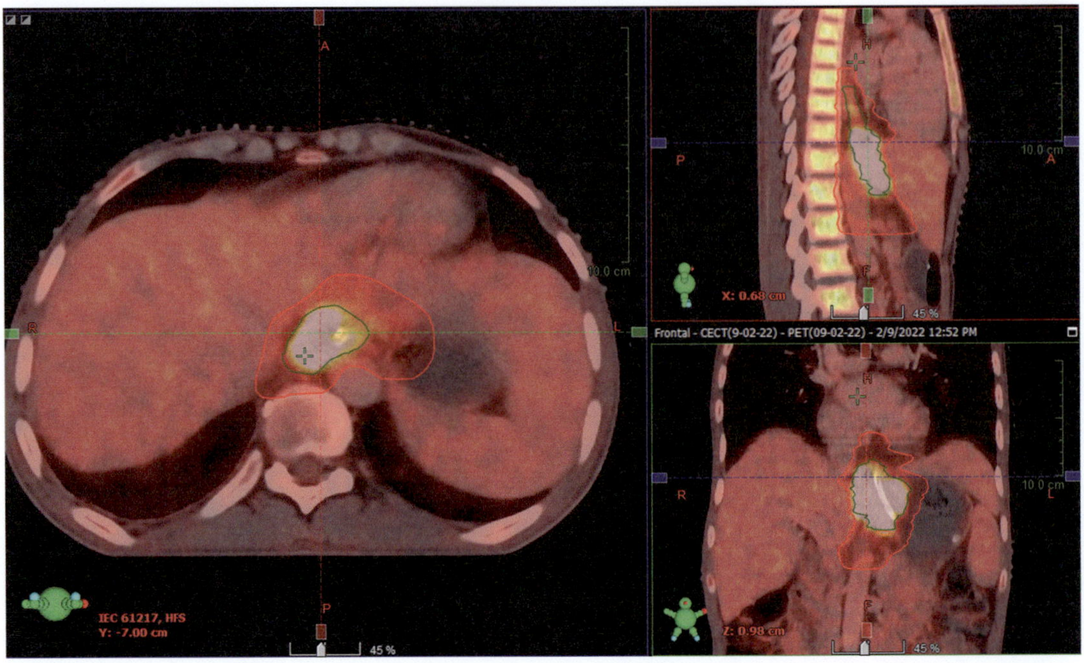

Fig. 17 PET-CT based contouring of GEJ tumor (Green = Gross tumor volume, Red = Planning tumor volume)

Table 8 RT prescription dose

RT dose	Notes
50 Gy in 25 fractions	Concurrent chemo-radiotherapy (external beam) followed by ILRT 6 Gy × 2 sessions (without concurrent chemo)
60 Gy in 30 fraction	External RT alone or in combination with concurrent chemotherapy as a radical treatment
41.4 Gy in 23 fractions	Neo-adjuvant chemo-radiotherapy
45 Gy in 25 fractions	Neo-adjuvant chemo-radiotherapy

Gy = Gray

Table 9 Dose constraints for organs at risk

OAR	Dose constraints
Combined lung	D mean ≤ 20 Gy; V20 Gy ≤ 35%
Heart	D mean ≤ 26 Gy; V25 Gy ≤ 50%
Liver	D mean ≤ 20 Gy; V30 Gy ≤ 40%
Spinal cord	D max ≤ 45 Gy
Breast	V10 Gy ≤ 20%

patients had a significantly greater risk of dying (72.6% vs. 52.9%, $p < 0.0001$) and of loco-regional recurrence (LRR; $p = 0.0038$). No difference was seen in cancer-specific mortality or distant failure rates. There was increased cumulative incidence of cardiac death in 3D-CRT group ($p = 0.049$). Thus they concluded that IMRT can be considered in the treatment of esophageal cancer.

Yaremko et al. in 2013 [97] evaluated the effectiveness of adjuvant CTRT using IMRT and SIB for resected high-risk adenoCA of the distal esophagus and GEJ (T3 and/or N1 adenocarcinoma). The median dose to 95% of PTV1 was 3747 cGy and to 95% of PTV2 was 4876 cGy. All RT was given in a median of 28 daily fractions. Adjuvant concurrent chemoRT with IMRT and SIB is feasible for resected high-risk adenocarcinoma of the distal esophagus and GEJ.

Although the conformity in the dose delivery is achievable with IMRT techniques, yet IMRT comes with a price that we have to pay- a low-dose bath. The proximity of the esophagus to the lung makes radiation pneumonitis (RP) one of the most dreaded complications of esophageal IMRT. Tonison et al. [98] undertook an analysis in 2019 to investigate the incidence of RP after radiochemotherapy with IMR Ttechnique in patients with esophageal cancer and correlate the incidence with dose volume histogram (DVH) related parameters. The data from 73 institution patients and their EBRT plans were extracted. In addition, a systematic review on PubMed identified 493 titles of which 19 studies reported 874 patients evaluated for the final analysis. No grade IV or V RP after radiochemotherapy with IMRT for esophageal cancer was reported in the literature. Grade II or higher RP is reported in 6.6% of the patients. A higher incidence can be seen with increasing values for lung V20. This analysis recommended keeping a target of V20 <23% and to exercise caution in patients with pre-existing lung conditions. Delivering higher radiation doses and achieving better disease control for upper esophageal cancer patients has been established with the use of the IGIMRT technique [99].

15.1 Proton Therapy

Proton therapy in the setting of thoracic tumors, including esophageal cancer, remains investigational. The rationale for using Proton therapy is the ability to achieve a high conformality in the high dose region via the SOBP (spread our Bragg Peak) and the feasibility of delivering higher doses to the tumor.

However, the study by Lin et al. [100] is the first published randomized study of proton vs. photon irradiation. It was a Phase IIB randomized trial of PBT or IMRT (50.4 Gy) in unresectable and potentially resectable cases included, including stages II to III, and eligible to receive concurrent CHT.

The posterior mean TTB was 2.3 times higher for IMRT than PBT. The mean POC score was 7.6 times higher than IMRT vs. PBT. The posterior probability that mean TTB was lower for PBT compared with IMRT was 0.9989. The 3-year PFS (51%) and OS (44.5%) were essentially identical in both arms. Thus, PBT for neoadjuvant or definitive treatment of locally advanced EC produced a lower toxicity profile, but similar PFS, compared to IMRT.

15.2 PET CT-Based Planning

Since 2010 [101] the feasibility of a PET/CT-based tumor (GTV) delineation, further to define a sub-volume within the GTV for dose escalation to attain superior local control rate have been studied. However, the limited spatial resolution of 5–7 mm with PET CT and the related partial volume effects result in an underestimation of activity and an overestimation of small-size objects.

In 2021, Fan et al. [102] undertook a study to assess the feasibility of dose escalation guided by 18F-FDG PET/CT for esophageal cancer. Threshold of 50% of SUVmax was used to define the high FDG uptake region of the GTV (GTVPET). Three intensity-modulated radiation therapy (IMRT) plans were generated, delivering three dose levels to three different planning target volumes (PTV). Normal tissue complication probability (NTCP) modeling. showed that selective boosting of sub-volumes based on 18F-FDG PET/CT (50.4 Gy, 63 Gy, 70GY) could be feasible with a modest increase in the risk of cardiac and lung toxicities. The use of FDG-PET-CT in EC patients receiving concurrent chemoradiotherapy, either as non-surgical therapy or, as NACRT, at different dose levels, for example at 36 Gy, 45 Gy, 50 Gy, to improve GTV/PTV delineation will need larger prospective studies.

16 4D-CT-Based Respiratory Motion Management

Patel et al. in 2009 [103] conducted a retrospective study to evaluate the respiratory motion of esophageal tumors and involved celiac-region lymph nodes using 4D CT during quiet breathing in 30 patients. It was noted that primary esophageal tumors and celiac-region lymph nodes could move substantially with respiration and that the magnitude of motion can vary significantly from patient to patient. Distal primary tumors seemed to have greater respiratory motion than proximal or mid-esophageal tumors, and the motion was the greatest in the superior-inferior (SI, craniocaudal) direction. They proposed margin expansions to account for the motion of >95% of primary esophageal tumors: 1.5 cm SI, 0.75 cm (antero-posterior (AP), and 0.75 cm left to right (LR). To account for the motion of 100% of primary esophageal tumors, the following margins would be necessary: 2.5 cm SI, 1.25 cm AP, and 0.75 cm LR. For celiac-region lymph nodes, the following ITV margins would be reasonable: 2.25 cm SI, 1.0 cm AP, and 0.75 cm LR.

Roos et al. in 2021 [104] undertook a comprehensive comparative analysis of motion in esophageal cancer radiotherapy. This study aimed to evaluate the magnitude and dosimetric impact of breathing motion. Diaphragm breathing amplitudes and off-sets (changes in position concerning the planning CT) were determined from delineated left diaphragm structures in weekly 4D CT scans. It was noted that despite relatively constant breathing amplitudes, the variation in the diaphragm position (off-set), and consequently tumor position, was clinically relevant. These motion effects may result in either treatment that misses the target volume, or dose deviations in the form of highly localized over- or underdosed regions.

17 Follow-Up

All esophageal cancer patient should be followed up systematically after the completion of treatment course, based upon patient's age, disease stage, use of treatment modalities balancing the benefits and risks. It is dictated by the clinical knowledge that 90% of the recurrences occur within the first 2 years after completion of the curative treatment. Therefore, routine surveillance is recommended for 5 years. All the patients should be followed-up with complete history and routine physical examination in every 3–6 months for the first 2 years, every 6–12 months for 3–5 years and annually. Upper GI endoscopy and imaging (CECT or PET-CT) are indicated in symptomatic patients. For advanced and inoperable disease at presentation, which constitute more than 60% of diagnosed patients in LMIC, the palliative therapy by short courses of radiotherapy or, chemo-radiotherapy would provide tumor progression restraint and dysphagia relief between 3 months to 9 months, depending upon the response and physical status. These patients would need more frequent follow-up at one to 2 months, so that a satisfactory transition to palliative care can be counselled and instituted.

18 Prognosis and Survival Outcomes

The long-term outcomes of the esopahgeal cancer patient depend on multiple factors. These factors can be related to the patient herself/himself, tumor, and treatment. Elderly patients are associated poor outcomes. Other factors like a higher stage, poorly differentiated tumors, and poor tolerance to the treatment are associated with poor prognosis.

Survival of the patients depends on the stage and histological subtypes. The 5 years overall survival is shown as approximately 20% across all the stages. Patients with node-positive disease have poor outcomes compared to node-negative patients. As per the national cancer database, localized esophageal cancer has a 5- year survival rate of 47%, and regional node positive disease has 5-yr. survival of 25%.

Percepts Box

1. Esophageal cancer is seventh most common cancer and sixth leading cause of cancer-related mortality.
2. Squamous cell carcinoma comprises vast majority of esophageal cancers globally and in India, although there is increase in incidence of adenocarcinoma in last decade.
3. Squamous cell carcinomas arise from small polypoid excrescences, denuded epithelium, or plaques. Early lesions are usually subtle, whereas advanced lesions are characterized by infiltrating and ulcerated masses, which may be circumferential.
4. The majority of adenocarcinomas are located near the GEJ and are associated with Barrett's esophagus. Lesions are characterized by infiltrating and ulcer-

(continued)

ated masses, which may be circumferential with involvement of celiac and perihepatic nodes.
5. Advanced cases usually present with progressive dysphagia and weight loss.
6. Diagnosis of esophageal cancer is confirmed by endoscopic biopsy. After establishing a diagnosis, evaluation of both locoregional extent and distant metastases is done for an appropriate therapeutic approach.
7. Treatment: There is a difference in management of cervical esophageal cancers, thoracic esophageal cancers, and GE jn esophageal cancers. Management is also guided by squamous versus adenocarcinoma histology. Surgery remains the primary modality for disease control, chemotherapy regimes and radiotherapy dose and techniques have been added successfully to improve treatment approaches.
8. Locally advanced, unresectable, or inoperable esophageal cancer is incurable in the majority of patients. A major goal of treatment is improvement in quality of life by restoring and/or maintaining the ability to swallow.

Multiple Choice Questions

1. As per Globocan 2020, what is overall incidence of esophageal cancer
   (a) Just above 200,000
   (b) Just above 300,000
   (c) Just above 400,000
   (d) Just above 600,000
2. What is extent of upper esophagus
   (a) Cricopharynx to azygous
   (b) Azygous vein to inferior pulmonary vein
   (c) Inferior pulmonary vein to GEj
   (d) Larynx to cricopharynx
3. Barret's esophagus is associated with which histology of esophageal malignancy
   (a) Squamous cell carcinoma
   (b) Adenocarcinoma
   (c) Small cell carcinoma
   (d) Neuroendocrine carcinoma
4. A 50 years male presents with dysphagia for sold food, but can take semisolid. What is grade of dysphagia
   (a) Grade 1
   (b) Grade 2
   (c) Grade 3
   (d) Grade 4
5. PERCIST stands for
   (a) Patient response criteria in solid tumors
   (b) Physician response criteria in solid tumors
   (c) PET response criteria in solid tumors
   (d) Pathological response criteria in solid tumors
6. Which investigation is preferred for both depth of infiltration (T stage) and nodal involvement (N stage) in esophageal cancers
   (a) PET-CT
   (b) Contrast enhanced CT
   (c) Endoscopic ultrasound
   (d) Upper GI scopy
7. A 70 years male presented to OPD with c/o dysphagia for semisolid food. On Upper GI scopy an ulcerative lesion is seen starting from GEJ extending to 3 cm beyond the GEJ. What is the Siewert type?
   (a) Type I
   (b) Type II
   (c) Type III
   (d) Type IV
8. What is indication for upfront surgery in Carcinoma esophagus
   (a) Well differentiated tumor
   (b) Size <3 cm
   (c) No evidence of nodal mets
   (d) All the above
9. Transthoracic esophagectomy with removal of entire intra-thoracic esophagus with cervical anastomosis is referred as
   (a) McKeown's tri-incision method
   (b) Ivor Lewis esophagectomy
   (c) Left thoraco-abdominal approach
   (d) Transhiatal approach
10. What is preferred longitudinal margin esophageal specimen in post operative histopathology

(a) 2 cm
(b) 3 cm
(c) 4 cm
(d) 5 cm

11. What is the largest and practice-defining landmark trial in support of NACT-RT
    (a) CALGB 9781
    (b) Dutch CROSS trial
    (c) NEOCRTEC 5010
    (d) NEOCRTEC 5000

Answer Key

1. (d)
2. (a)
3. (b)
4. (a)
5. (c)
6. (c)
7. (c)
8. (d)
9. (a)
10. (d)
11. (b)

References

1. Sung H, Ferlay J, Siegel RL, Laversanne M, Soerjomataram I, Jemal A, Bray F. Global cancer statistics 2020: GLOBOCAN estimates of incidence and mortality worldwide for 36 cancers in 185 countries. CA Cancer J Clin. 2021;71:209–49.
2. Mathur P, Sathishkumar K, Chaturvedi M, Das P, Sudarshan KL, Santhappan S, Nallasamy V, John A, Narasimhan S, Roselind FS, ICMR-NCDIR-NCRP Investigator Group. Cancer statistics, 2020: report from National Cancer Registry Programme, India. JCO Glob Oncol. 2020;6:1063–75.
3. Chang-Claude J, Becher H, Blettner M, Qiu S, Yang G, Wahrendorf J. Familial aggregation of oesophageal cancer in a high incidence area in China. Int J Epidemiol. 1997;26:1159–65.
4. Chak A, Lee T, Kinnard MF, Brock W, Faulx A, Willis J, Cooper GS, Sivak MV Jr, Goddard KA. Familial aggregation of Barrett's oesophagus, oesophageal adenocarcinoma, and oesophagogastric junctional adenocarcinoma in Caucasian adults. Gut. 2002;51:323–8.
5. Jemal A, Bray F, Center MM, Ferlay J, Ward E, Forman D. Global cancer statistics. CA Cancer J Clin. 2011;61:69–90. Erratum in: CA Cancer J Clin. 2011;61:134.
6. Siddiqi M, Tricker AR, Preussmann R. The occurrence of preformed N-nitroso compounds in food samples from a high risk area of esophageal cancer in Kashmir, India. Cancer Lett. 1988;39:37–43.
7. Li X, Gao C, Yang Y, Zhou F, Li M, Jin Q, Gao L. Systematic review with meta-analysis: the association between human papillomavirus infection and oesophageal cancer. Aliment Pharmacol Ther. 2014;39:270–81.
8. Cui R, Kamatani Y, Takahashi A, Usami M, Hosono N, Kawaguchi T, Tsunoda T, Kamatani N, Kubo M, Nakamura Y, Matsuda K. Functional variants in ADH1B and ALDH2 coupled with alcohol and smoking synergistically enhance esophageal cancer risk. Gastroenterology. 2009;137:1768–75.
9. Graham DY, Schwartz JT, Cain GD, Gyorkey F. Prospective evaluation of biopsy number in the diagnosis of esophageal and gastric carcinoma. Gastroenterology. 1982;82:228–31.
10. Kumar N, Deo S, Bhoriwal S, Sharma A, Pramanik R, Kumar R, Das P, Arora S, Kumar S. Comparison of treatment response assessed by 18F-FDG PET/CT with the histopathological response using tumor regression grading on surgically resected specimen following neoadjuvant chemotherapy in squamous cell carcinoma of esophagus. Nucl Med Commun. 2021;42(8):928–34.
11. Luo LN, He LJ, Gao XY, et al. Endoscopic ultrasound for preoperative esophageal squamous cell carcinoma: a meta-analysis. PLoS One. 2016;11:e0158373.
12. Vazquez-Sequeiros E, Wiersema MJ, Clain JE, Norton ID, Levy MJ, Romero Y, Salomao D, Dierkhising R, Zinsmeister AR. Impact of lymph node staging on therapy of esophageal carcinoma. Gastroenterology. 2003;125:1626–35.
13. Ancona E, Rampado S, Cassaro M, et al. Prediction of lymph node status in superficial esophageal carcinoma. Ann Surg Oncol. 2008;15:3278–88.
14. Rice TW, Kelsen D, Blackstone EH, et al. Esophagus and esophagogastric junction. In: Amin MB, editor. AJCC cancer staging manual. 8th ed. Chicago: AJCC; 2017. p. 185. Corrected at 4th printing, 2018.
15. Siewert JR, Stein HJ. Carcinoma of the cardia: carcinoma of the gastroesophageal junction—classification, pathology and extent of resection. Dis Esophagus. 1996;9:173–82.
16. Sun F, Yuan P, Chen T, Hu J. Efficacy and complication of endoscopic submucosal dissection for superficial esophageal carcinoma: a systematic review and meta-analysis. J Cardiothorac Surg. 2014;7(9):78.
17. Pech O, Behrens A, May A, Nachbar L, Gossner L, Rabenstein T, Manner H, Guenter E, Huijsmans J, Vieth M, Stolte M, Ell C. Long-term results and risk factor analysis for recurrence after curative endoscopic therapy in 349 patients with high-grade intraepithelial neoplasia and mucosal adenocarcinoma in Barrett's oesophagus. Gut. 2008;57:1200–6.
18. Boshier PR, Anderson O, Hanna GB. Transthoracic versus transhiatal esophagectomy for the treatment

of esophagogastric cancer: a meta-analysis. Ann Surg. 2011;254:894–906.
19. Li B, Zhang Y, Miao L, Ma L, Luo X, Zhang Y, et al. Esophagectomy with three-field versus two-field lymphadenectomy for middle and lower thoracic esophageal cancer: long-term outcomes of a randomized clinical trial. J Thorac Oncol. 2021;16:310–7.
20. Moertel CG. Carcinoma of the esophagus: is there a role for surgery? The case against surgery. Am J Dig Dis. 1978;23:735–6.
21. Ries LAG, Melbert D, Krapcho M, et al. SEER cancer statistics review, 1975–2005. Bethesda: National Cancer Institute; 2008. Available at: http://seer.cancer.gov/csr/1975_2005/, based on November 2007 SEER data submission, posted to the SEER web site, 2008.
22. Exner A. Veber die behandlung von oesophagus karzinomen mit ardiumstrahlen. Wien Klin Wochenschr. 1904;17:514.
23. Launois B, Delarue D, Campion JP, Kerbaol M. Preoperative radiotherapy for carcinoma of the esophagus. Surg Gynecol Obstet. 1981;153:690–2.
24. Gignoux M, Roussel A, Paillot B, Gillet M, Schlag P, Dalesio O, Buyse M, Duez N. The value of preoperative radiotherapy in esophageal cancer: results of a study by the EORTC. Recent Results Cancer Res. 1988;110:1–13.
25. Arnott SJ, Duncan W, Kerr GR, Walbaum PR, Cameron E, Jack WJL, MacKillop WJ. Low dose preoperative radiotherapy for carcinoma of the oesophagus: results of a randomized clinical trial. Radiother Oncol. 1992;24:108–13.
26. Wang M, Gu XZ, Yin WB, Huang GJ, Wang LJ, Zhang DW. Randomized clinical trial on the combination of preoperative irradiation and surgery in the treatment of esophageal carcinoma: report on 206 patients. Int J Radiat Oncol Biol Phys. 1989;16:325–7.
27. Arnott SJ, Duncan W, Gignoux M, Hansen HS, Launois B, Nygaard K, Parmar MK, Rousell A, Spilopoulos G, Stewart G, Tierney JF, Wang M, Rhugang Z. Preoperative radiotherapy for esophageal carcinoma [Internet]. Cochrane Database Syst Rev. 2005;2005:CD001799. Available from: https://pubmed.ncbi.nlm.nih.gov/16235286/.
28. Kelsen DP, Winter KA, Gunderson LL, et al. Long-term results of RTOG trial 8911 (USA Intergroup 113): a random assignment trial comparison of chemotherapy followed by surgery compared with surgery alone for esophageal cancer. J Clin Oncol. 2007;25:3719–25.
29. Wayman J, Forman D, Griffin SM. Monitoring the changing pattern of esophagogastric cancer: data from a UK regional cancer registry. Cancer Causes Control. 2001;12:943–9.
30. Fiorica F, Di Bona D, Schepis F, Licata A, Shahied L, et al. Preoperative chemoradiotherapy for oesophageal cancer: a systematic review and meta-analysis. Gut. 2004;53:925–30.
31. Urschel JD, Vasan H. A meta-analysis of randomized controlled trials that compared neoadjuvant chemoradiation and surgery to surgery alone for resectable esophageal cancer. Am J Surg. 2003;185:538–43.
32. Mariette C, Taillier G, Van Seuningen I, Triboulet JP. Factors affecting postoperative course and survival after en bloc resection for esophageal carcinoma. Ann Thorac Surg. 2004;78:1177–83.
33. Bosset JF, Gignoux M, Triboulet JP, Tiret E, Mantion G, Elias D, Lozach P, Ollier JC, Pavy JJ, Mercier M, Sahmoud T. Chemoradiotherapy followed by surgery compared with surgery alone in squamous-cell cancer of the esophagus. N Engl J Med. 1997;337:161–7.
34. Bedenne L, Michel P, Bouché O, Milan C, Mariette C, Conroy T, Pezet D, Roullet B, Seitz JF, Herr JP, Paillot B. Chemoradiation followed by surgery compared with chemoradiation alone in squamous cancer of the esophagus: FFCD 9102. J Clin Oncol. 2007;25:1160–8.
35. Stahl M, Stuschke M, Lehmann N, Meyer HJ, Walz MK, Seeber S, Klump B, Budach W, Teichmann R, Schmitt M, Schmitt G. Chemoradiation with and without surgery in patients with locally advanced squamous cell carcinoma of the esophagus. J Clin Oncol. 2005;23:2310–7.
36. Stahl M, Walz MK, Riera-Knorrenschild J, Stuschke M, Sandermann A, Bitzer M, Wilke H, Budach W, et al. Preoperative chemotherapy versus chemoradiotherapy in locally advanced adenocarcinomas of the oesophagogastric junction (POET): long-term results of a controlled randomised trial. Eur J Cancer. 2017;81:183–90.
37. Tepper J, Krasna MJ, Niedzwiecki D, et al. Phase III trial of trimodality therapy with cisplatin, fluorouracil, radiotherapy, and surgery compared with surgery alone for esophageal cancer: CALGB 9781. J Clin Oncol. 2008;26:1086–92.
38. Shapiro J, Van Lanschot JJ, Hulshof MC, van Hagen P, van Berge Henegouwen MI, Wijnhoven BP, van Laarhoven HW, Nieuwenhuijzen GA, Hospers GA, Bonenkamp JJ, Cuesta MA. Neoadjuvant chemoradiotherapy plus surgery versus surgery alone for oesophageal or junctional cancer (CROSS): long-term results of a randomised controlled trial. Lancet Oncol. 2015;16:1090–8.
39. Yang H, Liu H, Chen Y, Zhu C, Fang W, Yu Z, Mao W, Xiang J, Han Y, Chen Z, Yang H. Long-term efficacy of neoadjuvant chemoradiotherapy plus surgery for the treatment of locally advanced esophageal squamous cell carcinoma: the NEOCRTEC5010 randomized clinical trial. JAMA Surg. 2021;156:721–9.
40. Chan KKW, Saluja R, Delos Santos K, et al. Neoadjuvant treatments for locally advanced, resectable esophageal cancer: a network meta-analysis. Int J Cancer. 2018;143:430–7.
41. Pasquali S, Yim G, Vohra RS, Mocellin S, Nyanhongo D, Marriott P, Geh JI, Griffiths EA. Survival after neoadjuvant and adjuvant treatments compared to surgery alone for resectable esophageal carcinoma. Ann Surg. 2017;265:481–91.
42. Sjoquist KM, Burmeister BH, Smithers BM, Zalcberg JR, Simes RJ, Barbour A, Gebski V, Australasian

Gastro-Intestinal Trials Group. Survival after neoadjuvant chemotherapy or chemoradiotherapy for resectable oesophageal carcinoma: an updated meta-analysis. Lancet Oncol. 2011;12:681–92.
43. Messager M, Mirabel X, Tresch E, Paumier A, Vendrely V, Dahan L, Glehen O, Vasseur F, Lacornerie T, Piessen G, El Hajbi F. Preoperative chemoradiation with paclitaxel-carboplatin or with fluorouracil-oxaliplatin—folinic acid (FOLFOX) for resectable esophageal and junctional cancer: the PROTECT-1402, randomized phase 2 trial. BMC Cancer. 2016;16:1–7.
44. Herskovic A, Leichman L, Lattin P, Han I, Ahmad K, Leichman CG, et al. Chemo/radiation with and without surgery in the thoracic esophagus: the Wayne State experience. Int J Radiat Oncol Biol Phys. 1988;15:655–62.
45. Forastiere AA, Orringer MB, Perez-Tamayo C, Urba SG, Husted S, Takasugi BJ, Zahurak M. Concurrent chemotherapy and radiation therapy followed by transhiatal esophagectomy for local-regional cancer of the esophagus. J Clin Oncol. 1990;8:119–27.
46. Bedenne L, Seitz JF, Milan C, et al. Cisplatin, 5-FU and preoperative radiotherapy in esophageal epidermoid cancer: multicenter phase II FFCD 8804 study. Gastroenterol Clin Biol. 1998;22:273–81.
47. Urba SG, Orringer MB, Turrisi A, et al. Randomized trial of preoperative chemoradiation versus surgery alone in patients with locoregional esophageal carcinoma. J Clin Oncol. 2001;19:305–13.
48. Posner MC, Gooding WE, Lew JI, Rosenstein MM, Lembersky BC. Complete 5-year follow-up of a prospective phase II trial of preoperative chemoradiotherapy for esophageal cancer. Surgery. 2001;130:620–8.
49. Kleinberg L, Knisely JP, Heitmiller R, Zahurak M, Salem R, Burtness B, Heath EI, Forastiere AA. Mature survival results with preoperative cisplatin, protracted infusion 5-fluorouracil, and 44-Gy radiotherapy for esophageal cancer. Int J Radiat Oncol Biol Phys. 2003;56:328–34.
50. Tepper J, Krasna MJ, Niedzwiecki D, Hollis D, Reed CE, Goldberg R, Kiel K, Willett C, Sugarbaker D, Mayer R. Phase III trial of trimodality therapy with cisplatin, fluorouracil, radiotherapy, and surgery compared with surgery alone for esophageal cancer: CALGB 9781. J Clin Oncol Off J Am Soc Clin Oncol. 2008;26:1086.
51. Allum WH, Stenning SP, Bancewicz J, Clark PI, Langley RE. Long-term results of a randomized trial of surgery with or without preoperative chemotherapy in esophageal cancer. J Clin Oncol. 2009;27:5062–7.
52. Ychou M, Boige V, Pignon JP, et al. Perioperative chemotherapy compared with surgery alone for resectable gastroesophageal adenocarcinoma: an FNCLCC and FFCD multicenter phase III trial. J Clin Oncol. 2011;29(13):1715–21.
53. Reynolds JV, Preston SR, O'Neill B, Lowery MA, Baeksgaard L, Crosby T, et al. Neo-AEGIS (Neoadjuvant trial in Adenocarcinoma of the Esophagus and Esophago-Gastric Junction International Study): preliminary results of phase III RCT of CROSS versus perioperative chemotherapy (Modified MAGIC or FLOT protocol). J Clin Oncol. 2021;39:4004.
54. Ando N, Kato H, Igaki H, Shinoda M, Ozawa S, Shimizu H, et al. A randomized trial comparing postoperative adjuvant chemotherapy with cisplatin and 5-fluorouracil versus preoperative chemotherapy for localized advanced squamous cell carcinoma of the thoracic esophagus (JCOG9907). Ann Surg Oncol. 2012;19:68–74.
55. Kato K, Machida R, Ito Y, Daiko H, et al; JCOG1109 investigators. Doublet chemotherapy, triplet chemotherapy, or doublet chemotherapy combined with radiotherapy as neoadjuvant treatment for locally advanced oesophageal cancer (JCOG1109 NExT): a randomised, controlled, open-label, phase 3 trial. Lancet. 2024;404(10447):55–66. https://doi.org/10.1016/S0140-6736(24)00745-1.
56. von Döbeln GA, Klevebro F, Jacobsen AB, Johannessen HO, Nielsen NH, Johnsen G, Hatlevoll I, Glenjen NI, Friesland S, Lundell L, Yu J, Nilsson M. Neoadjuvant chemotherapy versus neoadjuvant chemoradiotherapy for cancer of the esophagus or gastroesophageal junction: long-term results of a randomized clinical trial. Dis Esophagus. 2019;1:32.
57. Jing SW, Qin JJ, Liu Q, Zhai C, Wu YJ, Cheng YJ, Czito BG, Wang J. Comparison of neoadjuvant chemoradiotherapy and neoadjuvant chemotherapy for esophageal cancer: a meta-analysis. Future Oncol. 2019;15:2413–22.
58. Herskovic A, Martz K, Al-Sarraf M, Leichman L, Brindle J, Vaitkevicius V, Cooper J, Byhardt R, Davis L, Emami B. Combined chemotherapy and radiotherapy compared with radiotherapy alone in patients with cancer of the esophagus. N Engl J Med. 1992;326:1593–8.
59. Cooper JS, Guo MD, Herskovic A, Macdonald JS, Martenson JA Jr, Al-Sarraf M, Byhardt R, Russell AH, Beitler JJ, Spencer S, Asbell SO. Chemoradiotherapy of locally advanced esophageal cancer: long-term follow-up of a prospective randomized trial (RTOG 85-01). JAMA. 1999;281:1623–7.
60. Noronha V, Prabhash K, Joshi A, et al. Clinical outcome in definitive concurrent chemoradiation with weekly paclitaxel and carboplatin for locally advanced esophageal and junctional cancer. Oncol Res. 2016;23:183–95.
61. Minsky BD, Neuberg D, Kelsen DP, Pisansky TM, Ginsberg R, Benson A 3rd. Neoadjuvant chemotherapy plus concurrent chemotherapy and high-dose radiation for squamous cell carcinoma of the esophagus: a preliminary analysis of the phase II intergroup trial 0122. J Clin Oncol. 1996;14:149–55.
62. Xu Y, Dong B, Zhu W, Li J, Huang R, Sun Z, et al. A phase III multicenter randomized clinical trial of 60 Gy versus 50 Gy radiation dose in concurrent chemoradiotherapy for inoperable esopha-

geal squamous cell carcinoma. Clin Cancer Res. 2022;28:1792–9.
63. Hulshof MCCM, Geijsen ED, Rozema T, Oppedijk V, Buijsen J, Neelis KJ, et al. Randomized study on dose escalation in definitive chemoradiation for patients with locally advanced esophageal cancer (ARTDECO study). J Clin Oncol. 2021;39:2816–24.
64. Liu M, Zhao K, Chen Y, Jiang GL. Evaluation of the value of ENI in radiotherapy for cervical and upper thoracic esophageal cancer: a retrospective analysis. Radiat Oncol. 2014;9:1–6.
65. Zhu H, Rivin Del Campo E, Ye J, Simone CB 2nd, Zhu Z, Zhao W, et al. Involved-field irradiation in definitive chemoradiotherapy for locoregional esophageal squamous cell carcinoma: results from the ESO-Shanghai 1 trial. Int J Radiat Oncol Biol Phys. 2021;110:1396–406.
66. Williams MV, Denekamp J, Fowler JF. A review of αβ ratios for experimental tumors: implications for clinical studies of altered fractionation. Int J Radiat Oncol Biol Phys. 1985;11:87–96.
67. Marcu LG, Bezak E. Radiobiological modeling of interplay between accelerated repopulation and altered fractionation schedules in head and neck cancer. J Med Phys. 2009;34:206.
68. Choi N, Park SD, Lynch T, Wright C, Ancukiewicz M, Wain J, Donahue D, Mathisen D. Twice-daily radiotherapy as concurrent boost technique during two chemotherapy cycles in neoadjuvant chemoradiotherapy for resectable esophageal carcinoma: mature results of phase II study. Int J Radiat Oncol Biol Phys. 2004;60:111–22.
69. Samuels SE, Stenmark MH, Lee JY, McHugh JB, Hayman JA, Orringer MB, Urba SG, Sun L, Xie C, Kong FM, Cuneo KC. Neoadjuvant twice daily chemoradiotherapy for esophageal cancer: treatment-related mortality and long-term outcomes. Adv Radiat Oncol. 2017;2:308–15.
70. Conroy T, Galais MP, Raoul JL, Bouche O, Gourgou-Bourgade S, Douillard JY, Etienne PL, Boige V, Martel-Lafay I, Michel P, Llacer-Moscardo C. Phase III randomized trial of definitive chemoradiotherapy (CRT) with FOLFOX or cisplatin and fluorouracil in esophageal cancer (EC): final results of the PRODIGE 5/ACCORD 17 trial. Lancet Oncol. 2014;15:305–14. https://doi.org/10.1016/S1470-2045(14)70028-2.
71. Alexandrou A, Davis PA, Law S, Whooley BP, Murthy SC, Wong J. Esophageal cancer in patients with a history of distal gastrectomy. Arch Surg. 2002;137:1238–42.
72. Koppert LB, Lemmens VE, Coebergh JW, Steyerberg EW, Wijnhoven BP, Tilanus HW, Janssen-Heijnen ML. Impact of age and co-morbidity on surgical resection rate and survival in patients with oesophageal and gastric cancer. J Br Surg. 2012;99:1693–700.
73. Vellayappan BA, Soon YY, Ku GY, Leong CN, Lu JJ, Tey JC. Chemoradiotherapy versus chemoradiotherapy plus surgery for esophageal cancer. Cochrane Database Syst Rev. 2017;8(8):CD010511. https://doi.org/10.1002/14651858.CD010511.
74. Vincent J, Mariette C, Pezet D, Huet E, Bonnetain F, Bouché O, Conroy T, Roullet B, Seitz JF, Herr JP, Di Fiore F. Early surgery for failure after chemoradiation in operable thoracic oesophageal cancer. Analysis of the non-randomised patients in FFCD 9102 phase III trial: chemoradiation followed by surgery versus chemoradiation alone. Eur J Cancer. 2015;51:1683–93.
75. Ajani JA, Winter K, Komaki R, Kelsen DP, Minsky BD, Liao Z, Bradley J, Fromm M, Hornback D, Willett CG. Phase II randomized trial of two non-operative regimens of induction chemotherapy followed by chemoradiation in patients with localized carcinoma of the esophagus: RTOG 0113. J Clin Oncol. 2008;26:4551.
76. Gaspar LE, Winter K, Kocha WI, Coia LR, Herskovic A, Graham M. A phase I/II study of external beam radiation, brachytherapy, and concurrent chemotherapy for patients with localized carcinoma of the esophagus (Radiation Therapy Oncology Group Study 9207): final report. Cancer. 2000;88:988–95.
77. Okawa T, Dokiya T, Nishio M, Hishikawa Y, Morita K. Multi-institutional randomized trial of external radiotherapy with and without intraluminal brachytherapy for esophageal cancer in Japan. Int J Radiat Oncol Biol Phys. 1999;45:623–8.
78. Gaspar LE, Nag S, Herskovic A, Mantravadi R, Speiser B. American Brachytherapy Society (ABS) consensus guidelines for brachytherapy of esophageal cancer. Clinical Research Committee, American Brachytherapy Society, Philadelphia, PA. Int J Radiat Oncol Biol Phys. 1997;38:127–32.
79. Schreiber D, Rineer J, Vongtama D, Wortham A, Han P, Schwartz D, Choi K, Rotman M. Impact of postoperative radiation after esophagectomy for esophageal cancer. J Thorac Oncol. 2010;5:244–50.
80. Deng W, Yang J, Ni W, Li C, Chang X, Han W, Zhou Z, Chen D, Feng Q, Liang J, Lv J. Postoperative radiotherapy in pathological T2–3N0M0 thoracic esophageal squamous cell carcinoma: interim report of a prospective, phase III, randomized controlled study. Oncologist. 2020;25(4):e701–8.
81. Ni W, Yu S, Xiao Z, Zhou Z, Chen D, Feng Q, Liang J, Lv J, Gao S, Mao Y, Xue Q. Postoperative adjuvant therapy versus surgery alone for stage IIB–III esophageal squamous cell carcinoma: a phase III randomized controlled trial. Oncologist. 2021;26:e2151–60.
82. Mummudi N, Jiwnani S, Niyogi D, et al. Salvage radiotherapy for postoperative locoregional failure in esophageal cancer: a systematic review and meta-analysis. Dis Esophagus. 2022;35(3):doab020.
83. Zafirellis K, Dolan K, Fountoulakis A, Dexter SP, Martin IG, Sue-Ling HM. Multivariate analysis of clinical, operative and pathologic features of esophageal cancer: who needs adjuvant therapy? Dis Esophagus. 2002;15:155–9.

84. Hofstetter W, Swisher SG, Correa AM, et al. Treatment outcomes of resected esophageal cancer. Ann Surg. 2002;236:376–85.
85. Mulligan CR. Multidisciplinary management of esophageal cancer. Surg Oncol Clin. 2013;22:217–46.
86. Kelsen DP, Ginsberg R, Pajak T, et al. Chemotherapy followed by surgery compared with surgery alone for localized esophageal cancer. N Engl J Med. 1998;339:1979–84.
87. Murray LJ, Din OS, Kumar VS, Dixon LM, Wadsley JC. Palliative radiotherapy in patients with esophageal carcinoma: a retrospective review. Pract Radiat Oncol. 2012;2:257–64.
88. Welsch J, Kup PG, Nieder C, Khosrawipour V, Bühler H, Adamietz IA, Fakhrian K. Survival and symptom relief after palliative radiotherapy for esophageal cancer. J Cancer. 2016;7:125.
89. Laskar SG, Lewis S, Agarwal JP, Mishra S, Mehta S, Patil P. Combined brachytherapy and external beam radiation: an effective approach for palliation in esophageal cancer. J Contemp Brachytherapy. 2015;7:453–61.
90. Vivekanandam S, Reddy KS, Velavan K, et al. External beam radiotherapy and intraluminal brachytherapy in advanced inoperable esophageal cancer: JIPMER experience. Am J Clin Oncol. 2001;24:128–30.
91. Homs MY, Steyerberg EW, Eijkenboom WM, Tilanus HW, Stalpers LJ, Bartelsman JF, et al. Single-dose brachytherapy versus metal stent placement for the palliation of dysphagia from oesophageal cancer: multicentre randomised trial. Lancet. 2004;364:1497–504.
92. Amdal CD, Jacobsen AB, Sandstad B, Warloe T, Bjordal K. Palliative brachytherapy with or without primary stent placement in patients with oesophageal cancer, a randomised phase III trial. Radiother Oncol. 2013;107:428–33.
93. Martin EJ, Bruggeman AR, Nalawade VV, Sarkar RR, Qiao EM, Rose BS, Murphy JD. Palliative radiotherapy versus esophageal stent placement in the management of patients with metastatic esophageal cancer. J Natl Compr Cancer Netw. 2020;18:569–74.
94. Wu AJ, Bosch WR, Chang DT, Hong TS, Jabbour SK, Kleinberg LR, Mamon HJ, Thomas CR, Goodman KA. Expert consensus contouring guidelines for intensity modulated radiation therapy in esophageal and gastroesophageal junction cancer. Int J Radiat Oncol Biol Phys. 2015;92:911–20.
95. Ajani JA, D'Amico TA, Bentrem DJ, Chao J, Corvera C, Das P, Denlinger CS, Enzinger PC, Fanta P, Farjah F, Gerdes H. Esophageal and esophagogastric junction cancers, version 2.2019, NCCN clinical practice guidelines in oncology. J Natl Compr Cancer Netw. 2019;17:855–83.
96. Lin SH, Wang L, Myles B, Thall PF, Hofstetter WL, Swisher SG, Ajani JA, Cox JD, Komaki R, Liao Z. Propensity score-based comparison of long-term outcomes with 3-dimensional conformal radiotherapy vs intensity-modulated radiotherapy for esophageal cancer. Int J Radiat Oncol Biol Phys. 2012;84:1078–85.
97. Yaremko BP, Palma DA, Erickson AL, Pierce G, Malthaner RA, Inculet RI, Dar AR, Rodrigues GB, Yu E. Adjuvant concurrent chemoradiation using intensity-modulated radiotherapy and simultaneous integrated boost for resected high-risk adenocarcinoma of the distal esophagus and gastro-esophageal junction. Radiat Oncol. 2013;8:1–1.
98. Tonison JJ, Fischer SG, Viehrig M, Welz S, Boeke S, Zwirner K, Klumpp B, Braun LH, Zips D, Gani C. Radiation pneumonitis after intensity-modulated radiotherapy for esophageal cancer: institutional data and a systematic review. Sci Rep. 2019;19(9):1–8.
99. Laskar SG, Sinha S, Singh M, et al. Post-cricoid and upper oesophagus cancers treated with organ preservation using intensity-modulated image-guided radiotherapy: a phase II prospective study of outcomes, toxicity and quality of life. Clin Oncol (R Coll Radiol). 2022;34:220–9.
100. Lin SH, Hobbs BP, Verma V, Tidwell RS, Smith GL, Lei X, Corsini EM, Mok I, Wei X, Yao L, Wang X. Randomized phase IIB trial of proton beam therapy versus intensity-modulated radiation therapy for locally advanced esophageal cancer. J Clin Oncol. 2020;38:1569.
101. Thorwarth D, Geets X, Paiusco M. Physical radiotherapy treatment planning based on functional PET/CT data. Radiother Oncol. 2010;96:317–24.
102. Fan B, Li C, Mu F, Qin W, Wang L, Sun X, Wang C, Zou B, Wang S, Li W, Hu M. Dose escalation guided by 18F-FDG PET/CT for esophageal cancer. Radiat Med Prot. 2021;2:55–60.
103. Patel AA, Wolfgang JA, Niemierko A, Hong TS, Yock T, Choi NC. Implications of respiratory motion as measured by four-dimensional computed tomography for radiation treatment planning of esophageal cancer. Int J Radiat Oncol Biol Phys. 2009;74:290–6.
104. Roos CT, Faiz Z, Visser S, Dieters M, van der Laan HP, den Otter LA, Plukker JT, Langendijk JA, Knopf AC, Muijs CT, Sijtsema NM. A comprehensive motion analysis–consequences for high precision image-guided radiotherapy of esophageal cancer patients. Acta Oncol. 2021;60:277–84.

Online Links

Contouring upper esophagus: https://econtour.org/cases/129

Contouring-GEJ: https://econtour.org/cases/60

https://www.youtube.com/watch?v=42-OxFyTKDU

https://www.youtube.com/watch?v=bte-P7lQxFw

https://www.youtube.com/watch?v=gAq-S0u4MX8

Gastric Cancer

S. V. S. Deo, Bidhu K. Mohanti, Atul Sharma, Naveen Kumar, Punita Lal, and Pooja Nandwani

1 Introduction

Gastric cancer is ranked among the top five most common cancers in the world, and it contributes to significant cancer-related mortality burden. Global trends indicate a higher prevalence of gastric cancer in specific geographic regions like Japan, Southeast Asia and China. Aetiology of gastric cancer is multifactorial, mostly related to infections and dietary habits. Epidemiological trends also indicate a migration from distal gastric to proximal gastric cancer globally. The majority present with locally advanced stage and early gastric cancers are mostly seen in countries like Japan with a screening program. Traditionally, radical surgery has been the mainstay of therapy along with adjuvant systemic chemotherapy. Radiotherapy has very limited role and indication in gastric cancer management. Recently, advances in molecular and genetic fields are opening new therapeutic avenues in the management of gastric cancer.

S. V. S. Deo (✉) · N. Kumar
Department of Surgical Oncology, MAX Hospital, Saket, New Delhi, Delhi, India

B. K. Mohanti
Department of Radiation Oncology, Bagchi Sri Shankara Cancer Centre & Research Institute, Bhubaneswar, Odisha, India

A. Sharma
Medical Oncology, MAX Hospital, New Delhi, India

P. Lal
Department of Radiotherapy, SGPGI, Lucknow, India

P. Nandwani
Radiation Oncology, GCRI, Ahmedabad, India

2 Surgical Anatomy of the Stomach

The stomach is a dilated structure of foregut. It extends from the left costal margin region into the epigastric and umbilical regions. It is relatively fixed on both ends, but it is very mobile. The stomach is grossly divided into four parts:

- Cardia
- Fundus
- Body
- Anteropyloric region

The stomach has two openings: Cardia and pylorus; two curvatures: The greater and lesser curvature; and two surfaces: anterior and posterior.

1. Cardia: Cardia is the junction between oesophagus and the stomach. It is the first portion of the stomach that receives the food.
2. Fundus: Fundus is a superior dilated structure of the stomach, which is located superior to a horizontal line of the cardiac junction.
3. Body: It is the largest portion of the stomach. It extends from the cardiac orifice to the incisura angularis. The food stays for a longer period for digestion.

B. K. Mohanti et al. (eds.), *Radiation Oncology – Principles, Precepts and Practice*,
https://doi.org/10.1007/978-981-95-5171-2_10

4. Anteropyloric region: It is a distal tubular structure. It extends from the incisura angularis to the pyloric sphincter.

2.1 Blood Supply

The stomach is primarily supplied by four arteries.

1. Left gastric artery: It is a direct branch of the celiac artery. It supplies the lower end of oesophagus and the right upper stomach.
2. Right gastric artery: It is a branch of hepatic artery and supplies the right lower part of the stomach.
3. Left gastric artery: It arises from the splenic artery. It supplies the greater curvature.
4. Right gastroepiploic artery: It is a branch of gastroduodenal artery and it supplies to the lower part of the greater curvature.
5. Short gastric artery: These are the direct branches of the splenic artery and supply the proximal stomach.

2.2 Venous Supply

1. Left and Right gastric veins: These veins drain directly into the portal veins.
2. Left gastroepiploic vein and short gastric veins: Both veins drain in the splenic vein.
3. Right gastroepiploic veins: This vein joins in the superior mesenteric vein.

Lymphatic draining of stomach is shown in Table 1.

Table 1 Lymphatic supply

Station.1	Right paracardial LN
Station.2	Left paracardial LN
Station.3	LN along the lesser curvature
Station.4sa	LN along the short gastric vessels
Station.4sb	LN along the left gastroepiploic vessels
Station.4d	LN along the right gastroepiploic vessels
Station.5	Suprapyloric LN
Station.6	Infrapyloric LN
Station.7	LN along the left gastric artery
Station.8a	LN along the common hepatic artery (anterosuperior group)
Station.8p	LN along the common hepatic (posterior group)
Station.9	LN around the celiac artery
Station.10	LN at the splenic hilum
Station.11p	LN along the proximal splenic artery
Station.11d	LN along the distal splenic artery
Station.12a	LN in the hepatoduodenal ligament (along the hepatic artery)
Station.12b	LN in the hepatoduodenal ligament (along the bile duct)
Station.12p	LN in the hepatoduodenal ligament (behind the portal vein)
Station.13	LN on the posterior surface of the pancreatic head
Station.14v	LN along the superior mesenteric vein
Station.14a	LN along the superior mesenteric artery
Station.15	LN along the middle colic vessels
Station.16a1	LN in the aortic hiatus
Station16a2	LN around the abdominal aorta (from the upper margin of the celiac trunk to the lower margin of the left renal vein)
Station.16b1	LN around the abdominal aorta (from the lower margin of the left renal vein to the upper margin of the inferior mesenteric artery)
Station.16b2	LN around the abdominal aorta

3 Clinical Presentation

Gastric cancer presents with vague symptoms, which frequently lead to late diagnosis at advanced stages of the disease. Common symptoms include upper abdominal pain or discomfort, anorexia, early satiety, and weight loss. Patients may also experience heartburn, nausea, vomiting, hematemesis, melena and fatigue. All these are non-specific symptoms and are often mistaken to have a benign cause. The pain associated with gastric cancer is continuous and non-radiating. It is not relieved by eating. The patients may also present with dysphagia in tumours involving the cardia and GE junction (GEJ). Gastric outlet obstruction may be seen in distal tumours involving the antrum and pylorus [1, 2].

The patient may have poor nutrition, cachexia, dehydration, and anaemia on general examination. Patients may present with metastatic disease in the form of supraclavicular lymph node

(Virchow's node), axillary lymph node (Irish node), peri-umbilical (Sister Mary Joseph nodule), drop metastasis to ovaries (Krukenberg tumour) or a peritoneal implant in pouch of Douglas (Blumer shelf) felt on per-rectal examination. A palpable abdominal mass, ascites, jaundice are indicative of advanced disease. Patients may even present with peritonitis if the tumour perforates. One may find abdominal distension and succussion splash in patients with gastric outlet obstruction [3].

Rarely, the patients may even present with paraneoplastic syndromes like diffuse seborrheic keratosis or acanthosis nigricans (dermatological), microangiopathic hemolytic anaemia and hypercoagulable state, i.e. Trousseau's sign (haematological); membranous nephropathy (renal) or polyarteritis nodosa (autoimmune) [3].

4 Histopathology, Classification Systems and Molecular Subtyping

Gastric cancers can be divided into early and advanced. Early gastric cancer is defined to be confined to mucosa/submucosa with or without lymph node involvement. These can be classified according to the Japanese classification based on gross appearance or the more recent Paris classification based on gross or endoscopic appearance (Tables 2 and 3) [4].

Table 2 Japanese classification

I	Protruding
IIa	Superficial elevated
IIb	Superficial flat
IIc	Superficial excavated
III	Excavated

Table 3 Paris classification

0–I	Protruding
0–IIa	Superficial elevated
0–IIb	Flat
0–IIc	Superficial depressed
0–III	Ulcerated

Advanced gastric cancer involves the muscularis and is classified using Borrmann's classification into four types. Type I (Polypoid), Type II (Fungating), Type III (Ulcerating) and Type IV (Diffusely infiltrating).

The most commonly used histologic classification is the Lauren classification, which classifies gastric cancer into diffuse and intestinal types. The intestinal type has a tendency to form glands and is better differentiated. It usually arises in the setting of a precancerous condition. It is more prevalent in areas where gastric cancer is epidemic and more common in men and old age. The diffuse type is poorly differentiated and consists of signet ring cells. It affects a relatively younger age group and affects males and females equally. It has an association with familial occurrence pointing to an underlying genetic cause. The diffuse type has a poorer prognosis than the intestinal type [1]. A third type is called mixed type of above two combined.

The WHO gave a classification system in 2010, dividing gastric cancer into four main types—papillary, tubular, mucinous and poorly cohesive. This classification is based on morphologic features.

Molecular subtypes of gastric cancer have also been described by The Cancer Genome Atlas (TCGA) and the Asian Cancer Research Group (ACRG). TCGA has subdivided gastric cancer into genetically stable, chromosomally unstable, microsatellite unstable, and EBV positive. ACRG subtypes include MSS/EMT (epithelial to mesenchymal transition), MSS/TP53 negative, MSS/TP53 positive and microsatellite unstable [2]. **Multimodality treatment of gastric cancer** is shown in Fig. 1.

5 Surgical Management

5.1 General Considerations

The standard of care for curative treatment is still resection with wide negative margins. The extent of resection varies with the site of the tumour in the stomach and the stage of the tumour. Patients with early gastric cancer (T1/T2–N0) can be

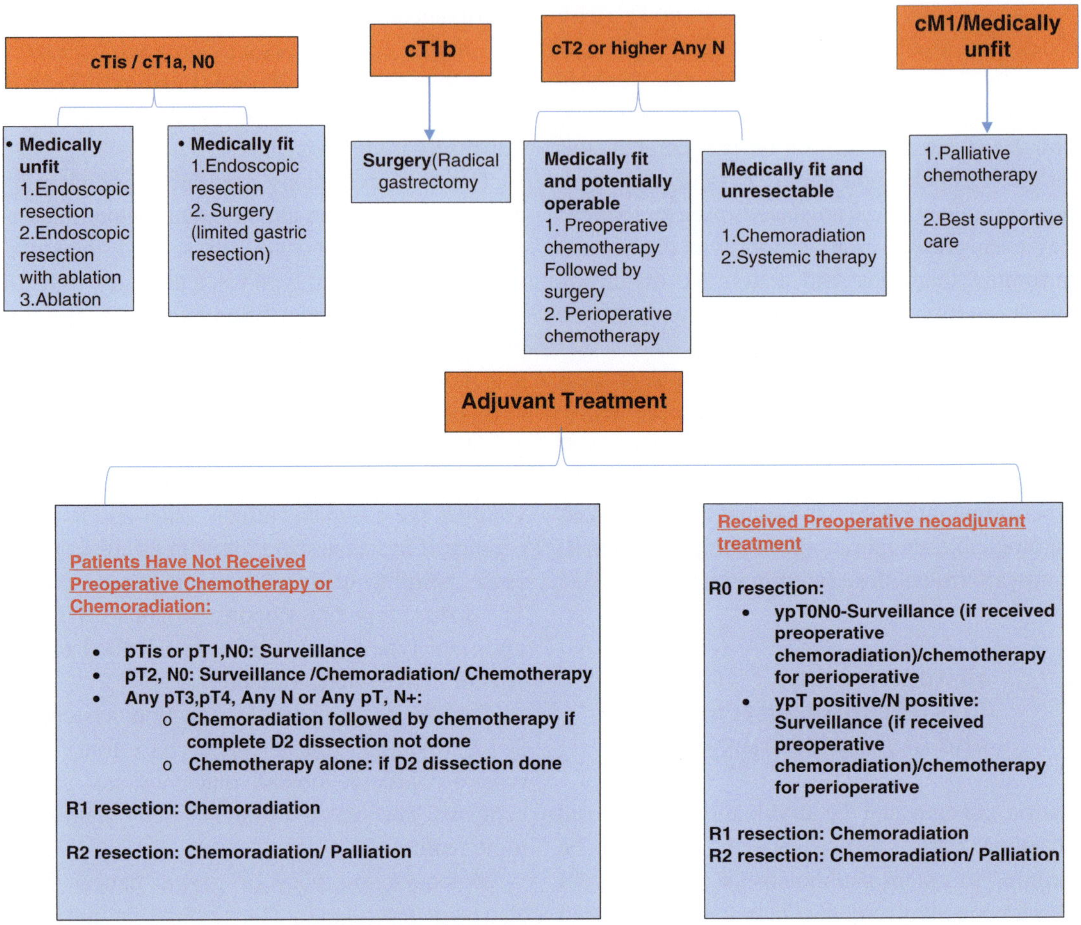

Fig. 1 Multimodality management approach of gastric cancer

considered for upfront surgery with curative intent. Upfront surgery may also indicate palliation in patients presenting with bleeding or luminal obstruction due to tumour, but the perioperative morbidity and mortality are considerably high in this group of patients.

While traditional teachings favoured upfront radical surgery followed by adjuvant chemotherapy or chemoradiation for locally advanced gastric cancer (T3/T4 N+), current management guidelines recommend perioperative chemotherapy along with surgery based on the outcomes of landmark MAGIC trial (2006). Where perioperative chemotherapy involves Epirubicin, Cisplatin and 5FU—ECF; 3 cycles before and 3 cycles after surgery [1, 5].

5.2 Resection of Primary

A. Endoscopic resection—In selected patients with early gastric cancer, endoscopic resections with curative intent can achieve adequate oncological outcomes. Standard patient selection criteria for endoscopic gastric cancer resection—intestinal type tumour, confined to mucosa, no LVI, non-ulcerated, less than 2 cm diameter.

Modalities for endoscopic resection:

1. EMR (Endoscopic Mucosal Resection)—EMR involves elevating the tumour using saline injection, using a snare to encircle the affected mucosa and excising it with electrocautery.

   2. ESD (Endoscopic Submucosal Dissection)—Useful for larger tumours with limited submucosal involvement. ESD involves injecting epinephrine with indigocarmine to hydrodissect the lesion, and then dissection is done in the submucosal plane deep to the tumour using an insulation-tipped knife [1].
B. Surgical resection:
   1. Distal gastric cancers—A 5 cm gross margin with R0 resection is the goal of surgery. Intraoperative frozen section to ensure negative margins may be used. Partial gastrectomy (Distal radical gastrectomy/Subtotal gastrectomy) is preferred over total gastrectomy due to better quality of life with partial gastrectomy.
   2. Proximal gastric cancers—For proximal cancers not involving the GE junction, total gastrectomy and proximal gastrectomy have equal oncologic outcomes, but the rates of reflux esophagitis and anastomotic stenosis are higher with the latter; thus, total gastrectomy is preferred by most surgeons.

Minimally invasive approaches are being explored for gastric cancer with smaller studies showing feasibility of laparoscopic and robotic resection for even locally advanced gastric cancer, but long-term data is limited [1, 5].

6 Types of Gastrectomy

1. Distal radical gastrectomy: This procedure is performed for distal stomach tumours. Herein, half to two-third of the stomach is resected preserving the cardia.
2. Proximal gastrectomy: Proximal third of the stomach is resected, preserving the pylorus and antrum.
3. Pylorus-preserving gastrectomy: The stomach is resected preserving the upper third of the stomach and pylorus along with the antrum.
4. Local resection (Limited Gatsrectomy): It is non-anatomical and wedge resection of the stomach. It is done for early gastric cancer.

6.1 Lymphadenectomy for Gastric Cancer

The lymph nodes around stomach have been classified into stations based on their location (Table 1). For adequate staging, AJCC recommends an excision of at least 16 nodes in gastric resections. The extent of dissection can be classified into:

1. D1 lymphadenectomy—Only perigastric nodes; stations 1–7
2. D2 lymphadenectomy—Celiac axis clearance +/− splenectomy; stations 1–12a
3. D3 lymphadenectomy—Periaortic nodal clearance; stations 1–16

While pancreatectomy and splenectomy were considered routine as part of surgery for gastric cancer, this is now avoided, with resection of pancreas or spleen being undertaken only if directly involved.

Currently, most centres prefer radical total/partial gastrectomy conserving pancreas and spleen + D2 lymphadenectomy sparing station 10 lymph nodes [1, 6, 7].

6.2 Reconstruction

1. Billroth 1 gastroduodenostomy—Involves direct anastomosis of duodenum and the gastric remnant. While it is a good option for distal radical gastrectomy, it is not a feasible option for subtotal or total gastrectomy.
2. Billroth 2 loop gastrojejunostomy—A loop of jejunum is brought up in an antecolic (in front of transverse colon) or retrocolic (through the transverse mesocolon) fashion and side to side gastrojejunal anastomosis is done in an isoperistaltic fashion.
3. Roux-en-y gastrojejunostomy—Jejunum is cut 20 cm distal to ligament of Trietz and brought up through the transverse mesocolon for anastomosis with the gastric pouch. The proximal cut end of jejunum is anastomosed to a jejunal loop at least 45–50 cm distal to the gastrojejunostomy to prevent reflux of biliary

Table 4 Landmark clinical trials on gastric cancer [2, 7]

Trial	Details
MAGIC trial	503 patients, stage II or higher, perioperative chemo (ECF) + surgery (250) vs surgery alone (253). Overall 5 5-year survival 36% versus 23%. Local recurrence and distant metastasis significantly less in chemotherapy arm.
FLOT4	716 patients, perioperative ECF vs FLOT4. Median overall survival (35 versus 50 months) and progression-free survival (18 versus 30 months) better in FLOT4 group
JCOG-0110	Compared D2 LND +/− splenectomy. No benefit of splenectomy routinely with LND.
JCOG-9501	D2 versus D2+ (Para-aortic LND) in patients with R0 resection. PAND does not improve survival.

and pancreatic secretions. This is the standard reconstruction after total gastrectomy [5]. Landmark clinical trials of gastric cancer is shown in Table 4.

7 Complications of Gastrectomy

7.1 Mechanical

1. Afferent limb syndrome—Partial or complete obstruction in the biliopancreatic limb after construction of loop gastrojejunostomy or roux-en-y gastrojejunostomy due to anastomotic stricture, adhesions, internal hernia or cancer recurrence.
2. Efferent limb syndrome—Obstruction in the efferent limb, i.e., the limb which receives food from the stomach (may be the roux loop). It is a rare phenomenon and may occur due to cancer recurrence.
3. Peterson's hernia—There is a potential space posterior to the gastrojejunostomy. Herniation of small bowel into this space through the defect in the transverse mesocolon posterior to the cut edge of mesentery when a retrocolic gastrojejunostomy is done can present with small bowel obstruction.
4. Stomal ulcer—Ulcer at site of gastrojejunostomy may occur due to tumour recurrence, increased acid production by the gastric pouch, and NSAID intake.

7.2 Functional

1. Dumping syndrome—This occurs due to early rapid gastric emptying. Dumping syndromes can be early or late and have different aetiologies.
   (a) Early dumping—Due to rapid emptying of food from stomach to small bowel, there is fluid sequestration in the gut secondary to high osmolarity of small bowel contents. This leads to abdominal and vasomotor symptoms. It occurs almost immediately after meals and responds to dietary manipulation. Small frequent meals based on fat and protein are advised.
   (b) Late dumping—Occurs due to reactive hypoglycemia secondary to a surge in insulin secretion caused by a sudden rise in plasma glucose after meals. This usually occurs after an hour of meal intake. Treatment is the same as early dumping. Octreotide is also effective.
2. Gastroparesis—It occurs due to loss of antropyloric coordination and presents with early satiety, vomiting of meals 6 h after ingestion and weight loss.
3. Postvagotomy diarrhoea—It is a diagnosis of exclusion and presents with postprandial watery diarrhoea 15–30 min after meals.
4. Roux stasis syndrome—Functional obstruction in the efferent limb after Roux-en-Y reconstruction. It is a diagnosis of exclusion.

7.3 Metabolic Complications

Loss of stomach and bypass of proximal small bowel due to Roux-en-Y reconstruction leads to micronutrient deficiencies, such as that of vitamins A, B, D, E, K, and deficiency of minerals such as iron and copper. The patient may present with iron deficiency anaemia or megaloblastic anaemia secondary to vitamin B12 deficiency [1, 5].

8 Role of Systemic Therapy in Gastric Cancer

8.1 Introduction

In the year 2020, more than one million new cases and approximately 0.76 million deaths due to gastric cancer were estimated worldwide, ranking it the fourth and fifth globally for incidence and mortality among all cancers [8]. Nearly 90% of patients present with locally advanced or metastatic disease owing to late presentation [9]. Randomised clinical trials (RCTs) provide evidence that the addition of systemic therapy to surgical resection improves overall survival (OS) in non-metastatic gastric cancer, perioperative chemotherapy being the preferred approach in current guidelines. In patient who undergoes primary surgery, post-operative chemotherapy and/or radiation are among other options. Moreover, in metastatic disease, systemic therapy is known to reduce symptom burden, improve health-related quality of life and prolong OS as compared to the best supportive care [10].

Herein, we review the systemic therapy strategies currently in use for the treatment of gastric cancer.

8.2 Perioperative Chemotherapy

In clinical stage T2NO or more, surgery alone is inadequate and inherently leads to decreased survival. To downstage the locally advanced disease, enhance the probability of R0 resection, address micro-metastatic disease and maximise the delivery of systemic therapy, neoadjuvant or perioperative systemic therapy is typically given.

The MRC MAGIC was a seminal study published in the year 2006 that established that the addition of six cycles (three pre-operatively and three post-operatively) of ECF regimen (epirubicin, cisplatin, 5-fluorouracil) to surgery improved 5-year OS compared to surgery alone (36% versus 23%; 95% confidence interval (CI) 0.60–0.93, $P = 0.009$) in locally advanced resectable gastric cancer (≥T1b N0 M0) despite only 42% patients completing surgery and all three cycles of post-operative chemotherapy. Notably, patients receiving chemotherapy in a neoadjuvant setting had more patients with T1/T2 tumours and less extensive nodal disease at the time of surgery, leading to higher rates of curative resection (79% versus 70%) as compared to surgery alone [11]. The anthracycline epirubicin is now known to add additional toxicity without OS benefit, as shown in a similarly designed phase 3 French trial that used cisplatin-5FU in place of ECF as a perioperative regimen [12]. A German phase 2/3 FLOT4-AIO trial demonstrated that a perioperative FLOT (fluorouracil plus leucovorin, oxaliplatin and docetaxel) regimen led to a 9% improvement in 5-year OS rates (45% versus 36%) over ECF regimen, making it the current standard of care. FLOT regimen was associated with significantly higher grade ≥3 neutropenia, infections, diarrhoea and sensory neuropathy [13]. Therefore, in less fit patients in terms of performance status and presence of comorbidities, fluoropyrimidine plus platinum doublet (Cisplatin-5-FU) is typically administered. Ongoing trials are evaluating the role of immunotherapy, anti-HER2 (human epidermal receptor 2) target therapy and VEGF (vascular endothelial growth factor) inhibition in the perioperative setting in resectable gastric cancer.

8.3 Adjuvant Chemotherapy and/or Radiation

The CLASSIC trial showed the benefit of adding adjuvant CAPOX (capecitabine plus oxaliplatin) in stage II-IIIB gastric adenocarcinoma patients from China, Taiwan and South Korea after D2 gastrectomy in terms of 3-year disease-free survival (DFS) (74% versus 59% [HR] 0.56, 95% CI 0.44–0.72) and 5-year OS (78% versus 69%, HR 0.66, 95% CI 0.51–0.85). This benefit was observed despite one-third not completing the planned adjuvant treatment and 90% requiring dose reduction due to adverse events [14, 15]. Adjuvant S1 (tegafur, gemeracil and oteracil combination) with or without docetaxel has been shown to improve survival in phase 3 trials over surgery alone in the countries where this drug is available [16, 17]. An individual patient-level meta-analysis of adjuvant chemotherapy in gastric cancer demonstrated a 6% absolute benefit in 5-year OS with 5-FU-based chemotherapy as compared to surgery alone (HR 0.82, 95% CI 0.76–0.90, $p < 0.001$) [18].

To further improve the outcomes after upfront surgery, the role of adjuvant chemoradiotherapy has been investigated in multiple studies. The INT-0116 is the most influential trial in this setting [19]. In this study, after curative resection, patients were randomised to observation versus 5-FU (5-fluorouracil) with leucovorin (5FU/LV) for 5 days, followed by radiotherapy (RT) (4500 cGy) with concurrent 5FU/LV on the first 4 and last 3 days of RT. In the experimental arm, patients were subsequently given two 5-day cycles of 5FU/LV starting 1 month after the end of RT. The use of adjuvant chemoradiation significantly improved 5-year OS over surgery alone (43% versus 28%). Notably, only 10% had undergone D2 lymph node dissection, and 54% did not have adequate clearance of the D1 nodal region in this study. Additionally, more than half of the patients had grade 3 or more haematological toxicities. The use of additional chemotherapy (ECF regimen in place of 5FU/LV) before and after concurrent chemoradiation in CALGB 80801 trial did not improve OS [20].

Multiple studies have compared adjuvant chemotherapy with adjuvant chemoradiation, but no OS benefit has been shown by one strategy over another to date [21, 22]. Current guidelines recommend that post-operative chemoradiation should not be added following R0 resection or for patients who have undergone upfront D2 gastrectomy. In patients who have undergone gastrectomy with involved margins and are not candidates for more surgery, post-operative RT or chemoradiation should be discussed by a multidisciplinary tumour board [23].

8.4 Systemic Therapy in Unresectable or Metastatic Gastric Cancer

Cytotoxic chemotherapy The chemotherapy regimen of choice depends upon patient characteristics like performance status or comorbidities and treatment characteristics like toxicity profile. The combination regimen of fluoropyrimidine plus platin (CAPOX or FOLFOX) leads to better response rates and OS as compared to single-agent chemotherapy and is typically preferred. In patients who are less fit, single-agent treatment with fluoropyrimidine, irinotecan or paclitaxel may be considered. In very fit patients who are willing to tolerate toxicity for a higher response rate and longer progression-free survival, docetaxel may be added to fluoropyrimidine plus platin doublet in the first-line treatment. In the second-line treatment, the cytotoxic agents which are not already used in the first line may be considered. The oral cytotoxic agent trifluridine-tipiracil is approved as a third-line regimen. It is a combination of an anti-metabolite (trifluridine) plus thymidine phosphorylase inhibitor (tipiracil) and has shown survival benefit over a placebo in a phase III RCT (5.7 months versus 3.6 months) [24].

Immunotherapy The presence of a higher number of neoantigens secondary to significantly more mutations, coupled with higher PD-L1-positive T cell infiltration in tumours with defective DNA mismatch repair system, a good response to PD-1 blockage is expected. The incidence of MSI-H variety is 22% in untreated gastric cancer cases, while it is a meagre 3% in metastatic cases [25]. Pembrolizumab is an anti-PD-1 antibody that shows high response rates and excellent long-term outcomes in MSI-H gastric adenocarcinoma [26]. It is FDA-approved in dMMR (mismatch repair-deficient)/MSI-H (microsatellite instability-high) solid tumours that have progressed on previous therapies, including gastric adenocarcinoma. In HER2-positive unresectable or metastatic gastric adenocarcinoma, pembrolizumab has received accelerated FDA approval with trastuzumab and fluoropyrimidine-oxaliplatin-based chemotherapy. In the last 10 years, immune check-point inhibitor (ICI) drugs, like Pembrolizumab, have transformed the management because of high response rates. Recent European task force recommendation is to use systemic chemotherapy plus ICI drug as standard of treatment for untreated gastro-esophageal adenocarcinoma (GEA), in both early and advanced stages. The high pathologic response rate seen after neo-adjuvant ICI followed by surgery, in early stage GEA tumors, has given rise to the prospect of organ preservation [27].

Nivolumab with ipilimumab has been contrasted with chemotherapy alone in the first-line treatment of metastatic HER2-negative gastric adenocarcinoma. In patients with PDL-L1 CPS (combined positive score) ≥5, nivolumab plus chemotherapy improved progression-free survival (PFS) (7.7 versus 6.1 months) and OS (14.4 versus 11.1 months) compared with chemotherapy alone. Patients were enrolled regardless of their PDL1 status initially but later stratified on individual CPS scores [28]. Due to these data, FDA approved nivolumab or pembrolizumab in combination with platinum and fluoropyrimidine-based regimen regardless of PD-1 status.

Targeted therapy The human epidermal growth factor receptor 2 (HER2) is a transmembrane glycoprotein receptor with kinase activity that promotes cell growth, differentiation, and angiogenesis. HER2 overexpression confirmed by immunohistochemistry (IHC) 3+ or IHC 2+ with fluorescent in-situ hybridisation positivity is seen in 15–20% of GEA, especially intestinal-type cancers compared to diffuse or mixed variety tumors [29]. Trastuzumab (anti-HER2 antibody) is FDA-approved in combination with cytotoxic chemotherapy in the first-line setting in HER2+ advanced/metastatic gastric adenocarcinoma based on a large phase 3 trial that demonstrated OS benefit (13.8 vs 11.1 months) of adding trastuzumab to fluoropyrimidine plus platin-based chemotherapy [30]. There is no benefit of continuing trastuzumab beyond disease progression [31]. Also, there is no benefit of adding other anti-HER2 agents like pertuzumab, lapatinib and trastuzumab emtansine to cytotoxic chemotherapy in HER+ metastatic gastric cancer [32–34]. However, trastuzumab deruxtecan (antibody-drug conjugate, ADC) is FDA-approved in trastuzumab-exposed metastatic HER2 amplified gastric cancer based on a phase 2 RCT where it showed high response rates and longer survival compared to standard-of-care treatment [35].

Claudin 18.2 is a cell surface protein expressed in a subset of gastric adenocarcinomas. Zolbetuximab is a chimeric monoclonal antibody that targets claudin 18.2 and induces antibody-dependent cell cytotoxicity or complement-dependent cytotoxicity. These combinations are yet to receive FDA approval at the time of writing this manuscript.

Antiangiogenic therapy Ramucirumab is a recombinant anti-VEGFR2 monoclonal antibody which is approved as monotherapy or in combination with paclitaxel in the second-line setting in unresectable/metastatic gastric adenocarcinoma based on multiple RCTs that demonstrated OS benefit with ramucirumab as a single agent or in combination with paclitaxel [36, 37]. The addition of bevacizumab to cytotoxic chemotherapy in gastric cancer did not prolong survival, and it is therefore not used in this subsite of gastrointestinal cancers [38, 39]. General scheme of systemic therapy in gastric adenocarcinoma is shown in Fig. 2.

9 Role of Radiotherapy in Gastric Cancer

9.1 Radiation Therapy in Gastric Cancer

Gastrectomy with a D2 lymphadenectomy is the mainstay of curative treatment for localised Gastric Cancer. However, survival rates are limited with surgery alone in patients with stages II and III GC. To increase survival, perioperative and adjuvant treatments have been established as standard of care, based on the results of randomised controlled trials. Despite this, mortality

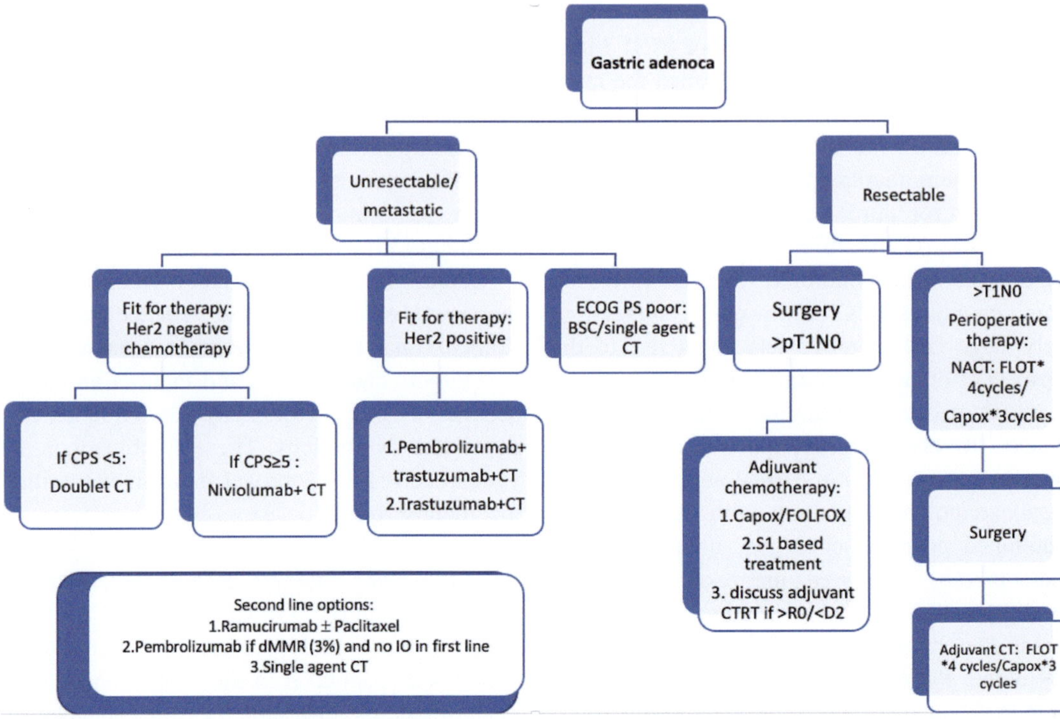

Fig. 2 General scheme of systemic therapy in gastric adenocarcinoma. Abbreviations: her2 human epidermal receptor 2, ECOG Eastern Cooperative Oncology Group, PS performance status, CT chemotherapy, NACT neoadjuvant chemotherapy, FLOT fluorouracil, leucovorin, oxaliplatin and taxane, CAPOX capecitabine oxaliplatin, CPS combined positive score, FOLFOX fluorouracil leucovorin oxaliplatin, CTRT chemoradiotherapy, dMMR deficient mismatch repair

in patients with localised disease at diagnosis remains high, with 5-year overall survival of only 40%. The value of adding adjuvant radiotherapy to perioperative CT in patients undergoing D2 gastrectomy has remained controversial.

In the US Intergroup-0116 (INT-0116) trial, postoperative chemoradiotherapy (CRT) significantly improved survival compared with surgery alone (40% versus 28% at 5 years) [12]. INT-0116 was, however, criticised for the fact that only 10% of all patients had an adequate D2 lymph node dissection. It has been suggested by some researchers that adjuvant CRT compensated for poor locoregional control resulting from inadequate surgery. The UK MAGIC study showed that the addition of perioperative CT to surgery improves survival for patients with resectable oesophagogastric adenocarcinoma compared with surgery alone [4].

9.2 Radiotherapy in Patients with D2 Dissection

Recent trials investigating adjuvant treatment of localised gastric cancer (GC) have come to nearly similar results. The conclusions from the Korean ARTIST-2 and Swedish CRITICS trials are that postoperative radiotherapy following D2 gastrectomy confers no additional benefit compared with chemotherapy (CT) alone.

In the CRITICS trial, 478 were randomised to CT versus CRT, 5-year OS CT versus CRT, 57.9% versus 45.9% [HR: CRT versus CT 1.62 (1.24–2.12; *P* 1/4 0.0004)] [40–42]. The intent-to-treat analysis of the CRITICS trial data did not show a survival benefit for patients in the CRT versus the CT arm. However, in the PP analysis (defined as those patients who actually started postoperative treatment), the CT group had a better 5-year overall and event-free survival as compared with the CRT group. The results of the PP analysis rejected the hypothesis that postoperative CRT would improve survival compared with postoperative CT by 10%

In the ARTIST-2 trial, the addition of RT to CT did not significantly reduce the rate of recurrence after D2 gastrectomy. DFS rates between patients treated with adjuvant CT and CRT were similar across all subgroups [15]. The ARTIST-2 report could be criticised in that little information is provided on RT delivery, and there was no RT quality assurance program to monitor RT quality, which has been shown to be critically important in optimising outcomes in GC. Nevertheless, as the results are in line with previously reported randomised clinical trials involving adjuvant CRT. In a related meta-analysis, although adjuvant CRT showed superior outcomes compared with adjuvant chemotherapy alone in terms of DFS (HR, 0.85; 95% CI, 0.713–0.98; $P = 0.03$) in the analysis conducted in all patients, this difference was not significant when platinum-based combination chemotherapy was administered (HR, 0.91; 95% CI, 0.78–1.07; $P = 0.24$) [43].

According to the outcomes of the above 2 large-scale multi-centre studies and/or meta-analyses, adjuvant RT cannot be recommended in patients who underwent GC after complete gastrectomy with D2 resection, at least when adjuvant platinum-based combination chemotherapy is administered.

In view of above evidence, CRT should not be considered as the standard of care for patients with D2-resected, node-positive GC when adjuvant therapy is indicated. As previously demonstrated for rectal cancer, sequencing of treatment matters. As postoperative treatment is often difficult to deliver, we are convinced that the future of improving cure rates in localised GC is treatment in the preoperative period. Several trials with this focus are currently accruing patients, including the TOPGEAR (NCT02661971) and the CRITICS-2 trials (NCT02661971) in which CT or CRT or a combination is given preoperatively [44].

9.3 Radiotherapy in Patients with Less Than D2 Dissection

In GC patients who have undergone less than D2 resection, adjuvant RT with concurrent chemotherapy (CRT) is generally recommended to improve the oncologic outcomes, including the local control rates [45, 46]. Intergroup Study 0116 (INT-0116), a randomised phase III study conducted under the leadership of the Southwest Oncology Group published in 2001, confirmed the superiority of surgery with adjuvant CRT in improving the recurrence-free survival and overall survival (OS) rates compared with surgery alone [47]. Although D2 lymphadenectomy was recommended in the INT-0116 trial, D1 or less resection was performed in >90% of enrolled patients. Additionally, the beneficial effect of adjuvant CRT was not seen in the subgroup that underwent D2 lymphadenectomy [48].

In patients who underwent micro- or macroscopically incomplete resection of localised GC, which is not generally indicated in clinical trials, and/or less than D2 resection of GC, adjuvant CRT before or after standard chemotherapy may still be considered as part of adjuvant treatment, based on the results of INT-0116 [49].

Some studies have indicated that the addition of adjuvant CRT is particularly effective in patients with complete D2-resected GC who do not have preoperative sarcopenia, have a non-mesenchymal subtype, are older than 45 years at diagnosis and have an adequate absolute lymphocyte count prior to surgery [50–52].

The classification of cancer has recently changed and is determined based on molecular characteristics, including human epidermal growth factor receptor 2 overexpression, mismatch repair deficiency, microsatellite instability, and Epstein-Barr virus infection status. Additionally, these characteristics are strongly related to the effects of chemotherapy, immunotherapy, and RT [50–52].

Hence, future studies should continue the application of RT as a tailored adjuvant treatment, according to the molecular characteristics of patients with GC.

9.4 Target Volumes

Rationale: The target of adjuvant RT is defined based on the postoperative recurrence pattern, especially that of loco-regional recurrence (LRR). Although several studies have evaluated the pattern of tumour recurrence after curative surgery in GC patients, the pattern has varied widely depending on the extent of the disease, geographic region, and adjuvant treatment used. The extent of lymphadenectomy especially affects the rates and patterns of LRR.

In general, RT for GC targets the tumour bed, remnant stomach, resection and/or anastomosis site, duodenal stump and regional LNs. In patients with T4b stage (infiltration of the surrounding organs), the tumour bed should be included as an RT target volume. The resection and/or anastomosis site could be included if the resection margin was not sufficient. Whether to include the remnant stomach remains controversial. Recent studies have reported that the risk of recurrence in this area is extremely low (1–2%) after complete resection, even if it is not included in the target of adjuvant RT. Additionally, the ARTIST and retrospective single-institutional Korean studies showed that the most common sites of LRR after D2 lymphadenectomy were the para-aortic (LN station Nos. 16a2 and 16b1, and the upper part of 16b2), celiac (No. 9), hepatoduodenal (No. 12), retropancreatic (No. 13), and superior mesenteric vessels (No. 14). Based on the results of these studies, adjuvant RT generally included the secondary and tertiary LN stations after the perigastric LNs.

9.5 General CTV Recommendations for Stomach Radiotherapy

For proximal gastric cancers undergoing esophagectomy with intrathoracic anastomosis, CTV includes:

- Tumour bed (including medial 2/3rd of the left hemidiaphragm)
- 3–4 cm of the mucosa of the oesophagus and distal stomach
- Lymph node stations 1 to 4, 7, and 9 to 11 (11, 12; if GEJ involved then stations 20, 110, 111)

For middle third patients undergoing total gasrectomy with Roux-en-Y EJ anastomosis, the CTV includes:

- Tumour bed
- 3–4 cm of the mucosa of the oesophagus and jejunum
- Lymph node stations 3–11 [12, 13] and 1, 2 in case of proximal third involvement

For distal third tumours undergoing distal gastrectomy with gastrojejunal anastomosis, CTV includes:

- Tumour bed
- 3–4 cm of the mucosa of the proximal stomach and jejunum
- 3–4 cm of duodenal stamp
- Lymph node stations 3–9 and 11–13

Generally, dose of 45–50 Gy in 25 fractions is recommended in adjuvant radiotherapy for stomach cancer. There may be benefit in using techniques such as IMRT for sparing of critical structures like the liver and kidneys. Sequelae of radiotherapy for stomach region are given in Table 5

10 Conclusion

Advances in multimodality treatment employing surgery, systemic therapy and radiotherapy has increased the survival of early and locally advanced gastric cancer patients worldwide. Optimisation of current treatment modalities and identification of newer therapeutic targets and novel biomarker-driven therapies will go a long way in further improving the outcomes of this highly morbid and fatal disease. In 2025, American Society for Radiation Oncology (ASTRO) has published a consensus-based guideline, 'Radiation Therapy in Gastric Cancer' [53]. The broad aspects for different clinical stages would be useful to utilize the radiation therapy practice in multidisciplinary GC man-

Table 5 Sequelae of radiotherapy for stomach region

Early	Late
Anorexia	Dyspepsia
Nausea, vomiting	Radiation gastritis
Fatigue	Gastric ulcer
Esophagitis	Complicated gastric ulcer (with perforation or obstruction)
Skin pigmentation	Nephrotoxicity
Weight loss	Cardiotoxicity (pericarditis, coronary artery disease, effusion)

agement. A. chemo-radiotherapy (CRT) should be considered: (i) upfront for patient who has borderline resectable disease, (ii) patient's performance status may not be suitable to tolerate and complete perioperative chemotherapy cycles; B. in patients who have undergone surgery, postoperative radiotherapy (PORT) should be considered: (i) who have shown <D2 nodal resection, R1 & R2 status, (ii) who would be unable to tolerate and complete peri-operative chemotherapy cycles; C. inoperable GC patients with good general health and nutrition status who would benefit from CRT to reduce disease progression for a reasonable time; D. palliative RT is considered for oligometastatic disease, for pain, bleeding and obstruction. RT dose and fractionation for (a) upfront CRT and PORT settings should be 45 Gy in 25 fractions, (b) palliative RT should be 30 Gy to 36 Gy in 10 to 12 fractions. A recent publication has given a detailed bibliometric analysis of published literature and trials from 2014 to 2023 [54]. These evidence-based recommendations would guide the current role and indications of RT in gastric cancer.

Percepts Box

1. The prevalence of stomach cancer varies by geographical area. Eastern Asia, South America's Andean areas, and Eastern Europe have the greatest occurrence rates, whereas North America, Northern Europe, and the majority of African and South-Eastern Asian nations have the lowest.
2. The worldwide incidence of stomach cancer has decreased dramatically over the last several decades, although the degree of reduction differs by country and location. This decrease might be attributed to the identification of specific risk factors such as H. pylori and other dietary and environmental hazards. Migration patterns and other geographical variables all have an influence on incidence.
3. Key trends in stomach cancer incidence.
   (a) Histology—When compared to diffuse-type gastric cancer, the global incidence of intestinal type is declining more dramatically. The incidence of the intestinal form has declined in tandem with the overall incidence of gastric cancer; the incidence of the diffuse type, on the other hand, has decreased more gradually.
   (b) Location—The prevalence of stomach cardia cancer has increased. The shift from distal to proximal stomach may be attributed to a reduction in distal malignancies.
   (c) Incidence of stomach cancer (cardia and non-cardiac) is increasing in young people (aged <50 years) in both low and high-incidence nations.
   (d) Gastric cancer is the fourth biggest cause of cancer deaths globally. The majority of stomach cancer patients have advanced illness, hence mortality rates are significant. However, stomach cancer mortality has been steadily declining globally, with rates differing by area.

(continued)

4. Risk factors—Bacterial, host, and environmental variables interact to cause gastric cancer in individuals deemed to be at average risk. Up to half of all stomach cancers are likely caused by lifestyle factors, including smoking and alcohol usage, as well as dietary variables such high salt diets lacking in vegetables and nitroso compounds. Infection with Helicobacter pylori, particularly with certain genotypes (vacAs1, vacAm1, and cagA positive), continues to be a significant risk factor. Those hosts with certain cytokine polymorphisms are at far greater danger.
5. Clinical features and diagnosis—The majority of people suffering from stomach cancer have symptoms, with weight loss and abdominal discomfort being the most typical ones. Results from upper GI endoscopy or radiographic investigations may raise the possibility of a stomach cancer diagnosis, but a histologic evaluation of tumour tissue—typically obtained endoscopically—is necessary to confirm the diagnosis.
6. Surgery could be necessary for palliation in situations of advanced illness, as part of the staging assessment for stomach cancer, or for possibly curative treatment of localised disease. The optimal treatment strategy for a stomach tumour is complete surgical removal along with the excision of surrounding lymph nodes. A neoadjuvant approach should be considered, or abdominal exploration (preferably with an initial laparoscopic approach) with curative-intent resection should be carried out, unless there is unmistakable evidence of disseminated disease, major vascular invasion, or other contraindications to surgery.
7. Several approaches, including adjuvant chemoradiotherapy (as used in two US intergroup trials—Intergroup [INT] 0116 and Cancer and Leukemia Group B [CALGB] 80101) and perioperative (preoperative plus postoperative) chemotherapy, have shown a significant survival benefit over surgery alone for patients with potentially resectable non-cardia gastric cancer.
8. Chemotherapy, either with or without chemoradiotherapy, is one option for adjuvant therapy. Recent evidence-based guideline for RT in gastric cancer (ASTRO, 2025) should become part of multi-disciplinary management either in potentially curable stage or in palliative setting.

Multiple Choice Questions

1. A 42-year-old female underwent partial gastrectomy and had pathological T1 gastric adenocarcinoma in postoperative histopathology report with negative margins and 0/17 lymph nodes involved. What should be offered as adjuvant treatment?
   (a) Chemoradiation
   (b) FOLFOX × 6 cycles
   (c) Observation
   (d) ECF × 3 cycles
2. A 60-year-old female was diagnosed with non-metastatic gastric adenocarcinoma and underwent partial gastrectomy with D1 lymph node dissection. The post-operative histopathology report revealed stage IIB disease (T3N1). What is the preferred adjuvant treatment strategy in this case?
   (a) mFOLFOX × 6 months
   (b) Observation
   (c) ECF × 6 cycles
   (d) 5-FU + Leucovorin × 1 cycle, 5FU/LV based chemoradiation + 2 cycles of 5FU/LV
3. A 48-year-old male was diagnosed with gastric adenocarcinoma 1 year ago and underwent only surgery at that time. He now presented with metastasis to liver and lungs,

and his clinical oncologist prescribed six cycles of paclitaxel-carboplatin. He comes to you for a second opinion. His ECOG performance status is one and has no comorbidities. What would you recommend?
   (a) Single agent capecitabine
   (b) CAPOX
   (c) Docetaxel, cisplatin, and 5-FU
   (d) Analyse the tumour for predictive biomarkers
4. A 54-year-old gentleman presented to the gastrointestinal oncology clinic with a diagnosis of stage 4 gastric adenocarcinoma (lung metastasis). In the biopsy report from the large mass in the gastric antrum, the CPS score was 0 and IHC 3+ for HER2. The patient has ECOG performance status of one and has controlled hypertension. Which therapy do you offer?
   (a) FOLFOX + Trastuzumab +/− pembrolizumab
   (b) FOLFOX + Nivolumab + Trastuzumab
   (c) CAPOX
   (d) Docetaxel, Cisplatin, and 5-FU
5. A 68-year-old female was diagnosed with stage 4 gastric cancer (lung and liver metastasis) 1.5 years back. The profiling of her tumour revealed IHC1+ for HER2, PD-L1 CPS 0%, MSS. In the first line, she was treated with FOLFOX and received paclitaxel + ramucirumab in the second-line treatment. She is not interested in a clinical trial and has good performance status. What would you offer?
   (a) Pembrolizumab
   (b) Trastuzumab
   (c) Trifluridine/tipiracil
   (d) Nivolumab
6. The criteria used by the Japanese to classify gastric carcinoma as D1, D2, and D3 are as follows:
   (a) The stage of the disease
   (b) The kind of anastamosis after surgical resection
   (c) The degree of nodal dissection during surgery resection
   (d) The degree of mucosal serosal involvement
7. Chemoradiotherapy after Induction Chemotherapy in Cancer of the Stomach (CRITICS) trial describes the following procedures for D1+ nodal dissection:
   (a) Dissection of lymph node stations 1–12
   (b) Dissection of lymph node stations 1–10
   (c) Dissection of lymph node stations 1–8
   (d) Dissection of lymph node stations 1–9 and 11
8. In the historic MAGIC experiment, the medication regimen was
   (a) Paclitaxel, carboplatin
   (b) Epirubicin, Cisplatin, and 5FU (ECF infusional)
   (c) Capecitabine, oxaloplatin
   (d) Folinic acid, 5-Flurouracil, oxaloplatin
9. Which trial suggests that CRT should not be considered as the standard of care for patients with D2-resected, node-positive GC when adjuvant therapy is indicated
   (a) CRITICS
   (b) INT0116
   (c) CALGB80101
   (d) FLOT-4
10. Nodal areas of risk for radiotherapy to distal third of stomach include
   (a) Perigastric, celiac, left gastric artery, splenic artery, splenic hilar, hepatic artery, porta hepatic, suprapyloric, subpyloric and pancreaticoduodenal lymph nodes
   (b) Perigastric, left gastric artery, celiac, hepatic artery, porta hepatic, suprapyloric, subpyloric and pancreaticoduodenal lymph nodes.
   (c) Perigastric, celiac, left gastric artery, splenic artery, splenic hilar, hepatic artery, and porta hepatic lymph nodes
   (d) Para-oesophageal, lesser curvature, splenic nodes and celiac axis nodal regions

Answer Key

1. (c)
2. (d)
3. (d)

4. (a)
5. (a)
6. (c)
7. (d)
8. (b)
9. (a)
10. (b)

References

1. Townsend CM, Evers M, Beauchamp RD, Mattox K. Sabiston's textbook of surgery: the biological basis of modern surgical practice. 21st ed. Missouri: Elsevier; 2022.
2. Devita VT, Lawrence TS, Rosenberg SA. Devita, Hellman and Rosenberg's cancer principles and practice of oncology. 12th ed. Philadelphia: Wolters Kluwer; 2023.
3. Mukkamalla SKR, Recio-Boiles A, Babiker HM. Gastric cancer. In: StatPearls [Internet]. Treasure Island: StatPearls Publishing; 2022 [cited 2023 Jan 15]. Available from: http://www.ncbi.nlm.nih.gov/books/NBK459142/.
4. Hu B, El Hajj N, Sittler S, Lammert N, Barnes R, Meloni-Ehrig A. Gastric cancer: classification, histology and application of molecular pathology. J Gastrointest Oncol. 2012;3(3):251–61.
5. Fischer JE. Mastery of surgery. 7th ed. Philadelphia: Wolters Kluwer; 2019.
6. Williams NS, O'Connell PR, McCaskie AW. Bailey and Love's short practice of surgery. 27th ed. Florida: Taylor and Francis Group; 2018.
7. Faiz Z, Hayashi T, Yoshikawa T. Lymph node dissection for gastric cancer: establishment of D2 and the current position of splenectomy in Europe and Japan. Eur J Surg Oncol. 2021;47(9):2233–6.
8. Ferlay J, Colombet M, Soerjomataram I, Parkin DM, Piñeros M, Znaor A, et al. Cancer statistics for the year 2020: an overview. Int J Cancer. 2021. https://doi.org/10.1002/ijc.33588.
9. Wanebo HJ, Kennedy BJ, Chmiel J, Steele G, Winchester D, Osteen R. Cancer of the stomach. A patient care study by the American College of Surgeons. Ann Surg. 1993;218(5):583–92.
10. Ajani JA, D'Amico TA, Bentrem DJ, Chao J, Cooke D, Corvera C, et al. Gastric cancer, version 2.2022, NCCN clinical practice guidelines in oncology. J Natl Compr Cancer Netw. 2022;20(2):167–92.
11. Cunningham D, Allum WH, Stenning SP, Thompson JN, Van de Velde CJH, Nicolson M, et al. Perioperative chemotherapy versus surgery alone for resectable gastroesophageal cancer. N Engl J Med. 2006;355(1):11–20.
12. Ychou M, Boige V, Pignon JP, Conroy T, Bouché O, Lebreton G, et al. Perioperative chemotherapy compared with surgery alone for resectable gastroesophageal adenocarcinoma: an FNCLCC and FFCD multicenter phase III trial. J Clin Oncol. 2011;29(13):1715–21.
13. Al-Batran SE, Homann N, Pauligk C, Goetze TO, Meiler J, Kasper S, et al. Perioperative chemotherapy with fluorouracil plus leucovorin, oxaliplatin, and docetaxel versus fluorouracil or capecitabine plus cisplatin and epirubicin for locally advanced, resectable gastric or gastro-oesophageal junction adenocarcinoma (FLOT4): a randomised, phase 2/3 trial. Lancet. 2019;393(10184):1948–57.
14. Bang YJ, Kim YW, Yang HK, Chung HC, Park YK, Lee KH, et al. Adjuvant capecitabine and oxaliplatin for gastric cancer after D2 gastrectomy (CLASSIC): a phase 3 open-label, randomised controlled trial. Lancet. 2012;379(9813):315–21.
15. Noh SH, Park SR, Yang HK, Chung HC, Chung IJ, Kim SW, et al. Adjuvant capecitabine plus oxaliplatin for gastric cancer after D2 gastrectomy (CLASSIC): 5-year follow-up of an open-label, randomised phase 3 trial. Lancet Oncol. 2014;15(12):1389–96.
16. Sakuramoto S, Sasako M, Yamaguchi T, Kinoshita T, Fujii M, Nashimoto A, et al. Adjuvant chemotherapy for gastric cancer with S-1, an oral fluoropyrimidine. N Engl J Med. 2007;357(18):1810–20.
17. Kakeji Y, Yoshida K, Kodera Y, Kochi M, Sano T, Ichikawa W, et al. Three-year outcomes of a randomized phase III trial comparing adjuvant chemotherapy with S-1 plus docetaxel versus S-1 alone in stage III gastric cancer: JACCRO GC-07. Gastric Cancer. 2022;25(1):188–96.
18. GASTRIC (Global Advanced/Adjuvant Stomach Tumor Research International Collaboration) Group, Paoletti X, Oba K, Burzykowski T, Michiels S, Ohashi Y, et al. Benefit of adjuvant chemotherapy for resectable gastric cancer: a meta-analysis. JAMA. 2010;303(17):1729–37.
19. Macdonald JS, Smalley SR, Benedetti J, Hundahl SA, Estes NC, Stemmermann GN, et al. Chemoradiotherapy after surgery compared with surgery alone for adenocarcinoma of the stomach or gastroesophageal junction. N Engl J Med. 2001;345(10):725–30.
20. Fuchs CS, Niedzwiecki D, Mamon HJ, Tepper JE, Ye X, Swanson RS, et al. Adjuvant chemoradiotherapy with epirubicin, cisplatin, and fluorouracil compared with adjuvant chemoradiotherapy with fluorouracil and leucovorin after curative resection of gastric cancer: results from CALGB 80101 (Alliance). J Clin Oncol. 2017;35(32):3671–7.
21. Park SH, Sohn TS, Lee J, Lim DH, Hong ME, Kim KM, et al. Phase III trial to compare adjuvant chemotherapy with capecitabine and cisplatin versus concurrent chemoradiotherapy in gastric cancer: final report of the adjuvant chemoradiotherapy in stomach tumors trial, including survival and subset analyses. J Clin Oncol. 2015;33(28):3130–6.
22. Park SH, Lim DH, Sohn TS, Lee J, Zang DY, Kim ST, et al. A randomized phase III trial comparing adjuvant single-agent S1, S-1 with oxaliplatin, and

postoperative chemoradiation with S-1 and oxaliplatin in patients with node-positive gastric cancer after D2 resection: the ARTIST 2 trial☆. Ann Oncol. 2021;32(3):368–74.
23. Lordick F, Carneiro F, Cascinu S, Fleitas T, Haustermans K, Piessen G, et al. Gastric cancer: ESMO clinical practice guideline for diagnosis, treatment and follow-up. Ann Oncol. 2022;33(10):1005–20.
24. Shitara K, Doi T, Dvorkin M, Mansoor W, Arkenau HT, Prokharau A, et al. Trifluridine/tipiracil versus placebo in patients with heavily pretreated metastatic gastric cancer (TAGS): a randomised, double-blind, placebo-controlled, phase 3 trial. Lancet Oncol. 2018;19(11):1437–48.
25. Janjigian YY, Sanchez-Vega F, Jonsson P, Chatila WK, Hechtman JF, Ku GY, et al. Genetic predictors of response to systemic therapy in esophagogastric cancer. Cancer Discov. 2018;8(1):49–58.
26. Marabelle A, Le DT, Ascierto PA, Di Giacomo AM, De Jesus-Acosta A, Delord JP, et al. Efficacy of pembrolizumab in patients with noncolorectal high microsatellite instability/mismatch repair-deficient cancer: results from the Phase II KEYNOTE-158 study. J Clin Oncol. 2020;38(1):1–10.
27. de la Fouchardière C, Cammarota A, Svrcek M, Alsina M, et al. How do I treat dMMR/MSI gastro-oesophageal adenocarcinoma in 2025? A position paper from the EORTC-GITCG gastro-esophageal task force. Cancer Treat Rev. 2025;134:102890. https://doi.org/10.1016/j.ctrv.2025.102890.
28. Janjigian YY, Shitara K, Moehler M, Garrido M, Salman P, Shen L, et al. First-line nivolumab plus chemotherapy versus chemotherapy alone for advanced gastric, gastro-oesophageal junction, and oesophageal adenocarcinoma (CheckMate 649): a randomised, open-label, phase 3 trial. Lancet. 2021;398(10294):27–40.
29. Cancer Genome Atlas Research Network. Comprehensive molecular characterization of gastric adenocarcinoma. Nature. 2014;513(7517):202–9.
30. Bang YJ, Van Cutsem E, Feyereislova A, Chung HC, Shen L, Sawaki A, et al. Trastuzumab in combination with chemotherapy versus chemotherapy alone for treatment of HER2-positive advanced gastric or gastro-oesophageal junction cancer (ToGA): a phase 3, open-label, randomised controlled trial. Lancet. 2010;376(9742):687–97.
31. Makiyama A, Sukawa Y, Kashiwada T, Kawada J, Hosokawa A, Horie Y, et al. Randomized, phase II study of trastuzumab beyond progression in patients with HER2-positive advanced gastric or gastroesophageal junction cancer: WJOG7112G (T-ACT Study). J Clin Oncol. 2020;38(17):1919–27.
32. Satoh T, Xu RH, Chung HC, Sun GP, Doi T, Xu JM, et al. Lapatinib plus paclitaxel versus paclitaxel alone in the second-line treatment of HER2-amplified advanced gastric cancer in Asian populations: TyTAN—a randomized, phase III study. J Clin Oncol. 2014;32(19):2039–49.
33. Thuss-Patience PC, Shah MA, Ohtsu A, Van Cutsem E, Ajani JA, Castro H, et al. Trastuzumab emtansine versus taxane use for previously treated HER2-positive locally advanced or metastatic gastric or gastro-oesophageal junction adenocarcinoma (GATSBY): an international randomised, open-label, adaptive, phase 2/3 study. Lancet Oncol. 2017;18(5):640–53.
34. Tabernero J, Hoff PM, Shen L, Ohtsu A, Shah MA, Cheng K, et al. Pertuzumab plus trastuzumab and chemotherapy for HER2-positive metastatic gastric or gastro-oesophageal junction cancer (JACOB): final analysis of a double-blind, randomised, placebo-controlled phase 3 study. Lancet Oncol. 2018;19(10):1372–84.
35. Shitara K, Bang YJ, Iwasa S, Sugimoto N, Ryu MH, Sakai D, et al. Trastuzumab deruxtecan in previously treated HER2-positive gastric cancer. N Engl J Med. 2020;382(25):2419–30.
36. Fuchs CS, Tomasek J, Yong CJ, Dumitru F, Passalacqua R, Goswami C, et al. Ramucirumab monotherapy for previously treated advanced gastric or gastro-oesophageal junction adenocarcinoma (REGARD): an international, randomised, multicentre, placebo-controlled, phase 3 trial. Lancet. 2014;383(9911):31–9.
37. Wilke H, Muro K, Van Cutsem E, Oh SC, Bodoky G, Shimada Y, et al. Ramucirumab plus paclitaxel versus placebo plus paclitaxel in patients with previously treated advanced gastric or gastro-oesophageal junction adenocarcinoma (RAINBOW): a double-blind, randomised phase 3 trial. Lancet Oncol. 2014;15(11):1224–35.
38. Ohtsu A, Shah MA, Van Cutsem E, Rha SY, Sawaki A, Park SR, et al. Bevacizumab in combination with chemotherapy as first-line therapy in advanced gastric cancer: a randomized, double-blind, placebo-controlled phase III study. J Clin Oncol. 2011;29(30):3968–76.
39. Chen Z, Yuan J, Xu Y, Zhang C, Li Z, Gong J, et al. From AVATAR mice to patients: RC48-ADC exerted promising efficacy in advanced gastric cancer with HER2 expression. Front Pharmacol. 2021;12:757994.
40. De Steur WO, van Amelsfoort RM, Hartgrink HH, et al. Adjuvant chemotherapy is superior to chemoradiation after D2 surgery for gastric cancer in the per-protocol analysis of the randomized CRITICS trial. Ann Oncol. 2021;32:360–7.
41. Cats A, Jansen EPM, van Grieken NCT, et al. Chemotherapy versus chemoradiotherapy after surgery and preoperative chemotherapy for resectable gastric cancer (CRITICS): an international, open-label, randomised phase 3 trial. Lancet Oncol. 2018;19:616–28.
42. Slagter AE, Jansen EPM, van Laarhoven HWM, et al. CRITICS-II: a multicentre randomised phase II trial of neo-adjuvant chemotherapy followed by surgery versus neoadjuvant chemotherapy and subsequent chemoradiotherapy followed by surgery versus neoadjuvant chemoradiotherapy followed by surgery in resectable gastric cancer. BMC Cancer. 2018;18:877.

43. Kim TH, Kim IH, Kang SJ, Choi M, Kim BH, Eom BW, et al. Korean Practice Guidelines for Gastric Cancer 2022: an evidence-based, multidisciplinary approach. J Gastric Cancer. 2023;23:3–106.
44. Leong T, Smithers BM, Haustermans K, et al. TOPGEAR: a randomized, phase III trial of perioperative ECF chemotherapy with or without preoperative chemoradiation for resectable gastric cancer: interim results from an international, intergroup trial of the AGITG, TROG, EORTC and CCTG. Ann Surg Oncol. 2017;24:2252–8.
45. Eom SS, Choi W, Eom BW, Park SH, Kim SJ, Kim YI, et al. A comprehensive and comparative review of global gastric cancer treatment guidelines. J Gastric Cancer. 2022;22:3–23.
46. Guideline Committee of the Korean Gastric Cancer Association (KGCA), Development Working Group & Review Panel. Korean practice guideline for gastric cancer 2018: an evidence-based, multi-disciplinary approach. J Gastric Cancer. 2019;19:1–48.
47. Malley SR, Benedetti JK, Haller DG, Hundahl SA, Estes NC, Ajani JA, et al. Updated analysis of SWOG- directed intergroup study 0116: a phase III trial of adjuvant radiochemotherapy versus observation after curative gastric cancer resection. J Clin Oncol. 2012;30:2327–33.
48. Park JS, Yu JI, Lim DH, Nam H, Kim YI, Lee J, et al. Clinical significance of preoperative hematological parameters in patients with D2-resected, node-positive stomach cancer. Biomedicine. 2022;10:1565.
49. Yu JI. Role of adjuvant radiotherapy in gastric cancer. J Gastric Cancer. 2023;23:194–206.
50. Kim ST, Sa JK, Oh SY, Kim K, Hong JY, Kang WK, et al. Comprehensive molecular characterization of gastric cancer patients from phase II second-line ramucirumab plus paclitaxel therapy trial. Genome Med. 2021;13:11.
51. Oh SC, Sohn BH, Cheong JH, Kim SB, Lee JE, Park KC, et al. Clinical and genomic landscape of gastric cancer with a mesenchymal phenotype. Nat Commun. 2018;9:1777.
52. Lee J, An JY, Choi MG, Park SH, Kim ST, Lee JH, et al. Deep learning-based survival analysis identified associations between molecular subtype and optimal adjuvant treatment of patients with gastric cancer. JCO Clin Cancer Inform. 2018;2:1–14.
53. Anker CJ, Arshad J, Cellini F, Dehal A, et al. Radiation therapy for gastric cancer: An ASTRO clinical practice guideline. Pract Radiat Oncol. 2025;S1879-8500(25)00270-X. https://doi.org/10.1016/j.prro.2025.10.010.
54. Weng ZH, Chen BB, Lin JR, Xu MM, Yuan JP, Hu HK. Gastric cancer radiation therapy: a bibliometric analysis of the scientific literature. Front Oncol. 2025;15:1513255. https://doi.org/10.3389/fonc.2025.1513255.

Online Links

https://www.youtube.com/watch?v=3qgkCsYSeVc
https://www.youtube.com/watch?v=CSx9p7VHIkI
https://www.youtube.com/watch?v=_AKUA1oGh5g

Hepatobiliary and Pancreatic Cancers

Indranil Mallick, Rahul Krishnatry, Anusheel Munshi, Amir Mushtaq Parray, Rakesh Sharma, Nitesh Rohatgi, and Sailesh Srikhande

1 Hepatocellular Carcinoma

1.1 Anatomy

The liver is the largest solid organ and is traditionally divided into left and right lobes separated by the falciform ligament (Fig. 1). It is important to determine resectability by understanding the spatial relationship of a tumor to the hepatic vascular system (portal and hepatic veins) to the segments. The most common segmentation scheme proposed by Couinaud divides the liver parenchyma into the right and left lobes with four segments each (Fig. 2). The left lobe of the liver consists of the caudate lobe (segment I), lateral segment (segments II and III), and medial segment (segment IV). The anatomic landmark between the medial segment and lateral segment is drawn between the gallbladder and inferior vena cava (the falciform ligament). The right lobe of the liver consists of anterior segments (segments V and VIII) and posterior segments (segments VI and VII), where the right hepatic vein separates them from each other. It is critical to spare about 700 cc of functional liver post- local treatment in the form of surgery or radiotherapy, or others, for adequate liver function recovery.

Of all primary liver tumors, benign tumors comprise 6–12% including hepatocellular hyperplasia, adenomas, hepatic cysts, mesenchymal hamartomas or hemangiomas, lipomas, and fibromas. Of all malignant primary tumors, 85–95% are of epithelial origin (including HCC, fibrolamellar HCC, cholangiocarcinoma, and hepatoblastoma), whereas 1–3% are malignant mesenchymal tumors. The HCC is commonly known to invade adjacent vascular structures such as the portal vein, the inferior vena cava (IVC), and sometimes the hepatic vein. It may also invade the diaphragm. Portal nodes are the most likely regional nodes to be involved, but spread to celiac, gastric, and peritoneal nodes

I. Mallick (✉)
Department of Radiation Oncology, Tata Medical Center, Kolkata, India
e-mail: indranil.mallick@tmckolkata.com

R. Krishnatry
Department of Radiation Oncology, Tata Memorial Center, Mumbai, India

A. Munshi
Department of Radiation Oncology, BLK-MAX Hospital, New Delhi, Delhi, India

A. M. Parray
BLK-MAX Super Speciality Hospital, New Delhi, India

R. Sharma
Institute of Liver and Biliary Sciences, New Delhi, India

N. Rohatgi
Medical Oncology, Fortis Memorial Research Institute, Gurugram, India

S. Srikhande
Gastrointestinal and Hepatobiliary Surgery, Tata Memorial Center, Mumbai, India

B. K. Mohanti et al. (eds.), *Radiation Oncology – Principles, Precepts and Practice*,
https://doi.org/10.1007/978-981-95-5171-2_11

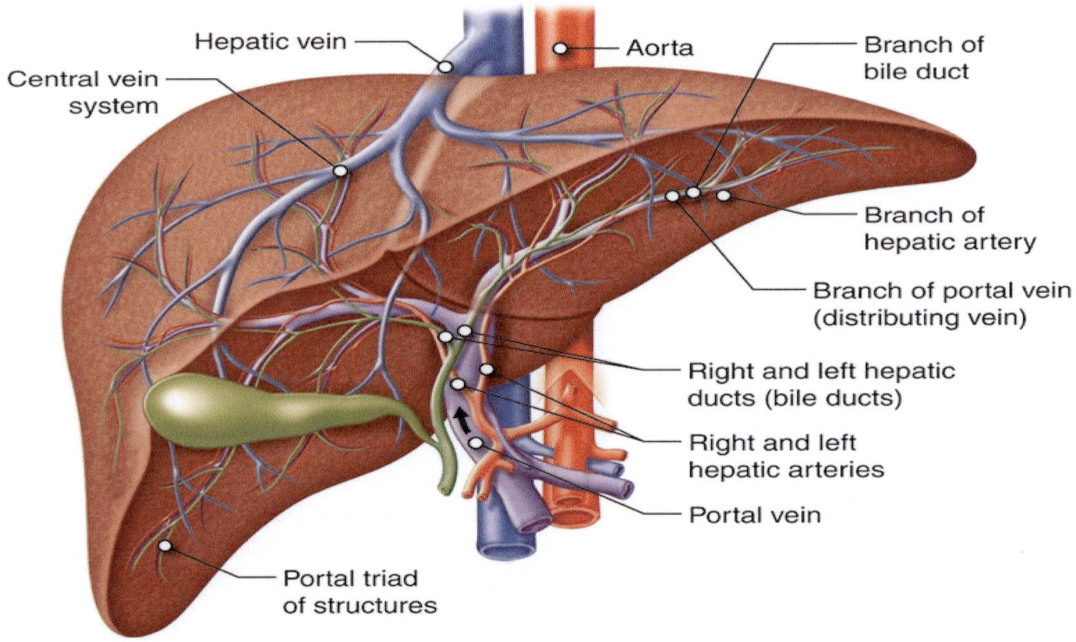

Fig. 1 Anatomy of the liver and the biliary tract. (Source: "Cenveo—Drawing Liver anatomy and vascularisation—English labels" at AnatomyTOOL.org by Cenveo, license: Creative Commons Attribution)

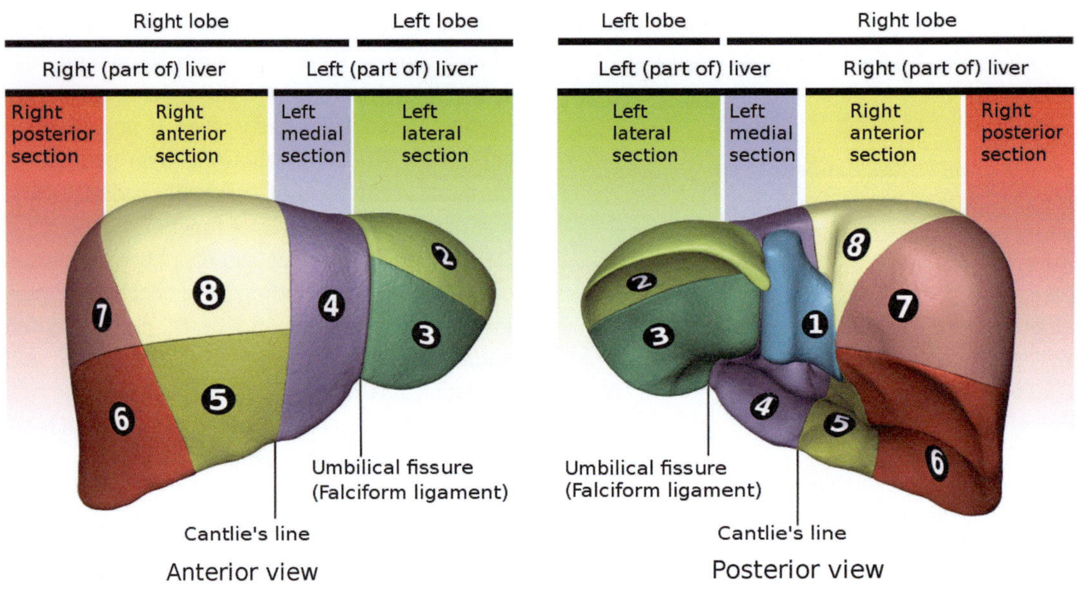

Fig. 2 Liver segment classification by Couinaud. This file is licensed under the Creative Commons Attribution-Share Alike 2.1 Japan license

may also occur. The distant metastases, although uncommon at presentation, mostly involve the abdominal cavity, the lungs, or bone.

1.2 Epidemiological Aspects and Risk Factors

Globally, hepatobiliary carcinoma is the sixth most common cause of cancer and the third most frequent cause of cancer death, as reported by GLOBOCAN 2020. HCC is twice as common in men as in women, where eastern and southeast Asia and middle Africa are high-risk regions. There is a worldwide trend in the increase in the incidence of HCC due to the hepatitis C epidemic, obesity, and nonalcoholic steatohepatitis (NASH) [1].

The primary risk factor for HCC is chronic viral hepatitis infection. In developing countries, approximately 60% of HCC is caused by the hepatitis B virus (HBV), and 33% is caused by the hepatitis C virus (HCV). The HBV and HCV carriers have a 200 and 17 to 20-fold increase in relative risk for HCC, respectively [2]. There also exists a synergistic interaction in patients having HBV and HCV combined infection. Universal HBV vaccination in many countries, such as Taiwan, has shown a significant decrease in the incidence of HCC, from 0.70 to 0.36 per 100,000. In patients with evidence of HBV or HCV infection, oral antiviral agents should be chosen to effectively control the progression of infection, which in turn reduces recurrence and improves survival for HBV-related HCC [3].

Cirrhosis from non-viral etiologies (alcohol, NASH, autoimmune chronic active hepatitis, hemochromatosis, and alpha-1-antitrypsin deficiency) is responsible for a substantial proportion of HCC in Western countries [4]. Chronic alcohol use of >80 g/day for >10 years increases the risk by approximately fivefold. In patients with HCV, alcohol use doubles the risk. NASH results from metabolic syndrome, obesity, insulin resistance, hypertriglyceridemia, and low high-density lipoprotein. Aflatoxin B, a metabolite of Aspergillus flavus found in stored grain and peanuts in humid parts of Africa and Asia, has been linked with HCC development. Patients with hereditary liver diseases, such as hemochromatosis, Wilson disease, hereditary tyrosinemia, and type I glycogen storage disease, are also at higher risk of developing HCC.

1.3 Clinical Symptoms and Signs, Pathology

HCC detection is generally an incidental finding on evaluation for unrelated issues for early-stage cancer and for cirrhosis in advanced stages. Symptoms in HCC patients are usually related to their chronic hepatitis and liver cirrhosis, which include general fatigue, poor appetite, ascites, jaundice, upper gastrointestinal bleeding, splenomegaly, dilated abdominal veins, palmar erythema, gynecomastia, testicular atrophy, leg oedema, and weight loss. Tumor-related symptoms include dragging pain, palpable mass in the abdomen, acute pain due to bleeding or rupture, abdominal fullness, low-grade fever, obstructive jaundice, and splenomegaly. Paraneoplastic syndromes, although rare, can also occur and include hypercholesterolemia, erythrocytosis, hypercalcemia, and hypoglycemia. The history of risk factors associated with HCC should be elicited along with a detailed clinical examination to document the signs of underlying liver disease, such as jaundice, ascites, ankle oedema, spider angiomata on the anterior chest wall, palmar erythema, splenomegaly, increasing abdominal girth, and weight loss. Evaluation of the abdomen for liver size, the existence of tumor masses, tenderness, and abdominal bruit should also be included.

1.3.1 Pathology

Three gross morphologic types of HCC have been identified: nodular, massive, and diffuse. Nodular HCC is often associated with cirrhosis and is characterized by well-circumscribed nodules. The massive type of HCC, usually associated with a non-cirrhotic liver, occupies a large area with or without satellite nodules in the surrounding liver. The less common diffuse type is characterized by diffuse hepatic involvement with many small, indistinct tumour nodules throughout the liver.

Histologic classification of malignant tumors of the liver includes HCC (conventional type), HCC (fibrolamellar variant), cholangiocarcinoma (intrahepatic bile duct carcinoma), mixed hepatocellular cholangiocarcinoma, undifferentiated carcinoma, and hepatoblastoma. The fibrolamellar variant of HCC has a relatively better prognosis. It occurs more frequently in adolescents or young adults and has a more indolent clinical course than conventional HCC. Hepatoblastoma occurs most commonly in young children (median age, 13–16 months) and usually presents in an advanced stage.

1.4 Diagnostic Tests and Staging

The workup includes investigations of the etiologic origin of liver disease, a hepatitis panel for detection of hepatitis B and/or C viral infection (i.e., HBsAg, hepatitis B surface antibody, hepatitis B core antibody [HBcAb], HBcAb IgM) an assessment of the presence of comorbidity; imaging studies to detect the presence of metastatic disease, and an evaluation of hepatic function, including a determination of whether portal hypertension is present. A summary of various tests and staging is described in Table 1.

Table 1 Diagnostic workup and staging

Diagnostic workup
Blood tests
HBsAg, HBcAb IgG, and HCV antibodies, and estimation of viral load if positive
Complete blood count (pancytopenia, especially low platelet count, is a surrogate of portal hypertension)
Urea and creatinine
Liver function tests, prothrombin time (PT), and international normalized ratio (INR)
Alfa fetoprotein (AFP)
Radiology
Contrast-enhanced multi-phasic liver protocol CT scan
Contrast-enhanced MRI (complementary to CT for equivocal CT findings)
CT Thorax
Bone scan if clinically indicated.
Histopathological assessment
A biopsy confirmation is not required unless the radiological and biochemical findings are equivocal

1.4.1 Alfa-Fetoprotein (AFP)

Although routinely used as a tumor marker, it is not a sensitive or specific diagnostic test for HCC.

Serum levels >400 ng/mL are observed only in a small percentage of patients with HCC, and in some series, close to half of the patients can have normal serum AFP levels <20 ng/mL. In patients with chronic liver disease, an elevated AFP could be more indicative of HCC than in non-infected patients. When used in conjunction with imaging results showing the presence of a growing liver mass has been shown to have a high positive predictive value for HCC. The diagnostic accuracy of an absolute AFP cutoff value has not been validated in this setting, and such values may vary by institution and patient population. Other conditions with elevated AFP include pregnancy, intrahepatic cholangiocarcinoma, some metastases from colon cancer, lymphoma, and germ cell tumors.

1.4.2 Imaging

The diagnostic HCC imaging involves the use of multiphasic liver protocol CT with multiphasic (e.g., pre-contrast, arterial phase, portal venous phase, delayed) intravenous contrast-enhanced (Gadolinium) MRI. The classic imaging profile associated with an HCC lesion is characterized by intense arterial uptake or enhancement followed by contrast washout or hypointensity in the delayed nonperipheral venous phase.

The LI-RADS (Liver imaging and Reporting Data Systems) criteria and scoring are used for radiological diagnosis of HCC [5]. The LI-RADS criteria are applicable only to those with cirrhosis, and a biopsy may be necessary for patients without any history of liver disease. Finding classical arterial enhancement using a single imaging technique is sufficient to diagnose HCC in patients with cirrhosis and liver nodules between 1 and 2 cm detected during surveillance, thereby reducing the need for a biopsy. It also considers enhancing capsule appearance and threshold growth compared to previous imaging as part of the diagnosis using CT or MRI imaging.

Positron emission tomography (PET)/CT has been used to evaluate extrahepatic metastases;

however, it is not as sensitive as multiphasic liver CT or MR for evaluating the hepatic extent of the disease.

1.4.3 Evaluation of Hepatic Reserve

The Child-Pugh (CP) classification incorporates laboratory measurements (i.e. serum albumin, bilirubin, PT) as well as more subjective clinical assessments of encephalopathy and ascites and classifies cirrhosis as compensated (class A) or decompensated (classes B and C) cirrhosis [6]. The CP scores are used for treatment decision making on appropriateness of local therapy (surgical resection radiotherapy, or interventional chemoembolization or radioembolization).

The Model for End-Stage Liver Disease (MELD) is a numerical scale ranging from 6 (less ill) to 40 (gravely ill) for individuals 12 years or older, derived from serum bilirubin, creatinine, and INR [7]. It allows a wider score range and takes into account renal function. However, it is currently unclear whether the MELD score is superior to the Child-Pugh score as a predictor of survival in patients with liver cirrhosis.

For local therapies, the future liver remnant can be calculated on a diagnostic CT. Hepatic functional reserve before hepatic resection in patients with cirrhosis may also be performed with different tools such as US and MRI elastography (which may provide and quantify the degree of cirrhosis-related fibrosis), non-focal liver biopsy, and transjugular liver biopsy with pressure measurements.

The indocyanine green (ICG) clearance test is used for the assessment of liver function before hepatic resection in patients with cirrhosis [8]. The ICG retention rate at 15 min (ICGR-15) after intravenous injection for the assessment of liver function prior to surgery is generally recommended.

1.4.4 Staging Systems

Several staging systems include all parameters from other staging systems as well as additional parameters. The AJCC staging system provides information on the pathologic characteristics of resected specimens only. The Okuda system incorporates aspects of liver function and tumour characteristics [9]. The Barcelona Clinic Liver Cancer (BCLC) staging system is the most widely used system for HCC, incorporating the Okuda system, Child-Pugh Score and performance status (Table 2).

Table 2 The Barcelona- Clinic Liver Cancer (BCLC) Staging System

Stage	Criteria
0—Very early	Child-Pugh class A Single <2 cm nodule ECOG PS 0
A—Early	Child-Pugh class A–B Single or two to three nodules <3 cm ECOG PS 0
B—Intermediate	Child-Pugh class A–B Multinodular ECOG PS 0
C—Advanced	Child-Pugh class A–B Portal vein invasion, N1, M1 ECOG PS 0–2
D—Terminal	Child-Pugh class C Any T, N, or M ECOG PS > 2

ECOG PS Eastern Cooperative Oncology Group Performance Status

1.5 Integrated Management Plan

1.5.1 Surgical Aspects

The treatment of choice for resectable HCC in patients without cirrhosis is surgical resection [10]. This is also the favored treatment for patients without clinically significant portal hypertension in Child-Pugh class A liver disease. For those patients with clinically significant portal hypertension and some hepatic decompensation, but with tumors within the Milan criteria (1 tumor up to 5 cm or up to 3 lesions with largest <3 cm), liver transplantation is the preferred option [11, 12].

Resectability is determined by anatomical considerations (the number and location of lesions), the hepatic reserve (volume of liver that will remain after the anticipated resection), and underlying hepatic function. There is no strict size cutoff if the other criteria are satisfactory. If the residual liver volume is anticipated to be small, preoperative portal vein embolization can be considered to increase the size of the contralateral lobe by 20–25% in 4–6 weeks and reduce the risk of hepatic insufficiency [13].

For tumors less than 2 cm, resection is associated with better overall and recurrence-free survival compared to ablation, as demonstrated in the meta-analysis of randomized controlled trials. Ablation may be preferable in patients with borderline functional status with deeply located tumors [14].

The risk of recurrence following resection depends on multiple factors: differentiation, vascular invasion, and presence of satellite nodules, but not independently on the size of tumor [15]. Direct-acting antiviral therapy may reduce recurrence after resection, but no other adjuvant systemic therapy is known to reduce recurrence after surgical treatment. The risk of recurrence following liver transplant is approximately 70% at 5 years. The results of liver transplant are very encouraging, but the difficulty in finding a donor limits the wider applicability of this treatment.

1.5.2 Percutaneous Ablation

Percutaneous ablation is a method of destroying tumor cells modifying the temperature (with radiofrequency, microwave, laser, or cryotherapy) or by the injection of chemical substances (e.g. ethanol or acetic acid). For HCCs <2 cm, percutaneous ethanol injection achieves a necrosis rate greater than 90% but this method is much less effective for larger lesions [16]. Radiofrequency ablation (RFA) involves the local application of radiofrequency thermal energy to the lesion. Optimal candidates are those with a single tumor >2 and <4 cm in diameter. RFA provides superior local disease control and survival compared to ethanol [14, 17].

1.5.3 Transcatheter Arterial Chemoembolization

The excellent arterial supply of HCCs not only serves as the basis for its radiological diagnosis, it can also be translated into a therapeutic option in the form of arterial embolization. Transarterial chemoembolization (TACE) involves, first, the selective injection of chemotherapeutic agents through arteries feeding the tumor followed by intra-arterial embolization of tumor-feeding arteries with lipiodol (an iodized oily contrast agent), Gelfoam, or plastic particles. TACE has been shown to improve survival outcomes, and has currently been accepted as a standard treatment for unresectable multicentric or relapsed disease [18]. Another advantage is that it can be used selectively in different segments and can be performed in a phased manner.

1.5.4 Systemic Therapy Aspects

Systemic therapy plays an important role in the management of HCC. Patients with transplant ineligible or not amenable for locoregional therapy including unresectable HCC constitutes BCLC (Barcelona Clinic Liver Cancer) stage--C/D and of these those with BCLC stage-C are potential candidates for systemic therapy in first line. Sorafenib was the first drug approved for the management of HCC, based on the results of SHARP trial demonstrating a survival benefit over placebo (median: 10.7 vs 7.9 months; Hazard ratio [HR]: 0.69; 95% Confidence interval [CI]: 0.55–0.87; $p < 0.001$) [19]. In 2018, Lenvatinib was approved in the first line based on a non-inferiority trial with a different adverse event profile [20]. However, in the era of immunotherapy, HCC being no exception, combination of Atezolizumab (immune check-point inhibitor, specifically PD-L1 inhibitor drug) with bevacizumab (anti-angiogenic VEGF inhibitor drug) was found to have superior median survival over sorafenib (19.2 vs 13.4 months; HR: 0.66, 95% CI: 0.52–0.85) [21].

Second-line therapy can be offered to patients progressing on first-line treatment with preserved performance status. Sequencing of agents in the second line is governed by agents used in the first line setting. Options available include multikinase inhibitors (Regorafenib, Cabozantinib, Ramucirumab, and Apatinib) and immunotherapy (Nivolumab plus Ipilimumab and Pembrolizumab) [22].

Chemotherapy usage in advanced HCC is obsolete nowadays. However, patients progressing on second-line therapy with preserved hepatic functions can be given an option of combination chemotherapy [22]. Various combination regimens tried include gemcitabine-based regimen, fluoropyrimidines-based regimens, and cisplatin-based regimens. However, benefit derived with chemotherapy if any at all is short-lived.

In the adjuvant setting, currently there is no role of systemic therapy following hepatic resection, liver transplant or locoregional therapy and observation is the current standard of care [23]. Following encouraging results in advanced disease, immunotherapeutic agents are being explored in the adjuvant setting. Checkmate 9DX trial is evaluating the potential role of adjuvant nivolumab following surgical resection or ablative therapy. Similarly, IMbrave-050 trial is exploring the role of a combination of atezolizumab and bevacizumab in the adjuvant setting.

1.6 Radiation Therapy

HCC is a radiosensitive tumor. The major drawback is the poor radiation tolerance of the adjacent normal liver and the difficulty of tumor localization. Recent technological and conceptual developments in the field of radiation therapy, such as intensity-modulated radiation therapy, image-guided radiation therapy, respiratory gating, and stereotactic body radiation therapy (SBRT), have raised the potential and feasibility of radiation treatment. By conforming the delivery of radiation dose distribution closer to the tumor or target volume outlined more accurately, radiotherapy can result in sparing more normal liver tissue from high-dose radiation. For patients with liver-confined disease treated with conformal radiotherapy with or without TACE, local control response rates ranged from 40% to 90%, and the median survival ranged from 10 to 25 months.

1.6.1 Dose-Limiting Organs

The tumor response to radiotherapy and survival of patients with HCC are related to the dose delivered. Before the era of conformal radiotherapy, the dose of radiation treatment was limited to <30 to 40 Gy for hepatic toxicity; as a result, partial response was usually <30%. Seong et al. reported an objective tumor-specific response rate of 67% after a mean dose of 51.8 ± 7.9 Gy for patients who failed TACE and were treated with conformal radiotherapy [24].

Dawson et al. escalated radiation doses for unresectable hepatobiliary cancer and observed that patients who received radiation doses >70 Gy had better median survival (>16.4 months) [25]. It appears that the higher the radiation doses given, the better the tumor response seen. However, caution should be given in HBV-related HCC, and local radiotherapy may cause deterioration of liver function by radiation-induced liver disease (RILD), portal hypertension, and HBV reactivation. To fend off HBV reactivation, prophylactic anti-HBV treatment should be considered. The optimal dose and fractionation are based on the volume of liver irradiated, nonirradiated liver reserve, baseline liver function, and proximity of tumor to luminal gastrointestinal tissues. The major dose-limiting organ for RT to the hepatobiliary system is the liver.

Radiation-induced liver disease (RILD) is separated into "classic" and "nonclassic" RILD. Classic RILD presents with anicteric hepatomegaly and ascites, typically occurring between 2 weeks and 3 months after RT or CRT, with an elevated alkaline phosphatase. Nonclassic RILD is more challenging to prevent and includes any liver toxicity occurring within 3 months of radiation (e.g., decline in Child-Pugh score or elevated liver enzymes). It is more likely in patients with baseline cirrhosis or CP-B or CP-C liver disease. For patients with RILD, restaging, possible paracentesis of the ascitic fluid to rule out disease relapse, and referral to hepatology are recommended. RILD has been treated with diuretics, steroids, and occasionally anticoagulation.

The risk for RILD is dependent on the volume of liver irradiated (or volume of liver spared from RT). For CP-A patients, whole-liver RT to a total dose less than 28 Gy in 2-Gy fractions has a low risk of toxicity, whereas 36 Gy in 2-Gy fractions is associated with a 50% risk of toxicity [26]. With conformal RT planning, far higher doses can be delivered to partial liver volumes safely. For standard fractionation, it is recommended that the mean liver dose be less than 28 Gy for patients with CP-A liver function. For SBRT, it has been recommended to maximize the volume of liver spared from RT (e.g., >700 cc to receive <15 Gy in three to five fractions) [27]. Effective liver volume irradiated (Veff) or mean dose to the liver (minus the GTV) has also been used to allocate dose for SBRT.

Patients with CP-B or CP-C are at far higher risk for liver toxicity given their baseline liver dysfunction and expected poor liver reserve. For patients with CP-B treated with four to six fractions, the mean liver dose should be kept as low as possible (very conservative threshold of <6 Gy, absolute dose constraint <16 Gy) [27]. Patients with CP-B7 fare better than those who are CP-B8 or higher. As previously noted, median survival after radiation for greater than or equal to CP-B8 was less than 3 months; radiation should be used with extreme caution for these patients.

Lawrence et al. developed a normal tissue Complication probability (NTCP) model of radiotherapy for intrahepatic malignancy [28]. Based on this model, authors have designed a protocol in which each patient receives maximum tolerated doses of radiation with no more than 10% risk of RILD. Thus, the mean doses that can be delivered according to this protocol are 56.6 ± 2.31 Gy (range, 40.5–81 Gy). Using this dosing range, they observed a reduction of radiation injury to 4.8% (95% confidence interval, 0–23.8%). This model, however, was derived using patients with relatively normal liver function, and only 4 of 21 in their study population had HCC. The NTCP model for patients with impaired liver function still requires further evaluation. For patients with cirrhosis but within Child-Pugh grade A functional classification, the mean dose of hepatic radiation tolerated for a normal liver is 23 Gy [29]. The authors suggested a dose–volume histogram for irradiation to normal liver where the irradiated hepatic volume over 10, 20, 30, and 40 Gy should be <68%, 49%, 28%, and 20%, respectively. Multivariate analyses demonstrated that the severity of hepatic cirrhosis was the only independent predictor for radiation-induced liver disease.

The QUANTEC guidelines recommend 28 and 32 Gy as mean dose to the liver for therapeutic partial liver RT using standard fractionation. For SBRT in three fractions, the corresponding doses are 13 and 15 Gy. For SBRT in five fractions, these doses are 18 and 20 Gy. The dose constraints should be tighter for patients with CP-B disease, where a mean dose of 6 Gy is recommended. Critical volume-based constraints recommended are that more than 700 cc of the liver should receive ≤15 Gy in three to five fractions [27]. These recommendations have since been validated by more recent reports and summaries [30].

The luminal gastrointestinal structures, such as bowel, stomach, and duodenum, often limit the safe dose that may be delivered to hepatobiliary cancers in proximity to them, and usual constraints may be followed for safe delivery as usual. Biliary radiation toxicity is more common in cholangiocarcinoma and may lead to biloma and/or cholangitis as a late complication. There are increased risks of strictures with SBRT or brachytherapy to the central biliary tract (contoured as a 1.5-cm expansion of the porta). Dose constraints to biliary tract are an evolving domain, and practitioners should use current guidelines based on consensus documents or ongoing clinical trials to select appropriate values [31, 32].

1.6.2 Planning and Delivery

For proper target delineation, triphasic arterial, venous, and delayed phase CT or MR images should be obtained and fused if possible with deformable systems. The gross target volume (GTV) should include the entire enhancing parenchymal tumor and vascular lesion. The clinical target volume (CTV) should include the GTV as well as any immediately adjacent regions at risk, such as a prior ablation cavity or prior TACE zone. Care is needed to ensure delineation of the entire extent of vascular involvement, if present, often best seen on delayed-phase imaging. Respiratory motion should be assessed at the time of simulation, either via four-dimensional CT or fluoroscopic assessment. Lesions with movement greater than 1 cm in any direction should be strongly considered for respiratory motion management to allow the planning target volume (PTV) to be reduced, sparing more non-tumor liver and reducing the risk of toxicity. Voluntary breath-hold, active breathing control (ABC), gating the beam to a specified phase of the respiration cycle, respiratory tracking, and abdominal compression are common strategies used to reduce the impact of respiratory motion. Measuring the reproducibility of breath-hold or patient-specific tumor motion is important for individualized ITV creation. Four-dimensional CT, kV fluoroscopy, and cine MR can be used to measure liver (or tumor) motion. Typical PTV margins for breath-hold or gated patients treated with image-guided radiotherapy (IGRT) are 5–10 mm but depend on patient and setup factors, including the reliability of immobilization and respiratory management.

Three-dimensional conformal RT, arc therapy, IMRT, volumetric arc therapy (VMAT), and particle therapy have all been used to treat intrahepatic tumors, including HCC and IHCC. Planning goals are a conformal plan that covers the PTV with the prescription isodose (e.g., to 95% PTV) and maintains dose limits to the luminal GI structures and other critical organs as discussed in previous sections. Less conformality may be acceptable in situations in which dose reduction to a cirrhotic liver takes precedence.

IGRT is crucial to account for shifts in the liver position that may occur day to day, despite the use of breathing motion management. Such shifts occur even when breathing motion is of a small magnitude, providing rationale for the use of daily soft-tissue-guided IGRT. Radiopaque fiducial markers (if placed) or serendipitous Lipiodol from prior TACE treatment may be used with two-dimensional planar kV imaging, fluoroscopy, or cone beam CT (CBCT) for targeting. The liver contour itself can be used for guidance using CBCT; accuracy is improved with breath-hold and four-dimensional respiratory sorted CBCT.

1.6.3 Acute and Late Complications

The dose-limiting tissue injuries in radiation treatment for HCC include the liver, stomach, duodenum, bowels, and kidneys. Acute complications include general fatigue, transient elevation of liver function test, and nausea and vomiting (mainly for tumors in the left lobe of the liver), fever, and pancytopenia. Subacute and late complications include hepatic failure, radiation pneumonitis, and gastrointestinal bleeding (caution should especially be given in tumor located in the inferior portion of the right lobe of the liver where the duodenum and jejunum are nearby and radiation doses plan to give more than 50 Gy). Hepatic failure can be avoided by limiting the radiation dose to the organs at risk as mentioned above.

1.7 Follow-Up

After transplant, partial hepatectomy, or locoregional therapy, imaging, and AFP are recommended every 3–6 months for 2 years, and then every 6–12 months. Imaging should be triphasic, in the same modality (CT or MRI) from diagnosis, so that changes can be followed longitudinally. Given the often multifocal nature of HCC, the treated lesion should be assessed and there should be careful vigilance for new liver lesions. Response Evaluation Criteria InSolid Tumors (RECIST) or a modified version of RECIST (mRECIST) is commonly used; special attention is needed in post-SBRT, as there are complex changes in the tumor and surrounding liver parenchyma expected [33]. The treated lesion may not measurably shrink but is expected to no longer arterially enhance. RECIST and mRECIST systems have positive predicted value >76% but poor negative predictive value. This is similar for other response grading systems, such as the World Health Organization (WHO) and European Association for the Study of the Liver (EASL) criteria.

1.8 Prognosis, Results and Outcome, Survival

Survival of HCC with various treatments depends largely on the clinical stage and liver function. Five-year survival in resectable HCC after partial hepatectomy is 50–73% in stage I patients, 30–56% in stage II patients, 10–29% in stage III patients, and approximately 10% in stage IV patients. The 5-year survival for patients with unresectable HCC is usually <10%. The major cause of failure after resection is tumor recurrence within the liver. Extrahepatic metastasis in advanced HCC has become more frequently encountered in recent years, probably related to improvements in control and survival from intrahepatic disease.

1.9 Future Research Needed

Modern treatment advances—including complex dose calculations, homogeneity corrections, target delineation, respiratory motion assessment/management, image-guided treatment, and highly conformal treatment planning—permit the delivery of higher doses of RT for hepatobiliary cancers than would have been possible using standard techniques. However, there remain many unanswered questions and research opportunities to improve the management of these aggressive cancers.

The appropriate balance of tumor control with liver toxicity in a background of cirrhosis may require improved functional liver imaging and enhanced posttreatment evaluation techniques. Novel treatments for liver toxicity and regeneration medicine are the next frontier for collaboration between oncologists, basic scientists, and hepatologists. Striving for the minimum RT dose required for LC with a low chance of toxicity is an important goal. Although it is becoming apparent that HCC is a relatively RT-sensitive tumor, the most appropriate doses and dose fractionations are still not well defined. Collaborative efforts will be required to obtain evidence demonstrating the best treatment options for patients, risk factors for relapse and toxicity, optimal doses and fractionation schedules, and how to most appropriately combine RT with other regional and systemic therapies. Despite the growing literature on the use of RT for hepatobiliary cancer, there is a dearth of level 1 evidence. Multiple ongoing randomized trials are enrolling to provide evidence for the changing treatment paradigm of hepatobiliary cancer. Results from these studies will help guide treatment decisions for a wide range of patients, from locally advanced HCC (RTOG 1112) to unresectable IHCC (NRG G1001) and palliative liver radiation (NCT02511522).

2 Biliary Cancers

Gallbladder cancer (GBC) is the most common cancer of the biliary tract region. It ranks sixth among gastrointestinal cancers.

In 2020, there were an estimated 115,949 new cases of GBC worldwide (ranking 25th out of 36 cancers in 185 countries) [1]. GBC incidence also increases with age. In Delhi, India, the age-adjusted incidence rates increased from less than 1/100,000 in individuals below 30 years of age to a peak of 43.7 and 24.0/100,000 in women and men, respectively, aged 70–74 years. The average age at diagnosis is ~20 years younger in India than in Western countries [34].

2.1 Anatomical Concepts for GBC

The gallbladder lies on the undersurface of the liver. It drains via the cystic duct into the common hepatic duct and then forms the common bile duct. The gallbladder consists of a discontinuous muscle layer with no muscular mucosa, and ~30% of its surface is attached to the liver; the peritoneum covers the rest. The wall of the gallbladder has a mucosa, a smooth muscle layer, perimuscular connective tissue, and serosa. There is an absence of serosa along the attachment to the liver. In this region, the perimuscular connective tissue is continuous with the connective tissue of the liver. For GBC, the T stage classification depends on the depth of tumor penetration into the wall of the GB, tumor invasion into the liver, hepatic artery, or portal vein, and on adjacent organ involvement.

2.2 Pathology and Risk Factors

Adenocarcinoma is the most frequent histological type, representing 90% of cases. Other subtypes, such as squamous, undifferentiated, mucinous, and neuroendocrine carcinomas, are less common. Most gallbladder cancers (GBCs) develop in the setting of cholelithiasis following a metaplasia–dysplasia–carcinoma sequence. Gallstones and pro-inflammatory lithogenic bile, and possibly bacterial infections, enable continuous cycles of epithelium destruction and regeneration, leading to a long-standing chronic inflammatory response that promotes malignant transformation and tumor progression. Risk factors for GBC include age (max in seventh decade of life) and women gender. GBC also has an association with GB stones [35]. Body mass index (BMI) has also been associated with an increased risk of gallbladder cancer. An important driver of GBC is Long-standing chronic inflammation, regardless of the lithiasis or non-lithiasis origin. Gallbladder cancer is also associated with a shorter median survival duration, a much shorter time to recurrence, and a shorter survival duration after recurrence than hilar cholangiocarcinoma [36].

2.3 Symptoms

GBC does not have an effective screening strategy, nor do patients generally have early or specific Often, right hypochondrial pain may be the only symptom. Some patients present with obstructive jaundice. A significant portion of patients are diagnosed with incidental malignancy after cholecystectomy.

2.4 Diagnosis and Imaging

Ultrasonography (USG) is the most frequently utilized imaging modality for biliary pathology. The main disadvantage is user dependency. Suggestive features include gallbladder wall thickening, calcifications, mass or soft tissue density interrupting the mucosa, and architectural ambiguity at the gallbladder-liver interface. Endoscopic ultrasound is a technique modification, which can also be used to do fine needle aspiration cytology (FNAC) of a suspicious area. Computed tomography (CT) may provide specific information about the extent of local disease and define the advanced or distant disease. Magnetic resonance imaging (MRI) is another useful diagnostic modality in the preoperative evaluation of suspected GBC. This modality is especially good in outlining carcinoma invasion into adjacent live and surrounding soft tissues. Specifically, MRI can help distinguish the extent of invasion of adjacent biliary structures, obstruction or dilation of these, and also help define the extrahepatic disease. For patients presenting with jaundice, additional workup should include Magnetic resonance cholangiopancreatography (MRCP) may better clarify the extent of biliary pathology and help guide operative management. Noninvasive magnetic resonance cholangiography (MRCP) is preferred over endoscopic retrograde cholangiopancreatography (ERCP). Fluorodeoxyglucose positron emission tomography (PET) has evolved to become an important modality in GBC. It is capable of confirming the extent of local and regional disease, including nodal involvement and distant metastasis. CEA and CA 19-9 testing could be considered as part of the initial workup (in conjunction with imaging studies). Elevated serum CEA levels (>4.0 ng/mL) or CA 19-9 levels (>20.0 units/mL) could be suggestive of gallbladder cancer [37]. However, these markers are not specific to gallbladder cancer, and CA 19-9 could also be elevated in patients with jaundice from other causes.

2.5 Staging and Prognosis

In the current AJCC (8th edition) staging system, gallbladder cancer is classified into four stages based on the depth of invasion into the gallbladder wall and the extent of spread to surrounding organs and lymph nodes. T2 gallbladder carcinoma has now been subdivided into two groups: tumors on the peritoneal side (T2a) and tumors on the hepatic side (T2b). This is based on retrospective studies suggesting worse outcomes for GBC located on the hepatic side as compared to the peritoneal side [38]. Gallbladder cancer (GBC) is characterized by a very poor prognosis when diagnosed at advanced stages. This is related to several factors, including its insidious nature, late presentation, intrinsic aggressive nature, as well as limited treatment options [39]. Further, GBC spreads early by (1) lymphatic or (2) hematogenous metastasis and by direct invasion into the liver.

3 Management

3.1 Surgery

3.1.1 Surgical Aspects

Margin-negative surgical resection is the only potentially curative treatment; most of these patients are locally unresectable or have distant disease at the time of diagnosis.

The surgical management of gallbladder cancer is significantly dependent on the circumstances in which it is diagnosed [40–42]. Whereas the majority of these patients are diagnosed incidentally, the final histopathological stage dictates the further resection strategy.

In T1a lesions, the cholecystectomy suffices with 5-year survival in the range of 97–99%, whereas in T1b lesions the incidence of residual disease in periportal nodes and gallbladder bed is in the range of 15–20%, mandating completion cholecystectomy with portal lymphadenectomy. Bile duct resection is required if the cystic duct margin is positive to attain a negative margin resection. T2 lesions are managed similarly to T1b lesions.

In locally advanced gallbladder cancer patients, a selected subset of patients with non-progression of local disease following neoadjuvant treatment may benefit from surgical resections that may include major hepatic and/or bile duct resections to achieve margin-negative resections. In patients where there is intraoperative suspicion of gallbladder cancer, the diagnosis should be confirmed on frozen section examination, and if skill permits, a complete en bloc resection of the gallbladder with segment IVb and V of the liver, and a portal lymphadenectomy should be done at the same operation. Sometimes more extensive liver resection or bile duct resection may be needed to obtain a margin-negative resection.

For perihilar cholangiocarcinomas, despite staging refinements, up to a third are either unresectable or metastatic. Only patients in whom both arterial and portal inflow to the hepatic remnant can be preserved should proceed with resection. Individualized patients with limited vascular involvement of the inflow to the hepatic remnant, particularly involvement of the portal vein, are selected for concomitant resection and reconstruction at experienced and high-volume cholangiocarcinoma centers. The role of arterial resection and reconstruction is controversial, and consistent success has been reported only at select high-volume centers. Complete tumor extirpation usually consists of complete hepatoduodenal ligament lymphadenectomy (including cystic, peri-choledochal, peri-portal, and retroportal, hepatic artery, hilar, and superior pancreaticoduodenal lymph nodes), resection of the entire extrahepatic bile duct from the hepatic hilus to the pancreas with the attached gallbladder, and concomitant liver resection of the ipsilateral hepatic lobe. The biliary system is subsequently reconstructed using a Roux-en-Y hepaticojejunostomy [43–45].

Right- or left-sided hemihepatectomy is indicated in hilar cholangiocarcinoma- type IIIa tumors and IV tumors based on the location [46]. Concomitant caudate lobe resection yields better R0 resection rates and higher cumulative survival rates. Wider resection margins (margins greater than 5 mm) are associated with better disease-free and overall survival as compared to patients with R1 resection [47]. Patients with certain unresectability criteria are candidates for liver transplantation [48].

Distal cholangiocarcinoma involves the pancreatic portion of the common bile duct and accounts for 30–40% of cholangiocarcinomas. Given the location, pancreaticoduodenectomy is the treatment of choice. Among the periampullary cancers, distal cholangiocarcinomas are associated with higher rates of locoregional failure and relatively poorer prognosis. Pancreaticoduodenectomy with mesopancreatic triangle resection is recommended to optimize the locoregional clearance [49].

3.1.2 Systemic Therapy Aspects

Surgical resection remains the mainstay of management of biliary tract cancers with curative potential. In general, bile duct cancer is more aggressive with poorer survival compared to GBC. For patients of gallbladder cancer with tumor ≥T1b adjuvant chemotherapy is recommended. Whereas, all patients with cholangiocarcinoma should receive adjuvant chemotherapy. For adjuvant setting approved agents include single agent capecitabine, gemcitabine, or a combination of the two [50, 51]. Patients with locally advanced unresectable disease can be converted to resectable disease with platinum-based neoadjuvant chemotherapy.

Management principles of unresectable and metastatic disease are similar for both gallbladder cancer and cholangiocarcinoma. A combination of gemcitabine with either cisplatin or oxaliplatin is the usual first line chemotherapy choice [52, 53]. In cases with biliary obstruction fluoro-pyrimidine-based chemotherapy is an alternative [54]. TOPAZ-1 trial demonstrated a marginal survival benefit (median overall survival [OS]: 12.8 vs. 11.5 months, hazard ratio [HR]: 0.8, 95% confidence interval [CI] 0.66–0.97) of the addition of Durvalumab to chemotherapy in first-line setting [55].

Following progression on first-line treatment, further treatment is governed by previous agents used and availability of targetable markers and performance status of the patient [56]. All patients should be offered next-generation sequencing (NGS) and mismatch repair status testing. Patients with mismatch repair-deficient (dMMR) can benefit with Pembrolizumab [57]. Ivosidenib an isocitrate dehydrogenase-1 (IDH-1) inhibitor is approved in IDH-1 mutated cholangiocarcinoma in second line or beyond setting [58]. Other potentially targetable markers include TRK fusions, BRAF V600E mutation, HER2 over-expression, and EGFR mutations.

3.2 Radiotherapy

The main sites of isolated locoregional recurrence in GBC are hilum, anastomotic site, resection margin of the liver, and the retroperitoneal lymph nodes. The postoperative radiotherapy volumes must include the tumor bed and the regional lymph nodes. The regional lymph nodes must include the porta hepatis, celiac, para-aortic, and pancreaticoduodenal nodes. The CTV primary includes the GB fossa as evident in the preoperative CECT image and the surgical clips with 1 cm isotropic expansion. A dose of 45 Gy/25#/5 weeks is acceptable. A boost of 5.4 Gy may be considered in an R1 resection. A boost of 15 Gy may be given in cases of gross residual lesions.

Hyder et al. analyzed the SEER database to define the role of adjuvant radiotherapy for GBC. The authors identified 5011 patients with GBC who underwent surgical resection. 75% had localized disease. Only 17.9% of patients received adjuvant radiation. Adjuvant radiation was generally used for a younger age, tumor extension beyond the serosa, intermediate to poorly differentiated tumors, and patients with lymph node metastasis. In a propensity-matched multivariate analysis, the authors reported significantly improved 1-year survival with the use of adjuvant radiotherapy. The survival benefit was more pronounced for N1 disease and moderately-poorly differentiated tumors. However, the benefit was not significant at 5 years [59].

For patient with a positive surgical margin, the options include (1) Fluoropyrimidine-based chemoradiation and (2) Fluoropyrimidine- or gemcitabine-based chemotherapy followed by fluoropyrimidine-based chemoradiation. In routine post-operative cases, the role of radiation therapy as adjuvant therapy for GBC is not well defined. A series of 21 patients from a high-volume center concluded that the addition of EBRT to 5-FU following R0 resection, with no evidence of residual disease, exhibited a 5-year survival (all stages of disease included) of 64%, whereas 5-year survival was 0% in patients with evidence of residual disease. Additionally, these authors reported 100% 5-year local control rates with high-dose EBRT (>54 Gy) [60]. These studies do not provide definitive evidence for everyday use. High-quality randomized trials are needed to evaluate the benefit of adjuvant radiation for GBC.

The phase II SWOG S0809 trial included patients with extrahepatic cholangiocarcinoma or gallbladder cancer (*N* = 79). This trial provided prospective data for adjuvant chemotherapy/chemoradiotherapy (concurrent chemoradiotherapy with capecitabine after capecitabine/gemcitabine chemotherapy). The 2-year survival rate was 65%, with a median survival time of 35 months. Most patients (86%) who participated in the trial completed the treatment, indicating that the regimen was generally tolerable [61, 62]. But gemcitabine concurrent chemoradiotherapy is not recommended because of its limited experience and side effects. A prospective study including 28 patients with locally advanced gallbladder cancer showed that an R0 resection was achieved in 14 patients, with good local control (93%) and 5-year survival (47%), following treatment with gemcitabine with concurrent RT [63].

In the absence of phase III data, it is challenging to get level-I evidence for adjuvant radiotherapy. Radiotherapy may be used as an adjuvant therapy in resected cases of GBC when the surgical margins are involved, or in cases of locoregionally advanced disease. It must be combined with chemotherapy in all feasible patients to strengthen local control and reduce distant recurrences.

MSI, mismatch repair (MMR), and tumor mutational burden (TMB) (defined as ≥10 mutations/megabase), 554 testing should be performed on biopsied tumor tissue, as cancers with MSI-H, dMMR, and TMB-high (TMB-H) may benefit from programmed death receptor-1 (PD-1) blockade such as pembrolizumab [57].

For unresectable diseases, the treatment options include palliative chemotherapy, palliative radiotherapy, and best supportive care, based on the general condition of the patient and liver function parameters.

3.3 Follow-Up

For follow-up of patients, one can consider imaging every 3–6 months for 2 years and with increasing intervals. CEA and CA 19-9 analyses can be considered clinically indicated.

3.4 Future

Further work needs to be done to understand next-generation sequencing and multidisciplinary care for GBC. Neoadjuvant and adjuvant strategies need to be pragmatically designed. Novel systemic therapies, including chemotherapy and immunotherapies, are changing the treatment paradigm and prognosis of this challenging disease.

Cholangiocarcinoma

Cholangiocarcinoma (CCA) is a malignant epithelial tumor arising from the biliary tract and represents one of the most aggressive hepatobiliary malignancies. Although historically considered rare, the global incidence and mortality of CCA have increased steadily over the past two decades, particularly for intrahepatic cholangiocarcinoma (iCCA) [64, 65]. CCA accounts for approximately 10–15% of primary liver cancers and nearly 3% of gastrointestinal malignancies, with marked geographic variation in incidence and etiology [64].

Classification and Epidemiology

According to the current World Health Organization and ICD-11 classification, CCA is categorized based on anatomical origin into intrahepatic (iCCA), perihilar (pCCA), and distal (dCCA) subtypes [64]. This classification reflects differences in risk factors, molecular profiles, clinical behaviour, and therapeutic strategies. iCCA arises from bile ducts proximal to the second-order branches within the liver, whereas pCCA and dCCA originate from the extrahepatic biliary tree. Despite anatomical and biological differences, all subtypes share an overall poor prognosis, largely due to late-stage diagnosis and limited curative treatment options [64, 66].

In Western countries, the majority of cases are sporadic, with no identifiable predisposing condition. In contrast, in Southeast Asia, chronic infection with liver flukes such as Opisthorchis viverrini and Clonorchis sinensis remains a major aetiological factor [64, 65]. Other established risk factors include primary sclerosing cholangitis (PSC), choledochal cysts, hepatolithiasis, chronic viral hepatitis (HBV and HCV), cirrhosis, and metabolic dysfunction–associated steatotic liver disease [64, 67]. Patients with PSC carry a particularly high lifetime risk, and CCA is a leading cause of mortality in this population [64].

Clinical Presentation and Diagnosis

CCA often develops insidiously and remains asymptomatic until advanced stages. Common presenting symptoms include weight loss, fatigue, abdominal pain, and anorexia, while obstructive jaundice is more frequently observed in pCCA and dCCA due to bile duct involvement [64, 66]. Laboratory findings typically demonstrate cholestatic liver enzyme elevation and increased serum carbohydrate antigen 19-9 (CA19-9) levels; however, CA19-9 lacks sensitivity for early-stage disease and specificity in the presence of biliary obstruction [64].

Radiological imaging is central to diagnosis and staging. Contrast-enhanced magnetic resonance imaging (MRI) with magnetic resonance cholangiopancreatography (MRCP) as the preferred modality for tumor characterization, assessment of biliary involvement, and surgical planning [64, 68]. Histological confirmation is generally required, particularly in unresectable or advanced disease, and adequate tissue sampling is essential to enable molecular profiling and for guiding targeted therapy [64].

Molecular Pathogenesis

CCA is characterized by marked molecular heterogeneity. iCCA frequently harbors potentially actionable genetic alterations, including isocitrate dehydrogenase 1/2 (IDH1/2) mutations and fibroblast growth factor receptor 2 (FGFR2) fusions, whereas KRAS, TP53, and ERBB2 alterations are more commonly identified in extrahepatic tumors [64, 69]. These molecular differences have important prognostic and therapeutic implications. Consequently, comprehensive next-generation sequencing is now recommended in patients with advanced disease to identify targetable alterations and guide precision treatment strategies [64].

Management

Surgical resection remains the only potentially curative treatment for CCA; however, only 20–30% of patients are eligible at diagnosis due to locally advanced or metastatic disease [64, 66]. Stage at presentation depends on the location of the cancer. Even in patients with no documented metastatic disease, futile surgeries are common [70]. Published outcomes from India demonstrate poor treatment completion rates and poor prognosis irrespective of location [71]. Liver transplantation has emerged as a curative option in highly selected patients with early-stage iCCA or unresectable pCCA under strict protocols [64]. For patients undergoing curative-intent resection, adjuvant chemotherapy with capecitabine is currently recommended [64].

For unresectable or metastatic disease, systemic therapy is the mainstay of treatment. Combination chemotherapy with gemcitabine and cisplatin, increasingly combined with immune checkpoint inhibitors, constitutes the current first-line standard of care [64, 72]. The current standard of care is gemcitabine and durvalumab following the survival benefit demonstrated in the TOPAZ-1 trial [55]. Second-line therapy typically includes FOLFOX in patients without actionable molecular alterations [64]. Targeted therapies, including FGFR inhibitors and IDH1 inhibitors, have demonstrated clinically meaningful benefits in molecularly selected populations and represent a major advance in the management of advanced CCA [64, 69].

Radiation therapy is an important adjunct in the multidisciplinary management of cholangiocarcinoma, particularly for patients with unresectable disease or high-risk features after surgery, including margin positive status. External beam radiation therapy (EBRT), including advanced techniques such as intensity-modulated radiation therapy (IMRT) and stereotactic body radiation therapy (SBRT), allows for improved local tumor control while minimizing radiation exposure to surrounding liver and gastrointestinal structures [73, 74]. Typical dose schedule used in CCA are 50-60 Gy (for inoperable cases as well as adjuvant after surgery), with or without concurrent chemotherapy. Adjuvant chemoradiation is often considered in patients with positive surgical margins or nodal involvement, while definitive radiation combined with chemotherapy may provide local control and symptom relief in non-surgical candidates [74].

In suitable cases, doses of 30-50 Gy in 3-5 fractions have been used in SBRT for this site with progression free survival ranging from 6-9 months. Duodenal exposure to higher doses has been associated with risk of duodenal stenosis. The following dose constraints are suggested (Liver ≥ 700 mL of normal liver should receive < 15 Gy; Duodenum: Dmax < 24-30 Gy in 3 fractions); Central Hepatobiliary Tract: Mean dose < 14 Gy).

Although randomized data are limited due to the rarity of the disease, multiple retrospective studies and clinical guidelines support the selective use of radiation therapy to improve local disease control and potentially extend overall survival when integrated with systemic therapy and surgery.

Prognosis and Future Directions

Despite recent advances, the prognosis of CCA remains poor, with 5-year survival rates below 20% [64, 66]. Early-stage detection, improved biomarkers, refinement of molecular classification, and integration of targeted and immune-based therapies are critical unmet needs. Ongoing international collaborative efforts aim to improve outcomes through multidisciplinary care and precision medicine approaches.

4 Pancreatic Carcinoma

4.1 Anatomy

The pancreas is a retroperitoneal structure. The pancreatic head rests in the C-loop of the duodenum, while the tail extends laterally into the splenic hilum.

The common hepatic duct and the main pancreatic excretory duct (duct of Wirsung) traverse the head and enter the second part of the duodenum to excrete their contents. Occasionally, an accessory duct (duct of Santorini) is also present and drains in the same way. The junction between the head and the body of the pancreas is referred to as the neck. The body of the pancreas lies posterior to the stomach and ends in the pancreatic tail in the splenic hilum near the origin of the splenic vein.

The superior mesenteric artery (SMA) and the vein (SMV) are in close relation to the pancreatic neck. The splenic vein lies posterior to the pancreas and joins with the SMV to form the portal vein. The abdominal aorta and inferior vena cava (IVC) lie posterior to the pancreas. The celiac artery exits the abdominal aorta superior to the pancreatic head, and branches into the common hepatic artery, right gastric artery, and splenic artery. The latter traverses superiorly along the body and tail of the pancreas to reach the splenic hilum.

The location of cancers in the pancreas and their relationship with the vascular structures determine prognosis and treatment. Majority of pancreatic cancer is located at head (40–50%), body and tail (10–15% each location), and tumors originating from pancreatic duct and Islets of Langerhans together in <2%.

4.2 Epidemiological Aspects

According to the GLOBOCAN, there were close to half a million new cases of pancreatic cancer diagnoses worldwide in 2020. This made it the 12th most common cancer when both sexes were combined. Age-standardized incidence rates are the highest in China and countries with a higher human development index. Unfortunately, nearly half a million people also die of pancreatic cancer annually, making it one of the most lethal malignancies and the seventh leading cause of cancer deaths [75]. Pancreatic carcinoma is the most lethal solid tumor among all human cancers.

4.3 Risk Factors

The most consistently identified factor associated with pancreatic cancer is smoking [76]. Other factors include Type 2 diabetes mellitus and obesity. High alcohol consumption, hepatitis B or C, history of cholecystectomy are also associated with a small increased risk [77].

Family history of pancreatic cancer is a known risk factor, with nearly one in 10 cases demonstrating hereditary pancreatic and non-pancreatic cancers. The risk of pancreatic cancer increases with the number of first-degree relatives affected. Pancreatic cancer is associated with hereditary breast and ovarian cancer syndrome and BRCA1 and 2 mutations. Other germline mutations like CDKN2A/p16, STK11, MLH1/MSH2, APC and PRSS1 have also been associated an increased risk [78].

4.4 Genetic Basis of Disease

The most common proto-oncogene mutation in pancreatic cancer is KRAS, which is mutated in more than 90% of cancers. Similarly, the tumor suppressor gene CDKN2A is inactivated in the vast majority of patients. P53 mutations are also prevalent. Prognostically, SMAD4 inactivating mutations, present in about half of the tumors represent a more aggressive disease with a poor prognosis.

4.5 Pathology

The histopathological subtypes of pancreatic neoplasms are shown in Table 3. Pancreatic intraepithelial neoplasia (PanIN) is identified as a non-invasive precursor lesion of the infiltrating ductal adenocarcinoma, the predominant pathological variant. Pancreatic neoplasms are often described as solid or cystic. Most of the pancreatic cancers are the ductal adenocarcinomas arising out of the cells that normally differentiate into the epithelial lining of the ducts. The next most common histology is the pancreatic neuroendocrine tumors arising from the endocrine cells within the islets of Langerhans. They have a better prognosis compared to the ductal adenocarcinomas. Cystic neoplasms are much less common and also usually have a better prognosis than solid adenocarcinomas.

Table 3 Histopathological subtypes of pancreatic neoplasms

Histopathological subtypes
Precursor lesion
Pancreatic intraepithelial neoplasia (PanIN)
Solid neoplasms
Infiltrating ductal adenocarcinoma
Variants of ductal adenocarcinoma: Adenosquamous carcinoma, anaplastic carcinoma
Pancreatic neuroendocrine tumors (PanNETs)
Acinar cell carcinoma
Cystic lesions
Intraductal papillary mucinous neoplasms (IPMN) and papillary mucinous carcinoma
Serous cystadenoma or cystadenocarcinoma
Mucinous cystadenoma or cystadenocarcinoma

4.6 Clinical Symptoms and Signs

Presenting symptoms of pancreatic neoplasms are related to the histology and location. The common adenocarcinomas often arise in the head, neck, or uncinate process of pancreas in the periampullary region and therefore give rise to symptoms of biliary obstruction—jaundice, pruritus, and steatorrhea. As they grow larger, they can obstruct or infiltrate the duodenum or the celiac plexus, leading to symptoms and signs of gastric outlet obstruction. About one in four individuals also has a new onset of diabetes. Symptoms and signs of pancreatitis and cholangitis may also rarely be the presenting symptoms in these cancers. On the other hand, tumors arising from the pancreatic tail usually do not produce symptoms early, often resulting in a late presentation with back pain from celiac plexus involvement, bleeding from gastric erosion, or splenomegaly from splenic vein thrombosis.

4.7 Initial Evaluation

Initial evaluation for the common presenting symptoms usually involves liver function tests, which demonstrate an obstructive biliary pathology, including elevation of serum conjugated bilirubin and gamma-glutamyl transpeptidase, followed by elevations in alkaline phosphatase and aminotransferases.

The serum carbohydrate antigen 19-9 (CA 19-9) serves as a tumor marker for the diagnosis and prognostication of pancreatic adenocarcinomas. The sensitivity and specificity of this test are approximately 80% each [79]. CA 19-9 levels more than 100–200 U/mL have been shown in studies to predict for unresectable disease and/or poor survival outcomes [80, 81]. However, this marker may also be elevated as a result of other causes of pancreaticobiliary obstruction, cholangitis, and pancreatitis, or even uncontrolled diabetes. It may also be undetectable in patients who lack the Lewis antigens. In a patient with a confirmed diagnosis of adenocarcinoma, CA 19-9 can be used for prognostication and surveillance following therapy.

Radiological evaluation focuses on confirming the presence of a neoplasm and identifying the extent of the cancer to determine stage and resectability. A multi-detector computed tomographic scan (CT) is the standard imaging modality for evaluation of the primary tumor and regional nodal metastases. Magnetic resonance imaging (MRI) is considered as accurate as a CT scan and in some cases, can offer advantages in visualization of soft-tissue planes and in the evaluation of patients in whom a contrast-enhanced CT scan cannot be performed.

Radiologic reporting of locoregional extent is done based on the consensus statement of the consensus statement of the Society of Abdominal Radiology and the American Pancreatic Association [82].

Cancers are classified radiologically into resectable, borderline resectable, and locally advanced pancreatic cancer by the American Hepato-Pancreatico-Biliary Association consensus report [83], adopted by the NCCN for defining treatment pathways (Table 4).

A biopsy is usually not performed if there is a radiologically apparent neoplastic, resectable lesion of the pancreas. This is because the primary treatment of all benign and malignant neoplasms is surgical, and also because there is a relatively high chance of false negatives on biopsy, as the radiological lesion is often composed of desmoplastic stromal reactions, where there can be a sampling error. If radiological findings are equivocal or if a non-surgical treatment is planned, then a biopsy is required, and is performed using either endoscopic ultrasound (EUS) or externally using CT-guidance.

EUS can also provide additional information on infiltration of surrounding mucosal structures and vasculature. It can also supplement CT/MRI in the evaluation of nodal metastases. However, EUS is not widely available and is operator-dependent, limiting its utility in most low-resource settings.

Additional metastatic workup is usually performed with a CT of the thorax. The role of positron-emission tomography (PET) with fluorodeoxyglucose (FDG) in the staging of pancre-

Table 4 Radiological classification of resectability (simplified from National Comprehensive Cancer Network guidelines)

	Arterial anatomy	Venous anatomy
Resectable	No tumor contact with CA, SMA, or CHA	No tumor contact of SMV or PV, or $\leq 180^\circ$ contact without vein contour irregularity
Borderline resectable	Solid tumor contact with CHA without extension to CA or hepatic artery bifurcation Solid tumor contact with the SMA or CA of $\leq 180^\circ$ Solid tumor contact with variant arterial anatomy	Solid tumor contact of SMV or PV, of $\geq 180^\circ$ Solid tumor contact of $\leq 180^\circ$ with vein contour irregularity Solid tumor contact with the IVC
Locally advanced/ unresectable	Solid tumor contact with the SMA or CA of $>180^\circ$[a] Solid tumor contact with CA with involvement of the aorta	SMV/PV unreconstructible due to involvement or occlusion.

[a]Solid tumor contact of >180 with the CA but without contact with the aorta and intact gastroduodenal artery may allow reconstruction using a modified Appleby procedure (and hence be classified as borderline resectable by some experts)

atic cancers is not well-defined and is not considered a standard of care. FDG avidity in pancreatic cancers is low, and there is only a marginal benefit in sensitivity and positive predictive value over CT scans alone [84].

4.8 Staging

The eight edition (2017) of the American Joint Committee on Cancer (AJCC) Staging Manual bases the T staging of pancreatic cancer primarily on tumor size, and N category on the number of nodes involved pathologically. Further details are provided in Tables 5 and 6 [85, 86].

Table 5 The American Joint Committee on Cancer (TNM) staging system for pancreatic cancer

T category	*T criteria*
Tx	Primary tumor cannot be assessed
T0	No evidence of primary tumor
Tis	Carcinoma in situ. This includes high-grade pancreatic intraepithelial neoplasia (PanIn-3), intraductal papillary mucinous neoplasm with high-grade dysplasia, intraductal tubulopapillary neoplasm with high-grade dysplasia, and mucinous cystic neoplasm with high-grade dysplasia.
T1	Tumor ≤2 cm in greatest dimension
T1a	Tumor ≤0.5 cm in greatest dimension
T1b	Tumor >0.5 cm and <1 cm in greatest dimension
T1c	Tumor 1–2 cm in greatest dimension
T2	Tumor >2 cm and ≤4 cm in greatest dimension
T3	Tumor >4 cm in greatest dimension
T4	Tumor involves celiac axis, superior mesenteric artery, and/or common hepatic artery, regardless of size.
N category	*N criteria*
Nx	Regional lymph nodes cannot be assessed
N0	No regional lymph node metastases
N1	Metastasis in one to three regional lymph nodes
N2	Metastasis in four or more regional lymph node
M category	*M criteria*
cM0	No distant metastasis
cM1	Distant metastasis
pM1	Distant metastasis, microscopically confirmed

Table 6 Pancreatic cancer prognostic stage grouping

Stage groups	Criteria
Stage IA	T1N0M0
Stage IB	T2N0M0
Stage IIA	T3N0M0
Stage IIB	T1-3N1M0
Stage III	T1-3N2M0 or T4NanyM0
Stage IV	TanyNanyM1

4.9 Treatment Options

4.9.1 Surgical Aspects

Resectability is a key determinant of curative intent treatment in pancreatic cancer. Unresectable cancers rarely demonstrate long-term survival. Unfortunately, even after R0 resection, the 5 year survival is low at approximately 20% [87].

The classic surgical treatment for a primary in the head of pancreas is the pancreaticoduodenectomy or Whipple procedure. This surgery involves the resection of the head of pancreas, the gallblader, the common bile duct, the second to fourth parts of the duodenum and the regional lymph nodes. In the traditional Whipple procedure, the stomach is divided proximal to the antrum. In a pylorus-preserving Whipple, the division is made distal to the pylorus in the first part of the duodenum. This is followed by three anatosmoses—the gastrojejunal, biliary-enteric, and pancreatico-enteric. After this complex procedure, morbidity rates are as high as 30–45%, while post-operative mortality rates are 2–3% [88]. The most common complications are pancreatic leaks and infections, pancreatic fistula, and delayed gastric emptying.

For primaries in the body or tail, the traditional surgical procedure is the distal pancreatectomy with an en bloc splenectomy.

There has been considerable advancement in the surgical treatment of pancreatic cancer, particularly in the last two decades. The surgical advances coupled with neoadjuvant treatment have led to significant improvements in historically meager resection rates [89]. There has been significant underutilization and variations in pancreatic cancer surgery as reported in population-based studies and Surveillance, Epidemiology, and End Results database analysis [90].

One of the important aspects of surgical advances in pancreatic cancer has been a considerable decrease in operative mortality. Centralization of pancreatic cancer surgery combines the positive impact of the center volume and the surgeon's experience. This aspect of pancreatic cancer surgery was initially addressed in the landmark study by Birkmeyer et al. and later addressed in numerous other studies. Studies also suggest that centralization impacts margin status and long-term mortality in pancreatic cancer patients [91, 92].

Pancreatic cancer has a strong propensity for perineural invasion that hinders complete surgical clearance, consequently resulting in significantly higher rates of local recurrence and poor long-term survival [93]. There is significant evidence to suggest the strong impact of the tumor-free margin on overall survival, with a clear detrimental outcome on those who have "direct R1" resections compared with those who have margins <1 and >1 mm [94, 95].

Traditional pancreatic resections don't address the tumor-infiltrated perineural and lymphatic tissue situated along the superior mesenteric artery and celiac axis. Modern pancreatic surgery has evolved into a vessel-oriented approach that has been variously addressed as systematic mesopancreas dissection, anatomical pancreaticoduodenectomy, vessel-oriented pancreatic oduodenectomy, and triangle operation. In contrast to the traditional medial-to-lateral approach, the vessel-oriented lateral-to-medial approach allows a structured approach to pancreatic head resection, decreased risk of vascular injuries, and removal of neural and lymphatics along the superior mesenteric artery and celiac axis up to their origins [96, 97]. Different SMA approaches allow a radical mesopancreatic and a vessel-oriented approach to the pancreaticoduodenectomy, increasing the likelihood of true R0 resection. Multiple center-specific retrospective studies have reported higher R0 resection rates and overall survival rates when compared to conventional resections. The benefits of the vessel-oriented approaches need to be weighed against the possibility of increased morbidity. Studies have suggested acceptable morbidity rates when these procedures are performed in high-volume centers.

There have been considerable advancements in minimally invasive approaches to pancreatic cancer resections. Whereas the feasibility and safety of minimally invasive approaches have been established, meta-analyses of randomized trials and comparative studies have not demonstrated meaningful benefits in morbidity or oncological outcomes [98, 99].

Apart from resection margins as described above, nodal metastases and pathological tumor size are important prognostic factors. Patients with nodal metastases have significantly poorer outcomes compared to those without [85]. The lymph node ratio is an independent predictor of local failure and metastases [100].

Patterns of failure after surgery suggest that the majority of failures occur in the abdominal cavity. Locoregional failures occur commonly around the proximal celiac axis and superior mesenteric artery. Liver, omental, and lung are the commonest sites of distant failure. Liver and omental failures often occur within the first year of surgery, while lung metastases often manifest later.

4.10 Adjuvant and Neoadjuvant Therapy

Pancreatic cancer is associated with a poor prognosis, and radiotherapy has been used both in the setting of operable, borderline operable, and inoperable pancreatic cancer, with mixed success. Indications for radiotherapy are evolving, and its exact role is still to be defined.

4.10.1 Operable Pancreatic Cancer

The traditional treatment of operable esophageal cancer is upfront surgery with a pancreaticoduodenectomy. Unfortunately, even in this setting, with surgery alone, recurrences are common with 5 year OS of 15–20% in most historical series. Approximately 25–30% of patients relapse in locoregionally, while the rest relapse with distant or combined relapse. Therefore the use of adjuvant or neoadjuvant therapy to improve locoregional control is justified in principle.

Studies investigating prognostic factors for recurrence after surgery have identified several factors affecting the risk of recurrence. In an analysis of a pooled cohort of 25,000 cases, tumor size >2 cm, poorly differentiated lesions, positive resection margins, perineural or vascular invasion, and lymph node metastases were independently associated with poorer survival [101]. Nodal metastases have special relevance, especially a higher ratio of involved vs. dissected nodes [100]. Other factors, like the post-operative CA-19-9 levels, have a known impact as well [81]. The prognostic impact of margins and CA19-9 has been demonstrated even after adjuvant chemoradiation therapy [102].

The benefit of adjuvant radiotherapy after pancreaticoduodenectomy has been reported both from institutional series and randomized controlled trials Table 7. In a combined analysis of patients from the Mayo Clinic and Johns Hopkins Hospitals in the USA, Hsu et al. reported that adjuvant radiotherapy was associated with an approximately 33% improvement in overall survival with adjuvant chemoradiation [113]. Unfortunately, this benefit has been more ambiguous in randomized controlled trials (Table 7). Apart from the older GITSG trial, we do not have any evidence of benefit from the addition of adjuvant radiotherapy.

Based on ESPAC-4 and the PRODIGE24/ CCTG PA.6 trial results, the current standard of care in the adjuvant setting is either gemcitabine and capecitabine-based doublet chemotherapy or a modified FOLFIRINOX regimen [110, 111].

The role of adjuvant radiotherapy is therefore hard to define. Currently, adjuvant radiotherapy can be considered in the presence of positive resection margins. However, considering that close to 50% of patients in the chemotherapy trials have a component of local relpase, the role of modern conformal adjuvant RT in addition to chemotherapy is being tested in the RTOG 0848 trial where 5FU-based chemoradiation is being tested against observation in patients who have not progressed after 5 cycles of adjuvant gemcitabine-based chemotherapy (NCT01013649).

4.10.2 Neoadjuvant Therapy for Operable and Borderline Operable Pancreatic Cancer

Neoadjuvant therapy is an alternative to adjuvant therapy for operable or borderline operable pancreatic cancer. While the goals of both approaches are similar, neoadjuvant therapy has certain advantages. First neoadjuvant chemotherapy potentially addresses micrometastatic disease earlier. This is important in pancreatic cancer where distant metastases is common. Radiotherapy and chemotherapy also potentially improves the rate of margin negative R0 resection, a known predictor of better outcomes. Compliance to adjuvant chemotherapy with or without radiation after pancreaticoduodenectomy has been poor. Neoadjuvant therapy in most gastointestinal solid tumors is also better tolerated than adjuvant therapy, and may offer a similar advantage in pancreatic cancer. Alongside these considerations, we must also appreciate in some patients, there may be development of metastases during the course of neoadjuvant therapy. This is generally understood to represent poor biology and may offer a pathway of optimal patient selection for major surgery like pancreaticoduodenectomy. Patients who have not progressed on neoadjuvant therapy may be the ones who derive the most benefit from surgery.

The initial use of neoadjuvant therapy has been reported for borderline resectable pancreatic cancer. In this scenario, the primary goal is to achieve operability and a margin negative resection. Neoadjuvant treatment with chemoradiation has been reported mainly in single institutional series. Typically a course of conventionally fractionated radiotherapy with concurrent gemcitabine or capecitabine along with additional cycles of gemcitabine have been used. Results have shown resection rates between 35% and 55%, with high rates of R0 resection (>75%) [114–116]. The overall survival of the resected patients ranged between 20 and 40 months. This provided proof of principle that neoadjuvant chemoradiation may play an important role in resectability and outcomes in this group.

Table 7 Randomized trials of adjuvant therapy regimens in resected pancreatic adenocarcinoma

Trial	Arms	Sample size	Overall survival	Comment
GITSG 1985 [103]	(Control) Surgery (Intervention) Surgery + Split course RT 40 Gy with concurrent and adjuvant 5FU bolus	40	Median OS 11 months vs. 20 months ($p = 0.035$)	Older techniques, parallel opposed portals, small sample size
EORTC 40891 [104]	(Control) Surgery (Intervention) Surgery + Split course RT 40 Gy with concurrent continuous infusion 5FU	218	Median OS 1.6 years vs. 1.8 years ($p = 0.5$)	Included peri-ampullary cancers also. Treatment fields 3–4
ESPAC-1 [105]	2 × 2 factorial design Observation Concurrent CRT Chemo alone Conc CRT + chemo RT: Split course 40 Gy Chemo: Bolus 5FU D1–3 with RT and/or D1–5q4weekly × 6	289	CRT vs no CRT 5 year OS (10% vs 20%) Chemo vs no chemo 5 year OS (21% vs 8%)	Poor RT QA and compliance are likely to have contributed to the detrimental effect of RT
RTOG 9704 [106]	(Control) Surgery + adjuvant CRT (5FU based) and adjuvant 5FU (Investigational) Surgery + adjuvant CRT (5FU based) and adjuvant gemcitabine	451	Median OS 16.9 months vs 20.5 months ($p = 0.09$) 3 year OS (22% vs 31%)	Gemcitabine considered standard of care as adjuvant
CapRI [107]	Surgery + adjuvant 5FU/leucovorin Surgery + 50.4 Gy/28 Fr RT with concurrent 5FU + cisplatin + IFα-2b	132	Median OS 28.5 months vs 26.5 months ($p = 0.99$)	Study underpowered to detect small differences
CONKO-001 [108]	Surgery Surgery + gemcitabine	368	5-year OS 10.4% vs 20.7% ($p = 0.01$)	
JASPAC-01 [109]	Surgery + gemcitabine Surgery + S1	385	5-year OS 24.4% vs. 44.1% ($p < 0.001$)	S1 is a superior option for Japanese patients compared to gemcitabine alone.
ESPAC-4 [110]	Surgery + gemcitabine Surgery + gemcitabine + Capecitabine	732	Median OS 25.5 months vs. 28.0 months ($p = 0.032$)	
PRODIGE24/ CCTG PA.6 [111]	Surgery + gemcitabine Surgery + mFOLFIRINOX	493	Median OS 35.0 months vs. 54.4 months ($p < 0.001$)	
APACT [112]	Surgery + gemcitabine Surgery + gemcitabine + nab-paclitaxel	866	Median OS 37.4 months vs 41.8 months ($p = 0.023$)	No significant difference in primary endpoint of DFS

GITSG Gastrointestinal Tumor Study Group, *RT* radiotherapy, *CRT* chemoradiotherapy, *DFS* disease-free survival, *OS* overall survival

However, the use of neoadjuvant therapy has now been expanded to upfront resectable tumors as well. The use of neoadjuvant chemoradiotherapy alone has been reported retrospectively from the MD Anderson Cancer Center [117]. A variety of chemoradiation regimens in 240 patients achieved a 3-year survival rate of 47%.

Several prospective studies are evaluating the role of regimens containing chemotherapy, with or without radiotherapy. The PREOPANC-I study compared neoadjuvant gemcitabine 1000 mg/m^2 D1,8,15 for 3 cycles along with radiotherapy course delivering 36 Gy/15 Fr/3 weeks on weeks 4–6, followed by surgery and a further 4 cycles of adjuvant gemcitabine vs upfront surgery followed by 6 cycles of adjuvant gemcitabine for resectable and borderline operable pancreatic cancer. Long-term results demonstrated improved overall survival, disease-free survival, and locoregional control l [118, 119]. PREOPANC-II is an ongoing study comparing a similar study arm to neoadjuvant mFOLFIRINOX [120]. The recent developments in neo-adjuvant chemo-radiotherapy [119, 120], with refinements in systemic therapy, RT technique and RT dose would require more robust clinical trials. Total neo-adjuvant treatment (TNT) regimen [119] for maximum non-surgical approach before surgery or even to avoid surgery needs to be safe and cost effective.

Several studies are also evaluating the role of chemotherapy alone in the neoadjuvant setting. The phase III PREP-02/JSAP-05 study in Japan compared adjuvant S1 vs neoadjuvant gemcitabine and S1 and adjuvant S1 and found improved survival in the neoadjuvant arm [121]. This has established the role of this regimen in the Far East. The SWOG S1505 phase II trial compared neoadjuvant mFOLFIRINOX with neoadjuvant gemcitabine and nab-paclitaxel and found equivalent outcomes with median survival of approx 22 months [122].

The ESPAC-5 trial was a small phase 2 randomized multi-arm trial comparing upfront surgery with 3 different neoadjuvant strategies in borderline resectable cancer (8 weeks of FOLFIRINOX-based chemotherapy, the same duration of gemcitabine and capecitabine-based chemotherapy and capecitabine-based concurrent chemoradiation) [123]. The neoadjuvant strategies did not yield a significantly higher rate of R0 resection. However, the combined group of patients receiving neoadjuvant therapy had longer disease free survival and the two neoadjuvant chemotherapy regimens led to an improved overall survival compared to the surgery-only arm.

Combination of aggressive multi-agent therapy with radiotherapy has been reported in prospective single-center studies. Results from Massachusetts General Hospital demonstrated excellent long-term outcomes with modified FOLFIRINOX followed by either short course radiotherapy 5 Gy × 5 fractions with protons or concurrent long-course chemoradiation with capecitabine, leading to a median overall survival of 37 months [124].

The Alliance A021501 Phase 2 trial, designed to establish the standard neoadjuvant therapy in borderline resectable disease, studied mFOLFIRINOX and mFOLFIRINOX and stereotactic radiotherapy prospectively [125]. The chemotherapy alone arm of this study performed better, and the stereotactic radiotherapy arm was stopped.

The results of these trials evaluating multiple neoadjuvant options with chemotherapy with or without radiation suggest a clear benefit of this approach in borderline resectable cancer. While the value of systemic therapy is apparent, the choice of agents and the role of radiotherapy still remain to be clarified.

4.11 Treatment of Unresectable but Non-Metastatic Pancreatic Cancer

The traditional treatment of locally advanced unresectable pancreatic cancer has been a combination of systemic therapy and radiotherapy.

The GITSG trial published in 1981 established a combination of moderate dose radiotherapy with 40 Gy split-course and 5FU as the standard treatment, as compared to high dose radiotherapy alone with or without concurrent 5FU [126]. Since then, further trials have sought to refine the use of both radiation (through more conformal techniques and higher doses without breaks) and chemotherapy (other agents like gemcitabine, combination therapies and determining the optimal concurrent regimen) with mixed results.

The French study 2000–01 FFCD/SFRO comparing addition of 60 Gy of radiation to gemcitabine-based chemotherapy showed poorer survival in the radiotherapy arm [127]. This study was also stopped early due to a perceived lack of benefit. The failure to show benefit was attributed to increased complication rates arising out of the regimen of high dose RT and gemcitabine.

The ECOG 4201 trial sought to compare gemcitabine-based chemotherapy with or without RT. Although the trial closed due to poor accrual, a comparison of outcomes in the 74 patients accrued demonstrated a survival benefit for radiotherapy [128].

THE SCALOP Phase II randomized controlled trial compared gemcitabine vs. capecitabine as concurrent chemotherapy with 50.4 Gy of radiation therapy after 4 cycles of systemic therapy with a combination of gemcitabine and capecitabine [129]. This study randomized 78 patients and demonstrated that median survival with concurrent capecitabine were better at 15.2 months compared to 13.4 months with gemcitabine.

The GERCOR LAP-07 trial comparing chemotherapy alone with 4 cycles of Gemcitabine with or without erlotinib, followed by two further cycles of the same chemotherapy versus chemoradiation with 50.4 Gy with concurrent capecitabine [130]. The concurrent chemoradiotherapy arm demonstrated improved progression-free survival, but no improvement in overall survival. Chemoradiotherapy did not result in increased grade 3 or 4 side-effects. There was no benefit of erlotinib or the chemoradiation in overall survival. Nearly 40% of patients had disease progression by the end of the first 4 cycles of systemic therapy, highlighting the resistant nature of the disease.

To summarize, the current evidence from randomized controlled trials on treatment of inoperable but non-metastatic pancreatic cancer is either single-agent or combination systemic therapy with gemcitabine followed by chemoradiation. The benefit of radiation therapy in improving overall survival is unclear due to conflicting results. However, the results from aggressive chemotherapy in metastatic pancreatic cancer have been impressive, and current clinical practice is shifting toward the use of these regimens in the locoregionally advanced setting.

4.12 Treatment of Metastatic Disease

Management of metastatic disease is governed by various factors, of which age and performance status are the most important [131]. Young patients with good performance status are the candidates for FOLFIRINOX regimen, resulting in overall survival of 11.1 months (Hazard ratio [HR]: 0.57; 95% Confidence interval [CI]: 0.45–0.73; $p < 0{\cdot}001$) as demonstrated in a phase-3 trial [132]. Patients with borderline or poor performance status and old age are usually managed with a combination of gemcitabine with nab-paclitaxel. This regimen has shown a superior overall survival compared to standard of care (8.7 vs 6.6 months, HR: 0.72, 95% CI: 0.62–0.83, $p < 0.001$) [133].

With the availability of various molecular techniques, 5–9% of pancreatic cancer cases can demonstrate germline or somatic mutations like BRCA1/2 genes [131]. These patients are candidates for maintenance olaparib post response to chemotherapy. POLO trial demonstrated a progression-free survival (PFS) of 7.4 months with olaparib maintenance vs 3.8 months with placebo (HR: 0.53, 95% CI: 0.35–0.82). However, no overall survival benefit was demonstrated, possibly because of crossover trial design [134, 135].

Patients with disease progression following first line chemotherapy, and in good performance status, should be offered next-generation sequencing and treatment should be governed by targetable mutation identified. Patients with preserved performance status without targetable mutation should be offered second line therapy guided by agents used in first-line setting.

4.13 Radiotherapy Treatment Planning

4.13.1 Patterns of Spread

Patterns of spread of pancreatic cancer and patterns of failure after surgery and radiation determine the target volumes for radiation therapy.

Locoregionally advanced pancreatic cancer often spreads to adjacent lymph nodes. The lymphatic drainage of the pancreas is complex. There are two systems of classification of the draining lymph nodes, the Japanese and the UICC [86, 136]. The former is more commonly used. The patterns of nodal involvement depend on the anatomical location of the primary tumor in the pancreas and therefore determine the extent of target volume delineation for elective nodal treatment.

Audits of patterns of locoregional failure after surgery demonstrate that common sites of local failure are the tissue around the SMA, the region between the celiac artery, SMA, and IVC, the pancreatic resection margins, and the tissue around the common hepatic artery. The majority of nodal recurrences after surgery occur around the mesenteric root close to the SMA and in the paraaortic region [137].

4.14 Simulation and Contouring

Positioning: The patient is positioned supine, with arms supported above the head, along with knee and ankle support. An alpha cradle or vacuum bag may be used. There is no role for thermoplastic sheets. Consistency in internal organ volumes may be aided by fasting for 2 h or more to ensure emptying of gastric contents.

Contrast: Ideally, a triple-phase protocol in exhalation breath-hold is recommended (arterial, pancreatic, and portal venous phase) to ensure optimal delineation of the pancreatic primary as well as the vascular structures. Additionally, oral contrast may help in the differentiation of the pancreas from the stomach and duodenum. As recommended in the ESTRO-ACROP guidelines, without bolus tracking, the delays are 25, 40, and 70 s from the start of contrast injection at 3 mL/s [138]. When using bolus tracking, the region of interest should be on the descending aorta with delays of 5, 20, and 50 s from the tracking signal at 80-100HU. Slice reconstruction should be less than 3 mm.

Motion management: When treatment is delivered in the definitive or neoadjuvant setting, the pancreas is prone to movement in the supero-inferior axis due to diaphragmatic motion. Motion management is an important consideration in SBRT planning. Motion restriction techniques include abdominal compression and either voluntary or assisted breath-hold. Other motion management methods include a motion-encompassing technique using an internal target volume (ITV) or an approach using respiratory-gating using 4DCT.

In MRI-based treatment planning, the superior soft-tissue delineation of the tumor boundaries on MRI can be used for more accurate target volume delineation. Modern MR-Linacs allow improved motion management by allowing real time tumor tracking with respiratory motion and gated delivery.

4.14.1 Target Volumes

Target Volumes for Neoadjuvant or Curative-Intent Treatment of Pancreatic Cancer:

Consensus recommendations for target delineation have been published by the ESTRO-ACROP [138]. The recommendations are to delineate the primary tumor and radiologically enlarged nodes >1 cm in size as gross tumor volume (GTV). It is acknowledged that radiologically apparent volumes do not always match with pathological tumor dimensions. This is most apparent for tumors <3 cm in diameter in the pancreatic head, where the pathological tumor dimensions are larger. Therefore, CTV margins of 7–10 mm are recommended for smaller tumors. When neoadjuvant systemic therapy is used, the CTV should encompass the pre-chemotherapy volumes anatomically. However, for upfront radiotherapy in larger (>3 cm) tumors in the head of the pancreas and tumors of the body and tail, CTV expansion is not routinely used.

The sensitivity and specificity of size-based determination of nodal metastases are also low. Usually, 3–5 mm CTV margins around suspicious nodes are adequate for conformal radiotherapy.

Elective nodal radiotherapy is not practiced as a standard in the setting of locally advanced or borderline resectable pancreatic cancer. Patterns of failure studies generally demonstrate in-field failures and a relatively low incidence of out-of-field nodal failures [139, 140]. In addition, given the common practice of neoadjuvant combination chemotherapy in the LA-PC setting, the micrometastatic disease in the lymph nodes is considered to be addressed with the chemotherapy. On the other hand, elective nodal radiotherapy can be considered when neoadjuvant radiotherapy is being considered for operable pancreatic cancer, where the chances of local control are much higher and nodal failure is the main concern. The target volumes for nodal regions are similar to the target volumes for adjuvant radiotherapy.

Nodal regions for elective nodal radiotherapy depend on the site of the primary. For pancreatic head tumors, the nodes to be covered are the celiac nodes, common hepatic nodes, hepatoduodenal, superior mesenteric, paraaortic, pancreaticoduodenal, and superior and inferior head nodes. For body and tail lesions, the subpancreatic and splenic hilar/arterial nodes are added, while the pancreaticoduodenal nodes are omitted.

4.14.2 Postoperative Target Volumes

Target volume delineation in the setting of adjuvant chemoradiotherapy follows the principles and recommendations broadly laid down in the RTOG study. The structures and the expansions are given in Table 8. The individual CTVs are merged and smoothed to get the final CTV for planning.

4.14.3 Planning Target Volume (PTV) Margins

PTV margins incorporate the uncertainty of positioning and verification of the CTV. Without motion management strategies, the ESTRO-ACROP guideline recommends supero-inferior margins of 20 mm and anteroposterior margins of 15 mm. With motion mitigation strategies and/or 4DCT, these margins can be reduced to 5–10 mm. For SBRT techniques, the published protocols use PTV margins of 0–5 mm with more robust daily image guidance.

4.15 Treatment Planning and Delivery

The traditional dose fractionation schema for pancreatic cancer has been 50–55.8 Gy in 1.8–2 Gy per fraction. Increasingly, stereotactic body radiation therapy (SBRT) is being utilized as an alternative approach, delivering two to five fractions at higher doses per fraction of 5 Gy or higher. The advantages of SBRT are that (a) the

Table 8 Recommendations for target volumes in the adjuvant setting in pancreatic cancer

	Structure delineation	CTV expansion
Tumor bed	Preoperative GTV after image fusion, including operative clips if relevant	5–10 mm
Pancreaticojejunostomy	From pancreatic remnant to the junction with jejunum (avoiding pancreatogastrostomy)	5–10 mm
Celiac artery	Proximal 10–15 mm up to first branching	10–15 mm isotropic
Superior mesenteric artery	Proximal 25–30 mm	10–15 mm isotropic
Portal vein	From confluence to hilar bifurcation	10–15 mm isotropic
Aorta	The uppermost contour of other structures to the bottom of the L2 vertebra	Anterior 20–25 mm Posterior 2 mm Right 25–30 mm Left 10 mm

course of treatment can be completed within 1–2 weeks, (b) the higher dose per fraction potentially allows dose escalation, (c) the schedule allows more flexibility for integration into a plan involving multi-agent systemic therapy. The disadvantages of SBRT are that doses to the stomach and duodenum need to be carefully controlled to minimize the risk of toxicities at a higher dose per fraction, and it can only be considered for relatively small target volumes confined to the pancreas alone. SBRT is becoming the preferred approach to pancreatic cancer radiotherapy, especially with the advent of magnetic resonance-based image guidance and adaptation [141, 142].

Table 9 lists the results of selected studies involving SBRT using several different fractionation schedules. Modeling studies have identified dose dependence with better outcomes above the equivalent of 24 Gy in three fractions [150]. Overall, SBRT studies show encouraging local control outcomes compared to older studies with conventional fractionation, but there are no randomized comparisons between the two. Grade 2 or higher toxicity rates are approximately 10% in modern multifraction series. Unfortunately, the ALLIANCE A021501trial testing the benefit of adding SBRT to multi-agent systemic chemotherapy did not demonstrate any benefit [125].

There is also interest in the use of proton and heavy ion therapy in pancreatic cancer. The results of prospective studies of proton therapy in the unresectable and borderline resectable patients show that it is safe and has good local control [151, 152]. A large multi-institutional analysis of patients treated with carbon-ion therapy in Japan of 72 patients (J-CROS 1403) demonstrated encouraging local control and overall survival (2-year rates of overall survival of 46% and local control of 76%), with low rates of late grade 3 toxicities [153]. The safety of this approach in older patients has also been published [154].

4.15.1 Organs at Risk Dose Constraints

The organs at risk and their dose constraints should be based on QUANTEC for conventionally fractionated treatment and UK SABR consortium guidelines for SBRT [155, 156].

Image Guidance: Verification of treatment is very important for conformal radiation techniques, especially ultrahypofractionated/stereotactic treatment. For pancreatic cancer treated

Table 9 Results of studies reporting on the use of stereotactic body radiation therapy (SBRT) for pancreatic cancer

Author (Institution)	n	Dose fractionation	Local control	Overall survival
Lin (Nebraska 2008–2013) [143]	39 borderline or unresectable	35 Gy in 5 fractions	1 year: 92%, 2 years: 83%	1 year: 69%, 2 years: 18%
Jung (Asan, Korea 2011–2017) [144]	95 unresectable	28 Gy in 4 fractions	1 year: 80%, 2 years: 40%	1 year: 67%, 2 years 20%
Bernard (Pittsburgh 2013–2018) [145]	49 adjuvant close or positive margins	36 Gy in 3 fractions	1 year: 85%, 2 years: 77%	1 year: 68%, 2 years: 50%
Zhu (Changai, China 2012–2016) [146]	419 unresectable	36 Gy in 5 fractions		1 year: 63%, 2 years: 14%
Sutera (Pittsburgh 2004–2014) [147]	291 resectable, borderline and unresectable	18–25 Gy in 1 Fr 24–36 Gy in 3 Fr	1 fraction: 1 year: 63%, 2 years: 53% 3 fractions: 1 year: 79% 2 years: 72%	1 fraction: 2 years: 31% 3 fractions: 2 years: 38%
Herman (multi-institutional prospective) [148]	49 unresectable	33 Gy in 5 Fr		1 year: 59%, 2 years: 18%
Pollom (Stanford 2002–2013) [149]	167 unresectable	25 Gy in 1 Fr 25–45 Gy in 5 Fr	1 fraction: 1 year: 90.5% 5 fractions: 1 year: 88.3%	1 fraction: 1 year: 30.8% 5 fractions: 1 year: 34.9%

with free-breathing techniques, this is an even greater challenge. The image guidance is most reproducibly achieved with implanted fiducials when CT-based or 2D kilovoltage imaging is used. Image-guidance without fiducials is a challenge with free-breathing techniques but can be used with motion-restricted techniques outlined above.

If a magnetic resonance (MR) linac is available, imaging verification becomes easier due to superior soft-tissue contrast, and adaptive techniques are available for daily adaptation.

Radiotherapy Quality Assurance: Pancreatic cancer radiotherapy workflows are plagued by poor quality assurance. In an analysis of patients treated on RTOG 9704 trial, protocol variance was measured on several parameters [157]. Nearly half of the patients had some variation. Patients with variation had worse survival, higher risk of failure, and higher rates of non-hematological toxicity. This emphasizes the need for clear and unambiguous protocols on target delineation, planning and image-guidance.

4.16 Radiotherapy Sequelae

Radiotherapy for pancreatic cancer is associated primarily with gastrointestinal side-effects related to doses received by the stomach, duodenum, and small intestine. Older studies before the use of conformal techniques often used anteroposterior fields with a relatively higher incidence of small bowel toxicities. Modern conformal and stereotactic techniques lead to an approximately 10% rate of grade 2 or higher late bowel toxicity related to doses received by the gastric and duodenal mucosa. The most concerning late effect is gastrointestinal bleeding which is reported to 1–5% of cases. Patient selection and plan evaluation are therefore very important.

4.17 Follow-Up

Follow-up in pancreatic cancer is usually done with a combination of CA 19-9 and CT scans of the abdomen and thorax. Usually, these would be performed every 2–4 months. There is no proven benefit of PET-CT scans in routine surveillance of pancreatic cancer.

4.17.1 Prognosis, Results, and Outcome, Survival

As has been described earlier, pancreatic cancer is most lethal of all solid tumors. Resectable pancreatic cancer followed by aggressive multi-agent chemotherapy has a median survival of 30–55 months in different trials. For unresectable but non-metastatic cancers, the median survival ranges from 10 to 20 months. In borderline resectable and locally advanced PC, the neoadjuvant chemo-radiotherapy (CRT) or total neoadjuvant therapy (TNT) with good patient selection extend the survival beyond 24 months. For metastatic pancreatic cancer, the median survival is 5–12 months. One neglected aspect of medical care in PC is the implementation of good palliative care and supportive care. Since majority of patients continue to present with locally advanced pancreatic cancer, patients have high symptom burden alongside the poor prognosis and limited survival. Symptom management for nausea, vomiting, weight loss, cachexia, constipation, abdominal pain, insomnia and for psychological distress require careful attention and optimal symptom relief measures right from the time of cancer diagnosis. Quality of life is to be considered an important parameter for clinical research along with the clinical trials to improve survival.

4.17.2 Future Research

Current pancreatic cancer research is focused on the potential use of immunotherapy alone or in combination with multi-agent chemotherapy. Radiation research is investigating the use of magnetic resonance-guided adaptive radiation to reduce toxicities and dose escalation through stereotactic body radiotherapy. Particle therapy, especially with carbon ions, may have a higher radiosensitivity. Molecular classification of pancreatic cancer may identify subgroups that are better candidates for radiation therapy than others.

Precepts Box

1. Globally, hepatobiliary cancer is the sixth most common cause of cancer and the third most common cause of cancer death.
2. Chronic hepatitis B or hepatitis C is the strongest risk factor for hepatocellular carcinoma (HCC)
3. Liver cirrhosis from any cause, such as fatty liver, also increases the risk.
4. Biopsy confirmation in HCC is only required for equivocal radiological features.
5. Alfa-fetoprotein is a useful tumor marker when it is raised alongside abnormal radiological findings in the liver.
6. Liver function must also be assessed using laboratory tests and clinical features, and scored using a standardized system like the Child-Pugh score or MELD score.
7. The most widely used staging system is the Barcelona Clinic Staging System which takes into account the Child-Pugh score, the size and stage, and the performance status.
8. Treatment of HCC involves surgical resection for small lesions when there is good liver function without portal hypertension. When liver function is compromised with limited liver lesions, a liver transplant produces the best overall disease control outcomes.
9. Unresectable or recurrent but liver-limited lesions are usually treated with trans-arterial chemo-embolization (TACE) and/or stereotactic body radiotherapy (SBRT). These techniques can also be used as bridge therapies for patients awaiting transplants.
10. For HCC that is metastatic or too locally advanced for local therapy, targeted therapies like sorafenib, lenvatinib, or immunotherapy with Atezolizumab are choices for therapy.
11. Primary sclerosing cholangitis is a strong risk factor for cholangiocarcinoma. Gallbladder cancer is related to cholelithiasis.
12. For operable gallbladder and biliary tract tumors, the best outcomes are with surgery. Adjuvant chemotherapy with capecitabine is the current standard of care.
13. Adjuvant radiotherapy is considered for positive margins. For inoperable cancers, prognosis is very poor. Concurrent chemoradiation is an option for patients with localized but inoperable cancers.
14. Recurrent or metastatic cancers are usually treated with systemic therapy with gemcitabine with or without cisplatin or capecitabine-based regimens. Trials with immunotherapy show marginal benefit.
15. Pancreatic cancer is the 12th most common cancer and the seventh leading cause of cancer death.
16. Smoking, Type 2 diabetes, and obesity are risk factors. Adenocarcinoma is the predominant histology.
17. Obstructive jaundice is the usual presenting feature for common pancreatic head cancers. Diagnosis is usually based on radiology.
18. High serum levels of CA 19.9 have been shown to be associated with more advanced disease and poorer outcomes.
19. Based on radiological evaluation of the relation of the tumor with the vascular anatomy, pancreatic cancers are classified as resectable, borderline resectable, and unresectable.
20. The majority of pancreatic cancers are unresectable or metastatic at diagnosis. For resectable tumors, the primary approach is surgical with a pancreaticoduodenectomy or distal pancreatectomy depending on the location of the tumor.

(continued)

21. Advances in surgical techniques have allowed more tumors with vascular encasement to be resected. Adjuvant systemic therapy with gemcitabine/capecitabine or modified FOLFIRINOX-based regimens is considered standard.
22. The role of adjuvant radiotherapy is uncertain, but it could be considered in patients with involved surgical margins. For borderline resectable cancers, neoadjuvant treatment with chemoradiation or stereotactic body radiation therapy, or multiagent systemic therapy can be considered and often results in microscopically negative resections.
23. For unresectable cancers, the current standard of care is systemic therapy with modified FOLFIRINOX or gemcitabine/nab-paclitaxel with or without additional radiotherapy/chemoradiotherapy. Immunotherapy is still experimental.
24. Metastatic pancreatic cancer is usually treated with systemic therapy but has a poor prognosis. Palliative and supportive care provide symptom relief and improve quality of life for all patients.

Multiple Choice Questions

1. The most common etiological factor for hepatocellular carcinoma in developing countries is
   (a) Chronic alcohol abuse
   (b) Aflatoxin B
   (c) Chronic viral hepatitis
   (d) Metabolic syndrome
2. Which of the following statements about alfa-fetoprotein (AFP) is true?
   (a) It is a highly sensitive and specific tumor marker for hepatocellular carcinoma
   (b) AFP has a high positive predictive value when there is a liver mass in the presence of chronic liver disease
   (c) AFP may be raised in most cases of cholangiocarcinoma
   (d) All patients with hepatocellular carcinoma do not need AFP test
3. The Child-Pugh Classification takes into account all of the following except:
   (a) Encephalopathy
   (b) Serum albumin
   (c) Prothrombin time
   (d) Alanine transaminase (ALT)
4. The most commonly used staging system for hepatocellular carcinoma is
   (a) Child-Pugh score
   (b) American Joint Committee for Cancer (AJCC)
   (c) Barcelona Clinic Liver Cancer (BCLC) Staging system
   (d) Karnofsky score
5. A 58-year-old patient has two lesions in the liver of size 1.5 and 2.5 cm consistent with hepatocellular carcinoma, with features of cirrhosis and portal hypertension. What would be the ideal plan of management?
   (a) Surgical resection
   (b) Liver transplantation
   (c) Sorafenib
   (d) Stereotactic body radiation therapy
6. Classic radiation induced liver disease has which of the following characteristics?
   (a) Jaundice
   (b) Raised levels of alkaline phosphatase
   (c) Onset between 2 and 12 weeks
   (d) Features of disseminated intravascular coagulation
7. The QUANTEC recommended mean dose constraint to the normal liver in a five fraction stereotactic radiotherapy regimen for primary liver tumors is
   (a) 28 Gy
   (b) 24 Gy
   (c) 20 Gy
   (d) 18 Gy
8. The most important risk factor for developing gallbladder cancer is
   (a) Viral hepatitis
   (b) Inherited mutations
   (c) Aflatoxin
   (d) Gallstones

9. The most useful radiological investigation for patients presenting with unexplained conjugated hyperbilirubinemia is
   (a) Non-contrast CT of the abdomen
   (b) Liver angiography
   (c) Magnetic resonance cholangiopancreatography (MRCP)
   (d) Triple phase CT of upper abdomen
10. Which proto-oncogene mutation is commonly associated with pancreatic cancer?
   (a) KRAS
   (b) NRAS
   (c) P53
   (d) SMAD4
11. Which of the following radiological criteria traditionally denotes an unresectable pancreatic cancer?
   (a) Solid tumor contact with superior mesenteric or celiac artery of >180°
   (b) Solid tumor contact with varian arterial anatomy
   (c) Solid tumor contact with with superior mesenteric vein or portal vein of >180°
   (d) Solid tumor contact with common hepatic artery away from bifurcation
12. The standard surgical treatment option for pancreatic head and body cancers is
   (a) Distal resection
   (b) Anterior resection
   (c) Pancreaticoduodenectomy
   (d) Pancreatotomy
13. Standard adjuvant therapy after pancreatic cancer after curative resection is
   (a) Postoperative radiation therapy
   (b) Adjuvant chemotherapy with 5-FU
   (c) Adjuvant chemotherapy with modified FOFIRINOX or Gemcitabine based doublet
   (d) Adjuvant atezolizumab
14. Stereotactic body radiotherapy in pancreatic cancer is meant for
   (a) Improvement in overall survival
   (b) Improvement in local control
   (c) Improvement in distant metastases rate
   (d) Improvement in long term toxicities compared to conventionally fractionated radiation

Answer Key

1. (c)
2. (b)
3. (d)
4. (c)
5. (b)
6. (b)
7. (d)
8. (d)
9. (c)
10. (a)
11. (a)
12. (c)
13. (c)
14. (b)

References

1. Sung H, Ferlay J, Siegel RL, Laversanne M, Soerjomataram I, Jemal A, et al. Global cancer statistics 2020: GLOBOCAN estimates of incidence and mortality worldwide for 36 cancers in 185 countries. CA Cancer J Clin. 2021;71:209–49. https://doi.org/10.3322/caac.21660.
2. Global Burden of Disease Liver Cancer Collaboration, Akinyemiju T, Abera S, Ahmed M, Alam N, Alemayohu MA, et al. The burden of primary liver cancer and underlying etiologies from 1990 to 2015 at the global, regional, and national level: results from the Global Burden of Disease Study 2015. JAMA Oncol. 2017;3:1683–91. https://doi.org/10.1001/jamaoncol.2017.3055.
3. Kanwal F, Kramer J, Asch SM, Chayanupatkul M, Cao Y, El-Serag HB. Risk of hepatocellular cancer in HCV patients treated with direct-acting antiviral agents. Gastroenterology. 2017;153:996–1005.e1. https://doi.org/10.1053/j.gastro.2017.06.012.
4. Estes C, Razavi H, Loomba R, Younossi Z, Sanyal AJ. Modeling the epidemic of nonalcoholic fatty liver disease demonstrates an exponential increase in burden of disease. Hepatology. 2018;67:123–33. https://doi.org/10.1002/hep.29466.
5. Elsayes KM, Kielar AZ, Elmohr MM, Chernyak V, Masch WR, Furlan A, et al. White paper of the Society of Abdominal Radiology hepatocellular carcinoma diagnosis disease-focused panel on LI-RADS v2018 for CT and MRI. Abdom Radiol (NY). 2018;43:2625–42. https://doi.org/10.1007/s00261-018-1744-4.
6. Tsoris A, Marlar CA. Use of the Child Pugh score in liver disease. Treasure Island: StatPearls Publishing; 2022.

7. Kamath PS, Kim WR, Advanced Liver Disease Study Group. The model for end-stage liver disease (MELD). Hepatology. 2007;45:797–805. https://doi.org/10.1002/hep.21563.
8. De Gasperi A, Mazza E, Prosperi M. Indocyanine green kinetics to assess liver function: ready for a clinical dynamic assessment in major liver surgery? World J Hepatol. 2016;8:355–67. https://doi.org/10.4254/wjh.v8.i7.355.
9. Okuda K, Ohtsuki T, Obata H, Tomimatsu M, Okazaki N, Hasegawa H, et al. Natural history of hepatocellular carcinoma and prognosis in relation to treatment. Study of 850 patients. Cancer. 1985;56:918–28. https://doi.org/10.1002/1097-0142(19850815)56:4<918::aid-cncr2820560437>3.0.co;2-e.
10. Marrero JA, Kulik LM, Sirlin CB, Zhu AX, Finn RS, Abecassis MM, et al. Diagnosis, staging, and management of hepatocellular carcinoma: 2018 practice guidance by the American Association for the Study of Liver Diseases. Hepatology. 2018;68:723–50. https://doi.org/10.1002/hep.29913.
11. Mazzaferro V, Regalia E, Doci R, Andreola S, Pulvirenti A, Bozzetti F, et al. Liver transplantation for the treatment of small hepatocellular carcinomas in patients with cirrhosis. N Engl J Med. 1996;334:693–9. https://doi.org/10.1056/NEJM199603143341104.
12. Li PJ, Shah S, Mehta N. Recent Advances in Liver Transplantation for Hepatocellular Carcinoma. Curr Treat Options Oncol. 2024;25:1153–1162. https://doi.org/10.1007/s11864-024-01247-8.
13. Denys A, Lacombe C, Schneider F, Madoff DC, Doenz F, Qanadli SD, et al. Portal vein embolization with N-butyl cyanoacrylate before partial hepatectomy in patients with hepatocellular carcinoma and underlying cirrhosis or advanced fibrosis. J Vasc Interv Radiol. 2005;16:1667–74. https://doi.org/10.1097/01.RVI.0000182183.28547.DC.
14. Qi X, Tang Y, An D, Bai M, Shi X, Wang J, et al. Radiofrequency ablation versus hepatic resection for small hepatocellular carcinoma: a meta-analysis of randomized controlled trials. J Clin Gastroenterol. 2014;48:450–7. https://doi.org/10.1097/MCG.0000000000000008.
15. Tabrizian P, Jibara G, Shrager B, Schwartz M, Roayaie S. Recurrence of hepatocellular cancer after resection: patterns, treatments, and prognosis. Ann Surg. 2015;261:947–55. https://doi.org/10.1097/SLA.0000000000000710.
16. Meloni F, Lazzaroni S, Livraghi T. Percutaneous ethanol injection: single session treatment. Eur J Ultrasound. 2001;13:107–15. https://doi.org/10.1016/s0929-8266(01)00124-0.
17. Lin S-M, Lin C-J, Lin C-C, Hsu C-W, Chen Y-C. Radiofrequency ablation improves prognosis compared with ethanol injection for hepatocellular carcinoma < or = 4 cm. Gastroenterology. 2004;127:1714–23. https://doi.org/10.1053/j.gastro.2004.09.003.
18. Llovet JM, Bruix J. Systematic review of randomized trials for unresectable hepatocellular carcinoma: chemoembolization improves survival. Hepatology. 2003;37:429–42. https://doi.org/10.1053/jhep.2003.50047.
19. Llovet JM, Ricci S, Mazzaferro V, Hilgard P, Gane E, Blanc J-F, et al. Sorafenib in advanced hepatocellular carcinoma. N Engl J Med. 2008;359:378–90. https://doi.org/10.1056/NEJMoa0708857.
20. Kudo M, Finn RS, Qin S, Han K-H, Ikeda K, Piscaglia F, et al. Lenvatinib versus sorafenib in first-line treatment of patients with unresectable hepatocellular carcinoma: a randomised phase 3 non-inferiority trial. Lancet. 2018;391:1163–73. https://doi.org/10.1016/S0140-6736(18)30207-1.
21. Finn RS, Qin S, Ikeda M, Galle PR, Ducreux M, Kim T-Y, et al. Atezolizumab plus bevacizumab in unresectable hepatocellular carcinoma. N Engl J Med. 2020;382:1894–905. https://doi.org/10.1056/NEJMoa1915745.
22. Llovet JM, Kelley RK, Villanueva A, Singal AG, Pikarsky E, Roayaie S, et al. Hepatocellular carcinoma. Nat Rev Dis Primers. 2021;7:6. https://doi.org/10.1038/s41572-020-00240-3.
23. Bruix J, Takayama T, Mazzaferro V, Chau G-Y, Yang J, Kudo M, et al. Adjuvant sorafenib for hepatocellular carcinoma after resection or ablation (STORM): a phase 3, randomised, double-blind, placebo-controlled trial. Lancet Oncol. 2015;16:1344–54. https://doi.org/10.1016/S1470-2045(15)00198-9.
24. Seong J, Park HC, Han KH, Lee DY, Lee JT, Chon CY, et al. Local radiotherapy for unresectable hepatocellular carcinoma patients who failed with transcatheter arterial chemoembolization. Int J Radiat Oncol Biol Phys. 2000;47:1331–5. https://doi.org/10.1016/s0360-3016(00)00519-8.
25. Dawson LA, McGinn CJ, Normolle D, Ten Haken RK, Walker S, Ensminger W, et al. Escalated focal liver radiation and concurrent hepatic artery fluorodeoxyuridine for unresectable intrahepatic malignancies. J Clin Oncol. 2000;18:2210–8. https://doi.org/10.1200/JCO.2000.18.11.2210.
26. Dawson LA, Ten Haken RK. Partial volume tolerance of the liver to radiation. Semin Radiat Oncol. 2005;15:279–83. https://doi.org/10.1016/j.semradonc.2005.04.005.
27. Pan CC, Kavanagh BD, Dawson LA, Li XA, Das SK, Miften M, et al. Radiation-associated liver injury. Int J Radiat Oncol Biol Phys. 2010;76:S94–100. https://doi.org/10.1016/j.ijrobp.2009.06.092.
28. McGinn CJ, Ten Haken RK, Ensminger WD, Walker S, Wang S, Lawrence TS. Treatment of intrahepatic cancers with radiation doses based on a normal tissue complication probability model. J Clin Oncol. 1998;16:2246–52. https://doi.org/10.1200/JCO.1998.16.6.2246.
29. Liang S-X, Zhu X-D, Xu Z-Y, Zhu J, Zhao J-D, Lu H-J, et al. Radiation-induced liver disease in three-dimensional conformal radiation therapy for primary liver carcinoma: the risk factors and

hepatic radiation tolerance. Int J Radiat Oncol Biol Phys. 2006;65:426–34. https://doi.org/10.1016/j.ijrobp.2005.12.031.
30. Miften M, Vinogradskiy Y, Moiseenko V, Grimm J, Yorke E, Jackson A, et al. Radiation dose-volume effects for liver SBRT. Int J Radiat Oncol Biol Phys. 2021;110:196–205. https://doi.org/10.1016/j.ijrobp.2017.12.290.
31. Diez P, Hanna GG, Aitken KL, van As N, Carver A, Colaco RJ, et al. UK 2022 consensus on normal tissue dose-volume constraints for oligometastatic, primary lung and hepatocellular carcinoma stereotactic ablative radiotherapy. Clin Oncol. 2022;34:288–300. https://doi.org/10.1016/j.clon.2022.02.010.
32. Gerhard SG, Palma DA, Arifin AJ, Louie AV, Li GJ, Al-Shafa F, et al. Organ at risk dose constraints in SABR: a systematic review of active clinical trials. Pract Radiat Oncol. 2021;11:e355–65. https://doi.org/10.1016/j.prro.2021.03.005.
33. Lencioni R, Llovet JM. Modified RECIST (mRECIST) assessment for hepatocellular carcinoma. Semin Liver Dis. 2010;30:52–60. https://doi.org/10.1055/s-0030-1247132.
34. Dutta U, Bush N, Kalsi D, Popli P, Kapoor VK. Epidemiology of gallbladder cancer in India. Chin Clin Oncol. 2019;8:33. https://doi.org/10.21037/cco.2019.08.03.
35. Siegel RL, Miller KD, Jemal A. Cancer statistics, 2015. CA Cancer J Clin. 2015;65:5–29. https://doi.org/10.3322/caac.21254.
36. Jarnagin WR, Ruo L, Little SA, Klimstra D, D'Angelica M, DeMatteo RP, et al. Patterns of initial disease recurrence after resection of gallbladder carcinoma and hilar cholangiocarcinoma: implications for adjuvant therapeutic strategies. Cancer. 2003;98:1689–700. https://doi.org/10.1002/cncr.11699.
37. Strom BL, Maislin G, West SL, Atkinson B, Herlyn M, Saul S, et al. Serum CEA and CA 19-9: potential future diagnostic or screening tests for gallbladder cancer? Int J Cancer. 1990;45:821–4. https://doi.org/10.1002/ijc.2910450505.
38. Shindoh J, de Aretxabala X, Aloia TA, Roa JC, Roa I, Zimmitti G, et al. Tumor location is a strong predictor of tumor progression and survival in T2 gallbladder cancer: an international multicenter study. Ann Surg. 2015;261:733–9. https://doi.org/10.1097/SLA.0000000000000728.
39. Roa JC, García P, Kapoor VK, Maithel SK, Javle M, Koshiol J. Gallbladder cancer. Nat Rev Dis Primers. 2022;8:69. https://doi.org/10.1038/s41572-022-00398-y.
40. You DD, Lee HG, Paik KY, Heo JS, Choi SH, Choi DW. What is an adequate extent of resection for T1 gallbladder cancers? Ann Surg. 2008;247:835–8. https://doi.org/10.1097/SLA.0b013e3181675842.
41. Wagholikar GD, Behari A, Krishnani N, Kumar A, Sikora SS, Saxena R, et al. Early gallbladder cancer. J Am Coll Surg. 2002;194:137–41. https://doi.org/10.1016/s1072-7515(01)01136-x.
42. Patkar S, Patel S, Gupta A, Ramaswamy A, Ostwal V, Goel M. Revision surgery for incidental gallbladder cancer-challenging the dogma: ideal timing and real-world applicability. Ann Surg Oncol. 2021;28:6758–66. https://doi.org/10.1245/s10434-021-09687-4.
43. Lee SG, Song GW, Hwang S, Ha TY, Moon DB, Jung DH, et al. Surgical treatment of hilar cholangiocarcinoma in the new era: the Asan experience. J Hepatobiliary Pancreat Sci. 2010;17:476–89. https://doi.org/10.1007/s00534-009-0204-5.
44. Nuzzo G, Giuliante F, Ardito F, Giovannini I, Aldrighetti L, Belli G, et al. Improvement in perioperative and long-term outcome after surgical treatment of hilar cholangiocarcinoma: results of an Italian multicenter analysis of 440 patients. Arch Surg. 2012;147:26–34. https://doi.org/10.1001/archsurg.2011.771.
45. DeOliveira ML, Cunningham SC, Cameron JL, Kamangar F, Winter JM, Lillemoe KD, et al. Cholangiocarcinoma: thirty-one-year experience with 564 patients at a single institution. Ann Surg. 2007;245:755–62. https://doi.org/10.1097/01.sla.0000251366.62632.d3.
46. Wu W, Cheng Q, Chen J, Chen D, Feng X, Wu J. Left-side vs. right-side hepatectomy for hilar cholangiocarcinoma: a meta-analysis. World J Surg Oncol. 2021;19:107. https://doi.org/10.1186/s12957-021-02213-6.
47. Han IW, Jang J-Y, Lee KB, Kang MJ, Kwon W, Park JW, et al. Clinicopathological analysis and prognosis of extrahepatic bile duct cancer with a microscopic positive ductal margin. HPB. 2014;16:575–81. https://doi.org/10.1111/hpb.12193.
48. Machairas N, Kostakis ID, Tsilimigras DI, Prodromidou A, Moris D. Liver transplantation for hilar cholangiocarcinoma: a systematic review. Transplant Rev. 2020;34:100516. https://doi.org/10.1016/j.trre.2019.100516.
49. Bhandare MS, Mondal A, Chaudhari V, Bal M, Yadav S, Ramaswamy A, et al. Factors influencing local and distant recurrence following resection of periampullary cancer. Br J Surg. 2021;108:427–34. https://doi.org/10.1093/bjs/znaa143.
50. Primrose JN, Fox RP, Palmer DH, Malik HZ, Prasad R, Mirza D, et al. Capecitabine compared with observation in resected biliary tract cancer (BILCAP): a randomised, controlled, multicentre, phase 3 study. Lancet Oncol. 2019;20:663–73. https://doi.org/10.1016/S1470-2045(18)30915-X.
51. Ben-Josef E, Guthrie KA, El-Khoueiry AB, Corless CL, Zalupski MM, Lowy AM, et al. SWOG S0809: a phase II intergroup trial of adjuvant capecitabine and gemcitabine followed by radiotherapy and concurrent capecitabine in extrahepatic cholangiocarcinoma and gallbladder carcinoma. J Clin Oncol. 2015;33:2617–22. https://doi.org/10.1200/JCO.2014.60.2219.
52. Valle J, Wasan H, Palmer DH, Cunningham D, Anthoney A, Maraveyas A, et al. Cisplatin plus

gemcitabine versus gemcitabine for biliary tract cancer. N Engl J Med. 2010;362:1273–81. https://doi.org/10.1056/NEJMoa0908721.
53. Sharma A, Kalyan Mohanti B, Pal Chaudhary S, Sreenivas V, et al. Modified gemcitabine and oxaliplatin or gemcitabine + cisplatin in unresectable gallbladder cancer: Results of a phase III randomised controlled trial. Eur J Cancer. 2019;123:162–170. https://doi.org/10.1016/j.ejca.2019.10.004.
54. Nehls O, Oettle H, Hartmann JT, Hofheinz R-D, Hass HG, Horger MS, et al. Capecitabine plus oxaliplatin as first-line treatment in patients with advanced biliary system adenocarcinoma: a prospective multicentre phase II trial. Br J Cancer. 2008;98:309–15. https://doi.org/10.1038/sj.bjc.6604178.
55. Oh D-Y, He AR, Qin S, Chen L-T, Okusaka T, Vogel A, et al. Durvalumab plus gemcitabine and cisplatin in advanced biliary tract cancer. NEJM Evid. 2022;1:EVIDoa2200015. https://doi.org/10.1056/EVIDoa2200015.
56. Tella SH, Kommalapati A, Borad MJ, Mahipal A. Second-line therapies in advanced biliary tract cancers. Lancet Oncol. 2020;21:e29–41. https://doi.org/10.1016/S1470-2045(19)30733-8.
57. Le DT, Durham JN, Smith KN, Wang H, Bartlett BR, Aulakh LK, et al. Mismatch repair deficiency predicts response of solid tumors to PD-1 blockade. Science. 2017;357:409–13. https://doi.org/10.1126/science.aan6733.
58. Zhu AX, Macarulla T, Javle MM, Kelley RK, Lubner SJ, Adeva J, et al. Final overall survival efficacy results of ivosidenib for patients with advanced cholangiocarcinoma with IDH1 mutation: the phase 3 randomized clinical ClarIDHy trial. JAMA Oncol. 2021;7:1669–77. https://doi.org/10.1001/jamaoncol.2021.3836.
59. Hyder O, Dodson RM, Sachs T, Weiss M, Mayo SC, Choti MA, et al. Impact of adjuvant external beam radiotherapy on survival in surgically resected gallbladder adenocarcinoma: a propensity score-matched Surveillance, Epidemiology, and End Results analysis. Surgery. 2014;155:85–93. https://doi.org/10.1016/j.surg.2013.06.001.
60. Kresl JJ, Schild SE, Henning GT, Gunderson LL, Donohue J, Pitot H, et al. Adjuvant external beam radiation therapy with concurrent chemotherapy in the management of gallbladder carcinoma. Int J Radiat Oncol Biol Phys. 2002;52:167–75. https://doi.org/10.1016/s0360-3016(01)01764-3.
61. Das P, Wolff RA, Abbruzzese JL, Varadhachary GR, Evans DB, Vauthey JN, et al. Concurrent capecitabine and upper abdominal radiation therapy is well tolerated. Radiat Oncol. 2006;1:41. https://doi.org/10.1186/1748-717X-1-41.
62. Lim K-H, Oh D-Y, Chie EK, Jang J-Y, Im S-A, Kim T-Y, et al. Adjuvant concurrent chemoradiation therapy (CCRT) alone versus CCRT followed by adjuvant chemotherapy: which is better in patients with radically resected extrahepatic biliary tract cancer?: a non-randomized, single center study. BMC Cancer. 2009;9:345. https://doi.org/10.1186/1471-2407-9-345.
63. Engineer R, Goel M, Chopra S, Patil P, Purandare N, Rangarajan V, et al. Neoadjuvant chemoradiation followed by surgery for locally advanced gallbladder cancers: a new paradigm. Ann Surg Oncol. 2016;23:3009–15. https://doi.org/10.1245/s10434-016-5197-0.
64. Banales JM, Rodrigues PM, Affò S, Andersen JB, Aspichueta P, Boulter L, et al. Cholangiocarcinoma 2026: status quo, unmet needs and priorities. Nat Rev Gastroenterol Hepatol. 2026;23(1):65–96.
65. Qurashi M, Vithayathil M, Khan SA. Epidemiology of cholangiocarcinoma. Eur J Surg Oncol. 2025; 51:107064.
66. Søreide K, Dopazo C, Berrevoet F, Carrion-Alvarez L, Diaz-Nieto R, Andersson B, et al. Biliary tract cancer. Eur J Surg Oncol. 2025;51:108489
67. Colangelo M, Di Martino M, Polidoro MA, Forti L, Tober N, Gennari A, et al. Management of intrahepatic cholangiocarcinoma: a review for clinicians. Gastroenterol Rep (Oxf). 2025;13:004. https://doi.org/10.1093/gastro/goaf005.
68. Zerunian M, Polidori T, Palmeri F, Nardacci S, Del Gaudio A, Masci B, et al Artificial intelligence and radiomics in cholangiocarcinoma: a comprehensive review. Diagnostics (Basel). 2025;15(2):148.
69. Banales JM, Marin JJG, Lamarca A, Rodrigues PM, Khan SA, Roberts LR, et al. Cholangiocarcinoma 2020: the next horizon in mechanisms and management. Nat Rev Gastroenterol Hepatol. 2020; 17:557–588.
70. Goel M, Varty GP, Patkar S, Meghana V, Kazi M, Nandy K, Ostwal V, Ramaswamy A, Gala KB, Shetty NS. Preventing futile surgery in Intrahepatic and Perihilar cholangiocarcinomas: can we identify preoperative factors to improve patient selection and optimize outcomes? Surg Oncol. 2024;55:102096. https://doi.org/10.1016/j.suronc.2024.102096. Epub 2024 Jun 29. PMID: 38964224.
71. Patkar S, Gupta V, Khobragade K, Goel M. The reality of cholangiocarcinoma in India – real world data from a tertiary referral centre. HPB (Oxford). 2022;24(9):1511–18. https://doi.org/10.1016/j.hpb.2022.03.007. Epub 2022 Mar 16. PMID: 35379594.
72. Valle JW, Lamarca A, Goyal L, Barriuso J, Zhu AX. New horizons for precision medicine in biliary tract cancers. Cancer Discov. 2017;7:943–962.
73. Shinohara ET, Mitra N, Guo M, Metz JM. Radiation therapy is associated with improved survival in the adjuvant and definitive treatment of intrahepatic cholangiocarcinoma. Int J Radiat Oncol Biol Phys. 2008;72:1495–501.
74. Kopek N, Holt MI, Hansen AT, Høyer M. Stereotactic body radiotherapy for unresectable cholangiocarcinoma. Radiother Oncol. 2010;94:47–52.

75. Huang J, Lok V, Ngai CH, Zhang L, Yuan J, Lao XQ, et al. Worldwide burden of, risk factors for, and trends in pancreatic cancer. Gastroenterology. 2021;160:744–54. https://doi.org/10.1053/j.gastro.2020.10.007.
76. Heinen MM, Verhage BAJ, Goldbohm RA, van den Brandt PA. Active and passive smoking and the risk of pancreatic cancer in the Netherlands Cohort Study. Cancer Epidemiol Biomarkers Prev. 2010;19:1612–22. https://doi.org/10.1158/1055-9965.EPI-10-0121.
77. Raimondi S, Maisonneuve P, Lowenfels AB. Epidemiology of pancreatic cancer: an overview. Nat Rev Gastroenterol Hepatol. 2009;6:699–708. https://doi.org/10.1038/nrgastro.2009.177.
78. Hruban RH, Canto MI, Goggins M, Schulick R, Klein AP. Update on familial pancreatic cancer. Adv Surg. 2010;44:293–311. https://doi.org/10.1016/j.yasu.2010.05.011.
79. Huang Z, Liu F. Diagnostic value of serum carbohydrate antigen 19-9 in pancreatic cancer: a meta-analysis. Tumour Biol. 2014;35:7459–65. https://doi.org/10.1007/s13277-014-1995-9.
80. Berger AC, Winter K, Hoffman JP, Regine WF, Abrams RA, Safran H, et al. Five year results of US intergroup/RTOG 9704 with postoperative CA 19-9 ≤90 U/mL and comparison to the CONKO-001 trial. Int J Radiat Oncol Biol Phys. 2012;84:e291–7. https://doi.org/10.1016/j.ijrobp.2012.04.035.
81. Hata S, Sakamoto Y, Yamamoto Y, Nara S, Esaki M, Shimada K, et al. Prognostic impact of postoperative serum CA 19-9 levels in patients with resectable pancreatic cancer. Ann Surg Oncol. 2012;19:636–41. https://doi.org/10.1245/s10434-011-2020-9.
82. Al-Hawary MM, Francis IR, Chari ST, Fishman EK, Hough DM, Lu DS, et al. Pancreatic ductal adenocarcinoma radiology reporting template: consensus statement of the Society of Abdominal Radiology and the American Pancreatic Association. Radiology. 2014;270:248–60. https://doi.org/10.1148/radiol.13131184.
83. Callery MP, Chang KJ, Fishman EK, Talamonti MS, William Traverso L, Linehan DC. Pretreatment assessment of resectable and borderline resectable pancreatic cancer: expert consensus statement. Ann Surg Oncol. 2009;16:1727–33. https://doi.org/10.1245/s10434-009-0408-6.
84. Kim HR, Seo M, Nah YW, Park HW, Park SH. Clinical impact of fluorine-18-fluorodeoxyglucose positron emission tomography/computed tomography in patients with resectable pancreatic cancer: diagnosing lymph node metastasis and predicting survival. Nucl Med Commun. 2018;39:691–8. https://doi.org/10.1097/MNM.0000000000000855.
85. Allen PJ, Kuk D, Castillo CF-D, Basturk O, Wolfgang CL, Cameron JL, et al. Multi-institutional validation study of the American Joint Commission on Cancer (8th edition) changes for T and N staging in patients with pancreatic adenocarcinoma. Ann Surg. 2017;265:185–91. https://doi.org/10.1097/SLA.0000000000001763.
86. Amin MB, Greene FL, Edge SB, Compton CC, Gershenwald JE, Brookland RK, et al. The eighth edition AJCC cancer staging manual: continuing to build a bridge from a population-based to a more "personalized" approach to cancer staging. CA Cancer J Clin. 2017;67:93–9. https://doi.org/10.3322/caac.21388.
87. Wagner M, Redaelli C, Lietz M, Seiler CA, Friess H, Büchler MW. Curative resection is the single most important factor determining outcome in patients with pancreatic adenocarcinoma. Br J Surg. 2004;91:586–94. https://doi.org/10.1002/bjs.4484.
88. Winter JM, Cameron JL, Campbell KA, Arnold MA, Chang DC, Coleman J, et al. 1423 pancreaticoduodenectomies for pancreatic cancer: a single-institution experience. J Gastrointest Surg. 2006;10:1199–210; discussion 1210–1. https://doi.org/10.1016/j.gassur.2006.08.018.
89. Unno M, Hata T, Motoi F. Long-term outcome following neoadjuvant therapy for resectable and borderline resectable pancreatic cancer compared to upfront surgery: a meta-analysis of comparative studies by intention-to-treat analysis. Surg Today. 2019;49:295–9. https://doi.org/10.1007/s00595-019-01786-w.
90. Huang L, Jansen L, Balavarca Y, Molina-Montes E, Babaei M, van der Geest L, et al. Resection of pancreatic cancer in Europe and USA: an international large-scale study highlighting large variations. Gut. 2019;68:130–9. https://doi.org/10.1136/gutjnl-2017-314828.
91. Birkmeyer JD, Siewers AE, Finlayson EVA, Stukel TA, Lucas FL, Batista I, et al. Hospital volume and surgical mortality in the United States. N Engl J Med. 2002;346:1128–37. https://doi.org/10.1056/NEJMsa012337.
92. Shrikhande SV, Shinde RS, Chaudhari VA, Kurunkar SR, Desouza AL, Agarwal V, et al. Twelve hundred consecutive pancreato-duodenectomies from single centre: impact of centre of excellence on pancreatic cancer surgery across India. World J Surg. 2020;44:2784–93. https://doi.org/10.1007/s00268-019-05235-0.
93. Gasparini G, Pellegatta M, Crippa S, Lena MS, Belfiori G, Doglioni C, et al. Nerves and pancreatic cancer: new insights into a dangerous relationship. Cancer. 2019;11:893. https://doi.org/10.3390/cancers11070893.
94. Ghaneh P, Kleeff J, Halloran CM, Raraty M, Jackson R, Melling J, et al. The impact of positive resection margins on survival and recurrence following resection and adjuvant chemotherapy for pancreatic ductal adenocarcinoma. Ann Surg. 2019;269:520–9. https://doi.org/10.1097/SLA.0000000000002557.
95. Strobel O, Hank T, Hinz U, Bergmann F, Schneider L, Springfeld C, et al. Pancreatic cancer surgery: the new R-status counts. Ann Surg. 2017;265:565–73. https://doi.org/10.1097/SLA.0000000000001731.

96. Sanjay P, Takaori K, Govil S, Shrikhande SV, Windsor JA. "Artery-first" approaches to pancreatoduodenectomy. Br J Surg. 2012;99:1027–35. https://doi.org/10.1002/bjs.8763.
97. Shrikhande SV, Barreto SG, Bodhankar YD, Suradkar K, Shetty G, Hawaldar R, et al. Superior mesenteric artery first combined with uncinate process approach versus uncinate process first approach in pancreatoduodenectomy: a comparative study evaluating perioperative outcomes. Langenbeck's Arch Surg. 2011;396:1205–12. https://doi.org/10.1007/s00423-011-0824-5.
98. Nickel F, Haney CM, Kowalewski KF, Probst P, Limen EF, Kalkum E, et al. Laparoscopic versus open pancreaticoduodenectomy: a systematic review and meta-analysis of randomized controlled trials. Ann Surg. 2020;271:54–66. https://doi.org/10.1097/SLA.0000000000003309.
99. Kamarajah SK, Bundred J, Marc OS, Jiao LR, Manas D, Abu Hilal M, et al. Robotic versus conventional laparoscopic pancreaticoduodenectomy a systematic review and meta-analysis. Eur J Surg Oncol. 2020;46:6–14. https://doi.org/10.1016/j.ejso.2019.08.007.
100. Pawlik TM, Gleisner AL, Cameron JL, Winter JM, Assumpcao L, Lillemoe KD, et al. Prognostic relevance of lymph node ratio following pancreaticoduodenectomy for pancreatic cancer. Surgery. 2007;141:610–8. https://doi.org/10.1016/j.surg.2006.12.013.
101. Garcea G, Dennison AR, Pattenden CJ, Neal CP, Sutton CD, Berry DP. Survival following curative resection for pancreatic ductal adenocarcinoma. A systematic review of the literature. JOP. 2008;9:99–132.
102. Kinsella TJ, Seo Y, Willis J, Stellato TA, Siegel CT, Harpp D, et al. The impact of resection margin status and postoperative CA19-9 levels on survival and patterns of recurrence after postoperative high-dose radiotherapy with 5-FU-based concurrent chemotherapy for resectable pancreatic cancer. Am J Clin Oncol. 2008;31:446–53. https://doi.org/10.1097/COC.0b013e318168f6c4.
103. Kalser MH, Ellenberg SS. Pancreatic cancer. Adjuvant combined radiation and chemotherapy following curative resection. Arch Surg. 1985;120:899–903.
104. Smeenk HG, van Eijck CHJ, Hop WC, Erdmann J, Tran KCK, Debois M, et al. Long-term survival and metastatic pattern of pancreatic and periampullary cancer after adjuvant chemoradiation or observation: long-term results of EORTC trial 40891. Ann Surg. 2007;246:734–40. https://doi.org/10.1097/SLA.0b013e318156eef3.
105. Neoptolemos JP, Stocken DD, Friess H, Bassi C, Dunn JA, Hickey H, et al. A randomized trial of chemoradiotherapy and chemotherapy after resection of pancreatic cancer. N Engl J Med. 2004;350:1200–10. https://doi.org/10.1056/NEJMoa032295.
106. Regine WF, Winter KA, Abrams RA, Safran H, Hoffman JP, Konski A, et al. Fluorouracil vs gemcitabine chemotherapy before and after fluorouracil-based chemoradiation following resection of pancreatic adenocarcinoma: a randomized controlled trial. JAMA. 2008;299:1019–26. https://doi.org/10.1001/jama.299.9.1019.
107. Schmidt J, Abel U, Debus J, Harig S, Hoffmann K, Herrmann T, et al. Open-label, multicenter, randomized phase III trial of adjuvant chemoradiation plus interferon Alfa-2b versus fluorouracil and folinic acid for patients with resected pancreatic adenocarcinoma. J Clin Oncol. 2012;30:4077–83. https://doi.org/10.1200/JCO.2011.38.2960.
108. Oettle H, Post S, Neuhaus P, Gellert K, Langrehr J, Ridwelski K, et al. Adjuvant chemotherapy with gemcitabine vs observation in patients undergoing curative-intent resection of pancreatic cancer: a randomized controlled trial. JAMA. 2007;297:267. https://doi.org/10.1001/jama.297.3.267.
109. Uesaka K, Boku N, Fukutomi A, Okamura Y, Konishi M, Matsumoto I, et al. Adjuvant chemotherapy of S-1 versus gemcitabine for resected pancreatic cancer: a phase 3, open-label, randomised, non-inferiority trial (JASPAC 01). Lancet. 2016;388:248–57. https://doi.org/10.1016/S0140-6736(16)30583-9.
110. Neoptolemos JP, Palmer DH, Ghaneh P, Psarelli EE, Valle JW, Halloran CM, et al. Comparison of adjuvant gemcitabine and capecitabine with gemcitabine monotherapy in patients with resected pancreatic cancer (ESPAC-4): a multicentre, open-label, randomised, phase 3 trial. Lancet. 2017;389:1011–24. https://doi.org/10.1016/S0140-6736(16)32409-6.
111. Conroy T, Hammel P, Hebbar M, Ben Abdelghani M, Wei AC, Raoul J-L, et al. FOLFIRINOX or gemcitabine as adjuvant therapy for pancreatic cancer. N Engl J Med. 2018;379:2395–406. https://doi.org/10.1056/NEJMoa1809775.
112. Tempero M, O'Reilly E, Van Cutsem E, Berlin J, Philip P, Goldstein D, et al. LBA-1 Phase 3 APACT trial of adjuvant nab-paclitaxel plus gemcitabine (nab-P + Gem) vs gemcitabine (Gem) alone in patients with resected pancreatic cancer (PC): updated 5-year overall survival. Ann Oncol. 2021;32:S226. https://doi.org/10.1016/j.annonc.2021.06.009.
113. Hsu CC, Herman JM, Corsini MM, Winter JM, Callister MD, Haddock MG, et al. Adjuvant chemoradiation for pancreatic adenocarcinoma: the Johns Hopkins Hospital-Mayo Clinic collaborative study. Ann Surg Oncol. 2010;17:981–90. https://doi.org/10.1245/s10434-009-0743-7.
114. Katz MHG, Pisters PWT, Evans DB, Sun CC, Lee JE, Fleming JB, et al. Borderline resectable pancreatic cancer: the importance of this emerging stage of disease. J Am Coll Surg. 2008;206:833–46; discussion 846–8. https://doi.org/10.1016/j.jamcollsurg.2007.12.020.
115. Takahashi H, Ohigashi H, Gotoh K, Marubashi S, Yamada T, Murata M, et al. Preoperative

gemcitabine-based chemoradiation therapy for resectable and borderline resectable pancreatic cancer. Ann Surg. 2013;258:1040–50. https://doi.org/10.1097/SLA.0b013e31829b3ce4.

116. Stokes JB, Nolan NJ, Stelow EB, Walters DM, Weiss GR, de Lange EE, et al. Preoperative capecitabine and concurrent radiation for borderline resectable pancreatic cancer. Ann Surg Oncol. 2011;18:619–27. https://doi.org/10.1245/s10434-010-1456-7.
117. Estrella JS, Rashid A, Fleming JB, Katz MH, Lee JE, Wolf RA, et al. Post-therapy pathologic stage and survival in patients with pancreatic ductal adenocarcinoma treated with neoadjuvant chemoradiation. Cancer. 2012;118:268–77. https://doi.org/10.1002/cncr.26243.
118. Versteijne E, Suker M, Groothuis K, Akkermans-Vogelaar JM, Besselink MG, Bonsing BA, et al. Preoperative chemoradiotherapy versus immediate surgery for resectable and borderline resectable pancreatic cancer: results of the Dutch randomized phase III PREOPANC trial. J Clin Oncol. 2020;38:1763–73. https://doi.org/10.1200/JCO.19.02274.
119. Saúde-Conde R, El Ghali B, Navez J, Bouchart C, Van Laethem JL. Total Neoadjuvant Therapy in Localized Pancreatic Cancer: Is More Better? Cancers (Basel). 2024;16(13):2423. https://doi.org/10.3390/cancers16132423.
120. Janssen QP, van Dam JL, Bonsing BA, Bos H, Bosscha KP, Coene PPLO, et al. Total neoadjuvant FOLFIRINOX versus neoadjuvant gemcitabine-based chemoradiotherapy and adjuvant gemcitabine for resectable and borderline resectable pancreatic cancer (PREOPANC-2 trial): study protocol for a nationwide multicenter randomized controlled trial. BMC Cancer. 2021;21:300. https://doi.org/10.1186/s12885-021-08031-z.
121. Unno M, Motoi F, Matsuyama Y, Satoi S, Matsumoto I, Aosasa S, et al. Randomized phase II/III trial of neoadjuvant chemotherapy with gemcitabine and S-1 versus upfront surgery for resectable pancreatic cancer (Prep-02/JSAP-05). J Clin Orthod. 2019;37:189. https://doi.org/10.1200/JCO.2019.37.4_suppl.189.
122. Sohal D, Duong MT, Ahmad SA, Gandhi N, Beg MS, Wang-Gillam A, et al. SWOG S1505: results of perioperative chemotherapy (peri-op CTx) with mfolfirinox versus gemcitabine/nab-paclitaxel (Gem/nabP) for resectable pancreatic ductal adenocarcinoma (PDA). J Clin Oncol. 2020;38:4504. https://doi.org/10.1200/JCO.2020.38.15_suppl.4504.
123. Ghaneh P, Palmer D, Cicconi S, Jackson R, Halloran CM, Rawcliffe C, et al. Immediate surgery compared with short-course neoadjuvant gemcitabine plus capecitabine, FOLFIRINOX, or chemoradiotherapy in patients with borderline resectable pancreatic cancer (ESPAC5): a four-arm, multicentre, randomised, phase 2 trial. Lancet Gastroenterol Hepatol. 2023;8:157–68. https://doi.org/10.1016/S2468-1253(22)00348-X.
124. Murphy JE, Wo JY, Ryan DP, Jiang W, Yeap BY, Drapek LC, et al. Total neoadjuvant therapy with FOLFIRINOX followed by individualized chemoradiotherapy for borderline resectable pancreatic adenocarcinoma: a phase 2 clinical trial. JAMA Oncol. 2018;4:963–9. https://doi.org/10.1001/jamaoncol.2018.0329.
125. Katz MHG, Shi Q, Meyers JP, Herman JM, Choung M, Wolpin BM, et al. Alliance A021501: preoperative mFOLFIRINOX or mFOLFIRINOX plus hypofractionated radiation therapy (RT) for borderline resectable (BR) adenocarcinoma of the pancreas. J Clin Oncol. 2021;39:377. https://doi.org/10.1200/JCO.2021.39.3_suppl.377.
126. Moertel CG, Frytak S, Hahn RG, O'Connell MJ, Reitemeier RJ, Rubin J, et al. Therapy of locally unresectable pancreatic carcinoma: a randomized comparison of high dose (6000 rads) radiation alone, moderate dose radiation (4000 rads + 5-fluorouracil), and high dose radiation + 5-fluorouracil: the Gastrointestinal Tumor Study Group. Cancer. 1981;48:1705–10.
127. Chauffert B, Mornex F, Bonnetain F, Rougier P, Mariette C, Bouché O, et al. Phase III trial comparing intensive induction chemoradiotherapy (60 Gy, infusional 5-FU and intermittent cisplatin) followed by maintenance gemcitabine with gemcitabine alone for locally advanced unresectable pancreatic cancer. Definitive results of the 2000-01 FFCD/SFRO study. Ann Oncol. 2008;19:1592–9. https://doi.org/10.1093/annonc/mdn281.
128. Loehrer PJ Sr, Feng Y, Cardenes H, Wagner L, Brell JM, Cella D, et al. Gemcitabine alone versus gemcitabine plus radiotherapy in patients with locally advanced pancreatic cancer: an Eastern Cooperative Oncology Group trial. J Clin Oncol. 2011;29:4105–12. https://doi.org/10.1200/JCO.2011.34.8904.
129. Mukherjee S, Hurt CN, Bridgewater J, Falk S, Cummins S, Wasan H, et al. Gemcitabine-based or capecitabine-based chemoradiotherapy for locally advanced pancreatic cancer (SCALOP): a multicentre, randomised, phase 2 trial. Lancet Oncol. 2013;14:317–26. https://doi.org/10.1016/S1470-2045(13)70021-4.
130. Hammel P, Huguet F, van Laethem J-L, Goldstein D, Glimelius B, Artru P, et al. Effect of chemoradiotherapy vs chemotherapy on survival in patients with locally advanced pancreatic cancer controlled after 4 months of gemcitabine with or without erlotinib: the LAP07 randomized clinical trial. JAMA. 2016;315:1844–53. https://doi.org/10.1001/jama.2016.4324.
131. Mizrahi JD, Surana R, Valle JW, Shroff RT. Pancreatic cancer. Lancet. 2020;395:2008–20. https://doi.org/10.1016/S0140-6736(20)30974-0.
132. Conroy T, Desseigne F, Ychou M, Bouché O, Guimbaud R, Bécouarn Y, et al. FOLFIRINOX versus gemcitabine for metastatic pancreatic cancer. N Engl J Med. 2011;364:1817–25. https://doi.org/10.1056/NEJMoa1011923.
133. Von Hoff DD, Ervin T, Arena FP, Chiorean EG, Infante J, Moore M, et al. Increased survival in pan-

creatic cancer with nab-paclitaxel plus gemcitabine. N Engl J Med. 2013;369:1691–703. https://doi.org/10.1056/NEJMoa1304369.
134. Golan T, Hammel P, Reni M, Van Cutsem E, Macarulla T, Hall MJ, et al. Maintenance olaparib for germline BRCA-mutated metastatic pancreatic cancer. N Engl J Med. 2019;381:317–27. https://doi.org/10.1056/NEJMoa1903387.
135. Kindler HL, Hammel P, Reni M, Van Cutsem E, Macarulla T, Hall MJ, et al. Overall survival results from the POLO trial: a phase III study of active maintenance olaparib versus placebo for germline BRCA-mutated metastatic pancreatic cancer. J Clin Oncol. 2022;40:3929–39. https://doi.org/10.1200/JCO.21.01604.
136. Isaji S, Murata Y, Kishiwada M. New Japanese classification of pancreatic cancer. In: Neoptolemos JP, Urrutia R, Abbruzzese JL, Büchler MW, editors. Pancreatic cancer. New York: Springer New York; 2018. p. 1021–37. https://doi.org/10.1007/978-1-4939-7193-0_84.
137. Dholakia AS, Kumar R, Raman SP, Moore JA, Ellsworth S, McNutt T, et al. Mapping patterns of local recurrence after pancreaticoduodenectomy for pancreatic adenocarcinoma: a new approach to adjuvant radiation field design. Int J Radiat Oncol Biol Phys. 2013;87:1007–15. https://doi.org/10.1016/j.ijrobp.2013.09.005.
138. Brunner TB, Haustermans K, Huguet F, Morganti AG, Mukherjee S, Belka C, et al. ESTRO ACROP guidelines for target volume definition in pancreatic cancer. Radiother Oncol. 2021;154:60–9. https://doi.org/10.1016/j.radonc.2020.07.052.
139. Ben-Josef E, Schipper M, Francis IR, Hadley S, Ten-Haken R, Lawrence T, et al. A phase I/II trial of intensity modulated radiation (IMRT) dose escalation with concurrent fixed-dose rate gemcitabine (FDR-G) in patients with unresectable pancreatic cancer. Int J Radiat Oncol Biol Phys. 2012;84:1166–71. https://doi.org/10.1016/j.ijrobp.2012.02.051.
140. Crane CH, Varadhachary GR, Yordy JS, Staerkel GA, Javle MM, Safran H, et al. Phase II trial of cetuximab, gemcitabine, and oxaliplatin followed by chemoradiation with cetuximab for locally advanced (T4) pancreatic adenocarcinoma: correlation of Smad4(Dpc4) immunostaining with pattern of disease progression. J Clin Oncol. 2011;29:3037–43. https://doi.org/10.1200/JCO.2010.33.8038.
141. Parekh A, Rosati LM, Chang DT, Goodman KA, Koong AC, Herman JM. Stereotactic body radiation for pancreatic cancer: results of an international survey of practice patterns. Int J Radiat Oncol Biol Phys. 2015;93:E132. https://doi.org/10.1016/j.ijrobp.2015.07.884.
142. Bryant JM, Palm RF, Liveringhouse C, Boyer E, Hodul P, Malafa M, et al. Surgical and pathologic outcomes of pancreatic adenocarcinoma (PA) after preoperative ablative stereotactic magnetic resonance image guided adaptive radiation therapy (A-SMART). Adv Radiat Oncol. 2022;7:101045. https://doi.org/10.1016/j.adro.2022.101045.
143. Lin C, Verma V, Ly QP, Lazenby A, Sasson A, Schwarz JK, et al. Phase I trial of concurrent stereotactic body radiotherapy and nelfinavir for locally advanced borderline or unresectable pancreatic adenocarcinoma. Radiother Oncol. 2019;132:55–62. https://doi.org/10.1016/j.radonc.2018.11.002.
144. Jung J, Yoon SM, Park J-H, Seo D-W, Lee SS, Kim M-H, et al. Stereotactic body radiation therapy for locally advanced pancreatic cancer. PLoS One. 2019;14:e0214970. https://doi.org/10.1371/journal.pone.0214970.
145. Bernard ME, Sutera PA, Iarrobino NA, Quan K, Burton SA, Bahary N, et al. Initial results of a prospective study of adjuvant pancreatic stereotactic body radiation therapy for close or positive margins. Adv Radiat Oncol. 2019;4:294–301. https://doi.org/10.1016/j.adro.2018.11.007.
146. Zhu X, Shi D, Li F, Ju X, Cao Y, Shen Y, et al. Prospective analysis of different combined regimens of stereotactic body radiation therapy and chemotherapy for locally advanced pancreatic cancer. Cancer Med. 2018;7:2913–24. https://doi.org/10.1002/cam4.1553.
147. Sutera PA, Bernard ME, Gill BS, Harper KK, Quan K, Bahary N, et al. One- vs. three-fraction pancreatic stereotactic body radiation therapy for pancreatic carcinoma: single institution retrospective review. Front Oncol. 2017;7:272. https://doi.org/10.3389/fonc.2017.00272.
148. Herman JM, Chang DT, Goodman KA, Dholakia AS, Raman SP, Hacker-Prietz A, et al. Phase 2 multi-institutional trial evaluating gemcitabine and stereotactic body radiotherapy for patients with locally advanced unresectable pancreatic adenocarcinoma. Cancer. 2015;121:1128–37. https://doi.org/10.1002/cncr.29161.
149. Pollom EL, Alagappan M, von Eyben R, Kunz PL, Fisher GA, Ford JA, et al. Single- versus multifraction stereotactic body radiation therapy for pancreatic adenocarcinoma: outcomes and toxicity. Int J Radiat Oncol Biol Phys. 2014;90:918–25. https://doi.org/10.1016/j.ijrobp.2014.06.066.
150. Mahadevan A, Moningi S, Grimm J, Li XA, Forster KM, Palta M, et al. Maximizing tumor control and limiting complications with stereotactic body radiation therapy for pancreatic cancer. Int J Radiat Oncol Biol Phys. 2021;110:206–16. https://doi.org/10.1016/j.ijrobp.2020.11.017.
151. Hiroshima Y, Fukumitsu N, Saito T, Numajiri H, Murofushi KN, Ohnishi K, et al. Concurrent chemoradiotherapy using proton beams for unresectable locally advanced pancreatic cancer. Radiother Oncol. 2019;136:37–43. https://doi.org/10.1016/j.radonc.2019.03.012.
152. Hong TS, Ryan DP, Borger DR, Blaszkowsky LS, Yeap BY, Ancukiewicz M, et al. A phase 1/2 and biomarker study of preoperative short course chemoradiation with proton beam therapy and capecitabine

followed by early surgery for resectable pancreatic ductal adenocarcinoma. Int J Radiat Oncol Biol Phys. 2014;89:830–8. https://doi.org/10.1016/j.ijrobp.2014.03.034.
153. Kawashiro S, Yamada S, Okamoto M, Ohno T, Nakano T, Shinoto M, et al. Multi-institutional study of carbon-ion radiotherapy for locally advanced pancreatic cancer: Japan Carbon-ion Radiation Oncology Study Group (J-CROS) Study 1403 Pancreas. Int J Radiat Oncol Biol Phys. 2018;101:1212–21. https://doi.org/10.1016/j.ijrobp.2018.04.057.
154. Bhattacharyya T, Shinoto M, Takiyama H, Nitta Y, Koto M, Imai R, et al. Long-term outcomes of octogenarian pancreatic cancer patients treated with carbon ion radiotherapy. Pancreatology. 2022;22:381–6. https://doi.org/10.1016/j.pan.2022.03.010.
155. Hanna GG, Murray L, Patel R, Jain S, Aitken KL, Franks KN, et al. UK consensus on normal tissue dose constraints for stereotactic radiotherapy. Clin Oncol. 2018;30:5–14. https://doi.org/10.1016/j.clon.2017.09.007.
156. Marks LB, Yorke ED, Jackson A, Ten Haken RK, Constine LS, Eisbruch A, et al. Use of normal tissue complication probability models in the clinic. Int J Radiat Oncol Biol Phys. 2010;76:S10–9. https://doi.org/10.1016/j.ijrobp.2009.07.1754.
157. Abrams RA, Winter KA, Regine WF, Safran H, Hoffman JP, Lustig R, et al. Failure to adhere to protocol specified radiation therapy guidelines was associated with decreased survival in RTOG 9704--a phase III trial of adjuvant chemotherapy and chemoradiotherapy for patients with resected adenocarcinoma of the pancreas. Int J Radiat Oncol Biol Phys. 2012;82:809–16. https://doi.org/10.1016/j.ijrobp.2010.11.039.

Online Links

https://econtour.org/ (radiotherapy contouring)
https://www.youtube.com/watch?v=1ctVxiIhT9E (SBRT for liver cancers)
https://www.youtube.com/watch?v=77jtiDlSks0 (Chang ing treatment landscape of HCC)

Colorectal and Anal Canal Cancers

Rahul Krishnatry, Debanjan Chakraborty,
Shakthivel Mani, and Reena Engineer

1 Introduction

Colorectal Carcinoma is the third most common cancer worldwide. It is the third most common cancer in men and the second most common cancer in women. There were more than 1.9 million new cases of colorectal cancer in 2020. In 2022, an estimated 151,030 new cases of CRC will be diagnosed, with rectal cancer accounting for 44,850 of these cases. Among Indian men, the rising incidence of colon and rectal cancer is noted with annual incidence rates (AIR) at 4.4 and 4.1 per 100,000 population, while the incidence of colon cancer among women is seen at 3.9 per 100,000 population. The projected annual incidence of CRC, reported by the National Cancer Registry Programme 2020 [1] is 36,000 patients approximately (21,000 in males and 15,000 in females gender). The incidence is steeply rising, mostly due to obesity, excess consumption of red meat, processed food, less fiber in the diet, and increased smoking and alcohol consumption. Incidence is higher in African and men, compared to Caucasian and women—taking into account—gender and ethnicity. In the USA, the lifetime average risk of colorectal cancer is 5% [2]. Anal canal is a continual part of the colo-rectal region, anatomically, but a rarer site of cancer. In this chapter, we will discuss rectal and anal cancer in further detail below.

R. Krishnatry (✉) · D. Chakraborty · S. Mani
R. Engineer
Department of Radiation Oncology, Tata Memorial Centre, Mumbai, India

HBNI University, Mumbai, India

2 Rectal Cancer

2.1 Biology and Behavior

The most important prognostic factor for survival is the loco-regional and distant extent of disease—depth of bowel wall involved, lymph nodal involvement, and presence of distant metastasis. Various biomarkers have been utilized for prognostic assessment and relevant correlation with outcomes, with very little robust evidence. Now, TNM staging by AJCC 8th is used for staging Rectal Cancer [3]. Diagnosis as per AJCC staging system is utilized to guide treatment; a general overview of the management of rectal cancer stage wise is summarized in Table 1.

3 Primary Therapy

The primary treatment modality is surgical excision of the tumor with adequate negative margins, sparing the post-surgical morbidity as much as possible, and maintaining the QoL as intact as feasible. The inception of TME has come from the concept of mesorectal radial lymphatic

B. K. Mohanti et al. (eds.), *Radiation Oncology – Principles, Precepts and Practice*,
https://doi.org/10.1007/978-981-95-5171-2_12

Table 1 General treatment overview in the management of rectal cancer

Stage	Treatment
Stage I	cT1N0–*Trans-anal local excision followed by observation* Selected group for local excision—*(pT1 lesion, <3 cm size, <30% bowel wall circumference, <8 cm from Anal Verge, margins minimum 3 mm, Grade 1 and 2, no LVSI)* If HPR shows high risk features—*Close/Positive margins, LVI, G3* tumors: TME/LAR followed by risk adapted adjuvant therapy Similar for pT2N0M0
Stage II and III	Preoperative long-course chemoradiation/Short course RT and induction chemotherapy, then LAR/APR with TME, then adjuvant Chemo if needed (all current Phase III evidences support total neoadjuvant approach) **If obstructed may** need diverting colostomy before induction therapy
Stage IVA-oligometastatic disease	*Neoadjuvant chemotherapy* followed by RT (short or long course), then staged or synchronous resection (primary with metastasis) and adjuvant chemotherapy Neoadjuvant chemo-radiation followed by staged/simultaneous resection (primary and metastasis) followed by adjuvant chemo
Poly-metastatic rectal cancer	Palliative Chemotherapy Stoma might be needed for bowel function/continuity Poor PS- Best Supportive and Palliative Care
Anastomotic/ Pelvic local recurrence	Resectable: Chemoradiation -f/b- Surgery Debatable role of IORT Unresectable: Definitive Chemoradiation In Re-irradiation setting: Twice daily, hyperfractionation is desirable

spread. The idea of total mesorectal excision (TME) [4].

Though It has increased local control to great extent, still it can be improved further with preoperative (neoadjuvant) radiation therapy. In the Dutch TME and Swedish Trial [5], it has shown a significant local control benefit.

4 Adjunct Therapy

The standard management for resectable locally advanced rectal cancer (T3-4 or Node positive) is neoadjuvant chemoradiation followed by surgery and adjuvant chemotherapy.

Pre-Op. chemoradiation has resulted in a significant reduction in rates of local failure, lower acute and late toxicity and also a significant increment in the rate of sphincter preservation in patients who were supposed to be undergoing APR on presurgical evaluation. This is validated in the German rectal Cancer trial by Sauer [6] and many other Phase III studies also. The completion rates of planned treatment and compliance are far better in patients receiving neoadjuvant chemoradiation. The primary disadvantage in such patients is: the theoretical overtreatment of possible lower-stage tumors with intensive treatment before surgery and failure to use specific subsequent pathological information, which might enable to make decisions in patients who might need less/no treatment. In the case of upfront surgery, the pathological stage can guide exact tailored adjuvant treatment in indicated selected patients who only need it esp. R1/R2 resections, multiple nodal involvements, T3/4 disease.

Despite preoperative chemoradiation in unresectable tumors, the local recurrence rates remain at 15–30% [7]. The addition of chemotherapy/IORT/brachytherapy boost in such a scenario may decrease the rate of local recurrence [8].

5 Palliation

Pelvic Radiotherapy offers effective palliation in terms of pain relief, hemostasis and incessant mucous secretion control. Short, hypofractionated schedules usually help to achieve the goal of palliation within a short period of time, albeit with corresponding acute toxicity. Usually, 6–8 Gray in a single fraction to 25 Gray in 5 fractions is usually effective to attain palliation [9].

6 Etiology

The etiopathogenesis of colorectal cancer appears to be multifactorial and includes both environmental and genetic factors. Approximately 75% are sporadic, whereas 20% develop in those with familial or a personal history of colorectal cancer or polyps. The remaining genetic risk/predisposition is seen in hereditary nonpolyposis colorectal cancer (HNPCC, Lynch syndrome; 2% to 4%) or familial adenomatous polyposis (FAP; 1%), or in people with inflammatory bowel disease, especially chronic ulcerative colitis (1%) as depicted in Table 2 [10].

7 Young Colorectal Cancers

7.1 Risk Factors

- Increasing age
- FAP/HNPCC/Peutz Jeghers Syndrome/ Juvenile polyposis -Higher risk in younger Age.
- Personal/family history of polyps
- Obesity
- Sedentary lifestyle, less exercise

Table 2 Certain hereditary syndromes associated with colorectal cancer

FAP	Autosomal dominant condition, germline mutation, APC gene in 5th chromosome. Usually younger age incidence, no genesis noted from adenoma Variants—Gardner's Syndrome, Turcot's Syndrome
HNPCC-Lynch Syndrome	Microsatellite instability. Deficient MMR genes. hMLH1, hMSH2,6, PMS2 Synchronous/Metachronous neoplasms possible Increased risk for Uterus, GI, Ovarian, and Hepatobiliary cancer

- Alcohol and tobacco consumption
- Low fiber, high trans-fat diet: red meat, canned and processed food*
- IBD

There are likely three pathways for rectal cancer—chromosomal instability (CIN), microsatellite instability (MSI), and CpG island methylator phenotype (CIMP).

Theoretically, protective factors are: *NSAID, Fiber, Vitamin B6.*

8 Pathology

Ninety percent of the tumors are adenocarcinoma. Approximately, 10–15% are mucinous, while signet ring tumours (Intracellular mucin pushing nucleus away) constitute 1–2% of all rectal cancer. They carry a poor prognosis and have a predilection of early distant metastasis with peritoneal deposits. Other rarer histologies include small cell, Carcinoid, Leiomyosarcoma, Lymphoma, and melanoma.

8.1 Prognostic Factors

- T and N Stage
- Circumferential resection margin (CRM) and LVI are the most important factors.
- Poor Performance status, AJCC stage, Higher grade, (CEA>5 ng/mL) have been associated with inferior RFS and OS [11].

9 Anatomy

The rectum is about 15–16 cm long hollow viscera in the pelvis, connected to the exterior via the anal opening. It begins at the rectosigmoid junction (~S3) and extends up to the anorectal ring, just above the dentate line. For surgical decisions, it is subdivided into three parts according to the distance of the lower edge of the tumor from the anal verge (assessed by rigid proctoscopy): upper third, 12–15 cm; middle third, 6–12 cm; and lower third, less than 6 cm. Tumors beyond 12 cm from the AV are considered a sigmoid colonic lesion. The anorectal ring is at the level of the puborectal sling and Levator Ani, representing the inner side of the pelvic floor. The point of anterior peritoneal reflection is where the rectum exits the peritoneal cavity (approximately 12–15 cm from the anal verge, at the level of upper rectum).

Mucosa, submucosa, muscularis propria, serosa are the layers of rectum and mesorectum is loose connective tissue containing terminal branches of IMA. The anorectal ring has crucial anatomical importance: it represents the internal anal sphincter, necessary for anal continence and also the inferior limit for functional sphincter preservation surgery.

9.1 Blood Supply and Lymphatics

The proximal third is peritonealised anteriorly and laterally, supplied by superior rectal arteries (Continuation of Inferior mesenteric artery). The Middle third rectum is peritonealized anteriorly and is supplied by the middle rectal branch from the internal iliac artery. The non-peritonealised lower rectum is supplied by inferior rectal arteries, branch from the internal pudendal artery as depicted in Fig. 1. Lymphatics: The Superior 50% of the rectum drains along the superior rectal artery to pararectal, presacral, sigmoidal, and inferior mesenteric nodes. Mid rectal Tumors above the dentate line tend to metastasize to internal iliac lymph nodes as compared to lower rectal tumors that may extend into the anal canal, involving eventually superficial inguinal nodes via nodes along the inferior rectal and external iliac pathways. Tumors that invade anteriorly into pelvic viscera mostly drain to external iliac nodes.

9.2 Metastasis

The liver is the most common site of distant metastasis in rectal cancer, but it has an increased propensity for lung metastasis too more than what is seen in Metastatic colon cancer. Upper rectal tumors reach to liver through portal circulation (via superior rectal vein). Middle and inferior rectal tumors spread into systemic circulation, leading to pulmonary metastases, accessing via middle and inferior rectal vein.

10 Early Detection

Screening aims at reducing rectal cancer-related mortality through earlier detection and treatment of benign or premalignant lesions and curable-early stage cancers [12].

Average-Risk Population Screening should begin at age 50 years for average risk people and one of the following testing options is advised: fecal occult blood testing (FOBT) or fecal immunochemical testing (FIT) every year, flexible sigmoidoscopy every 5 years, double-contrast barium enema every 5 years, CT colonography (virtual colonoscopy) every 5 years, or colonoscopy (preferably) every 10 years.

High-Risk Population Affected first-degree relatives, a family history of FAP or HNPCC, or a personal history of adenomatous polyps, colorectal cancer, or chronic IBD, screening should begin earlier (at age 40 years) or it should be done more frequently. Specifically, screening should start at age 40 or 10 years before the age of diagnosis of the youngest affected first-degree relative, whichever comes first, with colonoscopy repeated every 5 years thereafter. Patients with IBD should undergo annual colonoscopy beginning 8 to 10 years after the onset of symptoms. Once polyposis develops, elective colectomy or proctocolectomy is recommended in patients of FAP. For HNPCC patients, screen-

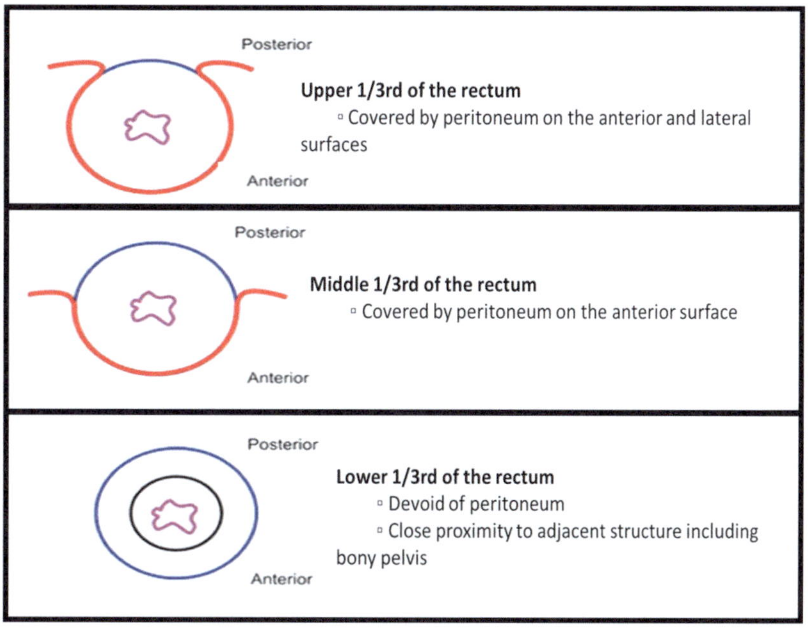

Fig. 1 Relationship of peritoneal reflection with different parts of rectum

ing colonoscopy should be performed every 1 to 2 years, starting at 20 to 25 years of age.

11 Clinical Presentation

Bleeding per rectum is the most common presenting symptom in rectal neoplasms. Abdominal pain is less common compared to colonic malignancy. Other symptoms are: constipation, diarrhea, or alternating episodes of loose stools and constipation. Also reduced stool calibre, tenesmus, rectal urgency, inadequate evacuation, in late stages: urinary symptoms, buttock and perineal pain. Recurrent and non-resolving Spurious Diarrhea, due to accumulated secreted mucus above the obstructive rectal tumor, is a distressing complaint and often required colostomy before starting neo-adjuvant therapies.

12 Evaluation

Pre-therapeutic Assessment in a patient of rectal adenocarcinoma should consist of a detailed history and clinical examination. Digital rectal examination (size, location, clock position, mobility, sphincter function) and pelvic exam in women is crucial for evaluation. Examination of groin nodes is important to detect nodal metastasis, esp. in lower rectal primaries.

The biopsy is done through Sigmoidoscopy/rigid proctoscopy.

Laboratory investigations include: Complete Blood count, Serum biochemical parameters incl. RFT and LFT, Serum electrolytes, coagulation profile, and viral markers. CEA is also done and has a proven adverse impact on survival independent of the stage—to differentiate secretors from non-secretors—helping to monitor therapy/treatment response.

Rigid proctoscopy allows direct visualization of the lesion, provides an estimation of the size of the lesion and the degree of obstruction, along with estimation of distance from anal verge and opportunity for biopsy.

A complete evaluation of the large bowel, preferably by colonoscopy, should be done to rule out synchronous neoplasms [13].

The primary imaging modalities for detecting the Local and regional extent of the primary tumor are endorectal ultrasound (ERUS), contrast-enhanced computed tomography (CECT), and magnetic resonance imaging (MRI) of the Abdomen and Pelvis. Both endorectal ultrasound (ERUS) and high-resolution pelvic MRI (Figs. 2 and 3) are accurate for assessing T-stage by evaluating bowel wall thickness and depth of tumor invasion. MRI is particularly reliable in detecting mesorectal fascia involvement and predicting circumferential resection margin (CRM) positivity. ERUS has limited utility in highly stenotic tumors or upper rectal lesions. On MRI, lymph node morphology—such as mixed signal intensity and irregular borders—is more dependable for assessment. Sub-staging of T3 tumors (T3a/b with ≤5 mm extramural spread) has been prospectively validated by the MERCURY study, demonstrating strong correlation between pretreatment MRI and histopathology. T2-weighted sequences, often combined with diffusion-weighted imaging, are most commonly used for optimal evaluation [14].

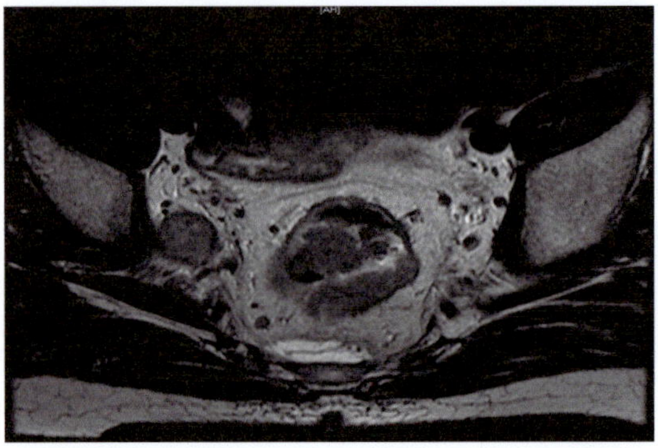

Fig. 2 Pelvic MRI showing tumor (T2 intermediate signal intensity) invading serosa and infiltrating mesorectal fat (T2 bright)

Detecting Nodal metastasis in CECT/MRI is mostly done using size criteria with higher sensitivity, but in FDG PET CT scan, the uptake (SUV Max) indicates the pathological involvement with more specificity. Also, the major advantage of a PET scan is to differentiate between recurrent tumor and scar tissue by measuring tissue metabolism of an injected glucose-based substance.

PET CT scan is chosen, If potentially surgically curable M1 disease in selected cases- esp. Oligo-metastatic Cases. If liver-directed therapy like RFA/SBRT or surgery is contemplated, a hepatic MRI with intravenous routine extracellular or hepatobiliary GBCA is selected as the imaging of choice to assess the exact number and distribution of metastatic foci for local treatment planning [15].

If liver-directed therapy or surgery is contemplated, a hepatic MRI with intravenous routine extracellular or hepatobiliary GBCA is preferred over CT to assess the exact number and distribution of metastatic foci for local treatment planning.

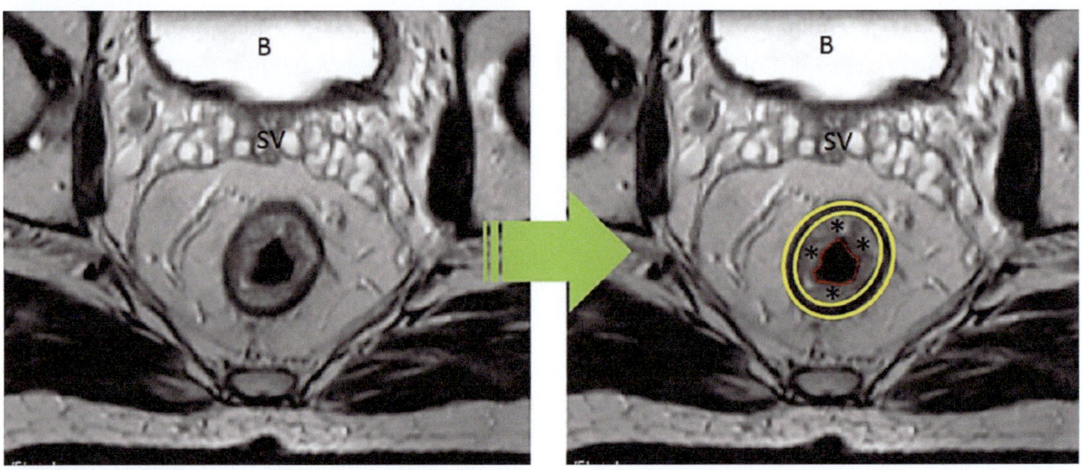

Fig. 3 T2-weighted MRI below anterior peritoneal reflection, Yellow elliptical boundary-Dark, muscular layer; Layer denoting * is Submucosa-Mild hyperintense signal; Red line: Dark- mucosa., SV- seminal vesicle, B- urinary Bladder, T2 Bright Fat in the mesorectum

13 STAGING—TNM Staging as per AJCC 8th Edition (Tables 3 and 4) [3]

Table 3 AJCC TNM classification

T stage	Definition
TX	Primary tumor cannot be assessed
T0	No evidence of primary tumor
Tis	Carcinoma in situ: intraepithelial or invasion of lamina propria
T1	Tumor invades submucosa
T2	Tumor invades muscularis propria
T3	Tumor invades through the muscularis propria into the subserosa or into non-peritonealized perirectal tissues without reaching the mesorectal fascia or adjacent organs (sub-classification of T3 is not included in AJCC 8th Edition) T3a: tumor extends <1 mm beyond muscularis propria 4 T3b: tumor extends 1–5 mm beyond muscularis propria 4 T3c: tumor extends 5–15 mm beyond muscularis propria 4 T3d: tumor extends 15 mm beyond muscularis propria 4
T4a	Tumor penetrates to the surface of the visceral peritoneum
T4b	Tumor directly invades or is adherent to other organs or structures

N stage	Definition
Nx	Regional nodes cannot be assessed
N0	No regional lymph node metastases
N1a	Metastasis in 1 regional lymph node
N1b	Metastasis in 2–3 regional lymph nodes
N1c	Tumor deposit(s) in the subserosa, mesentery, or non-peritonealized pericolic or perirectal tissues without regional nodal metastasis
N2a	Metastasis in 4–6 regional lymph nodes
N2b	Metastasis in 7 or more than 7 lymph nodes

M Stage	Definitions
Mx	Cannot be assessed
M0	No distant Metastasis
M1a	Metastasis confined to one organ or site (for example, liver, lung, ovary, non-regional node) without peritoneal metastases
M1b	Metastasis in more than one organ
M1c	Metastasis to the peritoneum with or without other organ involvement

Table 4 AJCC staging of rectal tumors

Stages	T/N/M criteria
0	TisN0M0
I	T1-2,N0M0
II	IIa T3N0M0 IIb T4aN0M0 IIc T4bN0M0
III	IIIa T1-2, N1, M0 IIIb T3-4, N1, M0 IIIc T3-4b, N2, M0
IV	Any T, ANy N, M1

14 Stage Grouping

15 Management

15.1 Patient Evaluation

The pre-treatment evaluation of a patient with rectal cancer should include a careful history, general physical examination and a meticulous digital rectal examination (the average finger can reach approximately 7–8 cm), which usually assesses for size, ulceration, and fixity to surrounding local structures. It also assesses sphincter continence and suitability for sphincter preservation surgery [16].

Rigid proctoscopy documents the size, position of the lesion and the degree of obstruction, visually, along with utility for biopsy.

A complete evaluation of the large bowel, preferably by colonoscopy, should be done to rule out synchrony.

15.2 Post Treatment Assessment

Surgical resection is classified as R0 (negative margins), R1 (microscopic margin involvement), or R2 (gross residual tumor). The most critical margin is the circumferential resection margin (CRM) surrounding the mesorectum. This margin can be threatened not only by direct tumor extension but also by incomplete removal of lymph nodes lying just beneath the mesorectal fascia (MRF). Even minor deviations from the correct surgical plane may breach this fascia, compromising local control.

Studies by Quirke [17] have shown that survival is lesser by 50% when the tumor can be demonstrated at or within 1 mm from the radial surgical plane of resection (CRM+).

15.3 Tumor Regression Grading

Neoadjuvant chemoradiation is able to induce T and N level downstaging where in 15–30% of cases, this can lead to the complete disappearance of tumor cells (i.e., a pathological complete response [pCR or ypT0N0]) indicating a higher rate of survival. Moreover, various tumor regression grading (TRG) systems, based on the relative amount of tumor cells and fibrosis have been proposed. A scale of 0 (complete response; no viable cancer cells) to 3 (poor response; minimal or no regression, extensive residual cancer) has been proposed by The College of American Pathologist's Guidelines to objectively grade the response, albeit with a issue of debatable standardization [18].

16 Surgery

16.1 Resectable Rectal Cancer-T1-3, N0-1

T1 tumors are usually managed by trans-anal excision. All other tumors usually undergo LAR or APR with sharp TME, with at least pelvic 12 lymph nodes resected for staging.

Local Excision (Trans-anal Excision or Trans-anal Endoscopic Microsurgery) Possible for T1 tumors that are <3 cm in greatest diameter, no more than 30% of rectal circumference, within 8 cm of dentate line or below the middle rectal valve, low-grade histology, and no LVSI.

Low Anterior Resection (LAR) Sphincter-sparing surgery with coloanal anastomosis (or colonic J-pouch). Distal margins of 2 cm or even less are now adequate, and the crucial margin is the circumferential resection margin (CRM).

Abdominoperineal Resection (APR) Historically for tumors <5 cm from the anal verge where sphincter sparing was not thought possible, requiring permanent colostomy and higher morbidity. Rectosigmoid is oversewn via abdominal incision and pulled out through anal canal via the perineal incision.

NSABP R-04 did not show worse QOL at 1 year between APR compared to sphincter-sparing surgery, but profiles of QOL were different [19].

Total Meso-rectal Excision Standard of Care Surgical Practice and mandatory for radical curative surgeries involving. Sharp dissection and en bloc removal of the mesorectum, including associated vascular and lymphatic structures, fatty tissue, and mesorectal fascia as a "package", designed to spare autonomic nerves [20].

TME improves LC and autonomic nerve damage (impotence, retrograde ejaculation, and urinary incontinence) compared with standard blunt dissection of conventional surgery, but with higher anastomotic leaks.

17 Additional Treatment

T1N0 Lesion A R0 local excision by the Trans-anal or Trans-abdominal route is sufficient. If Post-Op. HPR reveals a poorly differentiated histology, positive margins, invasion into the lower third of the submucosa (sm3 level), or LVI, or if the tumor is restaged to pT2, additional treatment is required.

If R+ resection, a trans-abdominal resection must be warranted. Results of a meta-analysis suggest that chemoradiation after transanal local excision without a transabdominal resection may be associated with higher rates of local recurrence.

17.1 Adjuvant Treatment Recommendations for cT1-2 N0 Rectal Cancer

Stage cT1–2 rectal cancers after Trans-abdominal resection are given further treatment based on the pathologic stage.

pT1–2, N0, M0—usually requires no further additional treatment.

If *pT3, N0, M0*—chemoradiotherapy, given either before or after chemotherapy, is one option.

Observation can also be considered in these patients if the tumor was well-differentiated or moderately well-differentiated carcinoma invading less than 2 mm into the mesorectum, without lymphatic or venous vessel involvement, and was located in the upper rectum.

Finally, chemotherapy with FOLFOX or CAPOX regimen alone is an option for margin-negative proximal tumors.

For pN+/or pT4 disease, chemotherapy and chemoradiation can be given sequentially with chemotherapy followed by concurrent chemoradiation or vice-versa. The recommended perioperative therapy is for a total duration of up to 6 months.

There are two general approaches in which radiation therapy has been utilized for management of rectal cancer: *Post-operative and Preoperative treatment.*

A third approach, known as the *Sandwich technique, which is no longer used*, includes a short preoperative course of radiation (5–15 Gray) followed by surgery, and in patients with pT3-4N1-2 disease, an additional 40 Gray to 45 Gray postoperatively [21].

Until 1990, most patients in the United States underwent surgery ± risk-adapted adjuvant radiotherapy.

The primary advantage of this approach was pathologic staging and avoiding overtreatment with preoperative therapy. NSABP trial R-01 (16% vs. 25%; $p = 0.06$) and the Medical Research Council (MRC) trial (21% vs 34%; $p = 0.001$) have shown improved local disease control in pT3/N+ rectal cancer [22, 23].

Preoperative Irradiation There are two approaches to preoperative therapy. The first, developed in Northern Europe, is short-course radiation (25 Gray in 5 fractions) therapy (SCRT), finished over a week. In contrast, majority of investigators recommended a standard long-course radiotherapy (LCRT) of (50.4 Gray in 28 fractions) combined with concurrent chemotherapy [24–26].

17.2 Preoperative SCRT

There are 12 modern randomized trials of short-course preoperative radiation therapy —all showing an increase in local control with a statistical significance. Although in some trials a subset analysis revealed a significant improvement in survival rates, the Swedish Rectal Cancer Trial is the only one that reported a survival advantage for the total treatment group, likely due to poorer local control by Non-TME surgeries in that Trial.

Despite an improved survival in meta-analysis by Chen et al. [26], but the Colorectal Cancer Collaborative Group analysis did not show any advantage. In the Swedish Rectal Cancer Trial, cT1-3 rectal cancer patients were randomized to short-course radiotherapy (25 Gy in 1 week) followed by surgery versus surgery alone. Preoperative RT significantly reduced local recurrence (12% vs 27%; p <0.001) and improved 5-year overall survival (58% vs 48%; p=0.004). The survival benefit persisted at 13 years (38% vs 30%; p=0.008).

The local recurrence rate in patients who are node positive and underwent surgery alone was 46%, particularly due to non TME surgeries. The Dutch CKVO 95-04 trial randomized [5] 1805 patients with the cT1-3 disease to TME or short-course RT before TME. Short course radiation meaningfully reduced the local relapse rate (8% vs 2%; $p < 0.0001$), but the almost equal 2-year OS. With longer follow-up, the 5-year local failure rate was 6% in arm containing TME with preoperative short course radiation. A subset analysis of 593 patients with R0 surgeries revealed that although there were 11% fewer deaths resulting from the disease in the preoperative radiation compared to TME alone arm (40% vs 51%, $p = 0.01$) there was equivalent OS in 2 arms, due to mortality related to other causes including treatment toxicity in Neo-adjuvant radiation +TME arm.

Despite the use of more conformal techniques, there was a substantial incidence of acute toxicity including neurotoxicity, perineal wound dehiscence, and anastomotic leaks in the radiation arm, which reflected that lower gap between radiation and surgery might cause this. Patients selected for treatment with short-course radiation historically have included those with cT1-3 disease, whereas those selected for chemoradiation include T3 or N+ disease.

18 Adjuvant Chemoradiation Node-Positive Disease

Patients who undergo high-quality TME, have at least 12 nodes examined, and have pT3N0 disease may not need the radiation component of chemoradiation, dependent on the adequacy of radial and distal resection margins. The small benefit of local control with irradiation may not be worth the risks, especially in women wishing to spare fertility. However, patients with pT3N0 tumors with adverse pathologic features, who undergo resection without TME, or who have fewer than 12 nodes examined should still receive postoperative chemoradiation to compensate for a higher risk of loco-regional failure [27].

18.1 Preoperative Chemoradiation

Based on the German CAO/ARO/AIO 94 trial, preoperative chemoradiation is the standard treatment for patients with cT3-4N0 or T-any N+ disease. It showed an increment in downstaging, resectability, and better adherence to completing full-dose systemic treatment. Possible overtreatment of patients with either early-stage disease (pT1-2N0) is the sole theoretical disadvantage [6].

19 Chemotherapy

Utilization of Chemotherapy leads to improved LC and OS as well as decreased risk of developing DM.

Adjuvant setting- Path. Stage T3/T4, N1/N2 disease, positive margins or at high risk for local recurrence (high-grade positive or close margin).

Concurrent setting- Esp. used with long-course Radiation.

1. *PVI 5-FU*: As per the Mayo Clinic/NCCTG study, protracted venous infusion (PVI) 5-FU with concurrent RT, with daily dose of 5 FU being 225 mg /sq m, throughout RT, when compared to concurrent bolus 5-FU, had a lower rate of recurrence and DM, with improvement in 4-years OS from 60% to 70%. [28].
2. *Capecitabine*: German phase III trials (including pre- and post-op chemoradiation) showed a significant reduction in DM and the trend toward OS and DFS benefit using concurrent Capecitabine. NSABP R-04 trial confirmed equivalency and showed the equivalence of capecitabine to PVI 5-FU. It is associated with more hand-foot syndrome, fatigue, proctitis, and less leukopenia compared to 5-FU. The concurrent dose is 825 mg/m^2 BID 5 days per week. Adjuvant chemotherapy dose is 1000–1250 mg/m^2 BID days 1–14, q3 weekly cycle [19].
3. *Oxaliplatin*: No benefit observed on multiple trials despite increased neuro-toxicity and neutropenia.

Adjuvant Chemo The role of adjuvant CHT is presently performed less given German rectal trial results. Common regimens included FOLFOX, CAPEOX, 5-FU, or 5-FU+LCV.

Adore trial [29] showed better 3-year disease-free survival with adjuvant FOLFOX (72% vs 63%). Similarly, the CAO/ARO/AIO-04 trial found that adding oxaliplatin to pre-operative chemoradiation and to post-operative chemotherapy (5 FU based) improved disease-free survival. In contrast, a recent patient-level meta-analysis showed no benefit of adjuvant chemotherapy over no adjuvant chemotherapy in patients who had already received pre- operative chemoradiation followed by surgery.

20 Radiation

Radiation improves loco-regional control, reduces disease-specific mortality as well as possible improvement in OS.

20.1 Pre-operative RT

Indications include cT3-4 or cN1-2. It enables downstaging, sphincter preservation, compliance, and reduced toxicity compared to Adjuvant RT.

20.2 Options

Short course radiotherapy-SCRT—(25 Gray/5 fractions with surgery within 1 week and adjuvant Chemo if node-positive).

Long course radiotherapy-LCRT—(50.4 Gray/28 fractions with concurrent Chemo followed by surgery 7–8 weeks later).

After SCRT, postoperative complications substantially increase if there is interval of 10 days between surgery and Radiation. Although waiting 4–6 weeks after a short course leads to improved downstaging (44% vs. 13%), higher pathological CR rates, there is no improvement in sphincter-sparing probability. Very early surgery can lead to anastomotic complications [30].

Post-operative RT: Indications are

- pT3-4
- pN1-2 (stage II–III)
- Positive margin
- PDAC/G3 tumor

Boosting should be considered up to 55–60 Gray for gross residual disease (R2 resection) to elevate the chance of local control, especially at the anastomosis site. The colostomy is planned prior to EBRT in select pts including pts with severe obstructive symptoms [31].

20.3 Contraindications for RT

- Active IBD- Crohns' disease, Ulcerative Colitis
- Pregnancy
- Collagen vascular disease

21 Locally Advanced Disease

Locally advanced rectal cancer is a heterogeneous group. Information, including the proximity/involvement of MRF surrounding the mesorectum and involvement of the sphincter, Extra-mural venous invasion, pelvic lymphadenopathy if any, is now considered a crucial factor in staging, prognostication and deciding management for locally advanced rectal cancers.

The choice of CT scan Thorax + Abdomen, or PET CT Whole body, depending on the patient's presenting symptoms, is crucial to rule out distant metastasis. Involvement of the sciatic notch indicates an inoperable situation and likely treatment for palliative intent.

21.1 Recommendations for Patients with T3, N Any Lesions with Clear CRM by MRI or with T1–2, N1–2 Lesions

Patients clinically staged as T3, N any, with the prediction of clear margins by MRI, have the same treatment options as those clinically staged as T1–2, N1–2. Prediction of CRM status by MRI is crucial and noted in MDJC. Two potential treatment courses are recommended for this group of patients, either TNT, total neoadjuvant treatment followed by TME, or a more traditional perioperative therapy approach, including both neoadjuvant and adjuvant therapy.

Of these two options, the preferred approach is TNT, consisting of chemotherapy with FOLFOX or CAPOX given either before or after chemoradiation [32].

Alternatively, short-course RT may be used when following a TNT approach after a multidisciplinary discussion of the need for downstaging, operability and the possibility of long-term toxicity. Following neoadjuvant therapy, restaging prior to transabdominal resection is mandatory.

The second option for the sequence of treatment in this population is chemoradiation or short-course RT followed by restaging, transabdominal resection, and then adjuvant chemotherapy.

In those patients who achieve a complete clinical response to neoadjuvant therapy before surgery, documented during re-staging, with no evidence of residual disease on digital rectal examination, rectal MRI, and direct endoscopic evaluation, a watch-and-wait nonoperative management approach may be considered in centers with experienced multidisciplinary care and informed discussion with patients (IWWD Consensus Guidelines) [33].

21.2 Recommendations for Patients with T3, N Any Lesions with Involved or Threatened CRM by MRI, with T4, N Any Lesions, with Locally Unresectable Disease, or Who Are Medically Inoperable

For patients with higher-risk stage II or III rectal cancer, including cT3 lesions with radiologically involved or threatened CRM, cT4 lesions, and locally unresectable or medically inoperable disease, TNT is the only recommended approach. This is because a pathologic complete response is less likely following an initial course of only chemoRT or short-course RT, and the full course of TNT is warranted prior to resection.

In the TNT approach, 12–16 weeks of chemotherapy are followed by chemoradiation or short-course RT, restaging, and transabdominal resection. Alternatively, a TNT approach may start with chemoRT or short-course RT, followed by 12–16 weeks of chemotherapy, then restaging and transabdominal resection. FOLFOX or CAPOX are generally used for chemotherapy, although FOLFIRINOX is also an option for T4, N+ disease, as noted in UNICANCER PRODIGE 23 trial [32, 34]. Figure 4 represents various TNT trials and their test arms.

Preoperative chemoradiation is necessary for patients with locally unresectable or MRF involved with primary or recurrent disease. After neoadjuvant chemoradiation, they have a higher R0 resection rate, pCR rate, and 5-year local control rate—a nonsignificant increment in the OS. Maximizing the delivery of systemic therapy upfront also enables early treatment of micrometastases with enhanced downstaging, with less interruption and more compliance compared to adjuvant chemotherapy, delivered after surgery.

The short course RT—5 Gray x 5 fractions and typical long course chemoradiation 50.4 Gray/28 fractions have been compared by Bujko et al., though the SCRT arm was not superior in terms of OS, DFS, or DMFS [35].

The interval between the start of radiation and surgery was 12 weeks in both groups. Even in non-responder patients, surgery should still be considered. Overall, approximately 10% of rectal cancers require extensive surgery like pelvic exenteration, to get an R0 resection as T4b tumors invading the prostate, bladder, or the uterus and vagina, where the disease can be resected en bloc with R0 margins. Midline posterior tumors invading the distal sacrum may be resectable for cure with APR extended to include the lower sacrum. Irrespective of the pre-op treatment, after neoadjuvant treatment finishes, the extent of surgery is decided after clinicoradiological restaging in the MDJC. The 5-year OS in such patients can go up to 50%.

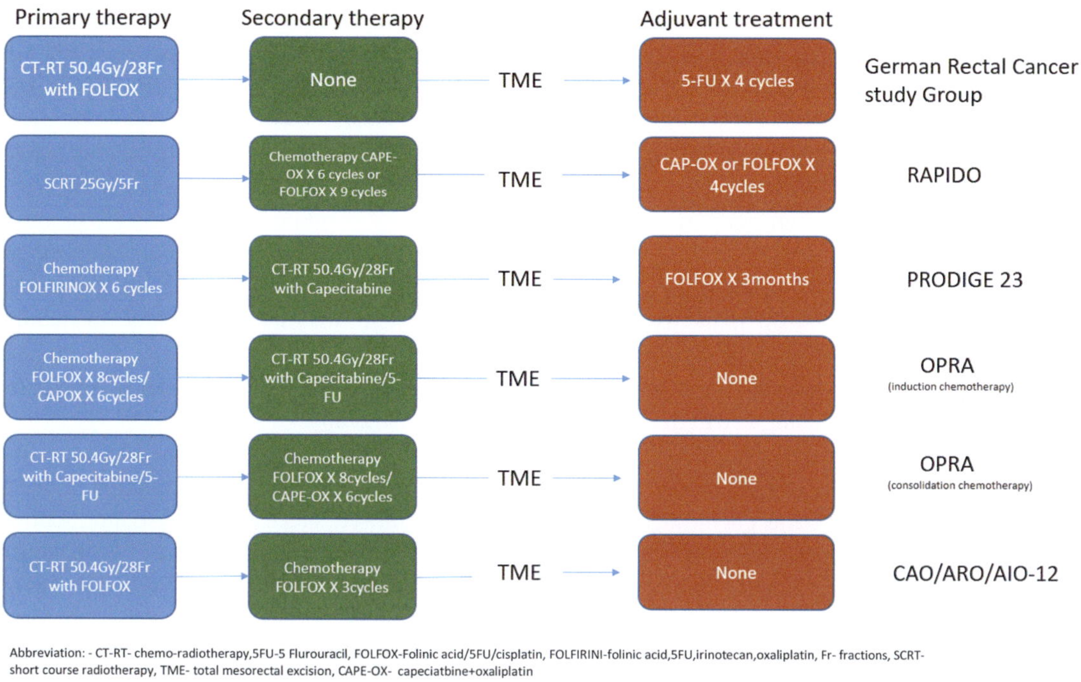

Fig. 4 TNT trials and their test arms for locally advanced rectal cancer

Improvements in patient selection, and surgical technique, Peri-operative care, such as vascularized tissue flaps to facilitate the healing of pelvic and perineal wounds, have improved the results. The 5-year OS ranges between 33% and 50%, with significant rates of morbidity and mortality up to 6%. In IORT institutions, an excellent alternative is marginal gross total resection-GTR (R0 or R1) plus IO RT [8].

Although sphincter preservation is a major goal for patients with primary resectable disease, this should be a lesser threshold in locally recurrent tumors [36].

In view of the high treatment morbidity from morbid surgery and/or often re-irradiation, and unfavorable outcomes, patients may have a better functional QoL with a permanent colostomy. Common local symptoms include pain, hemorrhages, infection, and obstructive symptoms. After recurrence, preoperative chemo-radiation to facilitate resectability can be used with accepted higher late toxicity, if suitable. However, some patients have limited opportunity for re-treatment in view of anticipated very high rates of intolerable toxicity and dismal outcomes.

22 Non Operative Management (Nom) of Rectal Cancer After NACTRT

In those patients who achieve a complete clinical response with no evidence of residual disease on digital rectal examination, rectal MRI, and direct endoscopic evaluation, a "watch and wait," non-operative (chemotherapy and/or RT) management approach may be considered in centres with an experienced multidisciplinary team.

In 1985–91, In a study by Haber Gamma, for approaching non-operative management of lower rectal cancers by neoadjuvant chemoradiation (50.4 Gy with 5FU), it was shown that 5-year OS and DFS in observation/NOM arm was 100 and 92%. Typically, T3/T4 resectable tumors of lower rectal, non-circumferential tumors, within <7 cm from the anal verge, non-signet-ring histology, and low/zero nodal burdens are typically selected for NOM [37].

Post therapy Surveillance recommendations include DRE, proctoscopy every 3–4 months for 2 years, then every 6 months for a total of 5 years. MRI rectum is recommended every 6 months for at least 3 years to monitor for extraluminal local recurrence. Then yearly up to 5 years is enough as summarized in Tables 4 and 5. CEA levels are important in secretory tumors, to monitor for relapse. Almost all relapses occur within the first 2 years, >80% in the first year. Local re-growth is usually salvaged early in an early stage due to strict surveillance.

In a recent Phase III randomized trial of OPRA, in a selected cohort of patients, chemotherapy followed by consolidation chemotherapy has been proven to preserve the organ and avoid any kind of surgery- reflecting in a higher GU, GI and Sexual QoL (Quality of Life) [38].

Also, other phase III trials like RAPIDO have shown SCRT with Induction chemotherapy has resulted in doubled pCR rates—from 14 to 28%—as compared to previous standard treatments, which consisted of NACTRT, subsequent surgery and Adjuvant chemotherapy [39].

22.1 Re-irradiation After Surgery

Even after R0 TME/APR, there is a subset of patients who will recur even after neoadjuvant or adjuvant RT/chemotherapy. Usually, these relapses are unresectable and re-treatment confers a high probability of normal tissue toxicity. Data from Mohiuddin et al. [40] suggest that reirradiation with doses of 30 Gy (40 Gy sometimes if excellent bowel sparing) can be used for limited volumes with a dismal 5-year median OS around 20%.

Another study from Italy has shown median doses around 50 Gray have enabled downstaging and R0 resection in locally recurrent tumors, with higher local control and DFS [41].

Data from Mayo Clinic and MDACC have shown similar outcomes but concurrent chemo and hyperfractionated regimens have shown better results, with lower late G3-4 toxicities. Disease-free interval >2 years indicates favorable biology and a modest increment in survival. Various combinations of EBRT, brachytherapy, and intracavitary irradiation has executed fruitful delivery of re-irradiation with acceptable acute and late toxicity. Especially medically inoperable rectal cancers should be treated aggressively with pelvic irradiation as a component of their therapy.

Effective palliation in terms of bleeding/discharge control, pain relief, and reduction of mass effect is achieved successfully by hypofractionated conformal EBRT. In a subset of 80 patients with metastatic disease who received pelvic irradiation, Crane et al. reported that 94% had complete relief of pelvic symptoms. In patients unfit for re-irradiation, laser treatment or stenting offers some palliative benefits for symptomatic relief [42].

23 Metastatic Disease

With the development of more effective systemic therapy, the median survival of patients with metastatic colorectal cancer is greater than 2 years. Approximately 50% to 60% of patients diagnosed with CRC will develop colorectal metastases, and 80% to 90% of these patients have unresectable metastatic liver disease. The liver was the only site of metastatic disease in one-third of patients. Synchronous presentations are usually more sinister, often with bi-lobar involvement, poor resectability, and worse prognosis.

Table 5 Follow-up strategy, IWWD consensus for follow-up of NOM patients

Year	Serum CEA	DRE	Endoscopy	Pelvic MRI	CECT chest abdomen pelvis
1st	3 months	3–4 months	3–4 months	3–4 months	6–12 months
2nd	3 months	3–4 months	3–4 months	3–4 months	Annually
3rd	3 months	6 months	6 months	6 months	Annually
4th	6 months	6 months	6 months	6 months	Annually
5th	6 months	6 months	6 months	6 months	Annually

Certain clinicopathologic factors, such as the presence of extrahepatic metastases, the presence of more than three tumors, and a disease-free interval of fewer than 12 months, have been associated with a poor prognosis in patients with CRC. Aggressive techniques to address liver metastasis with surgery and nonsurgical ablative techniques such as radiofrequency ablation, cryosurgery, microspheres, and EBRT have further improved median survival. Innovative radiation techniques such as stereotactic body radiotherapy-SBRT of liver metastases are under active investigation.

Ablative techniques include radiofrequency ablation (RFA), microwave (MW) ablation, cryoablation, and electrocoagulation (irreversible electroporation). A systematic review concluded that hepatic arterial infusion chemotherapy (HAIC) with Floxuridine + Dexamethasone, yttrium-90 microsphere radioembolization, and transcatheter arterial chemoembolization-drug eluting Irinotecan beads (TACE) have similar efficacy in patients with unresectable colorectal hepatic metastases [43].

With these advances, local therapy has become crucial in low-volume oligometastatic disease, depending on the site and number of extra-pelvic metastases, involved organs, if radically approached and especially in a good performance status. Good response to chemotherapy demands consolidation with chemoradiation for local disease, if low volume metastasis and performance status allows. Approximately 2–5% of colorectal cancers present with synchronous oligometastasis, usually in the liver and they are radically treated with curative intent. These patients can be treated with curative intent. Similar like colonic primary, R0 resection of both the primary tumor and metastases, either upfront or after induction therapy, is decided in a multidisciplinary team discussion for oligometastatic rectal cancer. Surgical resection of liver and lung metastases is potentially curative, with 5-year survival rates of 30–50%. The optimal timing of primary tumor surgery—whether simultaneous with metastasis resection or after chemoradiation—remains controversial and should be individualized by the multidisciplinary team discussing the sequence suitability. In patients with limited metastases usually FOLFOX and FOLFIRI are usually the most commonly used regimens in mCRC, sometimes combined with bevacizumab or with cetuximab/panitumumab for KRAS/NRAS/BRAF wild-type unresectable synchronous disease.

In addition, checkpoint inhibitors may be considered for MSI-high (MSI-H)/deficient mismatch repair (dMMR) disease as an alternative to chemotherapy-containing regimens.

24 Patterns of Relapse

The design of pelvic radiation fields is primarily guided by the patterns of local relapse after surgery alone. In locally advanced rectal cancer, recurrences commonly occur in the soft tissues of the pelvic sidewall, presacral space, bladder, prostate (in men), or vagina (in women), especially in tumors involving the mesorectal fascia or close (<1 mm) circumferential resection margins, increasing the likelihood of R1 resection. Lymphatic spread occurs mainly in a cephalad direction within the perirectal fascia and mesenteric vessels, being routinely removed during standard TME. However, mid and lower rectal tumors frequently spread laterally along the internal iliac and obturator nodes. The external iliac nodes are at risk only when there is involvement of anterior viscera. Tumors extending into the anal canal or lower third of the vagina, may warrant bilateral inguinal nodal coverage for regional control. A contemporary series by Hruby et al. of 269 patients showed that the majority of local failures occurred in the posterior central pelvis (47%) or at the anastomosis (21%), while anterior recurrences (11%) were largely limited to T4 tumors [44]. Following abdominoperineal resection, the presacral pelvis was the most common site of relapse. Similarly, analysis from the Dutch TME trial revealed that most cranial recurrences were located just above the sacral promontory, regardless of radiation volumes.

25 2D Radiotherapy Field Design

The whole-pelvic radiation field must cover the primary tumor, tumor bed, and at-risk nodal regions. The boost field targets only the primary tumor and tumor bed, with its size based on the tumor's location and extent. Whole-pelvic and boost fields are typically delivered using a three-field (PA + laterals) or four-field technique. Field shaping with blocks spares the small bowel antero-superiorly, tissues posterior to the sacrum, and the infra-pubic region.

26 Three-Dimensional Treatment Planning and Delineation Recommendations

Techniques using CT-based 3D treatment planning and MLC dependent field shaping have been used lately. Using a 3D planning system, Koelbl et al. found prone position plus a belly board decreased the dose to small bowel versus similar patients in the supine position.

The consensus guideline by Vincenzo Valentini et al. [45] for the delineation of rectal cancer target volumes is the most popular and informative guideline, guiding a proper and accurate delineation for RT worldwide.

First is the mesorectum. As per Valentini guidelines, in the superior pelvis, the anterior part of the mesorectal subsite does not have an anatomical boundary. In the presacral subsite space is small and it is often not visible on CT scan. It is usually delineated together with the mesorectum as only one subsite. Lastly, the internal iliac node area is represented by a triangular lymphovascular fat area located between the pelvic wall and the mesorectum behind the external iliac vessels. In some guidelines the obturator nerve is used to split it into two subsites: the obturator subsite encompassed by the external iliac vessels and the obturator nerves and the internal iliac subsite, posterior to the obturator nerve. The external iliac subsite is the easiest to identify, because of the external iliac arteries and veins, which are well visualized on CT scan.

For cT3 tumors the primary tumor, the entire mesorectum, presacral space, and internal iliac nodes should be included. In addition, the obturator nodes should be added in case of low and medium rectum MRF+, clearly positive internal iliac nodes, and posterior cT4 disease.

In cT4 tumors with anterior organ invasion, or for cT3 tumors with clear obturator node involvement, external iliac nodes are included in elective volumes.

The lower edge of the CTV may be modified according to tumor extension and invasion based on the lower edge of the tumor in sigmoidoscopy and DRE. For Tumors located at >1.5 cm above the anal-rectal ring, the lower border should be limited at the end of the mesorectum but if the lower edge of tumor is <1.5 cm from the anal-rectal ring, the lower border should extend to encompass 1 cm of the anal canal. If anal canal is involved, the entire anal canal and the sphincter complex should be included it is also recommended to contour 5 mm to 10 mm of fat around it. When the rectal fossa is directly infiltrated by the tumor, both ischiorectal fossa should be included. Inguinal nodes generally are not targeted in rectal cancer unless largely the anal canal and ischiorectal fossa is infiltrated [45].

27 Introduction to IMRT and IGRT

IMRT further improves dose conformality and homogeneity within the planning target volume (PTV). In addition to step-and-shoot delivery with a limited number of beam angles, IMRT can also be delivered continuously as intensity-modulated arc therapy (IMAT), during which collimator position, gantry rotation speed, and beam intensity are modulated in real time. The PTV margin is determined by geometrical uncertainties, which account for differences between the planned and actual treatment delivery.

The acquired IGRT images also enable accurate treatment delivery with visual verification. If External iliac lymph nodes needed to be included in the CTV, IMRT offered better sparing of organs and better coverage, keeping the bowel dose lower. With IMRT, it is possible to deliver

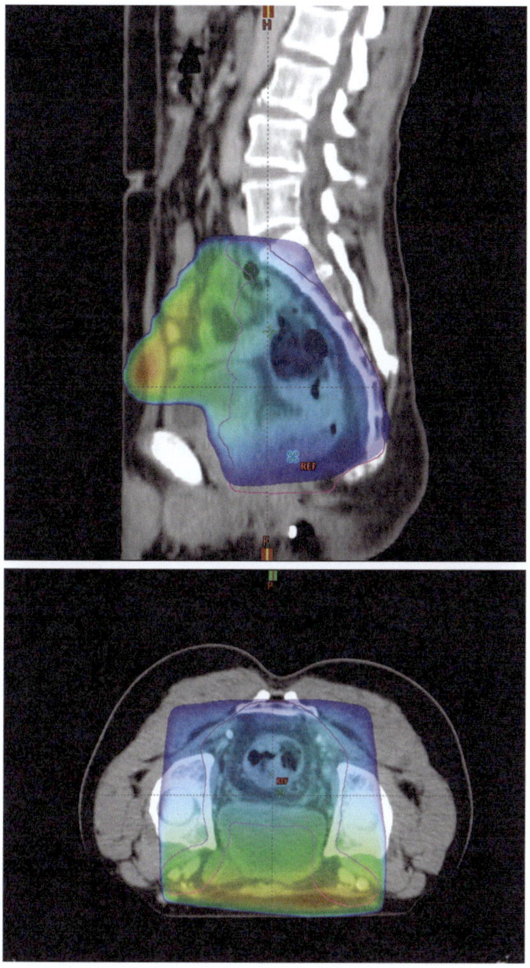

Fig. 5 Sagittal and axial section: 95% dose color wash showing coverage in 4 field conventional technique

more concave dose distributions, with uniformity and lower small intestine doses as illustrated in Figs. 5 and 6. Important parameters for prediction of acute and late bowel toxicity, such as the volume of small bowel receiving 45, 40, 30 and 15 Gy or more (V15) are significantly reduced using IMRT.

A study at MGH suggests that the volume of the small bowel in the radiation field in a 3DCRT plan is decreased with protons as compared with photons. IMRT treatment planning techniques can also decrease the volume of small bowel in the field when compared with 3D conformal techniques [46].

However, the clinical benefit of IMRT compared with 3D treatment delivery remains to be determined. Multiple large population dosimetric studies had already proven reduction in acute and late bowel toxicities, esp. acute enteritis by almost 50%. A simultaneous integrated boost to the gross disease delivering the standard dose to the CTV at same time without increasing normal tissue effects is a beneficial impact too. But better image guidance like Cone Beam CT are crucial to execute IMRT safely and accurately. Inter fraction and intrafraction set-up errors and target volume variation need to be compensated to ensure safe application of IMRT. Daily image guidance might enable to reduce PTV margin from 5 mm to 3 mm resulting into less toxicity. Online Corrections for set-up errors can be

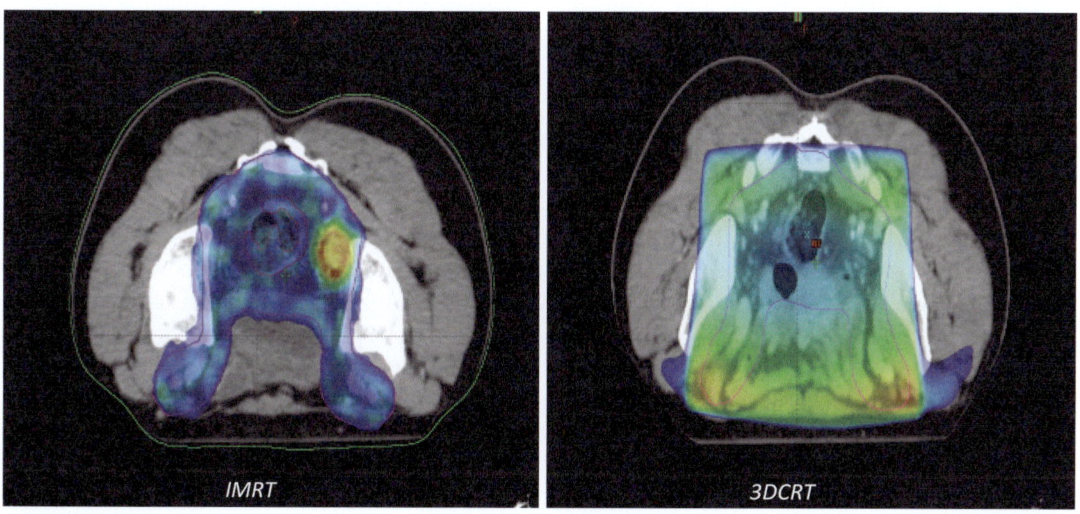

Fig. 6 IMRT and 3DCRT plans comparing dose coverage- superior conformity with a higher normal tissue sparing in IMRT

applied directly before treatment by applying couch shift.

Multiple studies, such as Nuyttens and Cookies [47], have demonstrated a reduction in PTV margins and the ability to online adaptation in a library of plans, with differential margins depending on organ size, shape, and bladder filling—Plan Of the Day approach, though not practiced routinely across the globe.

28 Irradiation Fractionation, Modality, and Dose

In Denmark, a study by Appelt confirmed a significant dose–response relationship for tumor regression after preoperative chemoradiation in locally advanced rectal cancer. Higher tumor doses (50.4 Gy to 70 Gy, including brachytherapy) produced better regression than standard doses. Preoperative biologically effective dose (BED) above 30 Gy was associated with a statistically significant reduction in locoregional recurrence. Doses required to achieve high local control for microscopic disease typically range from 45 Gy to 50.4 Gy delivered over 5–6 weeks [48].

A meta-analysis of individual patients included in European randomized trials published after 2000 showed that a radiation dose of more than 50 Gy improved local control and survival. The association between higher doses and improved local control but inferior sphincter function has been well recognized, although the impact of either factor, such as concomitant chemotherapy, continues to be debated. After the dose level of 45 Gy in 25 fractions over 5 weeks, a boost of 5.4–9 Gy may be delivered to the primary tumor or tumor bed may be delivered if the small bowel is excluded from the high-dose field. Higher preoperative doses up to 60 Gy are associated with increased pCR rates; however, they may also significantly increase acute and long-term morbidity rates.

The RTOG R-0012 [49] Phase II randomized trial compared twice-daily preoperative chemoradiation of up to 60 Gy (1.2 Gy to 45.6 Gy, with a boost of 9.6 Gy to 14.4 Gy) with conventional fractionation (1.8 Gy to 45 Gy, with a boost of 5.4 Gy to 9 Gy) plus 5-FU/irinotecan. Both regimens resulted in a 28% pCR rate but more than 40% rate of G3-4 acute toxicity.

In the postoperative setting, if there is incomplete resection (R1 or R2 resection), radiation doses of more than 60 Gy are required.

EBRT is limited by normal tissue tolerance, but, IORT may help to overcome this problem by direct visualization and irradiation of the persistent tumor.

29 Methods to Reduce Toxicity

Acute and late effects of pelvic radiation therapy are a function of radiation volumes, overall treatment time, fraction size, radiation beam energy, total dose, conformality, presence of image verification, and sequence of radiotherapy.

Acute side effects such as diarrhea and increased bowel frequency (small bowel), proctitis (large bowel), and dysuria are common during treatment, resolving within 2–3 weeks after radiation ends. They usually are function of the dose rate and fraction size rather than the total dose. More symptoms seen with concurrent chemotherapy. The bowel mucosa usually recovers completely by 3 months following irradiation.

Delayed complications are relatively rarer but substantially more serious. Occurring around 6–18 months following completion of irradiation, complications may include persistent diarrhea, frequency, proctitis and strictures at the anastomotic site, small bowel obstruction delayed perineal wound healing, urinary incontinence, and bladder atrophy and hematuria. Injury to the vascular and supporting stromal tissues is the presumed pathophysiology.

Serious late sequelae include small bowel enteritis, adhesions, and small bowel obstruction requiring surgery, especially in adjuvant EBRT setting around 4% to 12% in historical series. It was 2% in the preoperative chemoradiation arm of the German CAO/ARO/AIO-94 trial [6].

Even with appropriate doses and techniques of irradiation, approximately 1% of patients will have significant long-term toxicity of pelvic organs. Risk of pelvic fracture in the later half usually after 3 years is also supported in literature. Osteoporosis, female gender, and age older than 60 are usually independent risk factors for insufficiency fractures. In the Dutch CKVO trial, patients experienced new or worsening sexual dysfunction following treatment (men, 76%, and women, 62%). Surgical damage to nerve plexus is a more common scenario, compared to radiation [50].

Randomized trials have investigated the use of sucralfate enemas to decrease acute radiation proctitis, olsalazine, and mesalazine to decrease acute enteritis, and butyric acid to decrease chronic radiation proctitis. Per rectal amifostine is investigated as a radioprotector in rectal cancer patients, to try to control the rate of acute proctitis.

30 Multidisciplinary Teams

Cancer management using the multidisciplinary team (MDT) approach is robust and universal and practiced over all the world for better decision-making however often becomes vital for change in patient-specific treatment decisions. This is particularly relevant in rectal cancer, in which preoperative radiotherapy and chemoradiation are often delivered according to clinical findings and staging (particularly in terms of the MRI) and many different type of surgical options are available for future QoL in the patient. Like higher use of MRI in clinico-radiological staging leads to greater accuracy to select cases with a risk of threatened/positive CRM and enables the patient for neoadjuvant treatment.

Also, patients of lower rectal cancer, suitable for non-operative management, are selected in a MDJC and kept on stringent follow-up after treatment completion. Table 5 shows Follow Up Strategy, IWWD Consensus for Follow-Up of NOM patients and Table 6 shows Follow Up for Patients managed with Surgery- TME/APR.

31 Anal Canal Cancer

Anal carcinoma is considered a relatively rare disease and comprises 1–2% of large bowel cancers and over 2.5% of cancers of gastrointestinal cancers. Higher incidences are seen in age groups above 50 years, larger female preponderance, and high-risk sexual behavior [51]. There is an increased incidence of anal cancer in some populations, along with the identification of HPV DNA in most anal tumors [52]. Several prospective and randomized controlled trials over the years have established definitive radiotherapy along with concurrent chemotherapy as the current standard of care. This chapter will briefly cover the epidemiology risk factors, clinical features, staging, and management of anal cancer.

32 Etiology

Anal carcinoma can be considered as multifactorial, probably due to a summative effect of environmental and host factors such as:

HPV Infection Among sexually transmitted infections, HPV is strongly implicated as a potential causative agent of anal cancer. Most commonly, HPV 16,18,31,33 are associated with high-grade dysplasia or malignancy [53]. HPV-related proteins E6 and E7 oncogenes are involved in malignant cell transformation.

Table 6 Follow-up for patients managed with surgery—TME/APR

Year	Serum CEA	DRE	Endoscopy	CECT chest abdomen pelvis
1st	3–6 months	3–6 months	3–6 months	6–12 months
2nd	3–6 months	3–6 months	3–6 months	Annually
3rd	6 months	6 months	6 months	Annually
4th	6 months	6 months	6 months	Annually
5th	6 months	6 months	6 months	Annually

Oncoprotein E6 forms stable complexes with the p53 protein product of the tumor suppressor gene. The E7 protein forms complexes with the retinoblastoma gene products, subsequently resulting in the expression of Cyclin A and Cyclin E [54].

Sexual Behavior Studies have demonstrated a link between anal cancer and the number of sexual partners, receptive anal intercourse, and age at first sexual intercourse.

HIV Infection HIV is associated with a significantly increased risk for anal carcinoma and anal intraepithelial neoplasia, especially in homosexuality. The introduction of highly active antiretroviral therapy (HAART) has reduced the incidence of certain AIDS-associated malignancies, but the incidence of anal cancer has not declined [55].

Immunosuppressive Conditions Individuals on long-term immunosuppression, such as post-renal transplant, are associated with an increased relative risk of anal cancer.

Cigarette Smoking Several case-control studies have reported an association between anal cancer and cigarette smoking, which positively correlates with the number of cigarettes smoked per day.

33 Pathology and Pathways of Spread

Squamous carcinomas are the most common malignant anal canal tumors; other rare histopathological variants classified under the World Health Organization (WHO) include adenocarcinoma, mucinous adenocarcinoma, small cell carcinoma, undifferentiated carcinoma and melanoma. Most cases of adenocarcinomas are actually distal rectal adenocarcinoma with extension into anal canal and are managed as per distal rectal cancer guidelines.

34 Pattern of Spread

34.1 Anatomy of Anal Canal

Anal canal is approximately 3–4 cm in length. It begins where the rectum enters the puborectalis sling at the apex of the anal sphincter complex and ends where the squamous mucosa blends with the perianal skin. The anal canal is divided into superior and inferior parts by the dentate line due to its different embryological origin. Mucosa above dentate line originated from endodermal cloaca and is lined by columnar epithelium, and mucosa below the line originates from ectodermal proctodeum and is lined by stratified squamous epithelium [51].

Perianal cancers (Perianus)—tumors that arise distal to the squamous mucocutaneous junction that can be seen entirely with gentle traction on the buttocks and are within 5 cm of the anus are considered as perianal cancers and are treated as anal carcinoma

Anal cancer tumors spread by direct extension to surrounding structures, lymphatic dissemination to pelvic and inguinal lymph nodes, and hematogenous spread to distant viscera. Proximal canal above the dentate line is drained by the superior hemorrhoidal and perirectal lymph node, and around the line by the internal pudendal, hypogastric, obturator, and internal iliac lymph nodes. Below the dentate line, drainage is to the superficial and deep inguinal lymph nodes [56].

35 Clinical Features, Evaluation, and Staging

Bleeding per rectum is the most common presentation of anal malignant disease. Many patients with symptoms of early anal cancer are initially diagnosed with a benign condition such as fissures, hemorrhoids, or fistula. Anorectal pain, sensation of an anal mass, and altered bowel habits are also frequently reported.

36 Patient Evaluation

History and physical examination: A complete history and thorough physical examination. A digital rectal examination (DRE) and anoscopy should elaborate on tumor location, size, length of anal canal involvement, clock position of involvement, and sphincter tone. In women, a gynecologic examination should be done to rule out female genital tract involvement and presence of a second primary. Examination of inguinal lymph nodes and the supraclavicular lymph nodes in terms of size, location, and mobility of the tumor should be noted. Fertility risk discussion and counselling with experts should be considered in appropriate patients.

Investigations Laboratory and radiographic investigations are to be done as per recent guidelines such as NCCN 2025 and ESMO Guidelines. *Laboratory studies* should include a complete blood count, renal function tests, liver function tests, and viral markers, including HIV to assess patient fitness prior to starting treatment.
Radiographic imaging should include a CT scan of thorax, abdomen, and pelvis. MRI of the pelvis if available may be useful in locoregional staging (representative images shown in Fig. 7 of the primary and also in target volume delineation in radiotherapy planning [57].
Role of FDG-PET/CT: Role of FDG-PET/CT: FDG PETCECT is being routinely incorporated in the staging workup of anal cancer. PETCECT has shown a higher sensitivity of 99% in evaluating primary compared to 60% for CT and also in upstaging the disease [58].

37 Staging

The AJCC staging of anal canal cancer applies to all carcinomas that arise from the anal canal. The primary tumor size is classified on the basis of tumor size and lymph nodes, and regional lymph nodes are the anorectal, perirectal, lateral sacral, internal iliac (hypogastric), and superficial and deep inguinal lymph nodes, summarized in Table 7 and staging in Table 8. All other nodes are considered as distant metastases.

38 Treatment

38.1 Surgery

Prior to the mid-1970s, the standard of care was surgery, APR (abdominoperineal resection), which was associated with a permanent colostomy and severe long-term urinary and sexual dysfunction. Patients with APR have a reported

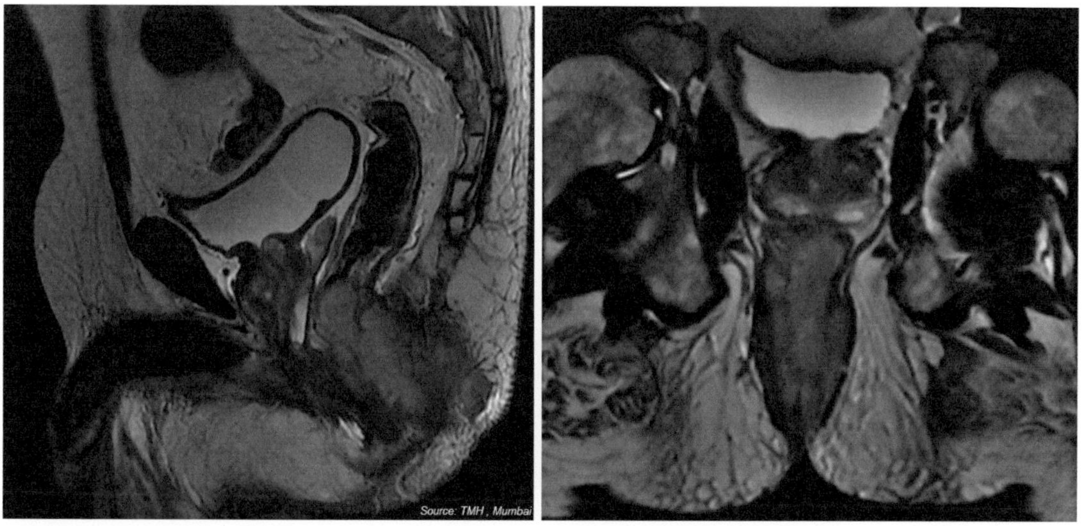

Fig. 7 Sagittal and coronal view in a case of locally advanced anal carcinoma

Table 7 Definition of T size and regional lymph nodes

T category	Criteria	N category	Criteria
TX	Primary tumor not assessed	NX	Regional lymph nodes not assessed
T0	No evidence of primary tumor	N0	No regional lymph node metastasis
Tis	High grade squamous intra-epithelial lesion [Previously termed carcinoma in-situ or Bowen disease]	N1	Metastasis in inguinal, mesorectal, internal iliac or external iliac nodes.
T1	Tumor ≤2 cm	N1a	Metastasis in inguinal, mesorectal or internal iliac nodes
T2	Tumor >2 cm but ≤5 cm	N1b	Metastasis in external iliac nodes
T3	Tumor >5 cm	N1c	Metastasis in external iliac with any one N1a nodes
T4 Tumor of any size invading adjacent organ(s), such as the vagina, urethra, or bladder		*M category*	*Criteria*
		M0	No distant metastasis
		M1	Distant metastasis

Adapted from 8th edition of AJCC

Table 8 TNM 8th Edition staging system of the AJCC

T	N	M	Stage
Tis	N0	M0	Stage 0
T1	N0	M0	Stage I
T2	N0	M0	Stage II A
T3	N0	M0	Stage II B
T1	N1	M0	Stage III A
T2	N1	M0	
T4	N0	M0	Stage III B
T3	N1	M0	Stage III C
T4	N1	M0	
Any T	Any N	M1	Stage IV

Adapted from AJCC manual

5-year OS of around 50% with a local recurrence rate ranging from 35% to 50% [59]. In the current era, the role of APR is reserved for patients with local recurrence after definitive radiotherapy with chemotherapy or for the management of complications of treatment [60]. However, there is no randomized controlled trial comparing surgery with radiotherapy.

38.2 Combined Modality Therapy

Definitive radiotherapy along with the concurrent use of chemotherapy remains the standard of care in the management of Stage I–III anal canal tumors. In 1974, surgeon Nigro et al. [59] along with radiation oncologist Gunter Seydel published a report on the use of preoperative radiation and chemotherapy in Anal Canal SCC followed by operation in three patients with cancer of the anal canal. This brief experience was successful enough to warrant further investigation. This series was updated by Buroker et at in 28 patients, (30 Gy) at 200 rad per day, 5 days a week, to the primary tumor with margin and to the pelvic and inguinal lymph nodes. 5-FU(Fluorouracil)—infusion 1000 mg/m^2 on days 1–4 and 29–32 of the treatment regimen. And Mitomycin C—intravenous bolus 15 mg/m^2 on day 1, complete response was seen in 57% of patients, the study concluded that definitive radiotherapy with chemotherapy is effective enough not to require APR if the lesion disappears and if the residual disease is present, proceed with radical APR. These studies laid the basis for definitive radiotherapy in anal carcinoma [59].

The evidence of radiotherapy along with chemotherapy is based on phase III randomized controlled trials EORTC [61] and UKCCCR trials which were further refined by the RTOG/ECOG study which established the role of Mitomycin C (MMC), results of these studies have been summarized in the below Table 8. The EORTC trial required a locally advanced anal canal tumor or involvement of regional lymph nodes, while

Table 9 Disease control and survival rates published across several randomized studies

After radiotherapy and 5-FU plus mitomycin c or cisplatin							
Study	**Number of patients**	**Colostomy free survival**		**Disease free survival**		**Overall survival**	
		%	*p* value	%	*p* value	%	*p* value
RTOG							
RT + FU/ MMC	325	71.9 (5 years)	**0.05**	67.8 (5 years)	0.006	78.3 (5 years)	**0.026**
RT + FU/ CDDP	324	65		57.8		70.7	
ACT II							
RT + FU/ MMC	472	68 (3 years)	0.94	69 (3 years)	0.63	79 (3 years)	0.7
RT + FU/ CDDP	468	67		69		77	

Comparing radiotherapy alone with radiation and chemotherapy (3 years disease free and survival)								
Study	**No. of. Patients**	**Complete response**		**Local control**		**Distant Mets (crude)**	**Overall survival%**	
		%	*p* value	%	*p* value	%	%	*p* value
EORTC								
RT	52	54		55		21	64	
RT plus 5-FU, MMC	51	80	**0.02**	69	0.02	18	69	0.17
UKCCR								
RT	285	30		39		17	58	
	292	39	0.08	61	<0.001	10	65	0.25

UKCCCR trial enrolled patients of any stage including distant metastasis. Assessment of complete response was at six weeks, no responders underwent APR, while responders underwent a further radiotherapy boost with EBRT or brachytherapy. The long-term 13-year follow-up results of UKCCR trial reported statistically significant better locoregional control rate and colostomy-free survival rates with combined modality treatment. Further refinement of concurrent chemotherapy regimen along with radiotherapy was established by the RTOG/ECOG trial in which patients receiving radiotherapy and 5-FU were randomized to receive MMC [62]. The MMC arm was associated with fewer colostomy rates (71% vs. 59%), higher local control rates and better disease-free survival rates, at the expense of increased Grade 4 toxicity (23% vs. 7%) and fatal neutropenic sepsis (4 vs. 1 patient) in the mitomycin group. The chemotherapy regimen differed from the European trial because two doses of MMC were given on Day 1 and Day 29 instead of a single dose of 12–15 mg/m^2 on day 1.

Table 9 shows disease control and survival rates published across several randomized studies

39 Replacement of Mitomycin with Cisplatin

Cisplatin as an alternative to Mitomycin C was not supported by the RTOG 9811 results. The use of induction chemotherapy (2 cycles of Cisplatin and 5-FU) along plus concurrent chemoradiotherapy using cisplatin with 5-FU was directly compared with the standard arm of mitomycin C and 5-FU, with the primary endpoint being 5-year DFS. The study results favored the standard arm of Mitomycin C and 5-FU, outcomes were significantly inferior in the cisplatin arm in terms of DFS (67.7% vs. 57.6%; $p = 0.0044$) and OS

(78.2% vs. 70.5%, respectively; $p = 0.02$), this was also associated with higher colostomy rates in the cisplatin arm. Hematological toxicity was worse with mitomycin, but compliance to both radiotherapy and chemotherapy in each arm suggests that the difference did not relate to excess toxicity.

The ACT II trial, a multicenter randomized controlled trial of 940 patients in the UK, enrolled non-metastatic SCCA without metastatic disease. Patients received 5-FU (1000 mg/m^2 on days 1–4; 29–32) and radiotherapy (50.4 Gy/28#) and were randomized to receive Mitomycin C (12 mg/m^2 on Day 1) or cisplatin 60 mg/m^2 on Day 1, 29, followed by a second randomization for consolidation therapy (5-FU/CDDP) 8 weeks after CRT. The 3-year recurrence-free survival rate was similar in both groups. Hence neither strategy was more effective in achieving a complete response. Acute hematological toxicity was lesser in the cisplatin arm (26% vs. 16%) but non-hematological rates were similar.

40 Oral Fluoropyrimidines

Capecitabine is an oral fluoropyrimidine which offers an equally effective alternative to 5-FU and the advantage in terms of ease of administration. The safety and efficacy of capecitabine are supported by phase II and several retrospective studies, the recommended dosage is 825 mg/m^2, PO BID on Day 1–Day 5. Capecitabine is currently recommended as a suitable alternative to 5-FU in NCCN, ESMO and UK IMRT anal canal guidelines [63, 64].

41 Radiotherapy Planning

The current radiotherapy target volumes and techniques have evolved through a better understanding of the natural history of anal cancer and correlation over the sites of failures. The most common site of failure is a local failure at the primary site followed by the regional nodes, subsequently distant metastasis.

General considerations

- Patients should be assessed for performance status, renal function, and comorbidities, prior to treatment. HIV testing and CD4 counting in HIV+ individuals is routinely recommended as it is associated with increased toxicity attributed to radiotherapy and cytotoxic chemotherapy.
- Sperm banking should be discussed prior to the commencement of treatment with patients who wish to preserve fertility. Testosterone levels may be reduced which may impair sexual function and have physical and psychosocial impacts after treatment.
- Premenopausal women should be counselled regarding loss of fertility and hormone replacement therapy may be required in those in whom early menopause is induced.
- A temporary (defunctioning stoma) could be considered in patients with transmural vaginal involvement due to the risk of fistula development or fecal incontinence.

Patient position, immobilization, simulation: Patients are usually treated in the supine position, since its more easily reproducible and more comfortable. A frog leg position may be considered in the individual scenario to reduce groin skin folds. A comfortably full bladder (>250 ml), usually based on the local bladder filling protocol, is recommended. There is no consensus on immobilization devices, but IMRT requires adequate immobilization of the patient for accurate treatment delivery. The use of a radio-opaque marker placed at the anal verge aids in target volume delineation. Contrast-enhanced CT scan of recommended slice thickness of 2–3 mm aids is recommended, extending superiorly from L2/L3 to at least 4–5 cm below the lesser trochanter.

42 Target Volume and Field Definitions

The target volume includes the disease primarily involving the anal canal with or without extension to the rectum and perianal skin, mesorectal space—to include the perirectal and mesorectal

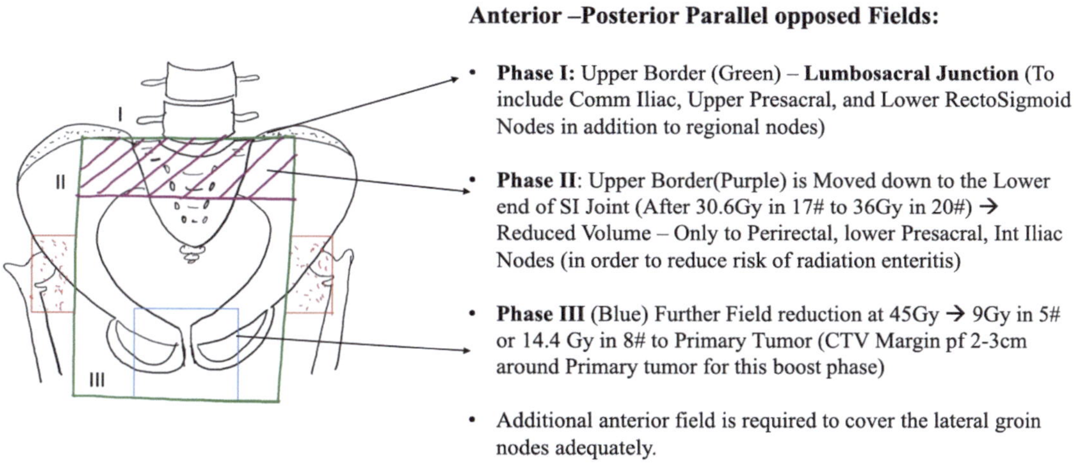

Fig. 8 Illustrative representation of radiotherapy portals in conventional planning

nodes. Lateral lymphatic group- Internal iliac Lymph node and obturator lymph node, external iliac lymph node, superficial and deep inguinal Lymph node- to include prophylactically [65].

Conventional field borders (illustrated in Fig. 8)—In conventional treatment planning, Phase I is parallel opposed fields, including all sites of GTV and all microscopic disease at risk in the inguino-femoral and pelvic lymph nodes. The phases are further modified in phases II and III based on baseline nodal burden.

43 Target Volume Delineation

GTV (Gross tumor volume)—GTV delineation should include all macroscopic disease. The use of radio-opaque markers at simulation, clinical examination findings are useful in determining the length of the tumor extent in the anal canal. The use of MRI fusion with CT helps in the measurement of tumor length in lateral, anterior and posterior directions.

CTV (Clinical target volume)—In RTOG 0529 [66, 67], CTV encompasses the gross tumor and plus a margin of at least 2.5 cm to the GTV primary (excluding from bone and air) and 1 cm to the nodal GTV. Then manually edited to avoid overlap into non-target muscles or bone, considered natural barriers to tumor infiltration. The recommendation of CTV delineation has evolved based on the refinement of radiotherapy techniques and disease status. The ACT (Anal Cancer Trial) study groups recommend the use GTV plus CTV margins of 1–1.5 cm and manually enlarged to ensure entire coverage of the entire anal canal, including the outer border, from the anorectal junction to the anal verge, including the internal and external sphinctors, excluding from anatomical barriers [68]. In node-positive tumors, the ACT V study recommends CTV node is generated by giving a margin of 5 mm to GTV node; nodes more than 3 cm in size are considered for boost [69].

PTV (Planning Target Volume)—PTV margin can be generated as per institutional practice, a margin of 5 mm to 1 cm isotropically is recommended; it is to be ensured that nodal PTV does not overlap the primary PTV.

Organs at risk—The following organs are to be delineated

1. Bladder
2. Small bowel
3. External genitalia
4. Right and Left Femoral Heads
5. Pelvic bone marrow

44 Radiotherapy Dose

The recommended dosage for SCC of the anal canal is based on the stage of the tumor. The principle of treatment is to deliver at least 50 Gy to gross macroscopic disease, and microscopic disease should receive a minimum of 30–40 Gy. The NCCN and the UK RCR recommended doses are summarized in below given Tables 10 and 11.

Table 10 Adopted from NCCN/RTOG 0529 guidelines

TNM stage	Primary tumor	Nodal PTV dose
T2, NO	50.4 Gy/28# at 1.8 Gy/#	42 Gy/28# at 1.5 Gy/#
T3-4, NO	54 Gy/30# at 1.8 Gy/#	45 Gy/30# at 1.5 Gy/#
T any N+ (lt;3 cm)	54 Gy/30# at 1.8 Gy/#	50.4 Gy/30# at 1.7 Gy/#
T any N + (gt;3 cm)	54 Gy/30# at 1.8 Gy/#	54 Gy/30# at 1.8 Gy/#

Table 11 Recommendation of radiotherapy dose proposed by UK RCR guidelines

Standard planned 2-phase radical chemoradiation	50.4 Gy in 28 daily fractions (Grade A)	
	Phase 1	30.6 Gy in 17 fractions over 3.5 weeks
	Phase 2	19.8 Gy in 11 fractions over 2.2 weeks
Radical inverse planned IMRT or arc radiotherapy	Dose to primary (early stage)	50.4 Gy in 28 fractions over 5.5 weeks (Grade D)
	Dose to primary and involved nodes (advanced stage)	53.2 Gy in 28 fractions over 5.5 weeks (Grade D)
	Dose to uninvolved nodes (prophylactic)	40 Gy in 28 fractions over 5.5 weeks (Grade D)
Palliative treatment (Grade D)	30 Gy in 10 fractions over 2 weeks	
	20 Gy in 5 fractions over 2 weeks	

45 Intensity-Modulated Radiotherapy (IMRT)

Although long-term survival rates are high in SCC of Anal canal, this survival is associated with long-term morbidity. The RTOG 0529 trial treated patients with inverse planning intensity-modulated radiotherapy and reported reduced toxicity as compared to that seen in RTOG 9811. IMRT provides the advantage of better dose conformality as illustrated in the below Figs. 9 and 10 resulting in the clinical benefit of reduced toxicity. IMRT is associated with a reduced treatment time of 49 (RTOG 9811) vs. 42 days (RTOG 0529) due to minimal treatment breaks, with studies suggesting reduced overall treatment time to be associated with improved overall survival [67].

46 Supportive Care During Radiotherapy

Patients should have their overall therapy tolerance and skin toxicity evaluated at least once per week. Checking full blood counts at least once is advised. weekly when receiving radiation therapy, especially if MMC is being administered. Additionally, it's crucial to employ straightforward antiemetics, antifungals, analgesics, skin care products, and nutritional assistance to enhance patient tolerance. Diarrhea, proctitis, frequent urination and dysuria, pubic hair loss, erythema, and moist desquamation of the skin in the groin and perineum are all anticipated acute adverse effects.

Before chemoradiation, patients should be made aware of the harmful effects of smoking. Smoking may exacerbate acute toxicity during therapy and result in a worse DFS and CFS outcome. Although there is little proof that vaginal dilators work, it has been suggested that sexually active ladies utilize them after treatment. Within two to three weeks after the end of the treatment, skin side effects usually resolve. Longer-lasting side effects are uncommon with external beams alone, although they were more frequent with a brachytherapy boost. Anal/rectal region ulcer-

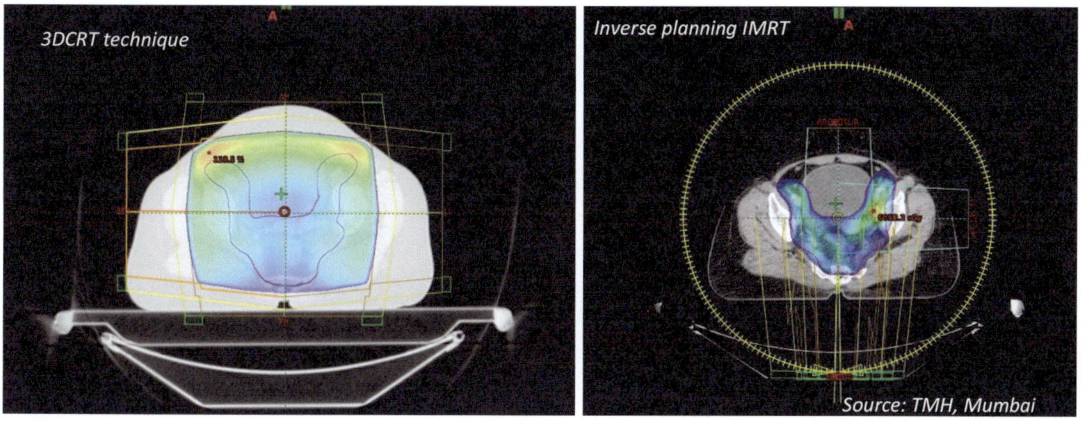

Fig. 9 95% coverage at mid pelvis level in 3DCRT (four field technique) vs. inverse planning IMRT. (Source: TMH, Mumbai)

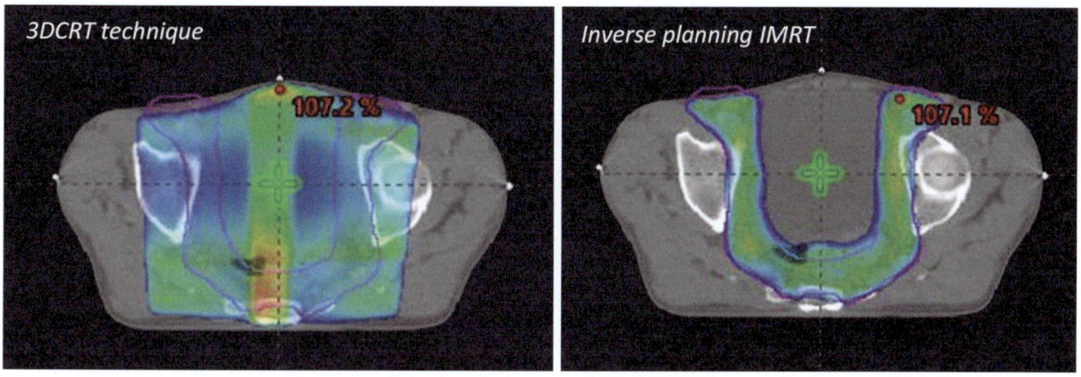

Fig. 10 95% coverage at inguinal nodes in 3DCRT vs. inverse planning IMRT

ation, small intestinal obstruction, urethral obstruction, and fistula development are examples of long-term morbidity.

46.1 Therapeutic Assessment and Follow-Up

Initial response assessment is done at 6–8 weeks post radiotherapy by clinical examination (DRE and inguinal nodal examination), some tumors maybe considered as late responders and may have residual disease and may not achieve a complete response even up to six months as suggested by a post hoc analysis results of ACT II study, provided there is no progressive disease elsewhere. Patients who do not respond to therapy are salvaged with abdomino-perineal resection surgery [70].

47 Palliative Treatment

A total of 10–15% of patients present with cancers spread beyond the pelvis at baseline and 10–30% of patients relapse after treatment. The most common site of metastasis is the liver followed by lungs, lymph nodes, skin, bones and even the brain have also been documented. Palliative chemotherapy with platinum-fluoropyrimidine or paclitaxel-based regimens has reported responses ranging from 34% to 53%, with a median survival time of 14 months. 115 In a recent Phase II study, patients with metastatic, chemotherapy-refractory anal cancer were assessed for the safety and effectiveness of immunotherapy with the single drug nivolumab or pembrolizumab can be considered (an anti-PD1 antibody). The median overall survival was 11.5 months, and the objective response rate was

24% (19% partial response and 5% complete response). No significant side effects were observed, and the treatment was well tolerated [71].

Palliative radiotherapy is delivered with the aim of alleviating symptoms and improving quality of life. The UK RCR guidelines recommend dose fractionation of 30 Gy/10# over 2 weeks or 20 Gy/5# over two weeks based on prognosis, disease burden, symptoms and performance status.

Percepts Box

1. Rectal Cancer
   - A multidisciplinary approach, including representation from gastroenterology, medical oncology, surgical oncology/colorectal surgery, radiation oncology, and radiology is necessary for treating patients with rectal cancer.
   - Patients with very-early-stage tumors that are node-negative by endorectal ultrasound or endorectal or pelvic MRI and who meet carefully defined criteria can be managed with a transanal local excision (T1-2, N0).
   - A transabdominal resection including TME, which is considered the current standard of care in all the other rectal lesions.
   - A TNT approach consisting of chemoRT/short-course RT and chemotherapy is preferred for the majority of patients with suspected or proven T3–4 disease and/or N+ disease.
   - Patient is with lower rectal cancer meeting the inclusion criteria as per IWWD can be offered rectal preservation strategies.
   - The recommended post-treatment surveillance program for patients following treatment for rectal cancer includes serial CEA in secretory rectal cancer tumors, as well as periodic chest, abdominal, and pelvic CT scans, and periodic evaluation by colonoscopy as per the follow up chart.
   - A patient with limited metastatic disease in the liver or lung should be considered for surgical resection or ablative therapy if safe and feasible. Preoperative systemic therapy, and sometimes chemoRT or short-course RT, are used in the synchronous setting, and perioperative chemotherapy is used in the metachronous setting. Recommendations for patients with disseminated, unresectable metastatic disease represent a continuum of care incorporating multiple approaches.
2. Anal Carcinoma
   - Anal canal squamous carcinoma is considered a rare entity, with risk factors such as high-risk sexual behavior, cigarette smoking, HIV, immunocompromised individuals.
   - Evaluation is done based on clinical examination, digital rectal examination, with investigations to support the diagnosis—MRI for local staging, FDG-PETCT is recommended especially in locally advanced cases, due to its high sensitivity and specificity in detected nodal and distant metastasis.
   - The current standard of care is Definitive radiotherapy and concomitant chemotherapy with 5-FU and Mitomycin C. Oral fluoropyrimidines can also be considered as an alternative to 5-FU.
   - IMRT is the preferred radiotherapy technique due to better conformality and lesser toxicities.

(continued)

- 5-year survival rates range from 40% to 80% and sphincter preservation rates of >90% in tumors less than 2 cm, and 60–75% with larger tumors.
- Palliative radiotherapy to hypo fractionated doses can be considered in metastatic cases and systemic chemotherapy -5-FU, platinum based and immunotherapy can be considered based on feasibility.

Multiple Choice Questions

1. Preferred Management of locally advanced rectal cancer is
   (a) Surgery f/b adjuvant chemoradiation
   (b) Neoadjuvant chemoradiation f/b surgery ± adjuvant chemotherapy
   (c) Surgery alone
   (d) Definitive chemoradiation
2. Most common histology observed in rectal cancers
   (a) Adenocarcinoma
   (b) Signet cell carcinoma
   (c) Squamous cell carcinoma
   (d) Melanoma
3. Which of the following is a tumor marker used for diagnosis, prognosis and monitoring response in rectal cancer?
   (a) CA-125
   (b) CA 19.9
   (c) S.CEA
   (d) AFP
4. As per the AJCC 8th edition, a rectal cancer cT2cN1, corresponds to which stage?
   (a) Stage I
   (b) Stage IIa
   (c) Stage IIb
   (d) Stage III
5. The standard dose regimen for Neoadjuvant short course radiotherapy in rectal cancer is
   (a) 20 Gy/5#
   (b) 25 Gy/5#
   (c) 30 Gy/5#
   (d) 30 Gy/10#
6. T3 N0 low volume lower rectal cancer, upper limit 3 cm from AV treatment plan
   (a) TME fb Adj Chemo and RT
   (b) NACTRT fb response assessment
   (c) NACTRT fb surgery and adj chemo
   (d) Def CTRT fb observation
7. Which of the following trial investigates incorporation of SCRT with induction chemotherapy in TNT
   (a) RAPIDO
   (b) ADORE
   (c) ACT II
   (d) ACCORD
8. T3N2M0 ca lower rectum, poor response after neoadjuvant chemoradiation, disease involving ext sphincter, treatment of choice
   (a) Second line chemotherapy
   (b) APR fb Adj chemo
   (c) Brachytherapy
   (d) Exenteration
9. All are criteria to select T1N0 rectal cancer for trans anal local excision alone, except
   (a) Less than 1/3 circumference involved
   (b) Less than 7 cm from AV
   (c) No LVSI
   (d) Int sphincter involved, but ext sphincter free
10. The anal canal embryologically originates from the
    (a) Endoderm
    (b) Enodermal cloaca and Ectodermal proctodeum
    (c) Mesoderm
    (d) All of the above
11. Which of the following is not considered a regional node in Anal canal cancer
    (a) Inguinal nodes
    (b) Common iliac nodes
    (c) External iliac nodes
    (d) Internal iliac nodes
12. Which of the following is considered as an oral alternative to 5-Fluorouracil?
    (a) Capecitabine
    (b) Methotrexate
    (c) Temozolomide
    (d) Cisplatin

13. On which of the following outcome does Mitomycin C have profound impact?
    (a) Overall survival
    (b) Colostomy free survival
    (c) Pathological complete response
    (d) Progression free survival
14. The preferred radiotherapy technique for management of Anal canal carcinoma
    (a) Conventional portals
    (b) 3DCRT technique
    (c) IMRT technique
15. How long would it be appropriate to wait to achieve complete clinical response post definitive radiotherapy and chemotherapy in anal carcinoma?
    (a) 4 weeks
    (b) 6 weeks
    (c) 3 months
    (d) 6 months

Answers Key

1. (b)
2. (a)
3. (c)
4. (d)
5. (b)
6. (b)
7. (b)
8. (b)
9. (d)
10. (b)
11. (b)
12. (a)
13. (b)
14. (c)
15. (d)

References

1. Cancer Statistics. Report From National Cancer Registry Programme, India. (National Centre for Disease Informatics and Research, Bengaluru, India) JCO Global Oncology, 6. 2020.
2. US Cancer statistics, 2021.
3. AJCC TNM Cancer staging 8th Edition.
4. Heald RJ, et al. Recurrence and survival after total mesorectal excision for rectal cancer. Lancet. 1986;1(8496):1479–82.
5. Preoperative radiotherapy combined with total mesorectal excision for resectable rectal cancer: 12-year follow-up of the multicentre, randomized controlled TME trial. Lancet Oncol. 2011;12(6):575–82.
6. Sauer, et al. Preoperative versus postoperative chemoradiotherapy for rectal cancer. N Engl J Med. 2004;2004(351):1731–40.
7. Yun, et al. Local recurrence after curative resection for rectal carcinoma. Medicine (Baltimore). 2016;95(27):e3942.
8. Alberda, et al. Intraoperative radiation therapy reduces local recurrence rates in patients with microscopically involved circumferential resection margins after resection of locally advanced rectal cancer. Int J Radiat Oncol Biol Phys. 2014;88(5):1032–40.
9. Cameron, et al. Palliative pelvic radiotherapy of symptomatic incurable rectal cancer – a systematic review. Acta Oncol. 2014;53(2):164–73.
10. Jasperson KW, Tuohy TM, Neklason DW, Burt RW. Hereditary and familial colon cancer. Gastroenterology. 2010;138(6):2044–58.
11. Zlobec I, Lugli A. Prognostic and predictive factors in colorectal cancer. J Clin Pathol. 2008;61(5):561–9.
12. NCCN Guidelines Insights: Colorectal Cancer Screening, Version 3. 2022.
13. NCCN Rectal cancer guidelines: Version 3.0. 2022.
14. Horvat N, et al. MRI of rectal cancer: tumor staging, imaging techniques, and management. RadioGraphics. 2019;15:2.
15. O'Connor OJ, McDermott S, Slattery J, Sahani D, Blake MA. The use of PET-CT in the assessment of patients with colorectal carcinoma. Int J Surg Oncol. 2011;2011:846512, 14 pages.
16. Brown G, Davies S, Williams G, et al. Effectiveness of preoperative staging in rectal cancer: digital rectal examination, endoluminal ultrasound or magnetic resonance imaging? Br J Cancer. 2004;91:23–9.
17. What is the role for the circumferential margin in the modern treatment of rectal cancer? J Clin Oncol 26(2):303–12. 2008.
18. Thies S, Langer R. Tumor regression grading of gastrointestinal carcinomas after neoadjuvant treatment. Front Oncol. 2013;3:262.
19. NSABP R04- Neoadjuvant chemoradiation (RT) comparing continuous infusion (CIV) 5-FU with capecitabine (Cape) with or without oxaliplatin (Ox) in patients with stage II and III rectal cancer. J Clin Oncol 32(15_suppl): 3603. 2014.
20. Parfitt JR, Driman DK. The total mesorectal excision specimen for rectal cancer: a review of its pathological assessment. J Clin Pathol. 2007;60(8):849–55.
21. Bayer I, Turani H, Lurie H, Chaimoff C. The sandwich approach: irradiation-surgery-irradiation in rectal cancer. Four years' experience. Dis Colon Rectum. 1985;28(4):222–4.
22. Fisher B, Wolmark N, Rockette H, Redmond C, Deutsch M, Wickerham DL, Fisher ER, Caplan R,

Jones J, Lerner H, et al. Postoperative adjuvant chemotherapy or radiation therapy for rectal cancer: results from NSABP protocol R-01. J Natl Cancer Inst. 1988;80(1):21–9.
23. Sebag-Montefiore D, Stephens RJ, Steele R, Monson J, Grieve R, Khanna S, Quirke P, Couture J, de Metz C, Myint AS, Bessell E, Griffiths G, Thompson LC, Parmar M. Preoperative radiotherapy versus selective postoperative chemoradiotherapy in patients with rectal cancer (MRC CR07 and NCIC-CTG C016): a multicentre, randomized trial. Lancet. 2009;373(9666):811–20.
24. Skóra T, Nowak-Sadzikowska J, Martynów D, Wszołek M, Sas-Korczyńska B. Preoperative short-course radiotherapy in rectal cancer patients: results and prognostic factors. J Radiat Oncol. 2018;7(1):77–84.
25. Long-course preoperative chemoradiation versus 5 × 5 Gy and consolidation chemotherapy for clinical T4 and fixed clinical T3 rectal cancer: long-term results of the randomized Polish II study.
26. Chen C, et al. Short course radiation in the treatment of localized rectal cancer: a systematic review and meta-analysis. Sci Rep. 5:10953.
27. Herzog T, Belyaev O, Chromik AM, Weyhe D, Mueller CA, Munding J, Tannapfel A, Uhl W, Seelig MH. TME quality in rectal cancer surgery. Eur J Med Res. 2010;15(7):292–6.
28. O'Connell MJ. A phase III trial of 5-fluorouracil and leucovorin in the treatment of advanced colorectal cancer. A Mayo Clinic/North Central Cancer Treatment Group study. Cancer. 1989;63(6 Suppl):1026–30.
29. Hong YS, Kim SY, Lee JS, Nam BH, Kim KP, Kim JE, Park YS, Park JO, Baek JY, Kim TY, Lee KW, Ahn JB, Lim SB, Yu CS, Kim JC, Yun SH, Kim JH, Park JH, Park HC, Jung KH, Kim TW. Oxaliplatin-based adjuvant chemotherapy for rectal cancer after preoperative chemoradiotherapy (ADORE): long-term results of a Randomized Controlled Trial. J Clin Oncol. 2019;37(33):3111–23.
30. Wu H, Fang C, Huang L, Fan C, Wang C, Yang L, Li Y, Zhou Z. Short-course radiotherapy with immediate or delayed surgery in rectal cancer: a meta-analysis. Int J Surg. 2018;56:195–202.
31. Krishnamurthi SS, Seo Y, Kinsella TJ. Adjuvant therapy for rectal cancer. Clin Colon Rectal Surg. 2007;20(3):167–81.
32. Liu S, Jiang T, Xiao L, Yang S, Liu Q, Gao Y, Chen G, Xiao W. Total Neoadjuvant Therapy (TNT) versus standard neoadjuvant chemoradiotherapy for locally advanced rectal cancer: a systematic review and meta-analysis. Oncologist. 2021;26(9):e1555–66.
33. Fokas E, Appelt A, Glynne-Jones R, et al. International consensus recommendations on key outcome measures for organ preservation after (chemo)radiotherapy in patients with rectal cancer. Nat Rev Clin Oncol. 2021;18:805–16.
34. Petrelli F, Trevisan F, Cabiddu M, Sgroi G, Bruchchieri L, Rausa E, Ghidini M, Turati L. Total neoadjuvant therapy in rectal cancer: a systematic review and meta-analysis of treatment outcomes. Ann Surg. 2020;271(3):440–8.
35. Bujko K, Nowacki MP, Nasierowska-Guttmejer A, Michalski W, Bebenek M, Kryj M. Long-term results of a randomized trial comparing preoperative short-course radiotherapy with preoperative conventionally fractionated chemoradiation for rectal cancer. Br J Surg. 2006;93(10):1215–23.
36. Rullier E, Laurent C, Carles J, Saric J, Michel P, Parneix M. Local recurrence of low rectal cancer after abdominoperineal and anterior resection. Br J Surg. 1997;84(4):525–8.
37. Habr-Gama A, São Julião GP, Perez RO. Nonoperative management of rectal cancer: identifying the ideal patients. Hematol Oncol Clin N Am. 2015;29(1):135–51.
38. Garcia-Aguilar J, Patil S, Gollub MJ, Kim JK, Yuval JB, Thompson HM, Verheij FS, Omer DM, Lee M, Dunne RF, Marcet J, Cataldo P, Polite B, Herzig DO, Liska D, Oommen S, Friel CM, Ternent C, Coveler AL, Hunt S, Gregory A, Varma MG, Bello BL, Carmichael JC, Krauss J, Gleisner A, Paty PB, Weiser MR, Nash GM, Pappou E, Guillem JG, Temple L, Wei IH, Widmar M, Lin S, Segal NH, Cercek A, Yaeger R, Smith JJ, Goodman KA, Wu AJ, Saltz LB. Organ preservation in patients with rectal adenocarcinoma treated with total neoadjuvant therapy. J Clin Oncol. 2022;40(23):2546–56.
39. Bahadoer RR, Dijkstra EA, van Etten B, Marijnen CAM, Putter H, Kranenbarg EM, Roodvoets AGH, Nagtegaal ID, Beets-Tan RGH, Blomqvist LK, Fokstuen T, Ten Tije AJ, Capdevila J, Hendriks MP, Edhemovic I, Cervantes A, Nilsson PJ, Glimelius B, van de Velde CJH, Hospers GAP. RAPIDO collaborative investigators. Short-course radiotherapy followed by chemotherapy before total mesorectal excision (TME) versus preoperative chemoradiotherapy, TME, and optional adjuvant chemotherapy in locally advanced rectal cancer (RAPIDO): a randomized, open-label, phase 3 trial. Lancet Oncol. 2021;22(1):29–42.
40. Mohiuddin MD, et al. Long-term results of reirradiation for patients with recurrent rectal carcinoma. Cancer. 2002;95(5)
41. Valentini V, Morganti AG, Gambacorta MA, Mohiuddin M, Doglietto GB, Coco C, De Paoli A, Rossi C, Di Russo A, Valvo F, Bolzicco G, Dalla Palma M. Study Group for Therapies of Rectal Malignancies (STORM). Preoperative hyperfractionated chemoradiation for locally recurrent rectal cancer in patients previously irradiated to the pelvis: a multicentric phase II study. Int J Radiat Oncol Biol Phys. 2006;64(4):1129–39.
42. Crane C, et al. Effective pelvic symptom control using initial chemoradiation without colostomy in metastatic rectal cancer. IJROBP. 2001;49(1):107–16.
43. Kwan J, Pua U. Review of intra-arterial therapies for colorectal cancer liver metastasis. Cancers (Basel). 2021;13(6):1371.

44. Hruby G, Barton M, Miles S, Carroll S, Nasser E, Stevens G. Sites of local recurrence after surgery, with or without chemotherapy, for rectal cancer: implications for radiotherapy field design. Int J Radiat Oncol Biol Phys. 2003;55(1):138–43.
45. Valentini V, Gambacorta MA, Barbaro B, Chiloiro G, Coco C, Das P, Fanfani F, Joye I, Kachnic L, Maingon P, Marijnen C, Ngan S, Haustermans K. International consensus guidelines on Clinical Target Volume delineation in rectal cancer. Radiother Oncol. 2016;120(2):195–201.
46. Hong TS, Moughan J, Garofalo MC, Bendell J, Berger AC, Oldenburg NB, Anne PR, Perera F, Lee RJ, Jabbour SK, Nowlan A, DeNittis A, Crane C. NRG Oncology Radiation Therapy Oncology Group 0822: a phase 2 study of preoperative chemoradiation therapy using intensity modulated radiation therapy in combination with capecitabine and oxaliplatin for patients with locally advanced rectal cancer. Int J Radiat Oncol Biol Phys. 2015;93(1):29–36.
47. Nuyttens JJ, Robertson JM, Yan D, Martinez A. The variability of the clinical target volume for rectal cancer due to internal organ motion during adjuvant treatment. Int J Radiat Oncol Biol Phys. 2002;53(2):497–503.
48. Appelt AL, Pløen J, Harling H, Jensen FS, Jensen LH, Jørgensen JC, Lindebjerg J, Rafaelsen SR, Jakobsen A. High-dose chemoradiotherapy and watchful waiting for distal rectal cancer: a prospective observational study. Lancet Oncol. 2015;16(8):919–27.
49. Mohiuddin M, Paulus R, Mitchell E, Hanna N, Yuen A, Nichols R, Yalavarthi S, Hayostek C, Willett C. Neoadjuvant chemoradiation for distal rectal cancer: 5-year updated results of a randomized phase 2 study of neoadjuvant combined modality chemoradiation for distal rectal cancer. Int J Radiat Oncol Biol Phys. 2013;86(3):523–8.
50. Wiltink LM, Chen TY, Nout RA, Kranenbarg EM, Fiocco M, Laurberg S, van de Velde CJ, Marijnen CA. Health-related quality of life 14 years after preoperative short-term radiotherapy and total mesorectal excision for rectal cancer: report of a multicenter randomized trial. Eur J Cancer. 2014;50(14):2390–8.
51. Valvo F, et al. Cancer of the anal region. Crit Rev Oncol Hematol. 2019;135:115–27.
52. Dunne EF, Park IU. HPV and HPV-associated diseases. Infect Dis Clin North Am. 2013;27:765–78.
53. Franceschi S, De Vuyst H. Human papillomavirus vaccines and anal carcinoma. Curr Opin HIV AIDS. 2009;4:57–63.
54. Skelin J, Sabol I, Tomaić V. Do or die: HPV E5, E6 and E7 in cell death evasion. Pathogens. 2022;11:1027.
55. Wang C-CJ, Palefsky JM. HPV-associated anal cancer in the HIV/Aids patient. Cancer Treat Res. 2019;177:183–209.
56. Pedersen CK, Babu AS. Understanding the lymphatics: review of the N category in the updated TNM staging of cancers of the digestive system. AJR Am J Roentgenol. 2020;215:58–68.
57. Kochhar R, Plumb AA, Carrington BM, Saunders M. Imaging of anal carcinoma. AJR Am J Roentgenol. 2012;199:W335–44.
58. Jones M, Hruby G, Solomon M, Rutherford N, Martin J. The role of FDG-PET in the initial staging and response assessment of anal cancer: a systematic review and meta-analysis. Ann Surg Oncol. 2015;22:3574–81.
59. Nigro ND, et al. Combined preoperative radiation and chemotherapy for squamous cell carcinoma of the anal canal. Cancer. 1983;51:1826–9.
60. Eng C, Messick C, Glynne-Jones R. The management and prevention of anal squamous cell carcinoma. Am Soc Clin Oncol Educ Book. 2019;39:216–25.
61. Bartelink H, et al. Concomitant radiotherapy and chemotherapy is superior to radiotherapy alone in the treatment of locally advanced anal cancer: results of a phase III randomized trial of the European Organization for Research and Treatment of Cancer Radiotherapy and Gastrointestinal Cooperative Groups. J Clin Oncol. 1997;15:2040–9.
62. Flam M, et al. Role of mitomycin in combination with fluorouracil and radiotherapy, and of salvage chemoradiation in the definitive nonsurgical treatment of epidermoid carcinoma of the anal canal: results of a phase III randomized intergroup study. J Clin Oncol. 1996;14:2527–39.
63. Astaras C, Bornand A, Koessler T. Squamous rectal carcinoma: a rare malignancy, literature review and management recommendations. ESMO Open. 2021;6:100180.
64. Martini G, Arrichiello G, Borrelli C, Poliero L, Martinelli E. How I treat anal squamous cell carcinoma. ESMO Open. 2020;4:e000711.
65. Gunderson LL, et al. Long-term update of US GI intergroup RTOG 98-11 Phase III Trial for anal carcinoma: survival, relapse, and colostomy failure with concurrent chemoradiation involving fluorouracil/mitomycin versus fluorouracil/cisplatin. J Clin Oncol. 2012;30:4344–51.
66. Kachnic LA, et al. RTOG 0529: a phase 2 evaluation of dose-painted intensity modulated radiation therapy in combination with 5-fluorouracil and mitomycin-C for the reduction of acute morbidity in carcinoma of the anal canal. Int J Radiat Oncol Biol Phys. 2013;86:27–33.
67. Kachnic LA, et al. Long-term outcomes of NRG oncology/RTOG 0529: a Phase 2 evaluation of dose-painted intensity modulated radiation therapy in combination with 5-fluorouracil and mitomycin-C for the reduction of acute morbidity in anal canal cancer. Int J Radiat Oncol Biol Phys. 2022;112:146–57.

68. Northover J, et al. Chemoradiation for the treatment of epidermoid anal cancer: 13-year follow-up of the first randomised UKCCCR Anal Cancer Trial (ACT I). Br J Cancer. 2010;102:1123–8.
69. ISRCTN – ISRCTN88455282: PLATO – Personalising anal cancer radiotherapy dose. https://www.isrctn.com/ISRCTN88455282. https://doi.org/10.1186/ISRCTN88455282
70. Glynne-Jones R, et al. Best time to assess complete clinical response after chemoradiotherapy in squamous cell carcinoma of the anus (ACT II): a post-hoc analysis of randomised controlled phase 3 trial. Lancet Oncol. 2017;18:347–56.
71. Symer MM, Yeo HL. Recent advances in the management of anal cancer. F1000Res. 2018;7:1572.

Online Links

Rectal cancer: ESMO clinical recommendations for diagnosis, treatment and follow-up.

Anal cancer: ESMO Clinical Recommendations for diagnosis, treatment and follow-up - Annals of Oncology.

https://www.rcr.ac.uk/publication/national-rectal-cancer-intensity-modulated-radiotherapy-imrt-guidance

Radiation Planning in Anal Canal Cancer_Dr Tanweer Shahid.

Target Volume Delineation in Rectal and Anal Cancers by Dr Indranil Mallick.

Uro-Oncology

Vedang Murthy, Gargee Mulye, Vasanthapriya Subramani, Amiya Agrawal, Shashank Srinivasan, Tanweer Shahid, Kushal Narang, Jiten Jaipuria, and Sanjai Addla

1 Prostate Cancer

1.1 Anatomy

The prostate gland comprises of three zones. The peripheral zone that forms the bulk of the gland (70%) is the most common site of cancer. The central zone is made up of 25% of the volume and includes the base of the prostate. The transition zone is the smallest (5% by volume) and is the most common site of benign prostatic hyperplasia.

V. Murthy (✉) · G. Mulye · V. Subramani
A. Agrawal · S. Srinivasan
Department of Radiation Oncology, Tata Memorial Centre, HBNI, Mumbai, India

T. Shahid
Department of Radiation Oncology, Apollo Hospital, Kolkata, India

K. Narang
Department of Radiation Oncology, Cancer Institute, Medanta, Gurugram, India

J. Jaipuria
Department of Surgical Oncology, Rajiv Gandhi Cancer Institute, Delhi, India

S. Addla
Department of Surgical Oncology, Apollo Hospitals, Hyderabad, India

1.2 Epidemiological Aspects and Risk Factors

Prostate cancer is the 5th most common cancer amongst men in India [1], with an incidence of 9–10/100,000 population [2]. Most cases (90%) are diagnosed with locoregional disease and are associated with overall survival at 5 yrs of >90%. Incidence rises with age, and the growth of the cancer is largely driven by androgen stimulation.

1.3 Screening

Screening for prostate cancer is an often-debated topic. Benefits of screening include detection and treatment of localised disease, thus reducing the morbidity of treatment and mortality associated with advanced or metastatic disease. On the other hand, screening causes overdiagnosis and overtreatment in many men who may never have required treatment for prostate cancer. Diagnostic procedures such as prostatic biopsy are associated with pain, infection, hematospermia, etc. Overtreatment may lead to urinary incontinence, erectile dysfunction and potential harms of hormone therapy. It is postulated that 1000 patients need to be screened to prevent 3 cases of metastatic prostate cancer and 1.3 deaths due to prostate cancer in patients aged 55–69 years of age. This benefit is not seen in patients 70 years and

B. K. Mohanti et al. (eds.), *Radiation Oncology – Principles, Precepts and Practice*,
https://doi.org/10.1007/978-981-95-5171-2_13

older, and the USPTF recommends against screening in these patients. In patients aged 55–69 years of age, it is recommended that PSA based screening should be initiated after a discussion of the pros and cons with the patient. Screening frequency may be every 2–4 years [3].

1.4 Clinical Symptoms and Signs, Pathology

Patients most commonly present with lower urinary tract symptoms in the form of urinary frequency, urgency, intermittency, straining, nocturia, weak stream. Hematuria may be present in cases of bladder invasion and local symptoms in case of metastatic disease. On prostate biopsy, grade is assigned using the Gleason's grade.

The predominant primary tumour pattern and secondary tumour pattern are graded from 1 to 5 (Table 1). The least Gleason's score is 3 + 3 and the maximum is 5 + 5.

Higher grade group is of worse prognostic outcomes [4].

Table 1 ISUP grade grouping

Gleason's score	ISUP grade
GS 3 + 3	1
GS 3 + 4	2
GS 4 + 3	3
GS 4 + 4, 5 + 3, 3 + 5	4
GS 9–10	5

1.5 Integrated Management Plan

1.5.1 Investigations

Clinical staging and risk stratification is determined by a combination digital rectal examination (DRE), serum PSA measurement, 12 core prostate biopsy showing Gleason score with estimation of cores involved, supplemented by multiparametric MRI of prostate and cross-sectional imaging like the newer Gallium 68 PSMA PET CT or conventional CECT thorax abdomen pelvis with Technitium 99 bone scan.

PSA is prostate specific and not cancer specific and may be raised in non-cancerous conditions like benign prostatic hyperplasia (BPH), prostatitis, tuberculosis or following instrumentation. Rise in age-specific PSA or PSA level >4 ng/mL can indicate malignancy of prostate. A ratio of free to total PSA of <0.1 is most likely associated with prostate cancer. While unreliable in isolation, as a general guide, PSA >10 ng/mL indicates capsular penetration in more than 50% patients while PSA >50 ng/mL is usually associated with metastatic disease.

Ultrasound (US)-guided biopsy is now the standard of care. A trans-rectal approach is most commonly used, though a trans-perineal approach is increasingly being preferred as it lowers the risk of faecal contamination and infection with comparable pain/discomfort and yield.

Multi-parametric MRI of prostate associates T2-weighted imaging with diffusion-weighted imaging, dynamic contrast-enhanced imaging, and/or H1-spectroscopy and has good sensitivity (93%) for the detection and localisation of Gleason score >7 cancers [5]. Ideally it should be performed prior to the biopsy [6]. Gallium 68-labelled PSMA PET-CT had a 27% greater accuracy than that of conventional imaging (92% vs 65%). Its sensitivity and specificity for detecting nodal and distant metastases is 85% and 98% respectively as shown in the proPSMA trial and should be the preferred imaging for metastatic work up in high-risk prostate cancer [7].

1.5.2 Management of Localised Prostate Cancer

Local treatment for prostate cancer could be surgery, radiotherapy, active surveillance or watchful waiting. The ProtecT trial randomised 1643 men with localised prostate cancer to active monitoring, surgery, or radiotherapy. At a median follow-up of 15-yrs there was no significant difference in the primary endpoint of prostate-cancer mortality or the number of deaths from any cause amongst the treatment groups. As expected, higher rates of disease progression were seen in the active monitoring arm. Metastases also developed in more men in the active monitoring group. The factors that were predictive of progression included age (65–69 Vs

50–64 yr), PSA level, Grade group, clinical stage, risk group, number of positive cores, tumour length and perineural invasion ($p < 0.005$).

1.5.3 Active Surveillance (AS)/ Watchful Waiting

The aim of AS for low and favourable-intermediate risk prostate cancer is that it reduces the risk of overtreatment of clinically insignificant prostate cancer while retaining the option of definitive therapy later for those patients who are reclassified over time as high risk. AS is a safe and viable option with a 10-year cause-specific survival of 98% [8]. The differences between active surveillance and watchful waiting are summarised in Table 2.

1.5.4 Surgery

Radical prostatectomy involves removal of prostate with an intact capsule and seminal vesicles followed by urethro-vesical anastomosis. The surgical approach for undertaking radical prostatectomy has changed with time from open perineal, open retropubic, laparoscopic to the current standard of Robotic assisted laparoscopic approach [9]. Though there is variability on immediate surgical outcomes with reduced re-admission rates and blood loss comparing open surgery to robotic approach, there is no level I evidence indicating long term superiority of one technique over the other. However, as with any surgical technique, there is good evidence to indicate lower margin positivity rates with better oncological outcomes for high volume surgeons [10], as well as high volume centres [11]. The role of pelvic lymph node dissection (PLND) is not well established in the management of prostate cancer [12]. It has failed to show any improvement in oncological outcomes or overall survival. However, extended PLND provides important information on staging and is a very valuable prognostic tool and better than any of the current imaging modalities in accurate staging [13].

Table 2 Differences between active surveillance and watchful waiting

	Active surveillance	Watchful waiting
Treatment intent	Radical	Palliative
Aim	To avoid overtreatment without compromising cure	To avoid treatment related toxicity
Patient characteristics	Fit for treatment, life expectancy >10 yrs	Frail, life expectancy <5 yrs
Tumour characteristics	Very low, low risk and favourable intermediate risk	Any risk category
Follow up	Predefined schedule	As per patient requirement or symptoms
Assessment	DRE, PSA, mpMRI, biopsy	As indicated clinically

1.6 Radiotherapy

1.6.1 Low/Intermediate Risk Prostate Cancer

Traditionally, prostate cancer has been treated with conventional doses of RT to the dose of 74–78 Gy in 37–39 #. However, in last decade, robust evidence from multiple randomised trials has made hypofractionation the standard of care for EBRT in prostate cancer.

Hypofractionation

The alpha–beta ratio of adenocarcinoma of the prostate is considered low compared to most other neoplasms, with several estimates derived from large populations in the range of 1.4–1.9 Gy. Unlike other solid tumours, the alpha–beta ratio of the adjacent dose-limiting normal structure, i.e. rectum, has been estimated to be greater than that of prostate cancer itself. An implication of this relationship is that hypofractionation may further improve the therapeutic ratio of EBRT. Moderate hypofractionation is defined as fraction size of 2.5–4 Gy/fraction.

The CHHiP, PROFIT, HYPRO trials and the trial by Arcangeli et al. established moderate hypofractionation as the standard of care in prostate cancer. The largest of the above, the CHHiP trial was a non-inferiority phase III trial that randomised 3216 men with predominantly intermediate-risk disease to one of three arms: 74 Gy/37 # (2 Gy/# over 7.4 weeks), 60 Gy/20# (3 Gy/# over 4 weeks), or 57 Gy/19# (3 Gy/# over 3.8 weeks). At a median follow-up of 5.2 years, the 60 Gy hypofractionated regimen had non-inferior biochemical and clinical failure compared to the 74 Gy conventionally fractionated regimen (HR 0.84 (90% CI 0.68–1.03), $p = 0.0018$). The 57 Gy hypofractionated regimen, however, was not non-inferior to the 74 Gy regimen with respect to this endpoint. There were no significant differences in either the proportion or cumulative incidence of side-effects 5 years after treatment using clinician-reported as well as patient-reported outcome measures [14–17].

Evolution of RT planning and delivery methods has enabled the use of very high doses per fraction (ultrahypofractionated RT/SBRT). Level I evidence for the use of SBRT in prostate cancer came from the HYPO RT PC trial. This multicentre non-inferiority study randomised 1200 men with majorly intermediate-risk prostate cancer to receive either 42.7 Gy/7# or 78 Gy/39#. At a median follow-up of 5 years, the estimated FFS was 84%. There was a marginal increase in acute physician-reported RTOG grade 2 or worse urinary toxicity in the SBRT group at end of RT, and an increase in urinary toxicity in the ultra-hypofractionation group compared to the conventional fractionation group at 1-year follow-up (6% vs 2%; ($p = 0{\cdot}0037$). Patient-reported outcome measures revealed significantly higher levels of acute urinary and bowel symptoms in the SBRT group and increased urinary symptoms at 1-year follow-up, consistent with the physician-evaluated toxicity [18]. In contrast, the PACE-B trial showed no difference in acute or late toxicity at 2 yrs in between the standard and SBRT arm. Moreover 70% patients in the standard arm received moderate hypofractionation, which is the current standard of care [19, 20].

Phase III randomised trials and several single-institution trials have confirmed the advantage of dose escalation for patients with localised prostate cancer. These trials have shown long-term biochemical control advantages especially among patients with intermediate- and high-risk disease. More recently, however, updates of some these studies have indicated a benefit for the application of higher radiation dose levels even for patients with favourable-risk disease. Zelefsky et al. reported their results in 2551 patients with T1–T3 prostate cancer treated with follow-up that extended beyond 20 years. The radiation dose was systematically increased from 64.8 to 86.4 Gy by increments of 5.4 Gy in consecutive groups of patients. Dose levels <70.2 Gy and 70.2–79.2 Gy were associated with 2.3- and 1.3-fold increased risks of PSA relapse compared with higher doses. Improved PSA relapse–free survival (PSA-RFS) outcomes with higher doses were observed for all risk groups.

The most common site of local recurrence post-RT is the dominant intraprostatic lesion (DIL). The FLAME trial randomised patients with localised prostate cancer to either standard RT (77 Gy to the entire prostate) or an additional integrated focal boost to the DIL to a dose of up to 95 Gy. The dose-escalation arm showed superior biochemical disease-free survival (92% vs 85%, $p < 0.001$) at 5 years, with no difference in overall survival or toxicity [21]. The four landmark trials addressing treatment intensification in high-risk prostate cancer are compared in Table 3.

Role of ADT

Short-term ADT of 4–6 months, along with RT improves biochemical relapse-free in intermediate risk prostate cancer [22, 23]. The benefit of ADT persists in spite of dose escalation to the prostate or DIL [24].

1.6.2 High-Risk and Very High-Risk Prostate Cancer

Patients with high-risk prostate cancer have a greater risk of pelvic lymph node involvement. Risk of nodal involvement can be estimated by the Roach formula. There had long been an equipoise regarding the role pelvic RT to the pelvis in high-risk patients. The GETUG-01 trial randomised patients with cT1b-T3N0M0 prostate cancer to RT to the prostate 66–70 Gy +/− RT to the pelvis (44 Gy). There was no difference in the event-free or overall survival between the two groups. Paradoxically, a post hoc subgroup analysis favoured pelvic radiotherapy in patients

Table 3 Treatment intensification in high-risk prostate cancer

	STAMPEDE [52]	POP-RT [27]	FLAME	ASCENDE-RT
Method of intensification	Abiraterone	Whole pelvic radiotherapy	Dose escalation by focal boost	Dose escalation by brachytherapy
Number of patients	1974	224	571	398
Stage cT3–T4	93%	46%	60%	30% (T3a)
Regional nodal involvement	39%	None	None	None
Gleason grade group 4–5	79%	48%	35%	40%
Staging investigations	CT, bone scan	PSMA-PET CT	CT, bone scan	CT, bone scan
Prostate dose EQD2 (a/b = 2)	74 Gy	78 Gy	108 Gy	115 Gy
Pelvic radiotherapy	None	50 Gy	None	46 Gy
5-year MFS (test vs standard arm)	82% vs 69% (6-year MFS)	96% vs 80%	90% vs 87% (approximately)	93% vs 93%

with <15% nodal risk [25]. The RTOG 9413 used a 2 × 2 factorial design to compare WPRT versus PORT and neoadjuvant or adjuvant ADT. Conventionally fractionated dose of 70.2 Gy was delivered to the prostate, with 50.4 Gy to the pelvic nodes in WPRT. All patients received only 4 months of ADT, before or after the radiotherapy as per assignment. Although initial results suggested improved biochemical control with WPRT, long-term outcomes have shown no clear difference between the PORT and WPRT.

These trials had lacunae in the form of inadequate ADT, heterogeneous patient selection, fractionation and treatment volumes; and clinicians were still divided between treating the pelvis or not [26]. The POP-RT trial has now produced some concrete answers. This Phase III trial randomised trial patients with high-risk and very high-risk prostate cancer with a risk of pelvic nodal involvement of at least 20% using the Roach formula. All patients were treated with hypofractionated IG-IMRT and received ADT for 2 years. The trial achieved its primary endpoint, showing significantly better 5-yr biochemical failure-free survival with WPRT (whole pelvic RT) compared to prostate-only RT (95.0% with WPRT versus 81.2% with PORT, with an unadjusted hazard ratio (HR) of 0.23 (95% CI, 0.10–0.52; *p*- 0.0001)). 5-yr DFS was also significantly better with WPRT (89.5% v 77.2%; HR, 0.40; 95% CI, 0.22–0.73; *p* 0.002). 5-yr OS did not differ, however 5-yr distant metastasis-free survival was better with WPRT [27].

The role of SBRT in high-risk prostate cancer is under evaluation and early results are promising. The Phase I/II SATURN trial evaluated 30 patients with high-risk prostate cancer. Grade 2 acute and late urinary toxicity were 47% and 52% respectively. Grade 2 acute and late gastro-intestinal toxicity were 3.3% and 32%, respectively. There were no Grade 3 or higher toxicities [28]. Murthy et al. reported 68 consecutively treated high-risk, very high-risk and node positive prostate cancer patients who were treated with SBRT All patients received long term ADT and node positive patients received pelvic RT. No grade 3 acute toxicities were recorded. Acute grade 2 genitourinary and gastrointestinal toxicity were 12% and 3%, respectively. Late grade 3 genitourinary and gastrointestinal toxicity was 3% and 0%, respectively. Prior transurethral resection of prostate did not increase toxicity [29]. The prospective Phase II SHORT trial from the Tata Medical Centre, Kolkata treated 30 patients with SBRT, a majority were high-risk. With a median follow-up of 41 months, there was low incidence of acute toxicities, the most common being urinary, which returned to near baseline at 3 months post-RT [30]. Another analysis of 220 patients treated with SBRT at TMC, Mumbai, had low rates of acute as well as late GU and GI toxicities. Even more importantly, 102 of these patients had received whole pelvic-SBRT. WPRT was associated with more late GU toxicity (45% vs 25%, $p = 0.003$), however rate of late Gr 3 toxicity was only 2.5%. No Gr 4/5 toxicities were seen in any patient [31]. The PRIME trial is a Phase III randomised trial addressing the role of SBRT in high-risk prostate cancer patients and has completed accrual [32].

Role of ADT

Long-term ADT is the standard of care in high-risk prostate cancer. The Phase III RTOG 85-31 established the role of ADT in high-risk prostate cancer. The EORTC 22863 and 22961 trials showed that longer ADT of 2–3 years was better than short-term ADT. There was no significant difference in cumulative risk of fatal cardiac events [33]. The recently published DART 01/05 trial too tested the role of short-term vs long term ADT with high dose radiotherapy. Though the trial could not establish statistical significance, the results showed a consistent and clinically relevant benefit with longer term ADT [34]. The FROGG 2019 guidelines give recommendations for the management of clinically and pathologically node positive prostate cancer [37]. In conclusion, high-risk patients should receive 18–24 months of ADT. A longer duration of at least 3 years should be considered in node positive patients.

1.6.3 Node-Positive Prostate Cancer

Node-positive prostate cancer was treated with ADT alone in the past. With the advent of conformal radiotherapy techniques, it became possible to safely treat the prostate and pelvic lymph nodes.

Post-radical prostatectomy for N0, about 15% patients are found to be pathologically node positive. Observation is not recommended due to the high rates of biochemical relapse (>60%). Individualised decisions may be made in patients with negative surgical margins and single nodal involvement. Adjuvant radiotherapy to the prostatic bed and pelvic lymph node gives biochemical recurrence-free survival outcomes to the tune of from 85% at 10 years. Adjuvant ADT alone adds toxicity and outcomes are inferior to adjuvant RT. Use of adjuvant RT is generally accompanied with use of ADT, though the duration has been variable across studies between 6 and 24 months [35].

Involvement of common iliac lymph nodes is staged as M1a disease in prostate cancer. Chopade et al. retrospectively analysed 130 patients with pelvic [86] and common iliac [42] lymph nodes. All patients received radiotherapy to the prostate and pelvis, with ADT for a minimum of 2-years. After a median follow-up of 61 months, both sets of patients had similar rates of biochemical failure, distant metastasis-free and overall survival [36]. There may thus be a case for treating patients with common iliac nodes (M1a) with curative radiotherapy to prostate and pelvis.

1.6.4 RT Post-transurethral Resection of the Prostate (TURP)

About 20% prostate cancer patients in India have a history of TURP prior to RT. Several case series have shown that TURP prior to RT increases risk of genitourinary toxicity in the form of urethral stricture and urinary incontinence [38]. However good patient selection and adequate gap between TURP and EBRT may allow for RT delivery lesser toxicity [29]. Prior TURP should not be a contra-indication for EBRT even with hypofractionation.

1.6.5 Salvage Post-loco-regional Failure

A. RT to prostate

About 3–10% patients experience local failure post-RT. Treatment options for locally recurrent prostate cancer post-RT include salvage prostatectomy, HIFU-high intensity focused ultrasound, cryotherapy or re-RT with brachytherapy. The MASTER systemic review and meta-analysis has analysed these options using the random-effects model. Outcomes and toxicities were evaluated by taking radical prostatectomy as the standard. Among the salvage therapies EBRT was associated with least incidence of late severe GU toxicity (4%), while HIFU was associated with the highest (23%). However, highest rates of severe late toxicity were seen in the standard treatment, i.e. radical prostatectomy. Overall rates of late GI toxicity were low across all treatments (0–2%). Two-year recurrence-free survival (RFS) was lower with HIFU compared to radical prostatectomy. Two- and four-year RFS was similar in all other salvage modalities [39].

B. RT to regional nodes

Salvage nodal RT and salvage lymph node dissection are treatment options in regional nodal recurrences in prostate cancer. A retrospective analysis by Kretschmer et al. which included 100 patients (67 receiving salvage RT and 33 undergoing salvage dissection) showed that on multivariable analysis that salvage RT was associated with significantly better 2-yr biochemical recurrence-free survival (92% vs 30%, $p = 0.001$) and significantly reduced rate of distant metastases (21% vs 52%, $p = 0.002$) [40]. The OLIGOPELVIS GETUG P07 is a Phase II trial involving 67 patients with nodal oligorecurrence (up to 5 pelvic nodes). Patients were treated with 6 months of ADT and RT to the pelvis and boost to the gross nodes. At 2 and 3 years, the biochemical recurrence-free survival rates were 58% and 46%, respectively. The dose of RT was 54 Gy/30# [41]. A higher dose and longer duration of ADT would possibly have improved the outcomes.

C. Salvage ADT

Another salvage option is the use of androgen deprivation therapy alone [42].

1.6.6 Post-operative RT

Based on the stage at diagnosis and post-operative histopathological features about half of the patients will experience a biochemical failure following radical prostatectomy [43]. American Urological Association defines biochemical recurrence post-surgery as a detectable or rising PSA value after surgery that is ≥0.2 ng/mL, supported by a second confirmatory level. Earlier trials such as the Finnish trial, the EORTC 22911 and ARO 96-02 showed that adjuvant RT was better than no RT in patients at high risk of recurrence [44–46]. However, the higher PSA cut-off value for initiating salvage RT have made these trials clinically obsolete. Trials such as the RAVES, RADICALS-RT, GETUG-AFU 17 and the Artistic meta-analysis showed the equivalence of salvage and adjuvant RT, thus preventing overtreatment and its associated side-effects. GETUG-AFU 16 and RTOG 96-01 showed that addition of ADT to salvage RT improved outcomes. Use of pelvic RT was inconsistent across these trials. The benefit of pelvic RT in the setting of ADT and that of ADT over PB RT alone was investigated in the SPPORT trial. The trial achieved its primary endpoint of improved freedom from progression with the addition of ADT to PBRT, addition of pelvic RT to ADT + PBRT or the addition of pelvic RT + ADT to PBRT alone. Grade 2 late adverse events were significantly higher in the arms with ADT and Pelvic RT [47–50]. Though above results suggest that early salvage RT should now become the standard of care following radical prostatectomy, there is still a role for adjuvant radiotherapy. Patients often seen in Indian practice, i.e. with multiple adverse features and a high-CAPRA-S score (calculated based on the preoperative PSA >20 ng/mL, Gleason score ≥8, positive surgical margins, extraprostatic extension, seminal vesicle involvement or lymph nodal involvement were under-represented in the three trials included in the ARTISTIC meta-analysis. It may be worthwhile to consider adjuvant RT in these patients.

1.7 Management for Metastatic Prostate Cancer

In metastatic disease, RT to primary or metastatic sites can be indicated with the goal of disease ablation or palliation.

1.7.1 Radiotherapy to the Primary

The rationale for treatment of the primary in metastatic cancer comes from the concept of the pre-metastatic niche. Animal studies have shown that compounds secreted by the primary tumour prime the metastatic site prior to the arrival of tumour cells in the distant organs and help in successful colonisation. Thus, RT to the primary may prevent further metastatic progression.

The HORRAD trial initially investigated the benefit of adding RT to the primary along with ADT. Median time to PSA progression was 15 months in RT arm vs 12 months in the control arm ($p = 0.02$) [51].

The STAMPEDE trial was a landmark study which demonstrated improvement in overall survival with prostate RT in low burden de novo oligometastatic prostate cancer. Patients were randomised to either standard of care (SOC) or SOC with radiotherapy. SOC was lifelong ADT with or without docetaxel. Radiotherapy improved failure-free survival (HR 0.76, 95% CI 0·68–0·84; $p < 0{\cdot}0001$) for the entire cohort. On subgroup analysis there was a significant OS advantage for radiotherapy for low volume disease (as defined by the CHAARTED trial) at 3 years (81% vs 73%, HR 0.68, 95% CI 0.52–0.90, $p = 0.0098$). PFS and PCSS was also significantly better with RT for the low burden group and the maximum benefit in FFS with RT was also seen in the low burden group [52].

1.7.2 Metastasis Directed Therapy

Intervention at the oligometastatic stage provides an opportunity for curative treatment by eradication of all disease sites with local therapy [53].

The Phase II STOMP trial randomised oligorecurrent prostate cancer (biochemical recurrence after previous curative intent therapy with <3 metastatic extracranial lesion on choline PET CT) to either surveillance or metastasis directed therapy (MDT) of all lesions (surgery or SBRT). The 5-year ADT free survival was 8% vs 34% in favour of the MDT group (HR – 0.57, 80% CI 0.38–0.85) [54]. Similarly, the ORIOLE trial randomised patients with recurrent hormone sensitive prostate-cancer and 1–3 metastases in a 2:1 ratio to receive stereotactic ablative radiotherapy (SABR) or observation. Treatment with SABR improved median progression-free survival [55]. Recently, the ESTRO-ACROP consensus guidelines recommend metastasis directed therapy to all sites in patients with 1–5 metastatic sites in the setting of de novo oligometastatic, oligorecurrent and oligoprogressive cancer [56].

Systemic Therapy in Metastatic Disease (Table 4)

Lifelong androgen suppression is the mainstay of treatment in metastatic prostate cancer. Median time to castration resistance is 12 months with ADT alone. Combined androgen blockade is now the standard of care in all patients with metastatic hormone sensitive prostate cancer.

Castration Resistant Prostate Cancer (CRPC)

Castration resistance is defined as either biochemical/clinical/radiological progression in the presence of serum testosterone <50 ng/dl. Biochemical progression is defined as three consecutive rises of PSA with PSA >2 ng/mL. Radiological progression is defined as appearance of ≥2 new lesions on bone scan/enlargement of soft tissue lesion. Patients may be treated with docetaxel or abiraterone acetate if not received previously. Newer agents can be used on further progression. Enzalutamide, darolutamide and apalutamide have shown improvement in metastasis-free survival and overall survival in Phase 3 trials- PROSPER, ARAMIS and SPARTAN, respectively.

Role of Radionuclide Therapy

Ra-223 dichloride is an α emitter that selectively targets bone metastases. The ALSYMPCA trial in 2013 randomised 917 m CRPC patients with bone metastases in a 2:1 ratio to receive 6 injections of Ra-223 (50 kBq/kg) every 4 weeks vs placebo. There was a significant improvement in overall survival with use Ra-223. The rates of Ra induced myelosuppression were low.

Lu-177-PSMA-617 is a radioligand that selectively targets PSMA- expressing cells and causes cell kill with ß emission. Unlike Ra-223 it targets all disease sites. The role of Lutetium was tested in mCRPC patients in the Phase III randomised VISION trial. Patients were randomised in a 2:1 ratio to receive either 6 weekly Lu-177-PSMA-617 for 4–6 cycles plus standard

Table 4 Systemic therapy in metastatic hormone sensitive prostate cancer

Drug	Trial	Outcomes	Median time to castration resistance in test arm
Docetaxel	CHAARTED (2015) Test Arm: 6 cycles Docetaxel ($75 mg/m^2$ 3 weekly + ADT) Std Arm: ADT alone	Median OS: 57 m vs 44 m ($p < 0.001$) favouring Docetaxel + ADT	20 months
Abiraterone	LATITUDE (2017) Test Arm: Abiraterone actetata (1000 mg OD) + Prednisone 5 mg OD Std Arm: ADT + Placebo	Median OS: NR in Test arm vs 35 m in Std arm ($p < 0.001$)	33 months
Enzalutamide	ENZAMET (2019) Test Arm: Enzalutamide 160 mg OD Std Arm: Bicalutamide/Nitutamide/Flutamide	3-yr OS: 80% in Test arm vs 72% in Std Arm ($p = 0.002$)	Not reached
Apalutamide	TITAN (2021) Test Arm: Apalutamide 240 mg OD + ADT Std Arm: ADT alone	2-yr OS: 82% in Test Arm, 73% in Std arm ($p = 0.005$)	Not reached
Darolutamide	ARASENS (2022) Test Arm: Darolutamide + ADT + Docetaxel Std Arm: ADT + Docetaxel	4-yr OS: 63% in Test arm and 50% in Std Arm	Not reached

of care or standard of care alone. With a median follow-up of 21 months, Lutetium significantly prolonged imaging-based progression-free survival and overall survival. Grade 3 or above toxicities were higher with Lutetium, but there was no difference in quality of life between the two arms.

Indian Perspective

In India, nearly 60% patients are metastatic at presentation. Amongst the patients with non-metastatic disease, 80% present with high-risk disease and <5% have low risk disease at presentation. In a nationwide survey of radiation oncologists, it was seen that nearly 60% patients receiving radical radiotherapy do so with moderate hypofractionation and up to 15% receive SBRT. Nearly all patients received image guided-IMRT. Use of brachytherapy is on a declining trend [2, 57].

1.7.3 Treatment Delivery

Radiation planning and delivery should be a stringent quality-controlled process, particularly in this era of conformal radiotherapy techniques.

RT Simulation

Patient positioning for prostate cancer should be supine with arms over chest/over head and a knee rest, fiducial placement at the pubic symphysis. Bladder and rectal filling contribute majorly to the change in position of the target organs thus leading to a need for large PTV margins. Change in bladder and rectal volumes also have an impact on RT induced toxicity. To minimise the variation in bladder and rectal volumes, patients should be simulated with a strict empty rectum and comfortably full bladder protocol.

Additional methods for reducing intra- and inter-fraction motion, or decreasing dose to critical normal tissues are being increasingly used as we shift towards moderately (Fig. 1) and ultrahypofractionated treatments. The anterior rectal wall is one of the most important OARs during prostate RT. The use of polyethylene glycol spacers injected into the retroprostatic space has shown statistically significant dosimetric improvements in the rectal volume receiving at least 50, 60, 70 and 80 Gy in a Phase III randomised controlled trial by Hamstra et al. With a median follow-up of three years, patients who

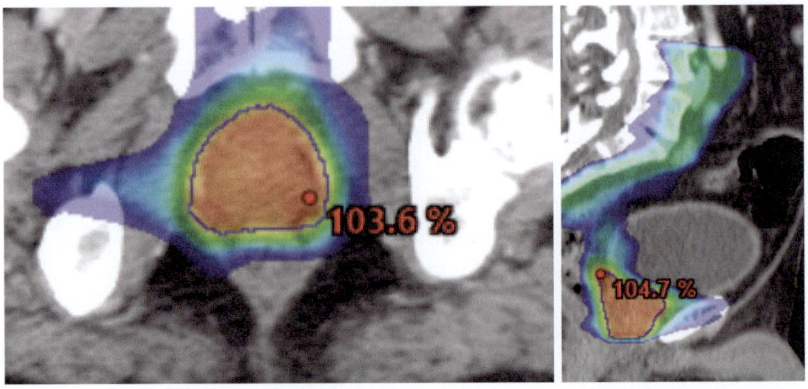

Fig. 1 50% isodose with moderate hypofractionation

received a rectal spacer experienced a significantly lower incidence of grade 1 and grade 2 rectal toxicity, as well as grade 1 urinary toxicity [58]. The rectal retractor is a device that unlike the endo-rectal balloon reduces anterior rectal wall doses (Fig. 2). When it retracts the rectum, it not only displaces the rectal wall from the prostate but also changes the rectal shape. This reduces the volume of anterior rectal wall receiving high doses of radiation [59]. Patient alignment based alone on skin marks or bony landmarks is not a reliable approach for the use of such precise technology. The use of fiducial markers implanted in the prostate for patient set up with verification on EPID has been shown to be superior to set up based on bony landmarks alone and it also allows for reduction of PTV margins [60]. This method is of particular use when on board CBCT is not available. Patients may also be simulated with a rectal balloon inflated with a pre-defined volume of air or water which helps to minimise intra-fraction prostate motion [61].

More conformal RT techniques have shown incremental benefit by allowing dose escalation while limiting OAR doses. Dearnaley et al. randomised men with prostate cancer to receive 64 Gy/32# using either conformal or conventional RT. In the 225 men treated, significantly fewer men developed radiation-induced proctitis and bleeding in the conformal group than in the conventional group [62]. Viani et al. randomised 215 men with localised prostate cancer to receive 70 Gy/35# by either IMRT or 3DCRT. The 3DCRT arm had a 27% rate of grade ≥2 acute GU toxicity compared with a 9% rate in the IMRT arm ($p = 0.001$) and a 24% rate of grade ≥2 acute GI toxicity compared with a 7% rate in the IMRT arm ($p = 0.001$). The maximal rate of grade ≥2 late GU toxicity during the entire period of follow-up was 3.7% in the IMRT group versus 12.3% in the 3DCRT group ($p = 0.02$). The maximal rate of grade ≥2 late GI toxicity during the entire follow-up was 6.4% in the IMRT group versus 21.7% in the 3DCRT group ($p = 0.001$). Disease outcomes were similar in both arms [63].

1.7.4 Contouring Guidelines (Table 5)

Nodal Contouring

Prophylactic nodal volumes for intact and post-operative should include the obturator, internal iliac, external iliac, presacral and the common iliac lymph nodal regions [65].

1.7.5 Prostate Brachytherapy

The prostate is an attractive target for brachytherapy due to the proximity to critical normal tissue—the anterior rectal wall and the bladder. Permanent seed brachytherary as well as temporary HDR brachytherapy are feasible options with appropriate patient selection. HDR brachytherapy is associated with fewer acute irritative symptoms, lower operator dependence and allows use of the same source for many patients.

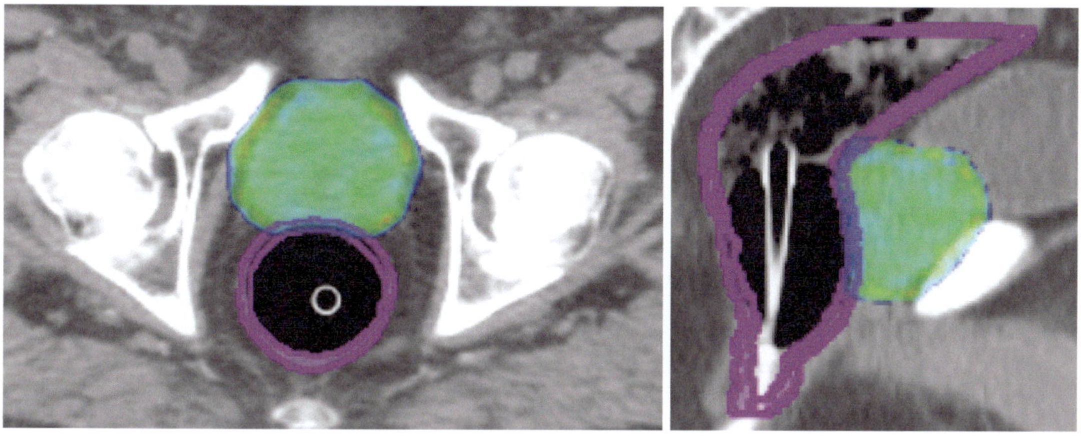

Fig. 2 Planning with endorectal balloon

LDR brachytherapy is associated with lower initial capital requirements, less shielding, completion of treatment in a single implant and more robust data from clinical trials. I-125 and Pd-103 are the commonest isotopes in use for permanent seed brachytherapy [66]. HDR/LDR monotherapy is adequate for low and intermediate risk prostate cancer. However, treatment for high-risk requires EBRT followed by a brachytherapy boost to the entire prostate. The ASCENDE-RT trial compared dose-escalated EBRT to EBRT + HDR boost in intermediate and high-risk prostate cancer. Though BT boost was associated with better biochemical control at 5 and 9-yrs, both acute and late GU as well as GI toxicities were significantly higher [67]. The more recent FLAME trial gives equivalent results with lesser toxicity using an EBRT boost to the DIL, making it a more attractive option [21]. However, brachytherapy still plays an essential role in low and favourable intermediate risk prostate cancer; and in patients requiring re-irradiation.

1.7.6 Radiotherapy Sequelae

Complications that occur during or after EBRT can be grouped mainly into GI, GU and sexual. Intestinal toxicity occurring during RT manifests as an acute enteritis because of irradiation of the small and large intestine with the probability and severity being proportional to the volume of bowel included in the treatment fields but is usually well controlled with antidiarrheal medications and local steroidal type preparations for proctitis. However, long-term injury may occur in a small proportion of patients, and this may manifest as persistent diarrhea, tenesmus, rectal/anal strictures or hematochezia; bowel ulceration, obstruction or perforation is more uncommon.

The symptoms of cystitis/urethritis are characterised by urinary frequency, urgency, hesitancy, decreased force of stream and dysuria. Significant long-term urinary sequelae are uncommon but may take the form of cystitis, hematuria, urethral stricture and/or bladder contracture.

1.7.7 Follow-Up and QOL

Follow-up post-treatment should include clinical examination, DRE and serial PSA monitoring. Frequency for Sr PSA can be 3 monthly for the first 2 yrs, 6 monthly thereafter for 5 yrs and annually thereafter. Trigger for imaging should be rise in PSA (>2 ng/mL for intact prostate, >0.2 ng mL for post-op prostate maintained on two separate occasions; or clinical signs of progression).

1.7.8 Prognosis, Results and Outcome, and Survival

Prostate cancer has across all stage groups (Table 6). This is largely due to high sensitivity to androgen deprivation and PSA as a biomarker for disease prognosis. Metastatic hormone sensitive prostate cancer too has a median survival beyond 5 years.

Table 5 Contouring of prostate [64]

		MRI based	CT based
Apex		Butterfly-shaped structure, excluding the urethra and starting above the penile bulb and genito-urinary diaphragm (Fig. 3)	Starts approximately 1 cm above the upper border of the penile bulb
Mid-prostate	Lateral border	Butterfly-shaped structure, excluding the urethra and starting above the penile bulb and genito-urinary diaphragm	After correct delineation of the rectum, the thickness of the musculus levator ani can be defined; the same thickness of the levator ani muscle defined at the level of the rectum can be extrapolated over the full length of the prostate. This forms the lateral border of the prostate
	Anterior border Posterior border	Exclude the retropubic space unless signs of invasion Anterior border of the rectum	Include the anterior fascia and exclude the fat area in front of the anterior fascia unless protrusion of the prostate is visible on CT Same as MRI
Base	In continuity with the bladder, to be controlled in the sagittal and coronal view		
ECE		To include area of suspicion of ECE	If high suspicion of ECE, to give a 3 mm margin around the prostate as part of CTV.
Seminal vesicles (Irrespective of imaging modality)	Low risk No inclusion	Int risk Inclusion of at least proximal 1.4 cm	High risk To include at least proximal 2.2 cm In case of involvement, to include the entire seminal vesicles
Target volumes			
Low risk Prostate only	*Intermediate risk* Prostate + Proximal 1–1.5 cm of seminal vesicles	*High risk* Prostate + Prox 1.5–2 cm of SV Include entire SV if involved	Pelvic LNs to be included in high risk, very high risk and node positive prostate cancer

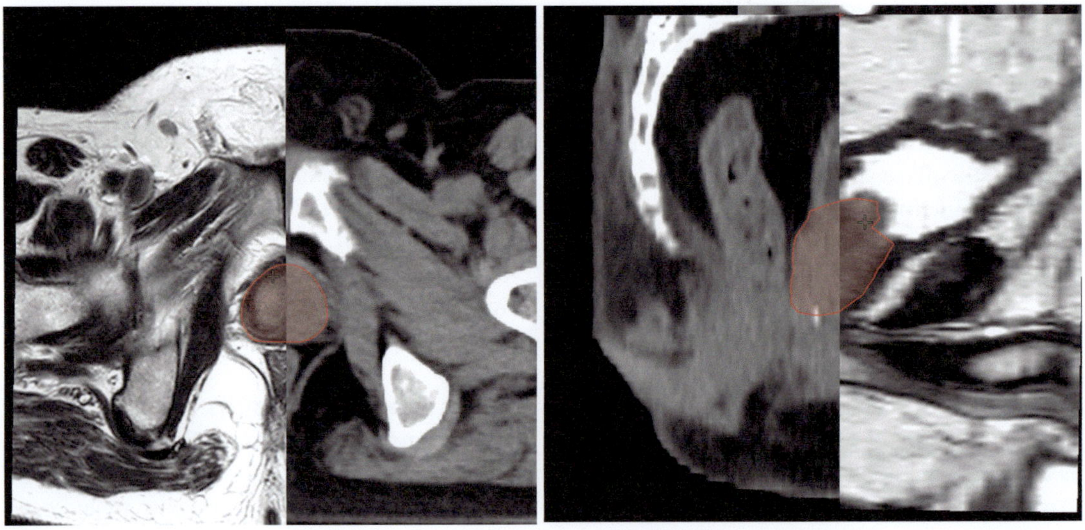

Fig. 3 MR/CT fusion

Table 6 SEER stage-wise 5-year relative survival rate

SEER stage	5-year relative survival rate
Localised	>99%
Regional	>99%
Distant	31%
All SEER stages combined	98%

Development of castration resistance leads to rapid disease progression and poor response to therapy.

1.8 Future Research

Recent advances in radiotherapy technology include advent of the MR-LINAC. It allows daily adaptive replanning and better ability to escalate dose by reducing PTV margins. Trials using MR-LINACs are ongoing. They are investigating the possibility of treating prostate cancer in 1–2 fractions.

1.9 Conclusion

Treatment of prostate cancer is a rapidly evolving landscape. The last decade has seen advancement in all aspects of management ranging from more sensitive PSA assays, emergence of newer radiopharmaceuticals for diagnosis and treatment, advances in robotic surgery, radiotherapy as well as systemic therapies. It is accompanied by increasing incidence probably due to regular PSA testing in elderly men. Use of these rapid enhancements must be tempered with appropriate case selection to improve outcomes and limit treatment related toxicity.

2 Bladder Cancer

2.1 Anatomy

The bladder has four anatomical parts: the apex or dome, body, fundus and neck. It is primarily made of smooth muscle called the detrusor with stratified transitional epithelium covering the luminal surface (Fig. 4). Its layers include transitional epithelium (lacks blood or lymphatic vessels), basement membrane, lamina propria (forms the submucous coat, contains nerves, blood vessels, and areolar connective tissue, a tumour needs to reach this layer to have the ability to spread), muscular coat (muscularis propria with three layers—inner longitudinal, middle circular and outer longitudinal), serosa in peritoneum lining the superior and lateral surfaces (or adventitia in other places) and peri-vesical fat. Lymphatics from bladder cancer primarily drain to the internal iliac, external iliac, obturator and presacral lymph nodes. Common iliac, para-aortic, interaortocaval and paracaval lymph nodes form secondary drainage sites.

2.2 Epidemiology and Risk Factors

According to GLOBOCAN 2020, bladder cancer is 10th in incidence among all cancers. It is four times more common in men, with the incidence in India being 2.5/100,000. Cigarette smoking (and tobacco exposure in general) is the most common risk factor. Environmental and occupational exposure to carcinogens is the 2nd most common factor. Particular carcinogens include aromatic amines, polycyclic aromatic hydrocarbons, chlorinated hydrocarbons, arsenic, disinfection by-products or nitrates. Schistosomiasis is another important risk factor in endemic areas and is associated with squamous cell carcinoma.

2.3 Clinical Symptoms and Signs, Pathology

Painless gross hematuria is considered a cardinal pathognomic sign and must be investigated in all. Other common clinical symptoms include pain or burning sensation during urination, increased urine frequency, urgency and lower back pain. Advanced disease may have signs and symptoms attributable to specific sites of metastasis.

Transitional cell carcinoma is the most common histological subtype, followed by squamous, adenocarcinoma, neuroendocrine and others (<1%). Muscle invasion and lymph nodal

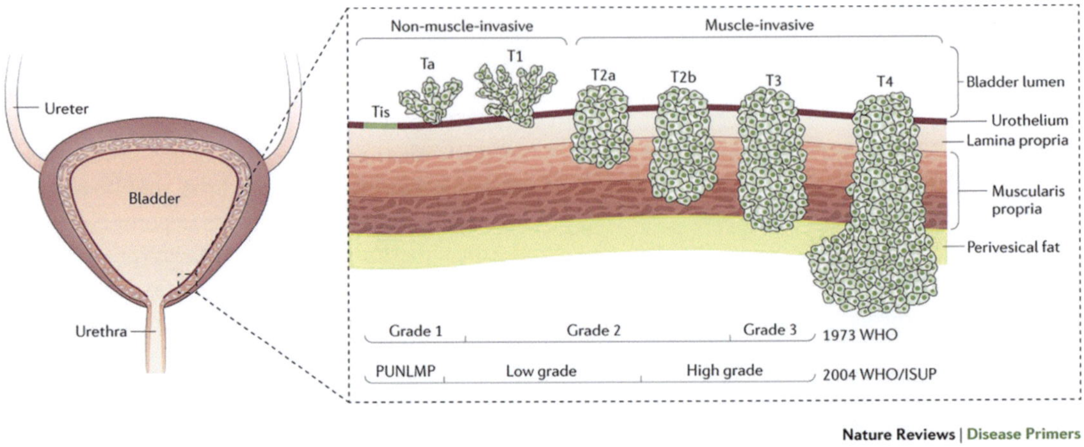

Fig. 4 Microscopic anatomy of the bladder

involvement are key prognostic factors. For non-muscle invasive disease (NMIBC), tumour grade and T sub-stage assumes primary importance influencing both treatment and prognosis. Variant histologies with poor prognosis include sarcomatoid, plasmacytoid and micropapillary variants.

2.4 Investigations

2.4.1 Surgery

TURBT

Transurethral resection of bladder tumour (TURBT) is the primary step in the diagnosis, staging, prognostication and management of bladder cancer. The standard components of a TURBT include examination under anaesthesia, complete visualisation of the urethra, inspection of the whole bladder lining and precise description of the location and the number of tumours and their relationship to the ureteric orifice and bladder neck. The objective is to excise the tumour completely when possible or resect a representative specimen including the underlying detrusor muscle.

2.4.2 Treatment

NMIBC

NMIBC patients are risk stratified into low, intermediate, high and very-high based on various factors including age of the patient, number of tumours, size of the tumour, grade of the tumour and most importantly presence or absence of CIS.

Adjuvant Treatment

Adjuvant intravesical chemotherapy following TURBT has been shown to decrease the risk of recurrence in low risk as well as some intermediate risk patients. No difference has been demonstrated between various intravesical chemotherapy regimens. This treatment is to be administered as soon as a TURBT is performed but definitely within the 24 hours following resection.

For high-risk patients and some intermediate risk patients intravesical BCG has been shown to decrease the risk of recurrence. However, it has been demonstrated that the efficacy is better when maintenance treatment is given following the initial induction with 6 weeks of intravesical BCG immunotherapy. A minimum period of 1 year of maintenance is advocated though the overall treatment regime is of 27 intravesical treatments given over a period of 3 years. BCG has been shown to be superior to intravesical chemotherapy with respect to overall and cancer specific survival. Patients with very high-risk disease should be considered for radical cystectomy [68].

2.4.3 MIBC

Surgery

Radical cystectomy with pelvic lymph node dissection is the surgical standard in muscle invasive bladder cancer. In men, radical cystectomy includes removal of the bladder, prostate, seminal vesicles, distal ureters and regional LNs. In women, standard RC includes removal of the bladder, entire urethra and adjacent vagina, uterus, distal ureters and regional LNs. The 5-year survival rates after radical cystectomy alone in T2, T3a, T3b and T4 disease are 63%, 57%, 31% and 18%, respectively. Urethrectomy may be done at the time of cystectomy or subsequently as a separate procedure if the tumour involves the bladder neck in women or the prostatic urethra in men, or if the urethral cut margin is positive at the end of cystectomy, or in cases of extensive prostatic involvement. Options for urinary diversion techniques include incontinent intestinal (ileal or colonic) conduit with an external stoma, continent catheterisable reservoirs with an abdominal stoma or bladder substitution (neobladder) procedures.

2.4.4 Neoadjuvant Chemotherapy

With radical cystectomy alone, the 5-year OS is around 50%. Thus, cisplatin-based chemotherapy regimens are used to improve survival outcomes in eligible patients [81]. Six cycles of dose-dense MVAC (methotrexate, vinblastine, adriamycin plus cisplatin) with primary GCSF is the preferred regimen; however, four cycles of cisplatin and gemcitabine is another suitable, more tolerable alternative. In the cisplatin ineligible, immune-checkpoint inhibitors have shown pCR rates ranging from 31% to 38%. Initial data on gene expression profiles suggest that patients with basal tumours have a more pronounced benefit.

2.4.5 Adjuvant Chemotherapy

Adjuvant cisplatin-based chemotherapy should be offered in patients with pT3-4 and or pN+ disease undergoing upfront surgery, as it confers an absolute OS benefit of 6% at 5 years, along with an improved recurrence-free and metastasis-free survival [69].

2.4.6 Metastatic Disease

Cisplatin combination therapies are the primary choice in fit patients. GC and MVAC are equally effective but GC is less toxic. For cisplatin ineligible, carboplatin-based combination chemotherapy can be used as a substitute. Evidence now supports the use of immune checkpoint inhibitors as a second line option after failure of platinum chemotherapy or first line in cisplatin unfit patients [70]. For patients who respond well or have stable disease throughout their full course of platinum-based first-line chemotherapy, maintenance therapy with the PD-L1 inhibitor, avelumab is recommended for better OS [71]. No robust biomarker exists as of today to predict response to ICIs.

2.5 Radiation Therapy

2.5.1 Role in Non-muscle Invasive Bladder Cancer

As elucidated previously, treatment of NMIBC consists of TURBT followed by risk adapted intravesical BCG or chemotherapy of appropriate duration. Radical cystectomy is required in a small population who are at a higher risk of progression to MIBC. These patients are often frail, old and may not be candidates or willing for cystectomy. Pessoa at al performed a meta-analysis of 746 high risk NMIBC patients who were treated radiotherapy. High risk features included high grade T1 lesions/Ta with associated risk factors such as CIS, multifocality, >5 cm diameter or multiple recurrences. The data were almost entirely retrospective. All patients underwent baseline TURBT. A total of 247 patients also received RT to the pelvis. The 5-yr RFS, CSS and OS were 54%, 86% and 72%, respectively. Salvage cystectomy was required in 13% patients [72]. The RTOG 0926 was single arm Phase II trial wherein patients with NMIBC (T1) underwent concurrent chemoradiotherapy following a TURBT. The 3-yr cystectomy-free survival was 90% [73]. Thus, radical radiotherapy is an alternative effective approach especially in patients who would otherwise require cystectomy.

2.5.2 Radical Radiotherapy for MIBC

Radical cystectomy and pelvic lymph node dissection are associated with significant post-operative morbidity. Most patients have a permanent stoma as a urinary diversion technique, significantly affecting their quality of life. Bladder preservation using tri-modality therapy is an effective alternative in well selected patients. Tri-modality therapy consists of maximal TURBT followed by concurrent chemo-radiotherapy. NACT is recommended in some patients to optimise outcomes. Previous history of pelvic radiotherapy is the only absolute contra-indication for bladder preservation. Patients with poor bladder function, carcinoma-in-situ, multifocal disease, and presence of hydronephrosis may be better treated with cystectomy. In the past, bladder preservation was exclusively practiced in patients not fit for or refusing cystectomy. However, continued evidence has shown that outcomes with bladder preservation are similar to those with cystectomy. SPARE was Phase III randomised controlled trial that aimed to randomise patients with T2-3N0M0 MIBC to undergo cystectomy or bladder preservation. The trial had to be closed prematurely due to slow accrual and large numbers of crossovers to the bladder preservation arm. It showed patient acceptance and preference for bladder preservation [75]. Though randomised evidence is scarce, multiple systematic reviews and meta-analyses provide evidence for bladder preservation. Kaushik et al. conducted a meta-analysis of nearly 10,000 bladder cancer patients treated in eight studies. There was no difference in the 5 yr (HR 0.96, favouring CMT, 95% CI 0.72–1.29; p = 0.778) or 10 yr (HR 1.02, favouring cystectomy, 95% CI 0.73–1.42; p = 0.905) overall survival. Disease-free survival and progression-free survival were also comparable at 5 and 10 years. As expected, cystectomy was associated with early major complications [76].

Use of concurrent radio sensitizers increases the potency of RT. The BCON trial published in 2010 investigated the role of concurrent carbogen and nicotinamide (CON) along with radiotherapy. Three hundred thirty-three patients were randomised to receive RT alone or RT + CON. Patients with T2-4a urothelial MIBC or T1 Gr 3 NMIBC were included. Radiation dose to the bladder was 55 Gy/20# or 64 Gy/32# treated with 3DCRT. Differences in OS, risk of death and local relapse were significantly in favour of RT+ CON. Greatest benefit in OS was seen in T2 tumours. Among the long-term survivors, 83% retained their bladder in the combined therapy arm and 60% in the RT arm. There was no difference in incidence of late toxicity in either arm [77]. The BC2001 randomised trial used 5-FU and Mitomycin-C as a radio sensitizer with RT. At 2 yrs, the rates of loco-regional disease-free survival were significantly higher in CTRT arm (67% vs 54%, p = 0.03.) The difference in survival was not statistically significantly. Rates of acute Gr 3–4 toxicities were higher in the combined therapy arm; however, incidence of late toxicity was similar [78]. An individual patient data meta-analysis of the above two trials showed that hypofractionated RT (55 Gy/20#) had superior invasive locoregional control compared to 64 Gy/32# [79]. HYBRID was a Phase II randomised trial in patients unfit for radical radiotherapy. All patients received 36 Gy/6# weekly radiotherapy. Randomisation was between standard planning and adaptive planning. The median age of the patients was 85 years. At 3 months, the local control rate was 81%. Adaptive radiotherapy reduced acute Grade 3 toxicity [80].

Radiation Technique

As in other disease sites, radiotherapy for bladder cancer has evolved from 2D-RT to 3DCRT and now IMRT, particularly VMAT. IMRT significantly reduces rectal and small bowel doses, resulting in clinically meaningful improvement in toxicity rates. Simulation for bladder cancer is done with the patient in the supine position with arms overhead/overchest with a knee rest. An empty bladder is preferred for better daily reproducibility. A distended rectum should be avoided to reduce proctitis.

Adaptive Radiotherapy

On account of the bladder being a distensible organ, there is considerable daily variability in spite of emptying before each fraction. This may be due to day-to-day variability of the time from bladder emptying to on-couch treatment delivery or variability in patient hydration, particularly on days of concurrent chemotherapy. Therefore, some form of adaptive radiotherapy is essential for safe delivery without a geographical miss (Table 7).

Table 7 Adaptive radiotherapy methods

Online	Offline	
Plan of the day [82] Involves creating a library of plans and selection of the appropriate plan using daily CBCT/MVCT (Fig. 5)	*Daily reoptimisation* Plan is reoptimised daily after acquisition of CBCT	*Comparative adaptive planning* A form of offline adaptation with individualised margins At baseline a large PTV margin (1.5 cm) is given to the baseline CTV Bladder from D1–4 CBCTs is contoured on the baseline Simulation scan. The D1–4 bladders are booleaned with the baseline CTV and new CTV volume is created. A smaller PTV margin (e.g. 5 mm) is given for remaining fractions (Fig. 6)
Population-based margins Standard isotropic or anisotropic margins are created around the CTV Anisotropic margins use a more generous margin in the anterosuperior direction as change in shape with bladder filling is along these directions Serially larger PTV margins are given and and a plan based on each margin is created. An appropriate plan based on bladder filling is selected at each fraction	*Individualised margins* A-POLO: Consists of taking serial CT simulation scans at various stages of bladder filling (e.g. at time zero, 15, 30 and 45 min post-bladder emptying. Individual plans are created based on the CTV derived at each time point (Fig. 7)	

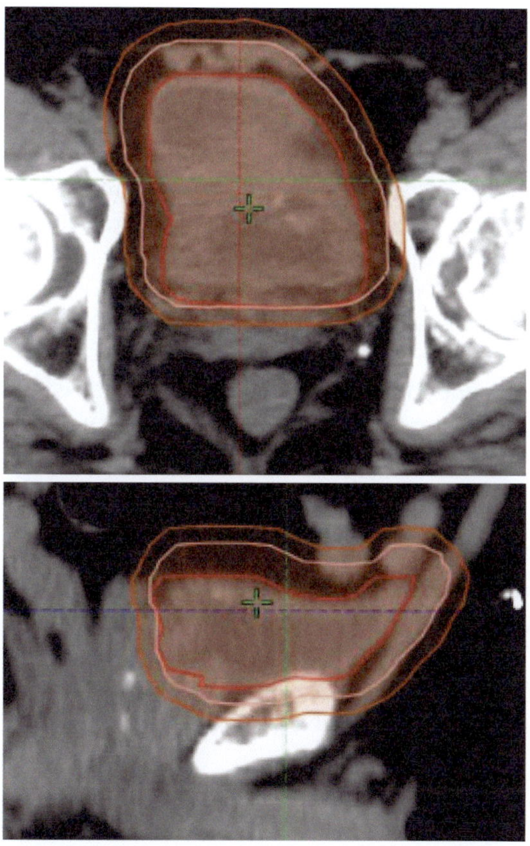

Fig. 5 Plan of the day with population-based margins

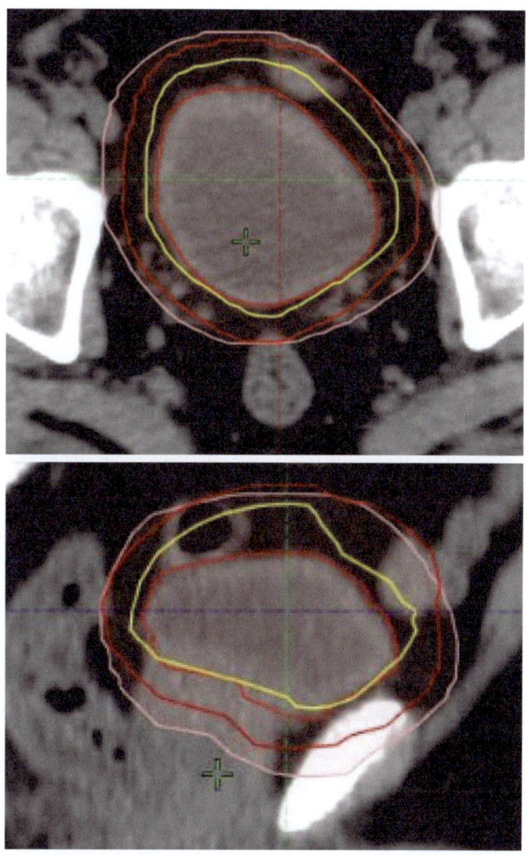

Fig. 6 Comparative adaptive planning with D1–4 CBCT

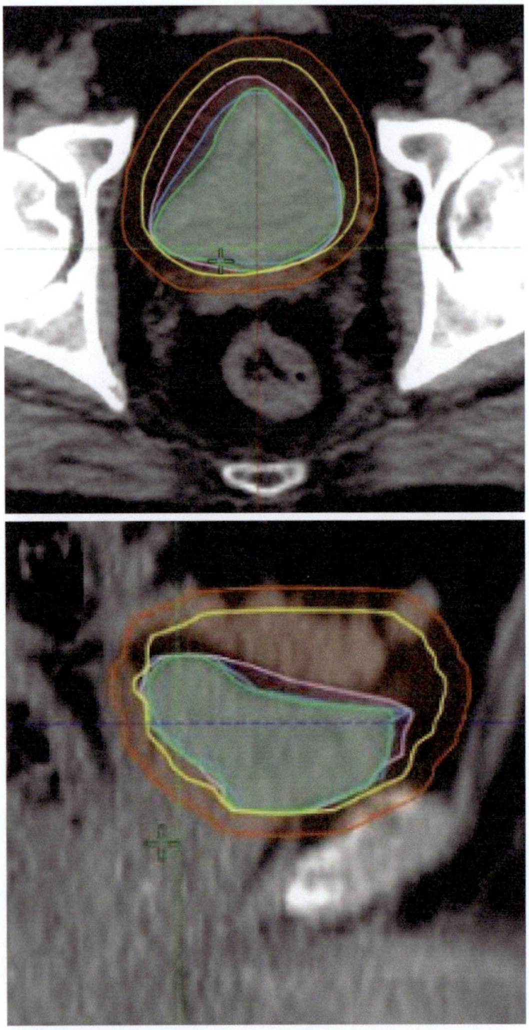

Fig. 7 Plan of the day with individualised margins (A-POLO Technique)

Pelvic RT

The role of pelvic nodal radiation in bladder preservation remains controversial, as a clear benefit in outcomes is yet to be proven [83]. Radiotherapy to the bladder alone results in significant dose to the obturator, external iliac and internal iliac lymph nodes [85]. However, given the high risk of nodal metastasis in bladder cancer and the routine use of lymph node dissection during cystectomy makes pelvic radiotherapy a desirable option.

Target Volume and Radiation Dose

Target volume for the primary consists of the entire bladder and perivesical extension if any. In cases of bladder neck involvement or extensive CIS, it is recommended that 1.5 cm of the prostatic urethra in males and 1 cm of the female urethra be taken in the treatment volume. Nodal volume consists of the obturator, external and iliac, and presacral nodes. In patients with lymph node involvement, common iliac nodes may also be included. Boost to the primary site of tumour did not improve outcomes in a study of 106 patients by Murthy et al. It is not routinely recommended [86].

Dose: Conventional fractionation and hypofractionation have been found have similar toxicities. However, as previously discussed an IPD meta-analysis of the BC-2001 and BCON trial showed superior locoregional control with hypofractionation.

Convention fractionation: 64 Gy/32# (Nodal dose: 55 Gy/32#)

Moderate hypofractionation: 55 Gy/20# (Nodal dose: 44 Gy/20#)

2.5.3 Adjuvant Radiotherapy

Radical cystectomy with peri-operative systemic chemotherapy is the standard of care in muscle invasive bladder cancer. However, approximately 35% patients still develop locoregional failure within the pelvis, with or without metastasis elsewhere. Therein lies an opportunity to escalate local therapy with RT in patients at high risk of recurrence. Christodouleas et al. stratified patients from the SWOG 8710 trial into low, intermediate and high-risk groups depending upon pathological tumour stage, surgical margin status and number of lymph nodes identified. They thus identified patients who would benefit with local RT [87]. Murthy et al. too classified patients post-cystectomy into low, intermediate and high risk based on probability of loco-regional recurrence (LRR). The cumulative incidence of LRR was 7.1%, 21.6% and 35% in the low, intermediate and high risk groups, respectively [88].

Target volumes and contouring guidelines were given by Baumann et al. and updated in 2022 [89]. Target volume comprised of cystectomy bed and pelvic nodal regions (common iliac, external iliac, internal iliac, obturator and presacral nodes. Indications for adjuvant RT are currently under investigation. Zagloul et al. conducted a Phase II randomised trial that included patients with *p* T3b, Grade 3 or node-positive prostate cancer. Of all, 53% had urothelial carcinoma and 47% had squamous carcinoma. Locoregional recurrence-free survival and disease-free survival were significantly better in the CT + RT arm. There was no significant difference in overall survival. Five patients in the RT arm had Grade 3 gastrointestinal toxicity [90]. BART is a randomised Phase III trial currently accrual at the Tata Memorial Centre, randomising locally advanced urothelial bladder cancer, randomising patients to receive RT or not after NACT -> Surgery Or Surgery -> adjuvant chemotherapy (NCT02951325).

2.5.4 Follow-Up and QOL Issues

Patients should be advised to follow up at 3-monthly intervals for the 1st 2 years, followed by 6-monthly intervals at 5-yrs and annually thereafter. Patients undergoing bladder preservation should be evaluated with a urine routine microscopy, cytology and a cystoscopy at each follow-up. A cross-sectional imaging may be done at 6 monthly intervals till 5 years post-treatment completion.

2.5.5 Prognosis, Results and Outcome, Survival (Table 8)

Table 8 SEER stage-wise 5-year relative survival rate

SEER stage	5-year relative survival rate
In situ alone	96%
Localised	70%
Regional	38%
Distant	6%
All SEER stages combined	77%

2.6 Future Research

An evolving molecular classification broadly classifies MIBC into three major subtypes:

1. Luminal—better prognosis, enriched for FGFR3 mutations found at high frequency in non-invasive tumours
2. Basal squamous—inferior prognosis, characterised by p53 mutations and alterations of DNA-damage repair pathways, more responsive to chemotherapy
3. Neuronal cluster subtype—associated with worst clinical outcomes

2.7 Conclusion

The role of radiation in bladder cancer is still evolving. Bladder preservation using trimodality therapy is now a credible option even in young, fit patients who may be particularly desirous of an intact bladder. The role of adjuvant radiotherapy is still under investigation, however, given the high incidence of locoregional recurrence may prove RT to be an integral part of treatment.

3 Testicular Cancer

3.1 Anatomy

Testes are paired glands located in the scrotum that produce sperm and the male sex hormone, testosterone. They are surrounded by membrane layers, the inner tunica albuginea and the outer tunica vaginalis. The regional lymph nodes for testicular cancer are the retroperitoneal nodes, with right-sided tumours spreading to inter-aortocaval nodes and left-sided tumours to para-aortic nodes [91] (Fig. 8). Retroperitoneal cross-over from right to left side is common due to natural lymphatic pathways. Inguinal nodes may be involved if drainage pathways are altered

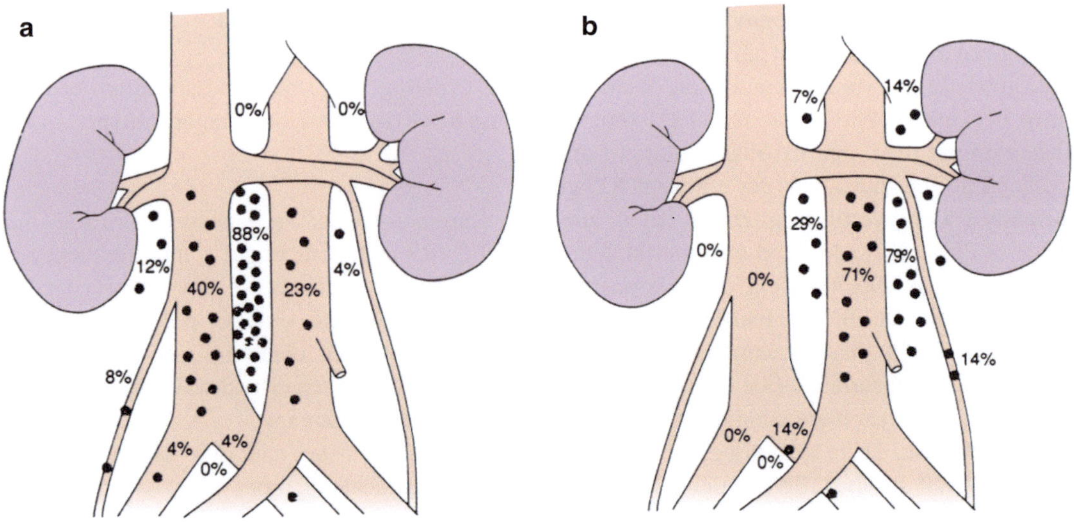

Fig. 8 Lymphatic drainage from testis

due to prior inguinal or scrotal surgery, or with epididymal or scrotal skin involvement.

3.2 Epidemiological Aspects and Risk Factors

The crude incidence of testicular cancer in India is 0.6/100,000 males [92]. There is a characteristic age distribution with a small peak in childhood around 2 years age and a second peak in adulthood around 25–40 years of age (GCT), and a final peak around 65–75 years of age (non germ cell tumours, mainly lymphomas). NSGCTs are more common in children and young adults, whereas seminomas usually present a decade later [93]. Risk factors include undescended testes (cryptorchidism), conditions of abnormal testicular development (e.g. Klinefelter syndrome), male infertility and family history [94]. The risk with cryptorchidism persists even after orchiopexy of the undescended testis. The contralateral testicle is also at risk in testicular cancer patients [95].

3.3 Clinical Symptoms and Signs, Pathology

Patients may present with a testicular lump (usually painless and unilateral), pain in the testicle or scrotum, heaviness or diffuse enlargement of the scrotum (fluid accumulation), dull ache in the abdomen, groin or back, breast enlargement, or, in advanced cases, an abdominal mass due to enlarged para-aortic nodes. Further spread occurs to the lung and lymph nodes in the mediastinum, pelvis and neck, and less commonly to liver and bones. Metastasis to the brain is rare and raises suspicion of choriocarcinoma [96]. The majority of testicular cancers are germ cell tumours (GCT) (Table 9), either seminoma (60%), nonseminoma (30–40%) or mixed (5–10%).

3.4 Integrated Management Plan

3.4.1 Investigations

Routine screening of young adult males is not recommended in view of the low incidence and high survival of testicular cancer [98].

Recommended workup includes a high-frequency (>10 MHz) ultrasound of the scrotum, which assesses size, nature (solid—likely malignant, or cystic—likely benign) and site of origin of the mass (testicular—malignant, or extra testicular), with a 92–98% sensitivity and 95–99.8% specificity for malignancy. Serum tumour markers (Table 10) like serum AFP, ß-HCG and LDH are reliable biomarkers for diagnosis, staging, prognosis, monitoring treatment response, and

Table 9 2016 Update of the World Health Organization (WHO) Pathological Classification of Testicular Tumours [97]

1. *Germ cell tumours (90–95%)*
Derived from germ cell neoplasia in situ (GCNIS)
Seminoma (60%) Nonseminomatous tumours (30–40%) Embryonal carcinoma Yolk sac tumour, post-pubertal type Trophoblastic tumours Teratoma, post-pubertal type Teratoma with somatic malignant components Mixed germ cell tumours (5–10%)
Unrelated to GCNIS
Spermatocytic tumour Yolk-sac tumour, pre-pubertal type Mixed germ cell tumour, pre-pubertal type
2. *Sex cord/stromal tumours (5–10%)*
Leydig cell tumour/malignant Leydig cell tumour Sertoli cell tumour/malignant Sertoli cell tumour/large cell calcifying Sertoli cell tumour/intratubular Large cell hyalinising Sertoli cell Neoplasia Granulosa cell tumour—adult type/Juvenile type Thecoma/fibroma group of tumours Other sex cord/gonadal stromal tumours—mixed/unclassified Tumours containing both germ cell and sex cord/gonadal stromal elements/Gonadoblastoma
3. *Miscellaneous non-specific stromal tumours*
Ovarian epithelial tumours Tumours of the collecting ducts and rete testis/Adenoma/Carcinoma Tumours of paratesticular structures/Adenomatoid tumour/Mesothelioma (Epithelioid/Biphasic) Epididymal tumours Cystadenoma of the epididymis Papillary cystadenoma Adenocarcinoma of the epididymis Mesenchymal tumours of the spermatic cord and testicular adnexae

Table 10 Properties of tumour markers relevant to testicular tumours

Tumour marker	Nature	Origin	Normal level	Half life	Elevated in
AFP	Protein	Liver, GIT, fetal yolk sac	<40 ug/L	5–7 days	NSGCT (yolk sac tumour, embryonal carcinoma, teratoma)
B-hCG	Glycoprotein	Placenta	<5 IU/L	24–36 hours	NSGCT (choriocarcinoma, embryonal carcinoma) Seminoma
LDH	Cellular enzyme	All body tissues	1.5–3.2 microkat/L	24 hours	Less specific for testicular cancer than AFP and b-hCG; mainly serves as a marker of aggressiveness of tumour

surveillance of seminomatous and nonseminomatous germ cell tumours [99]. These indicate the likely histology and are usually measured before and after orchiectomy for accurate staging. Biopsy of the suspected primary tumour is avoided to prevent scrotal seeding and, hence, upstaging [100]. Biopsy of the contralateral testis is only recommended in high-risk young patients with an atrophic testis and with history of cryptorchidism. CECT Thorax-Abdomen-Pelvis (TAP) is recommended for systemic staging. FDG PETCT is not recommended for initial staging but is useful for assessment of post-chemotherapy residual disease in GCTs [100].

Table 11 Staging of testicular tumours

Description	Stage
T Stage—clinical OR pathological[a]	
Primary tumour cannot be assessed	Tx
No evidence of primary tumour (e.g. histological scar in testis)	T0
Germ cell neoplasia in situ (GCNIS)/intratubular germ cell neoplasia/carcinoma in situ	Tis
Tumour involving testis (including tunica albuginea) and epididymis without LVI	T1 For pure seminoma, T1a if tumour is <3 cm in greatest dimension T1b if tumour is ≥3 cm in greatest dimension
Tumour involving testis and epididymis with LVI OR Tumour involving tunica vaginalis OR Tumour involving hilar soft tissue around epididymis	T2
Tumour involving spermatic cord[b] (with or without LVI)	T3
Tumour involving scrotum (with or without LVI)	T4
N Stage	
Regional lymph nodes cannot be assessed	Nx
No regional (retroperitoneal) lymph node metastasis[b]	N0
Lymph nodal mass ≤2 cm in size, or multiple (≤ 5) lymph nodes, none more than 2 cm	N1
Lymph nodal mass between 2 and 5 cm in size OR >5 positive nodes, none more than 5 cm OR evidence of extranodal extension of tumour	N2
Lymph nodal mass >5 cm in size	N3
M Stage (by imaging)[c]	
Distant metastases cannot be assessed	Mx
Non retroperitoneal nodal or pulmonary metastases	M1a
Non pulmonary visceral metastases	M1b
S stage (by serum tumour markers)	
Tumour markers not available/not performed	Sx
Tumour markers within normal limits	S0
LDH <1.5 times the upper limit of normal; OR AFP <1000; OR b-hCG <5000	S1
LDH 1.5–10 times the upper limit of normal; OR AFP 1000–10,000; OR b-hCG 5000–50,000	S2
LDH >10 times the upper limit of normal; OR AFP >10,000; OR b-hCG >50,000	S3

[a]The extent of the primary tumour is classified after radical orchidectomy (pT) in most cases. However, for clinico-radiologically evident Tis and T4 disease, radical orchidectomy is not always necessary for classification purposes. In the situation where no radical orchidectomy has been performed, it is staged as TX
[b]Positive lymph nodes are defined as lymph nodes 1.0 cm in their short axis on axial CT images
[c]Discontinuous involvements of the spermatic cord on orchidectomy specimen are considered as pM1

Seminoma is grossly well-circumscribed, homogenous, grey-white, lobulated cut surface without necrosis or haemorrhage. It has uniform tumour cells separated by fibrous septa containing lymphocytes which stains strongly for placental alkaline phosphatase (PLAP). IHC markers for seminoma are CD 117 (c-kit), OCT 3/4, SALL4. More than 80% have detectable isochromosome 12p.

Table 12 IGCCCG Prognostic System [103, 104]

Good-prognosis group	
Non-seminoma 5-year PFS 90% 5-year survival 96%	*All of the following criteria:* Testis/retro-peritoneal primary No non-pulmonary visceral metastases Post-orchidectomy AFP <1000 ng/mL hCG <5000 IU/L (1000 ng/mL) LDH <1.5 × upper limit of normal
Seminoma 5-year PFS 89% 5-year survival 95%	*All of the following criteria:* Any primary site No non-pulmonary visceral metastases Normal AFP Any hCG Any LDH
Intermediate-prognosis group	
Non-seminoma 5-year PFS 78% 5-year survival 89%	*Any of the following criteria:* Testis/retro-peritoneal primary No non-pulmonary visceral metastases Post-orchidectomy AFP 1000–10,000 ng/mL or hCG 5000–50,000 IU/L or LDH 1.5–10 × upper limit of normal
Seminoma 5-year PFS 79% 5-year survival 88%	*All of the following criteria:* Any primary site Non-pulmonary visceral metastases Normal AFP Any hCG Any LDH
Poor-prognosis group	
Non-seminoma 5-year PFS 54% 5-year survival 67%	*Any of the following criteria:* Mediastinal primary Non-pulmonary visceral metastases Post-orchidectomy AFP >10,000 ng/mL or hCG >50,000 IU/L (10,000 ng/mL) or LDH >10 × ULN
Seminoma	No patients classified as 'poor-prognosis'

The staging of testicular tumours and the prognostication for advanced disease by the International germ cell cancer collaborative group (IGCCCG) are mentioned in [101, 102] Tables 11 and 12, respectively.

3.4.2 Primary Treatment—High Inguinal Orchidectomy

High inguinal orchidectomy (HIO) including division of the spermatic cord at the internal inguinal ring is both a diagnostic and therapeutic procedure [105]. Trans-scrotal approach should be avoided when testicular cancer is suspected as it results in a higher local recurrence rate and altered pathways of metastatic dissemination. Certain special cases may warrant testis sparing surgery [106]. All patients planned for inguinal exploration with potential orchidectomy either U/L or B/L should be offered elective testicular prosthesis at time of surgery to preserve body image. Sperm banking if planned should be done prior to HIO.

3.4.3 Stage-Wise Management

Stage-wise management options vary as per histology and specific situations (Table 13).

Surveillance It is utilised for both germ cell neoplasia in situ (GCNIS) and Stage I seminoma/nonseminoma patients with no adverse features for relapse, and those who are likely to be compliant to follow-up [117]. It includes regular physical examination, monitoring of serum tumour markers and imaging (CT scans) 3–6 monthly for a year, and less often subsequently till 10 years. Optimum approach to surveillance has been investigated in the recently published TRISST trial [118]. Eligible patients were randomised 1:1:1:1 to either abdominal MRI or CT, at either 6-monthly intervals (7 scans) or at 6, 18 and 36 months (3 scans). It was seen that MRI was non-inferior to CT in both schedules, and less intensive imaging was non-inferior to 6-monthly imaging. Most recurrences occurred within the first 3 years, and all of them were salvaged with chemotherapy, with or without local radiotherapy or surgery. Five-year survival of 99% with no cancer-related deaths highlights the overall excellent prognosis in this group.

Tumour size >4 cm and rete testis invasion [119] are poor prognostic features and patients

Table 13 Stage-wise management of testicular cancers

Type	Stage	Surgery	Surveillance	Chemotherapy	Radiation therapy
Seminoma	*GCNIS*	*High inguinal orchiectomy*	*Preferred approach after surgery*; regular monitoring of serum tumour markers and USG testes if surgery not done; continued for up to 5 years after surgery	Only if tumour markers are persistently elevated after surgery (treating as IS disease)	To the testicle (Only if surgery not done)
Seminoma	*IA, IB or IS* (85% cases)	*High inguinal orchiectomy*	*Preferred approach after surgery (in 80–85%)* [107], *especially for patients likely to be compliant for follow-up* with regular physical examination, monitoring of serum tumour markers and imaging (CT scans) 3–6 monthly for a year, and less often subsequently till 10 years	For patients with doubtful compliance to follow-up or with risk factors like age, tumour size >4 cm, rete testis invasion, lymphovascular invasion, persistent high markers post-orchiectomy (Stage IS); preferred approach is 1–2 cycles carboplatin AUC 7 (less toxic than RT)	For patients with doubtful compliance to follow-up or with risk factors like age, tumour size >4 cm, rete-testis invasion, lymphovascular invasion, persistent high markers post-orchiectomy (stage IS); alternative to chemotherapy is *modified dog-leg RT* 20 Gy/10# [108, 109] for patients with history of inguinal surgery like inguinal herniorrhaphy or orchiopexy prior to orchiectomy, and *para-aortic RT* 20 Gy/10# for those with no such history [110]
Seminoma	*IIA or IIB* (11% cases)	*High inguinal orchiectomy*	–	For patients with *doubtful compliance to follow-up* after surgery or patients with *history of inguinal surgery* like inguinal herniorrhaphy or orchiopexy prior to orchidectomy,or with *horseshoe kidney* or *inflammatory bowel disease, preferred approach* as adjuvant treatment after surgery *(3 × BEP or 4 × EP)* [111, 112]. *Generally, preferred over RT for IIB seminoma*	*For patients compliant to follow-up* after surgery and with *no history of inguinal surgery* like inguinal herniorrhaphy or orchiopexy prior to orchidectomy, *preferred approach* as adjuvant treatment after surgery is *modified dog-leg RT* 20 Gy/10#, *followed by boost* to gross nodes to a dose of 10 Gy/5# for Stage IIA and 16 Gy/8# for Stage IIB. For those with prior *history of inguinal surgery, classic dog leg RT* in similar doses is utilised. *Generally, preferred over chemo for IIA seminoma*

(continued)

Table 13 (continued)

Type	Stage	Surgery	Surveillance	Chemotherapy	Radiation therapy
Seminoma	*IIC, IIIA, IIIB, IIIC*	High inguinal orchiectomy Salvage RPLND for residual lymph-nodal mass post-chemo	–	*3 × BEP; or 4 × EP; or 4 × VIP*	May be considered for residual lymph-nodal mass post-chemotherapy; SBRT has been utilised [113] Palliative radiation for abdominal mass not responding to chemo or relapsed scrotal mass
Non-seminoma	*GCNIS*	*High inguinal orchiectomy*	*Preferred approach after surgery*	If tumour markers are persistently elevated after surgery (treating as IS disease) OR if patient likely to be non-compliant to follow-up	–
	IA, IB or IS	*High inguinal orchiectomy* RPLND after orchiectomy (as alternative to chemotherapy) if risk factors for relapse present (vascular invasion, rete testis invasion, and embryonal carcinoma/ teratoma histology)	*Preferred approach after surgery if no risk factors for relapse present* [114]	*Preferred approach if risk factors for relapse present* (vascular invasion, and embryonal carcinoma/teratoma histology); *chemo preferred over RPLND* due to lower risk of relapse and avoidance of surgical complications [115] OR *if tumour markers are persistently elevated* after surgery (IS disease)	–
	IIA	*High inguinal orchiectomy RPLND preferred after orchiectomy if size of nodal mass upfront or of post-chemo residual is <1 cm*	–	*Preferred approach after surgery (cisplatin based), preferred over RPLND for nodal masses >1 cm* [116]	–
	IIB	*High inguinal orchiectomy* RPLND rarely if post-chemo residual nodal mass >1 cm	–	*Preferred approach after surgery (cisplatin based)*	–
	IIC IIIA IIIB IIIC	*High inguinal orchiectomy*	–	*Preferred approach after surgery (cisplatin based)*	Palliative radiation for abdominal mass not responding to chemo or relapsed scrotal mass

Table 14 BEP protocol

Chemotherapeutic drug	Dose	Route	Days
Bleomycin	30 IU	IV	D 1,8,15
Etoposide	100 mg/m^2	IV	D 1–5
Cisplatin (plus hydration)	20 mg/m^2	IV	D 1–5

with these features may benefit from adjuvant therapy.

Chemotherapy Stage I patients with risk factors like age, tumour size >4 cm, rete testis invasion, lymphovascular invasion, persistent high markers post-orchiectomy (Stage IS), or for those without risk-factors but with doubtful compliance to follow-up can be treated with SA carboplatin AUC 7. It is non-inferior to radiotherapy [120] and has additional benefit of reducing the risk of contralateral testicular malignancy.

For stage II, three cycles of 3 weekly BEP regimen [121] (Table 14) is an option in Stage IIa, and is the preferred treatment in stage IIb disease [122]. Bleomycin is known for its pulmonary toxicity and skin (Raynaud's phenomenon) and nail reactions, etoposide causes myelosuppression and mucositis, while cisplatin causes the characteristic triad of nephrotoxicity, ototoxicity and peripheral neuropathy. If patient is unfit for bleomycin, then four cycles of cisplatin and etoposide [EP] can be used as a suitable alternative.

Second-line chemotherapeutic options are ifosfamide, etoposide, cisplatin (VIP regimen) or substituting etoposide with paclitaxel (TIP regimen) or gemcitabine (GIP regimen).

Radiation Therapy For seminoma, it is utilised as an alternative to chemotherapy in Stage I patients with risk factors or with doubtful compliance. Prophylactic retroperitoneal nodal irradiation (PALN) to 20 Gy (MRC trial TE18) using 1.8–2 Gy/fraction is practiced. For stage IIA, RT is preferred over chemotherapy, and vice-versa for Stage IIB. For stage IIC and higher, RT may be considered for residual lymph-nodal mass post-chemotherapy. For Stage II A/B seminoma, the treatment options are RT to the retroperitoneal lymph nodes and pelvic lymph nodes (Dog-leg portal) 30–36 Gy/15–18# or chemotherapy 3 cycles BEP/4 cycles EP.

De-escalation of therapy is an area under investigation. The Phase II SAKK 01/10 trial [123] treated patients with Stage II A/B seminoma with SA Carboplatin AUC 7 followed by involved field RT (30–36 Gy). Results were promising with a 3 yr-PFS of 94%.

For Stage II C/ III seminoma response evaluation is preferably with a FDG PET CECT is recommended 10–12 weeks post-completion of chemotherapy. Treatment options for residual disease include salvage CTh/radiotherapy or RPLND. In a restrospective study of 69 patients from TMH, patients with residual mass with SUVmax >3 were more likely to benefit with RT. In this regard, a randomised trial from India, PROSem is ongoing (NCT05142982) to evaluate the role of FDG PET CT in identifying patients with residual viable tumour post-chemotherapy who would benefit with locoregional radiotherapy. The trial schema is shown in Fig. 9.

3.4.4 Management of NSGCT

The management of stage I is decided after careful consideration about exposure of patient to unnecessary adjuvant treatment vs need for salvage treatment at relapse. Therefore, patients should be actively involved in the decision-making after they are presented with the advantages and disadvantages of each treatment modality.

Unfortunately, 50% of the non-seminomas tend to relapse without adjuvant therapy. Active surveillance is an option in extremely few cases. Presence of lymphovascular invasion, embryonal predominance and invasion of spermatic cord are the strongest risk factors for relapse. Risk adapted approach (SWENOTECA) recommends 1 cycle of BEP (Bleomycin, Etoposide, Cisplatin) as the standard treatment in presence of vascular invasion as it reduces risk of relapse by 90–95% [124]. Alternate and a bit inferior option is primary nerve-sparing retroperitoneal lymph node dissection (RPLND) followed by chemotherapy based on nodal status [125]. In case of relapse post-surveillance or RPLND, 3–4 cycles of BEP

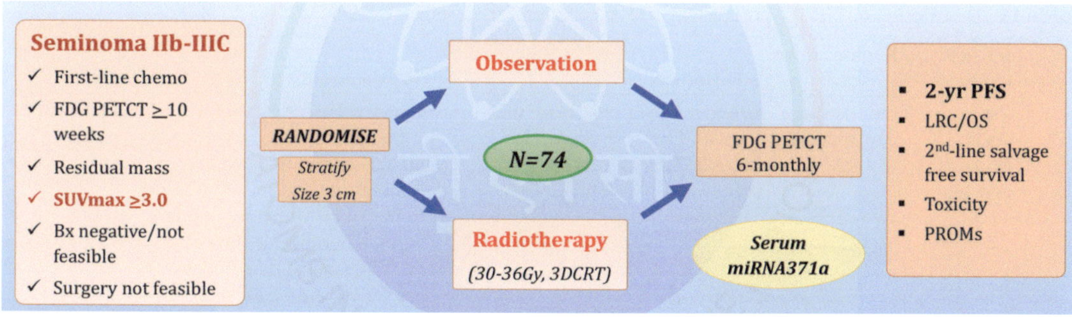

Fig. 9 PROSem trial schema

is administered. Surgery is offered in case of a single resectable lesion.

For stage II/III non-seminomas, patients are stratified as good, intermediate and poor risk (Table 4). For good risk cases, 3 cycles BEP (or EP × 4) is preferred over RPLND followed by adjuvant BEP. Intermediate and poor risk are treated with 4 cycles of BEP or VIP. Residual disease after primary chemotherapy is resected if more than 1 cm. Theories suggest that this residual disease may be either necrotic tissue or mature or immature teratoma. In contrast to seminomas, there are no imaging modalities including PET CT capable of distinguishing between necrosis/fibrosis, teratomas, or viable tumours in NSGCT [126]. In the event of relapse, salvage chemotherapy options include platinum containing regimens like VIP, TIP or GIP (etoposide, paclitaxel, gemicitabine with ifosfamide and cisplatin).

There is no established role of radiotherapy in NSGCT. There have been few case reports exploring stereotactic body radiation therapy (SBRT) as a salvage therapy in inoperable patients with recurrent chemo refractory NSGCT, with overall positive results. Currently, the use of radiation therapy should only be considered in chemo refractory inoperable disease or in patients with very high surgical risk as a salvage strategy [128, 129].

3.4.5 Radiation Therapy Planning

Doses and target volumes differ based on specific situations as described in Table 15. Prophylactic irradiation of mediastinal or left supraclavicular, contralateral iliac, inguinal nodes, or that of scrotal region for prior maldescended testis, inguinal or scrotal violation, or pT3/4 primary tumours is not indicated [130].

3.4.6 Simulation, 2-D Planning and Treatment Delivery

Patients are positioned supine with arms overhead to expose the abdomino-pelvic area. An abdominal thermoplastic cast or vacuum cushion may be used for immobilisation. A knee-rest is placed to stabilise the pelvis. The penis should be moved out of the radiation field, and a clamshell shield used to limit the dose to contralateral testis.

3.4.7 CT Acquisition, Contouring and 3-D Planning

After immobilisation, a contrast-enhanced CT scan extending from mid-thoracic spine to upper third of both femurs is acquired in 5 mm sections. Due to the close anatomical association of vasculature and lymphatics, blood vessels have been utilised as landmarks for accurate target delineation of nodal regions during 3-D planning [131]. The latter also ensures better sparing of normal tissues. For stage I seminoma, the nodal CTV includes the paracaval, precaval and interaortocaval lymph nodes for right-sided tumours and at least the lateroaortic and preaortic lymph nodes for left-sided tumours [132]. After contouring the IVC and aorta cranially from 2 cm below the top of the kidneys down to the point where the vessels bifurcate, a 1.2-cm expansion on the IVC [133] and a 1.9-cm expansion on the aorta is

Table 15 Description of 2-D RT portals and 3-D delineation for various RT fields

Stage	RT field name	Regions to be covered	2-D Borders	3-D delineation	Dose
IA, IB or IS	Para-aortic (Figs. 10 and 11)	Para-aortic, Aorto-caval	Cranial: Upper border of T12 Caudal: Lower border of L5 Lateral: Tips of transverse processes of vertebrae	Contour IVC & Aorta from 2 cm below the top of kidneys up to the level of vessel bifurcation, add 1.2 cm margin to IVC and 1.9 cm margin to aorta, edit off bone, bowel, muscle, fascia and bladder to get CTV1. Add PTV and penumbra margins.	20 Gy/10#
IIA	Modified dog-leg (Fig. 10)	Para-aortic, Aorto-caval, ipsilateral iliac	Upper straight part of portal is same as for Para-aortic RT noted above. Lower, curved part of portal: Lateral border: Line from the tip of the ipsilateral transverse process of L5 to the superolateral border of the ipsilateral acetabulum medial border: Line joining tip of the contralateral transverse process of L5 to the medial border of the ipsilateral obturator foramen. Caudal border: Just above ipsilateral acetabulum	In addition to above, the ipsilateral common, external, and proximal internal iliac veins and arteries down to the upper border of the acetabulum are contoured, 1.2 cm margin added and edited off bone and bowel to get CTV1.Gross nodes +0.8 cm margin, edited off bone and bowel, gives CTV2. 0.5 mm PTV and 0.7 mm penumbra margins added.	30 Gy/15#
IIB	Dog-leg or hockey stick	Para-aortic, aorto-caval, ipsilateral iliac and inguinal	Same as modified dog-leg, except that the lower border extends up to the lower border of ipsilateral lesser trochanter of femur	Vessels contoured up to lower end of lesser trochanter. Margins added similarly.	36 Gy/18#

given, and bone, bowel, muscle, fascia and bladder are edited out to create a nodal CTV1. A 0.5-cm margin is added to CTV1 to create a planning target volume (PTV1) to account for treatment setup errors. A uniform 0.7-cm margin should be provided on PTV1 to the block edge to account for beam penumbra (Fig. 11) [134].

For stage IIA or IIB, the ipsilateral common, external and proximal internal iliac veins and arteries down to the upper border of the acetabulum are additionally contoured. A 1.2-cm expansion on the iliac vessels, excluding bone and bowel, forms the CTV1. The gross nodes are contoured, and a uniform 0.8-cm expansion added to create CTV2. Respective PTVs and penumbra margins are added as described above. 3D conformal treatment planning and image guidance-based treatment delivery are desirable. Zilli et al. (Fig. 12) compared 3-D conformal 16 MV parallel-opposed AP-PA fields (Fig. 13) versus bone marrow-sparing intensity-modulated radiation therapy (BMS-IMRT, Fig. 14) utilising seven 6 MV non-opposed coplanar fields in patients with Stage I seminoma, and concluded that BMS-IMRT markedly reduces the dose to the critical structures. They postulated that this should help reduce acute and long-term toxicity, and the risk of secondary cancers.

3.4.8 Late Sequelae of Treatment

Second malignancies Patients receiving abdomino-pelvic radiotherapy are at a threefold higher risk of secondary leukemias, two-fold relative risk for solid cancers with radiation alone and 2.9 times for chemoradiation [135]. The commonest second cancers in this cohort are those of stomach, pancreas, pleura, bladder, colon, esophagus,

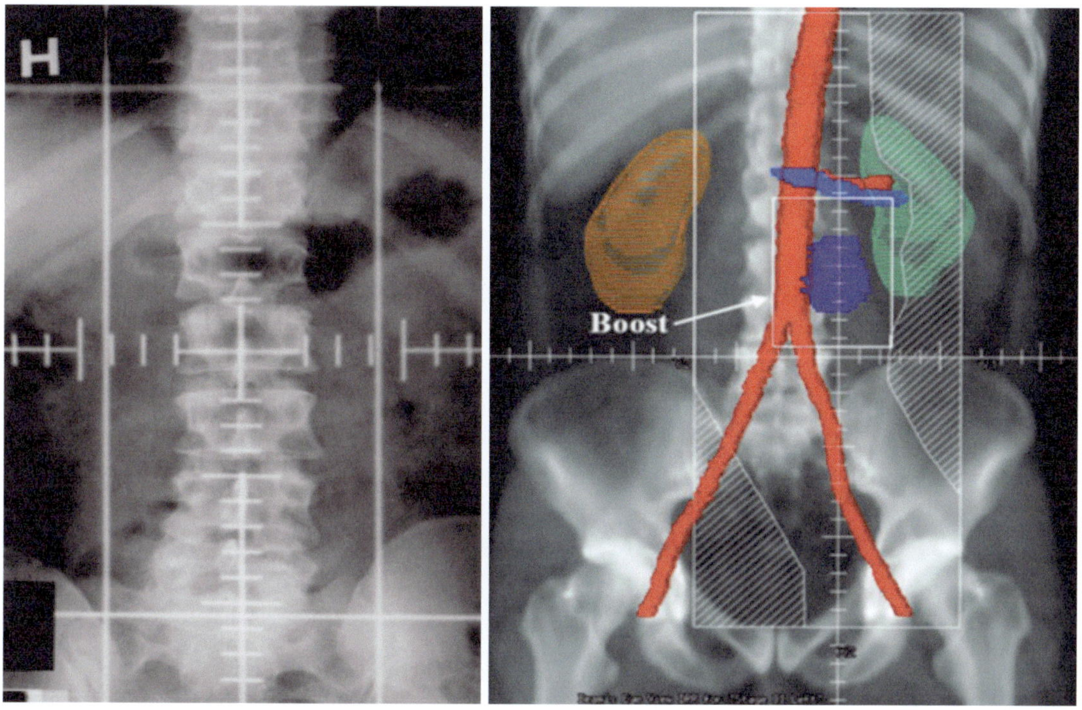

Fig. 10 2D representation of PALN and Hockey-stick portal

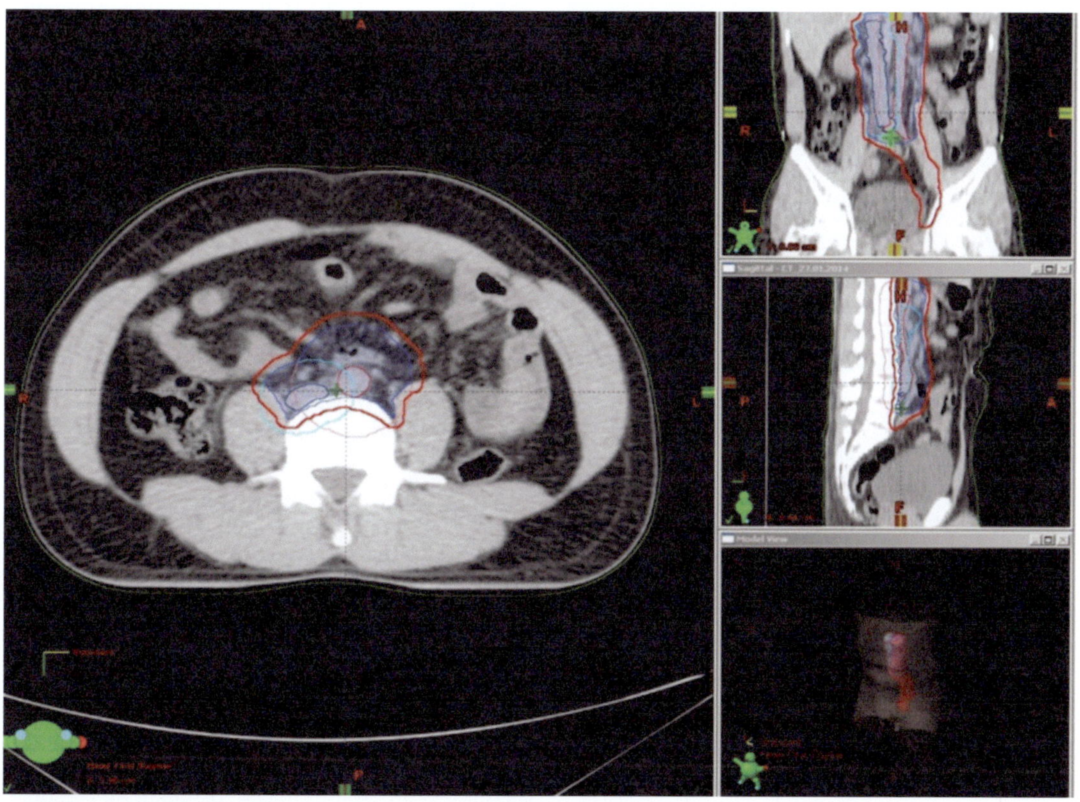

Fig. 11 Contouring of Aorta, IVC with margins and generated PTV for prophylactic RT to PALN

Structure	Constraints	Volume (%)	Dose in Gy (%)
CTV	Upper	0	22 (110%)
	D_{mean}	100	20 (100%)
PTV	Upper	1	21.4 (107%)
	Lower	100	19 (95%)
ABM	D_{mean}	100	< 7.5
Combined kidneys	Upper	1	20 (100%)
	Upper	20	15 (75%)
	Upper	33	10 (50%)
	D_{mean}	100	< 6.9
Bowel	Upper	50	10 (50%)
Stomach	Upper	50	5 (25%)
Pancreas	Upper	30	20 (100%)
	Upper	50	15 (75%)
Liver	Upper	33	10 (50%)
Spinal cord		No dose constraint	

Fig. 12 Dose constraints for BMS IMRT. (Adapted from Zili et al.)

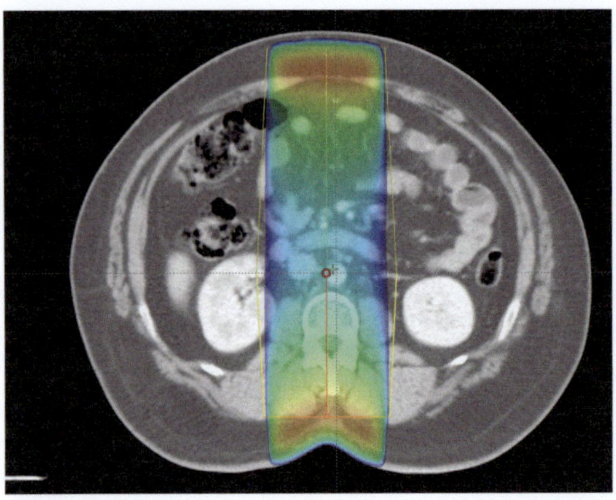

Fig. 13 95% dose coverage with AP/PA portal for PALN

melanoma, thyroid, kidney and connective tissue [136]. This is attributed to the delivery of a higher integral dose with IMRT/VMAT theoretically. However, practically less toxicity is observed using IMRT, and there is no concrete evidence to suggest that a high integral dose is causing second malignancies in the real world [137].

Infertility and Hypogonadism Semen abnormalities, infertility and hypogonadism may pre-exist in testicular cancer patients, or be induced by orchiectomy, chemotherapy and radiotherapy. Retroperitoneal lymph node dissection may lead to retrograde ejaculation or anejaculation due to nerve injuries.

Cardiovascular disease At 10 years post-treatment, abdomino-pelvic radiotherapy alone increases the risk of atherosclerotic disease by two-fold, while chemoradiation increases it by five-fold [138].

3.4.9 Follow-Up and QOL

Patients should be followed up for at least 5 years post-treatment to monitor for recurrence and late complications. It includes history and clinical examination, testicular ultrasound and serum tumour-markers (optional for stage I and IIA seminoma, but essential for higher stages of seminoma and all stages of nonseminoma). Chest X-Ray/CT Chest and CT abdomen may be done 2–6 monthly in first 2 years and 6–12 monthly till 5 years to rule out lung metastases and retroperitoneal or pelvic nodal recurrences. Commonest quality-of-life issues faced by testicular cancer

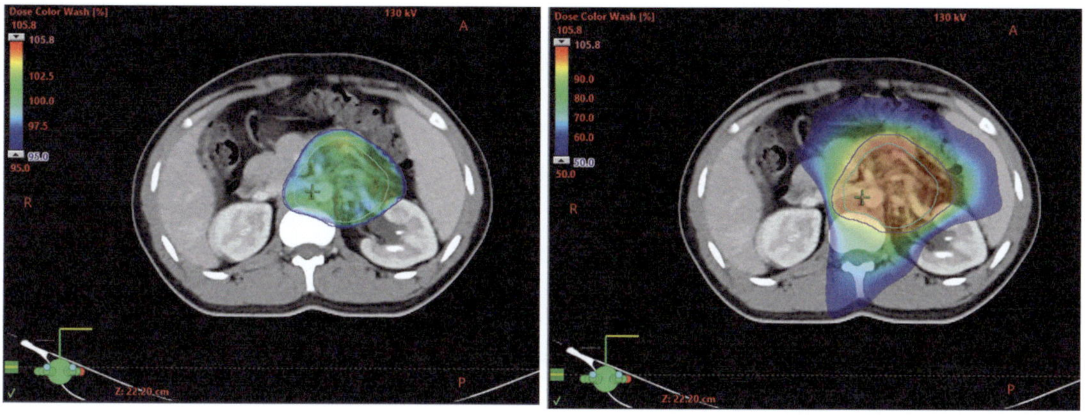

Fig. 14 Conformal VMAT plans with 95% and 50% dose wash

survivors include fatigue, anxiety, sexual problems and fear of cancer recurrence.

3.4.10 Prognosis, Results and Outcome, Survival

Overall, testicular cancers are curable, with a 5-year overall survival (OS) of 97%. Outcomes vary according to the histology, stage and the type of treatment modality employed (Table 6) [122, 139, 140]. The IGCCCG Update provides a more detailed estimate of survival based on prognostic-risk group. High-risk non-seminomatous tumours constitute the worst prognostic subgroup [141].

3.5 Future Research

Micro-RNAs, which are small molecules of RNA with biological activity that are released into biological fluids by testicular cancer cells, are increasingly being used as diagnostic and prognostic markers for testicular cancers [142]. There is a potential role of radiotherapy for residual PET-avid masses post-chemotherapy in seminoma. Treatment with scanning proton beam therapy has the potential to improve the therapeutic ratio over photons [143]. The advantageous dose deposition characteristics of proton beam allows much lower radiation doses to normal tissues, leading to much lesser acute toxicity, as well as five-fold lower risk of secondary malignancies compared with photon therapy [144]. High-dose chemotherapy followed by stem-cell transplant is an evolving treatment option for recurrent disease [145].

3.6 Conclusion

Testicular cancers are a success story for the oncologist because of favourable cure rates and long-term survival outcomes. Early detection and appropriate treatment are of paramount importance in ensuring a good quality of life and freedom from adverse effects.

4 Carcinoma Penis

4.1 Anatomy

Penis is composed of two major elements, corpora cavernosa and one corpus spongiosum (Fig. 15). Glans is the conical end of the corpus spongiosum and the urethra ends at its tip; corona marks the transition from corpus spongiosum to the corpus cavernosum. Superficial lymphatics from prepuce and skin of penile shaft converge dorsally and then split at the base of penis to drain into superficial inguinal nodes on either side. Deep lymphatics drain glans towards the frenulum, where large trunks are formed which encircle corona, and unite with others dorsally. Subsequently deep lymphatics

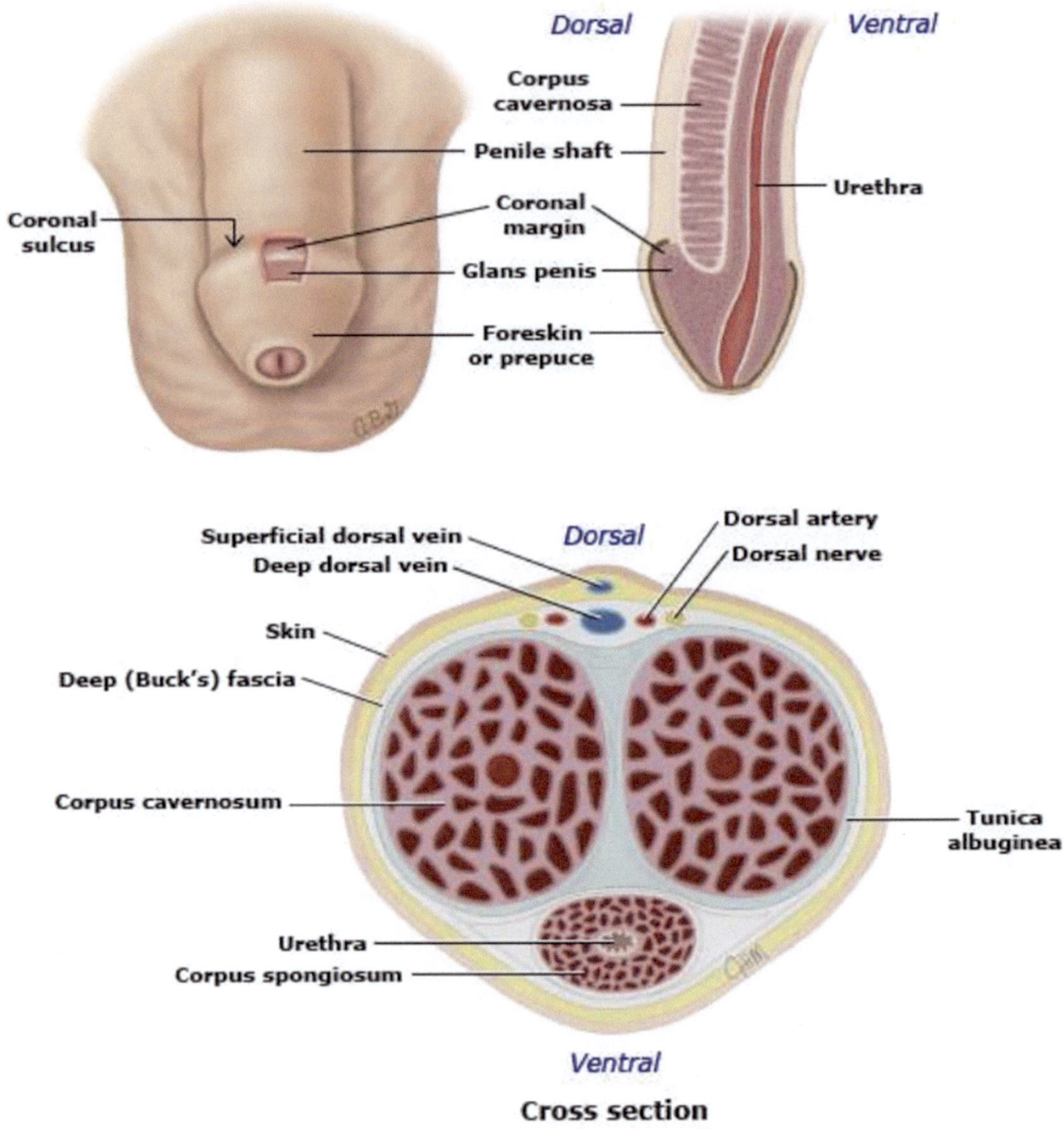

Fig. 15 Anatomy of penis

travel deep to the Buck's fascia and drain via presymphyseal lymphatics to the superficial and deep inguinal nodes on either side. Distal penile urethral lymphatics travel alongside those of glans. Bulbar urethral lymphatics may travel to femoral nodes, or sometimes course under the pubis towards anterior bladder wall to reach pelvic nodes [146].

4.2 Epidemiology Aspects and Risk Factors

Penile cancer is the fourth least cancer type according to incidence statistics estimated by the World Health Organization (WHO). However, there is a wide variation in its epidemiology with significantly higher incidence in countries with lower socioeconomic demographic profile (such as Africa, South America and South Asia) [147]. The impact is so profound that, lack of health insurance, black race, Hispanic ethnicity, low educational level, being divorced or never married, and living in nonmetropolitan areas have been identified as poor prognostic factors variously associated with advanced stage, treatment delay and poor overall survival (OS) [148]. Its age standardised incidence and mortality rate in India are 1.6 (world average is 0.8) and 0.72 per 100,000, respectively [149].

Risk factors include—human papilloma virus (HPV) infection (found in almost 50% penile cancers, especially types 16 and 18), not being circumcised as an infant or child, smoking and tobacco exposure in any form, ultraviolet light treatment for psoriasis, age, poor genital hygiene, obesity, and AIDS [150]. Premalignant lesions of the penis include cutaneous horn, balanitis xerotica obliterans (lichen sclerosis), and leukoplakia. Erythroplasia of Queyrat and Bowen's disease are histologically identical to in situ carcinoma and regularly evolve into invasive cancer. Malignant transformation of Buschke-Löwenstein tumour (giant condyloma) has also been reported.

4.3 Clinical Symptoms, Signs

Penile cancers involve obvious skin changes which can be any combination of change in skin thickness, colour, ulceration, a lump, rash, crusted lesions, proliferative growth, and discharge. Sometimes it presents with acquired phimosis and swelling of terminal shaft and glans. Malignant involvement of groin nodes is a feature of advanced disease and if untreated, can even lead to erosion and bleeding from the femoral vessels.

4.4 Pathology

The vast majority of penile cancers are squamous cell carcinomas (SCC). Other rare subtypes include basal cell carcinoma, extra-mammary Paget's disease, melanoma, lymphoma, metastasis from other cancers, and various mesenchymal tumours. The precursor lesion of SCC is Penile intraepithelial neoplasia (PeIN); a term that now replaces Erythroplasia of Queyrat, squamous cell carcinoma in-situ, Bowen's disease and Bowenoid papulosis [151]. The WHO classification of PeIN and invasive SCC to incorporate separate pathways of penile carcinogenesis based on the relationship with HPV. Differentiated PeIN is usually associated with nonviral factors and progresses to well-differentiated and keratinised SCC, while undifferentiated PeIN is usually associated with HPV infection that progresses to basaloid and warty subtypes of SCC [97]. It remains unclear whether cancers involving HPV infection have better survival than those without HPV infection, with contradictory evidence [152]. Lymph node invasion remains the principal prognostic factor for survival.

4.5 Staging (Table 16 and Fig. 16)

4.6 Integrated Management Plan

4.6.1 Surgery

Once the diagnosis is confirmed with biopsy, the treatment can be of four different gradations. Treatment of PeIN is by using topical 5-Fluorouracil or Imiquimod cream [153]. Laser therapy using Carbon dioxide, Neodymium YAG laser [154], KTP laser therapy have been described with excellent cosmetic results and preservation of sexual function though, long-term results have not be very encouraging with high local recurrences [155].

Radical circumcision excising fore skin upto the carona is sufficient primary curative treatment for low-stage (Tis, Ta, T1) and low grades (G1 and 2) disease limited to distal prepuce. This is also recommended before radiotherapy [156]. Glansectomy which can be either partial or total followed by skin graft gives good functional and oncological outcomes in well selected cases [157].

Table 16 TNM staging of penile carcinoma

T—Primary tumour	
TX	Primary tumour cannot be assessed
T0	No evidence of primary tumour
Tis	Carcinoma in situ
Ta	Non-invasive verrucous carcinoma
T1	Tumour invades subepithelial connective tissue T1a: Tumour invades subepithelial connective tissue without lympho- vascular invasion and is not poorly differentiated T1b: Tumour invades subepithelial connective tissue with lymphovascular invasion or is poorly differentiated
T2	Tumour invades corpus spongiosum with or without invasion of the urethra
T3	Tumour invades corpus cavernosum with or without invasion of the urethra
T4	Tumour invades other adjacent structures

N—Regional lymph nodes	
Nx	Regional lymph nodes cannot be assessed
N0	No palpable or visibly enlarged inguinal lymph nodes
N1	Palpable mobile unilateral inguinal lymph node
N2	Palpable mobile multiple or bilateral inguinal lymph nodes
N3	Fixed inguinal nodal mass or pelvic lymphadenopathy, unilateral or bilateral
M—Distant metastasis	
M0	No distant metastasis
M1	Distant metastasis

pN—Regional lymph nodes	
pNX	Regional lymph nodes cannot be assessed
pN0	No regional lymph node metastasis
pN1	Metastasis in one or two inguinal lymph nodes
pN2	Metastasis in more than two unilateral inguinal nodes or bilateral inguinal lymph nodes
pN3	Metastasis in pelvic lymph node(s), unilateral or bilateral extranodal or extension of regional lymph node metastasis

pM—Distant metastasis	
pM1	Distant metastasis microscopically confirmed
G—Histopathological grading	
GX	Grade of differentiation cannot be assessed
G1	Well differentiated
G2	Moderately differentiated
G3	Poorly differentiated
G4	Undifferentiated

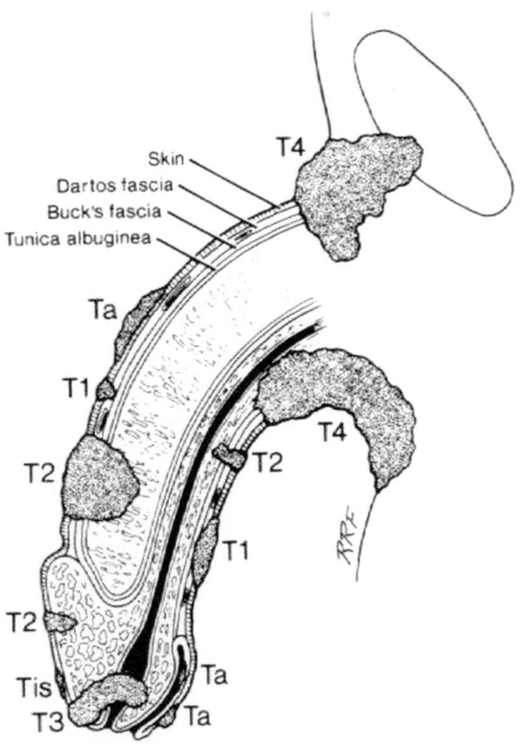

Fig. 16 Depiction of tumour staging

Partial penectomy is done when tumour can be excised with ~1 cm clear margin [158] whilst leaving a shaft 6–7 cm long, fit enough for voiding in standing posture and for sexual function. Radical penectomy comprises of amputation of the penis at or near the level of the suspensory ligament of the penis without removal of the corpora cavernosa more proximally. Perineal urethrostomy done for the urinary diversion. Long-term results show lower recurrences (4%) compared to organ preserving treatments [159].

Inguinal lymph node management is a critical component of penile cancer management. For low-risk patients (pTis, pTa, Grade 1pT1) groins can be kept under surveillance if there are no palpable lymph nodes. For any grade and stage more that pT1G1, there is at least 25% chance of lymph nodal metastasis even with non-palpable disease, in view of which they need surgical LN staging which could be a modified ILND or sentinel LND or standard radical ILND depending on the stage and surgical expertise available

[160]. Fine-needle aspiration cytology is not recommended.

Standard methods for histopathological diagnosis includes Dynamic sentinel-node biopsy (DSNB) which aims to detect affected sentinel nodes in both groins It has a sensitivity of 88% and a false-negative rate of 12–15% [161]. Modified inguinal lymphadenectomy (mILND) includes removal of medial superficial & central zone ILN bilaterally with preservation of greater saphenous vein. There is a lack of robust literature regarding the false-negative rate of mILND. Both methods may miss micro-metastatic disease. If lymph node metastasis is found, it is ideal to consider for ipsilateral radical inguinal lymphadenectomy. Superficial inguinal Lymphadenectomy (SILD) is performed via a 6–8 cm horizontal incision 1 cm inferior to the inguinal fold. In comparison with the MIL, this procedure involves excision of all the nodal basins superficial to the fascia lata from the adductor longus medially to the sartorius laterally. Like the MIL, the long saphenous vein is preserved [162]. Radical inguinal lymphadenopathy involves clearing the superficial and deep inguinal nodal basins. It is a life-saving procedure and should not be underused for fear of associated morbidity. There is associated significant morbidity of 25% with impaired lymph drainage from the legs and scrotum with increases by 50% with rising in body mass index (BMI). The most commonly reported complications in recent series are wound infections (1.2–1.4%), skin necrosis (0.6–4.7%), lymphoedema (5–13.9%) and lymphocele formation (2.1–4%) [163].

Ipsilateral pelvic lymphadenectomy is done when more than two inguinal nodes are involved on one side (pN2) or if extracapsular nodal metastasis (pN3) is confirmed [164]. Pelvic lymph node positivity is associated with a worse prognosis [165] than only inguinal nodal metastasis, with a five-year CSS of 71.0% vs 33.2%. It may be performed simultaneously with inguinal lymphadenectomy or as a secondary procedure.

4.6.2 Systemic Therapy

Neoadjuvant chemotherapy (NACT) can be considered in fixed (cN3) or relapsed inguinal nodes and when upfront complete surgical resection is unlikely. This allows for an early initiation of systemic therapy and helps in improving resectability in good responders. The TIP regimen (4 cycles of Paclitaxel, Ifosfamide and cisplatin) is the most preferred (but often poorly tolerated) with an ORR of 50%. Alternative platinum-based chemotherapy regimens include cisplatin with 5-FU, docetaxel and irinotecan. These agents may also be considered as rational in metastatic cases along with paclitaxel and gemcitabine [166].

Five-year survival in patients with a single involved inguinal lymph node treated with surgery alone is approximately 80%. However, with pelvic node involvement (N3), it ranges from 0% to 12%. Thus, adjuvant chemotherapy is recommended in pN2-3 but without much high-quality evidence. The role of multimodality management in pN3 disease was recently studied in a retrospective study of 128 patients by Khurud et al. wherein 24% patients had pelvic nodal involvement at diagnosis. Twenty-six patients (20.3%) received no adjuvant treatment, 40 (31.3%) received single modality adjuvant treatment and 62 (48.4%) received multimodality adjuvant treatment (a combination of chemotherapy and radiotherapy). After a median follow-up of 22 months, the DFS and OS were 55.4% and 62%, respectively. It shows that the sequence of adjuvant chemotherapy followed by concurrent chemo-radiation (C-CTRT) improves disease-free survival to 93% and gives the best outcomes [167].

An ongoing international penile advanced cancer trial (InPACT) is the first phase III trial for penile SCC with regional lymph node metastases, which aims to uncover all the unanswered questions regarding use of NACT and the role of prophylactic pelvic lymph nodal dissection with chemoradiation versus chemo-radiation alone in high-risk inguinal lymph nodal disease [168].

4.6.3 Radiation Therapy

Historically, radical surgery has been the mainstay of penile cancer management; however, treatment paradigm has evolved to include oncological, functional and cosmetic aspects with organ preservation methods [169]. Radiotherapy can be delivered with external beam radiation, interstitial brachytherapy or surface mold brachytherapy, providing organ preservation following circumcision [170].

4.6.4 External Beam Radiotherapy

Radiation may be used post-operatively after surgical resection when positive or close margins confer a high risk of local recurrence to a dose of 45–60 Gy. In cases with positive nodal disease post-operatively, chemoradiotherapy is recommended with EBRT to a dose of 50.4 Gy to inguinal/pelvic lymph node and boost to total dose of 56 Gy in case of extra capsular extension (Figs. 17 and 18).

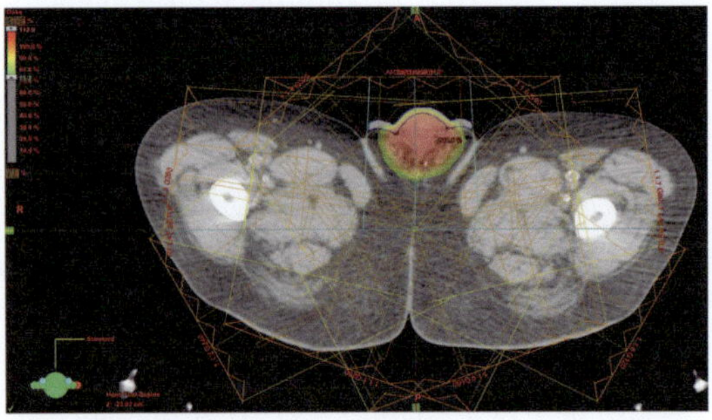

Fig. 17 Nine-field IMRT, axial image [15]. (Source: Smith et al. [210])

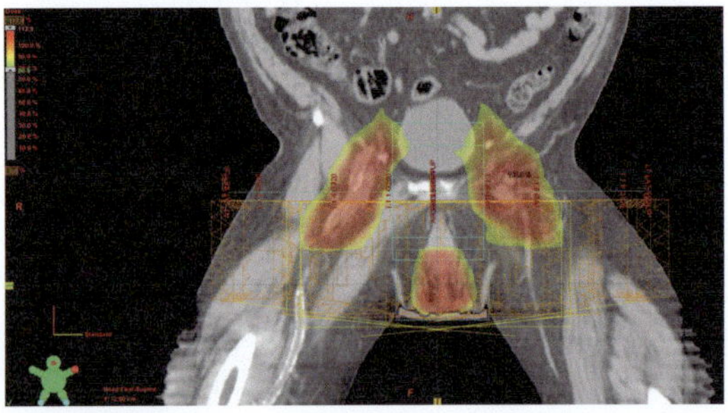

Fig. 18 Nine-field IMRT, coronal image [15]. (Source: Smith et al. [210])

4.6.5 Treatment Planning

Very small tumours on the glans or prepuce that are unsuitable for brachytherapy are treated using a direct appositional electron field (or 125–250 kV orthovoltage) and lead cut out. A 2-cm margin around the gross tumour is added to allow for penumbra and coverage of microscopic disease [171]. A layer of bolus material must be used to overcome skin-sparing.

Successful application of EBRT is technically challenging. It requires reproducible positioning of the penis along with patient comfort. Different immobilisation methods are in use like a wax block, plastic box, Perspex cylinder (Fig. 19), transparent Plexiglas or Lucite chambers [4, 8]. Tata Memorial Hospital developed an indigenous groin immobilisation board (Fig. 20) which has shown to improve the concordance between the pelvis and groin motion when comparing using conventional frog-leg position. This helped in reducing the PTV margins and may help in much better target coverage while avoiding dose unnecessary normal tissue [172].

4.6.6 Adjuvant Radiotherapy

The outcome of penile cancer is greatly influenced by involvement of regional lymph nodes, adversely affecting survival outcomes. Though

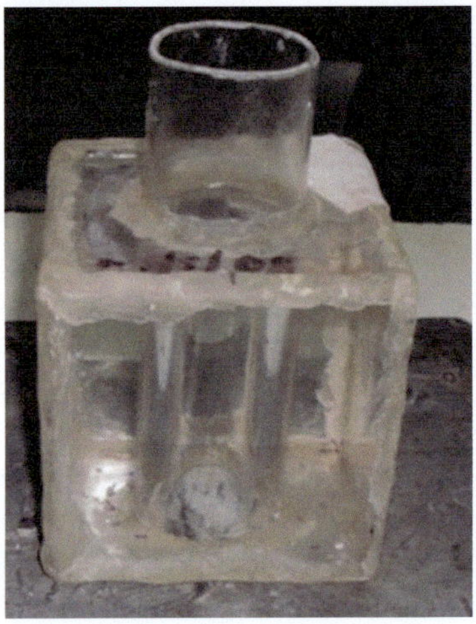

Fig. 19 Perspex cylinder with lead sheet

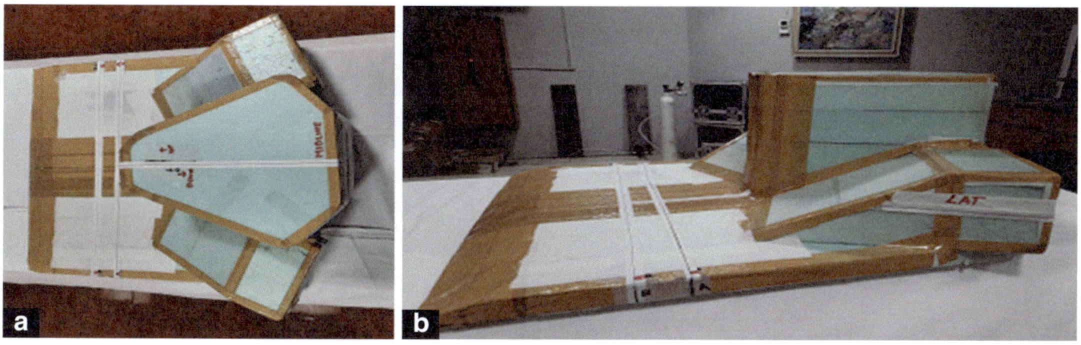

Fig. 20 Groin board for immobilisation

Table 17 Asymmetrical expansion to create inguinal CTVs [12]

Direction	Margin	
	Supra IPS	Infra IPS
Anterior	29 mm	21 mm
Medial	23 mm	23 mm
Lateral	21 mm	0 mm
Posterior	0 mm	0 mm
Cranial	48 mm	48 mm
Caudal	50 mm	50 mm

conventional radiotherapy portals for inguino femoral nodal region are defined by bony landmarks, which cause normal tissue toxicity and inadequate coverage. IMRT allows excellent coverage of target structures and relative sparing of healthy normal tissue. The contouring guidelines by Mittal et al. are specific to penile cancer (enumerated in Table 17 and Fig. 21) [173].

4.6.7 Definitive EBRT to the Groin

If there are palpable or radiologically evident inguinal nodes (clinically-positive [cN+]) or histologic confirmation on intra-operative assessment (pathologically-positive [pN+]), then a bilateral radical inguinal lymphadenectomy is often indicated. However, if these nodes are fixed or bulky, then neoadjuvant chemotherapy is commonly recommended, followed by consolidative surgery. Pelvic LN dissection is usually advised if there is evidence of >2 ILNs, extranodal extension (ENE), or obvious pelvic nodal disease [174].

Role of prophylactic groin EBRT in cN0 patients is unclear. In patients with cN+ or pN+ ILNs, inguinal EBRT may provide improved locoregional control. The NCCN guidelines (version 2.2021) recommend adjuvant EBRT if any of the following high-risk features are present: positive surgical margins, >2 pelvic nodal metastases, ENE, bilateral inguinal nodal involvement, or >4 cm tumour deposit in lymph nodes. In patients with pN3 disease post-operative adjuvant radiotherapy with Extended field (inguinal and pelvic nodal regions) improves disease-free and overall survival compared with involved-field radiation as given by Khurud et al. [175].

4.6.8 Brachytherapy [176, 177–181]

Aim

Organ preservation for urinary and sexual function while maintaining body image and quality of life without compromising survival outcomes.

Case Selection

(a) cT1-T2 Penile squamous carcinoma (<4 cm).
(b) Confined to glans penis.
(c) Locally recurrent lesion of distal penis.
(d) cT3 is not suitable due to higher risk of urethral stenosis and local failure.

Procedure of Implant

As a prerequisite, the patient should undergo circumcision to reduce tumour burden, ensure good exposure of lesion and to decrease the risk of late paraphimosis. Interstitial implant procedure takes place in 30–45 min and is done under general anaesthesia or penile block. First step is to cath-

Step 1: Contouring femoral vessels Identify IPS in 3D. Contour femoral vessels (artery + vein) in supra- and IIPS regions separately (craniocaudal length of vessels as per 95% nodal coverage in Table 1).				
Region	SIPS region		IIPS region	
Structure	SIPS_Rt_femoral_vessel	SIPS_Lt_femoral_vessel	IIPS_Rt_femoral_vessel	IIPS_Lt_femoral_vessel
	Cranially 48 mm superior from IPS 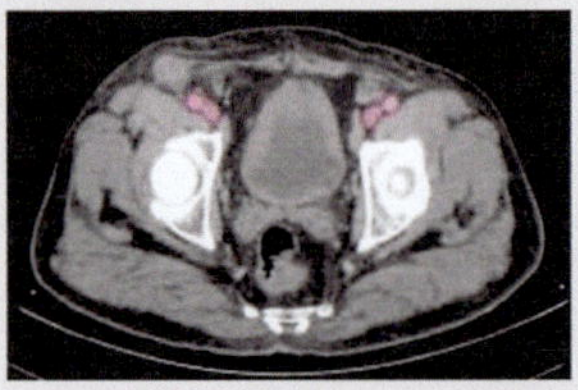		Caudally 50 mm inferior from IPS 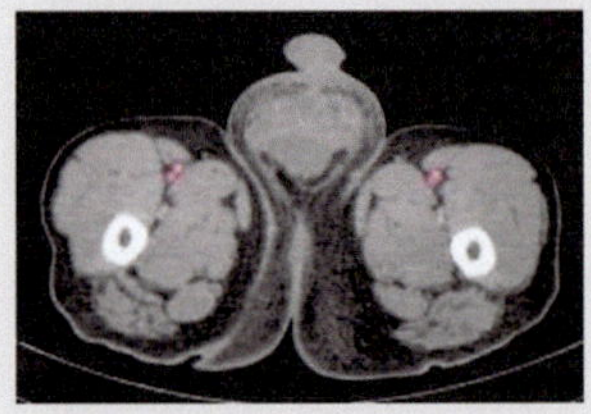	
Step 2: Delineating normal structures Bladder, rectum, femoral heads, spermatic cords				
Step 3: Generation of inguinal CTV Using 95% margins in Table 1, expand asymmetrically around the femoral vessels to generate separate CTVs in SIPS and IIPS regions (Fig. 3A,B)				
Region	SIPS region		IIPS region	
Structure	SIPS_Rt_inguinal_CTV	SIPS_Lt_inguinal_CTV	IIPS_Rt_inguinal_CTV	IIPS_Lt_inguinal_CTV
Step 4: Modification of inguinal CTV margins Inguinal CTV is edited from normal structures, muscles, and bones (Fig. 3A,B)				
Step 5: Boolean operations to generate final right and left inguinal CTV				
Structure	Rt_inguinal_CTV =	SIPS_Rt_inguinal_CTV + IIPS_Rt_inguinal_CTV	Lt_inguinal_CTV =	SIPS_Lt_inguinal_CTV + IIPS_Lt_inguinal_CTV

Abbreviations: 3D = 3-dimentional; CTV = clinical target volume; IIPS = infra-IPS; IPS = inferior edge of pubic symphysis; SIPS = supra-IPS.

Fig. 21 Step-wise delineation of inguinal CTV. (Adapted from Mittal et al.)

eterise the patient. The extent of the target lesion is identified as gross tumour volume (GTV) by inspection and palpation and marked with ink. The presumed clinical target volume (CTV) is the GTV with a margin of 8–10 mm (Fig. 22). For better radiological delineation of the tumour, 3–4 small silver markers can be placed at the boundaries. The orientation of the implant is decided based on the site of the tumour, its relation to the normal anatomic and functional position of the penis. Dorsal to ventral direction is most common for dorsal lesions and left to right direction is more feasible for ventral lesions.

The placement of the needles in accordance with the Paris system is the most important step in determining accurate dosimetry. Hollow steel needles are transfixed in such a way that it covers the entire CTV while being parallel and equidistant to each other with 12–18 mm spacing. The lateral-most needles are inserted at least 3 mm

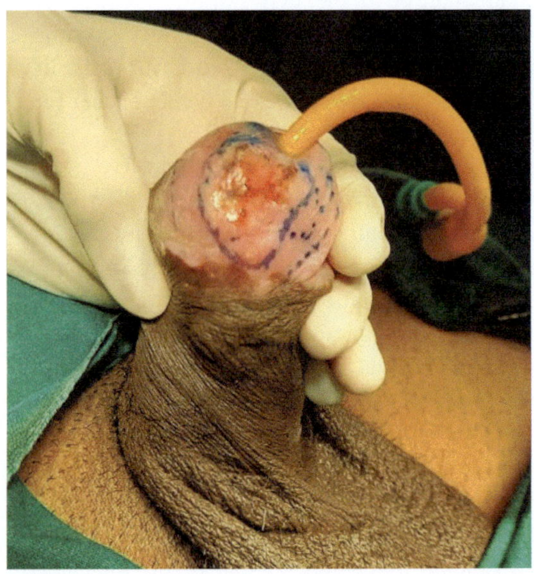

Fig. 22 Delineation of GTV and CTV in a ventrally placed lesion over glans penis with Foley's catheter in situ

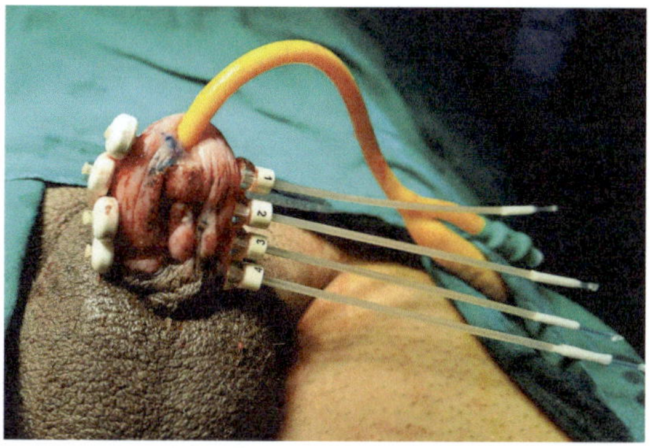

Fig. 23 Free-hand interstitial penile implant with dummy tubes inserted in the catheter

beyond the GTV. Based on the depth of the lesion, a free-hand single-plane implant or a template-based multiple-plane implant can be done. One must be careful to avoid inserting needles in the urethra or the dorsal vein of the penis. Expertise may be required in cases of circumferential and peri-meatal lesions. After a good needle placement, needles are replaced by catheter tubes using the Seldinger technique and fixed using silicon or metallic buttons (Fig. 23). The tubes are numbered in a defined sequence and measured for treatment delivery.

Planning and Delivery

After measurement of tubes is completed and a thin slice CT image is acquired, multiplanar reconstruction is done. Basal points and active dwell points are created for loading of the source. Optimisation of dwell time and position can be done for adequate coverage and to minimise confluence of high dose regions (Figs. 24 and 25). The dose is prescribed between 38 and 54 Gy at 3–4 Gy per fraction, twice daily, atleast 6 hours apart. CTV should be covered by 85–90% isodose line, while V115 and V125 should be away from urethra (<10%) and skin respectively. The diameter of the hyperdose sleeve (170%) should be less than 10 mm. The HDR brachytherapy with Iridium 192 or Cobalt 60 is delivered under physician supervision. After completion, the implant is removed bedside under analgesic cover and counselled for skin care.

Good cosmesis is achieved and penile conservation rates are 87% and 70% at 5 and 10 year, respectively. Five-year overall survival is 80%, alike with brachytherapy and surgery.

4.7 Radiotherapy Sequelae

4.7.1 Acute Reactions

Brisk erythema, dry or moist desquamation, and swelling of subcutaneous tissue of the shaft in virtually all patients. Often reversible with conservative treatment within a few weeks. Local hygiene is important, including frequent soaks in baking soda and water. Urethral adhesions in acute phase should be separated by meatal dilator or a foleys catheter to avoid development of chronic meatal stenosis.

4.7.2 Late Reactions

Soft-tissue ulceration and meatal stenosis are two most common and significant late complications of radiotherapy which peak time at 7–18 months after completion. High risk factors being dose above 60 Gy, stage T3 tumours, larger implant volume (>30 mL) and greater number of implant planes or needles. Telangiectasia is a common late consequence of radiation therapy and is usually asymptomatic Lymphoedema of the legs has been reported following inguinal and pelvic radiation therapy, but the role of irradiation in the development of this complication remains controversial as many patients with this symptom have active disease in the lymphatics that may be responsible for lymphatic blockage.

4.8 Quality of Life [182–184]

Small studies show encouraging data on the preservation of sexual and urinary functions and the quality of life after brachytherapy. Sexual outcomes with brachytherapy may be better than some of the organ sparing surgeries including glansectomy and partial penectomy. Common tools used are Post-Operative International Index of Erectile Function (IIEF)-5,15, SF36 Health

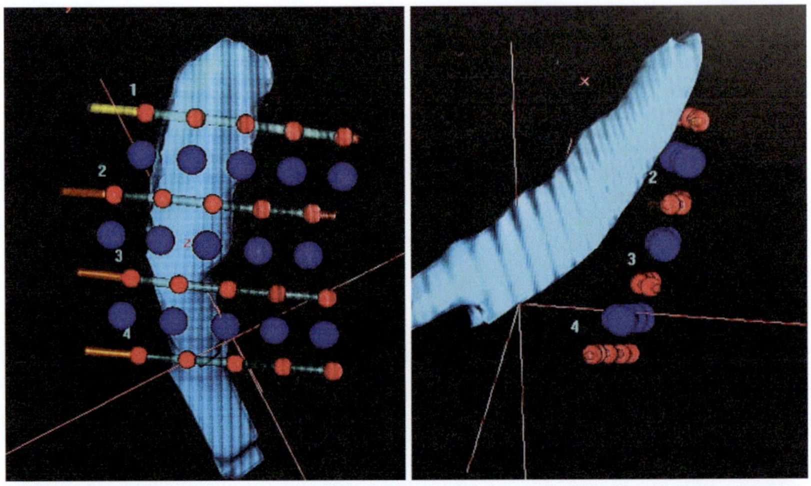

Fig. 24 Catheter reconstruction with active dwell points (red dots) and basal dose rate points (blue dots)

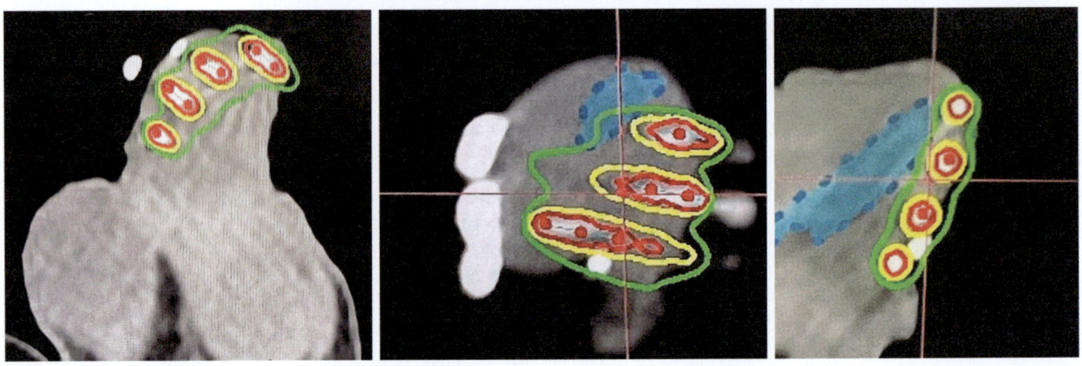

Fig. 25 Unoptimised isodoses showing 170% in red, 125% in yellow and 85% in green

Survey and the Impact of Cancer questionnaire, Overall Sexual Functioning Questionnaire, Quality of Erection Questionnaire (QEQ), Erectile Dysfunction Inventory of Treatment Satisfaction (EDITS) and Self-Esteem and Relationship (SEAR).

4.9 Follow-Up

Meticulous follow-up helps to assess the results and complications of the treatment. After penile conservation, patients should be taught and encouraged to do penile self-examination. After local treatment with negative inguinal nodes, a thorough physical examination must be done on follow-up. Additional imaging has no proven benefit. USG groin may be done when groin cannot be assessed due to obesity. Histology from the glans should be obtained to confirm disease-free status following laser ablation or topical chemotherapy. After potentially curative treatment for inguinal nodal metastases, CT or MRI or PET CT imaging must be done for the detection of the systemic disease every 3 monthly for the first 2 years then 6 monthly till 5 years.

4.10 Prognosis and Outcomes

The outcome of penile cancer is greatly influenced by the involvement of regional lymph nodes at presentation. The 5-year overall survival of >90% in localised disease, declines to 29–50% in patients with regional node-positive disease. Pelvic nodal involvement is a known prognostic factor in carcinoma penis, adversely affecting survival outcomes.

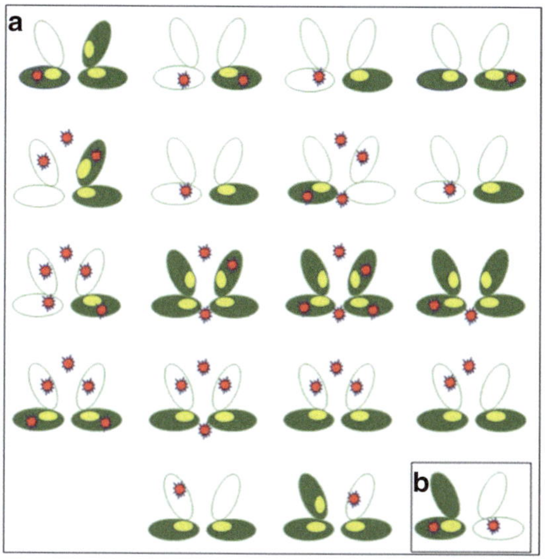

Fig. 26 Patterns of recurrence [175]. Represents the pattern of failure after (**a**), involved-field radiation therapy and (**b**), extended field radiation therapy (inset); pathologic nodal station of positivity (yellow), delivered radiation therapy target area (green), and (red) represents the respective pattern of failures- local, regional nodal area, distant, and mixed

Patterns of failure was studied at Tata Memorial Hospital by Khurud et al. [175]. At a median follow-up of 39 months, 38.6% (29/75) of patients had relapsed either locally, regionally, or at distant sites. Only 1 (4%) patient experienced relapse after extended field RT (EFRT) while Twenty-eight (55%) patients experienced relapse after involved-field radiation therapy (IFRT), of which 28.5% were regional-only relapses and 64% relapses were associated with a regional component (Fig. 26). The 2-year DFS and OS of the entire cohort were 62.2% and 70.8%, respectively. The 2-year DFS was 67.9% in patients who received IFRT and 94.1% in those who received EFRT with similar OS. They concluded that extended field radiation therapy significantly improves clinical outcomes compared with involved-field radiation in patients with pN3 penile cancer. Recent ongoing studies have demonstrated a high prevalence of high-risk human papilloma virus (HPV) subtypes and their association with improved survival outcomes in penile cancer. Adjuvant CRT and HPV + disease were independent predictors for improved locoregional control in pN + penile cancer in a study by Yuan et al. [185].

5 Renal Cell Carcinoma

5.1 Anatomy

The kidneys are paired retroperitoneal organs encased by a fibrous capsule, surrounded by perinephric fat that is enclosed by Gerota's fascia. Each kidney is 11–12 cm in length, lying at the level of T12-L3 vertebral bodies, with the right kidney being slightly more inferior than the left (Fig. 27).

5.2 Epidemiological Aspects and Risk Factors

Kidney cancers are rare, accounting for 2% of all malignancies [186]. The median age at diagnosis is 65 years, with a slight male preponderance in Asians. The most common risk factors associated are tobacco consumption, obesity and hypertension. Approximately 4–5% RCCs have a hereditary basis. Hereditary familial forms of kidney cancer are Von Hippel-Lindau disease (VHL), familial papillary renal cell carcinoma (HPRCC), hereditary leiomyoma RCC (HLRCC), Cowden syndrome, the Birt-Hogg-Dube Syndrome (BHD) and Tuberous Sclerosis (TS).

5.3 Clinical Signs, Symptoms and Pathology

The classical symptomatic triad of RCC consists of flank pain, gross hematuria and palpable abdominal mass, seen in less than 10% patients. With the utilisation of 3D abdominal imaging, incidental detection of a renal mass is the most common presentation. 25–30% patients present with metastatic disease. Paraneoplastic syndromes are seen in about 10–20% of patients with symptomatic RCC, mainly elevated ESR, hypertension, anaemia and weight loss.

Conventional clear cell RCC forms the most common pathology (75–80%) followed by papillary RCC and chromophobe RCC. It is recommended that Conventional RCC be graded by ISUP nuclear grading system instead of Fuhrman's grading as it is prognostically more relevant.

5.4 Investigations

1. USG: Can distinguish between solid and cystic lesions. It acts as basis to perform further radiological investigations.
2. CECT Thorax, abdomen, pelvis: RCC appears as a solid mass with heterogeneous post-contrast enhancement. CT assesses extent of the primary tumour, extra renal spread, venous involvement, and status of locoregional nodes. The Renal Nephrometry Score on CT is used to assess the complexity of the renal mass. CT Thorax is required to rule out lung metastases [187].
3. MRI Abdomen: MRI has better sensitivity than CT for evaluating venous extension and distinguishing between a tumour and a bland thrombus.
4. DTPA Renogram: To assess differential function of both kidneys.
5. Fine needle aspiration cytology/ biopsy (FNAC/FNAB) is rarely indicated only when a renal abscess or infected cyst is suspected and when RCC must be differentiated from metastatic malignant disease or renal lymphoma. Other indications are when surgery is not planned, before active surveillance (AS), SBRT, RFA and Cryosurgery. FNAB has excellent accuracy for detecting malignant masses, especially when combined with molecular analysis.
6. FDG PET CECT: Combining the FDG-PET and CT systems is helpful for detecting extra-renal metastasis rather than renal lesions as extrarenal lesions are not obscured by urinary FDG activity. In a recent meta-analysis, pooled sensitivity and specificity were reported to be 79% and 90%, respectively for detection of metastatic disease [188].

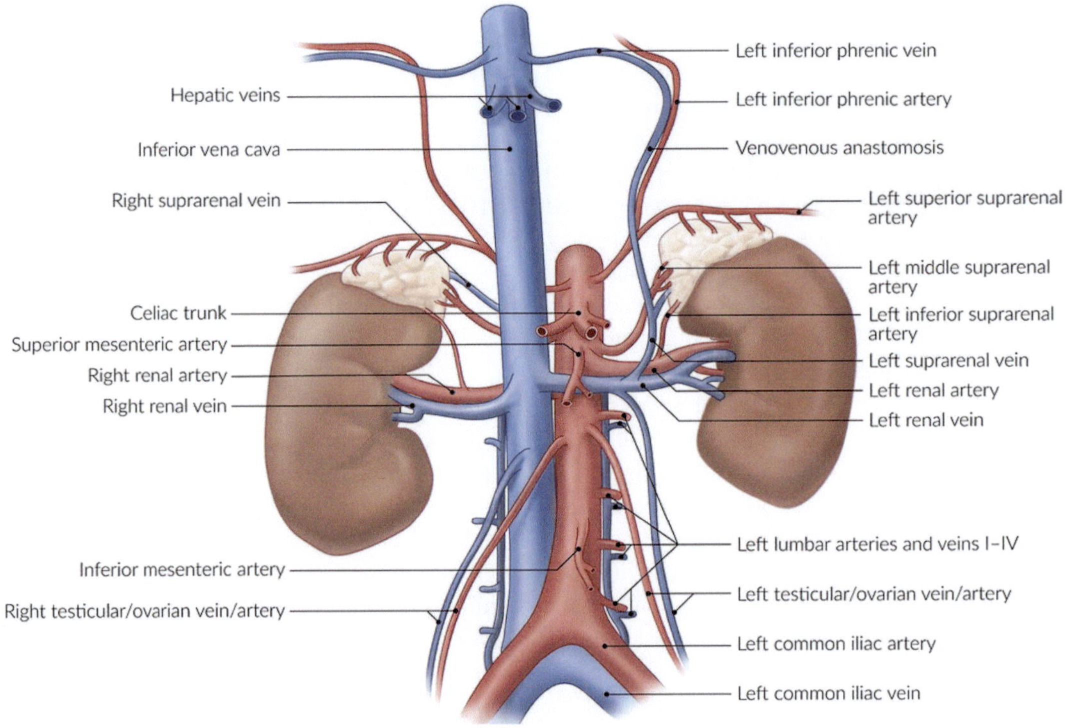

Fig. 27 Vascular anatomy of renal system

Table 18 Staging

Primary tumour (T)
TX Primary tumour cannot be assessed T0 No evidence of primary tumour
T1 Tumour 7 cm or less in greatest dimension confined to the kidney
T1a Tumour 4 cm or less in greatest dimension, confined to the kidney
T1b Tumour more than 4 cm but not more than 7 cm in greatest dimension, confined to the kidney
T2 Tumour more than 7 cm in greatest dimension limited to the kidney
T2a Tumour >7 cm but <10 cm
T2b Tumour >10 cm but limited to kidney
T3 Tumour extends into major veins or perinephric fat but not into the ipsilateral adrenal gland and not beyond Gerota's fascia
T3a Tumour grossly extends into the renal vein, or its segmental branches or tumour invades to perirenal and/or renal sinus fat but not beyond Gerota's fascia
T3b, tumour grossly extends into vena cava below the diaphragm
T3c Tumour grossly extends into vena cava above diaphragm or invades the wall of the vena cava
T4 Tumour invades beyond Gerota's fascia (including contagious extension to adrenal gland)
Regional lymph nodes (N)
Nx Regional lymph nodes cannot be assessed N0 No regional lymph node metastasisN1 Metastasis into regional lymph node
Distant metastasis (M)
MX Distant metastasis cannot be assessed M0 No distant metastasis M1 Distant metastasis

5.5 Staging

Currently, the AJCC TNM classification system (2018) is used, which gives a better differentiation of different prognostic groups (Table 18).

5.6 Stage Grouping (Table 19)

Table 19 Stage grouping

Stage I	T1	N0	M0
Stage II	T2	N0	M0
Stage III	T1 or T2	N1	M0
	T3 Any	N	M0
Stage IV	T4 Any	N	M0
	Any T	Any N	M1

5.7 Management

5.7.1 Local Therapy

Surgery

Surgery is the principal modality of treatment of renal tumours. There are three gradations in surgical treatment.

Nephron sparing surgery or partial nephrectomy (PN) is the standard of care for all Small (<4 cm) enhancing renal masses (SRM) and also in larger tumours when technically/anatomically feasible. The non-inferiority of PN compared to radical nephrectomy with regards oncological outcomes is well established with 10 yr follow-up observational studies and a RCT [189, 190].

Radical nephrectomy (RN) entails excision of kidney with all surrounding perirenal fat and any visible lymph node excision. The current standard approach is to do this laparoscopically with longterm studies showing oncological equivalence to open surgery with quicker recovery [191]. The 10-year cancer-specific survival is in excess of 95% following either PN or RN undertaken for SRM. Better overall survival secondary to better renal function preservation has been noted with PN compared to RN with decreased cardio and cerebro vascular risks.

The role of *debulking or cyto-reductive nephrectomy* in the presence of metastatic disease has decreased [192, 193] and currently only offered for symptomatic relief or when majority (>90%) of the tumour bulk removal can be achieved surgically. Regarding the timing of debulking, there is increasing evidence to suggest that the debulking operation is preferably done when there is a good response to systemic treatment [194].

Routine adrenalectomy and elective lymphadenectomy is no longer recommended. Adrenalectomy should be done when there is either abnormal radiographic appearance of adrenal gland or suspicious intraoperative findings, with no regard for primary tumour size.

Radiotherapy

Previously RCC was thought to be a radio resistant tumour. There is emerging data suggesting that the apparent radioresistance of RCC can be overcome with the use of higher dose per fraction treatments delivered by new high-precision radiotherapy such as SBRT. The rationale is attributed to the endothelial cell kill and subsequent activation of the acid sphingomyelinase and ceramide pathway, resulting in rapid cell death [195, 196].

Primary Lesion

SBRT is indicated in medically inoperable patients, those with a single functioning kidney, unfit for thermal ablation and operable but at risk for dialysis post-surgery. In a recent meta-analysis from IROCK, the incidence of local failure was 5.5% at 5-yrs with a mean fall in GFR of 14 mL/min. The median tumour diameter was 4 cm and single fraction SBRT has significantly better local control and progression-free survival compared to multi-fractionated treatment. Commonly used doses were 26 Gy in SF; 42 Gy/3# or 50 Gy/5# for fractionated treatment [197].

Oligoprogressive disease refers to the clinical scenario where there is progression of one or a few metastases, while the majority of other tumours are stable or responding to a systemic therapy strategy. With oligoprogression, the main goal of treating the progressive tumour(s) with SBRT is to delay the need to change the current systemic therapy [198]. A recently published randomised multicenter prospective phase II trial by Cheung et al. evaluated the use of SBRT in the setting of oligoprogressive mRCC while on TKI therapy. It demonstrated that the LC of irradiated oligoprogressive mRCC tumours was 93% and need to change systemic therapy was delayed for a median of >1 yr [199].

Other emerging indications for SBRT include neoadjuvant SBRT for IVC thrombus, neoadjuvant SBRT prior to cytoreductive nephrectomy or as a replacement for cytoreductive nephrectomy. The only potentially curative treatment for patients with an IVC thrombus is surgical resection, which is associated with a 35% rate of high-grade peri-operative morbidity and still has a 40% risk of relapse and metastasis even after curative resection. The hypothesis that neoadjuvant SBRT may reduce the risk of RCC recurrence that is due to positive surgical margins or presence of live tumour emboli is a matter of interesting research [200, 201].

Thus, the role of radiotherapy is gradually shifting from investigational to an alternative standard of care in selected therapy, with mature data now available for the safety and efficacy of SBRT.

Post-operative radiotherapy (PORT) is not standard in RCC. The role of adjuvant RT using modern technology & conventionally fractionated schedules is being revisited in a select group of patients. There is no standard role of neoadjuvant RT in patients with RCC. In the scenario of invasion of direct adjacent organ invasion and when complete resection may not be feasible, neoadjuvant irradiation can potentially downsize the tumour, increasing the likelihood of an adequate surgical resection but may not improve the overall survival based on two prospective clinical trials.

Radiotherapy Planning

CT Simulation is performed after positioning the patient in supine, arms overhead in a vacuum immobilisation using 1–3 mm slice thickness with or without IV contrast. For organ motion control, various techniques like 4DCT, abdominal compression and respiratory motion tracking/gating can be used. Registration (fusion) of diagnostic scans like contrast-enhanced CT or MRI or FDG PET CECT to treatment planning CT is done for accurate delineation of the gross target volume (GTV). Margin for microscopic disease (CTV) is not given, however an internal target volume (ITV) is generated in accordance to the MIP contour in 4DCT. A PTV expansion of 3–10 mm can be generated based on institutional on-board imaging facilities and it can be trimmed to avoid overlapping bowel structures (Fig. 28) [197]. The dose contraints for 42 Gy/3# and 26 Gy/SF are summarised in Table 20 [202].

Metastasis [203]

Palliative RT is an effective treatment for palliation of symptoms such as of bony pain, controlling the severity of neurological symptoms

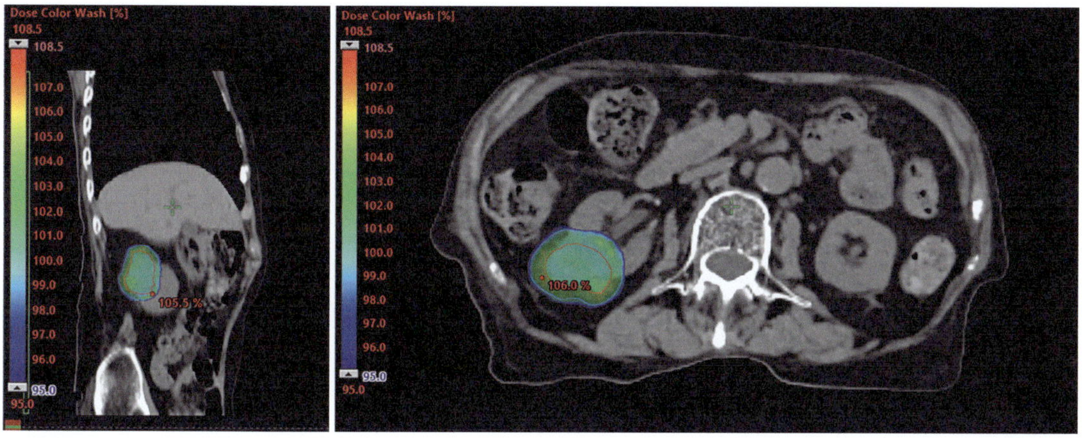

Fig. 28 Dose coverage and spill in SBRT

Table 20 Dose constraints for SBRT in RCC

Organ	Parameter	Dose/fractionation	
		26 Gy/1Fx	42 Gy/3Fx
Spinal canal	Maximum dose	0.03 cc <12 Gy point dose	0.03 cc <18 Gy point dose
Skin (5 mm subcutis)	Maximum dose (1.5 cc)	<18 Gy	<30 Gy
Small bowel	Maximum dose/volume	0.03 cc <26 Gy 5cc <22.5 Gy Aim for <13 Gy to full circumference of small bowel loop	0.03 cc <30 Gy 30cc ≤12.5 Gy
	Maximum dose covering full circumference of bowel wall	≤12.5 Gy	≤22.5 Gy
Large bowel	Maximum dose (1.5 cc)	ALARA, aim for <26 Gy	ALARA, aim for <42 Gy
Stomach	Maximum dose Maximum volume	1.5 cc <15.4 Gy 5 cc ≤22.5 Gy	0.03 cc <30 Gy 5 cc ≤22.5 Gy
Liver	Mean dose, maximum volume	No constraint, but mean dose and dose to 700 cc to be documented	700 cc <15 Gy
Ipsilateral kidney minus ITV	Maximum dose (1.5 cc), V10 Gy	ALARA: Minimise volume of high dose regions (>50% isodose)[a]	ALARA: Minimise volume of high dose regions (>50% isodose)
Contralateral kidney	V10 Gy	≤33%	≤33%

[a] Ipsilateral Kidney minus ITV should adhere to the ALARA principle. In particular, investigators should focus on minimising high dose regions (50% isodose) outside the ITV but within the ipsilateral kidney
Adapted from TROG 15.03 FASTRACK II

or to ameliorate hematuria using mainly SBRT. Response rates of >50% have been seen among patients with metastatic RCC receiving conventionally fractionated RT. The objective of SBRT should be to achieve maximum dose per fraction to target (7–15 Gy/#). Generally, 3–5# schedules are used. Some examples of dose schedule described in the literature include 25–26 Gy in single fraction, 42–45 Gy in 3 #, 44–48 Gy in 4 #, 30–50 Gy in 5#. Indications of radiotherapy in RCC with outcomes and toxicity are summarised in Table 21.

Table 21 Indications of radiotherapy in RCC with outcomes and toxicity

Indications	Local control	Grade III/IV toxicity
Primary RCC: Medically inoperable, nephron sparing surgery (NSS) not feasible, salvage post-NSS or RFA	>90%	0–9%
Brain metastasis: Definitive, post-operative cavity	1 yr LC: 90–97%	1–17%
Spinal metastasis: Definitive, post-operative	1 yr LC: 70–95%	1–10%
Extracranial oligometastatic disease: Definitive to defer/delay systemic therapy or in combination to improve outcomes	Definitive: 1 yr freedom from systemic therapy: 70–87% With systemic therapy: 1 yr LC: 75–98%	0–6% 0–73%
Oligoprogression	1 yr LC: 80–100% Time to change in systemic treatment: 11–14 month	0–5%

Adapted from Role of SBRT in RCC by Ali et al.

Combining SBRT with Immunotherapy

Based on preclinical and phase 2 clinical data, a particularly promising approach is the combination of RT and immunotherapy to augment the local efficacy of RT as well as to allow for improved and more durable systemic responses with immunotherapy. RT plays an important role in the potentiation and modulation of tumour immunity by orchestrating a spectrum of cellular and molecular alterations [204].

Radiofrequency Ablation (RFA)/ Cryoablation

RFA comprises percutaneously inserting electrodes into the tumour and causing thermal ablation. Cryoablation consists of a series of freezing and thawing cycles that cause tumour necrosis. Supercooled liquid is percutaneously inserted through a probe. Both RFA and cryoablation are limited by small tumour size, location (not feasible in tumours close to the pelvicalyceal system due to the risk of heat sink effects, stricture and/ or fistula development) and are ultimately invasive procedures. Treatment of larger tumours poses significant risks of haemorrhage, which can require a nephrectomy to control. Both these procedures are costly and dependent on user technician proficiency and availability [205].

5.7.2 Response Evaluation After SBRT

Response Evaluation criteria in Solid Tumors (RECIST) is the commonly utilised tool for measuring local control after SBRT. Persistent post-SABR stable masses are common findings immediately after treatment. Currently, arrest of radiological growth and subsequent slow regression on size criteria is considered a successful response to treatment. Functional MRI sequences show promise in detecting early response to therapy. Post-SABR biopsy is not recommended in routine clinical practice. Follow-up is done every 3–6 months with DTPA renogram and CT KUB renal protocol or MRI abdomen.

5.8 Systemic Therapy

5.8.1 Role of Adjuvant TKI/IO in Non-metastatic RCC

The rate of local recurrence or visceral metastases after nephrectomy is 25–40%. The understanding of benefit with adjuvant systemic therapy is still under way. Currently, only one RCT have shown significant improvement in disease free survival by adding Sunitinib 50 mg/ day [206] in cases with high risk of recurrence i.e. >T3 tumours, node positivity, higher Fuhrman grades [3, 4] and sarcomatoid features. Recent meta-analysis [207] including 5 major trials of RCC (S-TRAC, ASSURE, PROTECT, ATLAS, and SORCE) has concluded that TKIs did not improve OS and rather increased toxicity.

5.8.2 Systemic Therapy in Metastatic RCC

The ideal time to start systemic therapy is not well established yet. Observation is also considered as an option for selected patients who are asymptomatic with limited tumour burden. After stratification into favourable, intermediate and poor risk groups using the International Metastatic Renal Cell Carcinoma Database Consortium (IMDC) model, combinations of systemic agents like VEGFR inhibitors, mTOR inhibitors or PD-1/CTLA-4 immune checkpoint inhibitors (ICI) are planned.

For first-line therapy (Table 22), the combinations of axitinib-pembrolizumab, cabozantinib-nivolumab and lenvatinib-pembrolizumab are recommended irrespective of IMDC prognostic subgroup [208]. Alternatively, sunitinib, pazopanib [209] and cabozantinib can be considered if IO is contraindicated or not available (Table 23). ICIs can be stopped after 2 years in patients with good disease control. In case of progression with ICIs, VEGFR TKI therapy is considered standard of care despite poor evidence.

Table 22 First-line systemic therapy options

Preferred/standard regimens	Other options	Useful in select cases
Favourable risk		
Axitinib + Pembrolizumab	Axitinib + Avelumab	Active surveillance
Sunitinib		High dose IL-2
Pazopanib		Bevacizumab + IFN Axitinib, Sorafenib
Intermediate risk		
Nivolumab + Ipilimumab	Sunitinib	Axitinib
Axitinib + Pembrolizumab	Pazopanib	High dose IL-2
Cabozantinib	Axitinib + Avelumab	Temsirolimus
Poor risk		
Nivolumab + Ipilimumab	Sunitinib	Axitinib
Axitinib + Pembrolizumab	Pazopanib	Temsirolimus
Cabozantinib	Axitinib + Avelumab	

Table 23 Second-line options and beyond

Preferred regimens	Other recommended options	Useful in certain settings
Nivolumab	Lenvatinib + Everolimus	Bevacizumab
Axitinib	Everolimus	Sorafenib
Cabozantinib	Pazopanib	IL-2 (in select patients)
	Sunitinib	Temsirolimus

5.8.3 Follow-Up

Follow-up post-radiotherapy comprises of cross sectional imaging in the form of CECT A + P or PET CT scan at 3–4 monthly intervals for the first 2 years, 6 monthly till 5 years and annually thereafter. The tumour does not disappear, but remains stable post-radiotherapy. Role of a renal biopsy 1-yr post-RT is still under investigation.

5.8.4 Prognosis (Table 24)

5.8.5 Important Recent advances in Uro Radiation oncology:

Prostate cancer:

SBRT has evolved drastically across all stages of prostate cancer.

1. Low/Intermediate Risk Prostate Cancer: PACE-B is a phase III randomized trial comparing 5-fraction SBRT with conventional or moderate hypofractionated radiotherapy (MHRT) in low- and intermediate-risk localized prostate cancer without ADT. After a median follow-up of 74 months, SBRT was non-inferior for biochemical/clinical failure, with 5-year control rates of 95.8% (SBRT) vs 94.6% (control). Late GI toxicity was similar, while GU toxicity was modestly higher with SBRT, but overall quality-of-life outcomes were comparable, supporting SBRT as an effective and convenient standard option in this population [211].

2. High-Risk Prostate Cancer: PRIME Trial, interim analysis showed low rate of grade 3 acute toxicities for both MHRT and SBRT Schedules,

Table 24 SEER stage-wise 5-year relative survival rate

SEER stage	5-yr survival
Localised	93%
Regional	71%
Distant	14%
All stages combined	76%

with similar toxicities (Grade 2 GU: 33.1% vs 31.8%, p=0.5 and Grade 2 GI: 17.2% vs 15.2%, p=0.9) and QoL [212].

3. SBRT with Dominant Intraprostatic Lesion (DIL) boost: Implementing the concept of dose escalation to Dominant Intraprostatic Lesion (DIL) from FLAME trial, HypoFLAME (MRI-guided) and PROBE (PSMA PET + mpMRI–guided) trials demonstrate that intraprostatic focal boost can be safely combined with SBRT in prostate cancer. Despite differences in imaging-defined target volumes, both studies reported acceptable acute GU/GI toxicity with no grade ≥3 events, supporting the feasibility of biologically guided dose escalation with SBRT [213, 214].

4. SBRT with MR-LINAC: MRI-guided linear accelerators enable superior soft-tissue visualization, real-time motion monitoring, and reduced PTV margins. In the MIRAGE trial, MRI-guided SBRT significantly reduced acute grade ≥2 genitourinary (24.4% vs 43.4%) and gastrointestinal toxicity (0% vs 10.5%) compared with CT guidance [215].

5. SBRT with Prior TURP: Prior TURP is generally considered a relative contraindication to SBRT. Singh et al reported that in patients with prior TURP treated with SBRT, severe late urinary toxicity was transient and uncommon (<10%), predominantly hematuria or urinary obstruction [216].

6. Proton therapy: The PARTIQoL randomized trial showed no significant difference between proton and photon therapy for low- to intermediate-risk prostate cancer [217]. In contrast, the recent multicentric Pre-PROTO PRIME study from India evaluating stereotactic body proton therapy (SBPT) in high-risk and node-positive prostate cancer demonstrated substantial dosimetric sparing of the bowel and rectum, with a low acute toxicity (grade 2 GU and GI toxicities of 27% and 3.8%) [218].

7. Pelvic Oligorecurrent Prostate cancer: Management of oligorecurrent disease has evolved with improved imaging and targeted RT. The PEACE V–STORM trial showed superior 4-year metastasis-free survival with elective nodal radiotherapy compared with metastasis-directed therapy alone (76% vs 63%), along with improved biochemical and locoregional control [219].

8. Metastatic Directed Therapy (MDT): Recent data from India demonstrated that in patients with denovo oligometastatic prostate cancer, index metastatic sites are the most common sites of disease progression despite systemic therapy and emphasizes the need for MDT [220]. The WOLVERINE individual patient data meta-analysis, incorporating data from 5 randomized trials, demonstrated significant benefit with MDT in oligometastatic prostate cancer, with consistent improvements in PFS, rPFS and castration resistance–free survival, with an emerging signal toward overall survival benefit [221].

9. Local therapy in metastatic disease: Radiotherapy to prostate is the standard of care in low volume metastatic disease. Interestingly data is also evolving for high volume disease and radiotherapy to prostate is shown to prevent serious GU symptoms [222].

Bladder cancer:

1. Hypo fractionated radiotherapy in bladder preservation has been extensively investigated, with increasing adoption as an alternative to conventional fractionation. In a recent cohort of 221 patients treated with plan of the day adaptive radiotherapy, hypo fractionated RT (55Gy/20 fractions) achieved comparable oncologic outcomes to conventional RT, with an 85% 2-year overall survival and 90% local

control, despite higher acute grade ≥ GI toxicity (26.7% vs 13.7%) and no grade ≥3 acute events. Late toxicity events were similar between both the schedules, supporting the transition to hypo fractionated radiotherapy [223].

2. Bladder Adjuvant RadioTherapy (BART) trial, phase III multicentric study from India, evaluated adjuvant pelvic radiotherapy for patients with high-risk features after radical cystectomy (pT3/4, pN+, margin positive, < 10 nodes dissected). At a median follow up of 47 months, adjuvant radiotherapy (50.4 Gy/28 fractions) demonstrated a significantly improved 2-year LRFS, when compared with observation after radical cystectomy (87% vs 76%, HR: 0.43, p=0.04) [224]. Adjuvant radiotherapy had low serious adverse events, supporting its role in reducing pelvic relapse in high-risk post-cystectomy bladder cancer [225].
3. In a prospective study of 104 bladder cancer patients from Tata Memorial Centre, Mumbai, quality of life after radical cystectomy and bladder preservation with (chemo)radiotherapy was largely comparable for urinary, bowel, and global health domains. However, sexual quality of life was significantly better with bladder preservation (BCI sexual score 56.9 vs 41.5; p=0.01). Overall, both strategies achieved good long-term QoL, with bladder preservation offering an advantage in sexual outcomes [226].

Renal Cancer:

1. FASTRACK II, a multicentric phase II trial, evaluated SABR in localized primary renal cell carcinoma (T1–T2a, N0) in medically inoperable or high-risk patients. Tumours of ≤4 cm received 26 Gy in a single fraction, while tumours >4–10 cm received 42 Gy in 3 fractions. At a median follow-up of 43 months, 12-month local control and cancer-specific survival were 100%, with 97% freedom from distant failure, no local failures, and acceptable toxicity (10% grade ≥3, no grade 4 events), establishing the role of SABR in primary RCC [227].
2. The role of neoadjuvant SBRT in RCC with tumor thrombus is emerging. A recent review reported sustained disease control for 3 years in a patient with clear cell RCC and IVC thrombus, treated with SBRT 49 Gy in 7 fractions after progression on TKI therapy [228].

Adrenocortical Carcinoma (ACC):

1. Primary ACC is a rare malignancy with poor prognosis. Despite the complete resection with negative margin, which is the current standard in non-metastatic ACC, the rate of local recurrence is high. Guidelines recommend adjuvant radiotherapy in patients with high-risk features such as positive margin (R1), incomplete resection (R2), Ki-67 >10%, rupture of capsule, large tumor size, high grade or after salvage surgery for isolated local recurrence [229]. Limited retrospective literature established the benefit of adjuvant radiotherapy post-surgery in reducing recurrence. A recent study from India analyzed patients with ACC post-surgery and showed an improved LRFS (HR: 8.13, p=0.024) and DFS (HR: 3.40, p=0.029) in patients who received adjuvant RT. The study identified functional tumors, presence of venous invasion and high mitotic index (>5/50 HPF) as predictors of disease relapse while adjuvant RT emerged as an independent prognostic factor prolonging survival outcomes [230].

Percepts Box

Prostate Cancer

1. Active surveillance, surgery and radiotherapy are equivalent options in low and favourable intermediate-risk prostate cancer.
2. PSMA PET-CT improves metastatic yield in high-risk prostate cancer.
3. Moderate hypofractionation is the standard of care for radiotherapy across all risk groups. SBRT is under evaluation. Pelvic RT should be included in high-risk disease.

(continued)

4. Permanent castration is only indicated in metastatic disease. Node positive and metastatic patients benefit with complete androgen blockade.
5. SBRT to the prostate improves overall survival in low volume (as defined by CHAARTED) metastatic prostate cancer.

Bladder Cancer

1. Non-muscle invasive bladder cancer requires TURBT followed by intravesical chemotherapy or BCG. Select patients with very high-risk or recurrent disease require cystectomy.
2. NACT is the standard of care in MIBC. Adjuvant chemotherapy does not improve overall survival.
3. In well-selected patients, disease outcomes are equivalent with radical cystectomy and trimodality bladder preservation.
4. Bladder preservation should be done using some form of adaptive radiotherapy to reduce toxicity. Dose escalation to site of gross tumour does not improve local control.
5. Patients with SCC bladder with Stage III and above disease should receive adjuvant chemoradiotherapy.
6. Adjuvant radiotherapy in urothelial cancers is under investigation. Crucial factors responsible for locoregional recurrence are T stage, margin positivity, lymph node positivity and lymph node yield.

Testicular Cancer

1. Management of stage I germ cell tumours should be a matter of choice after a detailed discussion among options of surveillance (preferred), radiotherapy and chemotherapy.
2. Survival rates for seminoma have approached 100% for stage I disease for several decades, exceeded 90% for good-risk regional disease and 75–80% for those with disseminated disease.
3. Radiotherapy is the recommended treatment option for stage IIA, while chemotherapy is preferred for seminomas of stage IIB and above.
4. FDG PET CECT is an effective tool to identify post-chemotherapy residual viable disease in stage IIb-IIIC seminoma. The role of radiotherapy to decrease the risk of recurrence is under evaluation.
5. Survivorship issues are important to address as the treatment sequelae in patients with germ cell tumours.

Penile Cancer

1. Penile cancer is a rare disease with limited clinical trial data driving the majority of treatment decisions.
2. Brachytherapy is a suitable alternative as a functional penile-sparing modality, to penectomy in patients with localised penile SCC.
3. Combined-modality treatment approaches with radiotherapy and chemotherapy are used to achieve the highest probability of cure with the least morbidity.
4. Extended-field radiation therapy significantly improves clinical outcomes compared with involved-field radiation in patients with pN3 penile cancer.

RCC

1. The role of surgery in the management of renal cell carcinoma includes the use of nephron-sparing approaches, cytoreductive nephrectomy, and metastasectomy.
2. Stereotactic ablative radiotherapy is an emerging option for selected patients with biopsy-confirmed radiologically measurable primary RCC.
3. Other indications for SBRT include neoadjuvant SBRT for IVC thrombus, neoadjuvant SBRT prior to cytoreductive nephrectomy or as a replacement

(continued)

for cytoreductive nephrectomy. Palliative radiotherapy is the cornerstone of symptom relief for bone and brain metastases.

4. Numerous angiogenesis-directed therapies targeting VEGF, mTOR inhibitors and immunotherapy have led to a significant improvement in outcomes in patients with metastatic disease.

Multiple Choice Questions

1. Prostate cancer most commonly develops in the:
   (a) Transitional zone
   (b) Peripheral zone
   (c) Periurethral region
   (d) Prostatic apex
2. The following is true regarding watchful waiting:
   (a) Considered in patients unfit for treatment
   (b) Serial PSA monitoring done
   (c) Only suitable for Gleason grade ≤7
   (d) Treatment given at symptom progression
   (e) Both (a) and (d)
3. The rationale for moderate hypofractionation in prostate cancer is all except:
   (a) Low alpha/beta
   (b) Better therapeutic ratio
   (c) Shorter overall treatment time
   (d) Shorter duration of ADT required
4. The following are components of the CAPRA-S score except:
   (a) Pre-operative PSA
   (b) % of gland involved by tumour
   (c) Seminal vesicle involvement
   (d) Extra-prostatic extension
5. The benefit of radiotherapy to the prostate in metastatic prostate cancer was demonstrated by the following trial:
   (a) CHAARTED
   (b) LATITUDE
   (c) STAMPEDE
   (d) STOMP
6. Adequacy of TURBT is determined by:
   (a) Presence of detrusor muscle in the specimen
   (b) Presence of lamina propria in the specimen
   (c) Removal of at least 5 cc of tissue
   (d) Random biopsies to be included
7. Standard chemotherapy regimen in bladder cancer is:
   (a) Adjuvant ddMVAC
   (b) Neoadjuvant ddMVAC
   (c) Neoadjuvant Paclitaxel + Carboplatin
   (d) Adjuvant Paclitaxel + Carboplatin
8. The following are methods of Adaptive Radiotherapy in bladder cancer except:
   (a) A-POLO technique
   (b) Daily Reoptimisation method
   (c) Plan of the Approach
   (d) Elective weekly replanning
9. All of the following are factors affecting loco-regional recurrence in bladder cancer except:
   (a) Lymph node yield <10
   (b) Positive surgical margins
   (c) Tumour size >5 cm
   (d) Large tumour size
10. What is the dose of radiotherapy delivered to treat Germ cell Neoplasia in Situ (GCNIS)?
    (a) 16–20 Gy @ 2 Gy/#
    (b) 30–36 Gy @ 2 Gy/#
    (c) 12–16 Gy @ 4 Gy/#
    (d) 30–36 Gy @ 4 Gy/#
11. Risk factors for relapse in stage I seminoma managed by surveillance include
    (a) Tumour size ≥4 cm
    (b) Rete testis invasion
    (c) Both
    (d) None
12. Post-chemotherapy residual NSGCT of more than 1 cm with normal serum tumour markers can be either of the following
    (a) Fibrotic tissue
    (b) Mature teratoma
    (c) Immature teratoma
    (d) All of the above
13. What are the indications of adjuvant radiotherapy to primary site in penile carcinomas?

(a) R+ resection
(b) Node positivity
(c) Tumour size >4 cm
(d) All squamous cell carcinomas

14. Adjuvant external beam radiation therapy to inguinal region and/or chemotherapy is indicated if any of the following high-risk features is present
    (a) Pelvic nodal metastasis in ≥2 nodes
    (b) Extra capsular extension
    (c) Both a and b
    (d) None
15. For contouring post-operative groin to deliver adjuvant EBRT, the CTV should be edited from the surrounding muscles except
    (a) Sartorius muscle
    (b) Iliopsoas muscle
    (c) Pectineus muscle
    (d) Adductor group of muscles
16. The International Metastatic Renal Cell Carcinoma Database Consortium (IMDC) risk group classification does not include:
    (a) Low hemoglobin
    (b) KPS <80
    (c) Increased corrected calcium
    (d) Surgical status
17. SBRT to primary RCC is not indicated in the following:
    (a) Medically inoperable patients
    (b) Operable but at risk for dialysis post-surgery
    (c) Unfit for thermal ablation
    (d) History of connective tissue disorder
18. Which of the following statements with regard to SBRT to primary RCC is false
    (a) Unlike RFA or cryotherapy, SBRT does not have specific limitations relating to tumour size or position relative to pelvic calyceal structures.
    (b) Treatment of larger tumours poses significant risks of haemorrhage, which can require a nephrectomy to control.
    (c) Contrast enhancement on post-treatment CT is not a determinant of treatment failure and is expected after SBRT delivery.
    (d) All of the above.

Answer Key

1. (b)
2. (e)
3. (d)
4. (b)
5. (c)
6. (a)
7. (b)
8. (d)
9. (d)
10. (a)
11. (c)
12. (d)
13. (a)
14. (c)
15. (a)
16. (d)
17. (d)
18. (b)

References

1. Kulothungan V, Sathishkumar K, Leburu S, Ramamoorthy T, Stephen S, Basavarajappa D, et al. Burden of cancers in India – estimates of cancer crude incidence, YLLs, YLDs and DALYs for 2021 and 2025 based on National Cancer Registry Program. BMC Cancer. 2022;22(1):527.
2. Bakshi G, Tongaonkar H, Addla S, Menon S, Pradhan A, Kumar A, et al. Expert survey on management of prostate cancer in India: real-world insights into practice patterns. Indian J Cancer. 2022;59(Supplement):S19–45.
3. Grossman DC, Curry SJ, Owens DK, Bibbins-Domingo K, Caughey AB, Davidson KW, et al. Screening for prostate cancer: US Preventive Services Task Force recommendation statement. JAMA [Internet]. 2018 [cited 2022 Dec 28];319(18). Available from: https://pubmed.ncbi.nlm.nih.gov/29801017/.
4. Srigley JR, Delahunt B, Egevad L, Samaratunga H, Yaxley J, Evans AJ. One is the new six: the International Society of Urological Pathology (ISUP) patient-focused approach to Gleason grading. Can Urol Assoc J. 2016;10(9–10):339–41.
5. Ahmed HU, Bosaily AES, Brown LC, Gabe R, Kaplan R, Parmar MK, et al. Diagnostic accuracy of multi-parametric MRI and TRUS biopsy in prostate cancer (PROMIS): a paired validating confirmatory study. Lancet. 2017;389(10071):815–22.

6. Kasivisvanathan V, Rannikko AS, Borghi M, Panebianco V, Mynderse LA, Vaarala MH, et al. MRI-targeted or standard biopsy for prostate-cancer diagnosis. N Engl J Med. 2018;378(19):1767–77.
7. Hofman MS, Lawrentschuk N, Francis RJ, Tang C, Vela I, Thomas P, et al. Prostate-specific membrane antigen PET-CT in patients with high-risk prostate cancer before curative-intent surgery or radiotherapy (proPSMA): a prospective, randomised, multicentre study. Lancet. 2020;395(10231):1208–16.
8. Klotz L, Zhang L, Lam A, Nam R, Mamedov A, Loblaw A. Clinical results of long-term follow-up of a large, active surveillance cohort with localized prostate cancer. J Clin Oncol. 2010;28(1):126–31.
9. Allan C, Ilic D. Laparoscopic versus robotic-assisted radical prostatectomy for the treatment of localised prostate cancer: a systematic review. Urol Int. 2016;96(4):373–8.
10. Begg CB, Riedel ER, Bach PB, Kattan MW, Schrag D, Warren JL, et al. Variations in morbidity after radical prostatectomy. N Engl J Med. 2002;346(15):1138–44.
11. Gershman B, Meier SK, Jeffery MM, Moreira DM, Tollefson MK, Kim SP, et al. Redefining and contextualizing the hospital volume-outcome relationship for robot-assisted radical prostatectomy: implications for centralization of care. J Urol. 2017;198(1):92–9.
12. Fossati N, Willemse PPM, Van den Broeck T, van den Bergh RCN, Yuan CY, Briers E, et al. The benefits and harms of different extents of lymph node dissection during radical prostatectomy for prostate cancer: a systematic review. Eur Urol. 2017;72(1):84–109.
13. Yaxley JW, Raveenthiran S, Nouhaud FX, Samartunga H, Yaxley AJ, Coughlin G, et al. Outcomes of primary lymph node staging of intermediate and high risk prostate cancer with 68Ga-PSMA positron emission tomography/computerized tomography compared to histological correlation of pelvic lymph node pathology. J Urol. 2019;201(4):815–20.
14. Dearnaley D, Syndikus I, Mossop H, Khoo V, Birtle A, Bloomfield D, et al. Conventional versus hypofractionated high-dose intensity-modulated radiotherapy for prostate cancer: 5-year outcomes of the randomised, non-inferiority, phase 3 CHHiP trial. Lancet Oncol. 2016;17(8):1047–60.
15. Arcangeli G, Saracino B, Arcangeli S, Gomellini S, Petrongari MG, Sanguineti G, et al. Moderate hypofractionation in high-risk, organ-confined prostate cancer: final results of a phase III randomized trial. J Clin Oncol. 2017;35(17):1891–7.
16. Catton CN, Lukka H, Gu CS, Martin JM, Supiot S, Chung PWM, et al. Randomized trial of a hypofractionated radiation regimen for the treatment of localized prostate cancer. J Clin Oncol. 2017;35(17):1884–90.
17. Incrocci L, Wortel RC, Alemayehu WG, Aluwini S, Schimmel E, Krol S, et al. Hypofractionated versus conventionally fractionated radiotherapy for patients with localised prostate cancer (HYPRO): final efficacy results from a randomised, multicentre, open-label, phase 3 trial. Lancet Oncol. 2016;17(8):1061–9.
18. Widmark A, Gunnlaugsson A, Beckman L, Thellenberg-Karlsson C, Hoyer M, Lagerlund M, et al. Ultra-hypofractionated versus conventionally fractionated radiotherapy for prostate cancer: 5-year outcomes of the HYPO-RT-PC randomised, non-inferiority, phase 3 trial. Lancet Lond Engl. 2019;394(10196):385–95.
19. Brand DH, Tree AC, Ostler P, van der Voet H, Loblaw A, Chu W, et al. Intensity-modulated fractionated radiotherapy versus stereotactic body radiotherapy for prostate cancer (PACE-B): acute toxicity findings from an international, randomised, open-label, phase 3, non-inferiority trial. Lancet Oncol. 2019;20(11):1531–43.
20. Tree AC, Ostler P, van der Voet H, Chu W, Loblaw A, Ford D, et al. Intensity-modulated radiotherapy versus stereotactic body radiotherapy for prostate cancer (PACE-B): 2-year toxicity results from an open-label, randomised, phase 3, non-inferiority trial. Lancet Oncol. 2022;23(10):1308–20.
21. Kerkmeijer LGW, Groen VH, Pos FJ, Haustermans K, Monninkhof EM, Smeenk RJ, et al. Focal boost to the intraprostatic tumor in external beam radiotherapy for patients with localized prostate cancer: results from the FLAME randomized phase III trial. J Clin Oncol. 2021;39(7):787–96.
22. Dubray BM, Salleron J, Guerif SG, Le Prise E, Reynaud-Bougnoux A, Hannoun-Levi JM, et al. Does short-term androgen depletion add to high dose radiotherapy (80 Gy) in localized intermediate risk prostate cancer? Final analysis of GETUG 14 randomized trial (EU-20503/NCT00104741). J Clin Oncol. 2016;34(15_suppl):5021.
23. Bolla M, Neven A, Maingon P, Carrie C, Boladeras A, Andreopoulos D, et al. Short androgen suppression and radiation dose escalation in prostate cancer: 12-year results of EORTC trial 22991 in patients with localized intermediate-risk disease. J Clin Oncol. 2021;39(27):3022–33.
24. Nabid A, Carrier N, Vigneault E, Van Nguyen T, Vavassis P, Brassard MA, et al. Androgen deprivation therapy and radiotherapy in intermediate-risk prostate cancer: a randomised phase III trial. Eur J Cancer Oxf Engl 1990. 2021;143:64–74.
25. Pommier P, Chabaud S, Lagrange JL, Richaud P, Le Prise E, Wagner JP, et al. Is there a role for pelvic irradiation in localized prostate adenocarcinoma? Update of the long-term survival results of the GETUG-01 randomized study. Int J Radiat Oncol Biol Phys. 2016;96(4):759–69.
26. Roach M, Moughan J, Lawton CAF, Dicker AP, Zeitzer KL, Gore EM, et al. Sequence of hormonal therapy and radiotherapy field size in unfavourable, localised prostate cancer (NRG/RTOG 9413): long-

term results of a randomised, phase 3 trial. Lancet Oncol. 2018;19(11):1504–15.
27. Murthy V, Maitre P, Kannan S, Panigrahi G, Krishnatry R, Bakshi G, et al. Prostate-only versus whole-pelvic radiation therapy in high-risk and very high-risk prostate cancer (POP-RT): outcomes from phase III randomized controlled trial. J Clin Oncol. 2021;39(11):1234–42.
28. Musunuru HB, D'Alimonte L, Davidson M, Ho L, Cheung P, Vesprini D, et al. Phase 1–2 study of stereotactic ablative radiotherapy including regional lymph node irradiation in patients with high-risk prostate cancer (SATURN): early toxicity and quality of life. Int J Radiat Oncol Biol Phys. 2018;102(5):1438–47.
29. Murthy V, Sinha S, Kannan S, Datta D, Das R, Bakshi G, et al. Safety of prostate stereotactic body radiation therapy after transurethral resection of prostate (TURP): a propensity score matched pair analysis. Pract Radiat Oncol. 2019;9(5):347–53.
30. Mallick I, Arunsingh M, Chakraborty S, Arun B, Prasath S, Roy P, et al. A phase I/II study of stereotactic hypofractionated once-weekly radiation therapy (SHORT) for prostate cancer. Clin Oncol R Coll Radiol G B. 2020;32(2):e39–45.
31. Murthy V, Adsul K, Maitre P, Singla A, Singh P, Panigrahi G, et al. Acute and late adverse effects of prostate-only or pelvic stereotactic radiation therapy in prostate cancer: a comparative study. Int J Radiat Oncol Biol Phys. 2022;114(2):275–82.
32. Murthy V, Mallick I, Gavarraju A, Sinha S, Krishnatry R, Telkhade T, et al. Study protocol of a randomised controlled trial of prostate radiotherapy in high-risk and node-positive disease comparing moderate and extreme hypofractionation (PRIME TRIAL). BMJ Open. 2020;10(2):e034623.
33. Bolla M, de Reijke TM, Van Tienhoven G, Van den Bergh ACM, Oddens J, Poortmans PMP, et al. Duration of androgen suppression in the treatment of prostate cancer. N Engl J Med. 2009;360(24):2516–27.
34. Zapatero A, Guerrero A, Maldonado X, Álvarez A, San-Segundo CG, Rodríguez MÁC, et al. High-dose radiotherapy and risk-adapted androgen deprivation in localised prostate cancer (DART 01/05): 10-year results of a phase 3 randomised, controlled trial. Lancet Oncol. 2022;23(5):671–81.
35. Marra G, Valerio M, Heidegger I, Tsaur I, Mathieu R, Ceci F, et al. Management of patients with node-positive prostate cancer at radical prostatectomy and pelvic lymph node dissection: a systematic review. Eur Urol Oncol. 2020;3(5):565–81.
36. Chopade P, Maitre P, David S, Panigrahi G, Singh P, Phurailatpam R, et al. Common iliac node-positive prostate cancer treated with curative radiation therapy: N1 or M1a? Int J Radiat Oncol Biol Phys. 2022;114(4):711–7.
37. Lieng H, Kneebone A, Hayden AJ, Christie DRH, Davis BJ, Eade TN, et al. Radiotherapy for node-positive prostate cancer: 2019 recommendations of the Australian and New Zealand Radiation Oncology Genito-Urinary Group. Radiother Oncol J Eur Soc Ther Radiol Oncol. 2019;140:68–75.
38. Ishiyama H, Hirayama T, Jhaveri P, Satoh T, Paulino AC, Xu B, et al. Is there an increase in genitourinary toxicity in patients treated with transurethral resection of the prostate and radiotherapy? A systematic review. Am J Clin Oncol. 2014;37(3):297–304.
39. Valle LF, Lehrer EJ, Markovic D, Elashoff D, Levin-Epstein R, Karnes RJ, et al. A systematic review and meta-analysis of local salvage therapies after radiotherapy for prostate cancer (MASTER). Eur Urol. 2021;80(3):280–92.
40. Schmidt-Hegemann NS, Buchner A, Eze C, Rogowski P, Schaefer C, Ilhan H, et al. PSMA-positive nodal recurrence in prostate cancer. Strahlenther Onkol. 2020;196(7):637–46.
41. Supiot S, Vaugier L, Pasquier D, Buthaud X, Magné N, Peiffert D, et al. OLIGOPELVIS GETUG P07, a multicenter phase II trial of combined high-dose salvage radiotherapy and hormone therapy in oligorecurrent pelvic node relapses in prostate cancer. Eur Urol. 2021;80(4):405–14.
42. Tendulkar RD, Mian OY. Yes, nodal recurrence of prostate cancer is potentially curable. Int J Radiat Oncol Biol Phys. 2020;106(2):238.
43. Chalieopanyarwong V, Attawettayanon W, Kanchanawanichkul W, Pripatnanont C. The prognostic factors of biochemical recurrence-free survival following radical prostatectomy. Asian Pac J Cancer Prev APJCP. 2017;18(9):2555–9.
44. Bolla M, van Poppel H, Tombal B, Vekemans K, Pozzo LD, de Reijke TM, et al. Postoperative radiotherapy after radical prostatectomy for high-risk prostate cancer: long-term results of a randomised controlled trial (EORTC trial 22911). Lancet. 2012;380(9858):2018–27.
45. Hackman G, Taari K, Tammela TL, Matikainen M, Kouri M, Joensuu T, et al. Randomised trial of adjuvant radiotherapy following radical prostatectomy versus radical prostatectomy alone in prostate cancer patients with positive margins or extracapsular extension. Eur Urol. 2019;76(5):586–95.
46. Wiegel T, Bartkowiak D, Bottke D, Bronner C, Steiner U, Siegmann A, et al. Adjuvant radiotherapy versus wait-and-see after radical prostatectomy: 10-year follow-up of the ARO 96-02/AUO AP 09/95 trial. Eur Urol. 2014;66(2):243–50.
47. Kneebone A, Fraser-Browne C, Duchesne GM, Fisher R, Frydenberg M, Herschtal A, et al. Adjuvant radiotherapy versus early salvage radiotherapy following radical prostatectomy (TROG 08.03/ANZUP RAVES): a randomised, controlled, phase 3, non-inferiority trial. Lancet Oncol. 2020;21(10):1331–40.
48. Parker CC, Clarke NW, Cook AD, Kynaston HG, Petersen PM, Catton C, et al. Timing of radiotherapy after radical prostatectomy (RADICALS-RT): a randomised, controlled phase 3 trial. Lancet Lond Engl. 2020;396(10260):1413–21.

49. Sargos P, Chabaud S, Latorzeff I, Magné N, Benyoucef A, Supiot S, et al. Adjuvant radiotherapy versus early salvage radiotherapy plus short-term androgen deprivation therapy in men with localised prostate cancer after radical prostatectomy (GETUG-AFU 17): a randomised, phase 3 trial. Lancet Oncol. 2020;21(10):1341–52.
50. Pollack A, Karrison TG, Balogh AG, Gomella LG, Low DA, Bruner DW, et al. The addition of androgen deprivation therapy and pelvic lymph node treatment to prostate bed salvage radiotherapy (NRG Oncology/RTOG 0534 SPPORT): an international, multicentre, randomised phase 3 trial. Lancet Lond Engl. 2022;399(10338):1886–901.
51. Boevé LMS, Hulshof MCCM, Vis AN, Zwinderman AH, Twisk JWR, Witjes WPJ, et al. Effect on survival of androgen deprivation therapy alone compared to androgen deprivation therapy combined with concurrent radiation therapy to the prostate in patients with primary bone metastatic prostate cancer in a prospective randomised clinical trial: data from the HORRAD trial. Eur Urol. 2019;75(3):410–8.
52. Parker CC, James ND, Brawley CD, Clarke NW, Hoyle AP, Ali A, et al. Radiotherapy to the primary tumour for newly diagnosed, metastatic prostate cancer (STAMPEDE): a randomised controlled phase 3 trial. Lancet Lond Engl. 2018;392(10162):2353–66.
53. Hellman S, Weichselbaum RR. Oligometastases. J Clin Oncol. 1995;13(1):8–10.
54. Ost P, Reynders D, Decaestecker K, Fonteyne V, Lumen N, De Bruycker A, et al. Surveillance or metastasis-directed therapy for oligometastatic prostate cancer recurrence (STOMP): five-year results of a randomized phase II trial. J Clin Oncol. 2020;38(6_suppl):10.
55. Phillips R, Shi WY, Deek M, Radwan N, Lim SJ, Antonarakis ES, et al. Outcomes of observation vs stereotactic ablative radiation for oligometastatic prostate cancer: the ORIOLE phase 2 randomized clinical trial. JAMA Oncol. 2020;6(5):650–9.
56. Zilli T, Achard V, Dal Pra A, Schmidt-Hegemann N, Jereczek-Fossa BA, Lancia A, et al. Recommendations for radiation therapy in oligometastatic prostate cancer: an ESTRO-ACROP Delphi consensus. Radiother Oncol J Eur Soc Ther Radiol Oncol. 2022;176:199–207.
57. Murthy V, Mallick I, Arunsingh M, Gupta P. Prostate radiotherapy in India: evolution, practice and challenges in the 21st century. Clin Oncol R Coll Radiol G B. 2019;31(8):492–501.
58. Hamstra DA, Mariados N, Sylvester J, Shah D, Karsh L, Hudes R, et al. Continued benefit to rectal separation for prostate radiation therapy: final results of a phase III trial. Int J Radiat Oncol Biol Phys. 2017;97(5):976–85.
59. Ghaffari H, Mehrabian A. Rectal retractor in prostate radiotherapy: pros and cons. Radiat Oncol Lond Engl. 2022;17:204.
60. O'Neill AGM, Jain S, Hounsell AR, O'Sullivan JM. Fiducial marker guided prostate radiotherapy: a review. Br J Radiol. 2016;89(1068):20160296.
61. Hama Y, Tate E. Long-term follow-up results of endorectal balloon-assisted helical tomotherapy for localized prostate cancer patients in the high-risk group of gastrointestinal adverse events. Rep Pract Oncol Radiother J Gt Cancer Cent Poznan Pol Soc Radiat Oncol. 2022;27(5):842–7.
62. Dearnaley DP, Khoo VS, Norman AR, Meyer L, Nahum A, Tait D, et al. Comparison of radiation side-effects of conformal and conventional radiotherapy in prostate cancer: a randomised trial. Lancet Lond Engl. 1999;353(9149):267–72.
63. Viani GA, Viana BS, Martin JEC, Rossi BT, Zuliani G, Stefano EJ. Intensity-modulated radiotherapy reduces toxicity with similar biochemical control compared with 3-dimensional conformal radiotherapy for prostate cancer: a randomized clinical trial. Cancer. 2016;122(13):2004–11.
64. Salembier C, Villeirs G, De Bari B, Hoskin P, Pieters BR, Van Vulpen M, et al. ESTRO ACROP consensus guideline on CT- and MRI-based target volume delineation for primary radiation therapy of localized prostate cancer. Radiother Oncol J Eur Soc Ther Radiol Oncol. 2018;127(1):49–61.
65. Hall WA, Paulson E, Davis BJ, Spratt DE, Morgan TM, Dearnaley D, et al. NRG oncology updated international consensus atlas on pelvic lymph node volumes for intact and postoperative prostate cancer. Int J Radiat Oncol Biol Phys. 2021;109(1):174–85.
66. Zaorsky NG, Davis BJ, Nguyen PL, Showalter TN, Hoskin PJ, Yoshioka Y, et al. The evolution of brachytherapy for prostate cancer. Nat Rev Urol. 2017;14(7):415–39.
67. Morris WJ, Tyldesley S, Rodda S, Halperin R, Pai H, McKenzie M, et al. Androgen suppression combined with elective nodal and dose escalated radiation therapy (the ASCENDE-RT trial): an analysis of survival endpoints for a randomized trial comparing a low-dose-rate brachytherapy boost to a dose-escalated external beam boost for high- and intermediate-risk prostate cancer. Int J Radiat Oncol Biol Phys. 2017;98(2):275–85.
68. Schrier BP, Hollander MP, van Rhijn BWG, Kiemeney LALM, Witjes JA. Prognosis of muscle-invasive bladder cancer: difference between primary and progressive tumours and implications for therapy. Eur Urol. 2004;45(3):292–6.
69. Advanced Bladder Cancer (ABC) Meta-analysis Collaboration. Neoadjuvant chemotherapy in invasive bladder cancer: update of a systematic review and meta-analysis of individual patient data advanced bladder cancer (ABC) meta-analysis collaboration. Eur Urol. 2005;48(2):202–5; discussion 205–206.
70. Fradet Y, Bellmunt J, Vaughn DJ, Lee JL, Fong L, Vogelzang NJ, et al. Randomized phase III KEYNOTE-045 trial of pembrolizumab versus paclitaxel, docetaxel, or vinflunine in recurrent

advanced urothelial cancer: results of >2 years of follow-up. Ann Oncol. 2019;30(6):970–6.
71. Powles T, Park SH, Voog E, Caserta C, Valderrama BP, Gurney H, et al. Avelumab maintenance therapy for advanced or metastatic urothelial carcinoma. N Engl J Med. 2020;383(13):1218–30.
72. Rodrigues Pessoa R, Mueller AC, Boxley P, Flaig TW, Piper C, Konety B, et al. Systematic review and meta-analysis of radiation therapy for high-risk non-muscle invasive bladder cancer. Urol Oncol. 2021;39(11):786.e1–8.
73. Dahl DM, Rodgers J, Shipley WU, Michaelson D, Wu CL, Parker W, et al. NRG oncology/RTOG 0926: phase II protocol for patients with stage T1 bladder cancer to evaluate selective bladder preserving treatment by radiation therapy concurrent with radiosensitizing chemotherapy following a thorough transurethral surgical re-staging. Int J Radiat Oncol. 2021;111(3, Supplement):S133–4.
74. Mehta P, Sinha S, Kashid S, Chakraborty D, Mhatre R, Murthy V. Exploring texture analysis to optimize bladder preservation in muscle invasive bladder cancer. Clin Genitourin Cancer. 2022:S1558-7673(22)00241-5.
75. Huddart RA, Birtle A, Maynard L, Beresford M, Blazeby J, Donovan J, et al. Clinical and patient-reported outcomes of SPARE – a randomised feasibility study of selective bladder preservation versus radical cystectomy. BJU Int. 2017;120(5):639–50.
76. Vashistha V, Wang H, Mazzone A, Liss MA, Svatek RS, Schleicher M, et al. Radical cystectomy compared to combined modality treatment for muscle-invasive bladder cancer: a systematic review and meta-analysis. Int J Radiat Oncol Biol Phys. 2017;97(5):1002–20.
77. Song YP, Mistry H, Irlam J, Valentine H, Yang L, Lane B, et al. Long-term outcomes of radical radiation therapy with hypoxia modification with biomarker discovery for stratification: 10-year update of the BCON (bladder carbogen nicotinamide) phase 3 randomized trial (ISRCTN45938399). Int J Radiat Oncol Biol Phys. 2021;110(5):1407–15.
78. James ND, Hussain SA, Hall E, Jenkins P, Tremlett J, Rawlings C, et al. Radiotherapy with or without chemotherapy in muscle-invasive bladder cancer. N Engl J Med. 2012;366(16):1477–88.
79. Choudhury A, Porta N, Hall E, Song YP, Owen R, MacKay R, et al. Hypofractionated radiotherapy in locally advanced bladder cancer: an individual patient data meta-analysis of the BC2001 and BCON trials. Lancet Oncol. 2021;22(2):246–55.
80. Huddart R, Hafeez S, Lewis R, McNair H, Syndikus I, Henry A, et al. Clinical outcomes of a randomized trial of adaptive plan-of-the-day treatment in patients receiving ultra-hypofractionated weekly radiation therapy for bladder cancer. Int J Radiat Oncol Biol Phys. 2021;110(2):412–24.
81. Dracham CB, Kumar N, Kumar S, Elangovan A, Yadav BS, Mavuduru RS, et al. A phase II study of neoadjuvant chemotherapy followed by organ preservation in patients with muscle-invasive bladder cancer. Asian J Urol. 2022;9(3):318–28.
82. International Collaboration of Trialists, Medical Research Council Advanced Bladder Cancer Working Party (now the National Cancer Research Institute Bladder Cancer Clinical Studies Group), European Organisation for Research and Treatment of Cancer Genito-Urinary Tract Cancer Group, Australian Bladder Cancer Study Group, National Cancer Institute of Canada Clinical Trials Group, Finnbladder, et al. International phase III trial assessing neoadjuvant cisplatin, methotrexate, and vinblastine chemotherapy for muscle-invasive bladder cancer: long-term results of the BA06 30894 trial. J Clin Oncol. 2011;29(16):2171–7.
83. Murthy V, Master Z, Adurkar P, Mallick I, Mahantshetty U, Bakshi G, et al. "Plan of the day" adaptive radiotherapy for bladder cancer using helical tomotherapy. Radiother Oncol J Eur Soc Ther Radiol Oncol. 2011;99(1):55–60.
84. Tunio MA, Hashmi A, Qayyum A, Mohsin R, Zaeem A. Whole-pelvis or bladder-only chemoradiation for lymph node-negative invasive bladder cancer: single-institution experience. Int J Radiat Oncol Biol Phys. 2012;82(3):e457–62.
85. Lewis S, Murthy V, Mahantshetty U, Shrivastava SK. Incidental dose to pelvic nodes in bladder-only radiotherapy: is it clinically relevant? Technol Cancer Res Treat. 2017;16(3):382–7.
86. Murthy V, Gupta P, Baruah K, Krishnatry R, Joshi A, Prabhash K, et al. Adaptive radiotherapy for carcinoma of the urinary bladder: long-term outcomes with dose escalation. Clin Oncol R Coll Radiol G B. 2019;31(9):646–52.
87. Christodouleas JP, Baumann BC, He J, Hwang WT, Tucker KN, Bekelman JE, et al. Optimizing bladder cancer locoregional failure risk stratification after radical cystectomy using SWOG 8710. Cancer [Internet]. 2014 [cited 2023 Jan 7];120(8). Available from: https://pubmed.ncbi.nlm.nih.gov/24390799/.
88. Murthy V, Bakshi G, Manjali JJ, Prakash G, Pal M, Joshi A, et al. Locoregional recurrence after cystectomy in muscle invasive bladder cancer: implications for adjuvant radiotherapy. Urol Oncol. 2021;39(8):496.e9–496.e15.
89. Verghote F, Sargos P, Christodouleas JP, Murthy V, Baumann BC, Dirix P, et al. International consensus guidelines for adjuvant radiation therapy for bladder cancer after radical cystectomy: update from an IBIS Workgroup. Pract Radiat Oncol. 2022;12(6):524–32.
90. Zaghloul MS, Christodouleas JP, Smith A, Abdallah A, William H, Khaled HM, et al. Adjuvant sandwich chemotherapy plus radiotherapy vs adjuvant chemotherapy alone for locally advanced bladder cancer after radical cystectomy: a randomized phase 2 trial. JAMA Surg. 2018;53(1):e174591.
91. Yeh SD, Morse MJ, Grando R, Kleinert EL, Whitmore WF. Lymphoscintigraphic studies of

lymphatic drainage from the testes. Clin Nucl Med. 1986;11(12):823–7.
92. Mathur P, Sathishkumar K, Chaturvedi M, Das P, Sudarshan KL, Santhappan S, et al. Cancer statistics, 2020: report from National Cancer Registry Programme, India. JCO Glob Oncol. 2020;(6):1063–75.
93. Park JS, Kim J, Elghiaty A, Ham WS. Recent global trends in testicular cancer incidence and mortality. Medicine (Baltimore). 2018;97(37):e12390.
94. Testicular cancer: genes, environment, hormones. Frontiers [Internet]. [cited 2023 Jan 27]. Available from: https://www.frontiersin.org/articles/10.3389/fendo.2019.00408/full.
95. Risk of contralateral testicular cancer: a population-based study of 29 515 U.S. men. JNCI: J Natl Cancer Inst. Oxford Academic [Internet]. [cited 2023 Jan 27]. Available from: https://academic.oup.com/jnci/article/97/14/1056/2521308.
96. Smith ZL, Werntz RP, Eggener SE. Testicular cancer: epidemiology, diagnosis, and management. Med Clin North Am. 2018;102(2):251–64.
97. Moch H, Cubilla AL, Humphrey PA, Reuter VE, Ulbright TM. The 2016 WHO classification of tumours of the urinary system and male genital organs-part A: renal, penile, and testicular tumours. Eur Urol. 2016;70(1):93–105.
98. U.S. Preventive Services Task Force. Screening for testicular cancer: U.S. Preventive Services Task Force reaffirmation recommendation statement. Ann Intern Med. 2011;154(7):483–6.
99. Milose JC, Filson CP, Weizer AZ, Hafez KS, Montgomery JS. Role of biochemical markers in testicular cancer: diagnosis, staging, and surveillance. Open Access J Urol. 2011;4:1–8.
100. Albers P, Albrecht W, Algaba F, Bokemeyer C, Cohn-Cedermark G, Fizazi K, et al. Guidelines on testicular cancer: 2015 update. Eur Urol. 2015;68(6):1054–68.
101. TNM classification of malignant tumours. 8th ed. Wiley [Internet]. Wiley.com. [cited 2023 Jan 27]. Available from: https://www.wiley.com/en-us/TNM+Classification+of+Malignant+Tumours%2C+8th+Edition-p-9781119263579.
102. AJCC cancer staging manual. SpringerLink [Internet]. [cited 2023 Jan 27]. Available from: https://link.springer.com/book/9783319406176.
103. Predicting outcomes in men with metastatic non-seminomatous germ cell tumors (NSGCT): results from the IGCCCG Update Consortium [Internet]. [cited 2023 Jan 27]. Available from: https://www.researchgate.net/publication/350704336_Predicting_Outcomes_in_Men_With_Metastatic_Nonseminomatous_Germ_Cell_Tumors_NSGCT_Results_From_the_IGCCCG_Update_Consortium.
104. Beyer J, Collette L, Sauvé N, Daugaard G, Feldman DR, Tandstad T, et al. Survival and new prognosticators in metastatic seminoma: results from the IGCCCG-Update Consortium. J Clin Oncol. 2021;39(14):1553–62.
105. Radical inguinal orchidectomy: the gold standard for initial management of testicular cancer – PMC [Internet]. [cited 2023 Jan 27]. Available from: https://www.ncbi.nlm.nih.gov/pmc/articles/PMC7807348/.
106. Ory J et al. Outcomes of organ-sparing surgery for adult testicular tumors: A systematic review of the literature. BJUI Compass. 2021. Wiley Online Library [Internet]. [cited 2023 Jan 27]. Available from: https://bjui-journals.onlinelibrary.wiley.com/doi/full/10.1002/bco2.77.
107. Mead GM, Fossa SD, Oliver RTD, Joffe JK, Huddart RA, Roberts JT, et al. Randomized trials in 2466 patients with stage I seminoma: patterns of relapse and follow-up. J Natl Cancer Inst. 2011;103(3):241–9.
108. Fosså SD, Aass N, Kaalhus O. Radiotherapy for testicular seminoma stage I: treatment results and long-term post-irradiation morbidity in 365 patients. Int J Radiat Oncol Biol Phys. 1989;16(2):383–8.
109. Jones WG, Fossa SD, Mead GM, Roberts JT, Sokal M, Horwich A, et al. Randomized trial of 30 versus 20 Gy in the adjuvant treatment of stage I testicular seminoma: a report on Medical Research Council Trial TE18, European Organisation for the Research and Treatment of Cancer Trial 30942 (ISRCTN18525328). J Clin Oncol. 2005;23(6):1200–8.
110. Wilder RB, Buyyounouski MK, Efstathiou JA, Beard CJ. Radiotherapy treatment planning for testicular seminoma. Int J Radiat Oncol Biol Phys. 2012;83(4):e445–52.
111. Schmoll HJ, Souchon R, Krege S, Albers P, Beyer J, Kollmannsberger C, et al. European consensus on diagnosis and treatment of germ cell cancer: a report of the European Germ Cell Cancer Consensus Group (EGCCCG). Ann Oncol. 2004;15(9):1377–99.
112. Gilligan T, Lin DW, Aggarwal R, Chism D, Cost N, Derweesh IH, et al. Testicular cancer, version 2.2020, NCCN clinical practice guidelines in oncology. J Natl Compr Cancer Netw JNCCN. 2019;17(12):1529–54.
113. Murthy V, Karmakar S, Carlton J, Joshi A, Krishnatry R, Prabhash K, et al. Radiotherapy for post-chemotherapy residual mass in advanced seminoma: a Fluorodeoxyglucose positron emission tomography-computed tomography-based risk-adapted approach. Clin Oncol R Coll Radiol GB. 2021;33(7):e315–21.
114. Daugaard G, Gundgaard MG, Mortensen MS, Agerbæk M, Holm NV, Rørth M, et al. Surveillance for stage I nonseminoma testicular cancer: outcomes and long-term follow-up in a population-based cohort. J Clin Oncol. 2014;32(34):3817–23.
115. Gumus M, Bilici A, Odabas H, Ustaalioglu BBO, Kandemir N, Demirci U, et al. Outcomes of surveillance versus adjuvant chemotherapy for patients with stage IA and IB nonseminomatous testicular germ cell tumors. World J Urol. 2017;35(7):1103–10.

116. Horwich A, Norman A, Fisher C, Hendry WF, Nicholls J, Dearnaley DP. Primary chemotherapy for stage II nonseminomatous germ cell tumors of the testis. J Urol. 1994;151(1):72–7; discussion 77–78.
117. Aparicio J, Maroto P, García Del Muro X, Sánchez-Muñoz A, Gumà J, Margelí M, et al. Prognostic factors for relapse in stage I seminoma: a new nomogram derived from three consecutive, risk-adapted studies from the Spanish Germ Cell Cancer Group (SGCCG). Ann Oncol. 2014;25(11):2173–8.
118. Joffe JK, Cafferty FH, Murphy L, Rustin GJS, Sohaib SA, Swift S, et al. Imaging modality and frequency in surveillance of stage I seminoma testicular cancer: results from a randomized, phase III, factorial trial (TRISST). J Clin Oncol. 2021;39(6_suppl):374.
119. Warde P, Specht L, Horwich A, Oliver T, Panzarella T, Gospodarowicz M, et al. Prognostic factors for relapse in stage I seminoma managed by surveillance: a pooled analysis. J Clin Oncol. 2002;20(22):4448–52.
120. Oliver RTD, Mason MD, Mead GM, von der Maase H, Rustin GJS, Joffe JK, et al. Radiotherapy versus single-dose carboplatin in adjuvant treatment of stage I seminoma: a randomised trial. Lancet Lond Engl. 2005;366(9482):293–300.
121. de Wit R, Roberts JT, Wilkinson PM, de Mulder PHM, Mead GM, Fosså SD, et al. Equivalence of three or four cycles of bleomycin, etoposide, and cisplatin chemotherapy and of a 3- or 5-day schedule in good-prognosis germ cell Cancer: a randomized study of the European Organization for Research and Treatment of Cancer Genitourinary Tract Cancer Cooperative Group and the Medical Research Council. J Clin Oncol. 2001;19(6):1629–40.
122. Giannatempo P, Greco T, Mariani L, Nicolai N, Tana S, Farè E, et al. Radiotherapy or chemotherapy for clinical stage IIA and IIB seminoma: a systematic review and meta-analysis of patient outcomes. Ann Oncol. 2015;26(4):657–68.
123. Single-dose carboplatin followed by involved-node radiotherapy for stage IIA and stage IIB seminoma (SAKK 01/10): a single-arm, multicentre, phase 2 trial. Lancet Oncol [Internet]. [cited 2023 Jan 31]. Available from: https://www.thelancet.com/journals/lanonc/article/PIIS1470-2045(22)00564-2/fulltext.
124. Tandstad T, Cohn-Cedermark G, Dahl O, Stierner U, Cavallin-Stahl E, Bremnes RM, et al. Long-term follow-up after risk-adapted treatment in clinical stage 1 (CS1) nonseminomatous germ-cell testicular cancer (NSGCT) implementing adjuvant CVB chemotherapy. A SWENOTECA study. Ann Oncol. 2010;21(9):1858–63.
125. Albers P, Siener R, Krege S, Schmelz HU, Dieckmann KP, Heidenreich A, et al. Randomized phase III trial comparing retroperitoneal lymph node dissection with one course of bleomycin and etoposide plus cisplatin chemotherapy in the adjuvant treatment of clinical stage I Nonseminomatous testicular germ cell tumors: AUO trial AH 01/94 by the German Testicular Cancer Study Group. J Clin Oncol. 2008;26(18):2966–72.
126. Oechsle K, Hartmann M, Brenner W, Venz S, Weissbach L, Franzius C, et al. [18F] Fluorodeoxyglucose positron emission tomography in nonseminomatous germ cell tumors after chemotherapy: the German Multicenter Positron Emission Tomography Study Group. J Clin Oncol. 2008;26(36):5930–5.
127. Huddart RA, Gabe R, Cafferty FH, Pollock P, White JD, Shamash J, et al. A randomised phase 2 trial of intensive induction chemotherapy (CBOP/BEP) and standard BEP in poor-prognosis germ cell tumours (MRC TE23, CRUK 05/014, ISRCTN 53643604). Eur Urol. 2015;67(3):534–43.
128. Francolini G, Trodella LE, Marvaso G, Matrone F, Nicosia L, Timon G, et al. Radiotherapy role in nonseminomatous germ cell tumors, radiobiological and technical issues of an unexplored scenario. Int J Clin Oncol. 2021;26(10):1777–83.
129. Laflamme P, Doucet C, Sirois C, Kopek N, Vanhuyse M. Stereotactic radiation therapy for residual chemorefractory primary mediastinal nonseminomatous germ cell tumor after surgical thoracotomy. Pract Radiat Oncol. 2017;7(4):260–3.
130. Schmidberger H, Bamberg M, Meisner C, Classen J, Winkler C, Hartmann M, et al. Radiotherapy in stage IIA and IIB testicular seminoma with reduced portals: a prospective multicenter study. Int J Radiat Oncol Biol Phys. 1997;39(2):321–6.
131. Taylor A, Rockall AG, Reznek RH, Powell MEB. Mapping pelvic lymph nodes: guidelines for delineation in intensity-modulated radiotherapy. Int J Radiat Oncol Biol Phys. 2005;63(5):1604–12.
132. Pure seminoma: a review and update. Radiat Oncol | Full Text [Internet]. [cited 2023 Jan 31]. Available from: https://ro-journal.biomedcentral.com/articles/10.1186/1748-717X-6-90.
133. Dinniwell R, Chan P, Czarnota G, Haider MA, Jhaveri K, Jewett M, et al. Pelvic lymph node topography for radiotherapy treatment planning from ferumoxtran-10 contrast-enhanced magnetic resonance imaging. Int J Radiat Oncol Biol Phys. 2009;74(3):844–51.
134. Zilli T, Boudreau C, Doucet R, Alizadeh M, Lambert C, van Nguyen T, et al. Bone marrow-sparing intensity-modulated radiation therapy for Stage I seminoma. Acta Oncol Stockh Swed. 2011;50(4):555–62.
135. Fung C, Fossa SD, Williams A, Travis LB. Long-term morbidity of testicular cancer treatment. Urol Clin North Am. 2015;42(3):393–408.
136. Travis LB, Fosså SD, Schonfeld SJ, McMaster ML, Lynch CF, Storm H, et al. Second cancers among 40,576 testicular cancer patients: focus on long-term survivors. J Natl Cancer Inst. 2005;97(18):1354–65.
137. Xiang M, Chang DT, Pollom EL. Second cancer risk after primary cancer treatment with three-dimensional conformal, intensity-modulated,

or proton beam radiation therapy. Cancer. 2020;126(15):3560–8.
138. Haugnes HS, Wethal T, Aass N, Dahl O, Klepp O, Langberg CW, et al. Cardiovascular risk factors and morbidity in long-term survivors of testicular cancer: a 20-year follow-up study. J Clin Oncol. 2010;28(30):4649–57.
139. Baird DC, Meyers GJ, Hu JS. Testicular cancer: diagnosis and treatment. Am Fam Physician. 2018;97(4):261–8.
140. Petrelli F, Coinu A, Cabiddu M, Ghilardi M, Borgonovo K, Lonati V, et al. Surveillance or adjuvant treatment with chemotherapy or radiotherapy in stage I seminoma: a systematic review and meta-analysis of 13 studies. Clin Genitourin Cancer. 2015;13(5):428–34.
141. Nauman M, Leslie SW. Nonseminomatous testicular tumors. In: StatPearls [Internet]. Treasure Island: StatPearls Publishing; 2022 [cited 2023 Jan 31]. Available from: http://www.ncbi.nlm.nih.gov/books/NBK568754/.
142. De Martino M, Chieffi P, Esposito F. miRNAs and biomarkers in testicular germ cell tumors: an update. Int J Mol Sci. 2021;22(3):1380.
143. Pasalic D, Prajapati S, Ludmir EB, Tang C, Choi S, Kudchadker R, et al. Outcomes and toxicities of proton and photon radiation therapy for testicular seminoma. Int J Part Ther. 2020;7(2):11–20.
144. Simone CB, Kramer K, O'Meara WP, Bekelman JE, Belard A, McDonough J, et al. Predicted rates of secondary malignancies from proton versus photon radiation therapy for stage I seminoma. Int J Radiat Oncol Biol Phys. 2012;82(1):242–9.
145. Popovic L, Matovina-Brko G, Popovic M, Petrovic D, Cvetanovic A, Vukojevic J, et al. High dose chemotherapy with stem cell support in the treatment of testicular cancer. World J Stem Cells. 2015;7(11):1222–32.
146. Color Doppler US of the postoperative penis: anatomy and surgical complications [Internet]. [cited 2023 Jan 31]. Available from: https://www.researchgate.net/publication/7851905_Color_Doppler_US_of_the_Postoperative_Penis_Anatomy_and_Surgical_Complications1
147. Bandini M, Ahmed M, Basile G, Watkin N, Master V, Zhu Y, et al. A global approach to improving penile cancer care. Nat Rev Urol. 2022;19(4):231–9.
148. Attalla K, Paulucci DJ, Blum K, Anastos H, Moses KA, Badani KK, et al. Demographic and socioeconomic predictors of treatment delays, pathologic stage, and survival among patients with penile cancer: a report from the National Cancer Database. Urol Oncol. 2018;36(1):14.e17–24.
149. Fu L, Tian T, Yao K, Chen XF, Luo G, Gao Y, et al. Global pattern and trends in penile cancer incidence: population-based study. JMIR Public Health Surveill. 2022;8(7):e34874.
150. Morrison BF. Risk factors and prevalence of penile cancer. West Indian Med J. 2014;63(6):559–60.
151. Sewell A, Oxley J. An overview of benign and pre-malignant lesions of the foreskin. Diagn Histopathol. 2019;25(10):390–7.
152. Iorga L, Marcu RD, Diaconu CC, Stanescu AMA, Stoian AP, Mischianu DLD, et al. Penile carcinoma and HPV infection (Review). Exp Ther Med. 2020;20(1):91.
153. Alnajjar HM, Lam W, Bolgeri M, Rees RW, Perry MJA, Watkin NA. Treatment of carcinoma in situ of the glans penis with topical chemotherapy agents. Eur Urol. 2012;62(5):923–8.
154. Frimberger D, Hungerhuber E, Zaak D, Waidelich R, Hofstetter A, Schneede P. Penile carcinoma. Is Nd:YAG laser therapy radical enough. J Urol. 2002;168(6):2418–21; discussion 2421.
155. Meijer RP, Boon TA, van Venrooij GEPM, Wijburg CJ. Long-term follow-up after laser therapy for penile carcinoma. Urology. 2007;69(4):759–62.
156. Li J, Zhu Y, Zhang SL, Wang CF, Yao XD, Dai B, et al. Organ-sparing surgery for penile cancer: complications and outcomes. Urology. 2011;78(5):1121–4.
157. Philippou P, Shabbir M, Malone P, Nigam R, Muneer A, Ralph DJ, et al. Conservative surgery for squamous cell carcinoma of the penis: resection margins and long-term oncological control. J Urol. 2012;188(3):803–8.
158. Minhas S, Kayes O, Hegarty P, Kumar P, Freeman A, Ralph D. What surgical resection margins are required to achieve oncological control in men with primary penile cancer? BJU Int. 2005;96(7):1040–3.
159. Veeratterapillay R, Teo L, Asterling S, Greene D. Oncologic outcomes of penile cancer treatment at a UK Supraregional Center. Urology. 2015;85(5):1097–103.
160. Protzel C, Alcaraz A, Horenblas S, Pizzocaro G, Zlotta A, Hakenberg OW. Lymphadenectomy in the surgical management of penile cancer. Eur Urol. 2009;55(5):1075–88.
161. Kathiresan N, Raja A, Ramachandran KK, Sundersingh S. Role of dynamic sentinel node biopsy in carcinoma penis with or without palpable nodes. Indian J Urol IJU J Urol Soc India. 2016;32(1):57–60.
162. Inguinal lymph node dissection for penile cancer: a contemporary review – Teh. Transl Androl Urol [Internet]. [cited 2023 Jan 31]. Available from: https://tau.amegroups.com/article/view/29112/html.
163. Comparison of different surgical methods and strategies for inguinal lymph node dissection in patients with penile cancer. Sci Rep [Internet]. [cited 2023 Jan 31]. Available from: https://www.nature.com/articles/s41598-022-06494-z.
164. Djajadiningrat RS, van Werkhoven E, Horenblas S. Prophylactic pelvic lymph node dissection in patients with penile cancer. J Urol. 2015;193(6):1976–80.
165. Graafland NM, van Boven HH, van Werkhoven E, Moonen LMF, Horenblas S. Prognostic sig-

nificance of extranodal extension in patients with pathological node positive penile carcinoma. J Urol. 2010;184(4):1347–53.
166. Joshi VB, Chadha J, Chahoud J. Penile cancer: updates in systemic therapy. Asian J Urol. 2022;9(4):374–88.
167. Khurud P, Krishnatry R, Telkhade T, Patil A, Prakash G, Joshi A, et al. Impact of adjuvant treatment in pN3 penile cancer. Clin Oncol. 2022;34(3):172–8.
168. The International Penile Advanced Cancer Trial (InPACT): the first phase III trial for squamous carcinoma of the penis with regional lymph node metastases. J Clin Oncol [Internet]. [cited 2023 Jan 31]. Available from: https://ascopubs.org/doi/abs/10.1200/JCO.2022.40.6_suppl.TPS7.
169. Gerbaulet A, Lambin P. Radiation therapy of cancer of the penis. Indications, advantages, and pitfalls. Urol Clin North Am. 1992;19(2):325–32.
170. McLean M, Akl AM, Warde P, Bissett R, Panzarella T, Gospodarowicz M. The results of primary radiation therapy in the management of squamous cell carcinoma of the penis. Int J Radiat Oncol Biol Phys. 1993;25(4):623–8.
171. Sagerman RH, Yu WS, Chung CT, Puranik A. External-beam irradiation of carcinoma of the penis. Radiology. 1984;152(1):183–5.
172. Krishnatry R, Mangaj A, Bhajbhuje R, Murthy V. Indigenous groin board immobilization reduces planning target volume margins in groin radiotherapy. J Med Phys. 2021;46(2):88.
173. Mittal R, Krishnatry R, Maitre P, Murthy V. Recommendations and clinical validation of inguinal clinical target volume delineation in penile cancer. Int J Radiat Oncol Biol Phys. 2021;111(3):741–53.
174. Patel A, Naghavi AO, Johnstone PA, Spiess PE, Grass GD. Updates in the use of radiotherapy in the management of primary and locally-advanced penile cancer. Asian J Urol. 2022;9(4):389–406.
175. Khurud P, Gupta A, Krishnatry R, Panigrahi G, Phurailatpam RD, Menon S, Pal M, Bakshi G, Prakash G, Murthy V. Optimizing Target Volume for Adjuvant Radiation Therapy in Penile Cancer. Pract Radiat Oncol. 2023;13(3):e270–e277. https://doi.org/10.1016/j.prro.2022.11.001. Epub 2022 Nov 30. PMID: 36460183.
176. Korzeniowski MA, Crook JM. Contemporary role of radiotherapy in the management of penile cancer. Transl Androl Urol. 2017;6(5):855–67.
177. Crook JM, Haie-Meder C, Demanes DJ, Mazeron JJ, Martinez AA, Rivard MJ. American Brachytherapy Society–Groupe Européen de Curiethérapie–European Society of Therapeutic Radiation Oncology (ABS-GEC-ESTRO) consensus statement for penile brachytherapy. Brachytherapy. 2013;12(3):191–8.
178. Crook J, Grimard L, Tsihlias J, Morash C, Panzarella T. Interstitial brachytherapy for penile cancer: an alternative to amputation. J Urol. 2002;167(2 Part 1):506–11.
179. Crook J, Jezioranski J, Cygler JE. Penile brachytherapy: technical aspects and postimplant issues. Brachytherapy. 2010;9(2):151–8.
180. Chaudhary AJ, Ghosh S, Bhalavat RL, Kulkarni JN, Sequeira BVE. Interstitial brachytherapy in carcinoma of the penis. Strahlenther Onkol. 1999;175(1):17–20.
181. Hasan S, Francis A, Hagenauer A, Hirsh A, Kaminsky D, Traughber B, et al. The role of brachytherapy in organ preservation for penile cancer: a meta-analysis and review of the literature. Brachytherapy. 2015;14(4):517–24.
182. Soh PN, Delaunay B, Nasr EB, Delannes M, Soulie M, Huyghe E. Evaluation of sexual functions and sexual behaviors after penile brachytherapy in men treated for penile carcinoma. Basic Clin Androl. 2014;24:13.
183. Gambachidze D, Lebacle C, Maroun P, Escande A, Bossi A, Blanchard P, et al. Long-term evaluation of urinary, sexual, and quality of life outcomes after brachytherapy for penile carcinoma. Brachytherapy. 2018;17(1):221–6.
184. Brachytherapy for penile cancer: efficacy and impact on sexual function. ScienceDirect [Internet]. [cited 2023 Feb 1]. Available from: https://www.sciencedirect.com/science/article/pii/S1538472113002833.
185. The relationship between HPV status and chemoradiotherapy in the locoregional control of penile cancer. PMC [Internet]. [cited 2023 Feb 1]. Available from: https://www.ncbi.nlm.nih.gov/pmc/articles/PMC7771321/.
186. Jayson M, Sanders H. Increased incidence of serendipitously discovered renal cell carcinoma. Urology. 1998;51(2):203–5.
187. Davidson AJ, Hartman DS, Choyke PL, Wagner BJ. Radiologic assessment of renal masses: implications for patient care. Radiology. 1997;202(2):297–305.
188. Wang HY, Ding HJ, Chen JH, Chao CH, Lu YY, Lin WY, et al. Meta-analysis of the diagnostic performance of [18F]FDG-PET and PET/CT in renal cell carcinoma. Cancer Imaging. 2012;12(3):464–74.
189. A prospective, randomised EORTC intergroup phase 3 study comparing the oncologic outcome of elective nephron-sparing surgery and radical nephrectomy for low-stage renal cell carcinoma. PubMed [Internet]. [cited 2023 Jan 18]. Available from: https://pubmed.ncbi.nlm.nih.gov/21186077/.
190. Nephron-sparing techniques independently decrease the risk of cardiovascular events relative to radical nephrectomy in patients with a T1a-T1b renal mass and normal preoperative renal function. PubMed [Internet]. [cited 2023 Jan 18]. Available from: https://pubmed.ncbi.nlm.nih.gov/25282367/.
191. MacLennan S, Imamura M, Lapitan MC, Omar MI, Lam TBL, Hilvano-Cabungcal AM, et al. Systematic review of perioperative and quality-of-life outcomes following surgical management of localised renal cancer. Eur Urol. 2012;62(6):1097–117.

192. Bhindi B, Abel EJ, Albiges L, Bensalah K, Boorjian SA, Daneshmand S, et al. Systematic review of the role of cytoreductive nephrectomy in the targeted therapy era and beyond: an individualized approach to metastatic renal cell carcinoma. Eur Urol. 2019;75(1):111–28.
193. Sunitinib alone or after nephrectomy in metastatic renal-cell carcinoma. NEJM [Internet]. [cited 2023 Jan 18]. Available from: https://www.nejm.org/doi/full/10.1056/NEJMoa1803675.
194. Comparison of immediate vs deferred cytoreductive nephrectomy in patients with synchronous metastatic renal cell carcinoma receiving sunitinib: the SURTIME randomized clinical trial. Nephrology. JAMA Oncol. JAMA Netw [Internet]. [cited 2023 Jan 18]. Available from: https://jamanetwork.com/journals/jamaoncology/fullarticle/2718007.
195. Song CW, Glatstein E, Marks LB, Emami B, Grimm J, Sperduto PW, et al. Biological principles of stereotactic body radiation therapy (SBRT) and stereotactic radiation surgery (SRS): indirect cell death. Int J Radiat Oncol Biol Phys. 2021;110(1):21–34.
196. Garcia-Barros M, Paris F, Cordon-Cardo C, Lyden D, Rafii S, Haimovitz-Friedman A, et al. Tumor response to radiotherapy regulated by endothelial cell apoptosis. Science. 2003;300(5622):1155–9.
197. Siva S, Ellis RJ, Ponsky L, Teh BS, Mahadevan A, Muacevic A, et al. Consensus statement from the International Radiosurgery Oncology Consortium for Kidney for primary renal cell carcinoma. Future Oncol Lond Engl. 2016;12(5):637–45.
198. Ali M, Mooi J, Lawrentschuk N, McKay RR, Hannan R, Lo SS, et al. The role of stereotactic ablative body radiotherapy in renal cell carcinoma. Eur Urol. 2022;82(6):613–22.
199. Cheung P, Patel S, North SA, Sahgal A, Chu W, Soliman H, et al. Stereotactic radiotherapy for oligoprogression in metastatic renal cell cancer patients receiving tyrosine kinase inhibitor therapy: a phase 2 prospective multicenter study. Eur Urol. 2021;80(6):693–700.
200. Hannan R, Margulis V, Chun SG, Cannon N, Kim DWN, Abdulrahman RE, et al. Stereotactic radiation therapy of renal cancer inferior vena cava tumor thrombus. Cancer Biol Ther. 2015;16(5):657–61.
201. Freifeld Y, Pedrosa I, Mclaughlin M, Correa RM, Louie AV, Maldonado JA, et al. Stereotactic ablative radiation therapy for renal cell carcinoma with inferior vena cava tumor thrombus. Urol Oncol. 2022;40(4):166.e9–166.e13.
202. Siva S, Chesson B, Bressel M, Pryor D, Higgs B, Reynolds HM, et al. TROG 15.03 phase II clinical trial of Focal Ablative STereotactic Radiosurgery for Cancers of the Kidney – FASTRACK II. BMC Cancer. 2018;18(1):1030.
203. Kothari G, Foroudi F, Gill S, Corcoran NM, Siva S. Outcomes of stereotactic radiotherapy for cranial and extracranial metastatic renal cell carcinoma: a systematic review. Acta Oncol Stockh Swed. 2015;54(2):148–57.
204. Chow J, Hoffend NC, Abrams SI, Schwaab T, Singh AK, Muhitch JB. Radiation induces dynamic changes to the T cell repertoire in renal cell carcinoma patients. Proc Natl Acad Sci USA. 2020;117(38):23721–9.
205. Zagoria RJ, Hawkins AD, Clark PE, Hall MC, Matlaga BR, Dyer RB, et al. Percutaneous CT-guided radiofrequency ablation of renal neoplasms: factors influencing success. AJR Am J Roentgenol. 2004;183(1):201–7.
206. Ravaud A, Motzer RJ, Pandha HS, George DJ, Pantuck AJ, Patel A, et al. Adjuvant sunitinib in high-risk renal-cell carcinoma after nephrectomy. N Engl J Med. 2016;375(23):2246–54.
207. Laukhtina E, Quhal F, Mori K, Sari Motlagh R, Pradere B, Schuettfort VM, et al. Adjuvant therapy with tyrosine kinase inhibitors for localized and locally advanced renal cell carcinoma: an updated systematic review and meta-analysis. Urol Oncol Semin Orig Investig. 2021;39(11):764–73.
208. Deleuze A, Saout J, Dugay F, Peyronnet B, Mathieu R, Verhoest G, et al. Immunotherapy in renal cell carcinoma: the future is now. Int J Mol Sci. 2020;21(7):2532.
209. Pazopanib versus sunitinib in metastatic renal-cell carcinoma. NEJM [Internet]. [cited 2023 Feb 1]. Available from: https://www.nejm.org/doi/full/10.1056/nejmoa1303989.
210. Smith ML, Crook J, Algan O. Radiation therapy for the management of penile cancer. J Radiat Oncol. 2016;5(2):143–51.
211. Van As N, Griffin C, Tree A, et al. Phase 3 Trial of Stereotactic Body Radiotherapy in Localized Prostate Cancer. N Engl J Med. 2024;391:1413–25.
212. Murthy V, Maitre P, Arunsingh M, et al. OC-0924 Prostate RT In high risk or N+ Moderate vs Extreme hypofractionation (PRIME): An Interim analysis. Radiother Oncol. 2023;182:S770–S771.
213. Singh M, Katdare A, Ghosh S, et al. PSMA-PET Guided Intraprostatic Boost in Prostate SBRT (PROBE): A Phase 2 Trial. Int J Radiat Oncol. 2025;S0360301625002615. https://doi.org/10.1016/j.ijrobp.2025.03.033.
214. Draulans C, Haustermans K, Pos FJ, et al. Stereotactic body radiotherapy with a focal boost to the intraprostatic tumor for intermediate and high risk prostate cancer: 5-year efficacy and toxicity in the hypo-FLAME trial. Radiother Oncol. 2024;201:110568. https://doi.org/10.1016/j.radonc.2024.110568.
215. Kishan AU, Lamb JM, Wilhame H, et al. Magnetic Resonance Imaging-Guided vs. Computed Tomography-Guided Stereotactic Body Radiotherapy for Prostate Cancer: 2-Year Outcomes from the MIRAGE Randomized Clinical Trial. Int J Radiat Oncol. 2024;120:S124.
216. Singh M, Maitre P, Krishnan A, et al. Late Urinary Toxicity After Extreme or Moderate Hypofractionated Prostate Radiation Therapy in

Patients With Prior Transurethral Resection of Prostate. Int J Radiat Oncol. 2024;120:1011–20.
217. Wisdom AJ, Yeap BY, Michalski JM, et al. Setting the Stage: Feasibility and Baseline Characteristics in the PARTIQoL Trial Comparing Proton Therapy Versus Intensity Modulated Radiation Therapy for Localized Prostate Cancer. Int J Radiat Oncol. 2025;121:741–51.
218. Chilukuri S, Sundar SC, Subramani V, et al. Pre-PROTO-PRIME: stereotactic body proton therapy to the prostate and pelvic nodes for high-risk and node-positive prostate cancer — feasibility, acute toxicity and dosimetric insights. Clin Transl Radiat Oncol. 2026;56:101084.
219. Ost P, Siva S, Brabrand S, et al. Salvage metastasis-directed therapy versus elective nodal radiotherapy for oligorecurrent nodal prostate cancer metastases (PEACE V–STORM): a phase 2, open-label, randomised controlled trial. Lancet Oncol. 2025;26:695–706.
220. Verma P, Maitre P, Krishnasamy GS, et al. Progression of index metastases in oligometastatic hormone-sensitive prostate cancer: implications for metastases directed therapy? Prostate Cancer Prostatic Dis. 2025. https://doi.org/10.1038/s41391-025-01056-6.
221. Tang C, Sherry AD, Hwang H, et al. World-wide oligometastatic prostate cancer (omPC) meta-analysis leveraging individual patient data (IPD) from randomized trials (WOLVERINE): An analysis from the X-MET collaboration. J Clin Oncol 2025; 43:15–15.
222. Bossi A, Foulon S, Maldonado X, et al. Efficacy and safety of prostate radiotherapy in de novo metastatic castration-sensitive prostate cancer (PEACE-1): a multicentre, open-label, randomised, phase 3 study with a 2 × 2 factorial design. The Lancet. 2024;404:2065–76.
223. Krishnan A, Maitre P, Kashid S, et al. Online Adaptive Radiation Therapy for Bladder Preservation: Transitioning to Hypofractionation. Int J Radiat Oncol. 2025;122:995–1001.
224. Murthy V, Maitre P, Pal M, et al. Bladder Adjuvant RadioTherapy (BART): Clinical Outcomes from a Phase III Multicenter Randomized Controlled Trial. Int J Radiat Oncol. 2025;123:S32.
225. Murthy V, Maitre P, Bakshi G, et al. Bladder Adjuvant Radiation Therapy (BART): Acute and Late Toxicity From a Phase III Multicenter Randomized Controlled Trial. Int J Radiat Oncol Biol Phys. 2025;121:728–736.
226. Murthy V, Kashid SR, Pal M, et al. Prospective comparative study of quality of life in patients with bladder cancer undergoing cystectomy with ileal conduit or bladder preservation. BMJ Oncol. 2024;3:e000435.
227. Siva S, Bressel M, Sidhom M, et al. Stereotactic ablative body radiotherapy for primary kidney cancer (TROG 15.03 FASTRACK II): a non-randomised phase 2 trial. Lancet Oncol. 2024;25:308–316.
228. Jukaku S, Doshi J, Singh M, et al. Stereotactic body radiation therapy for inferior vena cava tumor thrombus in clear cell renal cell carcinoma: A case report and literature review. J UroOncology. 2026;1:38-44.
229. Fassnacht M, Dekkers OM, Else T, et al. European Society of Endocrinology Clinical Practice Guidelines on the management of adrenocortical carcinoma in adults, in collaboration with the European Network for the Study of Adrenal Tumors. Eur J Endocrinol. 2018;179:G1–G46.
230. Subramani V, Chauhan, H, David S, Maitre P, Menon S, Joshi A et al. Efficacy and safety of adjuvant radiotherapy in primary resected adrenocortical carcinoma – A comparative study. Journal of Uro-Oncology. 2026;1: 24–30.

Online Links

Target volume delineation in prostate:
https://youtu.be/Cydnkmpn9x0
Hypofractionation in Ca Prostate:
https://youtu.be/AZOpn3g9yeQ
https://youtu.be/faI3GsUlPag
Brachytherapy for prostate cancer:
https://youtu.be/Q0T3JikUDT0
High Risk prostate cancer:
https://youtu.be/YoXXdCVinWI
https://www.youtube.com/live/uWAiPEU9-6U?feature=share
Role of local RT in metastatic prostate cancer:
https://youtu.be/ApapSp4i53w
Management of bladder cancers:
https://youtu.be/d60d6X1-ABI
https://www.youtube.com/live/YlKwB_pFrA0?feature=share
Management of Testicular cancers:
https://youtu.be/AogA0J4ninI
https://youtu.be/qXheqPUvZbk
https://www.youtube.com/live/XMVdNyLPcJI?feature=share
Management of metastatic RCC:
https://youtu.be/M5P7Vrr0jN0

Gynaecological Cancers

Raviteja Miriyala, Andrew Keller, Kiriti Chiriki, Stephen Abel, K. K. Sreelakshmi, Ankur Patel, Umesh Mahantshetty, and Sushil Beriwal

1 Introduction

Gynaecological cancers contribute substantially to morbidity and mortality among women globally. Though the relative burden of HPV-associated gynaecological cancers (cervical, vaginal, and vulvar cancers) is decreasing in developed countries, they continue to be a significant public health problem in low- and low-middle-income countries. Simultaneous increase in the incidence of endometrial and ovarian cancers in the past few decades furthers the strain on the health infrastructure of developing economies. While multidisciplinary decision-making is paramount in the management of gynaecological cancers, radiation plays a crucial role in definitive, adjuvant, neo-adjuvant, as well as palliative settings in these patients. The following sections discuss the principles of management of gynaecological cancers with a special focus on evidence-based practice of Radiation Oncology.

R. Miriyala · K. Chiriki · U. Mahantshetty (✉)
Homi Bhabha Cancer Hospital and Research Centre, Visakhapatnam, India

A. Keller
Advent Health Cancer Institute, University of Central Florida College of Medicine, Orlando, FL, USA

S. Abel · K. K. Sreelakshmi · A. Patel · S. Beriwal (✉)
Allegheny Health Network Cancer Institute, Pittsburgh, PA, USA
e-mail: Stephen.abel@ahn.org; Ankur.Patel4@AHN.org

2 Cervical Cancer

2.1 Anatomy and Patterns of Spread

The uterus is a hollow muscular organ, about 7–8 cm long, located in the pelvis between the bladder and the rectum. The inverted pear-shaped organ has a corpus that is connected to the fallopian tubes superiorly, and a narrow cervix that communicates with the vagina inferiorly. The uterine cervix, which is about 3 cm long, is divided into a supra-vaginal and vaginal parts. Usually, the utero-cervical and cervico-vaginal axes have an anterior tilt (ante-flexion and ante-version, respectively).

The uterine fundus is supported laterally by the round ligaments and broad ligaments, while the uterine cervix is attached to the pelvic wall by uterosacral ligaments posteriorly and transverse cervical (cardinal) ligaments laterally. The lower part of the broad ligaments, which is lateral to the cervix and inferior to the uterine arteries, contains loose parametrial tissue and is a critical area for the spread of cervical cancer.

The uterus, and especially the uterine cervix, has a rich lymphatic network that drains initially into the para-cervical nodes, and thereafter to medial external iliac (obturator) nodes, internal iliac nodes, and presacral nodes, and eventually to common iliac and para-aortic nodal basins. Fundal lymphatics also have a direct drainage

B. K. Mohanti et al. (eds.), *Radiation Oncology – Principles, Precepts and Practice*,
https://doi.org/10.1007/978-981-95-5171-2_14

into the common iliac and para-aortic chains through the broad ligament along the ovarian vessels.

Histologically, the uterus has three distinct layers, the outer serosa, middle myometrium and inner endometrium. The endocervical canal connects the endometrial cavity through the internal os and with the vaginal cavity through the external os. The junction between the squamous epithelium of the ectocervix and the columnar epithelium of the endocervix, known as the squamo-columnar junction, recedes proximally from puberty to adulthood. This area of transition, between the original and final squamo-columnar junctions, known as the transformational zone, is considered highly active for the development of metaplasia and malignancy.

2.2 Epidemiology and Risk Factors

Cervical cancer is the fourth most common cancer and fourth leading cause of cancer-related mortality among women globally [1]. Significant disparities in incidence, stage at diagnosis and mortality exist across the world, largely due to differences in access to awareness, screening, and early detection programs. In most developing countries, cervical cancer continues to be the second most common cancer diagnosed in women [2]. Approximately 84% of cervical cancer incidence and 88% of cervical cancer mortality occur in countries with low Human Development Index (HDI), reflecting the importance of socioeconomic factors in addressing the global challenges associated with cervical cancer control [3].

Persistent infection with Human Papillomavirus (HPV) is the most significant factor associated with the development of invasive cervical cancer. Estimates indicate an association of HPV with more than 90% of cervical cancer cases, especially with high-risk subtypes 16 and 18 and less frequently with other subtypes like 31, 33, 35, 39, 45, 51, 52, 56, and 58, among others.

Consequently, risk factors for the development of invasive cervical cancer include those associated with persistent HPV infection, like initiation of sexual activity at a young age, multiple sexual partners, young age at first childbirth, multiparity, low socioeconomic status, poor genital hygiene, sexually transmitted infections, and immunocompromised state, among others. Other less frequently associated cofactors include active smoking and the use of oral contraceptive pills.

2.3 Clinical Presentation

In regions with effective screening programs, cervical cancer is frequently diagnosed in asymptomatic women during routine gynaecological examination. Postcoital bleeding, heavy menstrual bleeding, intermenstrual bleeding, and vaginal discharge are frequently reported in symptomatic women. Systemic symptoms like fatigue and breathlessness may indicate underlying anaemia. Pain is often an ominous symptom associated with advanced disease and may occur in the pelvic region due to involvement of utero-sacral ligaments or pelvic inflammation, and in the abdominal region due to retroperitoneal lymphadenopathy, hydronephrosis, or visceral metastases. Other symptoms of advanced disease include pedal oedema due to lymphadenopathy or venous thrombosis or renal dysfunction; cough due to lung metastases; or leakage of urine or faecal matter through the vagina due to fistulous communication.

2.4 Diagnostic and Staging Investigations

Complete physical and bimanual pelvic examinations that include per-speculum, per-vaginal and per-rectal examinations should be performed in all patients with suspected cervical cancer. Ideally, examination should be done under short general anaesthesia by two physicians—a Radiation Oncologist and a Gynaecological Oncologist—and findings corroborated, especially for early-stage cervical cancer before surgical management is offered, or when there is a discrepancy between clinical and imaging findings. Clinical examination findings should be documented in three dimensions on a scaled clinical drawing, especially when chemoradiation is offered; this helps in adapting the target volumes at the time of image-based brachytherapy [4].

Biopsy and histopathology of the primary lesion are mandatory to establish invasive cancer and for subtyping. Immunohistochemistry can be considered in selective cases. Large cell non-keratinizing squamous cell carcinoma is the most common histological variant, representing 70–80% of cases. Recently, cervical adenocarcinomas have been subclassified into various subtypes based on association with HPV [5].

Routine blood investigations should include a minimum of a complete hemogram, renal function tests, and HIV serology. Coagulation profile, liver function tests, serum electrolytes, and urine microscopy can be considered depending on the clinical scenario.

Clinical examination forms the crux of staging of cervical cancer. Previous reports by the International Federation of Gynaecology and Obstetrics (FIGO) recommend the use of chest radiographs, abdominal ultrasonography, and intravenous pyelography as the minimum investigations for staging of cervical cancer, considering the resource constraints in LMICs and LICs. The latest staging system (FIGO 2018) does not recommend any imaging modality over others. It allows the use of any available imaging modality and/or pathological findings in addition to clinical examination, for establishing the stage of the disease (Table 1).

Vaginal extension is best identified by clinical examination. Diagnostic CT often underestimates uterine extension and overestimates parametrial extension, except for very small tumours. Magnetic resonance imaging (MRI) is considered superior to computed tomography (CT) for identifying gross disease, uterine extension, and parametrial extension due to superior soft tissue resolution. Transrectal ultrasound has been found to be comparable to MRI for detecting parametrial extension, especially in early-stage cervical cancer [6].

Both CT and MRI are considered to have comparable sensitivity and specificity for evaluation of regional nodal metastases; however, the accuracy of MRI with dynamic sequences or PET-CT may be higher for smaller nodes that are indeterminate on CT. A recent pilot study reported that PET-MRI might have superior performance compared to PET-CT with a potential impact on treatment decision in 50% of patients [7]. Sensitivity and specificity of various imaging modalities for nodal staging in cervical cancer are summarized in Table 2 [8]. Functional MRI sequences such as diffusion-weighted imaging (DWI) and dynamic contrast enhancement (DCE) may assist with diagnosis and prognostication in cervical cancer and are currently being evaluated in prospective settings [9].

Cystoscopy and proctosigmoidoscopy should be considered in patients with suspicious symptoms or imaging findings suggestive of invasion into the bladder or rectum, respectively. Documentation of the extent of infiltration can be of assistance in determining the treatment intent, with infiltration less than 1 × 1 cm being considered as focal and more than that being diffuse [10]. Though biopsy from the bladder/rectal infiltration is recommended by FIGO for establishing stage IVA, concerns regarding increased risk of fistula formation with deep biopsies preclude widespread adaptation of this practice. Fine needle aspiration cytology can be considered for metastatic lesions in non-regional lymph nodes or visceral lesions, especially if it potentially upstages the disease.

2.5 General Principles of Management

2.5.1 Early Cervical Cancer

Early cervical cancer includes FIGO (2018) stages IA, IB1, IB2 and IIA1. Patients in these stages have excellent outcomes with single modality treatment (surgery or radiation). Combining surgery and radiation in these patients has been shown to increase treatment-related side effects, and hence all measures should be taken to avoid such scenarios [11].

Table 1 FIGO 2018 staging: Cervical cancer

Stage I:
The carcinoma is strictly confined to the cervix uteri (extension to the corpus should be disregarded)
IA Invasive carcinoma that can be diagnosed only by microscopy, with maximum depth of invasion <5 mm[a]
IA1 Measured stromal invasion <3 mm in depth
IA2 Measured stromal invasion ≥3 mm and <5 mm in depth
IB Invasive carcinoma with measured deepest invasion ≥5 mm (greater than stage IA), lesion limited to the cervix uteri[b]
IB1 Invasive carcinoma ≥5 mm depth of stromal invasion and <2 cm in greatest dimension
IB2 Invasive carcinoma ≥2 cm and <4 cm in greatest dimension
IB3 Invasive carcinoma ≥4 cm in the greatest dimension
Stage II:
The carcinoma invades beyond the uterus but has not extended onto the lower third of the vagina or to the pelvic wall
IIA Involvement limited to the upper two-thirds of the vagina without parametrial involvement
IIA1 Invasive carcinoma <4 cm in greatest dimension
IIA2 Invasive carcinoma ≥4 cm in greatest dimension
IIB With parametrial involvement but not up to the pelvic wall
Stage III:
The carcinoma involves the lower third of the vagina and/or extends to the pelvic wall and/or causes hydronephrosis or non-functioning kidney and/or involves pelvic and/or paraaortic lymph nodes[c]
IIIA Carcinoma involves the lower third of the vagina, with no extension to the pelvic wall
IIIB Extension to the pelvic wall and/or hydronephrosis or non-functioning kidney (unless known to be due to another cause)
IIIC Involvement of pelvic and/or paraaortic lymph nodes, irrespective of tumour size and extent (with r and p notations)[c]
IIIC1 Pelvic lymph node metastasis only
IIIC2 Paraaortic lymph node metastasis
Stage IV:
The carcinoma has extended beyond the true pelvis or has involved (biopsy-proven) the mucosa of the bladder or rectum. A bullous oedema, as such, does not permit a case to be allotted to stage IV
IVA Spread of the growth to adjacent organs
IVB Spread to distant organs

[a]Imaging and pathology can be used, when available, to supplement clinical findings with respect to tumour size and extent, in all stages

[b]The involvement of vascular/lymphatic spaces does not change the staging. The lateral extent of the lesion is no longer considered

[c]Adding notation of r (imaging) and p (pathology) to indicate the findings that are used to allocate the case to stage IIIC. For example, if imaging indicates pelvic lymph node metastasis, the stage allocation would be stage IIIC1r and, if confirmed by pathological findings, it would be stage IIIc1p. The type of imaging modality or pathology technique used should always be documented. When in doubt, the lower staging should be assigned

Table 2 Imaging modalities for pelvic nodal assessment

Imaging modality	Lymph node involvement	
	Sensitivity	Specificity
CT	31–58	92–97
MRI	37–71	83–93
DWI	86	84
PET-CT	34–82	93–100
PET-MRI	83–91	90–94

Historically, the presence of certain risk factors in the post-op histopathology has been shown to increase the risk of loco-regional recurrences, and they have been used in various combinations to decide on adjuvant treatment for such patients [12].

Intermediate risk factors for loco-regional recurrence include tumour dimension more than

4 cm (in histopathology), deep stromal invasion (extension to the outer third of the cervix) and presence of lympho-vascular space invasion. The presence of any two out of the three intermediate risk factors increases the risk of pelvic recurrences. In the landmark randomized controlled trial by Sedlis et al., the addition of adjuvant external beam radiotherapy was shown to reduce the rate of any recurrence from 28% to 15% [13]. Long-term follow-up of this study revealed improved progression-free survival and a trend towards improvement in overall survival, but it was underpowered for statistical significance [14]. Histology-specific nomograms may help predict recurrence risk in squamous cell carcinoma and adenocarcinoma based on different pathologic risk factors unique to each histology [15]. Addition of concurrent chemotherapy in this context has not yet been proven to be beneficial in a recent randomized controlled trial [16].

High risk factors include parametrial involvement, vaginal cuff margin positivity and nodal metastasis. The presence of even one high-risk factor is an indication for adjuvant radiotherapy with concurrent chemotherapy, which was shown to improve loco-regional control as well as overall survival [17]. Addition of chemotherapy after concurrent chemoradiotherapy did not improve outcomes in a recent randomized controlled trial [18].

There is no evidence-based consensus on the addition of vaginal cuff brachytherapy to adjuvant radiotherapy in intermediate or high-risk patients. It should be noted that the Sedlis trial did not mandate the use of vaginal cuff brachytherapy, and a substantial number of recurrences in the radiotherapy arm were observed in the vagina. Though contemporary clinical trials of adjuvant radiation use vaginal brachytherapy along with EBRT for all patients [19], patients with positive vaginal cuff margin and deep stromal invasion are likely to derive maximum benefit with the addition of vaginal cuff brachytherapy [20]. Unlike in endometrial cancer, there is no evidence to support vaginal cuff brachytherapy alone as an adjuvant treatment in cervical cancer, especially since the Sedlis criteria are considered risk factors for local as well as regional recurrences.

Among the histopathological risk factors for adjuvant treatment, parametrial invasion, pelvic node involvement and size of the tumour can be reliably predicted using pre-treatment MRI. While the presence of LVSI on deep biopsy or conization specimen can be reliably considered as an intermediate risk factor, absence of LVSI on biopsy may not correlate with the findings on surgical pathology. Hence, all possible information regarding the potential need for adjuvant treatment should be obtained before patients with early-stage cervical cancer are considered for surgical management, to avoid combined modality treatment.

2.5.2 Locally Advanced Cervical Cancer

Locally advanced cervical cancer includes the rest of the FIGO (2018) stages up to and including IVA. Historically, external beam radiotherapy followed by brachytherapy was considered the standard treatment for locally advanced cervical cancer. Several landmark clinical trials and meta-analyses have demonstrated improvement in survival outcomes when platinum-based chemotherapy is used concurrently with radiotherapy [21–27]. Following the National Cancer Institute (NCI) alerts of the late 1990s, concurrent chemoradiotherapy and brachytherapy became the standard of care for locally advanced cervical cancer [20, 28, 29]. While the initial trials reported maximum benefit of the addition of chemotherapy in stage II cervical cancer, subsequent studies demonstrated significant improvement in patients with stage III as well [30].

Traditionally, brachytherapy for cervical cancer was delivered with intracavitary applicators, and the dose prescription was point-based using two-dimensional (X-ray-based) planning. In the past few decades, the use of image-guided adaptive brachytherapy (IGABT) using MRI for target volume delineation and volume-based dose prescription has gained prominence. With such an approach, excellent 5-year local control rates of over 90% have been demonstrated in a large-scale prospective international multi-centre study

[31]. Use of alternate modalities like CT with or without TRUS has also been explored for image-guided adaptive brachytherapy, and recommendations have been published for target volume delineation in various environments [4]. However, MRI remains the preferred option for image-guided adaptive brachytherapy, and the use of alternative modalities for IGABT needs to be validated in large-scale prospective studies before it can be adopted in routine clinical practice [32].

Neoadjuvant chemotherapy followed by surgery has been tested as an alternative to radical chemoradiation in locally advanced cervical cancer, to cater to regions with limited access to radiation facilities. While such an approach was considered comparable to radical radiation alone, outcomes were reported to be significantly worse compared to concurrent chemoradiation in a large randomized controlled study, and thus a chemo-surgical approach should not be offered to patients in routine practice [33, 34].

Considering the patterns of failure after radical chemoradiation, adjuvant chemotherapy was tested in prospective clinical trials to improve distant control. While one prospective randomized study [35] evaluated the addition of gemcitabine to cisplatin in the concurrent and adjuvant settings and demonstrated modest improvements in outcomes, the other recent international multicentric trial using taxane and platinum-based adjuvant chemotherapy did not demonstrate clinically significant improvements in outcomes [36]. Consequently, current guidelines do not recommend routine use of adjuvant chemotherapy after radical chemoradiation in locally advanced cervical cancer [20, 28, 29]. While the addition of concurrent and adjuvant durvalumab failed to improve outcomes in locally advanced cervical cancer [37], the addition of concurrent and adjuvant pembrolizumab immunotherapy has recently been shown to improve outcomes in patients with 2+ pelvic lymph nodes or 1+ para-aortic lymph nodes or otherwise stage III-IVA disease [38].

2.5.3 Metastatic Cervical Cancer

Patients with limited metastases in non-regional nodes can be considered for treatment with curative intent, especially if the local disease is not extensive and responds well to chemotherapy. Addition of Stereotactic Body Radiotherapy (SBRT) to oligometastatic disease sites has been shown to improve survival outcomes in phase II studies and can be considered in selected patients [39].

Outcomes in patients with extensive or visceral metastases are generally poor, and treatment should be customized and symptom-directed [10]. Paclitaxel, carboplatin, cisplatin, gemcitabine, and 5-Flurouracil are active agents that can be considered alone or in combination. Modest improvement in survival has been reported with the addition of targeted agents like bevacizumab or immunotherapy with PD1/PDL1 inhibitors to platinum-based combination chemotherapy [20, 28, 29]. Short-course radiotherapy to the primary disease should be considered even for patients with metastatic cancer for effective palliation of symptoms [10].

2.6 Principles of Surgery

Surgical management of early-stage cervical cancer includes addressing the primary as well as elective nodal regions depending on the estimated risk of involvement. Prevalence of nodal metastases in pelvic and para-aortic nodal regions varies according to the stage of the primary disease. Conventionally, the risk of microscopic nodal metastases is deemed to be significant enough in patients with stage IA2 and above, and hence, elective addressal of pelvic nodal basins is recommended as part of curative surgery in such patients.

Historically, various classifications were used to describe the extent of surgery for cervical cancer. Piver–Rutledge–Smith (PRS) classification proposed in the late twentieth century divided hysterectomies into five distinct 'classes', I through V. Later, Surgeons Committee of the Gynaecologic Cancer Group of the European Organization of Research and Treatment of Cancer (GCG-EORTC) suggested an alternate classification into 5 'types', I through V, to standardize the surgical extent across European centres. More recently, the classification system proposed by Querleu and Morrow (QM) has been gaining wider acceptance, due to its inclusion of autonomic nerve sparing and paracervical lymphadenectomy in certain subtypes. QM classification of hysterectomies is summarized in Table 3.

For patients with incidentally detected malignancy after simple hysterectomy, various factors like size of the primary, presence of lymphovascular space invasion, stromal invasion, histology and grade, and status of margins need to be considered before offering completion surgery.

Fertility-preserving surgery in the form of radical trachelectomy can be offered to a very selected group of patients with early-stage cancer, with (IA2) or without (IA1) pelvic lymphadenectomy.

Table 3 Querleu and Morrow classification of hysterectomies

Type A (extra-fascial hysterectomy)	Para-cervix resected medial to ureter Vaginal resection as small as possible (less than 10 mm) without removal of para-colpos
Type B (modified radical hysterectomy)	Partial resection of vesico-uterine and uterosacral ligaments Unroofing of ureter Para-cervix transected at the level of ureteral tunnel Lateral para-cervical lymph nodes removed in Type B2 but not in Type B1 Removal of at least 1 cm of uninvolved vagina
Type C (classical radical hysterectomy)	Complete resection of vesico-uterine and uterosacral ligaments Ureters fully mobilized Para-cervix resected completely Autonomic nerves are spared in Type C1 but not in Type C2 Removal of 1.5–2 cm of uninvolved vagina, with corresponding para-colpos
Type D	Resection of tissues till pelvic side wall, including internal iliac vessels and exposure of sciatic nerve Lateral pelvic wall muscles and adjacent fascia also removed in type D2 (Laterally Extended Endopelvic Resection, LEER) but not in Type D1

Recently, minimally invasive surgical approaches (laparoscopic and robot-assisted) gained prominence due to their potential impact on peri-operative morbidity and hospital stay. However, such approaches have been shown to be inferior to open surgery in early-stage cervical cancer in a multi-centre randomized study [40]. Interestingly, no significant improvement in quality of life was observed after minimally invasive surgery, compared to open surgery [41]. Consequently, current guidelines do not recommend routine use of minimally invasive surgical approaches for cervical cancer, even for patients with small tumours [20, 28, 29].

Short-term complications may occur in one-third of patients after radical surgery for cervical cancer and include peri-operative blood loss, urinary retention requiring catheterization, ureteric injury, wound infection, deep vein thrombosis, or wound dehiscence among others [42]. Long-term complications like sexual dysfunction, urinary voiding dysfunction, pelvic lymphocele formation, and pedal lymphedema may occur depending on the extent of surgery [43].

2.7 Principles of Radiation Therapy

2.7.1 External Beam Radiotherapy

External beam radiotherapy is an integral part of the non-surgical management of cervical cancer (stage IB1 and above). Treatment volumes for EBRT traditionally included pelvic nodal regions electively, along with the primary disease, irrespective of the technique of radiation used. Two-dimensional planning using multiple coplanar fields based on skeletal landmarks is considered minimum, even in resource-constrained settings, while three-dimensional conformal radiation using volumetric data for target delineation and dosimetry-based forward planning is practiced at most centres and is considered optimal. Intensity-modulated radiotherapy (with or without image guidance) has been shown to improve some outcomes like haematological toxicity and can be considered desirable in specific contexts, for bone marrow sparing/delivering simultaneous integrated boost to involved lymph nodes/delivering extended field radiotherapy [44, 45]. A recent randomized trial in operated cervical cancer has demonstrated improved toxicity profile with IG-IMRT compared to 3DCRT, establishing a new standard of care for adjuvant treatment [19].

Pre-treatment Preparation, Patient Positioning and Immobilization

Irrespective of the technique of radiation used, appropriate positioning that is comfortable and reproducible over a period of 4–5 weeks is paramount for EBRT. Supine position with slight flexion at the hip and knee, using positioning devices like a knee-wedge, results in relaxation of lumbar lordosis and is considered optimal for simulation. Additional immobilization devices like abdominopelvic thermoplastic casts or vacuum devices may be used based on institutional protocols.

In addition, a standard departmental protocol for reproducible bladder and rectal filling is advised to reduce uncertainties due to internal motion. For example, at the author's institution, patients are asked to void the urine completely and drink 500 mL of water over a period of 45 minutes before simulation or treatment [46]. Similarly, evacuating the bowel within 3–4 hours prior to simulation or treatment, along with appropriate dietary advice to avoid flatulence, may help achieve reproducible rectal filling. Routine use of laxatives or enemas is not recommended.

Two-Dimensional Planning

Conventionally, the four-field box technique is considered standard for treatment of cervical cancer limited to the pelvis (Fig. 1). However, in patients with lower vaginal extension or inguinal lymphadenopathy, use of parallel opposed antero-posterior fields with a frog-leg position to open up the groin folds can be considered to avoid moist desquamation in the inguinal folds.

The superior border of the antero-posterior fields is usually placed at the junction of the L4 and L5 vertebrae. The inferior border is placed at the inferior edge of the obturator foramen (which usually covers the upper third to half of the vagina) or at least 2 cm below the distal extension of the vaginal disease (as determined by a radio-opaque marker), whichever is inferior. Lateral margins are placed 1.5–2 cm beyond the true pelvic brim to ensure adequate coverage of the parametrial and lateral pelvic regions. While superior and inferior borders remain the same for

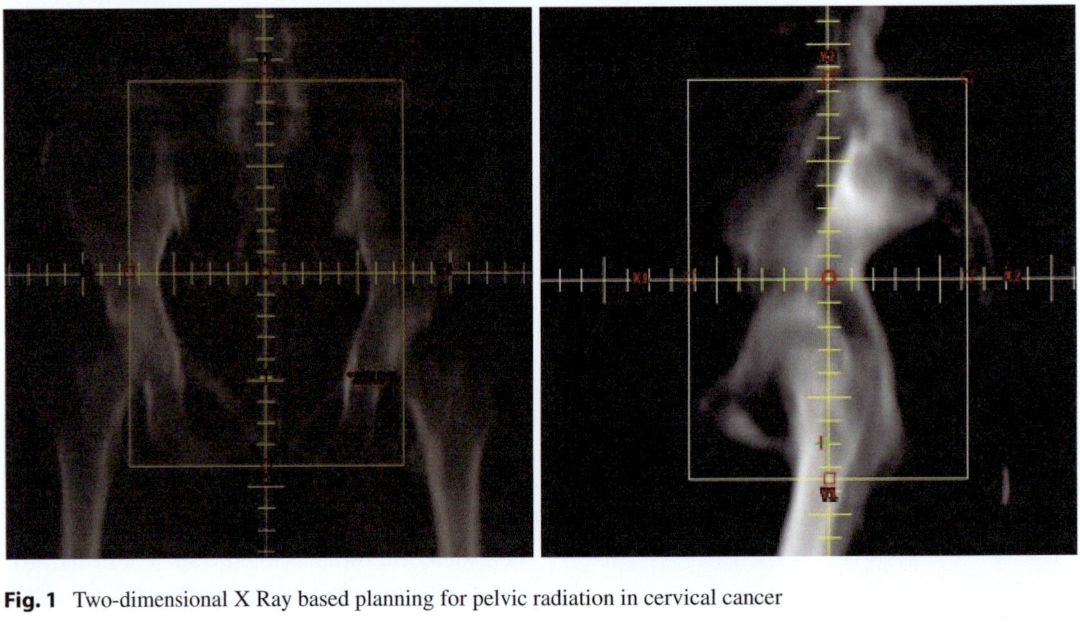

Fig. 1 Two-dimensional X Ray based planning for pelvic radiation in cervical cancer

the lateral fields, the anterior border is usually placed at the anterior cortex of the pubic symphysis. The posterior border is usually placed at the junction of the S2 and S3 vertebrae to ensure coverage of pre-sacral nodes while sparing the posterior rectal wall; it should be extended posteriorly to cover the entire sacral hollow in patients with uterosacral or meso-rectal involvement.

Corners of the box fields can be shielded to reduce the doses to the bowel, bone marrow and femoral heads. All fields are usually treated with equal weightage. Use of midline shielding for boosting of pelvic nodal or parametrial disease is strongly discouraged, and advanced techniques like conformal simultaneous/sequential boost for enlarged pelvic nodes and hybrid intracavitary-interstitial brachytherapy for parametrial coverage are preferred in such situations.

Alternatively, virtual simulation using volumetric data obtained from a planning CT scan can be used for EBRT planning. Though the field borders are usually similar to those for conventional planning, the upper border can be extended to include the aortic bifurcation [47]. Differential energies and field weightages can be used if appropriate dosimetric visualization is possible on the treatment planning systems.

Conformal Planning

Contrast-enhanced CT scan acquired in treatment position, with a 3–5 mm slice thickness, is recommended for target delineation. Organs at risk like the bladder, rectum, sigmoid, femoral heads and bowel are delineated as per standard recommendations. Numerous guidelines are available for delineation of nodal as well as primary target volumes [48–50]. Planning treatment volumes are generated by adding a department-specific margin for set-up uncertainties, and a dose of 45–50 Gy is prescribed at 1.8–2 Gy per fraction (Fig. 2a, b). Grossly enlarged lymph nodes are contoured, and an expansion margin of 0–5 mm is added for potential extra-nodal extension while planning simultaneous integrated boost, and a cumulative dose equivalent to 60 Gy (including contribution from BT) is prescribed to the planning target volume [51].

2.7.2 Brachytherapy

Brachytherapy has an indispensable role in the management of cervical cancer, with substantial evidence suggesting poorer outcomes in patients treated with EBRT alone [52]. Even with the use of advanced techniques like SBRT or Proton therapy, the dose heterogeneity inherent to brachytherapy could not be reproduced in dosimetric studies [53]. The importance of brachytherapy in curative treatment of cervical cancer is further reflected in the outcomes of a single-arm phase II study evaluating SBRT as a replacement for BT, wherein the study had to be terminated due to concerns of excessive toxicity with SBRT [54].

Traditionally, intracavitary brachytherapy using a combination of uterine tandem and vaginal ovoids was considered standard, and numerous systems like the Stockholm, Paris and Manchester systems were developed for guiding dose prescription. Recent technological advances in gynaecological brachytherapy including novel applicator design (ring-based applicators, hybrid intracavitary + interstitial applicators, MR compatible applicators, etc.), consolidation of high dose rate (HDR) treatment delivery, evolution of image-based brachytherapy and concepts of target volumes and the role of dose escalation have improved the precision and safety of brachytherapy and resulted in excellent local control rates [55].

Equivalence of HDR to LDR (low-dose rate) brachytherapy has been established in prospective randomized studies (including two large trials from India) and a Cochrane meta-analysis, while long-term follow-up from one of the Indian studies reported improved rectal toxicity with fractionated HDR compared to LDR. HDR is gradually expected to replace LDR as the preferred modality globally, due to the inherent logistical advantages and scope for optimization [55].

Strong dose–response relationships have always been theorized for local control in cervical cancer. However, dose escalation was cautiously practiced due to concerns regarding normal tissue toxicity and lack of robust clinical

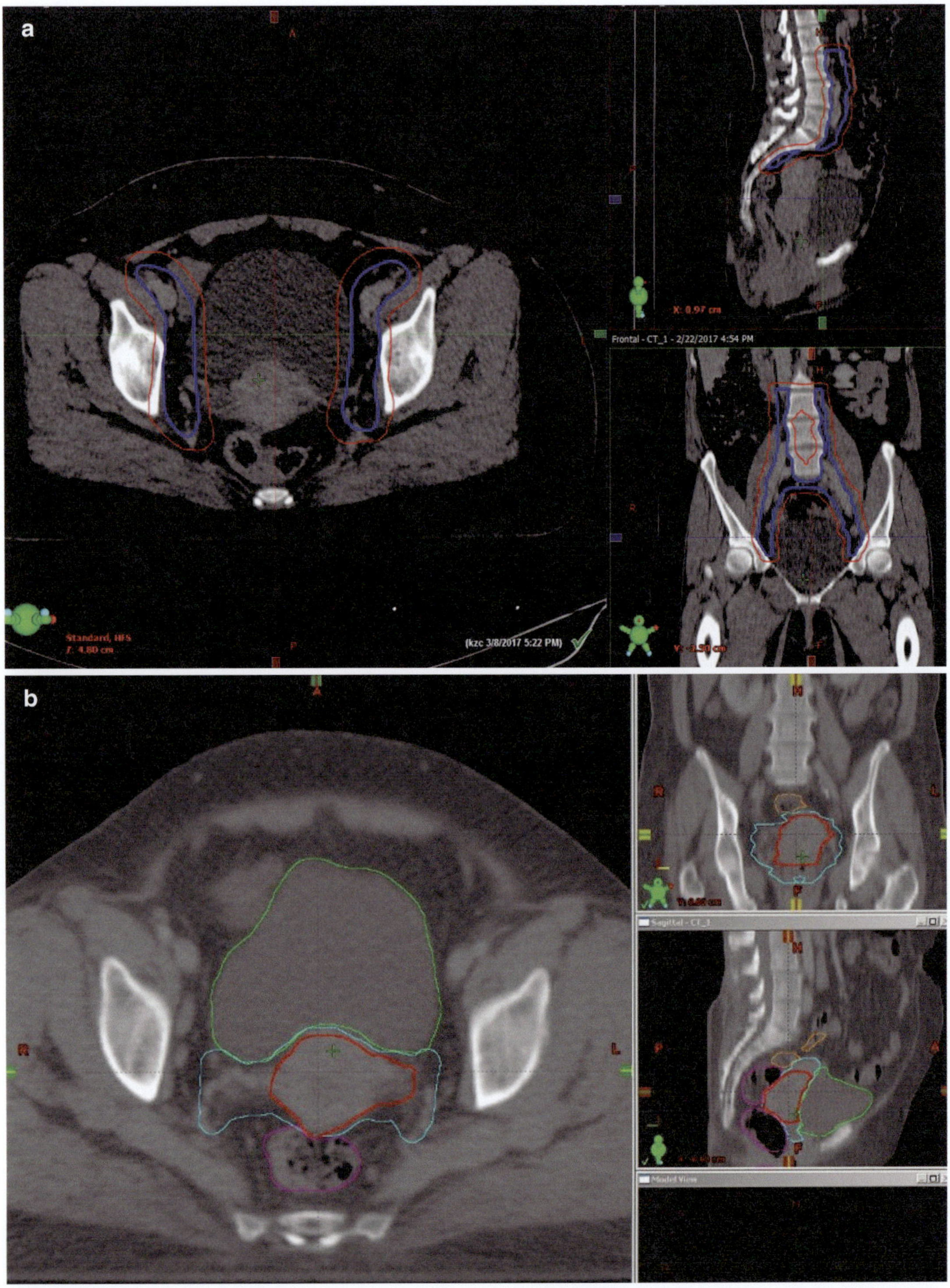

Fig. 2 (**a**) Nodal target delineation for conformal planning of cervical cancer (Blue: CTV; Red: PTV).(**b**) Primary target delineation for conformal planning of cervicalcancer(Red:GTV;Blue:CTV)

data. An international multi-centre prospective study by IAEA that randomized locally advanced cervical cancer patients in a 2 × 2 design, to 18 Gy in 2 fractions or 28 Gy in 4 fractions, with or without concurrent chemotherapy, established the role of dose escalation by demonstrating an improvement in local control from 78% to 88% in those receiving concurrent chemotherapy and 75% to 89% in those who did not receive concurrent chemotherapy. Though this improvement did not translate into a benefit in overall survival, a strong dose–response relationship for local control was confirmed with acceptable levels of toxicities, establishing a new standard of care [56].

Conventionally, orthogonal X-ray-based planning is done using the principles of the Manchester system, where doses are prescribed to predefined surrogate points that are anatomically comparable and reproducible. Principles of applicator design and source loading are such that a nearly constant dose rate is delivered at these points, irrespective of the variations in size and shape of the uterus and vagina. Recommendations for uniform reporting of doses and volumes in two-dimensional planning for intra-cavitary brachytherapy were described in the ICRU-38 report in 1985. Point A was described as a hypothetical point in the para-cervical triangle, 2 cm superior to the mucosa of the lateral vaginal fornix and 2 cm lateral to the central uterine canal, in the plane of the uterus. Point B was defined to be 5 cm lateral to the midline in the plane of point A and was theorized to represent the doses to the lateral pelvic wall. For documentation of doses received by the organs at risk, bladder and rectum points were defined. This report introduced the concept of reference volumes, in line with EBRT, and recommended doses designed to encompass these volumes for optimum outcomes. Universal acceptance of these recommendations was limited due to the complexity involved in the calculation of reference volumes. Moreover, there was significant variation in the correlation between these volumes and the reported outcomes, especially between the doses to OAR points and late toxicity.

With developments in imaging, applicator design and treatment planning, three-dimensional image-based brachytherapy was formalized by GEC-ESTRO in 2000. Brachytherapy in cervical cancer has evolved with imaging modalities to encompass the primary tumor and parametrial tissue infiltration by combining traditional intra-cavitary brachytherapy (IC-BT) with interstitial brachytherapy (IS-BT). Though various imaging modalities like CT, PET, MRI and Ultrasound were utilized for three-dimensional planning in gynaecological brachytherapy, MRI remains the gold standard due to superior soft tissue resolution, multi-planar imaging capability and potential for functional imaging. Detailed recommendations regarding the use of MRI for intra-cavitary brachytherapy, including the image parameters, sequences, technical parameters, target delineation, applicator reconstruction, co-registration, planning and quality assurance are published as a series of documents by GEC-ESTRO in the past decade. These were incorporated in the ICRU-89 report in 2016.

In MRI-based image-guided adaptive brachytherapy(IGABT), T2-weighted sequences are used in combination with clinical examination findings to define GTV, high-risk CTV and intermediate- risk CTV at the time of diagnosis and at brachytherapy [31]. Dose optimization at the time of brachytherapy is done to ensure adequate coverage of these volumes, instead of generic prescriptions to point A. Dose–volume parameters to target volumes (D98, D90 and V100) are reported in terms of cumulative EQD2 (equivalent doses at 2 Gy per fraction), combining both EBRT and brachytherapy doses, to allow easier comparison among different dose rates and fractionation schedules. Similarly, cumulative doses to organs at risk are also reported in volumetric terms (D0.1cc/D1cc/D2cc) as EQD2, for comparison and correlation with late toxicities (Fig. 3a–c). Details of principles, procedure and practice of cervical cancer brachytherapy have been described elsewhere [Volume 1 Chapter 13—Brachytherapy Technology and Principles].

Numerous retrospective dosimetric and prospective studies have established the significance of MR-guided adaptive brachytherapy for cervical cancer. Initial retrospective experience from

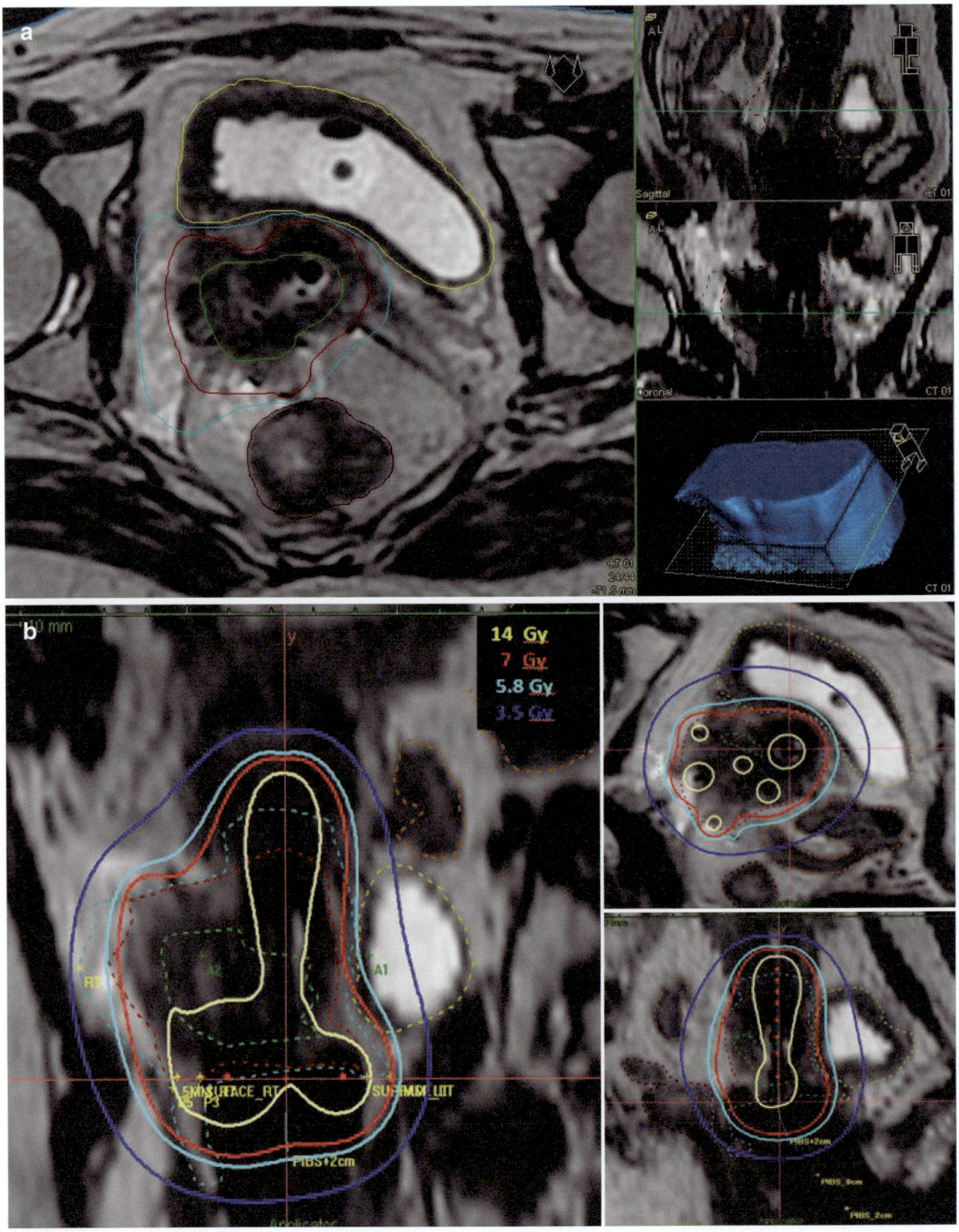

Fig. 3 (**a**) Target volume concepts for MR-IGABT. Green: GTV-B (macroscopic residual disease at the time of brachytherapy). Red: HR-CTV (macroscopic residual disease at the time of brachytherapy + whole cervix + presumed extra-cervical tumour extension). Blue: IR-CTV (HRCTV + macroscopic tumour extension at the time of diagnosis + minimum margin of 10 mm around the macroscopic residual disease at the time of brachytherapy in the direction of potential spread, after considering intact anatomical barriers). (**b**) Typical dose distribution with hybrid IC + IS application in MR-IGABT, for a prescription dose of 7 Gy per fraction. (**c**) Dose–volume parameters for plan evaluation in MR-IGABT

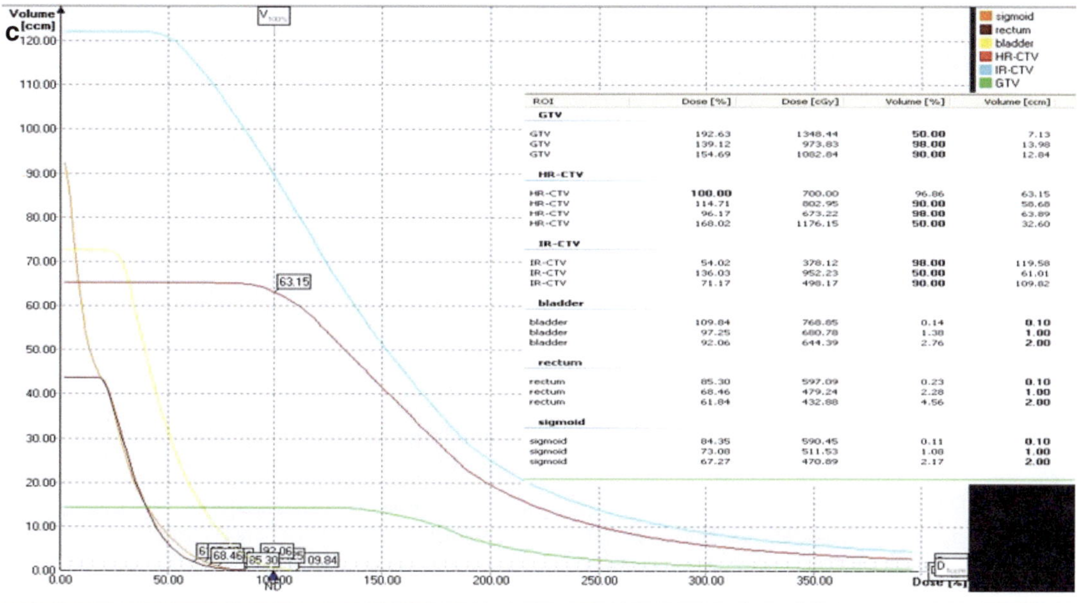

Fig. 14.3 (continued)

the Vienna group (Retro-EMBRACE) and the subsequent prospective international multicentric study of MRI-based image-guided adaptive brachytherapy (EMBRACE) have reported excellent disease-related outcomes with acceptable toxicities using dose-escalated IGABT. Additionally, the use of combined IC + IS applicators for those with large volume residual has been shown to be of significant benefit in terms of local control and toxicity. Recently reported 5-year outcomes of the EMBRACE study established a new benchmark for local control in cervical cancer. Apart from local control, various dose–volume parameters have been proven to correlate with normal tissue toxicities [31].

A non-statistical comparison of stage-wise local control and overall survival outcomes between two-dimensional planning and IGABT planning is presented in Table 4 [55]. Based on the existing non-randomized evidence, the National Cancer Grid of India has given an interim recommendation for transition to image-based brachytherapy [10]. However, it should be noted that the superiority of image-based brachytherapy over conventional point A-based brachytherapy has not yet been proven in a randomized trial; the ongoing COMBAT-Cx study comparing the both is expected to complete accrual in 2026 [57].

Recently, a phase-2 prospective dose escalation study delivering multiple fractions of image-based brachytherapy in a single application (SIMBRACE) demonstrated encouraging early disease-related outcomes with acceptable acute toxicities. Though long-term outcomes and late toxicities are awaited, such dose escalation protocols are expected to be beneficial for resource-limited, high-volume facilities [58, 59].

In a financial modelling study from India, it has been suggested that IGABT might be more cost -effective for developing countries [60]. However, owing to limited access to MRI and the antecedent costs of compatible applicators, alternative modalities like CT and ultrasound have been evaluated for image-based brachytherapy. Though CT has been shown to overestimate the width of HRCTV and underestimate the cranio-caudal extent of the disease compared to MRI, no significant differences were observed in the overall volumes and dose–volume parameters between these modalities. While PET-CT-based

Table 4 Outcomes with 2D and 3D planning for cervical cancer brachytherapy

Stage	Local control at 5 years		Overall survival at 5 years	
	Two-dimensional planning	Three-dimensional planning (MR-based)	Two-dimensional planning	Three-dimensional planning (MR-based)
IB	90%	92% for IB1 and 98% for IB2	85%	83% for IB1 and 73% for IB2
IIB	77%	91%	65–70%	78%
IIIB	44–66%	93%	34–52%	64%
IVA	18–48%	91%	0–20%	52%

brachytherapy has been reported to be clinically feasible, associated uncertainties in applicator reconstruction may have a detrimental impact. Studies have demonstrated a reasonable concordance in target delineation between TRUS-based and MRI-based brachytherapy for cervical cancer. Recently, recommendations for target volume delineation using alternate imaging modalities like CT with or without pre-brachytherapy MRI or TRUS were proposed by IBS ASTRO and ESTRO [4]. However, outcomes while using these modalities need to be benchmarked in large-scale prospective studies.

2.8 Recent updates in the Management of Cervical cancer

Surgical de-escalation has been evaluated in the ConCERV, LESSER and SHAPE trials for selected patients with early-stage cervical cancer (up to stage IB2, FIGO 2018), where simple hysterectomy combined with lymph nodal assessment is compared with radical hysterectomy [61–63]. Though the outcomes were found to be non-inferior, concerns regarding patient selection and quality assurance for wider adoption in routine clinical practice are reported [64].

Escalation of systemic therapy for improving survival outcomes has been evaluated in locally advanced cervical cancer. GCIG-INTERLACE study reported benefit in overall survival with six cycles of weekly dose-dense induction chemotherapy (paclitaxel and carboplatin), given before chemoradiotherapy for locally advanced cervical cancer [65]. However, the trial excluded patients with para-aortic disease, and brachytherapy utilization is considered suboptimal compared to the current standard of care (only one-third received IGABT and none received advanced IC+IS brachytherapy). Further, outcomes in the control arm are considered inferior to those reported with the current standard, especially for the relatively "lower risk" cases that were included in the INTERLACE study [66]. This led to concerns about the relevance of this approach in centres that have already adopted IGABT in their practice, especially for node-negative disease [67].

In contrast, the ENGOT-cx11/GOG-3047/KEYNOTE-A-18 study reported a survival advantage with the addition of pembrolizumab in concurrent as well as adjuvant contexts, in a predominantly node-positive patient population [38]. However, implementation in real-world practice is widely considered to be challenging due to financial constraints, especially in developing countries with resource limitations [68]. Moreover, outcomes of a similar cohort of patients treated with contemporary IGABT appear to be similar to those reported in the experimental arm of the KEYNOTE A-18 study [69]. While long-term outcomes with risk-adapted image-guided external beam radiotherapy and IGABT (EMBRACE II study) are awaited, early outcomes appear to be encouraging [70].

2.9 Follow-Up

With advances in techniques of EBRT as well as BT, a conspicuous change in patterns of failure has been observed. While locoregional 'in-field' failures have become less common, most treatment failures occur in the para-aortic region in patients treated with pelvic chemo-radiation, although distant metastases are also substantial. Current guidelines recommend routine pelvic examination and symptom-directed imaging during follow-up to identify potentially salvageable recurrences. Restaging CT or PET/CT can be considered 3 months after completion of EBRT and BT to assess for radiographic response in primary and nodal disease. Since most recurrences occur in the first 2 years after treatment, patients are typically followed up at shorter intervals of 3–4 months. Counselling the patients regarding late genitourinary, gastrointestinal, vaginal and musculoskeletal toxicity with appropriate rehabilitative measures should be integrated into survivorship care.

Percepts Box

1. Cervical cancer is predominantly a disease of the developing world.
2. Early-stage cervical cancer should preferably be managed with a single modality. While surgery and radiotherapy have equivalent efficacy for early-stage disease, management is largely decided by patterns of treatment-related morbidity, with surgery being the preferred option for younger women. Risk factors for adjuvant radio(chemo)therapy should be thoroughly discussed in a multi-disciplinary forum before offering surgical management, because combination therapy in this context has been shown to be detrimental in terms of treatment-related toxicity.
3. Radical chemoradiotherapy followed by brachytherapy is the standard of care for locally advanced cervical cancer. Brachytherapy forms an indispensable part of curative treatment and should not be replaced by alternative EBRT/SBRT regimens.
4. Image-guided adaptive brachytherapy with MR-defined target volume-based dose prescription is considered as the benchmark for local control and toxicity-related outcomes in cervical cancer brachytherapy. Use of alternative modalities like TRUS and CT for IGABT in cervical cancer needs to be validated in prospective studies and is an active area of research.
5. Supportive care forms an integral part of the management of cervical cancer, both in curative (for managing treatment-related toxicities during survivorship) as well as palliative contexts.

3 Endometrial Cancer

3.1 Introduction

Endometrial cancer is the second most common gynaecologic malignancy worldwide with an estimated incidence of greater than 417,000 cases per year worldwide [1]. It is the most common gynaecologic malignancy in western countries, with lower incidence within India [71]. Most cases of endometrial cancer are endometrioid type, with the majority of cases confined to the uterus at time of diagnosis [72]. More aggressive histologies include clear cell, serous and uterine carcinosarcoma, each of which have elevated risk of nodal involvement when compared to endometrioid cancers [72]. Localized endometrial cancer is primarily a surgically managed disease for medically operable patients, with standard management consisting of total hysterectomy and bilateral salpingo-oophorectomy with or without pelvic nodal sampling [73]. Adjuvant radiation therapy and chemotherapy are indicated for higher risk patients to reduce risk of disease recurrence, generally dictated by pathologic factors at present, with the recently-published PORTEC 4a trial seeking to validate the use of molecular factors to guide adjuvant treatment [74]. Definitive radiation therapy represents a reasonable treatment alternative for patients with medical comorbidities, which make them high risk for surgical intervention [75, 76]. Patients with metastatic disease are treated primarily with systemic therapy alone, with palliative radiation therapy indicated for symptomatic management [77].

3.2 Anatomy

Anatomically, the uterus is divided into the uterine corpus, defined as the upper 2/3rds (located above the internal cervical os), and lower uterine segment and cervix (located below the internal cervical os) [78, 79]. The wall of the uterus is divided into the innermost layer, known as the endometrium, followed by the middle muscular layer, known as the myometrium, followed by the outermost layer, known as the serosa [78]. Endometrial carcinoma arises from the endometrial layer, whereas uterine sarcoma arises from the myometrium or endometrial connective tissues [78]. Regional lymph nodes that the uterus can drain includes parametrial, obturator, internal iliac, external iliac, presacral, sacral, common iliac and para-aortic [79].

3.3 Epidemiological Aspects and Risk Factors

The majority of cases of endometrial carcinoma are oestrogen mediated, with conditions associated with excess oestrogen exposure resulting in increased risk, including obesity, diabetes, late menopause, early menarche and nulliparity. Other risk factors include older age, tamoxifen usage, oral contraceptive use and hormone replacement therapy [80–83]. Hereditary nonpolyposis colorectal cancer syndrome, also known as Lynch syndrome, is associated with a defect in mismatch repair genes, resulting in increased risk for multiple malignancies, including endometrial cancer, colorectal cancer, ovarian cancer and small bowel cancer [84]. Cowden syndrome is associated with a germline PTEN mutation and increases the risk of endometrial, breast and thyroid cancers [85].

3.4 Pathology

Traditional classification of endometrial carcinoma consists of type 1 and type 2 cancers. Type 1 cancers are oestrogen mediated, typically endometrioid subtype, low grade, developing following precancerous endometrial hyperplasia. Type 2 cancers are not associated with oestrogen exposure and include multiple different histologies including papillary serous carcinoma and clear cell carcinoma. Type 2 cancers have a worse prognosis when compared to type 1 cancers [86–89]. Uterine carcinosarcomas (previously known as Malignant mixed Mullerian tumour (MMMT)) consist of neoplasms with malignant epithelial and mesenchymal components, with high risk of nodal and distant progression [90]. Uterine sarcomas include leiomyosarcoma, endometrial stromal sarcoma, undifferentiated uterine sarcomas, SMARC4A-deficient uterine sarcoma and adenosarcoma [91].

A more recently developed classification of endometrial carcinoma from the Cancer Genome Atlas (TCGA) consists of four molecular subtypes: POLE ultramutated, microsatellite instability hypermutated, copy-number low (no specific molecular profile, p53 wildtype) and copy-number high (characterized by TP53 mutation). When comparing progression-free survival outcomes between these four subtypes, POLE ultramutated has the best outcomes, with microsatellite instability (MSI) hypermutated (mismatch repair deficient subtype) and copy-number low having intermediate outcomes and copy-number high having the worst progression-free survival outcomes [92]. PORTEC-4a has evaluated using molecular classification to adapt adjuvant radiation treatment recommendations for patients with high-intermediate-risk endometrial cancer [74]. A post hoc analysis of PORTEC 3 also demonstrated prognostic value for the TCGA classification in high-risk endometrial cancer, with benefit of addition of chemotherapy to adjuvant radiation therapy for patients with TP53 mutation [93].

3.5 Clinical Symptoms and Signs

Most cases of endometrial cancer present with postmenopausal vaginal bleeding, with additional symptoms including vaginal discharge, haematuria, rectal bleeding, constipation, abdominal/pelvic pain or discomfort and abdominal distention. The median age of diagnosis of endometrial cancer is 61 years old [94]. In pre-menopausal women who are diagnosed with endometrial cancer, heavy vaginal bleeding or bleeding between menstrual cycles may be present, although the absolute risk of endometrial cancer in premenopausal women presenting with vaginal bleeding is relatively low at less than 1% given the multitude of non-malignant aetiologies [95].

3.6 Integrated Management Plan, Including Diagnostic Tests and Staging

Following appropriate history and physical examination, including pelvic examination, in a patient presenting with symptoms concerning for endometrial cancer, particularly with post-menopausal bleeding, a transvaginal ultrasound should be performed, with thickened endometrial lining ≥5 mm in a post-menopausal female concerning for potential malignant aetiology [96]. Endometrial biopsy should then be performed for further evaluation if a thickened endometrial lining is noted. If the biopsy is negative or non-diagnostic and the patient has persistent symptoms, fractional dilatation and curettage should be performed under anaesthesia for further assessment [97]. Hysteroscopy can be utilized to better evaluate polyps, which may be cancerous in the setting of persistent vaginal bleeding without known aetiology [73, 98].

Staging of endometrial cancer is surgical (Table 5). The FIGO 2023 staging system incorporates histology, molecular profile, and extent of LVSI into staging, and is further discussed in the Recent Advances section of this chapter. In cases with high-grade/aggressive histologies or in instances where there is concern for locoregional or distant spread, preoperative imaging may be pursued. Pelvic MRI can be considered to evaluate the locoregional extent of disease in patients with high-grade histologies or non-operative candidates or to differentiate whether a mass seen on pelvic exam originates from the uterus or cervix. Pelvic MRI utilizing diffusion-weighting and dynamic contrast-enhancement is both effective at assessing the level of myome-

Table 5 2023 FIGO staging of cancer of the endometrium[a,b]

Stage	Description
Stage I	Confined to the uterine corpus and ovary[c]
IA	Disease limited to the endometrium OR non-aggressive histological type, i.e., low-grade endometroid, with invasion of less than half of myometrium with no or focal lymphovascular space involvement (LVSI) OR good prognosis disease
	IA1 Non-aggressive histological type limited to an endometrial polyp OR confined to the endometrium
	IA2 Non-aggressive histological types involving less than half of the myometrium with no or focal LVSI
	IA3 Low-grade endometrioid carcinomas limited to the uterus and ovary[c]
IB	Non-aggressive histological types with invasion of half or more of the myometrium, and with no or focal LVSI[d]
IC	Aggressive histological types[e] limited to a polyp or confined to the endometrium
Stage II	Invasion of cervical stroma without extrauterine extension OR with substantial LVSI OR aggressive histological types with myometrial invasion
IIA	Invasion of the cervical stroma of non-aggressive histological types
IIB	Substantial LVSI[d] of non-aggressive histological types
IIC	Aggressive histological types[e] with any myometrial involvement

(continued)

Table 5 (continued)

Stage	Description
Stage III	Local and/or regional spread of the tumor of any histological subtype
IIIA	Invasion of uterine serosa, adnexa, or both by direct extension or metastasis
	IIIA1 Spread to ovary or fallopian tube (except when meeting stage IA3 criteria)[c]
	IIIA2 Involvement of uterine subserosa or spread through the uterine serosa
IIIB	Metastasis or direct spread to the vagina and/or to the parametria or pelvic peritoneum
	IIIB1 Metastasis or direct spread to the vagina and/or the parametria
	IIIB2 Metastasis to the pelvic peritoneum
IIIC	Metastasis to the pelvic or para-aortic lymph nodes or both[f]
	IIIC1 Metastasis to the pelvic lymph nodes
	IIICli Micrometastasis
	IIIClii Macrometastasis
	IIIC2 Metastasis to para-aortic lymph nodes up to the renal vessels, with or without metastasis to the pelvic lymph nodes
	IIIC2i Micrometastasis
	IIIC2ii Macrometastasis
Stage IV	Spread to the bladder mucosa and/or intestinal mucosa and/or distance metastasis
IVA	Invasion of the bladder mucosa and/or the intestinal/bowel mucosa
IVB	Abdominal peritoneal metastasis beyond the pelvis
IVC	Distant metastasis, including metastasis to any extra- or intra-abdominal lymph nodes above the renal vessels, lungs, liver, brain, or bone

Abbreviations: *EEC* endometrioid carcinoma, *LVSI* lymphovascular space involvement

[a]Endometrial cancer is surgically staged and pathologically examined. In all stages, the grade of the lesion, the histological type and LVSI must be recorded. If available and feasible, molecular classification testing (*POLEmut*, MMRd, NSMP, p53abn) is encouraged in all patients with endometrial cancer for prognostic risk-group stratification and as factors that might influence adjuvant and systemic treatment decisions (Table 2)

[b]In early endometrial cancer, the standard surgery is a total hysterectomy with bilateral salpingo-oophorectomy via a minimally invasive laparoscopic approach. Staging procedures include infracolic omentectomy in specific histological subtypes, such as serous and undifferentiated endometrial carcinoma, as well as carcinosarcoma, due to the high risk of microscopic omental metastases. Lymph node staging should be performed in patients with intermediate-high/high-risk patients. Sentinel lymph node (SLN) biopsy is an adequate alternative to systematic lymphadenectomy for staging proposes. SLN biopsy can also be considered in low-/low-intermediate-risk patients to rule out occult lymph node metastases and to identify disease truly confined to the uterus. Thus, the ESGO-ESTRO-ESP guidelines allow an approach of SLN in all patients with endometrial carcinoma, which is endorsed by FIGO. In assumed early endometrial cancer, an SLN biopsy in an adequate alternative to systematic lymphadenectomy in high-intermediate and high-risk cases for the purpose of lymph node staging and can also be considered in low-/intermediate-risk disease to rule out occult lymph node metastases. An SLN biopsy should be done in association with thorough (ultrastaging) staging as it will increase the detection of low-volume disease in lymph nodes

[c]Low-grade EECs involving both the endometrium and the ovary are considered to have a good prognosis, and no adjuvant treatment is recommended if all the below criteria are met. Disease limited to low-grade endometrioid carcinomas involving the endometrium and ovaries (Stage IA3) must be distinguished from extensive spread of the endometrial carcinoma to the ovary (Stage IIIA1), by the following criteria: (1) no more than superficial myometrial invasion is present (<50%); (2) absence of extensive/substantial LVSI; (3) absence of additional metastases; and (4) the ovarian tumor is unilateral, limited to the ovary, without capsule invasion/rupture (equivalent to pT1a)

[d]LVSI as defined in WHO 2021: extensive/substantial, ≥5 vessels involved

[e]Grade and histological type

trial invasion, as well as cervical involvement [99, 100]. CT chest/abdomen/pelvis or FDG PET/CT scan is effective at assessing lymph node involvement and distant metastases in patients with high-grade or type 2 histologies, with higher sensitivity and specificity with PET/CT scan [101, 102]. In patients with suspected early stage endometrioid adenocarcinoma, systemic staging imaging is not always necessary in the absence of concerning symptoms and is per physician discretion. Chest imaging may be obtained to rule out lung metastases.

3.7 Surgical Aspects

Surgery remains the mainstay of treatment for patients with endometrial cancer who are surgical candidates, with treatment typically consisting of total hysterectomy and bilateral salpingo-oophorectomy with pelvic nodal sampling either in the form of sentinel lymph node biopsy or pelvic lymph node dissection. If there is no evidence of cervical involvement on examination, a type 1 simple hysterectomy is performed, with type III radical hysterectomy recommended for endometrial cancer with gross cervical involvement [73, 103]. Omental sampling is done for type 2 histologies. Pelvic washings are no longer required for surgical staging, though malignant peritoneal is a poor prognostic factor [104]. Laparoscopic hysterectomy is preferred to laparotomy to reduce morbidity [105, 106]. Robot-assisted laparoscopic surgery may reduce operative time and rates of conversion to laparotomy [107]. An alternative approach for patients with cervical involvement consists of neoadjuvant chemoradiation therapy with both external beam radiation therapy and high-dose rate brachytherapy, followed by extrafascial hysterectomy if feasible based on treatment response, with excellent outcomes demonstrated in some series [108–110].

GOG 33 demonstrated increased risk of nodal involvement with increasing FIGO grade and myometrial involvement in patients with presumed early-stage endometrial carcinoma who had undergone total abdominal hysterectomy and bilateral salpingo-oophorectomy with pelvic and para-aortic nodal dissection. Patients with grade 1 and inner 1/3rd myometrial involvement had <5% risk of pelvic and para-aortic nodal involvement, whereas those with grade 3 and outer 1/3rd myometrial involvement demonstrated approximately 35% risk of pelvic nodal involvement and approximately 25% risk of para-aortic nodal involvement [111].

The MRC ASTEC trial assessed patients with clinically uterine confined endometrial carcinoma who were randomized to standard surgery consisting of total hysterectomy and bilateral salpingo-oophorectomy vs. standard surgery plus lymphadenectomy. There was no demonstrated improvement in either overall survival or progression-free survival with the addition of lymphadenectomy, suggesting a potential lack of benefit for lymphadenectomy in the majority of patients [112]. However, with the less aggressive sentinel lymph node biopsy option now available, with high sensitivity and negative predictive value for patients with clinical stage I disease as demonstrated in the FIRES SLNB and SENTOR trials, nodal assessment is a reasonable option to consider for patients to provide more accurate surgical staging, which can better guide adjuvant therapies [113, 114].

The prognostic significance of micrometastases and isolated tumour cells identified on sentinel lymph node biopsy remains controversial, with multiple series suggesting a lower incidence of additional nodal involvement in non-sentinel lymph nodes on completion lymphadenectomy when compared to macrometastases identified on sentinel lymph node biopsy [115–118]. Patients with ITCs alone generally have favourable outcomes similar to node-negative disease; however, adjuvant therapy was delivered in the majority of series examining these patients, making it difficult to ascertain the true effect of isolated tumour cells on clinical outcome [119].

3.8 Systemic Therapy Aspects

Megesterol acetate (or other progestational agents), potentially combined with metformin, can be considered as fertility-sparing approaches for patients with stage IA, grade 1 endometrioid endometrial adenocarcinoma, with durable control possible in a subset of patients, although this approach may result in worsened oncologic outcomes [73, 120]. Progestational agents, tamoxifen, and aromatase inhibitors are also all options for patients with early-stage, low-grade endometrial cancer who are medically inoperable if definitive radiation therapy is not pursued [73].

For patients with early-stage, low-grade endometrioid endometrial carcinoma who undergo total hysterectomy and bilateral salpingo-oophorectomy, there is no indication for adjuvant systemic therapy, with the majority of patients cured by surgery alone. Regarding higher risk patients, in GOG 249, patients with FIGO stage I disease with endometrioid histology of age 70 or older with 1 intrauterine factor, age 50 or older with 2 intrauterine risk factors or age 18 or older with 3 intrauterine risk factors were enrolled, with intrauterine risk factors based on GOG 33 criteria of grade 2 or 3 tumour, outer half depth of invasion and lymphovascular space invasion. Patients with FIGO stage II disease with endometrioid histology, in addition to patients with FIGO stage I-II disease with serous or clear cell histology, were also included. Patients were randomized to pelvic radiation to 45–50.4 Gy over 5 weeks versus vaginal cuff brachytherapy followed by carboplatin/paclitaxel every 3 weeks × 3 cycles, with results demonstrating worse acute toxicity and increased pelvic/para-aortic recurrences in the brachytherapy/chemotherapy arm, with similar vaginal/distant recurrence rates between the two arms, suggesting potential lack of benefit of systemic therapy in this patient cohort [121].

PORTEC-3 enrolled patients following hysterectomy with FIGO stage I who were grade 3 endometrioid with deep myometrial invasion or lymphovascular space invasion, FIGO stage I serous or clear cell histology, or FIGO stage II-III disease and randomized patients to adjuvant radiation therapy alone to 48.6 Gy in 27 fractions vs. the addition of concurrent and adjuvant chemotherapy to the same radiation therapy. Chemotherapy in this trial consisted of 50 mg/m^2 cisplatin × 2 cycles every 3 weeks with external beam radiation therapy, followed by 4 cycles of adjuvant carboplatin/paclitaxel [122–124]. This trial demonstrated an approximate 10% improvement in overall survival with the addition of chemotherapy in patients with FIGO stage III or serous histology, at the cost of worsened acute toxicity, late toxicity, and quality of life with the addition of chemotherapy, including persistent peripheral neuropathy. As previously noted, a post hoc analysis of the trial also demonstrated improved recurrence-free survival, though p53-mutated tumours were the only type to benefit from the addition of chemotherapy [93]. Another adjuvant approach for high-risk patients would follow the GOG 258 protocol, utilizing six cycles of adjuvant carboplatin/paclitaxel following definitive surgical management, with the trial including patients with FIGO stage III or IVA endometrial carcinoma or those with FIGO stage I/II clear cell or serous histology and positive peritoneal washings [125].

In the recurrent or metastatic setting, GOG 209 defined the current standard of care of carboplatin/paclitaxel, which was shown to be non-inferior to paclitaxel-doxorubicin-cisplatin [126]. A phase II trial, which compared carboplatin-paclitaxel to carboplatin-paclitaxel-trastuzumab in FIGO stage III-IV or recurrent HER2/neu positive uterine papillary serous carcinoma, demonstrated improved overall survival and progression-free survival with the addition of trastuzumab [127]. KEYNOTE-775 examined patients with advanced endometrial cancer who had failed at least one platinum-based chemotherapy regimen, with randomization to lenvatinib plus pembrolizumab versus chemotherapy of the treating physician's choice. This trial demonstrated improved progression-free survival and overall survival with lenvatinib plus pembrolizumab [128]. Additional data suggests favourable response to pembrolizumab monotherapy for patients with microsatellite instability-high endometrial cancer [129].

3.9 Radiation Therapy: Indications and Selection

Currently, recommendations for adjuvant radiation therapy in endometrial carcinoma are based on FIGO stage and grade, with PORTEC 4a incorporating molecular classification to guide adjuvant radiation therapy recommendations [74]. Patients with FIGO stage IA and grade 1–2 endometrioid disease without lymphovascular space invasion can typically be spared adjuvant vaginal cuff brachytherapy, as demonstrated in the trial from Sweden, which did not reveal a significant local control benefit with the addition of vaginal cuff brachytherapy following hysterectomy [130].

For patients with endometrioid carcinoma of FIGO stage IA and grade 3, FIGO stage IB and grade 1–2 disease or FIGO IA and grade 1–2 disease with focal lymphovascular space invasion, adjuvant vaginal cuff brachytherapy should be considered to reduce the risk of local recurrence at the vaginal cuff. These recommendations stem from GOG 99 and PORTEC 1, which identified high intermediate risk subgroups that benefitted from adjuvant radiation therapy following hysterectomy, although the technique utilized in these 2 trials was external beam radiation therapy [131, 132]. In GOG 99, the high intermediate risk subgroup was defined based on the presence of grade 2–3 disease, LVSI, and outer third myometrial invasion. Patients of any age with all 3 risk factors, age 50 or greater with at least 2 of the above risk factors, or patients age 70 or greater with any of the above risk factors, comprised the high intermediate risk subgroup, which most benefitted from adjuvant radiation therapy [132]. PORTEC 1 identified a similar high intermediate risk subgroup of patients that significantly benefitted from adjuvant external beam radiation therapy, with patients having at least 2 of the following 3 risk factors: age ≥60, grade 3 disease or FIGO stage IB [131]. Adjuvant external beam radiation therapy in both of these trials demonstrated a reduction in locoregional recurrence without impact on overall survival in the identified high intermediate risk subgroups [131, 132]. PORTEC-2 demonstrated a similar risk of locoregional recurrence with vaginal cuff brachytherapy alone when compared to external beam radiation therapy in patients with high-intermediate risk disease based on PORTEC-1 criteria, with a reduction in toxicities in the vaginal brachytherapy arm, suggesting brachytherapy should be the standard of care for most patients who fit these high-intermediate risk criteria [133]. Select patients with FIGO stage II (based on microscopic cervical stromal involvement but no gross cervical involvement on examination) and grade 1–2 disease with surgical nodal assessment should also be considered for vaginal cuff brachytherapy alone as opposed to adjuvant external beam radiation therapy, given the low risk of failure in a multi-institutional analysis when external beam radiation therapy is omitted [134].

For patients with FIGO stage IB and grade 3 endometrioid disease or for patients with lower stage and grade disease with substantial lymphovascular space invasion, adjuvant external beam radiation therapy plus or minus vaginal cuff brachytherapy boost should be considered to reduce the risk of locoregional recurrence. Extent of lymphovascular space invasion was identified to be an independent risk factor of pelvic recurrence in a combined analysis of PORTEC 1 and PORTEC 2, demonstrating that patients with substantial lymphovascular space invasion derive greater locoregional control benefit with external beam radiation therapy as opposed to vaginal brachytherapy alone [135]. Brachytherapy boost after external beam radiation is often given for FIGO IB and II disease, but has wide variance in practice patterns and should be based on the risk of vaginal recurrence [136]. Presence of isolated tumour cells on nodal assessment remains an area of controversy, with most practitioners considering additional intrauterine risk factors when deciding to recommend adjuvant vaginal cuff brachytherapy alone or adjuvant external beam radiation therapy with vaginal cuff brachytherapy. For instance, a patient with otherwise favourable intrauterine factors such as minimal myometrial invasion with grade 2 disease with evidence of isolated tumour cells may be spared external beam radiation therapy, with treatment with vaginal cuff brachytherapy alone [119].

As previously discussed, GOG 258 enrolled patients with FIGO stage III-IVA disease or stage I-II with serous or clear cell histology with positive peritoneal washings, with randomization following hysterectomy and lymph node dissection to chemotherapy alone consisting of six cycles of carboplatin/paclitaxel versus chemoradiation therapy to 45 Gy in 25 fractions with brachytherapy boost if clinically indicated. Concurrent chemotherapy was cisplatin, with four cycles of adjuvant carboplatin/paclitaxel delivered in the chemoradiation arm, similar to the chemoradiation arm in PORTEC 3. The results of GOG 258 demonstrated a lack of overall survival or progression-free survival benefit with the addition of radiation therapy, with an increased rate of distant metastases in the chemoradiation therapy arm and increased rates of pelvic and para-aortic nodal failure in the chemotherapy alone arm [125]. Some would theorize that the less intensive chemotherapy delivered in the chemoradiation arm may explain the increased rate of distant metastases. Additionally, the regional nodal control benefit with the addition of radiation therapy may be greater in the sentinel lymph node biopsy era when completion lymph node dissection may not be performed as routinely. There are various institutional practices incorporating a combined modality approach, with some institutions beginning with chemotherapy given greater risk of metastatic recurrence in these patients, oftentimes six cycles of carboplatin/paclitaxel followed by restaging imaging, with external beam radiation therapy delivered to the pelvis plus or minus para-aortic lymph nodes based on surgical nodal assessment. A recent multi-institutional retrospective study did not demonstrate significant differences in overall survival or recurrence-free survival outcomes based on sequencing or type of adjuvant therapy for patients with FIGO stage IIIC disease [137].

For patients who are medically inoperable with FIGO stage I disease, definitive radiation therapy can be considered, either consisting of brachytherapy alone, typically with a tandem and cylinder applicator or a Y-applicator versus external beam radiation therapy plus brachytherapy boost if there is MRI evidence of deep myometrial invasion on pelvic MRI. If MRI is not available to assess myometrial invasion, a combined modality approach incorporating external beam radiation therapy and brachytherapy boost may be preferred. If patients have FIGO stage II-III disease and are medically inoperable, a combined external beam radiation therapy and brachytherapy approach would be favoured [75].

3.10 Simulation and Contouring

When treating postoperatively with external beam radiation therapy, patients should be simulated supine with their arms up, with utilization of an immobilization device like a Vac-Lok cushion. Prior to CT simulation, patients should be given bowel preparation instructions to minimize rectal distension at time of simulation. A CT with a minimum slice thickness of 2.5 mm should be performed, with both full and empty bladder scans performed to assess internal motion of vaginal cuff to allow for individualized patient-specific internal target volume (ITV). When contouring, both a vaginal CTV and nodal CTV should be created as outlined in the recently updated NRG atlas [138]. The vaginal CTV should be generated on both the full and empty bladder scans, beginning at the vaginal cuff, ensuring to extend laterally to include surrounding paravaginal and parametrial tissue. The vaginal CTV contour should include anteriorly to the posterior bladder wall, posteriorly to the anterior rectal wall, with inclusion of the anterior third of the mesorectum and consideration of additional coverage of the mesorectum and uterosacral ligaments if there was parametrial or substantial cervical involvement on pathology. The contour should extend inferiorly to include approximately 4 cm of the vaginal canal. The vaginal CTV contours from the full and empty bladder CT scans should be combined to generate a vaginal ITV. Pelvic nodal contours also should follow recommendations from the recently updated NRG atlas, ensuring to include common iliac, internal iliac, external iliac and obturator lymph nodes, with inclusion of presacral lymph nodes as well in cases of cervical involvement and inclusion of para-aortic lymph nodes if involved, with some institutions favouring prophylactic irradiation of para-aortic lymph nodes if they were not sampled in the setting of positive pelvic lymph nodes. Pelvic lymph nodes should be generated utilizing a 0.7–1 cm margin around the iliac vessels, beginning cranially at the bifurcation of the aorta into the common iliac vessels, extending inferiorly to the internal and external iliac vessels, with the presacral lymph nodes defined by a strip of tissue measuring 1–1.5 cm anterior to the sacrum and extending inferiorly to the level of the piriformis muscles. Obturator lymph nodes are defined as a strip of tissue measuring about 1.5–1.8 cm, located between the internal and external iliac vessels, extending inferiorly until the obturator vessels exit through the obturator foramen. If treated, para-aortic lymph nodes should be generated with a contour beginning 1–1.5 cm cranial to the left renal vessels, with contour extending from left psoas muscle to right psoas muscle [138, 139]. A 0.5–1.0 cm PTV margin should be added to the vaginal ITV and nodal CTV to create the PTV based on available daily image guidance.

When treating patients with medically inoperable disease or treating preoperatively for FIGO stage II disease, similar principles should be followed for the CTV nodal volume, with CTV primary generated by inclusion of entire uterus, cervix, parametrial tissue and upper vagina/paravaginal tissue, with ITV generated from full and empty bladder scans. A similar 0.5–1.0 cm PTV margin should be added to the ITV primary and CTV nodal volumes to create the final PTV based on daily image guidance.

When treating with HDR vaginal cuff brachytherapy alone or in combination with external beam radiation therapy, the maximum tolerated vaginal cylinder diameter should be utilized based on physical examination. When treating with brachytherapy alone, treatment should be initiated 6–8 weeks postoperatively following examination demonstrating that the vaginal cuff has fully healed. A CT scan should be performed with the cylinder in place, with the upper 3–5 cm of vagina typically treated based on institutional practices [140, 141]. Adjacent critical structures including the bladder, rectum, sigmoid, and small bowel should be contoured for the first fraction of HDR brachytherapy, with dose assessed utilizing a 3D-based treatment plan. Subsequent fractions can either be performed with an X-ray scout or CT scan, with CT scan offering three-dimensional detail to assess whether the vaginal cylinder is similarly positioned at the top of the vaginal cuff and for better assessment of bladder filling and rectal distension.

When treating patients with medically inoperable disease or for those treated neoadjuvantly with incorporation of HDR brachytherapy, a high-risk clinical target volume (HR-CTV) is generated by contouring the entire uterus, cervix and upper 1–2 cm of vagina. Similarly, nearby critical structures including the bladder, rectum, sigmoid and small bowel are contoured to assess dose. Utilization of MRI for each fraction of brachytherapy can allow for dose escalation to the GTV, which may be difficult to assess on a CT scan [75].

For patients with vaginal recurrence following hysterectomy in the setting of no prior radiation therapy, following pathologic confirmation and appropriate restaging imaging to rule out concomitant nodal or distant recurrence, external beam radiation therapy to the pelvis followed by HDR brachytherapy boost to the vaginal recurrence would be the favoured treatment option. Similar CTVs as described above would be generated for the external beam radiation component, with the vaginal CTV also including the area of gross recurrence and extending the vaginal CTV to include the entire vagina, rather than only including the upper 4 cm. If the distal vagina is involved by the recurrence, inguinal lymph nodes should also be included. Depending on the size and location of the recurrence, HDR brachytherapy boost would require either an intracavitary or interstitial applicator, with MRI-based planning favoured to help delineate gross tumour for each brachytherapy fraction [142]. The CTV in the recurrent setting for HDR brachytherapy varies between institutions, with the authors of this text treating the pre-treatment involved length of the vagina up to the mucosal surface, while also including the entire thickness of the involved vaginal wall plus any residual disease visualized on MRI [143]. Vaginal recurrences in the setting of prior radiation represent a more complex topic, with multiple series demonstrating favourable treatment outcomes utilizing HDR brachytherapy plus or minus external beam radiation therapy, adhering to strict cumulative dose constraints to reduce the risk of toxicity in the re-irradiation setting [144, 145].

3.11 Treatment Planning and Delivery (Options, Dose/Fractionation/OAR Constraints/Image Guidance in Delivery)

Various fractionation schedules exist for HDR vaginal cuff brachytherapy monotherapy, with the most common fractionation schemes being 7 Gy × 3 fractions prescribed to 5 mm from the cylinder surface and 6 Gy × 5 fractions prescribed to cylinder surface. Additional options include 4 Gy × 6 fractions prescribed to surface, 8.5 Gy × 4 fractions prescribed to surface and 5.5 Gy × 4 fractions prescribed to 5 mm [146]. When treating with HDR brachytherapy boost to the vaginal cuff following external beam radiation therapy, 5–6 Gy × 2–3 fractions prescribed to the cylinder surface is most commonly recommended [141]. In the setting of vaginal recurrence without prior radiation therapy, various doses can be utilized, with a more common regimen being 4.5–5.5 Gy × 5 fractions following 45 Gy in 25 fractions of pelvic external beam radiation while ensuring to limit cumulative rectal D2cc to 65 Gy EQD2, sigmoid D2cc to 70 Gy EQD2 and bladder D2cc to 80 Gy EQD2, with dose constraints based on cervical cancer literature [50, 142–146]. Retrospective data also suggests limiting the urethra 0.1 cc to 85 Gy EQD2 to reduce the risk of severe urethral toxicity [147].

When treating with HDR brachytherapy alone for patients with an intact uterus, typical fractionation regimens include 6 Gy × 6 fractions, 6.4 Gy × 6 fractions, 7.3 Gy × 5 fractions, and 8.5 Gy × 4 fractions, all prescribed to the HR-CTV. These regimens deliver an EQD2(10) of 48–52.4 Gy to the uterine outer surface, with a goal EQD2(10) of 80–90 Gy to the GTV if visible. When treating following external beam radiation therapy of 45 Gy in 25 fractions for an intact uterus, potential HDR brachytherapy boost fractionation regimens include 6.3–6.5 Gy × 3 fractions, 5.2 Gy × 4 fractions, 5 Gy × 5 fractions, and 8.5 Gy × 2 fractions, all prescribed to the HR-CTV [146]. These regimens after external beam radiation deliver a cumulative EQD2(10) of 70–75 Gy to the HR-CTV.

For adjuvant external beam radiation therapy, standard treatment involves 45–50.4 Gy in 25–28 fractions delivered to the pelvis plus or minus para-aortic lymph nodes. When delivering external beam radiation therapy, daily image guidance is recommended to better assess vaginal cuff or uterine displacement between fractions based on bladder filling and rectal distension to ensure adequate dose is delivered to target volumes.

Table 6 Dose constraints for external beam radiation therapy (at 1.8 Gy per fraction)

Organ at risk	Ideal dose constraints based on institutional practice
Bowel (contoured as bowel bag)	V40 Gy <30%; V45 Gy <200 cc (200 cc may not be achievable when treating para-aortic nodal chain)
Duodenum (important when boosting para-aortic lymph nodes)	V55 Gy <1 cc (can accept up to 5 cc)
Bladder	V45 Gy <50%
Rectum	V45 Gy <50%
Femoral heads	V30 Gy <15%; max dose of 50 Gy
Bone marrow	V20 Gy <80%; V10 Gy <90%; Mean dose <27 Gy
Spinal cord	Max dose 45 Gy

Various dose constraints exist to guide external beam radiation treatment planning, as demonstrated in Table 6. Based on RTOG 1203 and PARCER, IMRT would be favoured as the preferred treatment modality in the post-operative gynaecologic cancer setting, given demonstrated reductions in both acute and late GI and GU toxicities when compared to 3D-CRT [148–150]. A post hoc analysis of PORTEC 3 also demonstrated reduced grade 2+ diarrhoea and hematologic toxicity following completion of treatment, as well as reduced grade 3+ adverse events during treatment with the use of IMRT over 3D-CRT [151].

3.12 Radiotherapy Sequelae (Acute/Subacute and Late) Including Response Assessment

Some of the more common acute toxicities secondary to external beam radiation therapy to the pelvis include diarrhoea, dysuria, urinary frequency, urinary urgency, myelosuppression, and fatigue, with nausea also possible if para-aortic lymph nodes are treated. Potential late toxicities include vaginal stenosis, vaginal dryness, dyspareunia, sacral insufficiency fractures and small bowel obstruction. In patients treated with vaginal cylinder brachytherapy alone, the incidence of these side effects is greatly reduced given the lower dose delivered and smaller treated volume, as demonstrated by PORTEC-2 which compared the 2 treatment modalities, although modern radiation planning would likely reduce the incidence of side effects compared to historical data as demonstrated by PARCER and RTOG 1203 [148–150, 152, 153].

3.13 Follow-Up and QOL Issues

Routine follow-up imaging is not generally recommended for patients with endometrial cancer, with patients generally followed every 3–6 months following completion of treatment for the first 2 years, followed by every 6 months until 5 years post-treatment, assessing for symptoms/signs of recurrence and including gynaecologic examination to evaluate for vaginal recurrence. Imaging may be ordered as clinically indicated based on signs and symptoms concerning recurrence [73]. The recently published TOTEM study compared a more intensive versus a minimalist follow-up schedule for patients with FIGO stage I-IVA endometrial cancer treated with definitive surgery, with different schedules for low- and high-risk patients. This study demonstrated a non-significant increase in relapse detection in the more intensive follow-up arm, without differences in overall survival between arms in any subgroup analysed between the minimalist and intensive follow-up regimens [154].

In medically inoperable patients, a follow-up pelvic MRI allows for the best assessment of response to radiation treatment, with retrospective data demonstrating that follow-up MRI predicts for oncologic outcome [155]. Given the risk of vaginal stenosis following pelvic irradiation, a vaginal dilator is often recommended to reduce the risk of stenosis, typically initiated 2–4 weeks following completion of radiation treatment [156].

3.14 Prognosis, Results and Outcome, Survival

Overall prognosis for patients with operable early-stage endometrial cancer is excellent, with most patients cured following surgery alone. Patients with low-risk FIGO stage 1 disease who were enrolled in the Swedish study had <5% risk of any recurrence [130]. In PORTEC 2, long-term outcomes for patients with high-intermediate risk FIGO stage I disease were also excellent in both arms, with 10-year isolated pelvic relapse between 0.5% and 2.5%, 10-year distant metastasis rate between 8.9% and 10.4% and 10-year overall survival between 67.6% and 69.5% [157]. For patients with medically inoperable early-stage disease, radiation therapy generally results in high rates of local control and cancer-specific survival, as demonstrated by multiple series [155, 158]. As demonstrated by PORTEC-3, patients with higher risk disease have a 5-year failure-free survival of approximately 75% and a 5-year overall survival of approximately 80%, with lower recurrence-free survival noted in GOG 258 of approximately 60% given the inclusion of more locally advanced patients [123–125].

3.15 Recent Advances in Endometrial Cancer

Molecular profile has further defined prognosis and treatment recommendations [159]. PORTEC4a was a non-inferiority trial that randomized patients with high-intermediate risk endometrioid adenocarcinoma to standard treatment (vaginal brachytherapy) or molecular risk-adapted treatment [160]. In the molecular profile arm, patients with a favorable profile (POLE mutated or NSMP-CTNNB1 wild type) were observed, patients with an intermediate profile (MMR deficient or NSMP-CTNNB1 mutated) received vaginal brachytherapy, and patients with an unfavorable profile (p53 abnormal or substantial LVSI or L1CAM overexpression) received pelvic external beam radiotherapy. The 5-year cumulative incidence of vaginal recurrence was 1.6% in the standard arm and 4.5% in the molecular profile arm, which met the margin for non-inferiority, while sparing the favorable profile group (46% of patients) from adjuvant treatment. The 5-year cumulative incidence of vaginal recurrence in the favorable group was 0.9% in the standard arm and 4.1% in the molecular profile arm, which also met the margin for non-inferiority. Some may debate the appropriateness of a 7% non-inferiority margin for vaginal recurrence in the molecular risk-adapted group (and 8.5% non-inferiority margin for vaginal recurrence in the favorable group). Additionally, only 25% of patients in the trail had nodal staging, which calls into question the need for pelvic external beam radiotherapy in patients with substantial LVSI but a negative pathologic nodal assessment [161]. Immunotherapy has been shown to improve outcomes in patients with locally advanced non-metastatic endometrial cancer, particularly in patients with MMR deficiencies [162–167]. Recent consensus guidelines aim to incorporate molecular profile when deciding on adjuvant treatment [168].

In the setting of vaginal and/or lymph node recurrence of endometrial cancer, the addition of concurrent cisplatin to external beam radiation and brachytherapy boost did not improve outcomes in GOG 238 [169]. Utilization of hypofractionated external beam regimens is also being evaluated, with the recently published SPARTACUS trial demonstrating a favourable toxicity profile utilizing 30 Gy in 5 fractions to the whole pelvis following hysterectomy for FIGO stage I–III endometrial cancer [170].

3.16 Conclusion/Overview

Standard management for operable patients with endometrial cancer generally consists of total hysterectomy and bilateral salpingo-oophorectomy, with adjuvant therapies dictated by pathologic findings as detailed above, with either observation or vaginal brachytherapy alone favoured for the majority of early-stage patients based on risk factors. In early-stage disease, pelvic external beam radiation therapy is generally favoured in cases of FIGO stage IB and grade 3 endometrioid disease or for patients with lower stage and substantial lymphovascular space invasion. For patients with more locally advanced disease or aggressive histologies such as clear cell or serous cancers, a combined modality approach is typically favoured in the adjuvant setting. For medically inoperable patients, definitive radiation therapy, either consisting of brachytherapy alone or external beam radiation therapy plus brachytherapy boost, represents a reasonable treatment alternative.

Percepts Box

1. Endometrial cancer is primarily a surgical disease, with adjuvant therapy dictated by pathologic stage and additional risk factors for recurrence.
2. Most patients with endometrioid FIGO stage IA and grade 1 or 2 disease without additional risk factors should not receive adjuvant therapy due to the low risk of recurrence.
3. Most patients with FIGO stage IA and grade 3 or FIGO stage IB and grade 1–2 endometrioid disease should be considered for adjuvant vaginal cuff brachytherapy, given greatest risk of local recurrence is at the vaginal cuff.
4. Patients with FIGO stage IB and grade 3 endometrioid disease or lower stage with substantial lymphovascular space invasion should be considered for adjuvant external beam radiation therapy with vaginal cuff brachytherapy boost.
5. Select patients with grade 1–2 and FIGO stage II disease with microscopic cervical involvement and nodal sampling can be considered for adjuvant vaginal cuff brachytherapy alone.
6. Most patients with higher risk disease, including FIGO stage II-IVA and/or serous or clear cell histology, should be considered for adjuvant therapy incor-

porating both chemotherapy and external beam radiation therapy based on treatment arms of PORTEC 3 and GOG 258.
7. Patients with medically inoperable disease should be considered for definitive brachytherapy alone or in combination with external beam radiation therapy as an alternative to surgical management.
8. Patients with metastatic disease are primarily treated with chemotherapy or hormonal therapy if low-grade endometrioid histology, reserving radiation therapy for palliation of symptoms.

4 Vulvar Cancer

4.1 Introduction

Vulvar cancer is an uncommon malignancy representing <1% of all cancers in women [171]. Similar to other malignancies, treatment recommendations and oncologic outcomes relating to vulvar cancer are influenced by the stage of disease (Table 7) and adverse clinicopathologic factors, as well as patient functional status and comorbidities. FIGO staging from 2009 was updated in 2021 to include a new definition of depth of invasion and to allow the inclusion of cross-sectional imaging, and is discussed further in this chapter. Generally, early-stage vulvar cancer is managed surgically and tends to have more favourable outcomes; whereas locally advanced disease is managed with neoadjuvant/definitive chemoradiotherapy versus surgical resection followed by adjuvant (chemo)radiotherapy depending on the presence of risk factors. Selection of operative vs. non-operative management is typically a function of patient tolerance, extent of disease and anatomical location of disease. Metastatic disease is typically managed with systemic therapy and carries a far less favourable prognosis. Optimal treatment selection in vulvar cancer is critical, considering the physical as well as psychosocial impact treatment may have on the patient given the sensitive anatomic location of the vulva. As such, treatment recommendations and delivery should occur in a multidisciplinary setting involving an experienced team of oncologic providers and ancillary staff.

Table 7 FIGO 2021 vulvar cancer staging, adopted from Olawaiye et al. [172]

Stage	Description	
I	Tumor confined to the vulva	
	IA	Tumor size ≤2 cm and stromal invasion ≤1 mm[a]
	IB	Tumor size >2 cm or stromal invasion >1 mm[a]
II	Tumor of any size with extension to lower one-third of the urethra, lower one-third of the vagina, lower one-third of the anus with negative nodes	
III	Tumor of any size with extension to upper part of adjacent perineal structures, or with any number of nonfixed, nonulcerated lymph node	
	IIIA	Tumor of any size with disease extension to upper two-thirds of the urethra, upper two-thirds of the vagina, bladder mucosa, rectal mucosa, or regional lymph node metastases ≤5 mm
	IIIB	Regional[b] lymph node metastases >5 mm
	IIIC	Regional[b] lymph node metastases with extracapsular spread
IV	Tumor of any size fixed to bone, or fixed, ulcerated lymph node metastases, or distant metastases	
	IVA	Disease fixed to pelvic bone, or fixed or ulcerated regional[b] lymph node metastases
	IVB	Distant metastases

[a]Depth of invasion is measured from the basement membrane of the deepest, adjacent, dysplastic, tumor-free rete ridge (or nearest dysplastic rete peg) to the deepest point of invasion
[b]Regional refers to inguinal and femoral lymph nodes

4.2 Anatomy

Representing the most caudal portion of the female reproductive tract, the vulva describes the structures that comprise the female genitalia (Fig. 4). The structures that make up the vulva include mons pubis, labia majora, labia minora, clitoris, vestibular bulbs, vestibule, Bartholin's glands, Skene's glands, hymen, urethra and the vaginal orifice. Starting superiorly, the mons pubis is a mound of soft fatty tissue overlying the pubic bone and is typically covered by hair following puberty. The mons pubis carries a rich network of lymphatics and vasculature. Moving inferiorly, two sets of skin folds (i.e. labia) surround the vulvar vestibule: labia majora and labia minora. The labia majora represent the larger, outer folds and extend from the mons pubis anteriorly and meet posteriorly at the urogenital triangle (anterior portion of the perineum). The labia majora serve to protect the inner vulvar structures and are the most common location for vulvar cancer to develop. The smaller, inner set of folds are the labia minora which extend anteriorly to form the clitoral hood and merge posteriorly to form the posterior fourchette. Beneath the clitoral hood is the clitoris and vestibular bulbs. The clitoris is a vasculature, highly innervated structure that is homologous anatomically to the glans penis in males. Within the protective labia is the vulvar vestibule which contains the vaginal orifice, urethra and associated structures. The urethra is located between the clitoris anteriorly and the vaginal orifice posteriorly. Surrounding the urethra laterally are the lesser vestibular glands (Skene's glands) which secrete a lubricant into the urethral opening. The vaginal orifice is partially covered by the residual hymen and is surrounded posterolaterally by the greater vestibular glands (Bartholin's glands). Bartholin's glands are located in the posterior labia minora and secrete a lubricating fluid into the vaginal orifice during sexual arousal. The vulva receives innervation via the pudendal nerve (S2–4) and vascular supply from the internal pudendal artery (via internal iliac). Regarding lymphatic drainage, most vulvar structures drain to the inguinal lymph node basins. Typically, the lymphatic drainage sequence is from superficial inguinal lymph nodes to deep inguinal/femoral lymph nodes to external iliac lymph nodes. Of note, the most superiorly located deep inguinal lymph node has been described as the node of Cloquet and has historically been associated with additional pelvic nodal involvement. The perineum, clitoris and anterior labia often drain bilaterally. Additionally, the clitoris can often drain directly into pelvic nodal basins (obturator, internal and external iliac nodes).

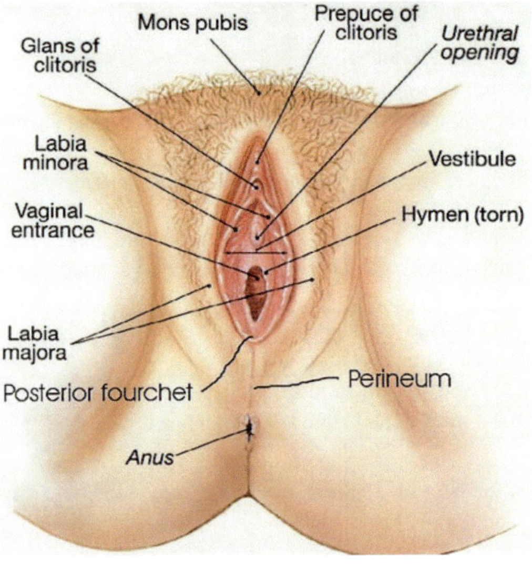

Fig. 4 External anatomy of the vulva

4.3 Epidemiology and Risk Factors

Vulvar cancer represents approximately 4% of all gynaecologic malignancies [171]. Predominantly, a disease of the elderly, over 75% of women who develop vulvar cancer are over the age of 50 years old, and upwards of 50% of women are over the age of 70 years old. While increasing age continues to be a risk factor for the development of vulvar cancer, the average age of diagnosis has decreased in recent years, likely a consequence of increased human papilloma virus (HPV) driven infections worldwide [173, 174]. In addition to HPV, infection with human immunodeficiency virus (HIV) has also been associated with the development of vulvar neoplasia [175]. Additional known risk factors associated with the development of vulvar cancer include smoking, immunosuppression, and inflammatory conditions such as vulvar intraepithelial neoplasia (VIN), extramammary Paget's disease (risk of invasive cancer estimated at 25%), Bowen's disease and lichen sclerosis (risk of malignant progression is approximately 5%). Particularly common in elderly patients, 30–60% of invasive vulvar cancer cases are associated with pre-existing lichen sclerosis. Similarly, nearly one-third of vulvar carcinoma cases develop on the background of pre-existing VIN. Risk of malignant progression in the setting of VIN varies, depending on the subset of VIN. For example, the risk of malignant progression for VIN 1 is approximately 5%, whereas the risk increases to upwards of 10% for cases of VIN 3 [176]. A particularly unfavourable subtype of VIN is differentiated VIN (dVIN), which is often associated with lichen sclerosis and a significant risk of invasive carcinoma progression (upwards of 50%) [177]. Of note, the International Society for Study of Vulvovaginal Disease (ISSVD) has modified the terminology for pre-invasive disease as of 2015 [178]. The 3 main categories are low-grade squamous intraepithelial lesion (LSIL) of the vulva (previously referred to as VIN1, vulvar LSIL, flat condyloma, or human papillomavirus [HPV] effect), high-grade squamous intraepithelial lesion (HSIL) of the vulva (previously referred to as VIN2 and VIN3, and includes vulvar HSIL, VIN usual type [uVIN]) and differentiated VIN (dVIN). dVIN lesions are not associated with HPV but are associated with vulvar dermatoses, mainly lichen sclerosis.

4.4 Clinical Symptoms and Signs, Pathology

In cases of early-stage vulvar cancer, the patient is often asymptomatic initially. However, signs and symptoms of vulvar cancer include palpable mass/nodule involving the vulva and or inguinal lymph node basins, pruritus or tenderness of the vulva, bleeding from the vulva/vagina, pelvic pain (particularly with urination and/or sexual intercourse), persistent vulvar skin changes including discoloration, changes in texture or appearance of verrucous/ulcerative growths.

4.5 Pathology

The vast majority of vulvar cancers are squamous cell carcinomas, representing nearly 90% of cases. In regard to squamous cell carcinomas, there are two general clinicopathologic entities. The first and most common (~70%) is keratinizing squamous cell carcinoma. Keratinizing squamous cell carcinoma is most commonly associated with older women, vulvar dystrophy, and lichen sclerosis, and is rarely associated with HPV. The second clinicopathologic entity (~30%) is that of basaloid squamous cell carcinoma. Basaloid squamous cell carcinoma is typically associated with younger women, HPV-driven disease, and presents clinically in a multifocal manner. Basaloid histologies are more commonly associated with other comorbid gynaecologic malignancies (i.e. cervical cancer). A less common verrucous subtype has also been reported, which typically has a less aggressive clinical course [179]. In addition to squamous cell carcinoma, the remaining histologies include melanoma (approximately 5–10%), sarcoma, basal cell carcinoma, adenocarcinoma (via Bartholin glands) and lymphoma.

Similar to squamous cell carcinomas of the cervix, anal canal and oropharynx, the oncogenic link between HPV and squamous cell carcinoma of the vulva is evident. An estimated 40–60% of invasive vulvar cancers are HPV-associated, likewise 70–80% of vulvar intraepithelial neoplasia (VIN) cases are related to HPV. The presence of p16 expression (i.e. p16 positive) is commonly reported as a surrogate marker for HPV-related disease. High risk HPV subtypes include HPV 16, 18, 31 and 33; however, over three-fourths of cases are linked to the HPV 16 subtype. Patients with HPV-related disease are often younger and interestingly have a more favourable response to treatment. For example, the clinical complete response (64% vs. 35%; $p = 0.014$) was significantly higher in p16 positive patients compared to p16 negative patients who were treated with neoadjuvant or definitive chemoradiotherapy [180]. This differential treatment response was found to translate to improvements in vulvar control at 2 years (76% vs. 50%; $p = 0.008$), favouring p16 positive disease. Furthermore, patients with p16 positive disease have also been found to have more favourable outcomes in terms of progression free survival (65% vs. 16% at 5 years; $p < 0.01$) and overall survival (65% vs. 22% at 5 years; $p = 0.01$) compared to p16 negative disease [181].

4.6 Management

The initial workup for cancer of the vulva starts with a comprehensive history and physical examination. Physical examination may need to be performed under sedation as patients may not be able to tolerate the exam due to pain. Internal gynaecologic examination should routinely be completed to assess the local extension of disease in addition to evaluation for a synchronous gynaecologic primary. Clinicians should also consider cervical HPV and cytology testing. Palpation of the bilateral inguinal lymph node basins should be performed routinely to assess for regional spread. Based on the initial clinical exam findings, cystoscopic and/or proctoscopic examination may be indicated. Patients who use tobacco should be counselled on smoking cessation and HIV testing should be considered in younger patients. Biopsy of the primary lesion and suspicious lymph nodes should be performed. Based on the clinicopathologic findings, further testing can be considered including complete blood count, comprehensive metabolic panel, and imaging studies to assess the local extent of disease (i.e. pelvic MRI) and/or to assess for metastatic disease (i.e. PET/CT or CT chest abdomen and pelvis). Generally speaking, early-stage disease (i.e. T1 N0 and small T2 N0) is managed primarily with surgical resection of the primary +/− exploration of the inguinal femoral lymph nodes depending on the pathologic features (Fig. 5). Locally advanced disease is often managed with surgical assessment of the inguinal femoral lymph nodes followed by neoadjuvant or definitive concurrent chemoradiotherapy (+/− surgical resection of the primary following neoadjuvant therapy). In patients treated with neoadjuvant or definitive concurrent chemoradiotherapy, upfront surgical assessment of lymph node status is often omitted to reduce morbidity and prevent delays in treatment. Metastatic disease is managed primarily with systemic therapy; however, palliative external beam radiotherapy is often recommended for locoregional control and/or symptom palliation.

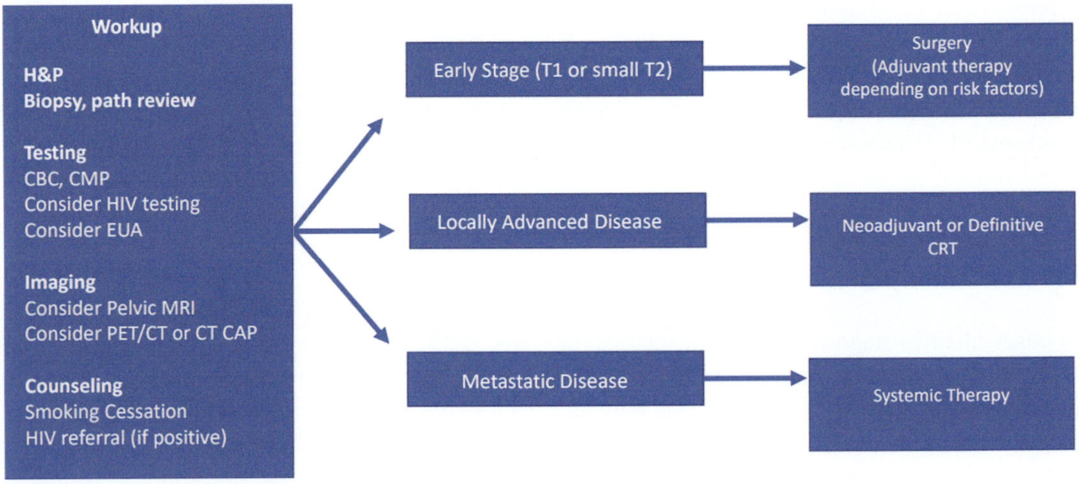

Fig. 5 Vulvar carcinoma treatment algorithm

4.7 Surgical Aspects

Surgical resection represents the primary treatment modality in cases of localized, early-stage disease. Wide local excision or modified radical vulvectomy (i.e. resection of involved parts of the vulva) is the current standard of care. Gross tumour should be excised to deep fascia and periosteum, and effort should be made to obtain negative surgical resection margins of at least 1 cm of fresh surgical tissue. Historically, ≥8 mm pathologic (formalin-fixed) margins of resection have been recommended, and re-excision (if possible) was to be considered in cases of close margins [182]. More recently, the recommended pathologic resection margin of 8 mm has been called into question and is an active area of investigation [183–185]. In patients with pathologic depth of invasion (DOI) ≤1 mm, assessment of the inguinal lymph nodes can be omitted as the risk of lymph node involvement is less than 5%. However, the vast majority of patients (i.e. >1 mm DOI) will require inguinal lymph node assessment given the high rate of occult nodal metastases. The resection of the vulva primary and inguinal evaluation should be performed through separate incisions. In patients with small (<4 cm), unifocal and well lateralized (≥2 cm from the midline) tumours with clinically-negative inguinofemoral lymph nodes, ipsilateral groin assessment is sufficient as the risk of contralateral groin involvement is <10% [186]. Of note, a negative unilateral inguinofemoral lymphadenectomy is associated with a less than 3% risk of contralateral metastasis [187]. However, in patients with tumours located within 2 cm of the midline and/or larger primary tumours, bilateral inguinofemoral lymph node evaluation is recommended. An optimal lymphadenectomy yields at least 10 lymph nodes total from bilateral dissection. In patients with a positive ipsilateral inguinofemoral lymphadenectomy, contralateral inguinofemoral lymphadenectomy (or radiotherapy) is recommended. Given the high rate of postoperative morbidity (wound healing and lymphedema) associated with inguinofemoral lymphadenectomy, sentinel lymph node biopsy has emerged as an alternative standard of care approach. Sentinel lymph node biopsy has been associated with decrements in postoperative morbidity without compromising detection of regional lymph node metastasis [188, 189]. Patients who are candidates for sentinel lymph node biopsy include those with a negative clinical groin examination, no prior vulvar surgery (i.e. disruption of lymphatics), and a primary unifocal vulvar tumour measuring less than 4 cm in diameter. Sentinel lymph node detection sensitivity has been reportedly increased when both radiocolloid and blue dye are used. In patients with a macrometastasis (i.e. lymph node metastases >2 mm) on sentinel lymph node biopsy, completion bilateral inguinofemoral lymphadenectomy is recommended with consideration of adjuvant radiotherapy +/− chemotherapy based on the extent of nodal burden. Conversely, if ipsilateral sentinel lymph node biopsy is positive for a micrometastases (i.e. >0.2 mm and ≤2 mm) or isolated tumour cells (ITC's), omission of completion inguinofemoral lymphadenectomy and adjuvant radiotherapy may be considered in an effort to reduce morbidity without compromising oncologic outcomes [190]. Patients meeting all criteria for sentinel lymph node biopsy eligibility who have negative sentinel lymph nodes may omit further groin treatment.

4.8 Systemic Therapy Aspects

Similar to more common gynaecologic malignancies, systemic therapy in vulvar cancer is primarily used concurrently with radiotherapy in definitive treatment for unresectable disease, postoperatively with radiotherapy in patients with risk factors (i.e. extracapsular extension, 2 or more positive lymph nodes, N3 disease, or high nodal burden), and as the primary treatment modality in cases of metastatic disease. Platinum-based chemotherapeutic agents (most commonly cisplatin) are often given at radiosensitizing doses (40 mg/m^2 weekly or 75 mg/m^2 every 3 weeks for cisplatin) concurrent with radiotherapy in both the definitive and postoperative setting. Given the rarity of vulvar cancer, much of the data regarding systemic therapy is based on extrapolations from cervical cancer. Single agent paclitaxel, as well as fluorouracil/mitomycin C may be considered in patients who are ineligible for platinum-based therapy; however, the data supporting their use is limited. More recently, the ongoing phase II GOG 279 study is evaluating the role of doublet chemotherapy (weekly gemcitabine 50 mg/m^2 and cisplatin 40 mg/m^2) in the setting of unresectable FIGO stage IIIA-IVA patients receiving preoperative/definitive dose escalated radiotherapy. The role of immunotherapy and targeted agents has primarily been reserved for patients who have progressed following prior treatment and in cases where there is no satisfactory alternative treatment available. For example, patients with potentially immunogenic tumours (i.e. mutational burden-high, microsatellite instability-high/mismatch repair-deficient or PD-L1 positive) who have progressed on prior therapy may be considered for immune checkpoint inhibitors as second-line therapy.

4.9 Radiation Therapy: Indications and Selection

Radiotherapy is utilized in the definitive, neoadjuvant, postoperative, and palliative settings. Definitive and neoadjuvant radiotherapy are employed in cases of unresectable disease and is often given with concurrent chemotherapy. Unresectable disease may include disease that involves the proximal vagina, urethra, anal canal, bladder, rectum, pubic bone and/or cases of fixed/ulcerative inguinal lymphadenopathy. Disease may be unresectable due to localized extent or due to a sensitive location where surgical resection with wide margins would be deemed morbid. Historically, indications for postoperative radiotherapy to the primary site include close/positive resection margins (i.e. less than 8 mm formalin-fixed margins, though adequate margin status is controversial as mentioned above) or the presence of two or more risk factors identified in the landmark retrospective study by *Heaps* et al and include: less than 8 mm surgical margin, depth of invasion greater than 9 mm, tumour thickness greater than 10 mm, LVSI, infiltrative growth pattern (spray vs. diffuse), greater than 25% keratinization and greater than 10 mitoses per 10 high power fields [182]. More recently, data suggests other factors, such as differentiated vulvar intraepithelial neoplasia (dVIN) and lichen sclerosis in the pathological margin rather than tumour free margin distance, are more predictive of local recurrence and should be considered for radiotherapy to the primary [184]. Indications for radiotherapy following lymph node dissection include: two or more positive inguinal lymph nodes, the presence of extracapsular extension, and inadequate lymph node assessment (no lymph node assessment, inappropriate sentinel lymph node biopsy, ipsilateral groin dissection only, and <10 lymph nodes removed bilaterally). In patients who completed sentinel lymph node biopsy, the presence of a macrometastasis or lymph node with extracapsular extension may be treated with completion bilateral inguinal lymph node dissection (preferred) or concurrent chemoradiotherapy, whereas patients with a micrometastases/isolated tumour cells can be managed with radiotherapy alone [191]. When adjuvant radiotherapy for the lymph nodes is indicated, the primary site is often treated as well due to the possibility of local failure, which may be difficult to salvage [192, 193].

4.10 Simulation and Contouring

Young patients should undergo pregnancy testing and discussion of fertility preservation if future childbearing is desired. Prior to simulation, clinical exam findings including the extent of disease should be documented, and the patient should be advised to arrive for the simulation with an empty rectum. In cases where the rectum is distended at simulation (i.e. greater than 3.5 cm in diameter), it is advisable to repeat the simulation after further bowel preparation. The patient should be placed in a supine, frog-leg position to minimize inguinal folds and aid in sparing the skin of the medial thighs. Immobilization with a vacuum bag is recommended. Radiopaque marker/wires should be applied to the patient's skin to delineate regions of gross disease, surgical scars, urethra and the anal verge. Additionally, palpable inguinal lymph nodes and/or regions of skin involvement should be delineated with a radiopaque marker. In cases of vaginal involvement, both full and empty bladder scans should be performed to account for internal motion of the vagina (i.e. generate an internal target volume). Scans should be obtained both with and without placement of bolus over the primary lesion. Alternatively, the patient may be simulated without bolus and a virtual bolus may be added at the time of planning and used to guide actual bolus placement. Typically, bolus over the inguinal nodal basins is not routinely recommended; however, in cases where lymph nodes are large/superficially located or demonstrate extracapsular extension/gross skin involvement bolus should be considered. Of note, it is important to ensure that only regions of concern are covered with bolus to limit excessive skin dose and toxicity. In vivo dosimetry with a thermoluminescent diode (TLD) at the time of treatment delivery is suggested to ensure the intended dose is delivered as prescribed. Prior diagnostic imaging such as PET-CT or CT may be co-registered with the planning CT.

In cases of locally advanced/unresectable disease, clinical examination (often under anaesthesia) is critical in defining the gross tumour volume (GTV), as well as, the clinical target volume (CTV). In addition to clinical exam, magnetic resonance imaging (MRI) with its superior soft tissue delineation may be helpful in defining the full extent of the disease as opposed to CT based imaging. The GTV should encompass all gross disease including disease that extends beyond the vulva and suspicious lymph nodes (i.e. PET avid, >1 cm in short axis, or those with a necrotic centre). The CTV should include GTV and the entire vulva, except in cases of posterior located lesions the mons pubis may be omitted. In cases where disease extends beyond the vulva, it is important to ensure that the CTV encompasses the GTV with a 2–3 cm margin.

In select patients with features such as extensive LVSI, satellite lesions or dermal lymphatic infiltration, additional margins of tissue surrounding the primary lesion can be encompassed within the CTV. If the tumour is seen invading muscle/soft tissue on the MRI or abutting muscle/tissue on CT, a portion of the muscle/tissue should be included in the CTV. In cases where the primary lesion involves the vagina, the GTV + 3.0 cm (into the vagina) should be included in the CTV. If uncertainty exists as to the extent of proximal invasion or in cases of LVSI, the entire vagina should be included in the CTV. Use of MRI in this setting can be helpful in delineating the extent of vaginal involvement and incorporated in the contouring process. As previously mentioned, in cases of vaginal involvement, an ITV using a full and empty bladder scan should be created to account for vaginal displacement. Similarly, in cases where the patient's rectum remains full after multiple attempts at bowel preparation and simulation, a vaginal ITV may be generated by combining vaginal contours from both full and empty rectal CT studies or alternatively, fiducials may be placed in the vagina to ensure target coverage. For posteriorly located lesions, the perineal space is to be included in the CTV [194]. In circumstances where the primary mass involves the anus, anal canal or bladder, the CTV should include the GTV expanded by at least 2 cm into the anorectum (and/or bladder). In cases of periurethral involvement such as disease involving the urethral meatus, the GTV plus at least 2 cm of urethra is included in the CTV. If the GTV extends into the mid or proximal urethra, the entire urethra and bladder neck should be included in the CTV. For clitoral lesions, the GTV plus at least 2 cm is included in the CTV, and in the majority of cases, the CTV should extend to the pubic bone, ensuring coverage of the suspensory ligament of the clitoris. The CTV (or ITV) to PTV margins should be 0.7–1 cm. In the postoperative setting, the CTV primary should cover the entire vulva resection bed if negative margins were obtained. If resection margins were close or positive, the resection bed plus a margin of at least 2 cm should be included in the CTV. Additionally, a wire should be placed on the surgical scar to identify regions to potentially boost.

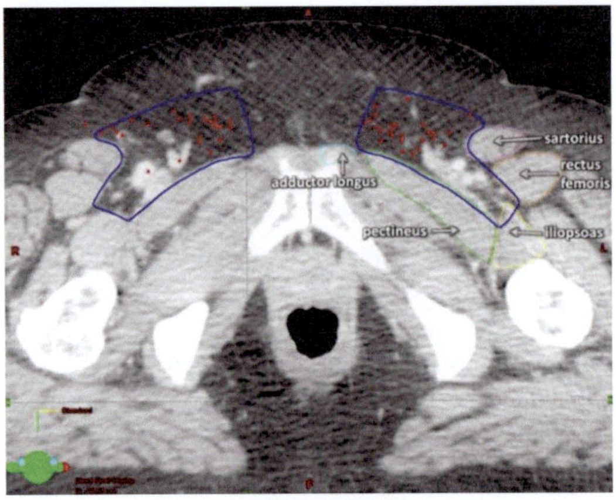

Fig. 6 Suggested anatomic boundaries for inguinal lymph node contouring as per Kim et al. [195]

In regard to nodal contouring in the undissected groin, any involved regional nodal basin should be included in the nodal contour. Grossly enlarged nodes are to be defined as a GTV. A PTV of 0.5–0.7 mm should be applied to each grossly enlarged nodal GTV. The CTV is to encompass the entire nodal bed (including the grossly enlarged node and its respective nodal PTV) to ensure that any extranodal spread (extracapsular extension) is covered. When contouring the pelvic lymph nodes, a 7–8 mm margin around the vessels should be included. When contouring the inguinofemoral lymph nodes, the groin compartment defined by the surrounding muscles should be contoured as shown in Fig. 6 [195]. Nodal basin anatomy is described further in Table 8. In cases of nodal involvement, the nodal echelon above the highest involved lymph node should be included in the nodal CTV. Additionally, in cases where the ipsilateral groin (inguinofemoral region) is involved, it is recommended to treat the contralateral groin as well (i.e. lymphatic flow disruption). In cases where the primary CTV involves the vulva only and/or the distal vagina (i.e. disease adjacent to the introitus), periurethral or periclitoral regions, the following nodal groups should be included in the nodal CTV: bilateral inguinofemoral, bilateral obturator, bilateral internal and external iliac groups. If the primary mass involves the proximal posterior vaginal wall, the pre-sacral nodes should be included in the nodal CTV. If the primary involves the anus/anal canal, the following nodal basins should be included in the CTV: bilateral inguinofemoral, bilateral obturator, bilateral internal and external iliac nodes, perirectal (including mesorectum) and presacral.

Table 8 Nodal anatomy

Lymph node basin	Superior border	Inferior border
Inguinofemoral	External iliac artery leaves the bony pelvis to become the femoral artery	2 cm below the sapheno-femoral junction; level of the lesser trochanter, in a plane perpendicular to the femur
External Iliac	Bifurcation of common iliac vessels; approximately L5/S1	External iliac artery leaves the bony pelvis to become the femoral artery
Internal Iliac	Bifurcation of common iliac vessels; approximately L5/S1	Levator ani inserts into obturator internus
Obturator	5 mm superior to the obturator canal, where the obturator artery is visible	Level of the obturator canal, where the obturator artery leaves the pelvis
Common Iliac	Bifurcation of the aorta	Bifurcation of the external and internal iliac vessels
Perirectal	Within mesorectum where rectum becomes sigmoid	Anorectal junction
Presacral	Superior aspect of S1	Inferior aspect of S3

4.11 Treatment Planning and Delivery

Given the proximity of sensitive organs at risk, image-guided intensity modulated radiotherapy is the preferred treatment technique for most cases of vulvar cancer. Dose and fractionation regimens depend on the goal of treatment (i.e.

neoadjuvant, definitive, adjuvant and palliative). In the neoadjuvant setting (as per GOG 205), 45–50.4 Gy (1.8 Gy fractions) is prescribed to the elective nodal basins and primary, with a sequential boost to 55.8 Gy–59.4 Gy to the primary. Additionally, large/suspicious nodes can be boosted to 55.8 Gy using a simultaneous integrated boost. Similarly, definitive treatment can be delivered in phases (i.e. sequentially) as follows: 45 Gy (1.8 Gy per day) to elective pelvic nodes, inguinal lymph nodes and entire vulva, and 50 Gy (2 Gy per day) to elective inguinal nodal basins and vulva primary (e.g. vulvar GTV + 1 cm). In cases of grossly enlarged nodes, a simultaneous integrated boost (SIB) to 55 Gy (2.2 Gy per day) can be considered. Following the initial phase, a sequential boost to the vulva primary (e.g., vulvar GTV + 1 cm) at 2 Gy per day (total dose: 66–70 Gy) is to be completed. In circumstances of markedly enlarged lymph nodes or nodes approximating the skin, a similar sequential boost (as an alternative or in addition to the aforementioned SIB) regimen should be considered. In the adjuvant setting, dosing to the primary in situations where the resection margins are negative is typically in the realm of 45–50 Gy [196]. In contrast, in the setting of close margins, at least 56 Gy is to be delivered, and positive margins should receive at least 60 Gy [197]. Clinically and/or radiographically uninvolved elective nodes are to receive a dose of 45–50 Gy. Postoperative dosing for the pathologically involved groin without evidence of extracapsular extension/gross residual disease is to receive a dose of 50 Gy, and in situations where extracapsular extension/gross residual disease is present, doses of 54–64 Gy are recommended. Lastly, in cases of unresectable gross nodal disease, doses of 60–70 are recommended. In regard to treatment planning, one must account for anatomic changes during treatment. For instance, patients will often experience significant acute dermatologic toxicity and vulvar/groin oedema over the course of treatment that can lead to treatment breaks and/or anatomic changes that drastically change the intended dose distribution. One strategy to pre-emptively attempt to address these challenges is to create a plan both with and without a 'virtual' 2–3 cm bolus in the event the non-bolus plan is needed. The virtual bolus is created in the treatment planning system (TPS) and should be placed where the PTV extends into air. Once the virtual bolus is added to the TPS, the PTV is extended into the bolus and the IMRT plan is created. The virtual bolus facilitates the TPS to flash dose distally (i.e. account for swelling/organ displacement during treatment) and allows the multi-leaf collimator leaves to remain open beyond the vulva. When treating, use a 0.5–1.0 cm physical bolus until grade III dermatitis/patient intolerance develops, then remove the bolus for the remainder of the treatment course. Nevertheless, adaptive therapy (i.e. replanning) should be strongly considered for some patients, especially when tumour shrinkage, vulvar oedema, or other developments such as lymphocyst formation during treatment change the position of either the tumour or a critical organ at risk.

GOG 279 was a single-arm phase II trial that attempted to improve outcomes with chemoradiation in locally advanced vulvar cancer, using dose-escalated IMRT (64 Gy in 34 fractions to gross vulvar disease) and concurrent cisplatin and gemcitabine [198]. Clinical and pathologic complete response rates were 71% and 73%, respectively. However, Grade 3 and higher toxicity was seen in 85% of patients, which may limit the applicability of this approach. A recent multi-institutional analysis of definitive IMRT to a median dose of 64 Gy to gross disease, with the majority receiving concurrent cisplatin, showed 94% compliance with planned treatment and a clinical complete response rate of 74% [199].

4.12 Organs at Risk (OARs)

Bladder, bowel (small bowel, sigmoid colon and large bowel), femoral heads, rectum and bone marrow should be contoured as organs at risk. The bowel OAR contour should exclude the rectum and anal canal and include the peritoneal cavity where the small bowel, sigmoid colon and large bowel (within the upper and lower boundaries of the treatment field) could potentially reside.

Table 9 Commonly employed dose constraints for vulvar cancer radiotherapy

OAR	Constraint
Bowel	V35 Gy <35%
	V40 Gy <30%
	V55 Gy < 5 cc
Bladder	Max <50 Gy
	V40 Gy <60%
Bone marrow	Max <60 Gy
	Mean <34 Gy
	V10 Gy <90%
	V20 Gy <80%
	V40 Gy < 37%
Kidneys	Max <25 Gy
	Mean <18 Gy
	V16 Gy <5%
Rectum	Max <50 Gy
	V40 Gy <40%
	V60 Gy <5%
Femoral heads	Max <45 Gy
	V35 Gy <5%
Spinal cord	Max <40 Gy
Ovaries	Mean <8 Gy

The bowel contour should extend at least 2 cm above the superior most aspect of the PTV. Table 9 outlines commonly employed dose constraints. The CTV nodal volume should be modified to exclude loops of small bowel on CT. The rectum should be contoured as an OAR with the inferior margin 2 cm above the anal verge and the superior margin where the rectum turns to become the sigmoid colon. The anus should be marked with a fiducial marker at the time of simulation, and the anal canal should be contoured separately.

4.13 Radiotherapy Sequelae

4.13.1 Acute/Subacute

Acute side effects in patients receiving a definitive course of radiotherapy are often significant. Most notably, radiation dermatitis of the vulva and/or groin is very common and can be severe (i.e. Grade 3+). Moist desquamation is not uncommon, particularly in area of skin folds; therefore, clinicians should be cognizant of superimposed infection. For instance, the rates of grade 3+ radiation dermatitis were 29% (radiation alone) and 56% (inguinofemoral dissection with adjuvant radiation) in the landmark GOG 88 trial [200]. In addition to dermatitis, symptoms related to bowel, vaginal and bladder irritation may be observed such as diarrhoea, increased urinary frequency, dysuria and vaginal discharge. Lastly, similar to other anatomic sites, acute/subacute fatigue may occur during and/or shortly after the radiotherapeutic course.

4.13.2 Late

Although many of the acute side effects resolve in the weeks following therapy, some side effects may present months to years after therapy is completed. Possible late effects include lymphedema of the vulva, groin, and/or lower extremities, bowel and bladder changes such as diarrhoea, small bowel obstruction, rectal bleeding, dysuria, or increased urinary frequency, vagina stenosis and menopause. Women should be counselled prior to and after therapy about vaginal dilator use to mitigate stenosis, as well as the utilization of moisturizers/lubricants during sexual intercourse.

4.14 Follow-Up and QOL Issues

After completion of therapy, patients should be evaluated every 3–6 months for the first 2 years with interval history and physical examination. From years 3–5 posttreatment, the patient should be evaluated every 6–12 months then annually thereafter. Surveillance imaging is currently not recommended; however, if there is suspicion for recurrence, appropriate imaging should be obtained. For patients treated with definitive radiotherapy and chemotherapy, PET/CT for response assessment is an option. Those with residual disease should be offered salvage surgery. Those with a complete response may be offered a biopsy at 3 months to confirm pathologic complete response, unless biopsy is felt to lead to complications. Gynaecologic survivorship should also include monitoring for physical and psychosocial effects related to cancer/therapy. For example, surgical and radiotherapeutic treatments significantly increase the risk of small bowel obstruction, urinary and/or gastrointestinal complications, in addition to issues with pelvic floor function. Chemotherapeutics may increase the risk of long-lasting side effects such as nephrotoxic city and/or neurotoxicity. Additional psychosocial factors may include depression and anxiety, financial concerns, as well as interpersonal (i.e. altered self-image, sexuality).

4.15 Prognosis, Results and Outcome, Survival

As is the case with many other malignancies, prognosis and outcomes in vulvar cancer are often a function of stage. Five-year overall survival rates are approximately 90%, 70–75%, 40–50% and 20% in patients with stage I, II, III, and IV disease, respectively [171]. With the exception of distant metastasis, lymph node involvement is the strongest predictor of outcome. In patients with lymph node involvement, five-year overall survival rates are 52% compared to 91% in patients with N0 disease. Predictors of lymph node involvement include depth of invasion (the strongest predictor), tumour size, grade and LVSI. Patients with a depth of invasion of 2 mm have approximately an 8% risk of lymph node involvement, whereas those with 3 mm have upwards of a 20% risk. In regard to patient selection for definitive therapy, there is limited evidence as to when to offer potentially curative therapy to patients with cephalad nodal involvement (i.e. iliac lymph nodes and/or lower para-aortic lymph nodes). Patients with pelvic-only lymph node metastasis may be potentially cured with aggressive locoregional therapy [201]. In some cases, clinicians may select patients for definitive treatment, whereas others may offer systemic therapy. In cases where definitive therapy is offered, intensity-modulated radiotherapy should be strongly considered. In patients with unresectable disease treated with preoperative or definitive chemoradiotherapy, there is a strong concordance between clinical complete response (cCR) and pathologic complete response (pCR), with reported concordance rates between 75% and 90%. In addition, lack of complete clinical response has been identified as a poor prognostic feature. In GOG 101, split-course BID radiotherapy (47.6 Gy) and cisplatin/5 FU were established as an effective preoperative regimen in which 48% and 31% of patients were found to have a cCR and pCR, respectively [202]. In contrast to GOG 101, GOG 205 utilized daily radiotherapy to a total dose of 57.6 Gy with weekly cisplatin [203]. Both cCR rates (64%) and pCR rates (50%) were improved in this trial compared to GOG 101, possibly due to increased dose and/or decreased overall treatment time. Further supporting a dose–response relationship, data from the University of Pittsburgh demonstrated a cCR rate of 63% and 88% in patients with unresectable disease receiving preoperative (median dose: 59.4 Gy) and definitive (median dose: 66 Gy) dose regimens [204]. Further study is ongoing (GOG 279) to elucidate the role of dose escalation in unresectable disease.

4.16 Future Research

While vulvar cancer represents a relatively rare malignancy, several phase II trials are ongoing in an attempt to further clarify several pertinent clinical questions. The recently-published GOG 279 phase 2 study assessed patients with unresectable FIGO stage IIIA-IVA disease who received upfront chemoradiotherapy with gemcitabine and cisplatin, and is discussed further in the Recent Advances section of this chapter. Another area of investigation is that of tailoring therapy based on the results of sentinel lymph node biopsy. The GROINNS-VIII, phase II trial, is assessing the role of chemoradiotherapy (56 Gy) to the groin in lieu of inguinofemoral dissection in early-stage vulvar patients who have a macrometastasis on SLNB. The primary endpoint is groin recurrence rate in the first 2 years following treatment.

Percepts Box

1. Vulvar cancer is an uncommon malignancy representing <1% of all cancers in women.
2. HPV driven vulvar cancer appears to have a more favourable response to therapy.
3. Selection of operative vs. non-operative management is typically a function of patient tolerance, extent of disease and anatomical location of disease.
4. Early-stage vulvar cancer is managed surgically and tends to have more favourable outcomes.
5. Locally advanced disease is managed with neoadjuvant/definitive chemoradiotherapy versus surgical resection followed by adjuvant (chemo)radiotherapy, depending on the presence of risk factors.
6. Radiotherapy is often an essential component of the treatment plan and may be utilized in the definitive, neoadjuvant, postoperative and palliative settings.
7. Clinical exam is paramount in delineating the CTV for radiation treatment planning.
8. Optimal treatment selection in vulvar cancer is critical, considering the physical as well as psychosocial impact treatment may have on the patient.
9. Acute and late side effects are often significant, and patients should be appropriately counselled before, during and after treatment is completed.
10. Ongoing studies are evaluating strategies of treatment escalation and de-escalation.

4.17 Conclusions

Vulvar cancer is a rare disease most commonly associated with the elderly and chronic inflammatory conditions, albeit there is an increasing number of HPV driven malignancies. Management is often surgical in early-stage cases, but often multidisciplinary in more advanced cases. Radiotherapy is often an essential component of the treatment plan and may be utilized in the definitive, neoadjuvant, postoperative and palliative settings. Acute and late side effects are often significant, and patients should be appropriately counselled before, during and after treatment is completed. Given the toxicities associated with treatment, ongoing studies are attempting to further identify which patient populations may safely undergo de-escalation of therapy, whereas others are attempting to determine who may benefit from treatment escalation.

5 Vaginal Cancer

5.1 Anatomy and Patterns of Spread

Vagina is the fibro-muscular passage extending from the uterine cervix superiorly to the vulva inferiorly. It is lined by stratified non-keratinizing mucosal epithelium, and a thin submucosal connective tissue separates the mucosa from the underlying muscular layer. Vagina has a rich and complex plexus of submucosal lymphatics while those from the proximal third of vagina follow the cervical lymphatics, distal third of vagina drains into superficial inguinal region.

5.2 Epidemiology and Risk Factors

Most malignant vaginal lesions are due to secondary involvement through local spread or metastases from other gynaecological cancers. There is no evidence-based consensus definition to differentiate primary vaginal cancer from vaginal recurrences of cervical or endometrial cancers. According to the definition by FIGO, involvement of cervix or vulva at the time of presentation excludes the diagnosis of primary vaginal cancer, and such cases are labelled as cervical or vulvar cancer, respectively [205]. Similarly, disease-free interval of 5 years in patients with prior gynaecological cancers is generally considered as the cut-off for differentiating primary vaginal cancer from recurrent vaginal cancer [206].

Clinical presentation, epidemiology and risk factors for primary vaginal cancer have a significant overlap with those for cervical and vulvar cancers, with incidence peaking in the sixth and seventh decade of life. Non-keratinizing squamous cell carcinoma is the most common histological variant, while others like basaloid, verrucous or sarcomatoid variants of squamous cell carcinoma, adenocarcinoma, clear cell carcinoma, melanoma and leiomyosarcoma are relatively rare [207].

5.3 Diagnostic and Staging Evaluation

Pre-treatment evaluation of patients with vaginal cancer is similar to that for cervical cancer, with thorough clinical examination and cross-sectional imaging of the thorax, abdomen and pelvis being the mainstay for staging. FIGO staging system (last revised in 2009) is commonly used for prognostication and deciding the treatment approaches and is presented in Table 10 [205].

Table 10 FIGO (2009) staging: Carcinoma of the vagina

Stage	Description
I	The carcinoma is limited to the vaginal wall
II	The carcinoma has involved the subvaginal tissue but has not extended to pelvic wall
III	The carcinoma has extended to the pelvic wall
IV	The carcinoma has extended beyond the true pelvis or has involved the mucosa of bladder or rectum; bullous oedema, such does not permit a case to be allotted to stage IV
IVA	Tumour invades bladder and/or rectal mucosa and/or direct extension beyond the true pelvis
IVB	Spread to distant organs

5.4 Principles of Management

Surgery has a limited role in the management of vaginal cancer and can be offered to a very selected group of patients with small, superficial, well-demarcated stage I lesions involving proximal vagina. Wide excision with adequate negative margins with or without hysterectomy and lymph node assessment is generally recommended for such patients. Adjuvant radiation may be considered in patients with close or positive margins and modality of delivery (EBRT or brachytherapy) should be individualized.

Surgical management of more advanced stages may necessitate radical procedures like total vaginectomy, vulvo-vaginectomy or pelvic exenteration in addition to lymph node assessment. Such procedures are not routinely recommended as primary treatment due to associated morbidity and are usually reserved for salvage of post-radiation recurrences.

Non-operative management with radiotherapy forms the mainstay of treatment for advanced non-metastatic vaginal cancer, both primary as well as recurrent. Though there is no randomized evidence supporting the benefit of adding concurrent chemotherapy in this setting, it is widely practiced based on extrapolation of benefits observed in cervical cancer patients.

Definitive radiotherapy should aim to deliver appropriate curative doses to the primary disease as well as elective nodal volumes, and the principles of management reflect those for cervical cancer. Brachytherapy forms an integral part of definitive management of vaginal cancer and often necessitates the use of interstitial component to deliver therapeutic doses to residual disease after EBRT. Appropriate brachytherapy applicators like single-channel vaginal cylinders, perineal template-based applicators or newer hybrid intracavitary-interstitial applicators or multichannel vaginal cylinders should be used based on the extent of residual disease and expertise available. Consensus recommendations for target volume delineation have been developed recently by GEC-ESTRO and ABS, with an aim to adapt the brachytherapy doses based on treatment response after EBRT [208].

Compared to cervical cancer stage-wise, survival outcomes are generally inferior for vaginal cancer [207]. Aggregated data from 13 centres reported 5-year survival rates of 74.3%, 53.5%, 34% and 15.3% for stage I, II, III and IV vaginal cancer, respectively [209]. Relatively better outcomes were reported in a recent retrospective analysis of patients treated with definitive radiation, with 5-year survival rates ranging from 96% for stage I patients to 53% for stage IVA patients [210].

Treatment of metastatic disease should be individualized based on the symptom burden and may include systemic therapies, palliative radiotherapy, or diversion surgery, among others, in appropriate combinations.

5.5 Follow-Up

Principles of follow-up after treatment of vaginal cancer are in parallel to those for cervical cancer, with clinical examination and symptom-directed imaging being the mainstay. Appropriate supportive and rehabilitative treatment should be offered concurrently, considering the morbidity associated with existing treatment options.

Multiple Choice Questions

1. High Risk CTV in MR-IGABT for cervical cancer includes all except
   (a) GTV residual at BT
   (b) Entire cervix
   (c) "Grey" areas
   (d) GTV at diagnosis
2. Wrong statement about endometrial cancer
   (a) Type 2 endometrial cancer is oestrogen-mediated.
   (b) Type 1 endometrial cancer has a better prognosis.
   (c) Clear cell carcinoma of the endometrium is considered type 2 histology.
   (d) The prognosis of endometrial carcinosarcoma is driven by the carcinomatous component.
3. A 42-year-old female was diagnosed with large cell non-keratinizing carcinoma of cervix, stage IIA1 (FIGO 2018). She underwent type II radical hysterectomy and histopathology revealed a 3 cm tumour arising from the anterior lip of the cervix and extending to anterior vaginal wall. Deep cervical stromal invasion, parametrial invasion were absent. Lympho-vascular space invasion and vaginal cuff margin were positive. All pelvic nodes were negative. Optimum adjuvant therapy for her would be.
   (a) Vaginal cuff brachytherapy alone
   (b) EBRT + Vaginal cuff brachytherapy
   (c) EBRT + concurrent chemotherapy
   (d) EBRT + concurrent chemotherapy + vaginal cuff brachytherapy
4. False statement regarding Lynch syndrome
   (a) Only females are affected.
   (b) Autosomal dominant pattern of inheritance.
   (c) Endometrial cancer is considered the commonest sentinel cancer among women with Lynch syndrome.
   (d) Increased risk of colorectal, ovarian and small bowel cancer.
5. True statement regarding systemic therapy for locally advanced cervical cancer (LACC)
   (a) Neoadjuvant chemotherapy followed by surgery is an effective strategy for FIGO (2018) stage IIB cervical cancer.
   (b) The addition of concurrent chemotherapy has no benefit in patients with stage IIIB cervical cancer.
   (c) The addition of Adjuvant chemotherapy has been shown to improve overall survival in LACC treated with concurrent chemoradiation.
   (d) Carboplatin is considered inferior to cisplatin for concurrent chemoradiation in LACC.
6. Lymph node regions included electively for EBRT in stage IIB (FIGO 2018) cervical cancer include all except
   (a) External iliac
   (b) Internal iliac
   (c) Presacral
   (d) Lower Para-aortic
7. False statement about landmark adjuvant therapy studies in endometrial cancer
   (a) PORTEC 1 compared (EBRT) to (Chemotherapy).

(b) PORTEC 2 compared (EBRT) to (Vaginal cuff BT).
(c) PORTEC 3 compared (EBRT) to (EBRT + Chemotherapy).
(d) GOG 258 compared (EBRT + Chemotherapy) to (Chemotherapy).

8. True statement regarding basaloid squamous cell carcinoma of the vulva
(a) Clinical behaviour is similar to basal cell carcinoma.
(b) Commonly associated with HPV.
(c) Older women are more frequently affected.
(d) Lichen sclerosus is a risk factor.

9. A 60-year-old lady was diagnosed with well-lateralized basaloid squamous cell cancer of the vulva. She underwent wide excision with ipsilateral inguinofemoral dissection; contralateral groin was not addressed surgically, since facilities for frozen section or sentinel nodal biopsy were not available. Post-op HPE revealed a 3 cm tumour in the right labia majora, well lateralised, with 1 cm surgical margins all around and 3 lymph nodes on the right side showing macrometastases with extracapsular extension. She was planned for adjuvant radiation therapy. False statement among the following
(a) Right inguinal region to be included in the target volume.
(b) Right pelvic region to be excluded from the target volume.
(c) Vulva to be included in the target volume.
(d) Left inguinal region to be included in the target volume.

10. False statement regarding lymph nodal management in vulvar cancer
(a) Bilateral inguinofemoral regions should be addressed in tumours within 2 cm of midline, when depth of invasion is more than 1 mm.
(b) In well lateralised tumours with negative nodes on ipsilateral inguinofemoral assessment, risk of microscopic nodal involvement in contralateral groin is >20%
(c) Nodal metastases >2 mm are considered as macro-metastases
(d) Nodal metastases >0.2 mm but ≤2 mm are considered as micro-metastases

11. Which among the following is the preferred strategy for patients with significant parametrial involvement after 5 weeks of concurrent chemoradiation in cervical cancer:
(a) Parametrial EBRT boost with midline shield followed by ICBT.
(b) EBRT boost/SBRT instead of brachytherapy.
(c) Hybrid IC + IS brachytherapy.
(d) Adjuvant chemotherapy after ICBT.

12. Image Guided Adaptive Brachytherapy for cervical cancer is discussed in detail in which of the following ICRU documents?
(a) ICRU 89
(b) ICRU 38
(c) ICRU 62
(d) ICRU 50

13. A 65-year-old female was diagnosed with high-grade serous endometrial cancer with deep myometrial invasion (FIGO stage IB), with extensive LVSI and negative pelvic lymph nodes on post-operative histopathology. The preferred management strategy would be
(a) Vaginal cuff brachytherapy.
(b) No adjuvant therapy needed.
(c) Chemotherapy + EBRT.
(d) EBRT alone.

14. A 40-year-old female was diagnosed with an infiltrative growth with epicentre in the mid vaginal region. Proximally, the growth was involving the posterior lip of cervix; distally, the growth was extending to the lower third of vagina, but 2 cm short of the introitus. Bilateral parametrium and paracolpos were free. No nodal/distant metastases were observed on imaging. According to FIGO, she should be classified as
(a) Vaginal Cancer, stage I
(b) Vaginal Cancer, stage II
(c) Cervical Cancer, stage IIIA
(d) Cervical Cancer, stage IIA

15. The presence of which marker among the following indicates the best prognosis in endometrial cancer
    (a) POL-E
    (b) P53
    (c) L1CAM
    (d) MMRd

Answer Key

1. (d)
2. (a)
3. (d)
4. (a)
5. (d)
6. (d)
7. (a)
8. (b)
9. (b)
10. (b)
11. (c)
12. (a)
13. (c)
14. (c)
15. (a)

References

1. Sung H, Ferlay J, Siegel RL, Laversanne M, Soerjomataram I, Jemal A, Bray F. Global cancer statistics 2020: GLOBOCAN estimates of incidence and mortality worldwide for 36 cancers in 185 countries. CA Cancer J Clin. 2021;71(3):209–49.
2. Bhatla N, Berek JS, Cuello Fredes M, Denny LA, Grenman S, Karunaratne K, Kehoe ST, Konishi I, Olawaiye AB, Prat J, Sankaranarayanan R. Revised FIGO staging for carcinoma of the cervix uteri. Int J Gynecol Obstet. 2019;145(1):129–35.
3. Mayadev JS, Ke G, Mahantshetty U, Pereira MD, Tarnawski R, Toita T. Global challenges of radiotherapy for the treatment of locally advanced cervical cancer. Int J Gynecol Cancer. 2022;32(3):436–45.
4. Mahantshetty U, Poetter R, Beriwal S, Grover S, Lavanya G, Rai B, Petric P, Tanderup K, Carvalho H, Hegazy N, Mohamed S. IBS-GEC ESTRO-ABS recommendations for CT based contouring in image guided adaptive brachytherapy for cervical cancer. Radiother Oncol. 2021;160:273–84.
5. Höhn AK, Brambs CE, Hiller GG, May D, Schmoeckel E, Horn LC. 2020 WHO classification of female genital tumors. Geburtshilfe Frauenheilkd. 2021;81(10):1145–53.
6. Fischerova D, Cibula D, Stenhova H, Vondrichova H, Calda P, Zikan M, Freitag P, Slama J, Dundr P, Belacek J. Transrectal ultrasound and magnetic resonance imaging in staging of early cervical cancer. Int J Gynecol Cancer. 2008;18(4):766–72.
7. Nguyen NC, Beriwal S, Moon CH, Furlan A, Mountz JM, Rangaswamy B. 18F-FDG PET/MRI primary staging of cervical cancer: a pilot study with PET/CT comparison. J Nucl Med Technol. 2020;48(4):331–5.
8. Haldorsen IS, Lura N, Blaakær J, Fischerova D, Werner HM. What is the role of imaging at primary diagnostic work-up in uterine cervical cancer? Curr Oncol Rep. 2019;21(9):1–5.
9. Matani H, Patel AK, Horne ZD, Beriwal S. Utilization of functional MRI in the diagnosis and management of cervical cancer. Front Oncol. 2022:6036.
10. Chopra SJ, Mathew A, Maheshwari A, Bhatla N, Singh S, Rai B, Surappa ST, Ghosh J, Sharma D, Bhaumik J, Biswas M. National cancer grid of India consensus guidelines on the management of cervical cancer. J Glob Oncol. 2018;4:1–5.
11. Landoni F, Maneo A, Colombo A, Placa F, Milani R, Perego P, Favini G, Ferri L, Mangioni C. Randomised study of radical surgery versus radiotherapy for stage Ib-IIa cervical cancer. Lancet. 1997;350(9077):535–40.
12. Delgado G, Bundy BN, Fowler WC Jr, Stehman FB, Sevin B, Creasman WT, Major F, DiSaia P, Zaino R. A prospective surgical pathological study of stage I squamous carcinoma of the cervix: a Gynecologic Oncology Group Study. Gynecol Oncol. 1989;35(3):314–20.
13. Sedlis A, Bundy BN, Rotman MZ, Lentz SS, Muderspach LI, Zaino RJ. A randomized trial of pelvic radiation therapy versus no further therapy in selected patients with stage IB carcinoma of the cervix after radical hysterectomy and pelvic lymphadenectomy: a Gynecologic Oncology Group Study. Gynecol Oncol. 1999;73(2):177–83.
14. Rotman M, Sedlis A, Piedmonte MR, Bundy B, Lentz SS, Muderspach LI, Zaino RJ. A phase III randomized trial of postoperative pelvic irradiation in Stage IB cervical carcinoma with poor prognostic features: follow-up of a gynecologic oncology group study. Int J Radiat Oncol Biol Phys. 2006;65(1):169–76.
15. Levinson K, Beavis AL, Purdy C, Rositch AF, Viswanathan A, Wolfson AH, Kelly MG, Tewari KS, McNally L, Guntupalli SR, Ragab O. Beyond Sedlis—a novel histology-specific nomogram for predicting cervical cancer recurrence risk: an NRG/GOG ancillary analysis. Gynecol Oncol. 2021;162(3):532–8.
16. Ryu SY, Deng W, Albuquerque K, Koh WJ, Mayadev J, Heugel A, Kim BJ, Kim DY, Cho CH, Kim JW, No JH, Mannel RS, Miller K, Fabian D, Chase DM,

Gil KM, Small W, Jr, Rodgers W, Leath CA, 3rd, & Monk, BJ. Randomized phase III trial of adjuvant radiation versus chemoradiation in intermediate-risk, early-stage cervical cancer following radical hysterectomy and lymphadenectomy: results from NRG Oncology/GOG-263/KGOG 1008. Annals of oncology: official journal of the European Society for Medical Oncol. 2025;36(12);1514–24. https://doi.org/10.1016/j.annonc.2025.09.003
17. Peters WA III, Liu PY, Barrett RJ, Stock RJ, Monk BJ, Berek JS, Souhami L, Grigsby P, Gordon W Jr, Alberts DS. Concurrent chemotherapy and pelvic radiation therapy compared with pelvic radiation therapy alone as adjuvant therapy after radical surgery in high-risk early-stage cancer of the cervix. Obstet Gynecol Surv. 2000;55(8):491–2.
18. Jhingran A. Adjuvant chemotherapy following concurrent chemoradiation (CRT) in patients with high-risk early-stage cervical carcinoma following radical hysterectomy: Results of NRG oncology/RTOG 0724/GOG-0724. J Clin Oncol. 2024;42(16_suppl):5504-5504. https://doi.org/10.1200/JCO.2024.42.16_SUPPL.5504
19. Chopra S, Dora T, Gupta S, Kannan S, Engineer R, Menachery S, Phurailatpam R, Mahantshetty UM, Swamidas J, Ghosh J, Maheshwari A. Phase III randomized trial of postoperative adjuvant conventional radiation (3DCRT) versus image guided intensity modulated radiotherapy (IG-IMRT) in cervical cancer (PARCER): final analysis. Int J Radiat Oncol Biol Phys. 2020;108(3):S1–2.
20. Abu-Rustum NR, Yashar CM, Bean S, Bradley K, Campos SM, Chon HS, Chu C, Cohn D, Crispens MA, Damast S, Fisher CM. NCCN guidelines insights: cervical cancer, version 1.2020: featured updates to the NCCN Guidelines. J Natl Compr Cancer Netw. 2020;18(6):660–6.
21. Morris M, Eifel PJ, Lu J, Grigsby PW, Levenback C, Stevens RE, Rotman M, Gershenson DM, Mutch DG. Pelvic radiation with concurrent chemotherapy compared with pelvic and para-aortic radiation for high-risk cervical cancer. N Engl J Med. 1999;340(15):1137–43.
22. Keys HM, Bundy BN, Stehman FB, Muderspach LI, Chafe WE, Suggs CL, Walker JL, Gersell D. Cisplatin, radiation, and adjuvant hysterectomy compared with radiation and adjuvant hysterectomy for bulky stage IB cervical carcinoma. N Engl J Med. 1999;340(15):1154–61.
23. Rose PG, Bundy BN, Watkins EB, Thigpen JT, Deppe G, Maiman MA, Clarke-Pearson DL, Insalaco S. Concurrent cisplatin-based radiotherapy and chemotherapy for locally advanced cervical cancer. N Engl J Med. 1999;340(15):1144–53.
24. Whitney CW, Sause W, Bundy BN, Malfetano JH, Hannigan EV, Fowler WC Jr, Clarke-Pearson DL, Liao SY. Randomized comparison of fluorouracil plus cisplatin versus hydroxyurea as an adjunct to radiation therapy in stage IIB-IVA carcinoma of the cervix with negative para-aortic lymph nodes: a Gynecologic Oncology Group and Southwest Oncology Group study. J Clin Oncol. 1999;17(5):1339–48.
25. Peters WA III, Liu PY, Barrett RJ II, Stock RJ, Monk BJ, Berek JS, Souhami L, Grigsby P, Gordon W Jr, Alberts DS. Concurrent chemotherapy and pelvic radiation therapy compared with pelvic radiation therapy alone as adjuvant therapy after radical surgery in high-risk early-stage cancer of the cervix. J Clin Oncol. 2000;18(8):1606–13.
26. Pearcey R, Brundage M, Drouin P, Jeffrey J, Johnston D, Lukka H, MacLean G, Souhami L, Stuart G, Tu D. Phase III trial comparing radical radiotherapy with and without cisplatin chemotherapy in patients with advanced squamous cell cancer of the cervix. J Clin Oncol. 2002;20(4):966–72.
27. Chemoradiotherapy for Cervical Cancer Meta-Analysis Collaboration. Reducing uncertainties about the effects of chemoradiotherapy for cervical cancer: a systematic review and meta-analysis of individual patient data from 18 randomized trials. J Clin Oncol. 2008;26(35):5802.
28. Chuang LT, Temin S, Camacho R, Dueñas-Gonzalez A, Feldman S, Gultekin M, Gupta V, Horton S, Jacob G, Kidd EA, Lishimpi K. Management and care of women with invasive cervical cancer: American Society of Clinical Oncology resource-stratified clinical practice guideline. J Glob Oncol. 2016;2(5):311–40.
29. Colombo N, Carinelli S, Colombo A, Marini C, Rollo D, Sessa C. Cervical cancer: ESMO Clinical Practice Guidelines for diagnosis, treatment and follow-up. Ann Oncol. 2012;23:vii27–32.
30. Shrivastava S, Mahantshetty U, Engineer R, Chopra S, Hawaldar R, Hande V, Kerkar RA, Maheshwari A, Shylasree TS, Ghosh J, Bajpai J. Cisplatin chemoradiotherapy vs radiotherapy in FIGO stage IIIB squamous cell carcinoma of the uterine cervix: a randomized clinical trial. JAMA Oncol. 2018;4(4):506–13.
31. Pötter R, Tanderup K, Schmid MP, Jürgenliemk-Schulz I, Haie-Meder C, Fokdal LU, Sturdza AE, Hoskin P, Mahantshetty U, Segedin B, Bruheim K. MRI-guided adaptive brachytherapy in locally advanced cervical cancer (EMBRACE-I): a multicentre prospective cohort study. Lancet Oncol. 2021;22(4):538–47.
32. Mahantshetty U, Gudi S, Singh R, Sasidharan A, Sastri SC, Gurram L, Sharma D, Ganeshrajah S, Mg J, Badakh D, Basu A. Indian Brachytherapy Society Guidelines for radiotherapeutic management of cervical cancer with special emphasis on high-dose-rate brachytherapy. J Contemp Brachytherapy. 2019;11(4):293.
33. Gupta S, Maheshwari A, Parab P, Mahantshetty U, Hawaldar R, Sastri S, Kerkar R, Engineer R, Tongaonkar H, Ghosh J, Gulia S. Neoadjuvant chemotherapy followed by radical surgery versus concomitant chemotherapy and radiotherapy in patients with stage IB2, IIA, or IIB squamous cervical can-

cer: a randomized controlled trial. J Clin Oncol. 2018;36(16):1548–55.
34. Miriyala R, Mahantshetty U, Maheshwari A, Gupta S. Neoadjuvant chemotherapy followed by surgery in cervical cancer: past, present and future. Int J Gynecol Cancer. 2022;32(3):260–5.
35. Duenas-González A, Zarbá JJ, Patel F, Alcedo JC, Beslija S, Casanova L, Pattaranutaporn P, Hameed S, Blair JM, Barraclough H, Orlando M. Phase III, open-label, randomized study comparing concurrent gemcitabine plus cisplatin and radiation followed by adjuvant gemcitabine and cisplatin versus concurrent cisplatin and radiation in patients with stage IIB to IVA carcinoma of the cervix. J Clin Oncol. 2011;29(13):1678–85.
36. Mileshkin LR, Moore KN, Barnes EH, Gebski V, Narayan K, King MT, Bradshaw N, Lee YC, Diamante K, Fyles AW, Small W. Adjuvant chemotherapy following chemoradiotherapy as primary treatment for locally advanced cervical cancer versus chemoradiotherapy alone (OUTBACK): an international, open-label, randomised, phase 3 trial. The Lancet Oncology. 2023;24(5):468–82.
37. Monk BJ, Toita T, Wu X, Vázquez Limón JC, Tarnawski R, Mandai M, Shapira-Frommer R, Mahantshetty U, Del Pilar Estevez-Diz M, Zhou Q, Limaye S, Godinez FJR, Oppermann Kussler C, Varga S, Valdiviezo N, Aoki D, Leiva M, Lee JY, Sulay R, Kreynina Y, … Mayadev J. Durvalumab versus placebo with chemoradiotherapy for locally advanced cervical cancer (CALLA): a randomised, double-blind, phase 3 trial. The Lancet. Oncology 2023;24(12), 1334–1348. https://doi.org/10.1016/S1470-2045(23)00479-5
38. Lorusso D, Xiang Y, Hasegawa K, Scambia G, Leiva M, Ramos-Elias P et al. Pembrolizumab or placebo with chemoradiotherapy followed by pembrolizumab or placebo for newly diagnosed, high-risk, locally advanced cervical cancer (ENGOT-cx11/GOG-3047/KEYNOTE-A18): overall survival results from a randomised, double-blind, placebo-controlled, phase 3 trial. The Lancet. 2024;404(10460):1321–32.
39. Mangaj A, Chopra S, Nout RA. Defining the role of high-dose radiation in oligometastatic & oligorecurrent cervical cancer. Indian J Med Res. 2021;154(2):303–18.
40. Ramirez PT, Frumovitz M, Pareja R, Lopez A, Vieira MA, Ribeiro R. Phase III randomized trial of laparoscopic or robotic versus abdominal radical hysterectomy in patients with early-stage cervical cancer: LACC Trial. Gynecol Oncol. 2018;149:245.
41. Frumovitz M, Obermair A, Coleman RL, Pareja R, Lopez A, Ribero R, Isla D, Rendon G, Bernardini MQ, Buda A, Moretti-Marquez R. Quality of life in patients with cervical cancer after open versus minimally invasive radical hysterectomy (LACC): a secondary outcome of a multicentre, randomised, open-label, phase 3, non-inferiority trial. Lancet Oncol. 2020;21(6):851–60.
42. Wenzel HH, Kruitwagen RF, Nijman HW, Bekkers RL, Van Gorp T, de Kroon CD, van Lonkhuijzen LR, Massuger LF, Smolders RG, van Trommel NE, Yigit R. Short-term surgical complications after radical hysterectomy—a nationwide cohort study. Acta Obstet Gynecol Scand. 2020;99(7):925–32.
43. Pieterse QD, Maas CP, Ter Kuile MM, Lowik M, Van Eijkeren MA, Trimbos JBMZ, Kenter GG. An observational longitudinal study to evaluate miction, defecation, and sexual function after radical hysterectomy with pelvic lymphadenectomy for early-stage cervical cancer. Int J Gynecol Cancer. 2006;16(3):1119–29.
44. Portelance L, Chao KC, Grigsby PW, Bennet H, Low D. Intensity-modulated radiation therapy (IMRT) reduces small bowel, rectum, and bladder doses in patients with cervical cancer receiving pelvic and para-aortic irradiation. Int J Radiat Oncol Biol Phys. 2001;51(1):261–6.
45. Mell LK, Sirák I, Wei L, Tarnawski R, Mahantshetty U, Yashar CM, McHale MT, Xu R, Honerkamp-Smith G, Carmona R, Wright M. Bone marrow-sparing intensity modulated radiation therapy with concurrent cisplatin for stage IB-IVA cervical cancer: an international multicenter phase II clinical trial (INTERTECC-2). Int J Radiat Oncol Biol Phys. 2017;97(3):536–45.
46. Mahantshetty U, Shetty S, Majumder D, Adurkar P, Swamidas J, Engineer R, Chopra S, Shrivastava S. Optimal bladder filling during high-dose-rate intracavitary brachytherapy for cervical cancer: a dosimetric study. J Contemp Brachytherapy. 2017;9(2):112–7.
47. Rai B, Bansal A, Patel F, Gulia A, Kapoor R, Sharma SC. Pelvic nodal CTV from L4–L5 or aortic bifurcation?—an audit of the patterns of regional failures in cervical cancer patients treated with pelvic radiotherapy. Jpn J Clin Oncol. 2014;44(10):941–7.
48. Taylor A, Rockall AG, Reznek RH, Powell ME. Mapping pelvic lymph nodes: guidelines for delineation in intensity-modulated radiotherapy. Int J Radiat Oncol Biol Phys. 2005;63(5):1604–12.
49. Lim K, Small JW, Portelance L, Creutzberg C, Jürgenliemk-Schulz IM, Mundt A, Mell LK, Mayr N, Viswanathan A, Jhingran A, Erickson B. Consensus guidelines for delineation of clinical target volume for intensity-modulated pelvic radiotherapy for the definitive treatment of cervix cancer. Int J Radiat Oncol Biol Phys. 2011;79(2):348–55.
50. Pötter R, Tanderup K, Kirisits C, de Leeuw A, Kirchheiner K, Nout R, Tan LT, Haie-Meder C, Mahantshetty U, Segedin B, Hoskin P. The EMBRACE II study: the outcome and prospect of two decades of evolution within the GEC-ESTRO GYN working group and the EMBRACE studies. Clin Transl Radiat Oncol. 2018;9:48–60.

51. Jürgenliemk-Schulz IM, Beriwal S, de Leeuw AA, Lindegaard JC, Nomden CN, Pötter R, Tanderup K, Viswanathan AN, Erickson B. Management of nodal disease in advanced cervical cancer. Semin Radiat Oncol. 2019;29(2):158–65. WB Saunders.
52. Gill BS, Lin JF, Krivak TC, Sukumvanich P, Laskey RA, Ross MS, Lesnock JL, Beriwal S. National Cancer Data Base analysis of radiation therapy consolidation modality for cervical cancer: the impact of new technological advancements. Int J Radiat Oncol Biol Phys. 2014;90(5):1083–90.
53. Georg D, Kirisits C, Hillbrand M, Dimopoulos J, Pötter R. Image-guided radiotherapy for cervix cancer: high-tech external beam therapy versus high-tech brachytherapy. Int J Radiat Oncol Biol Phys. 2008;71(4):1272–8.
54. Albuquerque K, Tumati V, Lea J, Ahn C, Richardson D, Miller D, Timmerman R. A phase II trial of stereotactic ablative radiation therapy as a boost for locally advanced cervical cancer. Int J Radiat Oncol Biol Phys. 2020;106(3):464–71.
55. Moiyadi AV. XIX annual conference on evidence based management of cancers in India "Technology and cancer care–promise and reality of the brave new world". 2021.
56. Hendry J, Jones GW, Mahantshetty UM, Sarria G, da Motta NW, Fidarova E, Abdel-Wahab M, Prasad RR. Radiobiological analysis of outcomes using external beam radiotherapy plus high dose-rate brachytherapy (4x7 Gy or 2x9 Gy) for cervical cancer in a multi-institution trial. Int J Radiat Oncol Biol Phys. 2017;99(5):1313–4.
57. https://beta.clinicaltrials.gov/study/NCT03005743.
58. Mahantshetty U, Gurram L, Bushra S, Ghadi Y, Aravindakshan D, Paul J, Hande V, Pilar A, Chopra S, Ghosh J, Shylasree TS. Single application multifractionated image guided adaptive high-dose-rate brachytherapy for cervical cancer: dosimetric and clinical outcomes. Int J Radiat Oncol Biol Phys. 2021;111(3):826–34.
59. Miriyala R, Mahantshetty U. Brachytherapy in cervical cancer radiotherapy during COVID-19 pandemic crisis: problems and prospects. J Contemp Brachytherapy. 2020;12(3):290–3.
60. Chakraborty S, Mahantshetty U, Chopra S, Lewis S, Hande V, Gudi S, Krishnatry R, Engineer R, Shrivastava SK. Income generated by women treated with magnetic resonance imaging-based brachytherapy: a simulation study evaluating the macroeconomic benefits of implementing a high-end technology in a public sector healthcare setting. Brachytherapy. 2017;16(5):981–7.
61. Schmeler KM, Pareja R, Blanco AL, Fregnani JH, Lopes A, Perrotta M, et al. ConCerv: a prospective trial of conservative surgery for low-risk early-stage cervical cancer. Int J Gynecol Cancer. 2021;31(10):1317–25.
62. Carneiro VC, Batista TP, Andrade MR, Barros AV, Câmara LH, Ramalho NM, et al. Proof-of-concept randomized phase II non-inferiority trial of simple versus type B2 hysterectomy in early-stage cervical cancer≤ 2 cm (LESSER). Int J Gynecol Cancer. 2023;33(4):498–503.
63. Plante M, Kwon JS, Ferguson S, Samouëlian V, Ferron G, Maulard A, et al. Simple versus radical hysterectomy in women with low-risk cervical cancer. N Engl J Med. 2024;390(9):819–29.
64. Takekuma M. Challenges and perspectives on less invasive surgery for early-stage cervical cancer: a critical analysis of the SHAPE trial and its implications. J Gynecol Oncol. 2024;35(2):e48.
65. McCormack M, Eminowicz G, Gallardo D, Diez P, Farrelly L, Kent C, et al. Induction chemotherapy followed by standard chemoradiotherapy versus standard chemoradiotherapy alone in patients with locally advanced cervical cancer (GCIG INTERLACE): an international, multicentre, randomised phase 3 trial. Lancet. 2024;404(10462):1525–35.
66. Lindegaard JC, Petric P, Tan LT, Hoskin P, Schmid MP, Jürgenliemk-Schulz I, et al. Are we making progress in curing advanced cervical cancer—again? Int J Gynecol Cancer. 2024;34(12):1940–5.
67. Petric P, Lindegaard JC, Schmid MP, Jürgenliemk-Schulz I, Mahantshetty U, Kirisits C, et al. INTERLACE: not a new standard for cervical cancer chemoradiation. Lancet. 2025;406(10505):806–7.
68. Courtney PT, Venkat PS, Shih YC, Chang AJ, Lee A, Steinberg ML, et al. Cost-effectiveness of pembrolizumab with chemoradiotherapy for locally advanced cervical cancer. JAMA Netw Open. 2025;8(3):e250033.
69. Schmid MP, Petric P, Mahantshetty U, Kirisits C, Tanderup K, Jürgenliemk-Schulz I, et al. Pembrolizumab for locally advanced cervical cancer. Lancet. 2024;404(10467):2050–1.
70. Pötter R, Tanderup K, Schmid MP, Ecker S, Kroon P, Lindegaard J, et al. EMBRACE II-a multicenter prospective interventional cohort study on IGRT-IMRT+ cisplatin+ MR-IGABT in locally advanced cervix cancer: overall results. Radiother Oncol. 2025;206:S837–40.
71. Lortet-Tieulent J, Ferlay J, Bray F, Jemal A. International patterns and trends in endometrial cancer incidence, 1978–2013. J Natl Cancer Inst. 2018;110(4):354–61.
72. Creasman WT, Ali S, Mutch DG, Zaino RJ, Powell MA, Mannel RS, et al. Surgical-pathological findings in type 1 and 2 endometrial cancer: an NRG Oncology/Gynecologic Oncology Group study on GOG-210 protocol. Gynecol Oncol. 2017;145(3):519–25.
73. Abu-Rustum NR, Yashar CM, Bradley K, Campos SM, Chino J, Chon HS, et al. NCCN guidelines(R) insights: uterine neoplasms, version 3.2021. J Natl Compr Canc Netw. 2021;19(8):888–95.
74. van den Heerik A, Horeweg N, Nout RA, Lutgens L, van der Steen-Banasik EM, Westerveld GH, et al. PORTEC-4a: international randomized trial

of molecular profile-based adjuvant treatment for women with high-intermediate risk endometrial cancer. Int J Gynecol Cancer. 2020;30(12):2002–7.
75. Schwarz JK, Beriwal S, Esthappan J, Erickson B, Feltmate C, Fyles A, et al. Consensus statement for brachytherapy for the treatment of medically inoperable endometrial cancer. Brachytherapy. 2015;14(5):587–99.
76. Gebhardt B, Gill B, Glaser S, Kim H, Houser C, Kelley J, et al. Image-guided tandem and cylinder brachytherapy as monotherapy for definitive treatment of inoperable endometrial carcinoma. Gynecol Oncol. 2017;147(2):302–8.
77. Lima J, Ali Z, Banerjee S. Immunotherapy and systemic therapy in metastatic/recurrent endometrial and cervical cancers. Clin Oncol (R Coll Radiol). 2021;33(9):608–15.
78. Koskas M, Amant F, Mirza MR, Creutzberg CL. Cancer of the corpus uteri: 2021 update. Int J Gynaecol Obstet. 2021;155(Suppl 1):45–60.
79. Powell MA, Olawaiye AB, Bermude A, Bhosale PR, Grigsby PW, Coepeland LJ, et al. Corpus uteri – carcinoma and carcinosarcoma. In: Amin MB, editor. AJCC cancer staging manual. 8th ed. Springer Nature; 2017.
80. Raglan O, Kalliala I, Markozannes G, Cividini S, Gunter MJ, Nautiyal J, et al. Risk factors for endometrial cancer: an umbrella review of the literature. Int J Cancer. 2019;145(7):1719–30.
81. Parslov M, Lidegaard O, Klintorp S, Pedersen B, Jonsson L, Eriksen PS, et al. Risk factors among young women with endometrial cancer: a Danish case-control study. Am J Obstet Gynecol. 2000;182(1 Pt 1):23–9.
82. Kaaks R, Lukanova A, Kurzer MS. Obesity, endogenous hormones, and endometrial cancer risk: a synthetic review. Cancer Epidemiol Biomarkers Prev. 2002;11(12):1531–43.
83. Gunter MJ, Hoover DR, Yu H, Wassertheil-Smoller S, Manson JE, Li J, et al. A prospective evaluation of insulin and insulin-like growth factor-I as risk factors for endometrial cancer. Cancer Epidemiol Biomarkers Prev. 2008;17(4):921–9.
84. Singh S, Resnick KE. Lynch syndrome and endometrial cancer. South Med J. 2017;110(4):265–9.
85. Tan MH, Mester JL, Ngeow J, Rybicki LA, Orloff MS, Eng C. Lifetime cancer risks in individuals with germline PTEN mutations. Clin Cancer Res. 2012;18(2):400–7.
86. Bokhman JV. Two pathogenetic types of endometrial carcinoma. Gynecol Oncol. 1983;15(1):10–7.
87. Slomovitz BM, Burke TW, Eifel PJ, Ramondetta LM, Silva EG, Jhingran A, et al. Uterine papillary serous carcinoma (UPSC): a single institution review of 129 cases. Gynecol Oncol. 2003;91(3):463–9.
88. Amant F, Moerman P, Neven P, Timmerman D, Van Limbergen E, Vergote I. Endometrial cancer. Lancet. 2005;366(9484):491–505.
89. Creasman WT, Kohler MF, Odicino F, Maisonneuve P, Boyle P. Prognosis of papillary serous, clear cell, and grade 3 stage I carcinoma of the endometrium. Gynecol Oncol. 2004;95(3):593–6.
90. Amant F, Cadron I, Fuso L, Berteloot P, de Jonge E, Jacomen G, et al. Endometrial carcinosarcomas have a different prognosis and pattern of spread compared to high-risk epithelial endometrial cancer. Gynecol Oncol. 2005;98(2):274–80.
91. Kolin DL, Quick CM, Dong F, Fletcher CDM, Stewart CJR, Soma A, et al. SMARCA4-deficient uterine sarcoma and undifferentiated endometrial carcinoma are distinct clinicopathologic entities. Am J Surg Pathol. 2020;44(2):263–70.
92. Cancer Genome Atlas Research N, Kandoth C, Schultz N, Cherniack AD, Akbani R, Liu Y, et al. Integrated genomic characterization of endometrial carcinoma. Nature. 2013;497(7447):67–73.
93. Leon-Castillo A, de Boer SM, Powell ME, Mileshkin LR, Mackay HJ, Leary A, et al. Molecular classification of the PORTEC-3 trial for high-risk endometrial cancer: impact on prognosis and benefit from adjuvant therapy. J Clin Oncol. 2020;38(29):3388–97.
94. Crosbie EJ, Kitson SJ, McAlpine JN, Mukhopadhyay A, Powell ME, Singh N. Endometrial cancer. Lancet. 2022;399(10333):1412–28.
95. Pennant ME, Mehta R, Moody P, Hackett G, Prentice A, Sharp SJ, et al. Premenopausal abnormal uterine bleeding and risk of endometrial cancer. BJOG. 2017;124(3):404–11.
96. Goldstein RB, Bree RL, Benson CB, Benacerraf BR, Bloss JD, Carlos R, et al. Evaluation of the woman with postmenopausal bleeding: Society of Radiologists in Ultrasound-Sponsored Consensus Conference statement. J Ultrasound Med. 2001;20(10):1025–36.
97. Leitao MM Jr, Kehoe S, Barakat RR, Alektiar K, Gattoc LP, Rabbitt C, et al. Comparison of D&C and office endometrial biopsy accuracy in patients with FIGO grade 1 endometrial adenocarcinoma. Gynecol Oncol. 2009;113(1):105–8.
98. Gimpelson RJ, Rappold HO. A comparative study between panoramic hysteroscopy with directed biopsies and dilatation and curettage. A review of 276 cases. Am J Obstet Gynecol. 1988;158(3 Pt 1):489–92.
99. Andreano A, Rechichi G, Rebora P, Sironi S, Valsecchi MG, Galimberti S. MR diffusion imaging for preoperative staging of myometrial invasion in patients with endometrial cancer: a systematic review and meta-analysis. Eur Radiol. 2014;24(6):1327–38.
100. Haldorsen IS, Salvesen HB. What is the best preoperative imaging for endometrial cancer? Curr Oncol Rep. 2016;18(4):25.
101. Kitajima K, Suzuki K, Senda M, Kita M, Nakamoto Y, Sakamoto S, et al. Preoperative nodal staging of uterine cancer: is contrast-enhanced PET/CT more accurate than non-enhanced PET/CT or enhanced CT alone? Ann Nucl Med. 2011;25(7):511–9.
102. Suzuki R, Miyagi E, Takahashi N, Sukegawa A, Suzuki A, Koike I, et al. Validity of positron emission tomography using fluoro-2-deoxyglucose for

the preoperative evaluation of endometrial cancer. Int J Gynecol Cancer. 2007;17(4):890–6.
103. Sartori E, Gadducci A, Landoni F, Lissoni A, Maggino T, Zola P, et al. Clinical behavior of 203 stage II endometrial cancer cases: the impact of primary surgical approach and of adjuvant radiation therapy. Int J Gynecol Cancer. 2001;11(6):430–7.
104. Matsuo K, Matsuzaki S, Nusbaum DJ, Machida H, Nagase Y, Grubbs BH, et al. Malignant peritoneal cytology and decreased survival of women with stage I endometrioid endometrial cancer. Eur J Cancer. 2020;133:33–46.
105. Janda M, Gebski V, Brand A, Hogg R, Jobling TW, Land R, et al. Quality of life after total laparoscopic hysterectomy versus total abdominal hysterectomy for stage I endometrial cancer (LACE): a randomised trial. Lancet Oncol. 2010;11(8):772–80.
106. Walker JL, Piedmonte MR, Spirtos NM, Eisenkop SM, Schlaerth JB, Mannel RS, et al. Laparoscopy compared with laparotomy for comprehensive surgical staging of uterine cancer: Gynecologic Oncology Group Study LAP2. J Clin Oncol. 2009;27(32):5331–6.
107. Maenpaa MM, Nieminen K, Tomas EI, Laurila M, Luukkaala TH, Maenpaa JU. Robotic-assisted vs traditional laparoscopic surgery for endometrial cancer: a randomized controlled trial. Am J Obstet Gynecol. 2016;215(5):588 e1–7.
108. Vargo JA, Boisen MM, Comerci JT, Kim H, Houser CJ, Sukumvanich P, et al. Neoadjuvant radiotherapy with or without chemotherapy followed by extrafascial hysterectomy for locally advanced endometrial cancer clinically extending to the cervix or parametria. Gynecol Oncol. 2014;135(2):190–5.
109. Boisen MM, Vargo JA, Beriwal S, Sukumvanich P, Olawaiye AB, Kelley JL, et al. Surgical outcomes of patients undergoing extrafascial hysterectomy after neoadjuvant radiotherapy with or without chemotherapy for locally advanced endometrial cancer clinically extending to the cervix or parametria. Int J Gynecol Cancer. 2017;27(6):1149–54.
110. Iheagwara UK, Vargo JA, Chen KS, Burton DR, Taylor SE, Berger JL, et al. Neoadjuvant chemoradiation therapy followed by extrafascial hysterectomy in locally advanced type II endometrial cancer clinically extending to cervix. Pract Radiat Oncol. 2019;9(4):248–56.
111. Creasman WT, Morrow CP, Bundy BN, Homesley HD, Graham JE, Heller PB. Surgical pathologic spread patterns of endometrial cancer. A Gynecologic Oncology Group Study. Cancer. 1987;60(8 Suppl):2035–41.
112. Group As, Kitchener H, Swart AM, Qian Q, Amos C, Parmar MK. Efficacy of systematic pelvic lymphadenectomy in endometrial cancer (MRC ASTEC trial): a randomised study. Lancet. 2009;373(9658):125–36.
113. Rossi EC, Kowalski LD, Scalici J, Cantrell L, Schuler K, Hanna RK, et al. A comparison of sentinel lymph node biopsy to lymphadenectomy for endometrial cancer staging (FIRES trial): a multicentre, prospective, cohort study. Lancet Oncol. 2017;18(3):384–92.
114. Cusimano MC, Vicus D, Pulman K, Maganti M, Bernardini MQ, Bouchard-Fortier G, et al. Assessment of sentinel lymph node biopsy vs lymphadenectomy for intermediate- and high-grade endometrial cancer staging. JAMA Surg. 2021;156(2):157–64.
115. Backes FJ, Felix AS, Plante M, Gregoire J, Sullivan SA, Rossi EC, et al. Sentinel lymph node (SLN) isolated tumor cells (ITCs) in otherwise stage I/II endometrioid endometrial cancer: to treat or not to treat? Gynecol Oncol. 2021;161(2):347–52.
116. Plante M, Stanleigh J, Renaud MC, Sebastianelli A, Grondin K, Gregoire J. Isolated tumor cells identified by sentinel lymph node mapping in endometrial cancer: does adjuvant treatment matter? Gynecol Oncol. 2017;146(2):240–6.
117. Altin D, Taskin S, Tokgozoglu N, Vatansever D, Guler AH, Gungor M, et al. Can risk groups accurately predict non-sentinel lymph node metastasis in sentinel lymph node-positive endometrial cancer patients? A Turkish Gynecologic Oncology Group Study (TRSGO-SLN-004). J Surg Oncol. 2021;123(2):638–45.
118. Kennard JA, Stephens AJ, Ahmad S, Zhu X, Singh C, McKenzie ND, et al. Sentinel lymph nodes (SLN) in endometrial cancer: the relationship between primary tumor histology, SLN metastasis size, and non-sentinel node metastasis. Gynecol Oncol. 2019;154(1):53–9.
119. Musunuru HB, Keller A, Olawaiye A, Sukumvanich P, Beriwal S. Indications for adjuvant radiation therapy in patients with pN0(i +) adenocarcinoma of the endometrium. Pract Radiat Oncol. 2022;12(4):348–53.
120. Garzon S, Uccella S, Zorzato PC, Bosco M, Franchi MP, Student V, et al. Fertility-sparing management for endometrial cancer: review of the literature. Minerva Med. 2021;112(1):55–69.
121. Randall ME, Filiaci V, McMeekin DS, von Gruenigen V, Huang H, Yashar CM, et al. Phase III trial: adjuvant pelvic radiation therapy versus vaginal brachytherapy plus paclitaxel/carboplatin in high-intermediate and high-risk early stage endometrial cancer. J Clin Oncol. 2019;37(21):1810–8.
122. Post CCB, de Boer SM, Powell ME, Mileshkin L, Katsaros D, Bessette P, et al. Long-term toxicity and health-related quality of life after adjuvant chemoradiation therapy or radiation therapy alone for high-risk endometrial cancer in the randomized PORTEC-3 trial. Int J Radiat Oncol Biol Phys. 2021;109(4):975–86.
123. de Boer SM, Powell ME, Mileshkin L, Katsaros D, Bessette P, Haie-Meder C, et al. Adjuvant chemoradiotherapy versus radiotherapy alone in women with high-risk endometrial cancer (PORTEC-3):

patterns of recurrence and post-hoc survival analysis of a randomised phase 3 trial. Lancet Oncol. 2019;20(9):1273–85.
124. de Boer SM, Powell ME, Mileshkin L, Katsaros D, Bessette P, Haie-Meder C, et al. Adjuvant chemoradiotherapy versus radiotherapy alone for women with high-risk endometrial cancer (PORTEC-3): final results of an international, open-label, multicentre, randomised, phase 3 trial. Lancet Oncol. 2018;19(3):295–309.
125. Matei D, Filiaci V, Randall ME, Mutch D, Steinhoff MM, DiSilvestro PA, et al. Adjuvant chemotherapy plus radiation for locally advanced endometrial cancer. N Engl J Med. 2019;380(24):2317–26.
126. Miller DS, Filiaci VL, Mannel RS, Cohn DE, Matsumoto T, Tewari KS, et al. Carboplatin and paclitaxel for advanced endometrial cancer: final overall survival and adverse event analysis of a phase III trial (NRG oncology/GOG0209). J Clin Oncol. 2020;38(33):3841–50.
127. Fader AN, Roque DM, Siegel E, Buza N, Hui P, Abdelghany O, et al. Randomized phase II trial of carboplatin-paclitaxel compared with carboplatin-paclitaxel-trastuzumab in advanced (stage III–IV) or recurrent uterine serous carcinomas that overexpress Her2/Neu (NCT01367002): updated overall survival analysis. Clin Cancer Res. 2020;26(15):3928–35.
128. Makker V, Colombo N, Casado Herraez A, Santin AD, Colomba E, Miller DS, et al. Lenvatinib plus pembrolizumab for advanced endometrial cancer. N Engl J Med. 2022;386(5):437–48.
129. O'Malley DM, Bariani GM, Cassier PA, Marabelle A, Hansen AR, De Jesus Acosta A, et al. Pembrolizumab in patients with microsatellite instability-high advanced endometrial cancer: results from the KEYNOTE-158 study. J Clin Oncol. 2022;40(7):752–61.
130. Sorbe B, Nordstrom B, Maenpaa J, Kuhelj J, Kuhelj D, Okkan S, et al. Intravaginal brachytherapy in FIGO stage I low-risk endometrial cancer: a controlled randomized study. Int J Gynecol Cancer. 2009;19(5):873–8.
131. Creutzberg CL, Nout RA, Lybeert ML, Warlam-Rodenhuis CC, Jobsen JJ, Mens JW, et al. Fifteen-year radiotherapy outcomes of the randomized PORTEC-1 trial for endometrial carcinoma. Int J Radiat Oncol Biol Phys. 2011;81(4):e631–8.
132. Keys HM, Roberts JA, Brunetto VL, Zaino RJ, Spirtos NM, Bloss JD, et al. A phase III trial of surgery with or without adjunctive external pelvic radiation therapy in intermediate risk endometrial adenocarcinoma: a Gynecologic Oncology Group study. Gynecol Oncol. 2004;92(3):744–51.
133. Nout RA, Smit VT, Putter H, Jurgenliemk-Schulz IM, Jobsen JJ, Lutgens LC, et al. Vaginal brachytherapy versus pelvic external beam radiotherapy for patients with endometrial cancer of high-intermediate risk (PORTEC-2): an open-label, non-inferiority, randomised trial. Lancet. 2010;375(9717):816–23.
134. Harkenrider MM, Martin B, Nieto K, Small C, Aref I, Bergman D, et al. Multi-institutional analysis of vaginal brachytherapy alone for women with stage II endometrial carcinoma. Int J Radiat Oncol Biol Phys. 2018;101(5):1069–77.
135. Bosse T, Peters EE, Creutzberg CL, Jurgenliemk-Schulz IM, Jobsen JJ, Mens JW, et al. Substantial lymph-vascular space invasion (LVSI) is a significant risk factor for recurrence in endometrial cancer–a pooled analysis of PORTEC 1 and 2 trials. Eur J Cancer. 2015;51(13):1742–50.
136. Mitra D, Klopp AH, Viswanathan AN. Pros and cons of vaginal brachytherapy after external beam radiation therapy in endometrial cancer. Gynecol Oncol. 2016;140(1):167–75.
137. Hathout L, Wang Y, Wang Q, Vergalasova I, Elshaikh MA, Dimitrova I, et al. A multi-institutional analysis of adjuvant chemotherapy and radiation sequence in women with stage IIIC endometrial cancer. Int J Radiat Oncol Biol Phys. 2021;110(5):1423–31.
138. Small W Jr, Bosch WR, Harkenrider MM, Strauss JB, Abu-Rustum N, Albuquerque KV, et al. NRG oncology/RTOG consensus guidelines for delineation of clinical target volume for intensity modulated pelvic radiation therapy in postoperative treatment of endometrial and cervical cancer: an update. Int J Radiat Oncol Biol Phys. 2021;109(2):413–24.
139. Kabolizadeh P, Fulay S, Beriwal S. Are Radiation Therapy Oncology Group Para-aortic Contouring Guidelines for Pancreatic Neoplasm applicable to other malignancies–assessment of nodal distribution in gynecological malignancies. Int J Radiat Oncol Biol Phys. 2013;87(1):106–10.
140. Small W Jr, Beriwal S, Demanes DJ, Dusenbery KE, Eifel P, Erickson B, et al. American Brachytherapy Society consensus guidelines for adjuvant vaginal cuff brachytherapy after hysterectomy. Brachytherapy. 2012;11(1):58–67.
141. Harkenrider MM, Grover S, Erickson BA, Viswanathan AN, Small C, Kliethermes S, et al. Vaginal brachytherapy for postoperative endometrial cancer: 2014 survey of the American Brachytherapy Society. Brachytherapy. 2016;15(1):23–9.
142. Beriwal S, Demanes DJ, Erickson B, Jones E, De Los Santos JF, Cormack RA, et al. American Brachytherapy Society consensus guidelines for interstitial brachytherapy for vaginal cancer. Brachytherapy. 2012;11(1):68–75.
143. Glaser SM, Beriwal S. Brachytherapy for malignancies of the vagina in the 3D era. J Contemp Brachytherapy. 2015;7(4):312–8.
144. Ling DC, Vargo JA, Glaser SM, Kim H, Beriwal S. Outcomes after definitive re-irradiation with 3D brachytherapy with or without external beam radiation therapy for vaginal recurrence of endometrial cancer. Gynecol Oncol. 2019;152(3):581–6.
145. Lee LJ, Alban GM, Cheng T, Buzurovic I, Pretz J, Singer L, et al. Clinical outcomes and dosimetric predictors of toxicity for re-irradiation of vaginal

recurrence of endometrial cancer. Brachytherapy. 2022;21(3):263–72.
146. Albuquerque K, Hrycushko BA, Harkenrider MM, Mayadev J, Klopp A, Beriwal S, et al. Compendium of fractionation choices for gynecologic HDR brachytherapy-an American Brachytherapy Society Task Group Report. Brachytherapy. 2019;18(4):429–36.
147. Rajagopalan MS, Kannan N, Kim H, Houser CJ, Beriwal S. Urethral dosimetry and toxicity with high-dose-rate interstitial brachytherapy for vaginal cancer. Brachytherapy. 2013;12(3):248–53.
148. Klopp AH, Yeung AR, Deshmukh S, Gil KM, Wenzel L, Westin SN, et al. Patient-reported toxicity during pelvic intensity-modulated radiation therapy: NRG Oncology-RTOG 1203. J Clin Oncol. 2018;36(24):2538–44.
149. Chopra S, Gupta S, Kannan S, Dora T, Engineer R, Mangaj A, et al. Late toxicity after adjuvant conventional radiation versus image-guided intensity-modulated radiotherapy for cervical cancer (PARCER): a randomized controlled trial. J Clin Oncol. 2021;39(33):3682–92.
150. Yeung AR, Deshmukh S, Klopp AH, Gil KM, Wenzel L, Westin SN, et al. Intensity-modulated radiation therapy reduces patient-reported chronic toxicity compared with conventional pelvic radiation therapy: updated results of a phase III trial. J Clin Oncol. 2022;40:JCO2102831.
151. Wortman BG, Post CCB, Powell ME, Khaw P, Fyles A, D'Amico R, et al. Radiation therapy techniques and treatment-related toxicity in the PORTEC-3 trial: comparison of 3-dimensional conformal radiation therapy versus intensity-modulated radiation therapy. Int J Radiat Oncol Biol Phys. 2022;112(2):390–9.
152. Nout RA, Putter H, Jurgenliemk-Schulz IM, Jobsen JJ, Lutgens LC, van der Steen-Banasik EM, et al. Five-year quality of life of endometrial cancer patients treated in the randomised Post Operative Radiation Therapy in Endometrial Cancer (PORTEC-2) trial and comparison with norm data. Eur J Cancer. 2012;48(11):1638–48.
153. de Boer SM, Nout RA, Jurgenliemk-Schulz IM, Jobsen JJ, Lutgens LC, van der Steen-Banasik EM, et al. Long-term impact of endometrial cancer diagnosis and treatment on health-related quality of life and cancer survivorship: results from the randomized PORTEC-2 trial. Int J Radiat Oncol Biol Phys. 2015;93(4):797–809.
154. Zola P, Ciccone G, Piovano E, Fuso L, Di Cuonzo D, Castiglione A, et al. Effectiveness of intensive versus minimalist follow-up regimen on survival in patients with endometrial cancer (TOTEM study): a randomized, pragmatic, parallel group, multicenter trial. J Clin Oncol. 2022;40:JCO2200471.
155. Gebhardt BJ, Rangaswamy B, Thomas J, Kelley J, Sukumvanich P, Edwards R, et al. Magnetic resonance imaging response in patients treated with definitive radiation therapy for medically inoperable endometrial cancer-does it predict treatment response? Brachytherapy. 2019;18(4):437–44.
156. Stahl JM, Qian JM, Tien CJ, Carlson DJ, Chen Z, Ratner ES, et al. Extended duration of dilator use beyond 1 year may reduce vaginal stenosis after intravaginal high-dose-rate brachytherapy. Support Care Cancer. 2019;27(4):1425–33.
157. Wortman BG, Creutzberg CL, Putter H, Jurgenliemk-Schulz IM, Jobsen JJ, Lutgens L, et al. Ten-year results of the PORTEC-2 trial for high-intermediate risk endometrial carcinoma: improving patient selection for adjuvant therapy. Br J Cancer. 2018;119(9):1067–74.
158. Mutyala S, Patel G, Rivera AC, Brodin PN, Saigal K, Thawani N, et al. High dose rate brachytherapy for inoperable endometrial cancer: a case series and systematic review of the literature. Clin Oncol (R Coll Radiol). 2021;33(9):e393–402.
159. Berek JS, Matias-Guiu X, Creutzberg C, Fotopoulou C, Gaffney D, Kehoe, Endometrial Cancer Staging Subcommittee, FIGO Women's Cancer Committee, et al. FIGO staging of endometrial cancer: 2023. Int J Gynaecol Obstetr. 2023;162(2):383–94. https://doi.org/10.1002/ijgo.14923.
160. van den Heerik ASVM, Horeweg N, Haverkort MAD, Kuijsters N, Kommoss S, Koppe FLA, et al. Molecular profile-based adjuvant treatment for women with high-intermediate risk endometrial cancer (PORTEC-4a): results of a randomised, open-label, phase 3, multicentre, non-inferiority trial. Lancet Oncol. 2026;27(1):23–35. https://doi.org/10.1016/S1470-2045(25)00612-6.
161. Pifer PM, Jaishankar S, Bhargava R, Schad MD, Keller A, Musunuru HB, et al. Is substantial Lymphovascular space invasion prognostic in patients with pathologically lymph node-negative endometrial cancer? Int J Radiat Oncol Biol Phys. 117(1):148–53. https://doi.org/10.1016/j.ijrobp.2023.02.053.
162. Eskander RN, Sill MW, Beffa L, Moore RG, Hope JM, Musa FB, et al. Pembrolizumab plus chemotherapy in advanced endometrial cancer. N Engl J Med. 2023;388(23):2159–70. https://doi.org/10.1056/NEJMoa2302312.
163. Eskander RN, Sill MW, Beffa L, Moore RG, Hope JM, Musa FB, et al. Pembrolizumab plus chemotherapy in advanced or recurrent endometrial cancer: overall survival and exploratory analyses of the NRG GY018 phase 3 randomized trial. Nat Med. 2025;31(5):1539–46. https://doi.org/10.1038/s41591-025-03566-1.
164. Mirza MR, Chase DM, Slomovitz BM, dePont CR, Novák Z, Black D, RUBY Investigators, et al. Dostarlimab for primary advanced or recurrent endometrial cancer. N Engl J Med. 2023;388(23):2145–58. https://doi.org/10.1056/NEJMoa2216334.
165. Powell MA, Bjørge L, Willmott L, Novák Z, Black D, Gilbert L, et al. Overall survival in patients

with endometrial cancer treated with dostarlimab plus carboplatin-paclitaxel in the randomized ENGOT-EN6/GOG-3031/RUBY trial. Ann Oncol. 2024;35(8):728–38. https://doi.org/10.1016/j.annonc.2024.05.546.
166. Van Gorp T, Cibula D, Lv W, Backes F, Ortaç F, Hasegawa K, et al. ENGOT-en11/GOG-3053/KEYNOTE-B21: a randomised, double-blind, phase III study of pembrolizumab or placebo plus adjuvant chemotherapy with or without radiotherapy in patients with newly diagnosed, high-risk endometrial cancer. Ann Oncol. 35(11):968–80. https://doi.org/10.1016/j.annonc.2024.08.2242.
167. Slomovitz BM, Cibula D, Lv W, Ortaç F, Hietanen S, Backes F, et al. Pembrolizumab or Placebo Plus adjuvant chemotherapy with or without radiotherapy for newly diagnosed, high-risk endometrial cancer: results in mismatch repair-deficient tumors. J Clin Oncol. 2024;43(3):251–9. https://doi.org/10.1200/JCO-24-0188.
168. Concin N, Matias-Guiu X, Cibula D, Colombo N, Creutzberg CL, Ledermann J, et al. ESGO-ESTRO-ESP guidelines for the management of patients with endometrial carcinoma: update 2025. Lancet Oncol. 2025;26(8):e423–35. https://doi.org/10.1016/S1470-2045(25)00167-6.
169. Klopp AH, Enserro D, Powell M, Randall M, Schink JC, Mannel RS, et al. Radiation therapy with or without Cisplatin for local recurrences of endometrial cancer: results from an NRG Oncology/GOG prospective randomized multicenter clinical trial. J Clin Oncol. 2024;42(20):2425–35. https://doi.org/10.1200/JCO.23.01279. Epub 2024 Apr 25. PMID: 38662968; PMCID: PMC11681946..
170. Leung E, Gladwish AP, Davidson M, Taggar A, Velker V, Barnes E, et al. Quality-of-life outcomes and toxic effects among patients with cancers of the uterus treated with stereotactic pelvic adjuvant radiation therapy: the SPARTACUS phase 1/2 nonrandomized controlled trial. JAMA Oncol. 2022;8(6):1–9.
171. Vulvar Cancer – Cancer Stat Facts. https://seer.cancer.gov/statfacts/html/vulva.html. Accessed 24 July 2022.
172. Olawaiye AB, Cotler J, Cuello MA, Bhatla N, Okamoto A, Wilailak S, et al. FIGO staging for carcinoma of the vulva: 2021 revision. Int J Gynaecol Obstetr. 2021;155(1):43–7. https://doi.org/10.1002/ijgo.13880
173. Barlow EL, Kang YJ, Hacker NF, Canfell K. Changing trends in vulvar cancer incidence and mortality rates in Australia since 1982. Int J Gynecol Cancer. 2015;25(9):1683–9. https://doi.org/10.1097/IGC.0000000000000547.
174. Bray F, Laversanne M, Weiderpass E, Arbyn M. Geographic and temporal variations in the incidence of vulvar and vaginal cancers. Int J Cancer. 2020;147(10):2764–71. https://doi.org/10.1002/ijc.33055.
175. Chiasson MA, Ellerbrock TV, Bush TJ, Sun XW, Wright TC. Increased prevalence of vulvovaginal condyloma and vulvar intraepithelial neoplasia in women infected with the human immunodeficiency virus. Obstet Gynecol. 1997;89(5 Pt 1):690–4. https://doi.org/10.1016/S0029-7844(97)00069-0.
176. Van Seters M, Van Beurden M, De Craen AJM. Is the assumed natural history of vulvar intraepithelial neoplasia III based on enough evidence? A systematic review of 3322 published patients. Gynecol Oncol. 2005;97(2):645–51. https://doi.org/10.1016/J.YGYNO.2005.02.012.
177. Thuijs NB, van Beurden M, Bruggink AH, Steenbergen RDM, Berkhof J, Bleeker MCG. Vulvar intraepithelial neoplasia: incidence and long-term risk of vulvar squamous cell carcinoma. Int J Cancer. 2021;148(1):90–8. https://doi.org/10.1002/IJC.33198.
178. Bornstein J, Bogliatto F, Haefner HK, et al. The 2015 International Society for the Study of Vulvovaginal Disease (ISSVD) terminology of vulvar squamous intraepithelial lesions. J Low Genit Tract Dis. 2016;20(1):11–4. https://doi.org/10.1097/LGT.0000000000000169.
179. Campaner AB, Cardoso F d A, Fernandes GL, Veasey JV. Verrucous carcinoma of the vulva: diagnosis and treatment. An Bras Dermatol. 2017;92(2):243. https://doi.org/10.1590/ABD1806-4841.20174929.
180. Horne ZD, Dohopolski MJ, Pradhan D, et al. Human papillomavirus infection mediates response and outcome of vulvar squamous cell carcinomas treated with radiation therapy. Gynecol Oncol. 2018;151(1):96–101. https://doi.org/10.1016/J.YGYNO.2018.08.002.
181. Lee LJ, Howitt B, Catalano P, et al. Prognostic importance of human papillomavirus (HPV) and p16 positivity in squamous cell carcinoma of the vulva treated with radiotherapy. Gynecol Oncol. 2016;142(2):293–8. https://doi.org/10.1016/J.YGYNO.2016.05.019.
182. Heaps JM, Fu YS, Montz FJ, Hacker NF, Berek JS. Surgical-pathologic variables predictive of local recurrence in squamous cell carcinoma of the vulva. Gynecol Oncol. 1990;38(3):309–14. https://doi.org/10.1016/0090-8258(90)90064-R.
183. Woelber L, Griebel LF, Eulenburg C, et al. Role of tumour-free margin distance for loco-regional control in vulvar cancer-a subset analysis of the Arbeitsgemeinschaft Gynäkologische Onkologie CaRE-1 multicenter study. Eur J Cancer. 2016;69:180–8. https://doi.org/10.1016/J.EJCA.2016.09.038.
184. Te Grootenhuis NC, Pouwer AW, de Bock GH, et al. Margin status revisited in vulvar squamous cell carcinoma. Gynecol Oncol. 2019;154(2):266–75. https://doi.org/10.1016/J.YGYNO.2019.05.010.
185. Raimond E, Delorme C, Ouldamer L, et al. Surgical treatment of vulvar cancer: impact of tumor-free margin distance on recurrence and survival. A mul-

ticentre cohort analysis from the francogyn study group. Eur J Surg Oncol. 2019;45(11):2109–14. https://doi.org/10.1016/J.EJSO.2019.07.005.
186. Homesley HD, Bundy BN, Sedlis A, et al. Prognostic factors for groin node metastasis in squamous cell carcinoma of the vulva (a Gynecologic Oncology Group study). Gynecol Oncol. 1993;49(3):279–83. https://doi.org/10.1006/GYNO.1993.1127.
187. Gonzalez Bosquet J, Magrina JF, Magtibay PM, et al. Patterns of inguinal groin metastases in squamous cell carcinoma of the vulva. Gynecol Oncol. 2007;105(3):742–6. https://doi.org/10.1016/J.YGYNO.2007.02.014.
188. Levenback CF, Ali S, Coleman RL, et al. Lymphatic mapping and sentinel lymph node biopsy in women with squamous cell carcinoma of the vulva: a Gynecologic Oncology Group study. J Clin Oncol. 2012;30(31):3786. https://doi.org/10.1200/JCO.2011.41.2528.
189. Oonk MH, van Hemel BM, Hollema H, et al. Size of sentinel-node metastasis and chances of non-sentinel-node involvement and survival in early stage vulvar cancer: results from GROINSS-V, a multicentre observational study. Lancet Oncol. 2010;11(7):646–52. https://doi.org/10.1016/S1470-2045(10)70104-2.
190. Te Grootenhuis NC, Van Der Zee AGJ, Van Doorn HC, et al. Sentinel nodes in vulvar cancer: long-term follow-up of the GROningen INternational Study on Sentinel nodes in Vulvar cancer (GROINSS-V) I. Gynecol Oncol. 2016;140(1):8–14. https://doi.org/10.1016/J.YGYNO.2015.09.077.
191. Oonk MHM, Slomovitz B, Baldwin PJW, et al. Radiotherapy versus inguinofemoral lymphadenectomy as treatment for vulvar cancer patients with micrometastases in the sentinel node: results of GROINSS-V II. J Clin Oncol. 2021;39(32):3623–32. https://doi.org/10.1200/JCO.21.00006.
192. Woelber L, Eulenburg C, Kosse J, et al. Predicting the course of disease in recurrent vulvar cancer – a subset analysis of the AGO-CaRE-1 study. Gynecol Oncol. 2019;154(3):571–6. https://doi.org/10.1016/J.YGYNO.2019.07.009.
193. Woelber L, Prieske K, Eulenburg C z, et al. Adjuvant radiotherapy and local recurrence in vulvar cancer – a subset analysis of the AGO-CaRE-1 study. Gynecol Oncol. 2022;164(1):68–75. https://doi.org/10.1016/J.YGYNO.2021.11.004.
194. Gaffney DK, King B, Viswanathan AN, et al. Consensus recommendations for radiation therapy contouring and treatment of vulvar carcinoma. Int J Radiat Oncol Biol Phys. 2016;95(4):1191–200. https://doi.org/10.1016/J.IJROBP.2016.02.043.
195. Kim CH, Olson AC, Kim H, Beriwal S. Contouring inguinal and femoral nodes; how much margin is needed around the vessels? Pract Radiat Oncol. 2012;2(4):274–8. https://doi.org/10.1016/J.PRRO.2011.12.005.
196. Rao YJ, Chundury A, Schwarz JK, et al. Intensity modulated radiation therapy for squamous cell carcinoma of the vulva: treatment technique and outcomes. Adv Radiat Oncol. 2017;2(2):148–58. https://doi.org/10.1016/J.ADRO.2017.02.006.
197. Viswanathan AN, Pinto AP, Schultz D, Berkowitz R, Crum CP. Relationship of margin status and radiation dose to recurrence in post-operative vulvar carcinoma. Gynecol Oncol. 2013;130(3):545–9. https://doi.org/10.1016/J.YGYNO.2013.05.036.
198. Horowitz NS, Deng W, Peterson I, Mannel RS, Thompson S, Lokich E, et al. Phase II trial of Cisplatin, Gemcitabine, and intensity-modulated radiation therapy for locally advanced vulvar squamous cell carcinoma: NRG Oncology/GOG study 279. J Clin Oncol. 2024;42(16):1914–21. https://doi.org/10.1200/JCO.23.02235
199. Rishi A, Albuquerque KV, Jhingran A, Donovan EK, Horne ZD, Ludwig MS, et al. Definitive intensity-modulated radiotherapy for organ preservation in vulvar cancer: A multicenter study. Gynecol Oncol. 2025;199:1–9. https://doi.org/10.1016/j.ygyno.2025.05.024
200. Stehman FB, Bundy BN, Thomas G, et al. Groin dissection versus groin radiation in carcinoma of the vulva: a Gynecologic Oncology Group study. Int J Radiat Oncol Biol Phys. 1992;24(2):389–96. https://doi.org/10.1016/0360-3016(92)90699-I.
201. Thaker NG, Klopp AH, Jhingran A, Frumovitz M, Iyer RB, Eifel PJ. Survival outcomes for patients with stage IVB vulvar cancer with grossly positive pelvic lymph nodes: time to reconsider the FIGO staging system? Gynecol Oncol. 2015;136(2):269–73. https://doi.org/10.1016/J.YGYNO.2014.12.013.
202. Moore DH, Thomas GM, Montana GS, Saxer A, Gallup DG, Olt G. Preoperative chemoradiation for advanced vulvar cancer: a phase II study of the Gynecologic Oncology Group. Int J Radiat Oncol Biol Phys. 1998;42(1):79–85. https://doi.org/10.1016/S0360-3016(98)00193-X.
203. Moore DH, Ali S, Koh WJ, et al. A phase II trial of radiation therapy and weekly cisplatin chemotherapy for the treatment of locally-advanced squamous cell carcinoma of the vulva: a gynecologic oncology group study. Gynecol Oncol. 2012;124(3):529–33. https://doi.org/10.1016/j.ygyno.2011.11.003.
204. Richman AH, Vargo JA, Ling DC, et al. Dose-escalated intensity modulated radiation therapy in patients with locally-advanced vulvar cancer – does it increase response rate? Gynecol Oncol. 2020;159(3):657–62. https://doi.org/10.1016/J.YGYNO.2020.09.019.
205. FIGO Committee on Gynecologic Oncology. Current FIGO staging for cancer of the vagina, fallopian tube, ovary, and gestational trophoblastic neoplasia. Int J Gynaecol Obstet. 2009;105(1):3–4.
206. Hacker NF, Eifel PJ, Van Der Velden J. Cancer of the vagina. Int J Gynecol Obstet. 2012;119:S97–9.

207. Rajaram S, Maheshwari A, Srivastava A. Staging for vaginal cancer. Best Pract Res Clin Obstet Gynaecol. 2015;29(6):822–32.
208. Kamrava M, Leung E, Bachand F, Beriwal S, Chargari C, D'Souza D, Erickson B, Fokdal L, Han K, Harkenrider M, Lin L. GEC-ESTRO (ACROP)–ABS–CBG consensus brachytherapy target definition guidelines for recurrent endometrial and cervical tumors in the vagina. Int J Radiat Oncol Biol Phys. 2023;115:654–63.
209. Di Donato V, Bellati F, Fischetti M, Plotti F, Perniola G, Panici PB. Vaginal cancer. Crit Rev Oncol Hematol. 2012;81(3):286–95.
210. Greenwalt JC, Amdur RJ, Morris CG, Morgan LS, Castagno J, Markham MJ, Rich S, Yeung AR. Outcomes of definitive radiation therapy for primary vaginal carcinoma. Am J Clin Oncol. 2015;38(6):583–7.

Online Links

https://www.youtube.com/watch?v=xBa3FhHhqmE (Radiotherapy planning for Ca Cervix)

https://www.youtube.com/watch?v=wVtL-oBDaKs (Treatment Options for Early-Stage Cervical Cancer)

https://youtu.be/xBa3FhHhqmE (Radiotherapy planning for Ca Cervix- Part 1)

https://youtu.be/kDmgZRAdvTQ (Radiotherapy planning for Ca Cervix- Part 2)

https://youtu.be/Xsb0Rkw7NOc (Radiotherapy planning for Ca Cervix- conventional brachytherapy)

https://youtu.be/uM5bUYi7k1A (Radiotherapy planning for Ca Cervix- MR based brachytherapy)

https://youtu.be/68el0IhuRqU (Radiotherapy planning for Ca Cervix- image guided brachytherapy)

Bone and Soft Tissue Tumors

Shah Alam Khan, Venkatesan Sampath Kumar,
Love Kapoor, Anusheel Munshi,
Vikas Kumar Pandey, and Bidhu K. Mohanti

1 Bone Tumors

1.1 Introduction

Bone tumors constitute a heterogenous group of malignant and benign types. Primary malignant bone tumors are uncommon and account for approximately 0.2% of global cancer burden. Diagnosis and treatment bone tumors require a multidisciplinary team of specialties-orthopedics, surgery, pathology, imaging, medical oncology, radiation oncology and physiotherapy. Advancements in the multimodality treatment approach have significantly enhanced the quality of life and survival of patients with bone sarcomas over the past two decades. In over 90% of patients, resection is performed instead of amputation, and the majority of patients with soft tissue and bone sarcomas can be cured through the use of limb-sparing surgery in conjunction with chemotherapy and radiation therapy. The 5-year survival rates of bone malignancies have increased from approximately 50% in 1970 to a range of 75–80% in the adolescent age group as a result of remarkable achievements in multimodality management. It is imperative to possess a comprehensive comprehension of the fundamental biology and pathology of soft tissue and bone tumors in order to effectively plan their treatment. This chapter examines the clinical presentation of bone malignancies, the principles of surgical management, numerous diagnostic modalities, and staging [1].

S. A. Khan (✉) · V. S. Kumar · L. Kapoor
Department of Orthopaedics, All India Institute of Medical Sciences, New Delhi, India

A. Munshi
Department of Radiation Oncology, BLK MAX Hospital, New Delhi, Delhi, India

V. K. Pandey
Department of Radiation Oncology, Cancer Care Manitoba, Winnipeg, Canada

B. K. Mohanti
Department of Radiation Oncology, Bagchi Sri Shankara Cancer Centre & Research Institute, Bhubaneswar, Odisha, India

1.2 Epidemiological Aspects

Primary bone sarcomas are uncommon lesions, accounting for approximately 0.2% of all malignancies. More frequently than primary bone sarcomas, benign bone tumors and tumor-like lesions are observed in both infants and adults. Due to their rarity, it is challenging to determine their actual prevalence. According to Western data, osteosarcoma, chondrosarcoma, and Ewing sarcoma/primitive neuroectodermal tumor (PNET) are the most prevalent bone sarcomas. The remaining subtypes include fibrosarcomas, chordomas, and undifferentiated pleomorphic sarcoma (UPS) [1]. The incidence and distribution of sarcomas in the Indian population have been assessed by a variety of hospital-based registries. Nevertheless, there is no recent, population-based assessment of the incidence of bone sarcomas in

B. K. Mohanti et al. (eds.), *Radiation Oncology – Principles, Precepts and Practice*,
https://doi.org/10.1007/978-981-95-5171-2_15

India [2]. Based on data from the Bombay Cancer Registry, Yeole and Jussawalla published the incidence of bone malignancy in Mumbai in 1998. According to that registry, bone malignancies accounted for 0.9% of all cancers, with Ewing sarcoma being the most prevalent bone malignancy [3]. As per the 2001 hospital-based cancer registry at Tata Memorial Hospital in Mumbai, osteosarcoma was identified as the most prevalent bone sarcoma, with Ewing sarcoma/PNET and chondrosarcoma following in that order [4]. According to Rao et al., 39% of the 523 bone tumors in Karnataka were malignant, with osteosarcoma and Ewing sarcoma accounting for 45.7% and 19.4% of malignant bone tumors, respectively, based on retrospectively collected data over 36 years [5]. The registry of JSS Medical College and Hospital, Mysore, Karnataka, India, provides more recent data. A review of 117 cases over an 8-year period revealed that osteosarcoma constituted the preponderance of malignant bone tumors (35.14%), with a median age of presentation of 26.87 years [6].

1.3 Classification of Bone Tumors

Bone tumors have a broad spectrum of morphology and biological behavior. Since the publication of the fourth edition of the World Health Organization (WHO) classification of tumors of soft tissue and bone in 2013 [7], considerable advances have been made in our understanding of the molecular biology, classification, prognostication, and treatment of many bone tumors. The fifth edition of the WHO classification of tumors of soft tissue and bone was published in April 2020 (Table 1) [8, 9].

1.4 Risk Factors

The etiology of most benign and malignant bone tumors is unknown and children are frequently affected. Risk factors for bone and soft tissue sarcomas include previous radiation therapy, exposure to chemicals (e.g., vinyl chloride, arsenic), immunodeficiency, prior injury (scars, burns), chronic tissue irritation (foreign body implants, lymphedema, chronic infection), neurofibromatosis, Paget disease, bone infarcts, and genetic cancer syndromes (e.g., hereditary retinoblastoma, Li-Fraumeni syndrome, Gardner syndrome, Rothmund-Thomson syndrome, Werner syndrome, Bloom syndrome), Marfucci syndrome, Ollier disease, multiple osteochondromatosis, and hereditary multiple exostoses.

1.5 Clinical Evaluation of Bone Tumors

A careful and systematic approach using a detailed history and physical examination with appropriate plain radiographs are the mainstay of the initial evaluation, which should lead to an accurate and brief differential diagnosis.

1.5.1 Presenting Symptoms

Mild pain relieved with medication is generally consistent with a benign condition. Pain associated with benign lesions is generally slow in onset and may be related to activity or trauma. Malignant bone tumors typically present with pain that starts as intermittent and progresses to a constant pain. Night pain often is a component. Pain typically is deep-seated and dull. Patients with high-grade tumors present with a history of several months of pain. Patients with low-grade tumors, by contrast, present with a history of mild pain of longer duration. Pain can be acute or sudden when lesions are associated with pathologic fracture. Systemic symptoms such as fatigue, malaise, and fever may be present.

Personal or family history of cancer or bone malignancy should be considered. Conditions such as retinoblastoma, Li-Fraumeni syndrome, and Rothmund-Thompson syndrome are known to predispose patients to primary bone malignancies such as osteosarcoma. Malignant transformations of benign conditions such as multiple enchondromatosis or osteochondromas are known entities. Bone malignancies are known to occur in the setting of Paget's disease, prior irradiation, chronic osteomyelitis, or bone infarct.

1.5.2 Physical Examination

Patients with suspected skeletal tumors should be examined thoroughly. The affected site is

Table 1 The 2020/2021 WHO classification of bone tumors

Predominant tissue	Benign	Intermediate (locally aggressive)	Malignant

Osteogenic	Osteoma
	Osteoid osteoma
		Osteoblastoma	Low-grade central osteosarcoma
			Osteosarcoma NOS
			  Conventional
			  Telangiectatic
			  Small cell
			Parosteal osteosarcoma
			Periosteal osteosarcoma
			High-grade surface osteosarcoma
			Secondary osteosarcoma

Chondrogenic	Subungual exostosis Bizarre parosteal osteochondromatous proliferation Periosteal chondroma Enchondroma Osteochondroma Chondroblastoma Chondromyxoid fibroma Osteochondromyxoma	Chondromatosis NOS Atypical cartilaginous tumor	Chondrosarcoma grade 1 Chondrosarcoma grade 2 Chondrosarcoma grade 3 Periosteal chondrosarcoma Clear cell chondrosarcoma Mesenchymal chondrosarcoma Dedifferentiated chondrosarcoma
Fibrogenic	Fibroma Fibromatosis	Desmoplastic fibroma	Fibrosarcoma
Mixed	Chondromyxoid fibroma		
Osteoclastic giant-cell rich tumors	Aneurysmal bone cyst Non-ossifying fibroma	Giant cell tumor of bone NOS	Giant cell tumor of bone, malignant
Marrow tumors			Ewing's sarcoma Myeloma
Vascular tissue	Hemangioma	Epithelioid hemangioma	Epithelioid hemangioendothelioma NOS Angiosarcoma
Notochordal tumors	Benign notochordal cell tumor		Chordoma NOS Chondroid chordoma Poorly differentiated chordoma Dedifferentiated chordoma
Other mesenchymal tumors of bone	Chondromesenchymal hamartoma of chest wall Simple bone cyst Fibrous dysplasia Osteofibrous dysplasia Lipoma NOS Hibernoma	Osteofibrous dysplasia-like adamantinoma Mesenchymoma NOS	Adamantinoma of long bones Dedifferentiated adamantinoma Leiomyosarcoma NOS Pleomorphic sarcoma, undifferentiated Bone metastases

Hematopoietic neoplasms of bone: Plasmacytoma of bone
- Malignant lymphoma, non-Hodgkin, NOS
- Hodgkin disease NOS
- Diffuse large B-cell lymphoma NOS
- Follicular lymphoma NOS
- Marginal zone B-cell lymphoma NOS
- T-cell lymphoma NOS
- Anaplastic large cell lymphoma NOS
- Malignant lymphoma, lymphoblastic, NOS
- Burkitt lymphoma NOS
- Langerhans cell histiocytosis NOS
- Langerhans cell histiocytosis, disseminated
- Erdheim-Chester disease
- Rosai-Dorfman disease

Abbreviations: *NOS* not otherwise specified

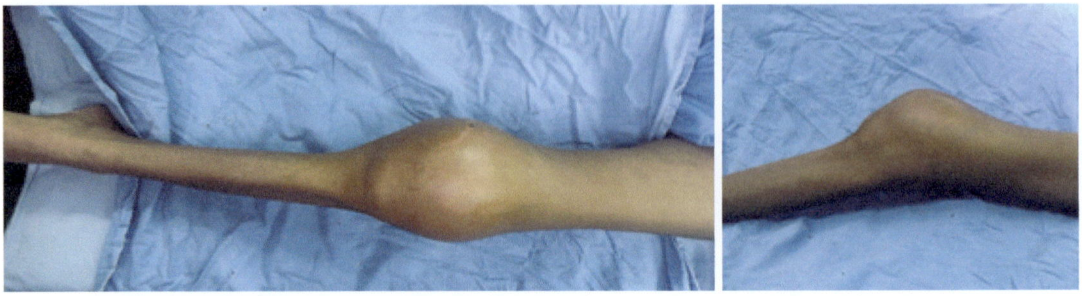

Fig. 1 A 14-year-old male presenting with a 2-month history of pain and swelling of the left distal thigh, with examination revealing a globular mass arising from the distal femur

inspected for bone swelling, overlying skin changes, lymphadenopathy, neurologic deficit, and vascular deficiency. An associated soft tissue mass and/or swelling is often seen, especially for extremity lesions (Fig. 1). Patients older than 40 years suspected to have a malignant bone lesion most commonly have metastatic carcinoma, multiple myeloma, or lymphoma. Appropriate history and clinical examination findings, including a breast or prostate examination, should be documented.

Variables such as patient age, location of the lesion within the bone, and plain radiograph characteristics can help guide the diagnosis (Tables 2 and 3).

Table 2 Common diagnosis by age

Age	Benign	Malignant
0–5 years	Histiocytosis Infection	Metastatic neuroblastoma
5–20 years	Nonossifying fibroma Aneurysmal bone cyst Simple bone cyst Osteoid osteoma Osteochondroma	Osteosarcoma Ewing sarcoma
20–40 years	Giant cell tumor Fibrous dysplasia Enchondroma	Lymphoma Ewing sarcoma
>40 years	Enchondroma Bone infarct Infection	Metastatic carcinoma Lymphoma Multiple myeloma Chondrosarcoma

1.6 Radiographic Evaluation of Bone Tumors

Characterization of the Lesion Radiographic evaluation should commence with plain radiographs of the entire bone containing the lesion in two perpendicular planes to describe osseous changes including location of lesion, pattern of destruction, zone of transition, margins, periosteal reaction, cortical integrity, and soft tissue component, which are important determinants of a lesion's biologic potential. Benign tumors typically are defined by a geographic radiological margin, with a narrow zone of transition and sclerotic border (Fig. 2).

Endosteal thinning can be seen with benign tumors. Cortical violation is rarely seen in benign tumors. Typical radiographic findings of malignant tumors include a pattern of permeative destruction

Table 3 Common diagnosis by location of lesion in long bones

Site	Benign	Malignant
Long bones		
Epiphyseal	Chondroblastoma Giant cell tumor	Clear cell chondrosarcoma
Metaphyseal	Nonossifying fibroma Aneurysmal bone cyst Simple/ unicameral bone cyst Enchondroma Osteochondroma	Osteosarcoma Chondrosarcoma Metastatic bone disease
Diaphyseal	Fibrous dysplasia Histiocytosis Osteoid osteoma	Ewing sarcoma Adamantinoma Lymphoma Metastatic bone disease

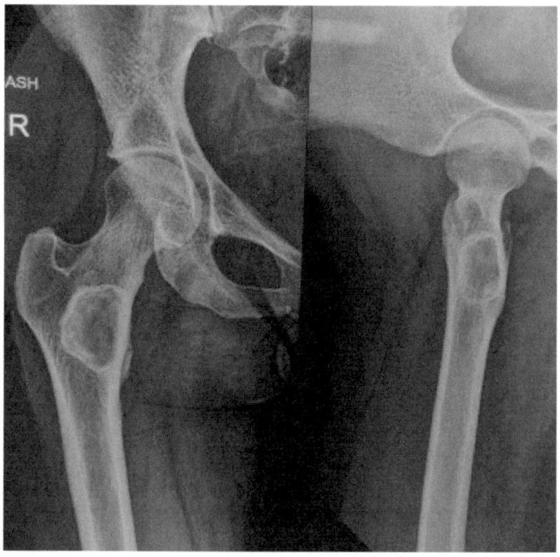

Fig. 2 Plain radiographs of the proximal femur showing a well-circumscribed lytic lesion with geographic margins, narrow zone of transition, and peripheral sclerosis, features suggestive of a benign process

with poorly defined borders, cortical destruction, periosteal elevation, and extraosseous extension (Fig. 3). As the neoplasm permeates the cortex, the periosteum may be elevated. This stimulates reactive bone formation and accounts for a distinctive radiologic feature called "Codman's triangle."

Defining the Local Extent of Tumor Magnetic Resonance Imaging (MRI) is the best imaging modality for defining the local extent of tumor. Whether a contrast enhanced MRI is required depends on the availability and surgeon's preference. It may be noted that MRI

- Should be performed prior to the biopsy.
- Should include the whole involved bone as well as the neighboring joints, so as to not miss skip lesions (intramedullary tumor foci without direct contact with the primary lesion).
- Should be evaluated for the intramedullary extent, soft tissue extension, relation to vessels and nerves, intra-articular extension, skip lesions, associated bone marrow edema, and signal characteristics of the lesion (Fig. 4).
- Post-chemotherapy MRI should be done at least 14 days after the completion of last cycle and within 2 weeks prior to surgery. Change in the size of the soft tissue mass confirms tumor response.

Computerized tomography (CT) scan provides information regarding matrix formation, calcification, endosteal erosion, and cortical thinning or violation.

Evaluation of Systemic Extent

1. Chest X-ray and non-contrast CT for lung metastasis: Since NCCT is better than 18F-FDG PET for detecting lung metastases smaller than 8 mm [10], NCCT chest remains an essential part of the staging process.
2. Whole body imaging: Radionuclide bone scan, PET scan, whole body MRI.
3. Bone marrow biopsy for Ewing sarcoma, myeloma.

Most patients with new bone lesions that elicit high suspicion of primary malignancy undergo bone scintigraphy with technetium Tc-99 methylene diphosphonate (99Tc MDP) to assess the primary mass and to look for additional bone lesions including metastases or synchronous sites of disease (Fig. 5). These bone scans, however, do not detect soft-tissue lesions or lesions exclusively involving bone marrow. Bone scintigraphy or technetium bone scanning is useful as a screening tool to assess multiple sites of bone involvement, as may occur in polyostotic fibrous dysplasia, multiple enchondromatosis, or histiocytosis. The appearance of a bone lesion in the flow and pool phases of a three-phase bone scan reflects its biologic activity. The presence of abnormal radiotracer uptake does not accurately characterize a lesion as benign or malignant. A negative or cold bone scan may indicate a latent or quiescent lesion. Notable exceptions include multiple myeloma or some types of metastatic carcinoma such as renal cell carcinoma. Conversely, many benign conditions such as giant cell tumor or enchondroma may indeed show abnormal radiotracer activity. Thus, the routine use of technetium bone scans is not recommended to evaluate a suspected benign bone lesion.

Positron emission tomography (PET) is a functional diagnostic imaging technique that provides information distinctly different from that obtained with other imaging modalities. The most widely used radiotracer is F-18 fluoro-2-deox:y-D-glucose (FDG), which is an analog of

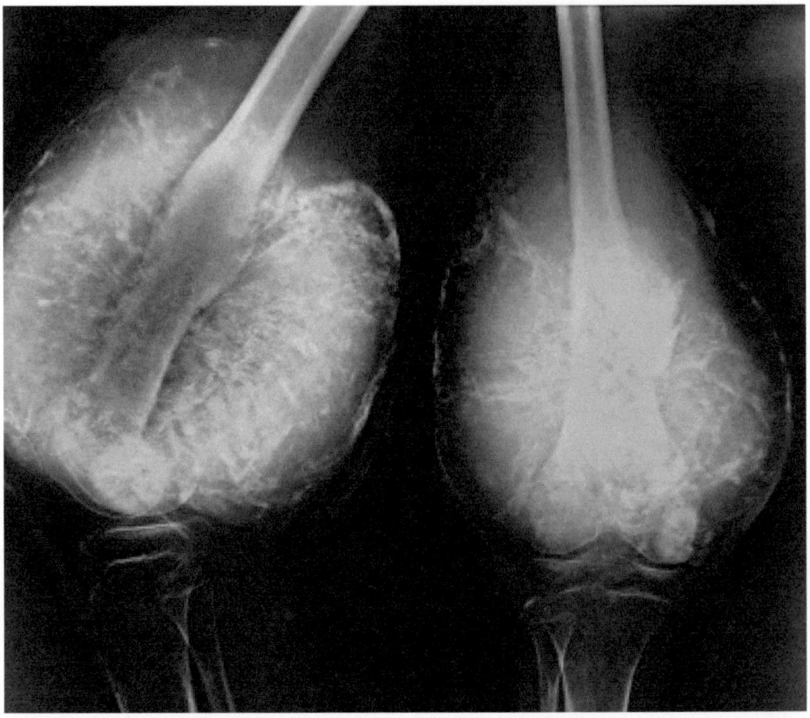

Fig. 3 Plain radiographs showing aggressive radiographic features of malignant bone tumors characterized by permeative destruction, ill-defined borders, cortical destruction, periosteal elevation, and extraosseous extension

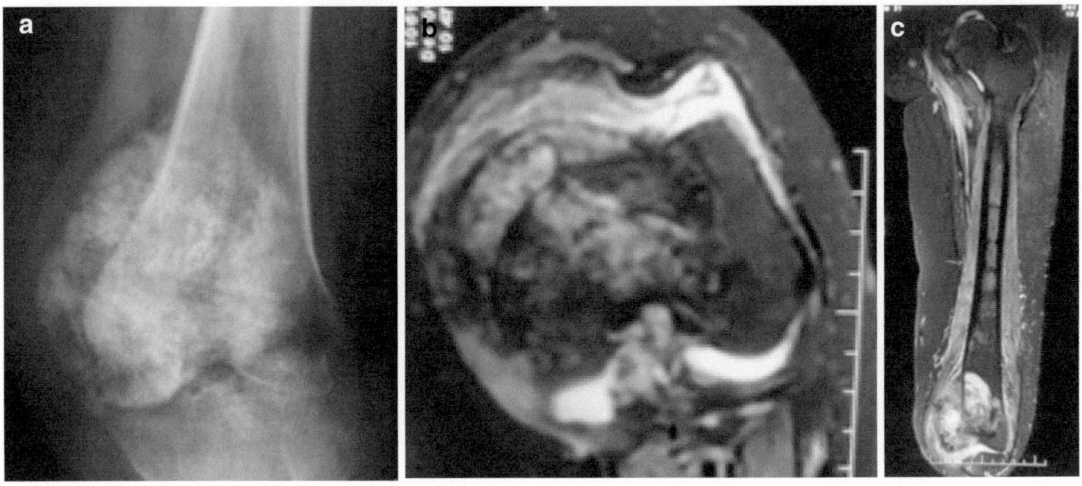

Fig. 4 (**a**) Plain radiograph shows a permeative, aggressive lesion within the metaphysis of the distal femur. (**b**, **c**) Axial and coronal sections MRI showing the intramedullary extent, soft tissue extension, and relation to vessels and nerves. Biopsy from the lesion revealed osteosarcoma

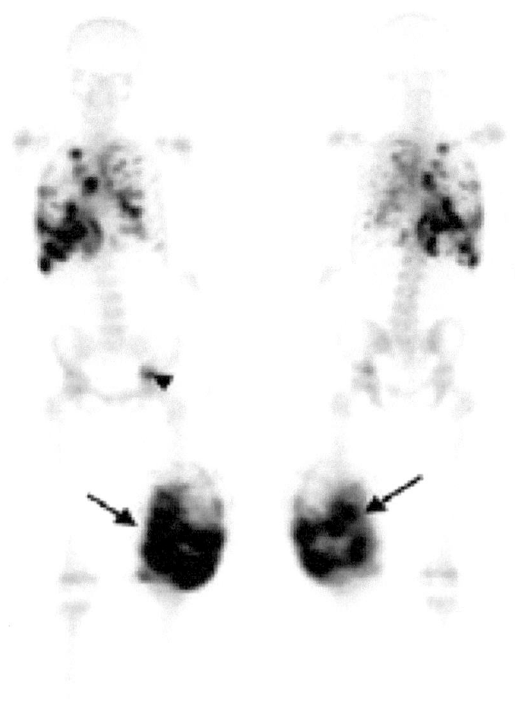

Fig. 5 99Tc-MDP whole body bone scan images of a 16-year-old male with osteosarcoma of left femur showing heterogeneous tracer uptake (arrow) consistent with primary tumor along with bone metastasis (arrowhead) and osteogenic pulmonary metastasis

glucose. The FDG uptake in cells is directly proportional to glucose metabolism, which is increased many times in malignant cells. FDG-PET now is the standard of care in initial staging, monitoring the response to therapy and management of various cancers. In many institutions, PET is replacing bone scans for the detection of distant metastasis and initial staging of bone tumors. PET has been most widely advocated for Ewing sarcoma, which has a fairly high (approximately 25%) incidence of metastases at diagnosis. In addition to metastatic survey, PET can provide physiologic information with regard to the primary tumor. The standardized uptake value (SUV) can provide a quantitative measure of metabolic activity, with malignant tumors generally having higher SUVs. The degree of overlap, however, between benign and malignant lesions, as well as inherent technical bias, prevents the use of a reliable threshold value. The introduction of combined PET-CT scanners, which provide not only functional but also structural information leading to a detection of subcentimeter lesions, has made this technique useful in the early detection of the disease process and in decreasing false-positive lesions.

Imaging Assessment of Therapeutic Response Some recent studies have evaluated the role of MRI as predictors of histological necrosis after chemotherapy as well as prognosis. In a study, more than 60% reduction in slope of curve on dynamic contrast enhanced MRI (DCE-MRI) proved to be an indicator of good histological response in osteosarcoma [11]. Another study group analyzed surrogates of tumor angiogenesis through radiological imaging by qualitative analysis of DCE-MRI in osteosarcoma and found that VEGF (vascular endothelial growth factor) expression correlated with CDE-MRI, thereby predicting the grade of tumor [12, 13].

Studies have shown that response to neoadjuvant chemotherapy (NACT) can be predicted reliably by PET-CT scan early in disease course and PET-CT parameters correlate well with histological necrosis after resection [14]. A retrospective study attempted to correlate fluorodeoxyglucose (FDG) uptake in PET scans with tumor behavior and to predict response to chemotherapy in Ewing sarcoma. They concluded that increased FDG uptake was indicative of metastatic potential of the tumor and that there was significant correlation between change in metabolic activity of the primary tumor and histopathological response after NACT, suggesting that FDG-PET might be an ideal noninvasive method to assess tumor behavior and response to therapy in Ewing sarcoma [15].

1.6.1 Surveillance Imaging

The mainstay of surveillance imaging for local recurrence following primary tumor resection remains standard radiography. Artifact associated with metallic hardware following skeletal reconstruction limits the utility of routine CT and MRI. Recent advances in MRI metallic susceptibility artifact reduction are promising and may offer high-quality local imaging follow-up in the near future [16]. Long-term surveillance imaging for distant metastases is an area of significant development in the last decade. Although detection of metastases was previously limited to identification of osseous metastasis by technetium scintigraphy and pulmonary metastasis with chest radiographs or chest CT, the advent of FDG PET, PET-CT, and whole-body MRI has enabled much broader and earlier detection. Hybrid PET-CT has been shown to have higher sensitivity and specificity than FDG PET alone for the detection of occult metastases [17, 18]. The ability to localize areas of increased FDG avidity to anatomic correlates has decreased the false-positive rates associated with PET imaging alone. For Ewing sarcoma, FDG PET-CT has been shown to be more sensitive than bone scanning for the detection of local and distant recurrence, and many experts advocate elimination of dedicated bone scintigraphy in this patient population [19]. Whole-body MRI has been used for several years to detect osseous metastases in patients with breast and lung cancer and is now being applied to musculoskeletal tumors with success. Several studies comparing whole-body MRI to PET-CT for metastatic disease tend to show similar sensitivities and specificities, each with their own advantages and limitations [20]. The lack of ionizing irradiation with whole-body MRI is an important advantage.

1.7 Laboratory Studies

Laboratory studies often are nonspecific. For patients younger than 40 years of age, they include a complete blood count with differential, peripheral blood smear, and erythrocyte sedimentation rate. Patients older than 40 years also need blood calcium and phosphate levels, serum and urine electrophoresis, and urinalysis. Serum alkaline phosphatase levels in primary osteosarcomas correlate with disease prognosis; therefore, pretreatment levels should be recorded.

1.8 Staging of Bone Tumors

Bone tumor staging provides a framework for patient evaluation, helps direct treatment, and stratifies risk or prognosis. Enneking proposed a simple and commonly used system for benign and malignant bone tumors (Tables 4 and 5). Variables used to assign stage to malignant bone tumors include tumor grade based on histology, extent of tumor as intra-compartmental or extra-compartmental, and presence or absence of metastatic disease based on appropriate imaging studies [21]. This system continues to be an easy and reproducible system for the assessment of malignant bone tumors.

The American Joint Committee on Cancer (AJCC) proposed a slightly different and more thorough system [22]. Four variables are used to assign stages using the AJCC system: tumor size, histologic grade, the presence or absence of regional (nodal) metastasis, and the presence or absence of distant metastasis. Beginning in 2003 with the sixth edition of the AJCC system [23], distant metastasis now receives a sub-classification based on the site of involvement. Pulmonary distant metastasis is designated Mla, whereas non-pulmonary distant metastasis is designated Mlb. The eighth and most recent edition of the AJCC system was released in 2017 [24].The only update from the sixth edition involves stage III. This stage is now reserved for noncontiguous G3 and G4 tumors (high-grade, poorly differentiated tumors, and high-grade, undifferentiated tumors, respectively). A brief outline to comprehend the details of AJCC staging of bone sarcoma is represented in Table 6.

1.9 Biopsy of Bone Tumors

An appropriately planned and performed biopsy is imperative for obtaining definitive diagnostic tissue in bone and soft-tissue tumors. The biopsy technique and approach are paramount for directing further treatment and

Table 4 Enneking staging system for benign bone lesions

Stage	Definition	Behavior	Radiographic findings	Examples
1	Latent	Remains static or heals spontaneously	Well-defined borders often with sclerotic edges without cortical disruption, permeative growth, and periosteal reaction	Non-ossifying fibroma, enchondroma, osteochondroma
2	Active	Progressive growth, limited by natural barriers	Varying amounts of bone destruction or cortical thinning	Osteoid osteoma, chondromyxoid fibroma, unicameral bone cysts
3	Aggressive	Progressive growth, not limited by natural barriers	Expansion of bone with cortical violation and soft-tissue extension, causing structural compromise	Giant cell tumor, aneurysmal bone cyst

Table 5 Enneking Surgical Staging System for malignant bone tumors

Stage	Grade[a]	Site[b]	Distant metastasis[c]
IA	Low (G1)	Intracompartmental (T1)	None (M0)
IB	Low (G1)	Extracompartmental (T2)	None (M0)
IIA	High (G2)	Intracompartmental (T1)	None (M0)
IIB	High (G2)	Extracompartmental (T2)	None (M0)
III	Any (G)	Any (T)	Regional or distant metastasis (M1)

[a]G1, low grade; G2, high grade
[b]T1, lesions that remain within an anatomic compartment (intraosseous for bone tumors): T2, lesions extending through or beyond the host cortex
[c]MO, no distant metastasis; M1, distant metastasis

Table 6 A brief outline of American Joint Committee on Cancer (AJCC) staging system for bone sarcoma

Stage IA- T1N0M0 with G1, GX (low grades)
Stage IB- T2-3N0M0 with G1, GX (low grades)
Stage IIA- T1N0M0 with G2, G3 (high grades)
Stage IIB T2N0M0 with G2, G3 (high grades)
Stage III T3N0M0 with G2, G3 (high grades)
Stage IVA AnyTN0M1a with any G
Stage IVB AnyTN1anyM with any grade or AnyTanyNM1b with any G

TX denotes primary tumor cannot be assessed; T0 denotes absence of primary tumor; T1 denotes a tumor 8 cm or less in greatest dimension; T2 denotes a tumor more than 8 cm in greatest dimension or more than one tumor in same bone; T3 denotes discontinuous tumors in the primary bone
NX denotes inaccessible primary regional lymph nodes, N0 denotes absence of regional lymph node involvement, and N1 denotes metastases to regional lymph nodes
MO denotes no distant metastasis; M1 denotes distant metastasis; M1a signifies lung metastases; M1b denotes other distant sites
GX, grade cannot be assessed; G1, well differentiated, low grade; G2, moderately differentiated, low grade; G3, poorly differentiated (earlier G1 to G4)

minimizing morbidity when definitive surgical intervention is appropriate. It is important to note that not all lesions require a biopsy for diagnosis. Particular lesions that may not necessitate a biopsy include some chondroid lesions and fibro-osseous lesions with characteristic radiographic findings. Referral to a musculoskeletal oncologist should be considered for biopsy of lesions that are suspected to be malignant or aggressive on imaging. Several key principles of the biopsy of musculoskeletal neoplasms, when followed appropriately, can help minimizing morbidity and contamination, maximizing diagnostic accuracy, and facilitating limb salvage surgery.

- The surgeon who will be carrying out the definitive procedure on the patient should do the biopsy.
- Before doing a biopsy, all the laboratory and imaging work-up of the patient should have been completed. Imaging studies indicate the most representative part of the lesion that should be targeted for tissue sampling.
- There should be no contamination of normal vital tissues such as neurovascular structures, tendons, ligaments, and joints. The biopsy

should be directed through one compartment to ensure that tissue planes are not violated.

- In the appendicular skeleton, the biopsy incision should be in the long axis of the bone. Avoid transverse incision.
- The surgeon should plan the biopsy scar such that it should fall in line with the scar of the definitive surgery when it is done at a later date (so that it could be excised) (Fig. 6).
- Core needle biopsy is the preferred method of biopsy in bone tumors, but open biopsy should be considered in patients with deep lying lesions or where a previous core biopsy has failed to give adequate tissue sample for diagnosis.
- Adequate homeostasis should be maintained at all times.
- Deep dissection in case of open biopsies should be sharp with avoidance of major neurovascular planes. In case a tourniquet is used, no exsanguination of the limb should be done. In case a drain is used, drain exit site should allow excision at the time of definitive surgery.
- Samples should be taken for microbiological culture as well as histology.
- All samples should be adequately stored and labeled (with patient's informed consent for the same).
- All clinical and radiological details should be made available to the pathologist on a biopsy requisition form.
- Samples should be interpreted by an experienced pathologist. There should be appropriate communication between surgeon, radiologist, and pathologist.
- Image-guided biopsies (using an image intensifier, CT scan, or navigation) should be used for deeper lesions like those in the pelvis.
- Fresh tissue is needed for molecular studies and should be taken before formalin fixation.
- Tumor banking should be considered wherever the facilities and the informed consent are available for later analysis as well as diagnosis and translational research into molecular pathology of cancer.

Historically, the most accurate method of obtaining diagnostic tissue was thought to be the open biopsy, followed by core biopsy and fine-needle aspiration (FNA) biopsy [25, 26]. In a study comparing the accuracy of the three biopsy

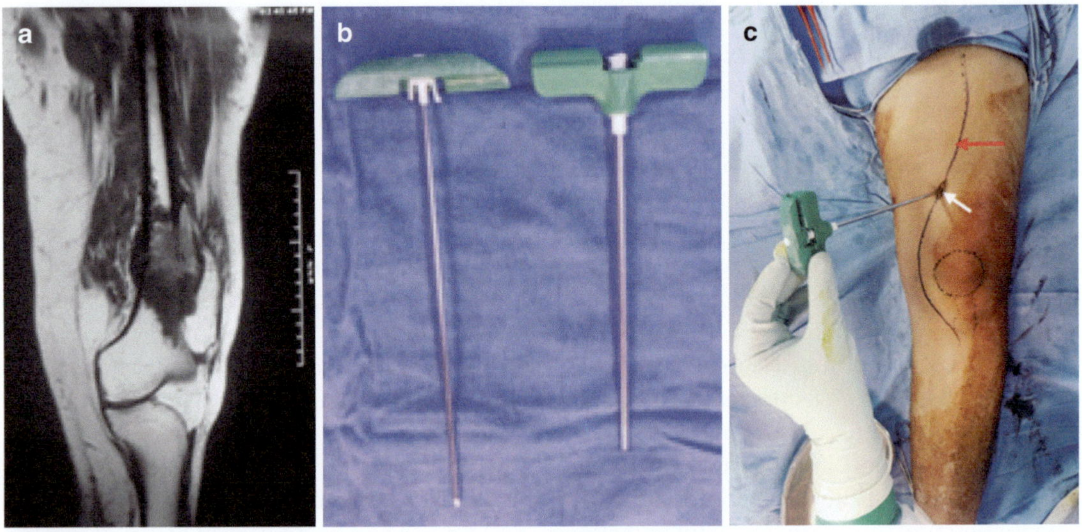

Fig. 6 (**a**) MRI of the femur depicting a lesion in the meta-diaphyseal region at the distal end of femur. (**b**) Core biopsy needles used for biopsy of bone tumors. (**c**) Biopsy technique using a longitudinal skin incision (white arrow) in line with the intended surgical incision of the definitive surgery (red arrow)

techniques, the authors found that all three modalities are acceptable biopsy techniques for soft tissue masses [27].

Percutaneous Techniques With the increasing popularity of the image-guided biopsy techniques using MRI, CT, and ultrasound, percutaneous biopsy techniques are preferred. These techniques can, theoretically, result in the least contamination of tissue, with minimal morbidity, and can usually be done with the use of local anesthesia, eliminating the risk of general or regional anesthesia often necessary in an incisional biopsy. These include fine-needle aspiration biopsy and core biopsy.

Fine-Needle Aspiration Biopsy FNA biopsy is a technique in which tissue is obtained by placing a needle (20-gauge or smaller) into the mass and aspirating tissue into the needle. Although historically regarded as less diagnostic than core and incisional biopsy, FNA biopsy is commonly used for both bone and soft-tissue neoplasms. In several studies, the diagnostic accuracy was approximately 90% [28, 29]. Lesions that contain myxoid or round cell neoplastic tissue, lesions accompanied by infection, and lesions in paraspinal anatomic locations have the lowest diagnostic accuracy with FNA biopsy [30]. Although FNA biopsy for primary diagnosis of sarcoma may be controversial, it clearly has a role in the diagnosis of local recurrence and of metastatic carcinoma in the musculoskeletal system.

Core Biopsy Core or trocar biopsy involves obtaining tissue from a bone or soft-tissue mass using a large-bore needle (commonly 14-gauge or larger). The diagnostic accuracy in percutaneous core biopsy of bone lesion, based on several studies, is from 75% to 95%, with most studies reporting greater than 90% accuracy [31, 32].

1.10 Fundamentals of Surgical Treatment of Bone Tumors

The armament of oncology surgeons has been expanded by surgical advancements, including the use of effective adjuncts (e.g., chemotherapy and radiation therapy), computer navigation, and enhanced biomaterials. In essence, bone lesions can be addressed through either limb-sacrificing or limb-sparing surgery. Despite the fact that each case is distinct, it is beneficial to comprehend the principles of surgical resection and the ways in which it affects the patient's function and the disease.

The selection of patients for limb salvage procedures is contingent upon the possibility of achieving a surgery with comparable oncologic control to amputation and the subsequent restoration of a limb with a modern prosthesis that is more functional than the amputated limb. Limb salvage should be considered for all patients with extremity sarcomas, provided that the tumor can be excised with a sufficient margin and limb function can be preserved. In certain situations, the aggressiveness of the lesion or the extent of surgical excision precludes limb-sparing alternatives and necessitates amputation. Examples of such indications for amputation include the inability to perform successful vascular bypass due to the encasement of main neurovascular structures, or extensive soft tissue involvement.

In 1951, Dallas Phemister at the University of Chicago was the first to perform limb-salvage surgery for osseous sarcoma in North America [33]. The objective of limb salvage surgery is to resect the entire tumor with negative margins and subsequently reconstruct the limb in the most functional manner possible. It comprises two distinct objectives: functional, durable reconstruction, and adequate resection.

The preoperative evaluation of surgical margins is a critical component of limb salvage surgery. Surgical margins are most accurately defined by the surgical staging system that was initially described by Enneking et al. in 1980 [21]. The relationship between the plane of dissection of the tumor and its pseudocapsular/reactive zone is the basis for the description of four categories of margins (Table 7). With the exception of low-grade chondrosarcoma, which may be treated with intralesional excision, nearly all malignant tumors and certain benign aggressive

Table 7 Classification of surgical margins

Intralesional excision	Plane of dissection passes within the lesion. Pseudocapsule of the tumor is entered (e.g., curettage)
Marginal excision	Pseudocapsule of the tumor is not entered. Plane of dissection passes through the reactive zone. Microscopic disease may be left behind
Wide excision	Plane of dissection passes through a cuff of normal tissue
Radical excision	Removal of entire compartment of origin; complete extirpation of an entire bone

Table 8 Evaluation method for surgical margins for bone tumors

Type	Plane of dissection
Intralesional	Curettage or debulking
Marginal	Pericapsular reactive zone
Wide (A) Inadequate (B) Adequate	Normal cuff of tissue 1 cm Normal cuff of tissue more than 1–4 cm
Curative	Normal cuff of tissue 5 cm or more

tumors necessitate wide excision, which involves the removal of the tumor with a margin of normal bone and soft tissue.

Nevertheless, Enneking did not specify the precise quantity of "normal" tissue that constitutes a wide margin. The Japanese Orthopedic Association's Evaluation Method for Surgical Margins was approved in 1989 (see Table 8) [34]. In this system, a surgical margin is classified into the four categories of curative, broad, marginal, or intralesional margin based on the distance of the margin from the tumor's reactive zone.

The concept of barrier in surgery for bone and soft tissue sarcoma was later described by Kawaguchi et al. [35]. Barriers encompass any tissue that exhibits resistance to tumor invasion, such as muscle fascia, joint capsule, tendon, tendon sheath, epineurium, vascular sheath, cartilage, pleura, and peritoneum. With the exception of joint cartilage, each of these tissues can be classified as either a dense barrier or a narrow barrier (Table 9). The equivalent thickness of normal tissue is achieved by converting barriers. Surgery can be performed at locations where barriers are present by utilizing a smaller margin than the actual physical distance by translating barrier effects into concrete distance equivalents. In other words, a surgical margin of at least 3 cm should be established when a patient with a high-grade musculoskeletal sarcoma is treated solely through surgery, whether initially or subsequently. The goal should be to use a 2 cm wide margin as the least margin during surgery when preoperative chemotherapy is efficacious, as evidenced by the somatic findings and imaging studies.

Table 9 Types of barrier

Barrier	Tissues	Equivalent Margin
Thin	Weaker membranous structure: muscle fascia, adult periosteum, vessel sheath, epineurium, thin growth plates in older children	2 cm
Thick	Strong membranous tissue with a white tendinous luster: iliotibial band, presacral fascia, joint capsule, infant periosteum, thin growth plate in older children	3 cm
Joint cartilage	–	5 cm

1.10.1 Reconstruction Considerations

The reconstruction options include endoprosthesis (modular and expandable), allograft, allograft-prosthesis composite, autograft (vascularized, non-vascularized, re-cycled tumor bearing), and arthrodesis. Endoprosthetic reconstructions offer the benefits of modularity, ease in assembly and insertion, immediate weight bearing, rapid rehabilitation, and excellent functional outcome (Fig. 7). However, prosthetic longevity is limited. In recent studies with proximal femoral replacements for tumor reconstruction, 10- and 20-year implant survivorships were 78–84%, and 55–56%, respectively [36, 37]. In the distal femoral endoprosthetic reconstructions, 10- and 20-year implant survivorships were 67–77% and 42–58%, respectively [38, 39]. Primary modes of failure of endoprosthesis are infection, aseptic loosening, and implant fracture [40].

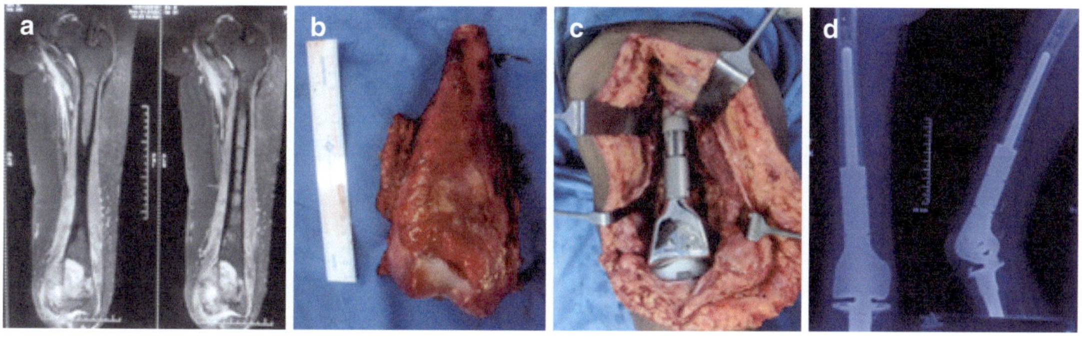

Fig. 7 Distal femoral osteosarcoma in a 17-year-old male demonstrating (**a**) MRI findings, (**b**) wide resection specimen, (**c**) intraoperative placement of endoprosthesis, and (**d**) postoperative radiographic appearance following limb-salvage surgery

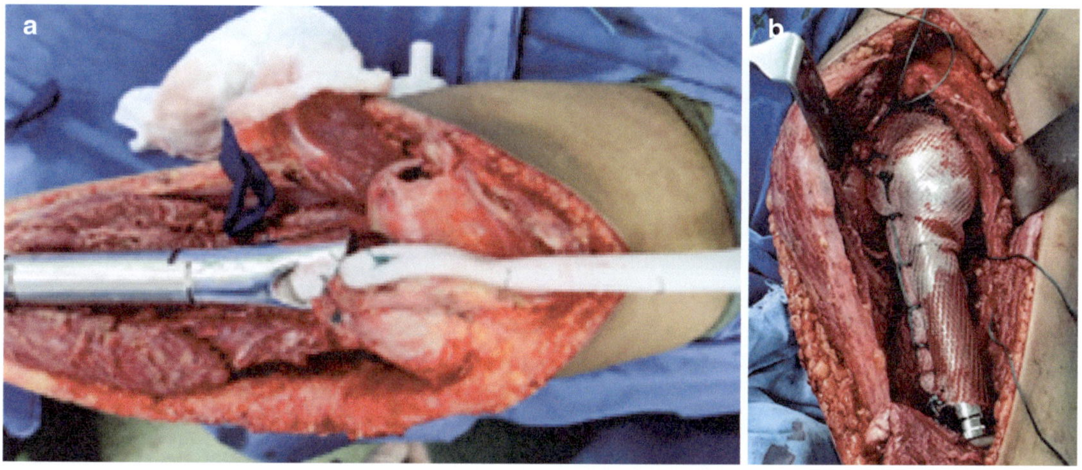

Fig. 8 Reconstruction with endoprosthesis and prolene mesh following resection of proximal tibia (**a**) and proximal humerus (**b**)

Wide excision of the bone tumors often necessitates removal of the surrounding soft tissue restraints of the joints (ligaments, tendons, muscles, joint capsule), which contribute to its stability. Wide excision of the proximal tibial tumors requires reconstruction of the extensor mechanism of the knee, as the insertion of the patella tendon on the tibial tubercle is usually resected with the tumor. Various modifications in surgical techniques and use of new biomaterials like prolene mesh have been described in literature for soft tissue reconstruction following bone tumor resection (Fig. 8) [41, 42].

In the skeletally immature patient, limb-salvage procedures present unique challenges that include the small size of the pediatric skeleton, the growth potential of the patient, the ensuing limb-length discrepancy, and the need for correction of the discrepancy. Expandable prostheses have been developed for skeletally immature patients to combat the ensuing limb-length discrepancy. The mechanism of expansion has shifted from modular systems that require open procedures to minimally invasive (telescoping using a gear device) and noninvasive (telescoping using electromagnetic induction) mechanisms. The most common complications are failure of the expansion mechanism, aseptic loosening, and infection [43, 44].

Intercalary resection for diaphyseal tumors allows preservation of adjacent joints wherein the skeletal defect can be reconstructed with intercalary endoprosthesis [45] or biological reconstructions using allografts [46], vascularized or free fibular autografts [47], and recycled tumor-bearing autograft [48, 49]. Intercalary and osteo-articular allografts offer a biologic reconstruction option. However, it is limited by the availability of bone bank facility and is associated with complications of graft fracture, infection, nonunion, and degeneration of the articular surface [50, 51].

Recycled autograft involves reimplantation of resected bone after it has been sterilized of the tumor cells. This can be achieved by autoclaving [52], pasteurization [53], liquid nitrogen [54], or irradiation [48, 49]. It provides biological reconstruction of large osseous defects, with the possibility of preserving native joints.

Extracorporeal radiation therapy (ECRT) has been reported as an oncologically safe and effective reconstruction technique for limb salvage in diaphyseal malignant tumors with promising functional results [48, 49]. This includes *en-bloc* removal of the tumor bearing bone segment, extracorporeal sterilization using single high dose irradiation with typical radiation dosage varying from 50 to 300 Gy, and re-implantation in the skeletal defect (Fig. 9). ECRT autografts grafts have also been used in combination with a vascularized or non-vascularized fibula. This reconstruction modality provides a "patient-specific" precise anatomic fit and offers the advantages of preservation of bone stock, low cost, and longevity. It obviates the need of bone bank facility for procurement of size-matched allografts and risk of viral transmission or immunologic reaction with allografts. Incorporation of the ECRT autograft occurs through creeping substitution which includes absorbance of the graft, crawling, and superseding with simultaneous deposition of new, viable bone. Chauhan et al. demonstrated loss in mechanical stiffness, with increased plastic deformation and indentation creep in compact bone of five patients suffering from Ewing's sarcoma [55]. Raman spectroscopy study in this patient group showed reduced mineralization and calcium content in the irradiated bone. These changes in biomechanical properties may result in graft resorption, stress fracture, or mechanical failure of the construct. Oike et al. in their analysis of long-term outcomes of extracorporeal irradiated autograft observed nonunion and infection in 37.5% and 16.6% of the patients, respectively [56]. Hayashi et al. [57] reported graft fracture in 11% of their patients, while Puri et al. [48] observed graft fracture in 6% of their patients. Jones et al. [58] and Puri et al. [48] reported 9% and 10% local recurrence rate using extracorporeal irradiation for limb salvage in bone tumors.

In cases of sarcomas of the extremities with extensive involvement of the bone and soft tissues which are resectable and yet necessitate amputations as these are not reconstructable with available limb salvage methods, surgical procedures, namely, rotationplasty (lower extremity) and surgical phocomelia or phoco-reduction (upper extremity), have been described as methods of limb salvage and prudent alternatives to severely incapacitating amputations [59, 60]. These procedures involve resection of a cylindrical segment of the limb comprising of the tumor-affected length of the bone along with soft tissues and the overlying skin while sparing the important nerves and vessels, with a subsequent attachment of the distal to the proximal segment, resulting in shortened limb with reasonable preservation of function (Fig. 9). Rotationplasty involves conversion of the ankle into the knee joint after shortening and 180° external rotation of the limb. Such procedures also offer good functional outcomes after failed limb salvage surgeries [61].

1.11 Pelvic Resections

The surgical treatment of pelvic tumors is quite challenging due to the complex anatomy, proximity to major neurovascular structures, the necessity for massive blood transfusions, and the absence of an optimal reconstruction technique. According to the literature available [62, 63], pelvic tumors are associated with high rates of local recurrence, which range from 7.4% to 48%.

In 1978, Enneking and Dunham characterized the conventional pelvic resections [64]. They identified four distinct categories of resections: Type I, which involves the iliac wing, Type II,

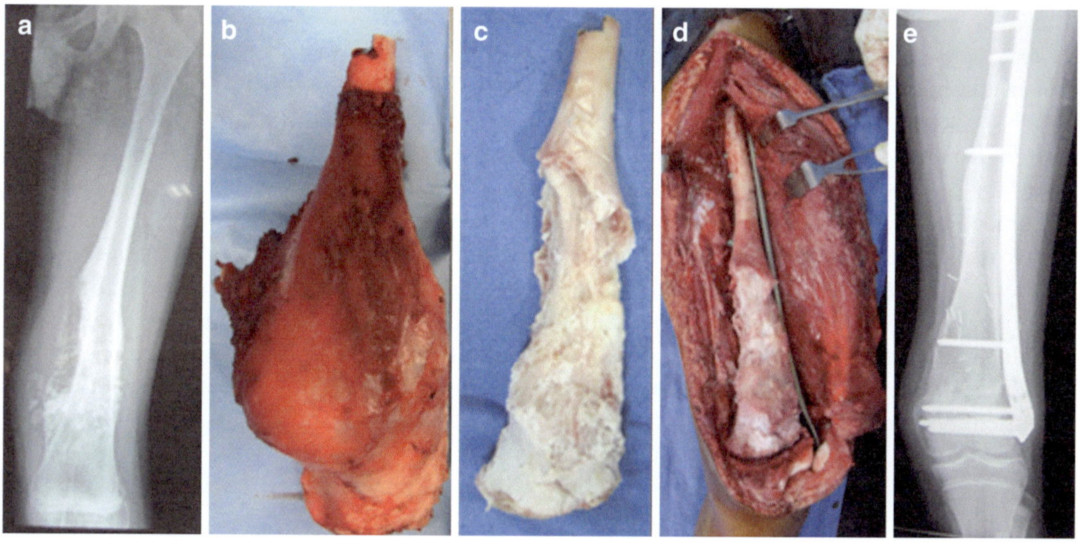

Fig. 9 Eleven year old male with osteosarcoma of femur (**a**), underwent wide resection (**b**), extracorporeal sterilization of the tumor bearing bone (**c**, **d**), and re-implantation in the skeletal defect (**e**)

which involves the periacetabular region, Type III, which involves the pubic rami, and Type IV, which involves the sacrum. A combination of these varieties is employed more frequently, contingent upon the presence of distinct oncological margins. Pring et al. found that patients who underwent Type I or Type III resections with preservation of the acetabulum had superior functional outcomes compared to those who underwent Type II resections [65, 66]. Kapoor et al. recently described Type I + half and Type III + half trans-acetabular pelvic resections in comparison to complete acetabular resection with conventional Type I + II and Type II + III pelvic resections according to Enneking [62]. Their findings indicated that transacetabular pelvic resections of this nature offer a functional advantage over conventional resections, without impairing oncological margins.

Pseudoarthrosis/hip transposition, ischio/iliofemoral arthrodesis, allograft or prosthetic or composite reconstruction, and reconstruction using treated (irradiated/pasteurized) autograft are among the numerous surgical reconstruction options [67, 68]. The rigidity that results from successful arthrodesis is intolerable to certain cultures where squatting is a necessity, despite the fact that the functional results are quite satisfactory [63] High rates of infection, nonunion, and graft fracture complicate allograft reconstruction [69, 70]. Despite having a similar complication profile to allografts, irradiated or pasteurized autografts have the advantage of being a size-matched graft and avoiding the danger of disease transmission [71]. Wound-related complications, dislocation, nerve dysfunction, and aseptic laxity are all associated with prosthetic reconstruction [68, 72].

Hip transposition is a safe and straightforward surgical procedure that can be implemented to obtain a favorable functional outcome in periacetabular tumors. The femoral head is affixed to the nearest available bone following tumor resection. It is a more advantageous alternative to other forms of reconstruction, as it involves fewer complications [72, 73]. In comparison to prosthetic reconstruction and hindquarter amputation, Hoffman et al. reported that patients who underwent hip transposition following acetabular resections obtained significantly improved functional outcomes and quality of life [74]. The reduction of wound-related complications may be facilitated by the absence of metallic hardware and tension-free closure. Kapoor et al. demonstrated favorable functional outcomes in their patients who underwent hip transposition with Prolene mesh [62].

Benign Tumors Intralesional excision may be employed to treat benign tumors and certain low-grade malignancies, such as low-grade chondrosarcoma of the extremities. Surgical intervention is necessary to prevent deformity, stabilize a pathologic fracture or impending pathologic fracture, and limit bone destruction. The cortical bone is exposed through the utilization of either a drill and osteotome or a pencil-tip burr. The cortical aperture should be sufficiently large to externalize the lesion and should be shaped in a circular or oval shape. Squared margins should be avoided due to the stress-raising effects and the challenge of achieving full exteriorization of the lesion, which is necessary for the complete eradication of the pathology. The bone lesion is subsequently removed using curettes, with caution taken to prevent contamination of the adjacent tissues. The curettage is prolonged by treating the cavity with adjuvants to mitigate the risk of local recurrence after all bulk tumors have been removed. Adjuvants are beneficial for treating microscopic cells that are believed to have evaded the initial curettage and are composed of a combination of chemical, thermal, or mechanical agents (Table 10). The structural support is provided by reconstructing the skeletal defect using bone graft (autograft or allograft) or PMMA (polymethylmethaacrylate) cement, or a combination of both (sandwich technique). The vacant cavity progressively fills with new bone that consolidates over time, allowing small defects to remain unfilled.

Table 10 Types of adjuvants that are used to extend the margins of an intralesional excision

Chemical	1. Hydrogen peroxide 2. Distilled water 3. Alcohol 4. Phenol
Mechanical	1. High-speed burr 2. Curettage
Thermal	1. Argon beam coagulator 2. Electrocautery 3. Polymethylmethacrylate (PMMA) 4. Liquid nitrogen 5. Cryoprobes

Following establishment of a benign diagnosis, appropriate treatment can be initiated. This may include observation and repeat imaging after an appropriate interval, usually 3–6 months, to ensure radiographic stability. Alternatively, surgical intervention may be warranted to limit bone destruction, stabilize a pathologic fracture or impending pathologic injury, and/or prevent deformity.

1.12 Prognosis and Survival

In the fields of osteosarcoma and Ewing's sarcoma, there have been numerous large-scale retrospective data from the All India Institute of Medical Sciences and Tata Memorial Hospital (TMH) that have reported outcomes that are comparable to Western data.

Osteosarcoma: The majority of cancer centers in India provide chemotherapy regimens that are not based on methotrexate in the treatment of osteosarcoma. In an effort to ascertain prognostic factors and report outcomes in a cohort of localized osteosarcoma patients who were treated pursuant to a uniform protocol, the study group from the All India Institute of Medical Sciences (AIIMS) published their data on 237 patients. They demonstrated a 5-year event-free survival (EFS) and overall survival (OS) rate of 36.6% and 50.3%, respectively. On multivariate analysis, they observed that a good performance status (PS) predicted a better EFS, while a good PS and normal serum alkaline phosphatase predicted a better OS [75]. Another study conducted by AIIMS assessed the potential of a high tumor volume at presentation as a predictor of local recurrence (LR) by utilizing MRI images to determine the baseline tumor volume. The findings of this retrospective analysis indicated that osteosarcomas do not exhibit a significant correlation with elevated tumor volume [76]. A meta-analysis conducted by a Chinese group recently revealed that a poor prognosis in osteosarcoma patients was associated with male patients, older age, large tumor size, non-extremity osteosarcoma, proximal osteosarcoma, poor chemotherapy response, no surgical treatment, and amputation surgery [77].

Ewing's sarcoma: In a large retrospective analysis conducted at AIIMS, which included 374 patients with localized and metastatic Ewing's sarcoma, the authors assessed potential prognostic factors. They suggested that patients with a combination of baseline white blood cell (WBC) count >11 × 10^9/L and spine/abdominopelvic region involvement had a significantly inferior OS, while patients with a combination of symptom duration >4 months, tumor diameter >8 cm, and baseline WBC count >11 × 10^9/L had a significantly inferior EFS [78]. These findings are in accordance with global data that has demonstrated inferior clinical outcomes in cases involving large volume disease (>200 mL) and pelvic primaries. In cases of metastatic tumor settings, hypoalbuminemia was identified as a distinctive prognostic factor associated with EFS in another study conducted by the same group [79]. They also published their data on prognostic factors and outcomes in extremity Ewing's sarcoma. Radiotherapy was found to be noninferior to surgery in the subset of patients with localized tumors with regard to tumor diameter or post-NACT response, despite the fact that metastases and radiotherapy alone (vs. surgery as primary local treatment) predicted poorer outcomes in the entire cohort of 158 patients. The total cohort's 5-year EFS, OS, and LC (local control) rates were 24.1%, 43.5%, and 55%, respectively. Patients without metastases had rates of 36.4%, 57.6%, and 58.2%, respectively. These findings indicate that radical radiation therapy alone leads to a suboptimal local control rate, despite a favorable post-neoadjuvant chemotherapy response. Additionally, patients who did not have metastases but exhibited a high white blood cell count had reduced event-free survival and local control rates. The outcomes of non-extremity have been the subject of data publication by numerous organizations. In comparison to head and neck, extraosseous, and mandible Ewing's sarcoma, pelvic and spinal Ewing's sarcoma appear to have inferior outcomes [80–85].

1.13 Conclusion

The treatment of bone tumors typically involves multidisciplinary input and cooperation. Referral to an established orthopedic oncology center is recommended. Adjuvant or neoadjuvant therapies including chemotherapy or radiation therapy may be coordinated with surgical intervention as deemed appropriate. Ongoing surveillance is indicated to assess for local recurrence and/or the presence of distant disease. The surgical treatment of bone tumors provides unique challenges for surgeons. Advances in preoperative imaging, intraoperative imaging (e.g., computer navigation) and surgical techniques, prosthetic design, and adjuvant treatments (chemotherapy and radiation) and improved understanding of the biologic behavior of these rare lesions continue to assist surgeons in improving functional outcomes.

2 Ewing's Sarcoma

Ewing's sarcoma is a highly malignant primary bone tumor (sometimes arising in soft tissue) that occurs mainly in children and adolescents, typically between 5 and 20 years of age.

Common sites of this disease include the diaphyses of long bones (femur, tibia, humerus), as well as the pelvis, ribs, and scapula (Fig. 10).

Typically, patients present with pain, swelling, fever, and weight loss (often mimicking infection). The disease is highly aggressive but chemo- and radiosensitive. The initial evaluation includes clinical assessment for pain, swelling, fever, and weight loss. X-ray imaging suggests a permeative lytic lesion, "onion-skin" periosteal reaction. MRI provides information on the local extent of disease and soft-tissue involvement. PET CT/CT chest is routinely suggested to rule out lung/bone/visceral metastasis.

The core biopsy, or open biopsy, is planned along the future surgical incision. The histopathology suggests small round blue cells. Cytogenetics often reveal the characteristic EWSR1–FLI1 translocation (t(11;22)).

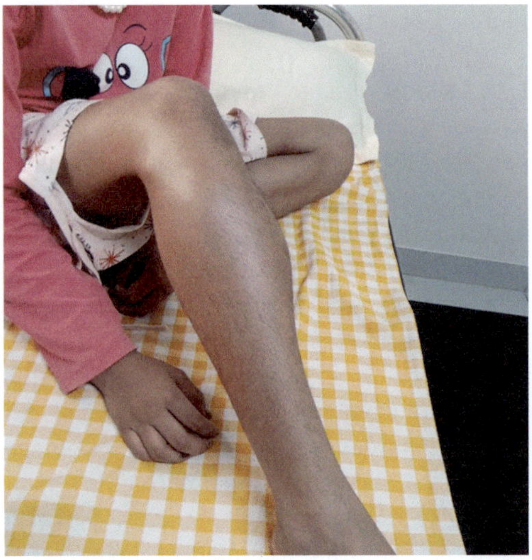

Fig. 10 Ewing's sarcoma of the right tibia in a 15 year old. (Courtesy: Dr Nehal Khanna, Department of Radiation Oncology, Tata Memorial Hospital, Parel, Mumbai, India)

Table 11 Use of surgery and RT in Ewing's sarcoma

	Surgery use	RT use
1	Wide excision with tumor-free margins in resectable sites	Tumor is unresectable
2	Limb-salvage surgery preferred	Margins are positive
3	–	Situations where surgery would cause unacceptable morbidity

Neo-adjuvant chemotherapy is generally given to all patients, even if the disease is localized. It aims to reduce tumor size and treat micrometastases. Standard regimens include Vincristine, Doxorubicin, Cyclophosphamide, Ifosfamide, and Etoposide. For local treatment, the two options are surgery and radiation therapy (Table 11).

Radiation therapy (RT) serves as an integral component of multidisciplinary management for Ewing sarcoma and plays a key role in achieving durable local control. Because Ewing sarcoma is a radiosensitive malignancy, RT becomes particularly important when the surgical team cannot achieve complete resection or when surgery would result in significant functional morbidity [86]. Careful integration of RT with systemic chemotherapy and surgery helps achieve optimal outcomes.

RT may be delivered as definitive treatment, postoperative adjuvant therapy, or preoperative therapy in selected cases. Definitive RT is indicated for unresectable tumors, including those arising in the pelvis, spine, skull base, or paraspinal regions. Standard definitive doses range from 54 to 60 Gy in conventional fractionation, targeting the pre-chemotherapy tumor volume with appropriate margins while respecting usual tissue constraints [87]. Adjuvant RT is recommended for patients with positive or close surgical margins, inadequate histologic response to induction chemotherapy, or tumor spillage during surgery, typically using doses of 45–54 Gy [86].

Accurate target delineation is critical in Ewing sarcoma. Magnetic resonance imaging is essential for defining tumor extent, while computed tomography is required for treatment planning. In addition, modern RT techniques, such as intensity-modulated radiation therapy (IMRT), improve conformality and reduce dose to adjacent organs at risk, particularly in pediatric and adolescent patients [88]. Furthermore, in specific situations, modalities such as proton beam therapy can offer additional normal tissue sparing. Overall, modern-day RT can significantly reduce long-term toxicity, including growth disturbances, cardiopulmonary injury, and secondary malignancies [89].

RT also has a well-established role in metastatic disease. For example, whole-lung irradiation (WLI) is commonly employed in patients with pulmonary metastases who respond to chemotherapy, typically to doses of 12–15 Gy (typically delivered as 1.5 Gy per fraction daily).

Bilateral lungs are irradiated with opposed fields and careful planning (CT-based) to minimize normal tissue dose. The fraction size of ~1.5 Gy helps reduce late lung toxicity compared with larger per-fraction doses. WLI is generally used in patients with exclusive pulmonary metastases at diagnosis or certain relapse settings who have responded well to chemotherapy. Pulmonary toxicities can be dose- and fraction-dependent, and combining WLI with high-dose chemotherapy (especially busulfan/melphalan) may increase risk, so timing and cumulative dose matter. WLI has been associated with improved pulmonary control and survival in selected patients [87].

RT, in appropriate patients, also provides effective palliation for painful bone metastases or spinal cord compression.

Given the young age of most patients with Ewing sarcoma, it is important to note that long-term surveillance for late effects is essential. Advances in imaging, planning, and delivery techniques continue to refine the therapeutic ratio of RT, reinforcing its central role in contemporary radiation oncology practice for Ewing sarcoma [88, 89].

3 Giant Cell Tumor of Bone

Giant cell tumor of bone is a benign but locally aggressive primary bone tumor that typically occurs in skeletally mature young adults (20–40 years) and characteristically involves the epiphysis of long bones, extending up to the subchondral bone. The disease, albeit generally benign, is locally aggressive. Common sites of disease include the distal femur, proximal tibia, and distal radius (Fig. 11).

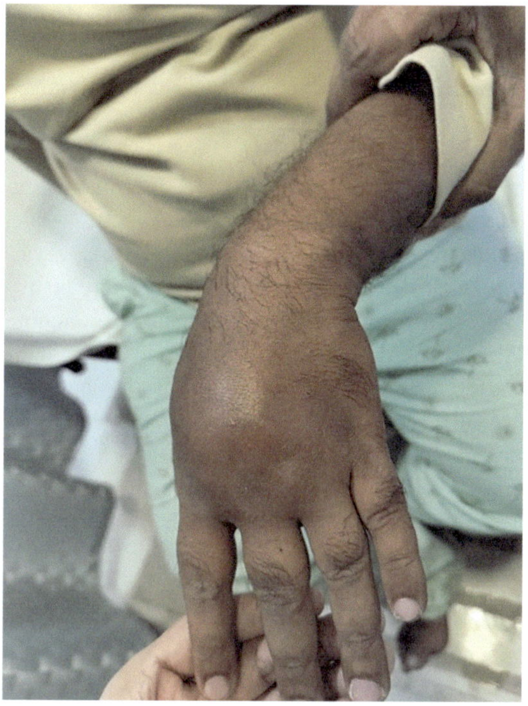

Fig. 11 Giant cell tumor of the metacarpal bone of the hand. (Courtesy: Dr Nehal Khanna, Department of Radiation Oncology, Tata Memorial Hospital, Parel, Mumbai, India)

Goals of treatment include achieving local tumor control, preserving maximum joint function, preventing local recurrence, and managing metastatic or aggressive disease (rare).

X-ray imaging typically suggests an eccentric, lytic lesion in the epiphysis/metaphysis. MRI is commonly done to see soft-tissue extension and articular involvement. A CT chest is sometimes done to rule out lung metastasis (rare but possible). The establishment of a diagnosis involves doing a biopsy (core or open biopsy) before definitive surgery.

The Campanacci grading system for Giant Cell Tumors (GCTs) categorizes them into three radiographic grades (I, II, III) reflecting increasing aggressiveness: Grade I (Latent) has well-defined borders with an intact cortex; Grade II (Active) shows a relatively defined margin with a thinned cortex and moderate expansion; and Grade III (Aggressive) has indistinct borders and cortical destruction, sometimes extending into soft tissues, guiding treatment from curettage (I, II) to wider resection (III).

Surgical management is the mainstay of treatment. An extended intralesional curettage is most commonly done. For Campanacci grade I and II, a thorough curettage is done. Local adjuvants to reduce recurrence include phenol, hydrogen peroxide, and liquid nitrogen (cryotherapy). The filling of the defect is done by bone graft or bone cement (PMMA).

Medical (adjuvant/neoadjuvant) therapy, such as denosumab (RANKL inhibitor), is used in occasional situations such as unresectable tumors and recurrent GCT or tumors where surgery would cause significant morbidity.

While surgery remains the primary treatment modality, radiation therapy (RT) plays a vital role in selected clinical scenarios where complete surgical excision is not feasible or would result in unacceptable morbidity. GCTB is considered radiosensitive, and durable local control can be achieved with appropriately delivered RT [90].

The principal indication for RT in GCTB is unresectable disease, particularly tumors involving the axial skeleton such as the sacrum, spine, skull base, or pelvis. In these locations, wide surgical resection may be associated with severe neurologic deficits, instability, or loss of organ function. Thus, definitive RT provides a noninvasive alternative capable of achieving long-term local control, with reported control rates ranging from 60% to 85% [90]. Typical doses range from 45 to 55 Gy in conventional fractionation, with higher doses reserved for bulky or recurrent disease.

RT may also be considered in the postoperative setting when residual disease is present or when surgical margins are positive, and re-excision is not possible. Additionally, RT has been used as salvage therapy for locally recurrent tumors after multiple surgical interventions. Careful target volume delineation using modern imaging is essential to encompass the gross tumor and areas at risk while minimizing dose to adjacent normal tissues [91].

Historically, concerns about radiation-induced malignant transformation have limited the use of RT in GCTB. Earlier series reported an increased risk of secondary sarcoma, primarily attributed to the use of orthovoltage techniques. With contemporary megavoltage RT, intensity-modulated radiation therapy (IMRT), and image guidance, the risk appears substantially lower, improving the therapeutic ratio [90, 91].

Metastasis of this disease generally involves the lungs. Management of lung metastasis can be done by surgery (metastasectomy) or the use of denosumab.

4 Soft Tissue Sarcoma

4.1 Introduction

Soft tissue sarcomas (STS) are a heterogeneous group of malignant tumors arising from mesenchymal tissues (such as muscle, fat, fibrous tissue, blood vessels, or peripheral nerves) in the adult population. Although they constitute only about 1% of adult malignancies, their diversity of histologic subtypes, anatomical locations, and clinical behavior make them a major challenge in oncology [85, 92–96].

4.2 Epidemiology and Classification

STS in adults represent an uncommon tumor group, with hundreds of histologic subtypes recognized (e.g., liposarcoma, leiomyosarcoma, synovial sarcoma, malignant peripheral nerve sheath tumor, etc.) [85, 92]. Their incidence ranges roughly around 5–7 per 100,000 persons per year in many developed countries [85]. Because of their rarity and heterogeneity, clinical trial data are limited compared to more common solid tumors.

The World Health Organization (WHO) classification of soft-tissue tumors divides them by lineage, grade, and site [92]. Important considerations in classification include tumor differentiation, mitotic rate, and necrosis (which influence grade), as well as site of origin (extremity, trunk, retroperitoneum, head and neck, visceral). For staging and prognostic purposes, the French Fédération Nationale des Centres de Lutte Contre le Cancer (FNCLCC) grading system is often used [93].

4.3 Pathology and Biological Features

Microscopically, STS display a wide variety of morphologies, depending on the subtype. Key pathological features that influence prognosis include: tumor grade (low grade vs high grade), mitotic count, extent of necrosis, resection margin status, depth (superficial vs deep), size, and anatomical site [93, 95].

From a biological standpoint, many STS subtypes harbor specific molecular alterations (for instance, translocations in synovial sarcoma, amplification of MDM2 in dedifferentiated liposarcoma, etc.) [94]. These molecular insights are increasingly important, both for diagnosis and for potential targeted therapies, although the vast majority of STS still rely primarily on conventional histology and immunohistochemistry [95, 96].

4.4 Clinical Presentation and Diagnostic Work-Up

4.4.1 Presentation

STS often present as a painless mass, commonly in the extremities or trunk. Because they can grow slowly, many patients may delay presentation or may be misdiagnosed as benign lesions. Features that should raise suspicion for a sarcoma include: size >5 cm, deep-to-fascia location, increasing size, pain or neurological symptoms (if adjacent to nerves), or working around major vessels. Retroperitoneal tumors may present late, often as vague abdominal discomfort, a palpable mass or mass effect symptoms.

4.4.2 Diagnostic Evaluation

Key components of the diagnostic work-up include:

Detailed history and physical examination: assessing size, depth, site, growth rate, relation to surrounding structures (nerves, vessels, organs, bone).

Imaging of the primary site: For extremity/trunk lesions, magnetic resonance imaging (MRI) is preferred to delineate tumor margins and involvement of neurovascular structures (Fig. 12). For retroperitoneal or intra-abdominal lesions, contrast-enhanced CT is often used.

Chest imaging (usually CT) is usually done to rule out pulmonary metastases (lungs being the commonest site of distant spread).

Other imaging (abdominal/pelvic CT or PET/CT) may be indicated depending on histology and suspicion for metastasis. Whenever there is high clinical suspicion of disease spread to chest or abdomen, more so in a high-grade sarcoma, the PET-CT scan before deciding the primary tumor management by surgery and/or RT is required (Fig. 13).

Biopsy: Core needle biopsy (preferably image-guided) is recommended before definitive surgery, since preoperative planning (extent of surgery, need for radiation, chemotherapy) depends on tumor subtype, grade, and size. Incisional biopsy should be done with caution, in a way that allows the biopsy tract to be excised during the definitive surgery.

Pathologic review: Grading (e.g., FNCLCC), assessment of margins, subtype, and if needed molecular testing for particular translocations or amplifications.

4.4.3 Staging and Prognostic Factors

The staging of STS is based on tumor size (T), nodal involvement (N), metastasis (M), and grade (G). The American Joint Committee on Cancer (AJCC) 8th edition has staging group-

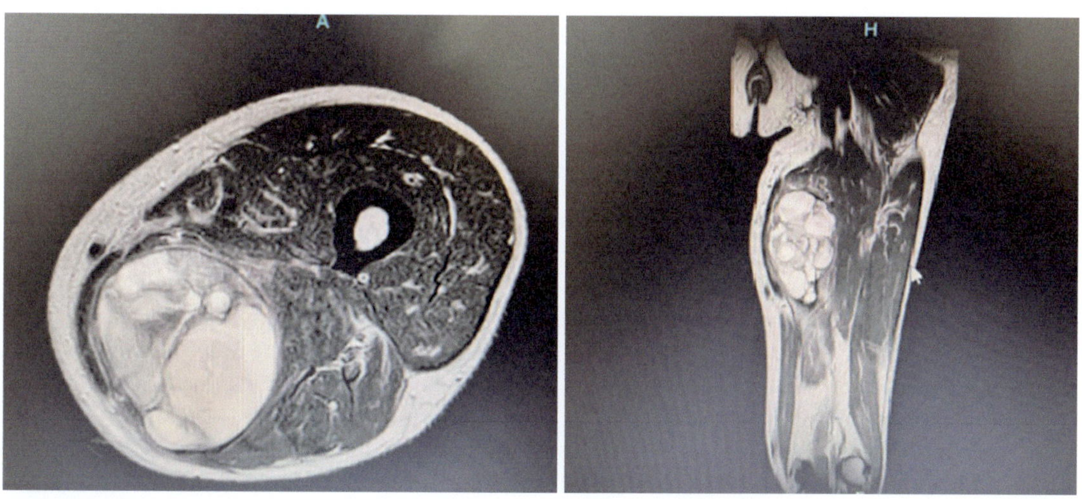

Fig. 12 MRI scan of soft tissue tumor in medial aspect of left thigh. (Courtesy Bagchi Sri Shankara Cancer Centre & Research Institute, Bhubaneswar)

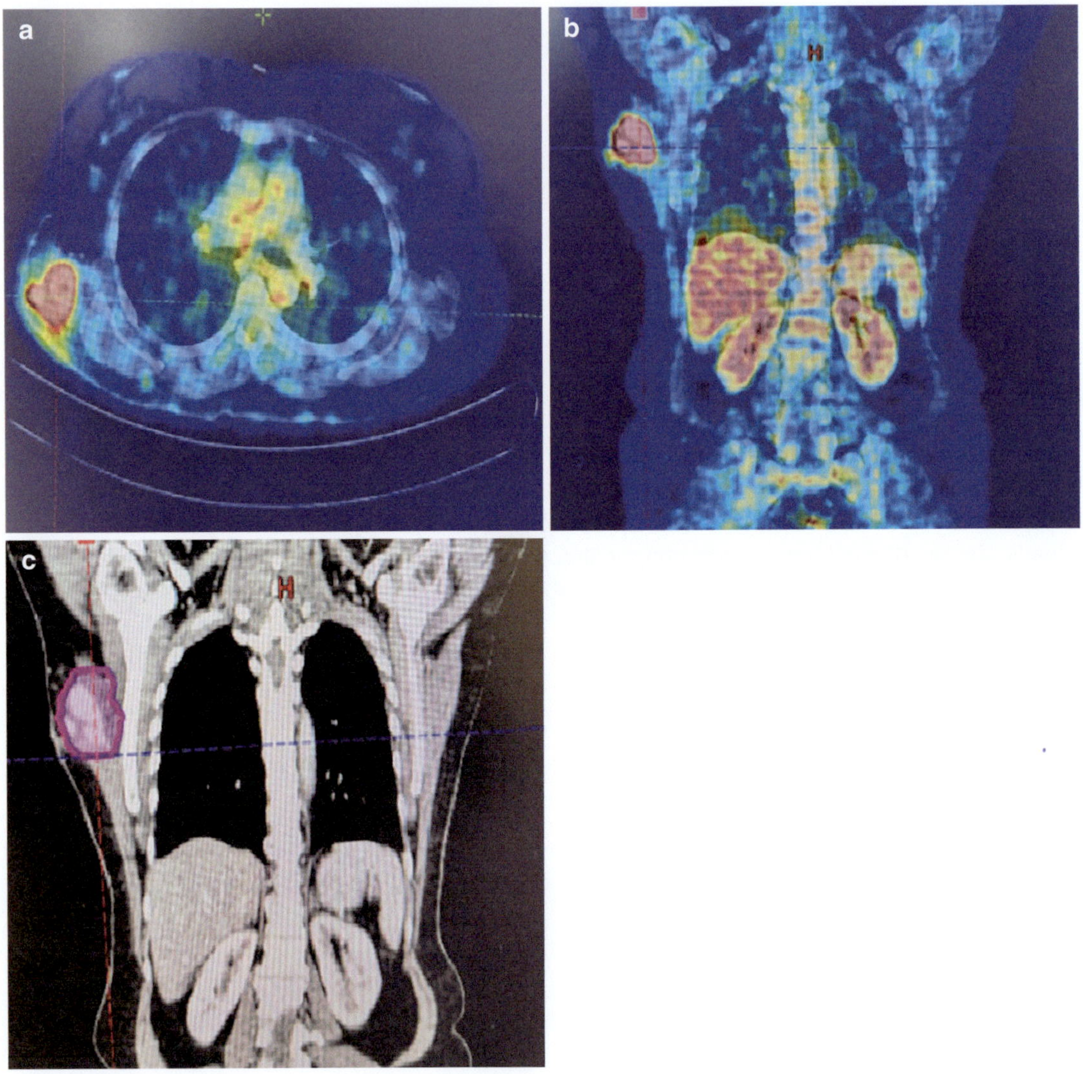

Fig. 13 PET-CT scan imaging of tumor and whole body in a biopsy-proven high-grade liposarcoma of right scapula region. (**a**) PET of the primary (right scapula). (**b**) PET-whole body. (**c**) Radiotherapy planning CT scan -tumor is delineated. (Courtesy Bagchi Sri Shankara Cancer Centre & Research Institute, Bhubaneswar)

ings specific to STS of the trunk, extremities, and retroperitoneum (Table 12, modified from AJCC staging manual) [97].

Important prognostic factors include:

(a) Tumor size: Larger tumors have worse outcomes.
(b) Depth (superficial vs deep): Tumors deep to fascia fare worse.
(c) Histologic grade: High-grade tumors (G2/G3) have higher risk of metastasis and recurrence.
(d) Resection margin status: Positive margins are associated with higher local recurrence.
(e) Primary site: Retroperitoneal tumors are more challenging and have worse outcomes compared to extremity lesions.
(f) Histologic subtype: Some subtypes (e.g., myxoid liposarcoma) may have specific behavior or sensitivity to therapy.
(g) Referral to a sarcoma-specialist center: Studies have shown that outcomes (especially local control) are improved when patients are

Table 12 TNM staging for STS of (Extremity/Trunk/Head/Neck)

Stage group	T (Tumor size)	N (Regional lymph nodes)	M (Distant metastasis)	FNCLCC grade	Stage description
Stage IA	T1 (≤5 cm)	N0	M0	G1–G2 (low grade)	Small, low-grade localized tumor
Stage IB	T2 (>5 cm)	N0	M0	G1–G2 (low grade)	Large, low-grade localized tumor
Stage IIA	T1 (≤5 cm)	N0	M0	G3 (high grade)	Small, high-grade localized tumor
Stage IIB	T2 (>5 cm ≤10 cm)	N0	M0	G3 (high grade)	Medium, high-grade localized tumor
Stage IIIA	T3 (>10 cm ≤15 cm)	N0	M0	G3 (high grade)	Large, high-grade localized tumor
Stage IIIB	T4 (>15 cm)	N0	M0	G3 (high grade)	Very large, high-grade localized tumor
Stage IIIC	Any T	N1	M0	Any G	Regional lymph node involvement
Stage IV	Any T	Any N	M1	Any G	Distant metastasis present

Modified from Ref. [24, 97]
Note: *Grade (FNCLCC System)*:
G1: Low grade (score 2–3)
G2: Intermediate grade (score 4–5)
G3: High grade (score 6–8)

managed at high-volume sarcoma centers rather than low-volume general hospitals.

4.5 Management Strategies

The management of adult STS is multidisciplinary and depends on the tumor size, grade, site, potential for resection, and metastasis status. The mainstays are surgery and radiation therapy, with systemic therapy used in selected cases. The approach must be individualized and often involves a sarcoma team (surgical oncologist/orthopedic oncologist, radiation oncologist, medical oncologist, pathologist, radiologist, and supportive care specialist).

4.6 Localized Disease (Resectable)

4.6.1 Surgery

Surgical resection remains the cornerstone of treatment for localized adult STS [98]. The goal is to achieve a complete (R0) resection with negative microscopic margins, while preserving function whenever possible. For extremity-based sarcomas, limb-sparing surgery is the standard, facilitated by adjuvant radiation when needed. In amputations or radical resections, the functional cost is high; in many cases, combining surgery plus radiation allows limb preservation without compromising oncologic outcomes. For retroperitoneal tumors, wide margins are harder to achieve; extended resections (including adjacent organs) may improve local control but must be balanced against increased morbidity.

4.6.2 Radiation Therapy

Radiation Therapy in Soft Tissue Sarcomas

Radiation therapy (RT) is a key component in the multidisciplinary management of *soft tissue sarcomas (STS)*, aimed primarily at improving local control following surgery. Surgery remains the cornerstone of treatment, but because STS often exhibit microscopic extension beyond gross tumor margins, RT helps eradicate residual disease and reduce local recurrence risk.

Rationale

The rationale for RT in STS arises from its ability to eliminate microscopic residual disease in tissues that have been surgically manipulated. Early randomized trials from the U.S. National Cancer Institute (NCI) and Memorial Sloan Kettering Cancer Center (MSKCC) demonstrated better local control with adjuvant RT compared to surgery alone [99, 100].

The NCI trial reported 5-year local control of 96% with limb-sparing surgery plus RT versus 77% with surgery alone [99]. The MSKCC brachytherapy study confirmed improved control in high-grade tumors (89% vs 66%) [100]. Both these studies conducted in 1990s set the benchmark for radiotherapy practice in STS.

These findings established RT as a vital complement to conservative surgery for extremity sarcomas.

RT can be given before surgery (neoadjuvant) or after (adjuvant), with the choice based on tumor size, location, resectability, and patient factors.

Indications of Radiotherapy

RT is indicated for patients with:

- High-grade histology
- Deep-seated or large (>5 cm) tumors
- Close or positive margins
- Anatomically constrained sites (e.g., head & neck, retroperitoneum) [98, 101]

All cases should be discussed at a specialized sarcoma tumor board, ideally at a high-volume center, to optimize sequencing and technique [98].

Preoperative Radiation Therapy

Preoperative RT is commonly delivered to a total dose of *50 Gy in 25 fractions* (2 Gy per fraction) over 5 weeks. The target volume includes the tumor with an appropriate margin to account for microscopic spread and setup uncertainties. The advantages of preoperative RT include smaller treatment fields, reduced total dose, and better sparing of normal tissues. It can also facilitate surgical resection by reducing tumor bulk. However, it carries a higher risk of acute wound-healing complications, particularly in lower extremity sarcomas.

Postoperative Radiation Therapy

Postoperative RT is generally administered when surgical margins are close or positive or when preoperative RT was not given. The typical regimen is *60–66 Gy*, delivered in *1.8–2 Gy fractions*, with an initial 50 Gy to a larger field followed by a boost to the tumor bed. Postoperative RT treats a larger volume due to the need to encompass surgical manipulation areas, which may increase the risk of late toxicities such as fibrosis, edema, and joint stiffness.

Modern Techniques and Outcomes

Advanced technologies like IMRT (intensity modulated radiotherapy) and IGRT (image guided radiotherapy) enable precise dose delivery, minimizing exposure to organs at risk. Brachytherapy, delivering 45–50 Gy via implanted catheters, is an option for selected extremity sarcomas. Overall, RT—combined with diligent surgery—achieves local control rates exceeding 85% for extremity STS while preserving limb function and quality of life.

Sequencing of Radiotherapy

RT may be delivered pre-operatively or post-operatively, with distinct advantages and limitations (Table 2). Multidisciplinary consensus and individualized planning are crucial [101–103]. The decision of timing is influenced by tumor size, site, and expected surgical morbidity. Current guidelines favor preoperative RT for most extremity and truncal STS because of smaller fields, better functional outcomes, and reduced late toxicity, accepting the higher acute wound risk [98, 102, 103].

The Combined-Modality Approach

For high-risk tumors (large size, high grade, deep location, close margins), the combination of surgery + RT is widely accepted to improve local control. Some series show that use of RT in such cases improves disease-specific survival. While deciding the combined modality, the comparison between pre-operative and post-operative RT approach from the published studies is valuable (Table 13).

Table 13 Comparison of pre-operative versus post-operative radiotherapy for soft tissue sarcoma

Feature	Pre-operative RT	Post-operative RT	References
Typical dose/ fractionation	50 Gy/25 fx (1.8–2 Gy per fx)	60–66 Gy/30–33 fx (often 50 Gy + 10–16 Gy boost)	[101, 103]
Target volume	Smaller, conforms to visible tumor	Larger, includes resection bed	[101, 103]
Wound complications	30–35% (esp. lower limb)	15–20%	[101, 102]
Late toxicities	Lower (fibrosis, stiffness, edema)	Higher (fibrosis, fracture risk)	[101, 103]
Functional outcome	Better limb function	Reduced flexibility	[101, 103]
Oncologic control	Equivalent local control	Equivalent local control, encompass larger high-dose volume	[101, 103]
Pathologic assessment	Margins unknown pre-RT	Pathology known	[101, 103]
Technical complexity	Requires MRI fusion and IGRT	Simpler volume definition	[101, 103]
Preferred use	Standard for extremity/ truncal STS	For unexpected high-risk pathology	[101, 103]

Table 14 Dose and fractionation for soft tissue sarcoma

Setting	Typical dose/fractionation	Total DOSE	Key reference
Pre-op	2 Gy × 25 fx	50 Gy	O'Sullivan et al. [105]
Post-op (R0)	1.8 Gy × 33 fx	60 Gy	Haas et al. [102]
Post-op (R1)	1.8 Gy × 36 fx	64–66 Gy	DeLaney et al. [104]
Brachytherapy boost	HDR 30–40 Gy (BID)	–	Campbell et al. [106]

4.7 Target Volume Delineation

4.7.1 Preoperative Volumes (Fig. 14)

- *Gross Tumor Volume (GTV)*: Defined by contrast-enhanced MRI fused with planning CT [102].
- *Clinical Target Volume (CTV)*: GTV + 4 cm longitudinally and 1.5 cm radially, modified along anatomic barriers [102, 104].
- *Planning Target Volume (PTV)*: CTV + 0.5–1.0 cm margin for setup uncertainties [102].

4.7.2 Postoperative Volumes

The postoperative target should encompass the entire operative bed and regions of surgical manipulation, with a 1–2 cm longitudinal and 1.5 cm radial margin. It is desirable to assess the pre-surgical imaging dimensions while deciding for the CTV volume. Surgical scars and drain sites may be included in a wider sub-clinical elective volume when appropriate [102, 104].

Dose and fractionation for STS is represented in Table 14.

Post-operative RT is more commonly the multi-disciplinary management approach in high-volume cancer centers (Figs. 15 and 16).

Modern radiotherapy planning for the 3-D dose plan evaluation and on-board imaging (OBI) combined together for the RT delivery can considerably reduce the tissue and organ doses providing improved disease control (Fig. 16).

4.7.3 Normal-Tissue Constraints

Careful adherence to constraints is crucial [98–102, 105]:

- *Bone*: V40 < 64%, V50 < 100% circumference for load-bearing bones.
- *Joint*: V50 ≤ 50%; V45 < 25–50%.
- *Skin*: Spare ≥2 cm circumferential strip; avoid bolus unless indicated.
- *Femoral head*: V50 < 5%.

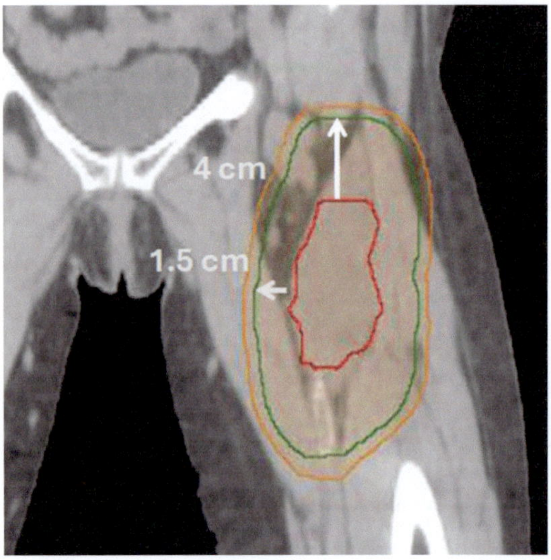

Fig. 14 CT-based preoperative radiotherapy planning demonstrating target volume delineation with gross tumor volume (GTV) in red, clinical target volume (CTV) in green, and planning target volume (PTV) in orange

Fracture risk is ~3%, predominantly in elderly females or after periosteal stripping [103].

4.7.4 Hypofractionation in Soft Tissue Sarcoma

Modern prospective studies have explored shorter hypo-fractionated regimens (Table 15) [107–110]:

Moderate hypofractionation (e.g., 42.75 Gy/15 fractions, @ 2.85 Gy per daily fraction) appears safe at experienced centers [110].

Ultra-hypofractionation (5 × 8 Gy) yields excellent control but would increase late morbidity and is best reserved for clinical trials [107–110].

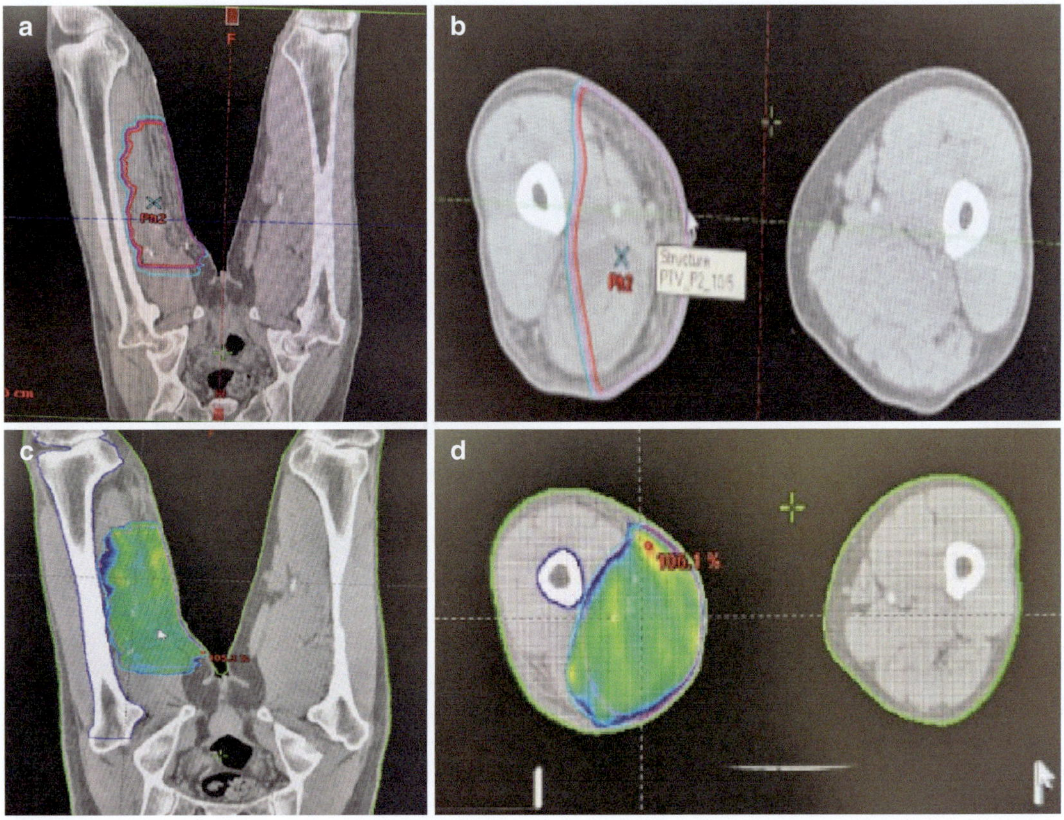

Fig. 15 Postoperative tumor volume contouring and the dose plan (95%) in extremity left thigh sarcoma. (**a**) Contouring (Red-CTV, sagittal) (**b**) Contouring (Red-CTV, axial). (**c**) Dose plan (Blue-95%, sagittal). (**d**) Dose plan (Blue-95%, axial)

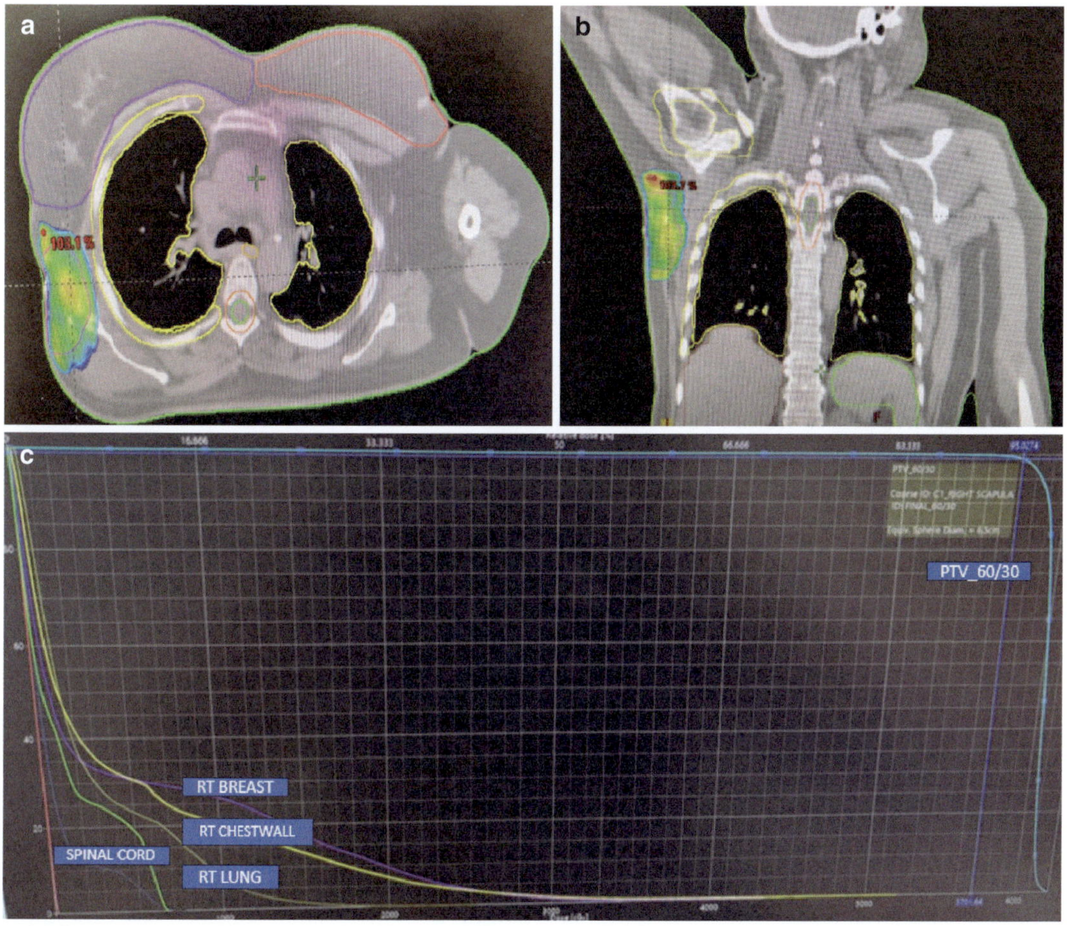

Fig. 16 Radiation therapy dose plan for proven high-grade liposarcoma of right scapula region. (**a**) Dose plan for the tumor site (95%). (**b**) Assessment of dose to surrounding OAR. (**c**) Dose-Volume Histogram (DVH) to assess dose to critical structures

Table 15 Hypo-fractionated RT trials on soft tissue sarcoma

Study	Regimen	Local control	Major wound complication
Kosela-Paterczyk et al., 2021 [107]	5 × 5 Gy	81% (5 yr)	24%
Kalbasi et al., 2020 [108]	5 × 6 Gy	94%	32%
Leite et al., 2021 [109]	5 X 8	100%	28% (16% amputation)
Guadagnolo et al., 2022 (HYPORT-STS) [110]	15 × 2.85 Gy	93% (4 yr)	31%

4.8 Toxicities

Acute

- Wound complications (25–35%), especially in distal extremities [101, 102]
- Seroma, infection, transient edema

Late

- Fibrosis (5–30%), lymphedema (3–15%), joint stiffness (10–20%), and fractures (2–4%) [101–103]

The 2025 ASTRO clinical practice guideline has emphasized limb-sparing field design and bone-dose optimization to mitigate these events [98].

4.8.1 Brachytherapy

The main rationale for using brachytherapy in STS lies in its ability to deliver a concentrated dose to the area most at risk for local recurrence—the surgical bed—while minimizing exposure to nearby healthy tissue. Studies have shown that brachytherapy can improve local control rates, particularly in high-grade or margin-positive sarcomas. Clinical series have demonstrated five-year local control rates ranging from 70% to 90%, comparable or superior to external beam radiotherapy (EBRT) in certain subsets [106, 111].

4.8.2 Indications

Brachytherapy is primarily indicated as an adjuvant therapy following surgical resection of soft tissue sarcomas, especially in cases with close or positive margins or when re-excision is not feasible. It is also used as a boost technique following EBRT or as a stand-alone modality in selected cases where the tumor is small, superficial, or anatomically suited for implantation. It is particularly advantageous in extremity sarcomas where function preservation is a priority.

4.8.3 Techniques

During surgery, flexible catheters or tubes are implanted into the tumor bed, often with radiopaque clips marking resection margins. Postoperative imaging assists in dosimetry and treatment planning. Both low-dose-rate (LDR) and high-dose-rate (HDR) brachytherapy techniques are used, with HDR offering logistical convenience and better dose control. The prescribed dose typically ranges between 18 and 32 Gy for HDR therapy, adjusted according to margin status and whether EBRT is also given. Brachytherapy can be done intr-operatively (IORT) or surface brachytherapy can be used for superficial tumors (Fig. 17). Figures 18 and 19 show technique of brachytherapy in flowchart and pictorial form, respectively.

4.8.4 Advantages

Brachytherapy offers several key benefits in the management of soft tissue sarcomas [111]. It enables high-dose delivery to the target while sparing surrounding tissues such as skin, bone, and neurovascular structures. The treatment duration is shorter compared with EBRT, reducing the overall burden on patients. It also supports limb-sparing surgery, preserving function and appearance. In pediatric cases, it helps minimize long-term radiation effects, such as growth disturbance and tissue fibrosis.

4.8.5 Limitations and Complications

Despite its advantages, brachytherapy has limitations. It requires specialized expertise and close coordination between surgical and radiation oncology teams. Wound complications are a notable concern, especially if catheters are placed in poorly vascularized or healing tissues. Other potential adverse effects include fibrosis, neuropathy, and bone fractures. Moreover, brachytherapy is less suitable for large or deep-seated tumors where uniform dose distribution is difficult to achieve.

4.8.6 Clinical Outcomes

Multiple retrospective studies have confirmed that brachytherapy provides excellent local control and survival rates comparable to EBRT, with the added benefit of improved functional outcomes. When combined with wide local excision, local control rates exceed 80–90% in many series [111]. Some data also suggest lower recurrence rates and reduced amputation rates in extremity sarcomas. However, randomized trials are limited, and ongoing research aims to refine patient selection and optimal dose protocols.

Brachytherapy remains an effective and valuable component in the multidisciplinary management of soft tissue sarcoma. When properly selected and performed at experienced centers, it enhances local control, preserves organ function, and shortens treatment time. Its success depends on careful patient selection, meticulous surgical technique, and precise radiotherapy planning within a coordinated multidisciplinary framework.

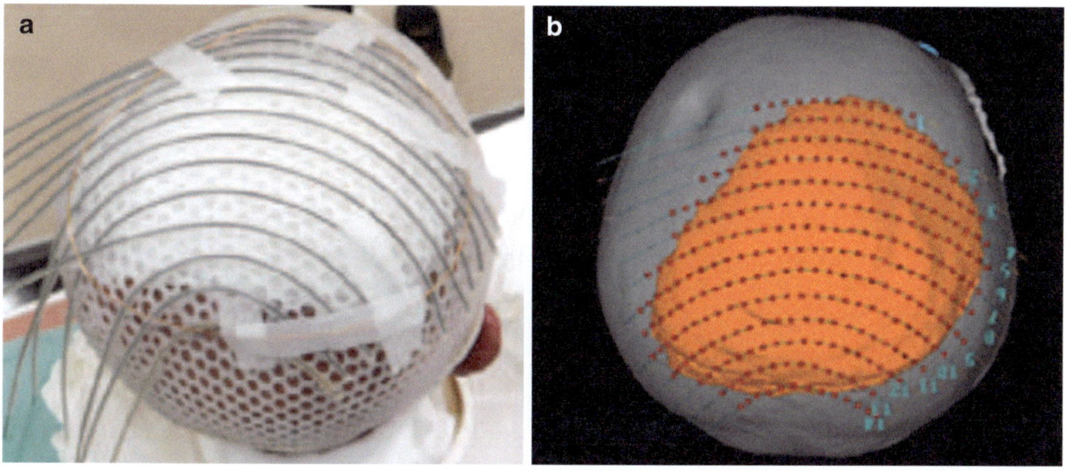

Fig. 17 Patient-specific surface mold for high-dose-rate brachytherapy in scalp angiosarcoma showing clinical applicator setup (**a**) and corresponding 3D treatment planning reconstruction (**b**)

Gross total resection (R0/R1) of the tumor.

↓

Measure the tumor bed

↓

Determine optimal catheter alignment

↓

Mark insertion ‡ exit (double button) positions on the skin surface ≥ 1 cm from the incision.

↓

Hollow needle guide is inserted and pushed out through the exit with the help of towel clips

↓

Tubing inserted into hollow needle guide and pushed through

↓

Needle is withdrawn leaving tubing intact Tubing secured on each end with buttons

↓

This is the BASIC / PULLING TECHNIQUE for Interstitial Brachytherapy

Catheters are inserted to a depth of approximately 5 mm into the tumor bed to avoid under dosage of the tumor bed.

Fig. 18 Flowchart illustrating technique of catheter placement in Interstitial Brachytherapy

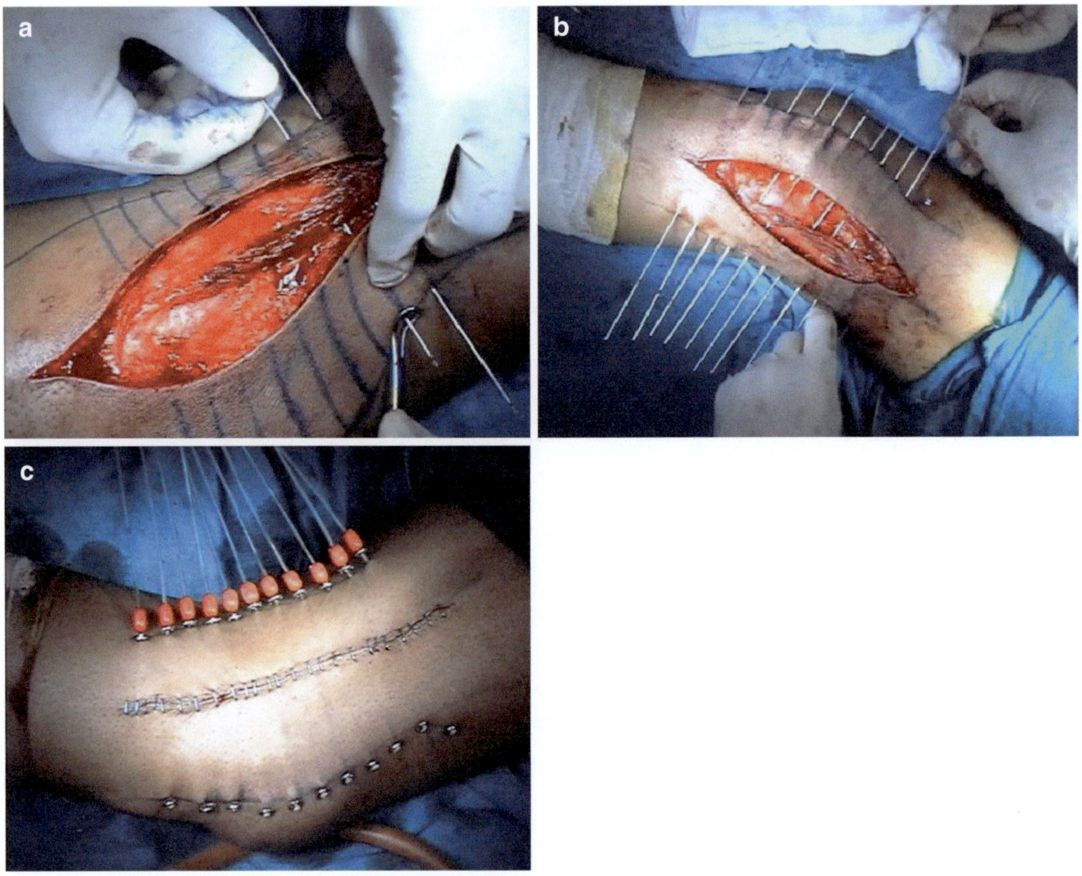

Fig. 19 Pictorial display of intra-operative tumor bed catheter placement for interstitial brachytherapy in soft tissue sarcoma. (**a**) Tumor bed marking on skin surface to decide catheter placement by radiation oncologist. (**b**) Tumor bed is covered adequately by intra-operative placement of catheters by radiation oncologist. (**c**) Tumor bed is sutured, and catheters are properly anchored by buttons at both ends for interstitial HDR brachytherapy. (Photos courtesy Tata Memorial Centre, Mumbai)

4.8.7 Systemic Therapy in Localized Disease

The use of adjuvant or neoadjuvant chemotherapy in STS has been explored in numerous trials, but the benefit has historically been modest and not uniform across subtypes. Meta-analyses suggest a small improvement in recurrence-free survival (RFS) but shows inconsistent overall survival (OS) benefit [112].

Some contemporary trials are exploring histology-tailored neoadjuvant chemotherapy [113].

Neoadjuvant chemotherapy (with or without RT) may be considered for large, high-grade tumors in selected patients (e.g., deep extremity STS >10 cm) to improve resectability and perhaps treat micro-metastases early. The decision requires multidisciplinary discussion—balancing toxicity, patient fitness, and expected benefit [114].

Systemic therapies have been explored in management of unresectable locally advanced or metastatic disease.

When STS are unresectable (locally advanced) or metastatic, the treatment shifts toward systemic therapy and palliative local therapies.

4.8.8 Surgery for Metastases

In selected patients with limited metastatic disease (e.g., lung only), surgical metastasectomy may provide survival benefit. Some retrospective studies suggest improved outcomes when metastases are resected.

4.8.9 Systemic Chemotherapy

The standard first-line systemic therapy for advanced/metastatic STS in adults has included anthracycline-based regimens, typically doxorubicin (with or without ifosfamide). However, the overall response rates are modest (generally ~20–30%) and median survival remains limited [115].

Beyond first line, a variety of agents have demonstrated activity in subtype-specific settings:

The multi-kinase inhibitor Pazopanib demonstrated benefit in non-adipocytic STS in the PALETTE trial [116]. Agents such as Trabectedin and Eribulin have shown benefit in liposarcomas and leiomyosarcomas. Newer systemic strategies and targeted therapies are emerging.

4.8.10 Radiation or Other Local Therapies

For locally advanced cases, RT may be used for palliation of symptoms (pain, bleeding, mass effect). In addition, ablative therapies such as radiofrequency ablation or stereotactic RT may be considered in selected metastases (e.g., lung, liver) within a multidisciplinary context.

4.9 Histology-Specific Considerations

Although this chapter is focused on adult STS broadly, it is important to recognize that specific histologic subtypes may have different behavior and require different therapeutic approaches.

For example, myxoid liposarcoma is unusually radiosensitive and has a propensity to fat-based metastases; this may influence preoperative RT decisions.

Well-differentiated/dedifferentiated liposarcoma of the retroperitoneum often harbors MDM2 gene amplification and require aggressive surgery given the high risk of local recurrence despite low metastatic potential in the well-differentiated component.

Synovial sarcoma (often in younger adults) has a characteristic translocation (SYT-SSX) and may be more chemo-sensitive than some other STS.

Some vascular sarcomas (e.g., angiosarcoma) or epithelioid sarcoma may spread to lymph nodes, which is uncommon in most STS.

Therefore, histology matters—not simply in diagnosis but also in planning treatment and considering systemic therapy options.

4.10 Emerging Therapies and Future Directions

The traditional approach of surgery + RT ± chemotherapy has limitations in loco-regional control. At the same time, many patients with high-grade STS eventually develop metastases (~40–50%) and the outcomes remain suboptimal. These limitations and natural behavior have become the agenda for research [96, 98].

This has driven the research agenda toward novel therapeutics including immunotherapy, targeted therapy, and novel combinations.

4.10.1 Immuno-Radiotherapy (Immuno-RT)

The *SU2C-SARC032* phase II trial [117] combined pembrolizumab with pre-op RT (50 Gy/25 fx) for stage III Un-differentiated Pleomorphic Sarcoma (UPS) and showed improved 2-year DFS (67% vs 52%) [117].

This trial represents the first positive randomized study supporting peri-operative immuno-RT in high-risk STS.

4.10.2 Molecularly Guided Radiotherapy

Research continues into radio-sensitivity signatures (e.g., myxoid liposarcoma) and radiomics-based adaptive planning to personalize dose [98, 102].

4.10.3 Targeted Therapy

With increasing understanding of molecular drivers in particular STS subtypes, targeted therapies are being explored, for example, MDM2 inhibitors in liposarcoma, CDK4/6 inhibitors, NTRK inhibitors in tumors with NTRK fusions, etc.

4.10.4 Immunotherapy

Although STS are often considered "cold" tumors with low immunogenicity, there is increasing interest in immune checkpoint inhibitors (e.g., anti-PD-1, anti-CTLA-4) either as monotherapy or in combination with chemotherapy, RT or targeted agents. Some histology-specific responses have been observed, though durability is still limited.

4.10.5 Multi-modality and Histology-Tailored Trials

Recent guidelines emphasize the importance of specialist referral and histology- and imaging-tailored management of STS. For example, an international phase III trial (ISG-STS 1001) compared standard neoadjuvant chemotherapy versus histology-tailored neoadjuvant chemotherapy in selected high-risk adult STS and further analyzed the radiologic responses reflecting the trend toward precision medicine [114].

4.10.6 Tumor Microenvironment, Biomarkers, and Novel Modalities

Clinical research and laboratory investigations on tumor microenvironment, biomarkers predictive of response, and new modalities (e.g., cell therapy, tumor vaccines, and radiomics) are underway. For instance, a recent review summarized studies from the 2024 American Society of Clinical Oncology (ASCO) meeting on STS including developments in cellular therapies [118].

4.11 Patterns of Relapse, Surveillance, and Survivorship

Following definitive treatment of localized STS, patients remain at risk of both local recurrence and distant metastases. Surveillance protocols vary by institution and risk category but typically include periodic clinical examination, imaging of the primary site (MRI or CT), and chest imaging (CT) for lung metastases.

The time-course of relapse depends on grade and site—higher-grade tumors and deep lesions tend to relapse earlier. Late relapses (after 5 years) can occur, especially in lower-grade or myxoid subtypes, underscoring the need for long-term follow-up.

Survivorship issues include: functional impairment (especially after surgery/RT in extremities), radiation late toxicities (fibrosis, joint stiffness, and secondary neoplasm), psychosocial aspects, and management of comorbidities. Decision-making about rehabilitation and quality of life is integral.

4.12 Special Site Considerations

4.12.1 Retroperitoneal Soft Tissue Sarcoma

STS arising in the retroperitoneum pose unique challenges due to late presentation (large size at diagnosis), difficulty obtaining wide margins, and high local recurrence rates. Aggressive surgical policies, with expert multidisciplinary care in high-volume centers, are associated with improved local control and survival.

Preoperative or adjuvant RT may play a role in selected patients, although evidence is less robust than for extremity STS. Preoperative RT (45–50.4 Gy) may reduce the risk of local recurrence but has not shown a survival advantage. The STRASS trial found no overall benefit in abdominal recurrence-free survival, although liposarcoma subgroups appeared to benefit [119].

4.12.2 Head and Neck, Thoracic Wall, and Visceral Soft Tissue Sarcomas

These anatomical sites often pose anatomical constraints to wide excision and may require a personalized approach balancing oncologic control and preservation of form and function. Multimodal therapy (surgery, RT, and sometimes chemotherapy) in specialist centers is required.

4.12.3 Rhabdomyosarcoma (RMS)

Rhabdomyosarcoma (RMS) is being covered in the chapter on Paediatric tumours (Vol 2, Chap. 16)

4.13 Key Decision Points and Management Algorithm

A simplified algorithm for adult STS is as follows:

Diagnosis: suspicious soft-tissue mass → imaging → biopsy at specialist center → histology + grade + molecular testing.

Staging: MRI/CT of primary site + chest CT (and additional PET-CT imaging as needed).

Multidisciplinary review: discuss resectability, functional outcome, need for RT/chemotherapy, referral to sarcoma expert center.

Treatment planning:

Low grade, small, superficial tumors: surgery with negative margins may suffice.

High grade, deep, large tumors: surgery + RT (pre- or post- surgery) with consideration of neoadjuvant/adjuvant chemotherapy.

Locally advanced/unresectable or metastatic disease: systemic chemotherapy (anthracycline-based) ± targeted therapies ± surgical metastasectomy ± palliative local therapy.

Follow-up/surveillance: regular clinical review + imaging, rehabilitation, survivorship support.

4.14 Outcomes and Prognosis

Outcomes in STS depend heavily on the previously mentioned prognostic factors. For example, 5-year overall survival (OS) for high-grade extremity STS treated with limb-sparing surgery + RT may range around 60–70% in selected series. For retroperitoneal STS, outcomes are poorer [96].

Local recurrence remains a major issue, particularly in cases with close or positive margins, deep location, and retroperitoneal site. Metastatic relapse (especially to the lung) remains the primary cause of death in STS patients.

4.15 Challenges in Management

Rarity and heterogeneity of STS make large randomized trials difficult and limit the subtype-specific evidence. Achieving wide margins remains a challenge. This is especially in certain anatomical sites (retroperitoneum, head/neck); achieving negative margins without unacceptable functional sacrifice is difficult. The role of adjuvant chemotherapy remains controversial; patient selection is key. Many patients will relapse and treatment options remain limited; improving systemic therapies is a key unmet need. Finally, non-specialist management is associated with worse outcomes; yet many patients may first present at general hospitals.

4.16 Best-Practice Recommendations

Based on current guidelines, all patients with suspected STS should be referred to a multidisciplinary sarcoma center before definitive surgery. Biopsy and staging imaging should be done prior to any surgical excision to allow optimal planning. Surgery with negative margins is the goal; functional preservation should be balanced with oncologic safety. RT should be delivered in high-risk disease (large size, high grade, close margins, deep location). Chemotherapy may be considered in selected high-risk patients or spe-

Percepts Box

1. Primary bone sarcomas are rare tumors, accounting for 0.2% of all cancers. Benign bone tumors and tumor-like lesions are encountered more often.
2. Osteosarcoma, chondrosarcoma, and Ewing sarcoma/primitive neuroectodermal tumor (PNET) are the common bone sarcomas.
3. Risk factors include previous radiation therapy, exposure to chemicals, immunodeficiency, prior injury (scars, burns),

(continued)

chronic tissue irritation, neurofibromatosis, Paget's disease, bone infarcts, and genetic cancer syndromes.
4. X-ray, NCCT, MRI, PET CT are the imaging used in the diagnosis of bone tumors. Bone biopsy is not always needed for a diagnosis, however when done should be done with extreme caution.
5. Staging is given by both the Enneking system and AJCC. AJCC concentrates on four variables to assign stages: tumor size, histologic grade, the presence or absence of regional metastasis, and the presence or absence of distant metastasis. Enneking, however, continues to be an easy and reproducible system for the assessment of malignant bone tumors.
6. Surgery is the mainstay of treatment which can be either limb sparing or limb sacrificing. Reconstruction could be by way of endoprosthesis, allograft, allograft-prosthesis composite, autograft, and arthrodesis.
7. Benign tumors can be treated with a simple excision and treating the cavity with adjuvants like chemical, thermal, or mechanical agents. Reconstructed is done by using bone graft or PMMA (polymethylmethaacrylate) cement or a combination of both (sandwich technique) to provide structural support.
8. Osteosarcomas are treated with adjuvant non methotrexate based chemotherapy regimens. High tumor volume is associated with a poorer outcome.
9. Ewings sarcoma has shown inferior clinical outcomes in cases with high volume disease (>200 mL) and pelvic primaries. Studies have shown a non-inferior outcome with RT in patients with localized disease and good response to NACT.
10. Extracorporeal radiation therapy (ECRT) has been reported as an oncologically safe and effective reconstruction technique for limb salvage in diaphyseal malignant tumors. This includes en-bloc removal of the tumor bearing bone segment, extracorporeal sterilization using single high dose irradiation varying from 50 to 300 Gy, and re-implantation in the skeletal defect.
11. Clinically one should suspect STS in any deep, enlarging, soft-tissue mass >5 cm or beneath fascia.
12. Imaging (CT, MRI, PET-CT), biopsy and staging before surgery are essential.
13. Surgery with negative margins is the cornerstone of curative treatment for sarcomas.
14. Radiation therapy improves local control in high-risk disease.
15. The role of systemic therapy in localized disease remains evolving; in metastatic disease anthracycline-based chemotherapy is standard, with newer agents for subsequent lines.
16. Management should be done in a specialist sarcoma center improves outcomes.
17. Long-term follow-up, rehabilitation, and survivorship care are important due to risk of late relapse and functional/quality-of-life issues.
18. Emerging therapies (targeted, immunotherapy, histotype-tailored) are promising and should be accessed via clinical trials when possible.

cific histologies (e.g., synovial sarcoma, myxoid liposarcoma) preferably within clinical trials. Emerging therapies should be considered within clinical trials whenever possible. Long-term follow-up including physical rehabilitation, psychosocial support, and monitoring for late toxicities is essential.

4.17 Conclusion

Adult soft tissue sarcomas are complex, because diverse tumor types would be requiring multidisciplinary care in specialized centers. Key pillars of management are complete surgical excision (when feasible), combined with radiation therapy in high-risk cases. Systemic therapy plays a role in selected patients and is evolving rapidly with newer targeted and immune-based approaches. Timely referral to expert centers, personalized treatment planning, and long-term follow-up are critical for optimal outcomes.

Ongoing research in molecular pathology, immunotherapy, histology-specific treatments, and radiologic responses holds promise for improving outcomes in this challenging group of malignancies.

Multiple Choice Questions

1. The most common bone tumor is
   (a) Osteoblastoma
   (b) Osteosarcoma
   (c) Chondrosarcoma
   (d) Leiomyosarcoma
2. Risk factors for bone tumors include
   (a) Prior radiation exposure
   (b) Vinyl chloride exposure
   (c) Paget disease
   (d) All of the above
3. All the following tumors are metaphyseal in origin except
   (a) Osteosarcoma
   (b) Chondrosarcoma
   (c) Ewings sarcoma
   (d) Giant Cell Tumor of bone
4. Radiographic features of a malignant tumor include
   (a) Permeative destruction with poorly defined borders
   (b) Cortical destruction
   (c) Periosteal elevation
   (d) All of the above
5. All of the following are latent benign lesions except
   (a) Non ossifying fibroma
   (b) Enchondroma
   (c) Chondromyxoid fibroma
   (d) Osteochondroma
6. Most preferred mode of biopsy for bone tumors
   (a) Core needle biopsy
   (b) Open biopsy
   (c) Excision biopsy
   (d) FNAC
7. When the plane of excision passes through a cuff of normal tissue, according to the Enneking classification, it is termed as
   (a) Wide excision
   (b) Marginal excision
   (c) Radical excision
   (d) Intralesional excision
8. When the plane of excision passes through the reactive zone, according to the Enneking classification, it is termed as
   (a) Wide excision
   (b) Marginal excision
   (c) Radical excision
   (d) Intralesional excision
9. Curative surgical margin according to the Japanese Orthopedic Association is defined as
   (a) Normal cuff of tissue 5 cm or more
   (b) Normal cuff of tissue 1 cm
   (c) Normal cuff of tissue more than 1–4 cm
   (d) Normal cuff of tissue of less than 1 cm
10. All of the following are considered as thick barrier except
    (a) Joint capsule
    (b) Infant periosteum
    (c) Adult periosteum
    (d) Presacral fascia
11. Radiation dose for ECRT is
    (a) 10–100 Gy
    (b) 20–200 Gy
    (c) 30–300 Gy
    (d) 50–300 Gy
12. External rotation in rotationplasty is
    (a) 270°
    (b) 180°
    (c) 90°
    (d) 360°

13. According to Enneking and Durham classification, Type III pelvic resections include removal of
    (a) Iliac wing
    (b) Periacetabular region
    (c) Pubic rami
    (d) Sacrum
14. Types of thermal adjuvants that are used to extend the margins of an intralesional excision include all except
    (a) Electrocautery
    (b) Liquid nitrogen
    (c) Cryoprobes
    (d) Hydrogen peroxide
15. A meta-analysis by Xin S et al. said all of the following are predictors of poor outcome in osteosarcoma except
    (a) Young age
    (b) Large tumor size
    (c) Poor chemotherapy response
    (d) Older age
16. Which of the following dose–fractionation schedules corresponds to the standard *preoperative* radiotherapy regimen for soft tissue sarcoma?
    (a) 60–66 Gy in 30–33 fractions
    (b) 50 Gy in 25 fractions
    (c) 45 Gy in 15 fractions
    (d) 64–66 Gy in 36 fractions.
17. In preoperative RT planning for STS, which of the following definitions is CORRECT for the Clinical Target Volume (CTV)?
    (a) GTV + 1 cm isotropic margin only
    (b) GTV + 4 cm longitudinally and 1.5 cm radially, respecting anatomic barriers
    (c) GTV + 0.5 cm isotropic margin
    (d) GTV + 2 cm longitudinally and 2 cm radially
18. Which of the following late toxicities is most commonly associated with *postoperative* radiotherapy in STS compared with preoperative RT?
    (a) Wound complications
    (b) Fibrosis and joint stiffness
    (c) Infection and seroma formation
    (d) Transient edema
19. Regarding hypofractionated RT for STS, which of the following regimens has demonstrated high local control (~93%) with acceptable toxicity in modern trials (e.g., HYPORT-STS)?
    (a) 5×5 Gy
    (b) 5×8 Gy
    (c) 15×2.85 Gy
    (d) 10×3.5 Gy
20. Which of the following statements regarding normal tissue constraints in extremity STS radiotherapy is TRUE?
    (a) Bone V40 > 70% is acceptable if fraction size <2 Gy.
    (b) Joint V50 $\leq$ 50% and bone V40 < 64% are recommended.
    (c) Skin sparing $\geq$0.5 cm circumferentially is adequate.
    (d) Femoral head constraint is irrelevant in extremity sarcoma RT.

Answer Key

1. (b)
2. (d)
3. (c)
4. (d)
5. (c)
6. (a)
7. (a)
8. (b)
9. (a)
10. (b)
11. (d)
12. (b)
13. (c)
14. (d)
15. (a)
16. (b)
17. (b)
18. (b)
19. (c)
20. (b)

References

1. Hosseini H, Heydari S, Hushmandi K, Daneshi S, Raesi R. Bone tumors: a systematic review of prevalence, risk determinants, and survival patterns. BMC Cancer. 2025;25(1):321. https://doi.org/10.1186/s12885-025-13720-035.
2. Ramaswamy A, Rekhi B, Bakhshi S, Hingmire S, Agarwal M. Indian data on bone and soft tissue sarcomas: a summary of published study results. South Asian J Cancer. 2016;5:138–45.
3. Yeole BB, Jussawalla DJ. Descriptive epidemiology of bone cancer in greater Bombay. Indian J Cancer. 1998;35:101–6.
4. Dinshaw KA, Ganesh B. Hospital based cancer registry. Annual report 2001. Mumbai: Tata Memorial Hospital; 2005. p. 90–1.
5. Rao VS, Pai MR, Rao RC, Adhikary MM. Incidence of primary bone tumours and tumour like lesions in and around Dakshina Kannada district of Karnataka. J Indian Med Assoc. 1996;94:103–4, 121.
6. Jain K, Sunila, Ravishankar R, Mruthyunjaya, Rupakumar CS, Gadiyar HB, et al. Bone tumors in a tertiary care hospital of South India: a review 117 cases. Indian J Med Paediatr Oncol. 2011;32:82–5.
7. Fletcher CD, Bridges AJ, Hogendoorn CW, et al. WHO classification of tumours of soft tissue and bone. 4th ed. Lyon: IARC Press; 2013.
8. The WHO Classification of Tumours Editorial Board. WHO classification of tumours soft tissue and bone tumours. 5th ed. Lyon: IARC Press; 2020.
9. Choi JH, Ro JY. The 2020 WHO classification of tumors of bone: an updated review. AdvAnat Pathol. 2021;28(3):119–38.
10. Volker T, Denecke T, Steffen I, et al. Positron emission tomography for staging of pediatric sarcoma patients: results of a prospective multicenter trial. J Clin Oncol. 2007;25:5435–41.
11. Amit P, Patro DK, Basu D, Elangovan S, Parathasarathy V. Role of dynamic MRI and clinical assessment in predicting histologic response to neoadjuvant chemotherapy in bone sarcomas. Am J Clin Oncol. 2014;37:384–90.
12. Bajpai J, Sharma M, Sreenivas V, Kumar R, Gamnagatti S, Khan SA, et al. VEGF expression as a prognostic marker in osteosarcoma. Pediatr Blood Cancer. 2009;53:1035–9.
13. Bajpai J, Gamanagatti S, Sharma MC, Kumar R, Vishnubhatla S, Khan SA, et al. Noninvasive imaging surrogate of angiogenesis in osteosarcoma. Pediatr Blood Cancer. 2010;54:526–31.
14. Bajpai J, Kumar R, Sreenivas V, Sharma MC, Khan SA, Rastogi S, et al. Prediction of chemotherapy response by PET-CT in osteosarcoma: correlation with histologic necrosis. J Pediatr Hematol Oncol. 2011;33:e271–8.
15. Gupta K, Pawaskar A, Basu S, Rajan MG, Asopa RV, Arora B, et al. Potential role of FDG PET imaging in predicting metastatic potential and assessment of therapeutic response to neoadjuvant chemotherapy in Ewing sarcoma family of tumors. Clin Nucl Med. 2011;36:973–7.
16. Ai T, Padua A, Goerner F, et al. SEMAC-VAT and MSVAT-SPACE sequence strategies for metal artifact reduction in 1.5T magnetic resonance imaging. Invest Radiol. 2012;47(5):267–76.
17. Treglia G, Salsano M, Stefanelli A, Mattoli MV, Giordano A, Bonomo L. Diagnostic accuracy of 18F-FDG-PET and PET/CT in patients with Ewing sarcoma family tumours: a systematic review and a metaanalysis. Skeletal Radiol. 2012;41(3):249–56.
18. Gerth HU, Juergens KU, Dirksen U, Gerss J, Schober O, Franzius C. Significant benefit of multimodal imaging: PET/CT compared with PET alone in staging and follow-up of patients with Ewing tumors. I Nucl Med. 2007;48(12):1932–9.
19. Walter F, Czernin J, Hall T, et al. Is there a need for dedicated bone imaging in addition to 18F-FDG PET/CT imaging in pediatric sarcoma patients? J Pediatr Hematol Oncol. 2012;34(2):131–6.
20. Aryal A, Kumar VS, Shamim SA, Gamanagatti S, Khan SA. What is the comparative ability of 18F-FDG PET/CT, 99mTc-MDP skeletal scintigraphy, and whole-body MRI as a staging investigation to detect skeletal metastases in patients with osteosarcoma and Ewing sarcoma? Clin Orthop Relat Res. 2021;479(8):1768–79.
21. Enneking WF, Spanier SS, Goodman MA. A system for the surgical staging of musculoskeletal sarcoma. Clin Orthop Relat Res. 1980;153:106–20.
22. American Joint Committee on Cancer: Bone. In: Fleming ID, Cooper JS, Henson DE, et al., editors. AJCC Cancer staging manual. Philadelphia: Lippincott Raven; 1997. p. 143–7.
23. American Joint Committee on Cancer: Bone. Chapter 1: Clinical presentation and staging of bone tumors. In: Fleming ID, Cooper JS, Henson DE, et al., editors. AJCC cancer staging manual. New York: Springer; 2002. p. 213–9. © 2014 American Academy of Orthopaedic Surgeons.
24. Amin MB, Edge SB, Greene FL, et al., editors. AJCC Cancer staging manual. 8th ed. New York: Springer; 2017.
25. Yeow KM, Tan CF, Chen JS, Hsueh C. Diagnostic sensitivity of ultrasound-guided needle biopsy in soft tissue masses about superficial bone lesions. Ultrasound Med. 2000;19(12):849–55.
26. Yang YJ, Damron TA. Comparison of needle core biopsy and fine-needle aspiration for diagnostic accuracy in musculoskeletal lesions. Arch Pathol Lab Med. 2004;128(7):759–64.
27. Rougraff BT, Aboulafia A, Biermann JS, Healey J. Biopsy of soft tissue masses: evidence-based medicine for the musculoskeletal tumor society. Clin Orthop Relat Res. 2009;467(11):2783–91.
28. Kilpatrick SE, Cappellari JO, Bos GD, Gold SH, Ward WG. Is fine -needle aspiration biopsy a practical alternative to open biopsy for the primary diagnosis

of sarcoma? Experience with 140 patients. Am J Clin Pathol. 2001;115(1):59–68.
29. Fleshman R, Mayerson J, Wakely PE Jr. Fine-needle aspiration biopsy of high-grade sarcoma: a report of 107 cases. Cancer. 2007;111(6):491–8.
30. Ogilvie CM, Torbert JT, Firlstein JL, Fox EJ, Lackman RD. Clinical utility of percutaneous biopsies of musculoskeletal tumors. Clin Orthop Relat Res. 2006;450:95–100.
31. Hryhorczuk AL, Strouse PJ, Biermann JS. Accuracy of CT-guided percutaneous core needle biopsy for assessment of pediatric musculoskeletal lesions. Pediatr Radiol. 2011;41(7):848–57.
32. Domanski HA, Akerman M, Carlen B, et al. Core needle biopsy performed by the cytopathologist: a technique to complement fine-needle aspiration of soft tissue and bone lesions. Cancer. 2005;105(4):229–39.
33. Phemister DB. Local resection of malignant tumors of bone. AMA Arch Surg. 1951;63:715–7.
34. Japanese Orthopaedic Association Musculoskeletal Tumor Committee. Evaluation method of surgical margin for musculoskeletal sarcoma. In: JOA Musculoskeletal Committee, editor. Evaluation method of surgical margin for musculoskeletal sarcoma. 1st ed. Tokyo: Kanehara; 1989. p. 3–22.
35. Kawaguchi N, Ahmed AR, Matsumoto S, Manabe J, Matsushita Y. The concept of curative margin in surgery for bone and soft tissue sarcoma. Clin Orthop Relat Res. 2004;419:165–72. https://doi.org/10.1097/00003086-200402000-00027.
36. Jeys LM, Kulkarni A, Grimer RJ, Carter SR, Tillman RM, Abudu A. Endoprosthetic reconstruction for the treatment of musculoskeletal tumors of the appendicular skeleton and pelvis. J Bone Joint Surg Am. 2008;90(6):1265–71.
37. Berntha l NM, Schwartz AJ, Oakes DA, Kabo JM, Eckardt JJ. How long do endoprosthetic reconstructions for proximal femoral tumors last? Clin Orthop Relat Res. 2010;468(11):2867–74.
38. Bergin PF, Noveau JB, Jelinek JS, Henshaw RM. Aseptic loosening rates in distal femoral endoprostheses: does stem size matter? Clin Orthop Relat Res. 2012;470(3):743–50.
39. Myers GJ, Abudu AT, Carter SR, Tillman RM, Grimer RJ. Endoprosthetic replacement of the distal femur for bone tumours: long-term results. J Bone Joint Surg Br. 2007;89(4):521–6.
40. Henderson ER, Groundland jS, Pala E, et al. Failure mode classification for tumor endoprostheses: retrospective review of five institutions and a literature review. J Bone Joint Surg Am. 2011;93(5):418–29.
41. Kapoor L, Banjara R, Khan SA, Majeed A. Extensor apparatus reconstruction using prolene mesh tube and medial gastrocnemius flap following proximal tibial endoprosthetic reconstruction. Tech Orthop. 2022;37(1):65–9.
42. Kapoor L, Banjara R, Ragase A, Majeed A, Kumar VS, Khan SA. Outcomes of major musculoskeletal oncological reconstructions using prolene mesh-a retrospective analysis from a tertiary referral centre. J Clin Orthop Trauma. 2021;16:195–201.
43. Gupta A, Meswania J, Pollock R, Cannon SR, Briggs TW, Taylor S, Blunn G. Non-invasive distal femoral expandable endoprosthesis for limb-salvage surgery in paediatric tumours. J Bone Joint Surg Br. 2006;88(5):649–54.
44. Lex JR, Adlan A, Tsoi K, Evans S, Stevenson JD. Frequency and reason for reoperation following non-invasive expandable endoprostheses: a systematic review. J Bone Oncol. 2021;31:100397.
45. Benevenia J, Kirchner R, Patterson F, et al. Outcomes of a modular intercalary endoprosthesis as treatment for segmental defects of the femur, tibia, and humerus. Clin Orthop Relat Res. 2016;474(2):539–48.
46. Aponte-Tinao LA, Ayerza MA, Albergo JI, Farfalli GL. Do massive allograft reconstructions for tumors of the femur and tibia survive 10 or more years after implantation? Clin Orthop Relat Res. 2020;478(3):517–24.
47. Li J, Chen G, Lu Y, Zhu H, Ji C, Wang Z. Factors influencing osseous union following surgical treatment of bone tumors with use of the Capanna technique. J Bone Joint Surg Am. 2019;101(22):2036–43.
48. Puri A, Byregowda S, Gulia A, Patil V, Crasto S, Laskar S. Reconstructing diaphyseal tumors using radiated (50 Gy) autogenous tumor bone graft. J Surg Oncol. 2018;118(1):138–43.
49. Sharma DN, Rastogi S, Bakhshi S, et al. Role of extracorporeal irradiation in malignant bone tumors. Indian J Cancer. 2013;50(4):306–9.
50. Sanders PTJ, Spierings JF, Albergo JI, et al. Long-term clinical outcomes of intercalary allograft reconstruction for lower-extremity bone tumors. J Bone Joint Surg Am. 2020;102(12):1042–9.
51. Aponte-Tinao LA, Albergo JI, Ayerza MA, Muscolo DL, Ing FM, Farfalli GL. What are the complications of allograft reconstructions for sarcoma resection in children younger than 10 years at long-term followup? Clin Orthop Relat Res. 2018;476(3):548–55.
52. Ikuta K, Nishida Y, Sugiura H, et al. Predictors of complications in heat-treated autograft reconstruction after intercalary resection for malignant musculoskeletal tumors of the extremity. J Surg Oncol. 2018;117(7):1469–78.
53. Lee SY, Jeon DG, Cho WH, Song WS, Kim BS. Are pasteurized autografts durable for reconstructions after bone tumor resections? Clin Orthop Relat Res. 2018;476(9):1728–37.
54. Garg SK, Aggarwal P, Virk J, Punia RPS, Dimri K, Jindal R. Limb salvage using liquid nitrogen-treated tumour-bearing autograft: a single institutional experience of 10 patients. Indian J Orthop. 2020;54(2):200–7.
55. Chauhan S, Manoj K, Rastogi S, Khan SA, Prasad A. Biomechanical investigation of the effect of extracorporeal irradiation on resected human bone. J Mech Behav Biomed Mater. 2017;65:791–800.
56. Oike N, Kawashima H, Ogose A, et al. Long-term outcomes of an extracorporeal irradiated autograft

for limb salvage operations in musculoskeletal tumours: over ten years' observation. Bone Joint J. 2019;101-B(9):1151–9.

57. Hayashi K, Araki N, Koizumi M, et al. Long-term results of intraoperative extracorporeal irradiation of autogenous bone grafts on primary bone and soft tissue malignancies. Acta Oncol. 2015;54(1):138–41.
58. Jones CW, Shatrov J, Jagiello JM, et al. Clinical, functional and radiological outcomes of extracorporeal irradiation in limb salvage surgery for bone tumours. Bone Joint J. 2017;99-B(12):1681–8.
59. Puri A, Agarwal M. Facilitating rotationplasty. J Surg Oncol. 2007;95(4):351–4.
60. Kapoor L, Banjara R, Kumar VS, Khan SA. Surgical phocomelia or phoco-reduction as a method of limb salvage for sarcomas of the upper limb: a suitable alternative to amputation. J Surg Oncol. 2021:1–10.
61. Gulia A, Prajapati A, Gupta S, Exner U, Puri A. Rotationplasty after failed limb salvage: an alternative to amputation. Eur J Orthop Surg Traumatol. 2023;33:1683–9.
62. Kapoor L, Sahoo B, Majeed A, et al. Leaving half the acetabulum in pelvic resections improves hip function. Is there a need to revisit conventional pelvic resections? J Surg Oncol. 2022:1–10.
63. Puri A, Pruthi M, Gulia A. Outcomes after limb sparing resection in primary malignant pelvic tumors. Eur J Surg Oncol. 2014;40(1):27–33.
64. Enneking WF, Dunham WK. Resection and reconstruction for primary neoplasms involving the innominate bone. J Bone Joint Surg Am. 1978;60(6):731–46.
65. Pring ME, Weber KL, Unni KK, Sim FH. Chondrosarcoma of the pelvis. A review of sixty-four cases. J Bone Joint Surg Am. 2001;83(11):1630–42.
66. Fuchs B, O'Connor MI, Kaufman KR, Padgett DJ, Sim FH. Iliofemoral arthrodesis and pseudarthrosis: a long-term functional outcome evaluation. Clin Orthop Relat Res. 2002;397:29–35.
67. Witte D, Bernd L, Bruns J, et al. Limb-salvage reconstruction with MUTARS hemipelvic endoprosthesis: a prospective multicenter study. Eur J Surg Oncol. 2009;35(12):1318–25.
68. Krieg AH, Mani M, Speth BM, Stalley PD. Extracorporeal irradiation for pelvic reconstruction in Ewing's sarcoma. J Bone Joint Surg Br. 2009;91(3):395–400.
69. Delloye C, Banse X, Brichard B, Docquier PL, Cornu O. Pelvic reconstruction with a structural pelvic allograft after resection of a malignant bone tumor. J Bone Joint Surg Am. 2007;89(3):579–87.
70. Zeifang F, Buchner M, Zahlten-Hinguranage A, Bernd L, Sabo D. Complications following operative treatment of primary malignant bone tumours in the pelvis. Eur J Surg Oncol. 2004;30(8):893–9.
71. Jaiswal PK, Aston WJ, Grimer RJ, et al. Periacetabular resection and endoprosthetic reconstruction for tumours of the acetabulum. J Bone Joint Surg Br. 2008;90(9):1222–7.
72. Gebert C, Wessling M, Hoffmann C, et al. Hip transposition as a limb salvage procedure following the resection of periacetabular tumors. J Surg Oncol. 2011;103(3):269–75.
73. Hoffmann C, Gosheger G, Gebert C, Jürgens H, Winkelmann W. Functional results and quality of life after treatment of pelvic sarcomas involving the acetabulum. J Bone Joint Surg Am. 2006;88(3):575–82.
74. Nataraj V, Batra A, Rastogi S, Khan SA, Sharma MC, Vishnubhatla S, et al. Developing a prognostic model for patients with localized osteosarcoma treated with uniform chemotherapy protocol without high dose methotrexate: a single-center experience of 237 patients. J Surg Oncol. 2015;112:662–8.
75. Poudel RR, Kumar VS, Bakhshi S, Gamanagatti S, Rastogi S, Khan SA. High tumor volume and local recurrence following surgery in osteosarcoma: a retrospective study. Indian J Orthop. 2014;48:285–8.
76. Xin S, Wei G. Prognostic factors in osteosarcoma: a study level meta-analysis and systematic review of current practice. J Bone Oncol. 2020;21:100281.
77. Biswas B, Rastogi S, Khan SA, Shukla NK, Deo SV, Agarwala S, et al. Developing a prognostic model for localized Ewing sarcoma family of tumors: a single institutional experience of 224 cases treated with uniform chemotherapy protocol. J Surg Oncol. 2015;111:683–9.
78. Biswas B, Rastogi S, Khan SA, Shukla NK, Deo SV, Agarwala S, et al. Hypoalbuminaemia is an independent predictor of poor outcome in metastatic Ewing's sarcoma family of tumours: a single institutional experience of 150 cases treated with uniform chemotherapy protocol. Clin Oncol (R Coll Radiol). 2014;26:722–9.
79. Biswas B, Rastogi S, Khan SA, Mohanti BK, Sharma DN, Sharma MC, et al. Outcomes and prognostic factors for Ewing-family tumors of the extremities. J Bone Joint Surg Am. 2014;96:841–9.
80. Biswas B, Agarwala S, Rastogi S, Khan SA, Mohanti BK, Sharma DN, et al. High burden of metastases and poor outcome in pelvic PNET. Pediatr Blood Cancer. 2013;60:E97–9.
81. Prabu R, Thulkar S, Chand Sharma M, Mohanti BK, Dhawan D, Bakhshi S. PNET spine: morbid and mortal, but ignored till late. J Pediatr Hematol Oncol. 2012;34:e164–9.
82. Biswas B, Shukla NK, Deo SV, Agarwala S, Sharma DN, Vishnubhatla S, et al. Evaluation of outcome and prognostic factors in extraosseous Ewing sarcoma. Pediatr Blood Cancer. 2014;61:1925–31.
83. Qureshi SS, Kembhavi S, Bhagat M, Laskar S, Chinnaswamy G, Vora T, et al. Primary non-metastatic Ewing sarcoma of the jaw in children: results of surgical resection and primary reconstruction. J Surg Oncol. 2014;110:689–95.
84. Biswas B, Thakar A, Mohanti BK, Vishnubhatla S, Bakhshi S. Prognostic factors in head and neck Ewing sarcoma family of tumors. Laryngoscope. 2015;125:E112–7.

85. Burningham Z, Hashibe M, Spector L, Schiffman JD. The epidemiology of sarcoma. Clin Sarcoma Res. 2012;2(1):14.
86. Paulussen M, Ahrens S, Dunst J, Craft AW, Lewis I, et al. Localized Ewing tumor of bone: final results of the cooperative Ewing's Sarcoma Study CESS 86. J Clin Oncol. 2001;19:1818–29.
87. Ahmed SK, Randall RL, DuBois SG, Krailo MD, Marcus KJ, et al. Identification of patients with localized Ewing sarcoma at higher risk for local failure. Int J Radiat Oncol Biol Phys. 2017;99:1286–94.
88. Krasin MJ, Rodriguez-Galindo C, Billups CA, Davidoff AM, Neel MD, et al. Definitive radiation therapy in the management of localized Ewing sarcoma. Cancer. 2004;
89. Merchant TE, Hua CH, Shukla H, Ying X, Nill S, et al. Proton versus photon radiotherapy for pediatric tumors: patterns of care and early outcomes. Int J Radiat Oncol Biol Phys. 2008;
90. Ruka W, Rutkowski P, Morysiński T, Nowecki ZI, Zdzienicki M, et al. The megavoltage radiation therapy in the treatment of patients with advanced or difficult giant cell tumors of bone. Int J Radiat Oncol Biol Phys. 2010;78:494–8.
91. Feigenberg SJ, Marcus RB, Zlotecki RA, Scarborough MT, Berrey BH, et al. Radiation therapy for giant cell tumors of bone. Clin Orthop Relat Res. 2003;(411):207–16.
92. Fletcher CDM, Bridge JA, Hogendoorn PCW, Mertens F, editors. WHO classification of tumours of soft tissue and bone. 5th ed. IARC: Lyon; 2020.
93. Coindre JM. Grading of soft tissue sarcomas: review and update. Arch Pathol Lab Med. 2006;130(10):1448–53.
94. Thway K, Jones RL, Noujaim J, Zaidi S, Miah AB, Fisher C. Dedifferentiated liposarcoma: updates on morphology, genetics, and therapeutic strategies. Adv Anat Pathol. 2016;23(1):30–40.
95. Doyle LA. Sarcoma immunohistochemistry update: diagnostic utility of markers old and new. Adv Anat Pathol. 2014;21(6):383–96.
96. Gronchi A, Miah AB, Dei Tos AP, et al. Soft tissue and visceral sarcomas: ESMO–EURACAN–GENTURIS Clinical Practice Guidelines for diagnosis, treatment and follow-up. Ann Oncol. 2021;32(11):1348–65.
97. Amin MB, Edge SB, Greene FL, et al., editors. AJCC cancer staging manual. 8th ed. New York: Springer; 2017.
98. Salerno KE, Alektiar KM, Baldini EH, Bedi M, Bishop AJ, Bradfield L, Chung P, DeLaney TF, Folpe A, Kane JM, Li XA, Petersen I, Powell J, Stolten M, Thorpe S, Trent JC, Voermans M, Guadagnolo BA. Radiation therapy for treatment of soft tissue sarcoma in adults: executive summary of an ASTRO clinical practice guideline. Pract Radiat Oncol. 2021;11(5):339–51. https://doi.org/10.1016/j.prro.2021.04.005.
99. Yang JC, Chang AE, Baker AR, Sindelar WF, Danforth DN, Topalian SL, DeLaney T, Glatstein E, Steinberg SM, Merino MJ, Rosenberg SA. Randomized prospective study of the benefit of adjuvant radiation therapy in the treatment of soft tissue sarcomas of the extremity. J Clin Oncol. 1998;16(1):197–203.
100. Harrison LB, Franzese F, Gaynor JJ, Brennan MF. Long-term results of a prospective randomized trial of adjuvant brachytherapy in the management of completely resected soft tissue sarcomas of the extremity and superficial trunk. Int J Radiat Oncol Biol Phys. 1993;27(2):259–65. https://doi.org/10.1016/0360-3016(93)90236-o. PMID: 8407399.
101. Tang C, Farooqi A, Hahn S, et al. Pocket notebook: pocket radiation oncology: the MD Anderson Cancer Center handbook of radiation oncology. 1st ed. Lippincott Williams & Wilkins; 2020.
102. Haas RL, Delaney TF, O'Sullivan B, Keus RB, Le Pechoux C, Olmi P, Poulsen JP, Seddon B, Wang D. Radiotherapy for management of extremity soft tissue sarcomas: why, when, and where? Int J Radiat Oncol Biol Phys. 2012;84(3):572–80.
103. Salerno KE. Radiation therapy for soft tissue sarcoma: indications, timing, benefits, and consequences. Surg Clin North Am. 2022;102(4):567–82.
104. DeLaney TF, Liebsch NJ, Pedlow FX, et al. Phase II study of combined proton and photon radiation therapy for retroperitoneal and pelvic sarcomas. Int J Radiat Oncol Biol Phys. 2007;67(1):153–61. https://doi.org/10.1016/j.ijrobp.2006.08.038.
105. O'Sullivan B, Davis AM, Turcotte R, Bell R, Catton C, Chabot P, Wunder J, Kandel R, Goddard K, Sadura A, Pater J, Zee B. Preoperative versus postoperative radiotherapy in soft-tissue sarcoma of the limbs: a randomised trial. Lancet. 2002;359(9325):2235–41.
106. Campbell BA, Herle P, Harris S, Kornaga EN, et al. High-dose-rate brachytherapy for soft tissue sarcoma: a single-institution experience and literature review. Brachytherapy. 2021;20(2):319–27. https://doi.org/10.1016/j.brachy.2020.11.003.
107. Koseła-Paterczyk H, Teterycz P, Spałek MJ, et al. Efficacy and safety of hypofractionated preoperative radiotherapy for primary locally advanced soft tissue sarcomas of limbs or trunk wall. Cancers (Basel). 2021;13(12):2981.
108. Kalbasi A, Kamrava M, Chu FI, et al. A phase II trial of 5-day neoadjuvant radiotherapy for patients with high-risk primary soft tissue sarcoma. Clin Cancer Res. 2020;26(8):1829–36.
109. Leite ET, Munhoz RR, de Camargo VP, et al. Neoadjuvant stereotactic ablative radiotherapy (SABR) for soft tissue sarcomas of the extremities. Radiother Oncol. 2021;161:222–9.
110. Guadagnolo BA, Bassett RL, Mitra D, et al. Hypofractionated, 3-week, preoperative radiotherapy for patients with soft tissue sarcomas (HYPORT-STS): a single-centre, open-label, single-arm, phase 2 trial. Lancet Oncol. 2022;23(12):1547–57.
111. Mayer C, Gasalberti DP, Kumar A. Brachytherapy. [Updated 2023 Jun 15]. In: StatPearls [Internet]. Treasure Island: StatPearls Publishing; 2025. Available from: https://www.ncbi.nlm.nih.gov/books/NBK562190/.

112. Pervaiz N, Colterjohn N, Farrokhyar F, Tozer R, Figueredo A, Ghert M. A systematic meta-analysis of randomized controlled trials of adjuvant chemotherapy for localized resectable soft-tissue sarcoma. Cancer. 2008;113(3):573–81.
113. Tap WD, Wagner AJ, Schöffski P, Martin-Broto J, Krarup-Hansen A, Ganjoo KN, et al. Effect of chemotherapy intensity and histology on outcome in localized soft-tissue sarcoma: a pooled analysis of contemporary neoadjuvant trials. J Clin Oncol. 2022;40(25):2909–20.
114. Vanzulli A, Vigorito R, Buonomenna C, Palmerini E, et al. Redefining radiologic responses in high-risk soft-tissue sarcomas treated with neoadjuvant chemotherapy: final results of ISG-STS 1001, a randomized clinical trial. ESMO Open. 2025;10:104299. https://doi.org/10.1016/j.esmoop.2025.104299.
115. Judson I, Verweij J, Gelderblom H, Hartmann JT, Schöffski P, Blay JY, et al. Doxorubicin alone versus intensified doxorubicin plus ifosfamide for first-line treatment of advanced or metastatic soft-tissue sarcoma: a randomised controlled phase 3 trial. Lancet Oncol. 2014;15(4):415–23.
116. van der Graaf WT, Blay JY, Chawla SP, et al. Pazopanib for metastatic soft-tissue sarcoma (PALETTE): a randomised, double-blind, placebo-controlled phase 3 trial. Lancet. 2012;379(9829):1879–86.
117. Mowery YM, Ballman KV, Hong AM, et al. Safety and efficacy of pembrolizumab, radiation therapy, and surgery versus radiation therapy and surgery for stage III soft tissue sarcoma of the extremity (SU2C-SARC032): an open-label, randomised clinical trial. Lancet. 2024;404(10467):2053–64.
118. D'Angelo SP, Tawbi HA, Kollar A, Patel SR. Novel immunologic and cellular approaches in soft tissue sarcoma: highlights from the 2024 ASCO Annual Meeting. J Clin Oncol. 2024;42(18_suppl):LBA11505.
119. Bonvalot S, Gronchi A, Le Péchoux C, et al. Preoperative radiotherapy plus surgery versus surgery alone for patients with primary retroperitoneal sarcoma (EORTC-62092: STRASS): a multicentre, open-label, randomised, phase 3 trial. Lancet Oncol. 2020;21(10):1366–77.

Online Links

https://www.youtube.com/watch?v=OlRWFf8M64o
https://www.youtube.com/watch?v=7J-WbzkeFRM
https://www.youtube.com/watch?v=otDM3-fHnzc
https://www.youtube.com/watch?v=iWJbL7E08vM
https://www.youtube.com/watch?v=bvScRuVmaJ0

Paediatric Tumours

Anusheel Munshi, Siddarth Laskar, Vikas Kumar Pandey, and Meenakshi Ravichandran

1 Introduction

Cancer may affect people of any age, including children. Although childhood cancers are rare, they are treatable if identified early and treated correctly. Childhood cancers are best treated in paediatric cancer units by specialized disease management teams. Paediatric age groups range from 0 to 14, with some centres accepting children as old as 18 years old.

Almost 280,000 children and adolescents (aged 0–19 years) were diagnosed with cancer globally in 2020, and almost 110,000 died as a result of cancer [1]. Estimated age-standardized childhood cancer incidence rates in the world in 2020 (Fig. 1), has brought to attention that the incidence is rising at 0.3% year-on-year. Hence, cancer epidemiologists and healthcare policy makers are projecting that facilities for specialized childhood cancer management in LMIC would need good planning and investment.

Variation has been observed in the childhood cancer incidence and mortality between high-income countries (HIC) and low and middle-income countries (LMIC) like India [2].

With substantial progress made in diagnosis and treatment of childhood cancers, most HIC have a 5-year net survival of approximately 80% [3]. Low and middle-income countries (LMICs) are home to up to 80% of children at risk of childhood cancer [2].

Inequality in healthcare access, a lack of sufficiently qualified personnel, treatment abandonment, and a variety of other issues are significant obstacles to improvement in children's cancer outcomes in LMICs compared to HICs [4].

According to the PBCR study (2012–2014), childhood cancer accounts for 0.7–4.4% of overall cancer cases in India [5]. Nearly 50,000 new paediatric malignancies are detected in India each year, which account for approximately 20% of all paediatric cancers diagnosed worldwide [6]. Childhood cancer is more common in males in India due to gender prejudice in seeking treatment. Children with cancer arrive late and at a more advanced stage, with inadequate awareness, delayed diagnosis, and therapy discontinuation being important management challenges. In the last few decades, forming collaborative organizations and training programmes has improved the outlook [7]. Access to radiation for cancer

A. Munshi (✉)
Department of Radiation Oncology, BLK MAX Hospital, New Delhi, Delhi, India

S. Laskar
Radiation Oncology, Tata Memorial Hospital, Mumbai, India

V. K. Pandey
Department of Radiation Oncology, Cancer Care Manitoba, Winnipeg, Canada

M. Ravichandran
Radiation Oncology, Sir H. N. Reliance Foundation Hospital and Research Centre, Mumbai, India

B. K. Mohanti et al. (eds.), *Radiation Oncology – Principles, Precepts and Practice*,
https://doi.org/10.1007/978-981-95-5171-2_16

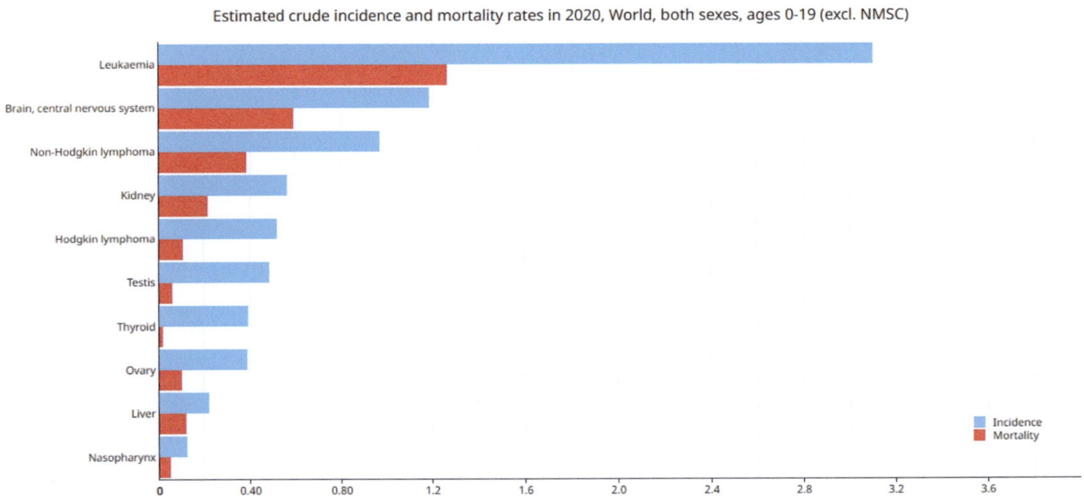

Fig. 1 Childhood cancers: incidence (blue bar) and mortality (red bar) for age group of 0 to 19 years, 2020. (open source: IARC Global Cancer Observatory)

patients in India is hampered by a number of variables, including the geographical closeness of the centre and the cost and availability of necessary technologies [8]. Improving accessibility, providing comprehensive support, forming of National Childhood Cancer Policy and finding overlooked instances should be priorities in the future (Table 1).

2 Importance of Early Diagnosis

A high degree of suspicion by the primary care practitioner and early referral to a paediatric oncologist are required for optimal therapy of children's cancer. Early identification and treatment can lessen disease-related morbidity and consequences [9].

Delays in diagnosis have been linked to the child's age (older children are more likely to be delayed), the kind of cancer, the presenting symptoms, the tumour location, the first medical specialty consulted, and access to health care. The duration between the beginning of symptoms and the diagnosis of paediatric cancer varies depending on the kind of cancer. The stated typical time to diagnosis for neuroblastoma is 2–5 weeks, 3–5 weeks for acute leukaemias, 7–10 weeks for lymphomas, 8–15 weeks for bone tumours, and 8–>20 weeks for brain tumours.

Blood and bone marrow, the brain and neurological system, lymph nodes, kidneys, bone and soft tissues are all common locations for juvenile cancers. The child's age determines the occurrence of a particular cancer. For example, neuroblastoma and Wilms tumour are more prevalent in children between the ages of one and four; leukaemia is most common in children below the age of ten; and Ewing sarcoma, Hodgkin lymphoma, and thyroid cancer are more common in children over the age of ten [10].

3 Presenting Signs and Symptoms

Paediatric cancer may exhibit signs and symptoms similar to other paediatric disorders. Although a single finding in isolation does not always necessitate a cancer evaluation, a combination of the multiple conclusions (Table 2) (e.g., weight loss, bone pain, and lymphadenopathy; easy bruising, abnormal blood counts, and hepatosplenomegaly) is concerning and warrants prompt referral to a paediatric oncologist and cancer evaluation. In addition, specific isolated

Table 1 Paediatric vs adult cancer

	Paediatric	Adult
Risk factors	Uncommon	Common
Biology	Embryonic: Derived from non-ectodermal embryonal tissue	Carcinoma: Derived from epithelial tissue
Average age at diagnosis	6 years	66 years
Tumour types	Embryonal	Carcinoma
Organ types	Both solid and liquid– a wide variety of unique tumours	Mostly solid tumours—Typically breast, gyn, colon
Diseases	Leukaemia / CNS	Breast /lung / prostate
Pathology clues	Associations are emerging, but not always linked- hypodiploid ALL (TPS3)	Several clear associations—Triple-negative breast (BRCA), MSI high CRC (Lynch)
Family history	Often don't see AD pattern; reduced penetrance, variable expressivity, de novo rate.	Often follows AD pattern
Somatic mutations	Limited	Abundant
Testing and management considerations	Testing guidelines not well established; screening guidelines not published for many syndromes (AACR 2017 Working Group)	Numerous clear consensus guidelines for testing and management (NCCN, ACS)
Survival rate	80%	50%
Research funding (% NCI budget in the US)	4% of overall budget	96% of overall budget
Outcomes	75–80% overall survival at 5 years	<60% overall survival at 5 years

AD Autosomal Dominant

abnormalities like abdominal or mediastinal masses, vision loss, headaches accompanied by morning vomiting, and blasts on a peripheral blood smear necessitate quick assessment and consultation.

4 Radiotherapy

Radiotherapy is an essential component in the multimodality approach for childhood malignancies. The best circumstances for radiation in young patients are still being shaped by multidisciplinary developments in cancer therapy and studies on the late effects of radiotherapy. According to institutional statistics, the percentage of newly diagnosed cases among children who get irradiation for any cancer has climbed from around 40% to over 60% in the last 18 years [11].

Because of their rarity, the significant variety of histological subtypes, and the complexity of therapy approaches that continue to advance, paediatric cancers pose a challenge for radiation oncologists (Table 3). Childhood cancer differs from adults in terms of rarity, high cure rates if diagnosed early, many unique requirements, and a high burden of late effects. Radiation therapy approaches, including technology and methodology, are continually being optimized. Intensity-modulated radiotherapy, proton therapy, and advanced imaging for treatment planning, localization, and verification aid in increasing precision. Interest in proton beam radiotherapy (PBRT) has been notably highlighted in CNS malignancies and sarcomas due to overwhelming dosimetric advantages favouring protons; convincing evidence supporting acute and late toxicity has encouraged technology-based centralized referral patterns [12]. There is, however, variation in access to PBRT worldwide. Almost 80% of childhood cancer patients reside in LMIC, where access to proton therapy is limited [13]. Paediatric brachytherapy is highly specialized, requiring special equipment and surgical skills.

Key radiation parameters are vital in paediatric treatment because the relative radiation sensitivities of paediatric malignancies compete with

Table 2 Symptoms and signs of paediatric tumours

Signs/symptoms	Initial evaluation	Associated malignancy	Role of radiotherapy
Constitutional symptoms-unexplained fever/weight loss/fatigue/pallor	CBC with differential, serum electrolytes, BUN, creatinine, LDH, uric acid, liver function tests Microbiological examinations Radiological investigations	Any malignancy	Site-specific
Symptoms of the nervous system: Headaches and vomiting in the early morning Papilledema Afebrile seizure Cranial nerves palsies Ataxia Deficits in focal motor function	Radiological investigations-including MRI brain with contrast +/− MRI whole spine	Brain tumour	Usually post-operative
Palpable abdominal and pelvic masses	CBC, serum electrolytes, BUN, creatinine, liver function tests, urinalysis Imaging of the abdomen and pelvis	Wilms tumour Neuroblastoma Adrenal gland tumours Germ cell tumours Hepatoblastoma Rhabdomyosarcoma Sarcoma of soft tissue	As indicated for the respective site in current protocols
Symptoms of the musculoskeletal system: Bony pains Limp/inability to walk Soft tissue mass	CBC Radiological investigations	Ewing's sarcoma Leukaemia Neuroblastoma Osteosarcoma Sarcoma of soft tissue	As indicated for respective sites in current protocols
Ophthalmologic findings: Leukocoria, acute visual impairment Proptosis, dual vision Intraorbital bleeding	Ophthalmology evaluation	Tumours of the brain Orbital RMS Metastatic neuroblastoma Retinoblastoma	As indicated for the respective site in current protocols

CBC complete blood counts, *MRI* magnetic resonance imaging, *CRP* c-reactive protein, *LDH* lactate dehydrogenase, *BUN* blood urea nitrogen, *RMS* Rhabdomyosarcoma

Table 3 Challenges for radiotherapy in paediatric population in LMIC

Challenges for radiotherapy
Access: 85% of the world's population lives in LMIC, where access to radiotherapy is limited.
Need: More than 70% of children present with advanced disease (and a large majority of them will therefore require radiotherapy for local control)
Children are treated on numerous different protocols with little audit of outcomes.
Lack of registries, coordinated research, and low publication combinedly means that outcomes are not recorded.
Paediatric radiotherapy is considered a specialized area and may not be the area of focus in small volume centres.
Sedation/paediatric anaesthesia for radiotherapy delivedry

the additional vulnerabilities of the growing, developing child or adolescent. More studies indicate disease control in most paediatric cancers using reduced target dose & fractionation, more conformal radiation, and three-dimensional treatment planning delivery to gain a competitive edge [14, 15]. Quality control becomes increasingly important when treatment volumes

(GTV, CTV, PTV) are reduced. Crucial knowledge for patient selection is equally important. For instance, consolidative irradiation for Hodgkin lymphoma patients may be safely avoided in some subpopulations of patients, similar to how we have shifted away from prophylactic cranial irradiation for ALL [11]. Molecularly targeted therapy in conjunction with radiation treatment is being investigated.

Children have increased vulnerability to radiotherapy due to developing tissues. If cured, children have years to live with radiation-related late effects, which are more pronounced than adults. They can have somatic (such as changes in musculoskeletal tissue growth and development) and functional (such as neurological, auditory, and endocrine) consequences and an increased risk of secondary malignancies on extended follow-up of long-term survivors [16, 17].

Just like Qualitative analysis of normal tissues in the clinic (QUANTEC), Paediatric normal tissue effect in the clinic (PENTEC, 2024) [18] provides 1. qualitative evidence-based dose/volume/risk guidelines. 2. Explore risk factors for toxicity; 3. Describe physics and dosimetric issues relevant to paediatric radiotherapy. 4. Propose dose-volume outcome reporting standards.

It is important for radiation oncologists treating childhood cancers to comprehend all aspects of PENTEC, 2024. In order to further quality assurance, investigators are looking for the possibility of artificial intelligence to assist in radiotherapy target delineation and planning [19].

5 Common Paediatric Tumours

- Leukaemias
- Lymphomas
- Brain tumours
- Neuroblastomas
- Wilms tumours
- Rhabdomyosarcoma
- Retinoblastoma
- Bone tumours (including osteosarcoma and Ewing sarcoma)
- Germ cell tumours

Leukaemia accounts for approximately 35% of all childhood cancers. Although it is more common in children under the age of 10, about 1 in 1000 children are diagnosed with leukaemia by the age of 1 year. Leukaemias are discussed in the relevant chapter 17 on Hematological Malignancies of this book.

Lymphomas are malignant neoplasms of the neck, axilla, and inguino-pelvic lymphatic system. Lymphomas are broadly classified as Hodgkin's and non-Hodgkin's. Hodgkin's lymphoma generally occurs in individuals between 15 and 40 years of age.

Since 1990s, childhood hematological malignancies (leukemias and lymphomas) are successfully achieving long-term cure with multiagent chemotherapy and bone marrow transplant. Historically, radiotherapy had played significant role for pediatric acute lymphoblastic leukemia (prophylactic cranial irradiation, PCI), Hodgkin's Lymphoma and Non-Hodgkin's Lymphoma (involved-field RT, consolidative RT). Because of the late effects of radiotherapy as enumerated earlier, and its synergistic deleterious effects when combined with systemic chemotherapy drugs, the indications for RT in ALL, HD, NHL in children are now judiciously decided. Whenever the disease is refractory to chemotherapy or shows relapse, the radiotherapy is delivered. The dose and fractions are now much reduced, for example (a) 18 Gy in 12-15 fractions for PCI; (b) 20 Gy to 25 Gy in 12 to 15 fractions; (c) 36 Gy to 45 Gy in 20 to 25 fractions in NHL (mediastinal DLBCL); (d) palliative radiotherapy for symptomatic skeletal or soft tissue lesions.

Brain Tumours

Brain tumours account for nearly 10–15% of paediatric cancers. The symptoms depend on the location of the tumour. Gliomas and medulloblastomas are the two main types of brain tumours affecting children. Medulloblastoma originates in the cerebellum or posterior fossa and may spread to other brain parts or the spinal cord. Most medulloblastomas occur before the age of 10. Brain tumours have been covered in detail in the relevant chapter in this book. (Chap. Central Nervous System Tumours).

6 Neuroblastoma

The term neuroblastoma (NB) refers to a group of neuroblastic tumours (including neuroblastomas, ganglioneuroblastomas, and ganglioneuromas) that originate from the primitive sympathetic ganglion cells and may secrete catecholamines. They are the most common extracranial tumours in infancy.

They are heterogeneous tumours in terms of location, histopathologic appearance, and clinical course, ranging from spontaneous regression in infants to highly aggressive disease with fatal outcomes in children >18 months [20].

Neuroblastomas constitute nearly 6–10% of paediatric malignancies worldwide. Children diagnosed with neuroblastoma (NB) at 18 months seldom achieve 5 years of overall survival better than 30% in India [21]. Most cases present at an advanced stage.

Neuroblastoma arises from nerve tissue of the adrenal gland, neck, chest, or spinal cord. It accounts for 5–7% of all childhood malignancies and usually occurs by the age of 5 years. Investigations in a case of neuroblastoma include 24 h of urinary vanillylmandelic acid (VMA), serum Lactate dehydrogenase (LDH), and serum ferritin. Whole-body PET CT/ CT / MRI imaging is typically used to diagnose and stage these lesions. A Metaiodobenzylguanidine (MIBG) scan (Level 1) is also recommended to complete staging. A PET/CT scan should be done if MIBG is non-avid. Bone scan is optional if more advanced tests have been done. Bone marrow aspiration (bilateral) and biopsy are required to complete staging. The presence of unequivocal tumour cells (adequate for histopathology and molecular pathology) in bone marrow biopsy, along with increased levels of urinary catecholamines, is sufficient for diagnosis.

Pathology examination should include routine histopathology and molecular pathology. The latter needs to include evaluation for N-MYC and chromosomal aberrations.

Life Threatening Symptoms (LTS) include a wide spectrum, namely pain requiring opioid treatment, gastrointestinal (feeding difficulty, not gaining weight) symptoms, respiratory distress, cardiovascular System (hypertension, inferior vena cava obstruction leading to pedal oedema) diseases, impaired renal function, hydronephrosis, hepatic dysfunction, bladder/bowel dysfunction, and neurological complications.

Aetiology

Little is known about the aetiology of Neuroblastoma. Due to the early age of onset, pre-conceptual or gestational environmental events (e.g., exposure to medicines like opiates, gestational diabetes, folate deficiency, hormones, toxins, or viruses) may have a role [22–24].

Genetic Predisposition

Most cases are sporadic. However, few genetic syndromes are associated with the disease. These include Congenital central hypoventilation syndrome/Hirschsprung's disease *(PHOX2B),* congenital *NB*- germline *ALK* mutation associated, familial paraganglioma/pheochromocytoma syndrome (*SDHB/C/D/AF2*), neurofibromatosis (*NF1*), Costello syndrome (*HRAS*), Noonan syndrome (*PTPN11*) and Li Fraumeni syndrome(*p53*). The molecular pathogenesis of neuroblastomas has been widely researched, and knowledge of individual anomalies is a critical component of defining prognostic risk categories [25, 26]. Molecular drivers of neuroblastoma are shown in Table 4.

Clinical Presentation

NB can be present throughout the sympathetic nervous system, the most common site being the adrenal (40%), followed by abdominal, thoracic, cervical, and pelvic sympathetic ganglion. These tumours typically metastasize to lymph nodes, bone marrow, dura, orbit, cortical bone, skin and liver [27]. Paraneoplastic syndromes associated with NB include Opsoclonus Myoclonus Syndrome and Kerner–Morrison Syndrome. Opsoclonus Myoclonus Syndrome is present in 4–5% of NB cases. The classical presentation includes rhythmic (myogenic) jerks and rapid, dancing eye movement with or without ataxia. The exact cause is unknown; it is generally hypothesized to be autoimmune. It may lead to

Table 4 Molecular drivers of neuroblastoma

Gene (%)	Alteration	Biologic role
NMYC (20%)	NMYC amplification and overexpression MYC overexpression	Oncogenic transcription factor
ATRX (13%)	Inactivating mutation Mutually exclusive with NMYC	Activates alternative lengthening of telomerase pathways Majority >5 years Smouldering clinical course
TERT (13%)	Activating re-arrangement	Telomerase complex Exclusive of NMYC and ATRX mutations
ALK (14%)	Amplification (4%) Gain of function mutation (15%)	Anaplastic lymphoma kinase receptor Occurs in setting of NMYC amplification Increased incidence of relapse Associated with congenital neuroblastoma
ARID 1a/b (11%)	Deletion and point mutation	Regulation of transcription by altering the chromatin structure

Table 5 Symptoms associated with NB

Symptoms associated with primary disease	Symptoms associated with metastatic disease
Abdominal mass	Constitutional symptoms- fever, irritability, anorexia, weight loss, fatigue, anaemia
Neck mass	Bone/bone marrow metastasis- ill-defined bone pain, limp, proptosis, ecchymosis
Shortness of breath (mediastinal mass)	Skin nodules
Horner syndrome	*Paraneoplastic syndromes:* - Opsoclonus myoclonus syndrome Kerner-Morrison syndrome
Urinary retention/constipation	
Neurologic abnormalities (paresis/paralysis)	
Hypertension	

the development of long-term neurocognitive deficits. Nevertheless, it predicts favourable biological features and excellent survival rates. Kerner-Morrison Syndrome is seen when the tumour secretes vasoactive intestinal polypeptide, causing intractable secretory diarrhoea. Tumour resection reduces secretion.

Common presenting symptoms are shown in Table 5.

Diagnosis

Imaging modalities are used for the evaluation of locoregional involvement and metastatic disease. After routine laboratory investigations (complete blood count, liver function, kidney function, and electrolytes), anatomic imaging is done using computed tomography (CT) or magnetic resonance imaging (MRI)—spine for primary and nodal metastatic sites. Radiolabelled Metaiodobenzylguanidine (I-123 MIBG, positive in 90% NB tumours). Whole-body positron emission CT(PET-CT) can be used in MIBG non-avid disease. Tecnicium-99 (Tc-99) Bone scan is obsolete and can be used at diagnosis but is no longer used to evaluate response.

Tissue diagnosis and determining tumour biology are mandatory for diagnosis to assist with risk stratification. NB appears as small round blue cell tumours with classical Homer Wright rosette patterns (tumour cells arranged around neuropils). Varying degrees of neuronal maturation, mitosis, karyorrhexis (MKI), and Schwannian stroma should be reported in pathology along with grade. Molecular/cytogenetic analysis of the disease should be done. Other tests include- bilateral bone marrow aspirate and biopsy (IHC staining S111, CD56, NSE, and synaptophysin), Urine homovanillic acid (HVA)-positive in 90% NB and nonspecific tumour markers (ferritin and LDH).

The use of urine catecholamines to screen newborns and infants for neuroblastoma is not

Table 6 International neuroblastoma staging system (INSS)

I	Localized GTR (R0)
IIA	Localized <GTR; N0
IIB	Localized; ipsilateral node positive (contralateral negative)
III	Unresectable disease crossing midline or contralateral node-positive
IV	Distant spread: Nodes, bone marrow/bone, liver, skin, or others
IVS	Localized dissemination is limited to skin, liver, or marrow (age < 1 year)

Table 7 International neuroblastoma risk group staging system (INRGSS)

Stage	Description
L1	Localized tumours not involving vital structures (without image-defined risk factors and confined to one body compartment)
L2	Locoregional tumour with one or more image-defined risk factor
M	Distant metastatic disease (except MS)
MS	Metastatic disease in children <18 months with illness confined to skin, liver, and bone marrow

suggested since statistics show that this strategy does not reduce mortality [28]. Medical complications associated with neuroblastoma include spinal cord compression, opsoclonus myoclonus, and tumour lysis syndrome.

Staging

Two staging systems exist for patients with neuroblastoma: The International Neuroblastoma Staging System (INSS) (Table 6) and the International Neuroblastoma Risk Group Staging System (INRGSS) (Table 7). The International Neuroblastoma Staging System (INSS) was the first staging system adopted in 1990. Staging is done according to resectability and lymph node involvement and spread to distant sites [29]. The International Neuroblastoma Risk Group staging system (INRGSS) is a new method created in 2009. It included pretreatment imaging characteristics rather than resection findings [30].

Prognostic Features of NB

Certain variables impact the biologic activity of these cancers and assist in predicting prognosis; some are patient-related (for example, age at diagnosis), while the majority are tumour-related (disease stage, tumour histology, molecular and cytogenetic characteristics) [30, 31].

The predictive features of NB are listed in Table 8.

Risk stratification is based on Prognostic factors. Low risk includes INSS Stage I, II, IVS; INRGSS L1, M; any age (IVS/MS < 18 months), no NMYC amplification. Intermediate risk includes- INSS stage III, INRGSSL2; INSS stage IV, INRGSS M, and age < 18 months; No NMYC amplification. High risk includes- NMYC amplification, INSS stage IV, INRGSS M, and age > 18 months, or 12–18 months with unfavourable histology or genomics.

Treatment

Improvements in outcomes for children with neuroblastoma have resulted from cooperative group, multicentre clinical studies incorporating mixed modality methods with an awareness of the predictive variables influencing success. Patients should be handled in a facility with suitable experience in neuroblastoma therapy. Treatment is based on risk categories.

Low-risk NB therapy They have favourable outcomes with 4 years event-free survival (EFS) and overall survival (OS) >90% [32]. Safe surgical resection is the mainstay of treatment. Surgery can be delayed for symptomatic INSS IVS/INRGSS MS. Complete resection is not mandatory. The goal is a 50% safe resection, reduction in primary tumours achieved by chemotherapy alone, surgery alone, or both.

Infants with small stage II/L1 adrenal tumours can be observed alone [32]. There are ongoing studies for additional non-adrenal small L1 tumours. Chemotherapy is reserved for acute life/organ-threatening symptoms or recurrence. Radiotherapy is reserved for acute life/organ-threatening symptoms.

Table 8 Prognostic features of NB

Features	Favourable	Unfavourable
Age	<18 months	>18 months
Stage	Lower	Higher
Pathology	Poorly differentiated/differentiating, low/intermediate MKI, age < 1.5 years Differentiating, low MKI, age 1.5–5 years Ganglioneuroblastoma, intermixed, regardless of age Ganglioneuroma, regardless of age	Undifferentiated high MKI of any age Poorly differentiated/intermediate MKI, 1.5–5 years Any differentiation, any MKI, 5 years or older Nodular ganglioneuroblastoma, regardless of age
Genetics	High expression of TRA-A/C Hyperdiploid DNA content	MYCN amplification Segmental chromosome aberration (1p and/or 11q) Diploid DNA content

Note: MKI reflects the degree of cell replication seen in a high-power microscope field and categorized as low (<2% or < 100/5000 mitotic and karyorrhectic cells), intermediate (2%–4% or 100–200/5000 mitotic and karyorrhectic cells), and high (>4% or > 200/5000 mitotic and karyorrhectic cells)

Intermediate Risk NB Therapy This group has a 4-year EFS of >85% and an OS of >90% [33]. Primary treatment options include intense multiagent chemotherapy with or without surgery [34]. Radiation is reserved for acute life/organ-threatening symptoms. An upfront biopsy is indicated for genetic and histology data. Response directed to 2–8 cycles of chemotherapy can be planned. Chemotherapy agents used are Vincristine, carboplatin, cyclophosphamide and doxorubicin. The goal is >50% reduction of primary tumour and resolution of metastatic disease. Longer duration of chemotherapy (at least four cycles up to 8 cycles, if combined with stage IV/INRGSS M disease) is preferred if unfavourable histology, tumour Segmental chromosome aberration, or tumour diploid. Complete resection is not mandatory- delayed resection is done to achieve >50% reduction in primary tumour size.

High-Risk NB Therapy

They have 4 years EFS of 30–50% and OS of 50–60% [35]. Multimodality treatment is recommended. Several chemotherapy regimens have been proposed, e.g., in Europe, rapid COJEC is used (a combination of cisplatin [C], vincristine [O], carboplatin [J], etoposide [E], and cyclophosphamide [C]) [36]. Treatment is done in three phases, starting with induction, followed by consolidation and post-consolidation phase. Induction chemotherapy is used to minimize primary and metastatic tumour burden and allow for attempts at local control in patients who have unresectable cancer. In the induction phase, multiagent chemotherapy is used, stem cell collection is done, and surgery can be done with the goal of complete resection of the tumour or > 90%, along with preserving critical organs.

Consolidation includes high-dose chemotherapy, autologous peripheral blood stem cell transplant (tandem superior to single) and radiotherapy.

Post-consolidation differentiation therapy with 13 cis-retinoic acid (BMT + cis RA-improves EFS/OS) and the addition of anti-GD2 immunotherapy increases EFS from 50–60%.

Novel approaches to the treatment of high-risk NB include ^{131}I MIBG therapy during induction, AntiGD-2 (early) during induction chemotherapy, the addition of Irinotecan in combination with temozolomide and Anti GD-2 for patients who fail to respond post induction [37–39]. Additionally, ALK inhibitors (lorlatinib) are used from induction throughout the three phases [40]. In post-consolidation, additional Irinotecan in combination with temozolomide and Anti GD-2 for patients has also been proposed. Some investigators have also investi-

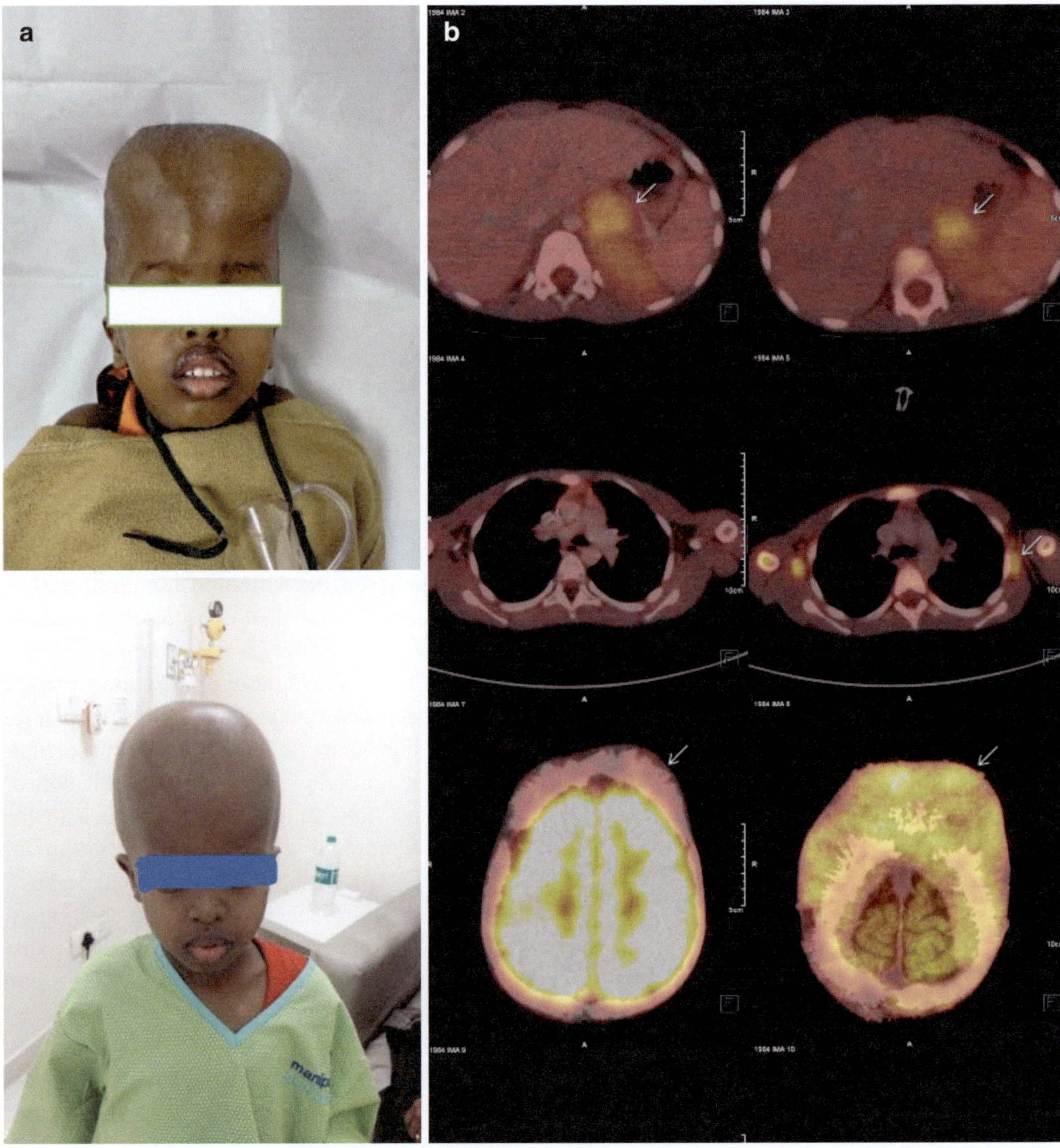

Fig. 2 Composite image showing (**a**) pre- and post-treatment clinical photographs of a child with neuroblastoma alongside corresponding (**b**) PET-CT scans demonstrating significant tumor regression; arrows highlight areas of disease

gated the role of ^{177}Lu- Dotatate in HR-NB. Immunotherapy techniques are being studied in people with relapsed and refractory neuroblastoma, like Chimeric antigen receptor (CAR) expressing T cells [41]. Figure 2 shows pre- and post-treatment pictures and corresponding radiology in a case of NB.

Radiotherapy

In low and intermediate-risk diseases, RT has a limited role. In high-risk diseases, RT is given during consolidation, following stem cell transplantation to the primary tumour to a dose of 21.6 Gray in 12 fractions (5 days a week) or 21Gray in 14 fractions (5 days a week). Boost to

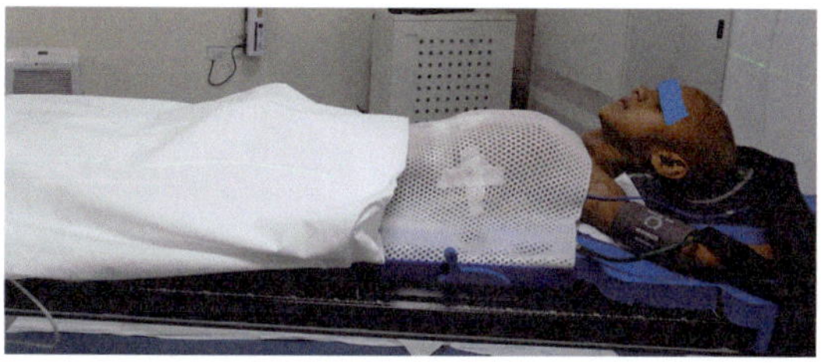

Fig. 3 Radiotherapy simulation setup demonstrating pediatric immobilization with thermoplastic mask for post-operative treatment of neuroblastoma

Table 9 Target volumes (as per COG)

Definition	Volume
GTV	Post-induction chemotherapy, pre-surgery residual disease
CTV	GTV + regional LN + 1–1.5 cm (edited off the anatomic border, edited off organs at risk, made sure surgical clips were adequately covered). Contour adjacent vertebrae on the bone window and Boolean with CTV (per physician discretion).
PTV	Depending on the site of tumour, as per institutional practice (e.g. 5 mm in neck and 1 cm in thorax and abdomen)

the residual gross tumour has not been shown to increase tumour control [42]. RT can be considered for metastatic soft tissue or bony sites that persist at the end of induction chemotherapy [27].

Simulation is done supine with arms overhead with/without anaesthesia. (Fig. 3) After immobilization, CT with or without contrast is planned with a slice thickness of not more than 3 mm—contouring as per standard guidelines (Table 9) [43].

Simple radiotherapy techniques with opposed anterior-posterior fields can be used in well-lateralized tumours (as it reduces the low-dose region exposure). VMAT/IMRT is preferred for centrally located tumours (Figs. 4 and 5). The main organs at risk (OARs) include the kidneys, spinal cord, and liver (Table 10). The prescribed dose is 21.6 Gy in 12 fractions to PTV. In the case of residual metastatic site post-induction therapy, 21.6 Gy in 12 fractions is prescribed. For symptomatic cord compression <3 years treat to 9Gy, if ≥3 years treat to 21.6 Gy (@1.8Gy/fraction). Symptomatic hepatomegaly is treated to 4.5–6 Gy (1.5 Gy x 3–4 fractions).

Survivors of neuroblastoma are at an elevated risk of long-term treatment-related morbidity and mortality [44]. Long-term follow-up as per the Children's Oncology Group (COG) recommendations for paediatric cancer survival is encouraged [45].

7 Wilms Tumour

Wilms tumour is considered the second most common abdominal tumour and constitutes 6% of all childhood cancers. Wilms tumour is the paradigm for the multidisciplinary treatment of paediatric malignant solid tumours. Wilms tumour develops as a result of abnormalities in the development of metanephric blastema. Wilms tumour is also known as nephroblastoma. It accounts for 6–8% of childhood cancer cases. This tumour occurs in about 8 in one million children under the age of 14 but is more common in children under the age of 5. Some children have a genetic tendency to develop Wilms tumour,

Wilms tumour has been reported to be associated with various anomalies. Genitourinary anomalies are the most common and account for an incidence of 4–8%. The anomalies include fused kidney, renal dysplasia, cryptorchidism, hypospadias, duplications of the collecting system, WAGR Syndrome (WT, aniridia, genitourinary abnormalities, and mental retardation). Wilms tumour is also featured in many disorders of overgrowth including Beckwith–Weildmann Syndrome, Perlman Syndrome, isolated hemihypertrophy. Although most patients with Wilms tumour are karyotypically average, genomic studies have led to the localization and subsequent cloning of WT genes in two regions — 11p13 and 11p15. The former is the *WT1* gene associated with WAGR Syndrome and the latter is the *WT2* gene associated with Beckwith-Wiedemann Syndrome.

Evaluation of patients should involve a proper history and physical Examination. One should look for the detection of an asymptomatic abdominal mass bulging in the flank. In addition,

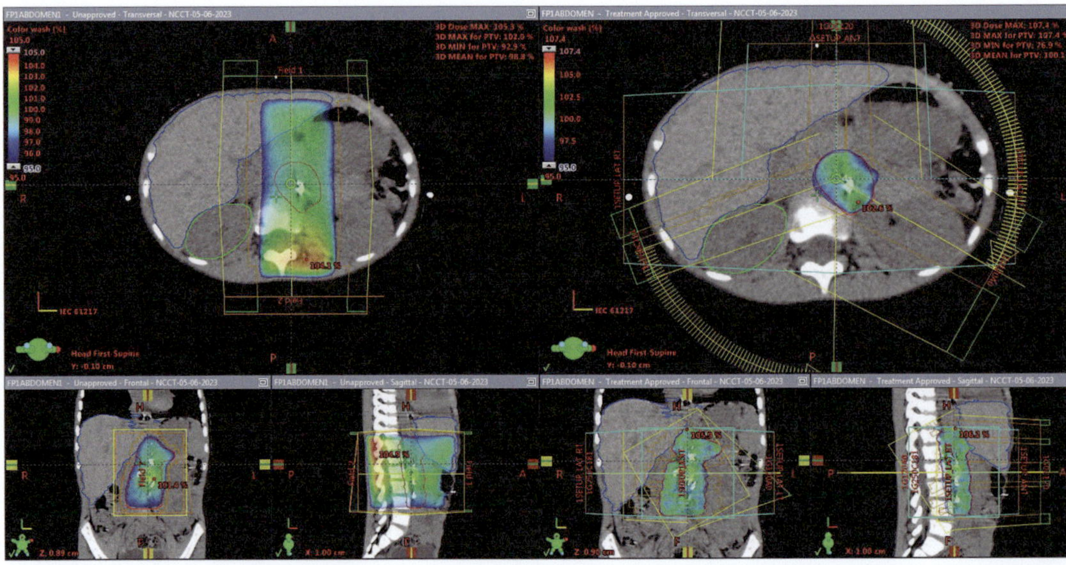

Fig. 4 CT-based dosimetric comparison of 95% isodose coverage between conventional AP–PA technique (**a**) and partial VMAT plan (**b**) in lateralized tumors

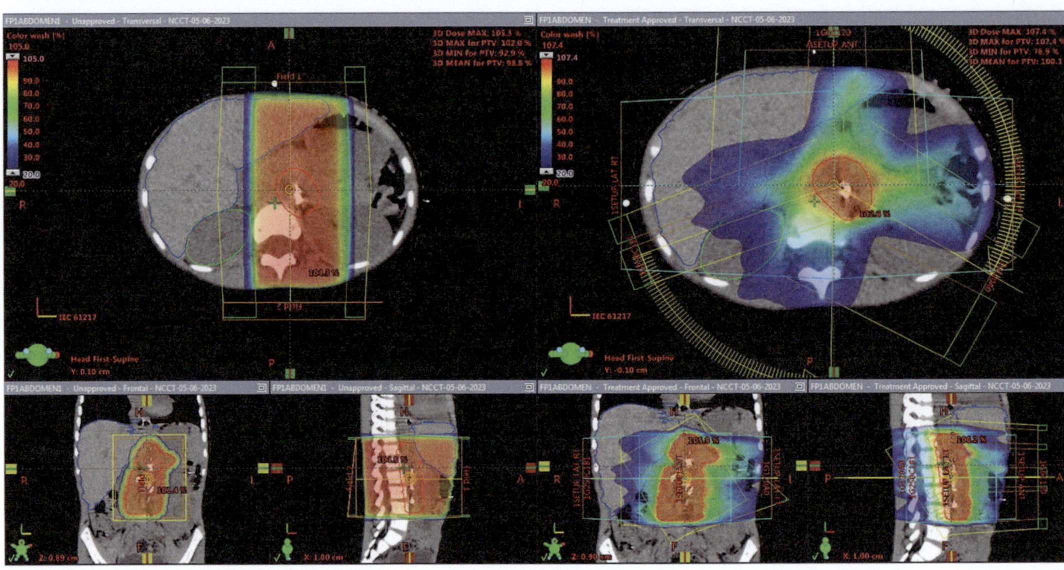

Fig. 5 CT Scan planning-based comparison of low dose distribution between AP-PA and partial VMAT plans for lateralized tumors; upper panel-antero-posterior dose distribution, lower panel- dose distribution in axial, coronal and sagittal planes

there can be nonspecific symptoms like abdominal pain, fatigue, and haematuria.

Investigation and their Purpose

1. Abdominal USG: To see the organ of origin, assess the contralateral kidney, evaluate the presence/absence of tumour thrombus in the IVC.
2. CT scan: To further evaluate the extent of the tumour. It helps see an extension into adjoining structures such as the liver, spleen and colon. It also aids in the visualization and

Table 10 Dose to OARs

OAR	Dose
Liver	Whole liver Dmean<19Gy 21.6 Gy is acceptable for 50% volume of liver
Spinal cord	Dmax<21.6Gy
Kidneys	Dmean<15Gy
Bone	Care must be taken to maintain the symmetry by irradiation of the whole vertebrae to around 21.6Gy. Limit gradient as per age group as follows 0–2 years- < △3 Gy 2–6 years- < △5Gy 6years to end of pubertal growth acceleration phase- < △ 5Gy After pubertal acceleration- all gradients are acceptable.

function of the contralateral kidney, ruling out metastatic disease.

3. Brain imaging (MRI/CT scan) Intracranial metastases in rhabdoid tumour of the kidney (RTK) and clear cell sarcoma pf the kidney (CCSK).
4. Fine needle aspiration cytology of mass: For cytological confirmation of diagnosis before nephrectomy/chemotherapy.

Surgery

Surgical staging includes the following components: (a) Examining the contralateral Kidney after opening Gerota's facia. (b) Retroperitoneal lymph node sampling (c) Palpation of the Liver surface.

The ideal pathology report should mention the clinical details, including age and gender. The gross specimen type (partial or radical nephrectomy) should be described, including laterality. Kidney size and weight needs to be specified. Tumour size, tumour characteristics, number of tumour nodules, and most significant dimensions of all nodules should be stated. If multiple, the location of these nodules, state of cortex and hilum—Gerota's fascia intact or disrupted, renal vein invasion present and adrenal involvement, if any, need to be stated. In microscopy, the pathologist needs to display the (a) type (Wilms tumour favourable histology, Wilms tumour with anaplasia, (unfavourable)-focal/diffuse), (b) Nephrogenic rests—type (intralobar, perilobar, unclassified), (c) Margins uninvolved/Cannot be assessed/involved—Distance of all margins, directions of Involved margins (Gerota's fascia, Renal vessels, Ureter) d) Renal sinus (whether involved or not) Regional lymph nodes (number and involvement) e) National Wilms tumour registry Stage.

Surgical Issues

Radical nephrectomy and lymph node sampling via a transabdominal or thoracoabdominal incision is the procedure of choice. Tumour removal should be complete and en bloc, not rupturing the capsule. Sampling and histological examination of all lymph nodes are critical. Renal-sparing surgery is recommended in children with bilateral WT or those predisposed to develop bilateral tumours (e.g., syndromes such as Denys–Drash or Frasier syndrome) and in children with single/horseshoe kidneys. Nephron sparing surgery or partial nephrectomy is not recommended in standard unilateral WT due to the increased risk of tumour spill leading to recurrence and the relatively low risk of developing end-stage renal disease.

Chemotherapy in Wilms Tumour

For Localized unilateral Wilms Tumour, the Optimal duration of pre-operative chemotherapy is 4 weeks. For Stage I and II diseases, 18 weeks of therapy with Vincristine and Actinomycin D is adequate for patients with FH.

For Stage I intermediate-risk and anaplastic Wilms tumour, post-operative treatment could be shortened to only 4 weeks from the standard 18 weeks.

For Stage III and IV FH, 6 months of therapy with Vincristine, Adriamycin, and Actinomycin D is optimal. For Stage II- III intermediate-risk histology (epithelial/stromal): 27 post-operative weeks of Vincristine, actinomycin D should be considered. The addition of Adriamycin improves EFS in large-volume (≥500 ml) stage II–III nonstromal, nonepithelial tumours. Intensification of treatment for post-chemotherapy blastemal predominant Wilms Tumour improves EFS and should be considered. The prognosis for patients with stage III FH is best when treatment includes either three-drug chemotherapy and 10.8 Gy of radiation therapy to the flank or two drugs of chemotherapy and 20 Gy of radiation therapy to the side. The outcome of patients with peritoneal implants treated with gross resection, three-drug chemotherapy, and whole abdominal radiation (10.5 Gy) is similar to that of other stage III patients.

Radiation Therapy in Wilms Tumour
Indications for radiotherapy in Wilms tumour include

- Stage I unfavourable histology (focal anaplasia/diffuse anaplasia) WT, rhabdoid tumour of the kidney (RTK) and clear cell sarcoma of the kidney (CCSK).
- Stage II unfavourable histology.
- Stage III and IV favourable and unfavourable histology.
- Local recurrence.
- Palliative radiotherapy for metastatic disease.

Radiotherapy should be started within 10 days of surgery. There is no change in radiotherapy dose for favourable and unfavourable histology, except for stage III Wilms tumour with diffuse anaplasia where dose is increased from 10.8 Gy to 19.8 Gy. Rhabdoid tumours should be treated as a separate entity.

Target volume: Volume should encompass tumour bed + site of excised kidney with a 2 cm margin—entire vertebral body to be contained in the RT portal. For Stage II, the volume is Tumour bed only. Volumes for stages III and IV are given in Table 11. Radiation doses are mentioned in Table 12.

Stage III and IV Disease
Positive hilar nodes Positive paraaortic nodes Gross or microscopic residuum Confined to flank Peritoneal seeding Gross residual abdominal disease Diffuse spillage at surgery Preoperative intraperitoneal rupture Lung Metastases. The indications of whole abdominal irradiation (WAI) include preoperative tumour rupture, intraoperative tumour spillage, diffuse peritoneal implants/seedings and malignant/haemorrhagic ascites. Figure 5 above shows dose distribution in a case of WT treated by partial abdomen irradiation can be improved by VMAT technique. Figure 6 shows a comparison of WAI versus a new concept of kidney-sparing WAI.

Treatment of Pulmonary Metastases
Pulmonary metastasis (single or multiple) may result from any paediatric malignancy, including Wilms tumour, Ewing Sarcoma, Rhabdomyosarcoma, or other sarcomas. Pulmonary metastases may occur at diagnosis or at relapse.

Table 11 Radiation volume in Wilms tumour

Extent of disease	Radiotherapy volume
Positive hilar nodes	Flank (operative bed) crossing midline to include bilateral paraaortic nodes.
Positive paraaortic nodes	Flank (operative bed) crossing midline to include bilateral paraaortic nodes.
Gross or microscopic residuum	Flank (operative bed) crossing midline to include bilateral paraaortic nodes
Confined to flank	Flank (operative bed) crossing midline to include bilateral paraaortic nodes
Peritoneal seeding	WAR with shielding of the acetabulum and bilateral femoral heads
Gross residual abdominal disease	Boost tumour >3 cm
Diffuse spillage at surgery	WAR with shield acetabulum and femoral heads
Preoperative intraperitoneal rupture	WAR with shield acetabulum and femoral heads
Lung metastases	Whole lung (bilateral)

WAR whole abdomen radiotherapy

Table 12 Radiation dose in Wilms tumour

Characteristics	Dose
Stage I and II FH,	No radiation therapy
Stage I anaplastic	10.8Gy
Stage III FH, stage IV FN with abdominal Stage III, stage II anaplastic, stage I-IV Clear cell sarcoma/ Rhabdoid tumour of Kidney	10.8 Gy to flank +10Gy Boost to gross residual disease (>3crn)
Stage III-IV WT with diffuse anaplasia	19.8Gy/11fractions
Stage IV (lung metastases)	12-Gy whole- lung Irradiation
Stage IV (liver metastases)	19.8 Gy to liver
Stage IV (brain metastases)	30.6 Gy to whole brain
Stage IV (bone metastases)	30.6 Gy to the tumour with 3 cm margin
Relapsed Wilms tumour	12.6–18Gy (< 12 months of age) and 21.6Gy in older Children if the previous radiation dose is 10.8Gy. Boost of up to 9Gy to gross Residual disease after surgery. Total dose Including previous radiation not to exceed 30.6Gy (< 1 year age) and 39.5Gy (* 2 year age)

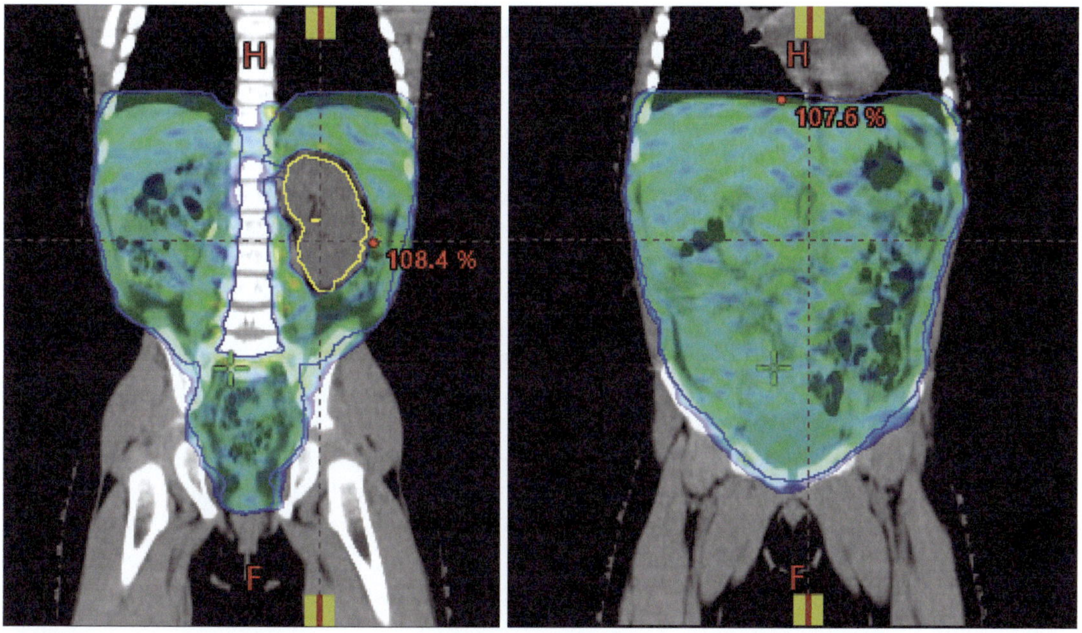

Fig. 6 CT-based treatment planning comparison of kidney-sparing whole abdomen irradiation (**a**) and conventional whole abdomen irradiation (**b**) (10.5 Gy in 7 fractions over 8 days); blue denotes the PTV and yellow outlines the left kidney

For stage IV Wilms tumour patients with lung metastasis, the current approach is to deliver whole lung irradiation (WLI) only when there is residual pulmonary disease after chemotherapy. This treatment increases the risk of radiation dose exposure to the thyroid gland. 12 Gy in 8 fractions to the lung, one fraction per day (with cardiac sparing), is a reasonable regime in indicated cases. However, Pulmonary RT can be omitted for patients with pulmonary metastasis and a complete response after induction chemotherapy with or without surgery.

The COG AREN0533 (NCT00379340) trial used a novel approach to enhance overall survival (EFS) and minimize lung irradiation in patients with FH Wilms tumour and isolated lung metastases, drawing on the European experience. The treatment was modified based on the response of the lung nodules and the particular loss of heterozygosity at 1p and 16q in the tumour [46].

Out of the total sample size of 292 participants included in the trial, 133 individuals (42%) exhibited a comprehensive response to lung nodules after a 6-week course of DD-4A (vincristine, dactinomycin, doxorubicin). These patients adhered to the same chemotherapy regimen without undergoing lung radiation treatment. The long-term survival rate was 80%, and overall survival rate was 96%.

A cohort of 145 patients had an inadequate response to lung nodules, while 18 patients experienced loss of heterozygosity at 1p/16q. These patients were administered lung radiation treatment along with four cycles of cyclophosphamide/etoposide, in addition to the DD-4A medicines (regimen M). The partial lung nodule response group without loss of heterozygosity had a 4-year EFS rate of 89% and an OS rate of 95%. The 4-year overall survival (EFS) and overall survival (OS) rates were 100% for patients with just lung metastases and loss of heterozygosity.

In a retrospective investigation of 1q gain in a cohort of 212 patients participating in AREN0533, wherein DNA data was accessible, it was shown that patients who had full remission of lung nodules and exhibited 1q gain demonstrated a substantially worse 4-year estimated survival rate (57% vs. 86%, $P = 0.001$) and a tendency towards poorer overall survival rates (89% vs. 97%). The relapses mostly affected the lungs. Patients with partial lung nodule response did not see any difference in outcome based on 1q gain.

Regimen M has an elevated propensity for late sequelae, namely, an augmented susceptibility to additional leukaemias and an increased likelihood of infertility, which may be attributed to a cumulative dosage of 8.8 g/m2 of cyclophosphamide.

The COG study showed that over 40% of patients might be spared from undergoing early lung radiation treatment. The overall performance (OS) was outstanding; yet, there was a tendency towards a higher number of incidents than anticipated (15%) and observed (20%) ($P = 0.052$).

While the COG experiment resulted in a lower number of patients receiving pulmonary radiation treatment compared to the European trials, it is crucial to acknowledge several disparities between the studies and the reasons why direct comparisons between them are not feasible. In Europe, patients are administered a higher dosage of dactinomycin and doxorubicin prior to reassessing their pulmonary metastases, in comparison to patients in North America. In Europe, patients receive a dosage of 135 ug/kg of dactinomycin and 100 mg/m^2 of doxorubicin, whereas in North America, patients receive a dosage of 45 ug/kg of dactinomycin and 45 mg/m^2 of doxorubicin. European studies permit the exclusion of lung radiation treatment for patients who have achieved full remission via chemotherapy or pulmonary metastasectomy, but in the United States, radiation therapy is only excluded for patients who have achieved complete remission alone by chemotherapy. The European trials did not undergo central review, unlike the United States, and the AREN0533 (NCT00379340) study may have had a more rigorous definition of full remission.

Treatment Outcomes Children diagnosed with a Wilms tumour have a 5-year relative survival rate of 93%.

The survival rates among paediatric patients diagnosed with a Wilms tumour exhibit variability due to many variables. These factors include the tumour's stage, an individual's age and overall health, and the efficacy of the treatment regimen. The recurrence rate of a Wilms tumour after therapy ranges from 15% to 50%, with the highest likelihood occurring during the first 2 years post-treatment.

Tumours classified as Stage I, II, and III, exhibiting good histology, have a relative survival rate of 95% to 100% over 4 years. Tumour histology refers to the microscopic appearance of its cells. Tumours classified as Stage IV and V, exhibiting good histology, have a relative survival rate of 85% to 100% over 4 years. Tumours with focal anaplastic histology often have reduced survival rates in each group, ranging from 70% to 100%. The survival rates for tumours with diffuse anaplastic histology vary between 30% and 85% across various stage groups. [https://www.cancer.net/cancer-types/wilms-tumor-childhood/statistics. Last assessed on 27.03.2024].

8 Rhabdomyosarcoma

Rhabdomyosarcoma (RMS) is a fast-growing, highly malignant soft-tissue sarcoma that develops in the muscle, mainly in the head, neck, bladder, and testes. It accounts for 5–8% of childhood cancers. It usually affects children aged 2–6 and 15–19. Most cases of RMS occur sporadically, and often, no recognized predisposing risk factor is found.

Some predisposing factors include

- Genetic factors include
  - Li-Fraumeni syndrome (with germline *TP53* mutations)
  - *DICER1* syndrome
  - Costello syndrome
  - Beckwith-Wiedemann syndrome
  - Neurofibromatosis type I (NF1)
- Higher weight at birth and large size for gestational age are occasionally associated with an increased incidence of embryonal RMS.

Investigations

PETCT/CT/MRI of the primary site (MRI is preferred in para meningeal, paraspinal, and pelvic masses, including bladder and prostate). Pathology examination includes a biopsy (or upfront excision where feasible) of the primary site. On immunohistochemistry they stain with MyoD1, myoglobin, myosin, desmin and vimentin.

Molecular studies for t(1:13) and t(2:13) should be done. Whole-body PET-CT or CT Chest, abdomen, whole-body bone scan, and bone marrow examination are indicated for metastatic staging.

CSF cytology needs to be done for parameningeal locations.

RMS patients need to be risk-stratified. This stratification depends on

1. Pretreatment TNM staging.
2. Surgical grouping.
3. Age and histology (molecular).

Types of RMS and their corresponding molecular features are as follows

Embryonal RMS Characterized by loss of heterozygosity (LOH) at 11p15 and by a high frequency of mutations in the RAS pathway.

Alveolar RMS Characterized by gene fusions involving *FOXO1* with either *PAX3* or *PAX7.*

Spindle cell/sclerosing RMS characterized by *NCOA2* gene rearrangements in young children.

Pleomorphic RMS Complex karyotypes with numerical and unbalanced structural changes.

The most common primary sites for RMS include

- Head and neck region (parameningeal) (25%).
- Genitourinary tract (approximately 30%).
- Extremities (approximately 15%). Within extremity tumours, tumours of the hand and foot occur more often in older patients and usually have an alveolar histology.

Other less common primary sites include the trunk, chest wall, perineal/anal region, and abdomen, including the retroperitoneum and biliary tract.

Site Implications

Favourable sites include orbit, non-para meningeal head and neck, genitourinary tract (other than bladder and prostate), and biliary tract.

Unfavourable sites include the rest of the sites. Parameningeal sites include the middle ear, nasal cavity, paranasal sinuses, nasopharynx, and pterygoid-infratemporal fossa.

Staging

T1—Confined to the anatomic site of origin (non-invasive).

T2a—With Tumour extension and fixation to surrounding tissues (invasive); Tumour less than or equal to 5 cm in maximum diameter.

T2b—Tumour extension and fixation to surrounding tissues (invasive); Tumour greater than 5 cm in maximum diameter.

N information N0—absence of nodal spread N1—presence of regional nodes beyond the primary disease NX—Unknown nodal status. M information M0—absence of metastatic spread M1—presence of metastatic spread beyond the prior site and regional lymph nodes.

Another system of Simplified Risk Stratification is sometimes used. In this system, three risk categories are considered [47].

1. High-risk: All Metastatic (M1) diseases, irrespective of histology.
2. Intermediate-risk: Locoregional ARMS, Unresectable ERMS at unfavourable site.
3. Low-risk: ERMS at favourable location, completely resected ERMS at damaging sites.

Surgery (Local Control Management)

Surgical removal of the entire tumour, if the same is possible, should be considered initially. However, surgery should be attempted only if there is no likely functional and cosmetic impairment [48]. Complete gross primary tumour removal, with a surrounding margin of normal tissue, is recommended. In some tumour sites, sampling of regional draining lymph nodes is recommended. In patients older than 10 years, Children's Oncology Group (COG) protocols require regional draining node sampling in extremity tumours and para testicular tumours. Important exceptions to achieving an R0 resection (negative margins) are in tumours of the genitourinary region and the orbit.

There is no evidence that debulking surgery improves outcomes compared with biopsy alone. Therefore, debulking surgery is not recommended for patients with rhabdomyosarcoma [49]. It is preferable to use induction chemotherapy to reduce tumour size and then attempt an R0 resection.

Chemotherapy in RMS

Rhabdomyosarcoma is a chemo-sensitive childhood neoplasm. For RMS, chemotherapy is usually given once a week during the initial months and less frequently. The total duration of treatment typically ranges from 6 months to a year.

A combination of drugs is used to treat RMS. The specific medicines depend on the patient's risk group:

For the Low-risk group, Common combinations include:

VA: Vincristine and dactinomycin (also known as actinomycin-D).

VAC: Vincristine, dactinomycin, and cyclophosphamide.

For the Intermediate-risk group, common regimens include:

VAC: Vincristine, dactinomycin, and cyclophosphamide.

VAC/VI: Alternating vincristine, dactinomycin and cyclophosphamide with vincristine and irinotecan. Researchers are studying whether adding the targeted drug temsirolimus to the VAC/VI regimen improves efficacy.

The VAC regimen is commonly used for the high-risk group (including metastatic disease). Intense chemotherapy with additional drugs (such as doxorubicin, ifosfamide and etoposide) has also been explored. Higher doses of chemotherapy followed by a stem cell transplant have also been considered, but their benefits are not yet clear. Clinical trials testing new drugs and combinations are recommended for high-risk patients.

RT (Local Control Management)

Despite improvement in the outcomes, the local failure remains a challenge. RT has always been an effective method for achieving local control of the tumour for patients with microscopic or gross residual disease after biopsy, surgical resection, or chemotherapy.

Group I: Patients with wholly resected *embryonal* RMS at diagnosis before initiation of chemotherapy do well without RT. However, because approximately 75% of embryonal rhabdomyosarcoma patients are Groups II to IV, RT is used in most patients. COG recommends the use of RT for all patients with *FOXO1* fusion–positive disease (these were previously called alveolar rhabdomyosarcoma).

Group II: In more than 50% of Group II rhabdomyosarcoma patients, local recurrence resulted from noncompliance with guidelines or omission of RT [49].

Group III: Approximately 35% of patients with Group III disease either do not achieve complete remission or relapse locally. Those patients who have =involved regional lymph nodes at diagnosis also have a higher risk of local and distant failure as compared to patients whose lymph nodes are uninvolved [50].

Treatment Volume

Several factors determine the treated radiation volume. These include the extent of the tumour at diagnosis before surgical resection and before chemotherapy, including clinically involved regional lymph nodes. Modern techniques may use a margin of 1 cm–1.5 cm for clinical target volume margins [49, 51]. This clinical tumour volume should be modified based on anatomical constraints. CTV needs consideration when the tumour is pushing rather than invading the adjacent normal tissues or when adjacent normal tissues are functionally critical (e.g., head and neck RMS). Planning target volume should be added as per institutional practice and protocols.

The volume irradiated may be further modified because of considerations for standard tissue tolerance. However, patients with gross residual disease at the time of RT should receive full-dose RT. A reduction in volume after 36 Gy is appropriate in chemoresponsive disease for patients with a regressed size of non-invasive displacement (T1). However, this should be avoided for invasive tumours (T2). Gross residual disease should receive the total RT dose (50.4–59.4 Gy, the higher dose if >5 cm at diagnosis). RT doses are tabulated in Table 13.

For involved nodal sites, the treated volume is defined as the extent of nodal involvement at diagnosis plus a 2–3 cm margin superiorly and inferiorly in the direction of lymphatic drainage. In cases of uncertainty, the inclusion of the entire nodal chain should be done.

For metastatic disease, the treated volume is the extent of metastases at diagnosis. In the case of lung or extensive brain metastases, the whole organ is irradiated. Similarly, the entire peritoneal cavity is included in the case of diffuse peritoneal metastases. The use of novel techniques, such as stereotactic body RT to appropriate sites (e.g., bone or small volume soft tissue metastases), can be considered.

Timing of RT

The general practice is to allow for chemotherapy to be given for up to 3 months before RT is initiated. RT is typically administered over 5–6 weeks (e.g., 1.8 Gy once per day, 5 days per week). During this time, chemotherapy is usually modified to avoid the radiosensitizing agents dactinomycin, doxorubicin, and temsirolimus. Another consideration related to radiation therapy is that the administration of RT before a planned second surgical excision may help achieve R0 resection. Pre-op RT might facilitate surgical resection to decrease the chances of loss of form or function. This approach is protocol-dependent or, as per institutional practice. Parameningeal RMS needs special attention and it is recommended to start RT as early as 6 to 9 weeks from Day1 of systemic chemotherapy.

For metastatic sites, RT is usually given after 16 to 20 weeks of chemotherapy or, rarely, as consolidation after planned chemotherapy.

Thus, conventional RT remains the standard for treating patients who have rhabdomyosarcoma with gross residual disease. The following

Table 13 Radiation Therapy (RT) Dose According to Rhabdomyosarcoma Group, Histology, and Site of Disease (Children's Oncology Group [COG]

Group	Treatment
Group I	
Fusion negative (embryonal)	RT is not required.
FOXO1 fusion-positive	36 Gy to involved (prechemotherapy) site.
Group II	
N0 (microscopic residual disease after surgery)	36 Gy dose to involved (prechemotherapy) site.
N1 (resected regional lymph node involvement)	36 Gy dose to the involved (prechemotherapy) site and 41.4 Gy dose to nodes.
Group III	
Orbital and nonorbital tumours	45 Gy dose for orbital tumours with complete response after chemotherapy. For other sites and orbital tumours in partial remission, 50.4 Gy with volume reduction after 36 Gy in patients with excellent response to chemotherapy (or complete remission after delayed re-excision) and non-invasive Pushing tumours; no volume reduction for invasive tumours. 59.4 Gy Boost to residual disease at 9 weeks for tumours >5 cm at diagnosis (if enrolled on the COG ARST1431 [NCT02567435]) protocol.
N1 with gross residual disease after surgery/chemotherapy	50.4 Gy
Group IV	
	As for other groups, including all metastatic sites, if safe and possible. Exception: Lung (pulmonary metastases) treated with 12 Gy to 15 Gy in 8–10 fractions, depending on age.

Table 14 General contours for RMS

Volumes	For 36Gy	For 50.4Gy
GTV	Initial disease	Post-chemotherapy volume (if no response, GTV = pre-chemo volume)
CTV	GTV + 0.5 to 1 cm	GTV + 0.5 to 1 cm
PTV	CTV + 0.3–0.5 cm	CTV + 0.3–0.5 cm
For LN involvement- 41.4Gy to involved nodal region		

factors are to be considered while planning: clinical group and dose, histology, surgical records, previous imaging, age, tumour location, organs at risk, and the cost of survival and optimal simulation and immobilization techniques.

General contours and site-specific for RMS and dose constraints for OAR's are shown in Tables 14, 15 and 16.

Brachytherapy

Brachytherapy in RMS can be used for appropriate cases in intracavitary applications or interstitial implants., is another effective method of local control that has been used in selected situations for children with RMS. The sites suitable for this treatment include the vaginal site and selected bladder/prostate sites [52]. Other sites, e.g., some head and neck subsites, have also been treated with brachytherapy.

Local Control Treatment of Children Aged Three Years and Younger

Rhabdomyosarcoma presents a therapeutic challenge in very young children (aged ≤36 months) due to their heightened risk of treatment-related complications. When delayed surgery can

Table 15 Site-specific contours

Parameningeal RMS A planning CT from vertex to clavicle is acquired using a head and neck mask with a 3 mm slice thickness with or without intravenous (IV) contrast. It is recommended to use pre-treatment imaging for registration with RT planning CT scan. GTV- initial disease CTV GTV+ 0.5 to 1 cm margin.
Orbital RMS CTV GTV+ 0.5 to 1 cm margin. PTV- as per institutional protocol. Recommended dose- 45Gy
Paratesticular RMS A body foam for immobilization in the frog-leg position may be used. CTV should include positive ipsilateral LN after lymph node dissection
Extremities Immobilization is essential for optimal beam arrangement. It includes oedema and can edit the PTV of bones and joints. It is better to spare a strip of tissue (lymphovascular corridor of 1–2 cm width) and not to irradiate the limb circumferentially.
Bladder and prostate RMS Contouring principles are the same as other sites—Bladder protocol should be adhered to.

Table 16 OAR dose constraints

Organ at risk	Primary criteria	Secondary criteria
Optic nerves	Dmax < 50Gy Dmax- < 54Gy	Dmax < 55Gy
Optic chiasm	Dmax < 52Gy Dmax < 54Gy V50Gy < 100%	Dmax < 55Gy
Hippocampus		V7.2Gy < 40% V20Gy < 20% Dmean < 30Gy
Cochlea	Dmean < 35Gy Dmean < 37Gy	Dmax < 40Gy
Brainstem	Dmax < 54Gy	Dmax < 60Gy V54-59Gy < 10 cc
Bladder	45Gy	
Heart	30Gy	
Liver- whole Liver- partial (50%)	23.4Gy 30.6Gy	
Spinal cord	45Gy	
Rectum	45Gy	
Peritoneum (whole abdomen pelvis)	24Gy	
Kidney- whole Kidney-partial (50%)	14.40Gy 19.8Gy	
Lung-whole Lung (when PTV >1/2 bilateral lung) Lung (when PTV <1/2 bilateral lung)	12Gy 15Gy 18Gy	

achieve negative margins, reduced radiation doses are employed. However, for patients where surgical resection is not feasible, higher doses of radiation therapy (RT) are administered.

Radiation techniques aim to spare normal tissues and often involve conformal approaches, including intensity-modulated radiation therapy (IMRT) or proton therapy. Even in Stage 1 disease, omitting radiation increases the risk of recurrence, particularly local recurrence, underscoring the importance of RT.

Delayed primary excision allows for a reduction in radiation dosage. However, concerns about normal tissue toxicity often lead to inadequate RT in the youngest patients. Surgical resection via delayed primary excision remains crucial for these patients.

Rates of local control from delayed primary excision and reduced-dose RT are comparable to those from RT alone.

Treatment Outcomes Prognosis depends upon the tumour site. Survival at 5 years is as follows

(a) Orbit- 97%.
(b) Head and Neck (Non parameningeal)- 83%.
(c) Cranial parameningeal- 69.5%.
(d) Genitourinary (excluding bladder/prostate)-89%.
(e) Localized bladder/prostate- 84%.
(f) Localized extremity- 67%.
(g) Trunk, abdomen, perineum- 67%.
(h) Biliary-76.5–78%.

Retinoblastoma is a type of orbital tumour in the retina of one or both eyes. It is the most common eye tumour in children. Retinoblastoma accounts for 3–5% of all childhood cancers. It usually occurs before the age of 5. Retinoblastoma has been covered in detail in the relevant chapter of this book, Orbital and Ocular tumors.

9 Osteosarcoma and Ewing's sarcoma

These tumours are the most common malignancies of bone tissues in children. Osteosarcoma usually presents in bones around the knee, whereas Ewing's sarcoma may affect the pelvis, femur, humerus, or ribs. Bone tumours are most common in ages 10–20, and they account for about 5–6% of all childhood cancers. More details of these tumours are given in the relevant chapter of this book, Bone and Soft Tissue Tumors.

10 Germ Cell Tumours

Germ cell tumours have been discussed in detail in the relevant chapter of this book, Uro-Oncology.

11 Immobilization and Planning for Paediatric Tumours

Immobilization cast preparation and simulation in a child-friendly environment should be done. The child should be treated on the same machine daily. In children not undergoing sedation, communication by the child in the treatment room with his parents outside is a good practice so that the child does not feel alone. In children who are borderline candidates for sedation/anaesthesia, it is a good practice to give a sedation-free trial after 4–5 sessions of radiotherapy. Using plans with fewer monitor units/treatment time and avoiding too many noncoplanar beams is a good practice.

Paediatric Anaesthesia for Radiotherapy
Radiation oncology is a cornerstone of paediatric cancer therapy. There are several challenges for anaesthesia and oncologists. Although painless, the children must lie still for radiation planning and treatment for several sessions. Anaesthesia or sedation is required in younger children (especially <5 years). Most of the time, younger children need sedation for cast-making/planning. A friendly atmosphere/play area may lessen the need for sedation/anaesthesia [52]. It is sometimes worthwhile for a child who initially required sedation to be challenged by sedation-free sessions.

Radiation therapy in paediatric oncology cases is now becoming more and more common. Even though most radiation therapies are painless, children often require sedation because of the fear and anxiety of being away from their parents. Most radiation procedures are of short-duration, feasible with short sedation, and never require complete general anaesthesia [53]. The following is a standard sedation protocol for paediatric oncology cases:

Child safety is increased by a thorough pre-anaesthesia evaluation and an integrated team approach. Once the radiation oncologist plans for the procedure, a paediatric sedation clearance is taken from the paediatric intensivist. The purpose of this is to anticipate and rule out any possible adverse event related to sedative drugs. The child is assessed for any problematic airway and the presence of any active chest infection (paediatric patients react abnormally to sedation drugs in the presence of upper or lower respiratory tract infections).

Once the paediatric intensivist clears the child, the patient is given an appointment for the procedure with the advice to bring the child in the fasting state (minimum 4 h fasting in case of a light meal and 6 h fasting if the child has taken a full meal).

The child is again assessed for signs of upper or lower respiratory infection during the procedure. The required preparation of the process includes checking all the equipment for paediatric resuscitation (Laryngoscope, Ambu bag, ET tubes of sizes needed, O2 and suction sources, O2 mask, suction apparatus, suction catheters) and preparation of sedative drugs (preferred drugs for short procedures in our unit are Ketamine and Midazolam).

At the start of the procedure, the child is connected to the monitor, and pre-procedure vitals are recorded on the paediatric sedation chart (including HR, RR, BP, and SpO2). Ketamine is used in a dose of 1 mg/kg along with Midazolam 0.1 mg/kg as slow i.v bolus. Most of the short sedation procedures do not require any premedication. Once the desired sedation is achieved, the radiation procedure is started.

Since radiation procedures are painless and of short duration (max time 10 min), usually single doses of Ketamine and Midazolam or propofol and midazolam are enough. In case the procedure gets prolonged (especially during PET CT/Mask preparation), Ketamine and Midazolam are used alternatively as a top-up to maintain the patient's position.

At the end of the procedure, an antiemetic (Inj Ondansetron @ 0.2 mg/kg) is given to prevent post-procedure nausea or vomiting. Post-procedure vitals are recorded, and the child is closely monitored for respiratory or hemodynamic compromise. Parents are counselled about the post-sedation precautions and observation period.

Once the child recovers from the sedation effect, is fully conscious, oriented and recognizing parents, the child is given sips of water. If there is no vomiting over the next 5–10 min, the child is discharged with the advice to continue with liquids for the next 2–3 h. Solids are usually allowed 4–6 h post-procedure.

The exact process is followed every day for the duration of the radiation therapy.

Table 17 First and corresponding second malignancies in paediatric patients

First malignancy	Second malignancy
RB, Ewing's sarcoma, STS, other bone tumours, ALL	Bone tumours
RB, STS, Wilms tumour, bone tumours, ALL, HD, brain tumours	Soft-tissue sarcoma
HD, bone tumours, STS, ALL, medulloblastoma, Wilms tumour, NHL	Breast cancer
ALL, HD, NB, STS, bone tumours, NHL	Thyroid cancer
ALL, brain tumours, HD	Brain tumours
ALL, NB, STS HD	Carcinomas
ALL HD, bone tumours	AML/ALL

Retinoblastoma (RB); heritable type. *STS* soft-tissue sarcoma, *HD* Hodgkin disease, *NB* neuroblastoma, *NHL* Non-Hodgkin lymphoma, *ALL* acute lymphocytic leukaemia, *AML* acute myelogenous leukaemia

SECOND MALIGNANCIES (SM)

- ❖ Overall rate 3-4% at 25 years
- ❖ Survivors of childhood cancer = 3 to 6 fold higher risk of SM than the general population
- ❖ Average latency period approximately 15 years
- ❖ Chemotherapy used along with RT increases risk
- ❖ Solid tumours 70-80% of all SM
- ❖ Bone & soft tissue sarcomas most common SM
- ❖ Risk dose linear relation; increases with time period

Fig. 7 Summary of long-term incidence, latency, and treatment-related risk factors for second malignancies in survivors of pediatric cancers

11.1 Palliative Care for Paediatric Tumours

Palliative care focuses on relieving symptoms caused by the illness, such as pain, nausea, and fatigue, and providing psychosocial support to patients and their families. Paediatric palliative care is considered a core component of comprehensive care, starting when the illness is diagnosed and continuing throughout treatment and care, regardless of whether or not a child receives therapy with curative intent. Palliative care programs can be delivered through community and home-based care, providing much-needed pain relief and psychosocial support to patients and their respective families. It is essential to ensure adequate access to oral morphine and other pain medicines for the treatment of moderate to severe cancer-related pain, which affects more than 80% of cancer patients in the terminal phase of their illness.

11.2 Toxicities of Treatment in Paediatric Tumours

Children have lower tolerance to radiation due to growing tissues and are consequently likely to suffer more damage. Treatment often involves a large treatment volume compared to their overall body volume. Immobilization issues, which can be challenging in children, too can have an impact on toxicity. Growing bones, pituitary, thyroid, heart, and lungs are organs that need special attention and protection during the radiotherapy course. Cognitive preservation is also a critical issue in patients undergoing cranial irradiation. Also, there is a risk of producing radiation-induced second malignancy. Many modern-day treatments, such as IMRT or arc therapy, may result in asymmetric organ doses leading to asymmetric growth patterns in children.

Issues related to sexual maturation can also arise from cranial irradiation or exposure of gonads to radiotherapy. In relevant cases, this counselling needs to be done before the start of the radiotherapy course. Methods include elimi-

Precepts Box

1. Constitutional symptoms like weight loss, unexplained fever, pallor and fatigue, neurological symptoms like headaches with vomiting in the morning, afebrile seizures, vision loss, or palpable abdominal or mediastinal mass, warrant an oncological workup
2. Paediatric cancer is treatable if identified early and treated correctly
3. Children with cancer arrive late and at a more advanced stage, with inadequate awareness, delayed diagnosis and therapy discontinuation being important management challenges, especially in low-income countries like India.
4. Childhood cancer differs from adults in terms of rarity, high cure rates if diagnosed early, many special requirements and high burden of late effects.
5. Common paediatric tumours are leukaemia, lymphoma, brain tumours, Wilms tumour, bone cancer among others.
6. Neuroblastomas (NB) are the most common extracranial malignancy in infancy with a heterogenous behaviour. Molecular drivers include NMYC and ALK amplification, ATRX and ARID mutations, TERT rearrangements. Diagnosis includes 24-h VMA, Serum LDH and Ferritin analysis. Radiologically, a PET-CT/ MRI/ MIBG scan is used to identify these tumours.
7. NBs are staged by INSS or INGRSS. Treatment is according to the stage and risk stratification. In low-risk NB, surgical excision may be sufficient treatment. Intermediate-risk NB are treated with chemotherapy and surgery. High-risk NB, treatment is given in three phases—induction with chemotherapy or surgery, consolidation with

(continued)

chemotherapy, BMT and RT and post-consolidation with cis-retinoic acid.

8. RT has a limited role in NB, given in the consolidation phase after stem cell transplant in high-risk patients or in persistent metastatic disease at the end of induction phase. Dose recommended is 21.6 Gy in 12 fractions.
9. Wilms tumour (WT) is the second most common abdominal tumour and constitutes 6 % of all childhood cancers.
10. Treatment of Wilms Tumor is multidisciplinary with surgery, chemotherapy and RT all playing important roles. Radical nephrectomy and lymph node sampling is the procedure of choice. Tumour removal should be complete and en bloc, taking care not to rupture the capsule.
11. Chemotherapy is started pre-operatively and is continued post-surgery, the duration of which varies according to the stage of WT.
12. In WT, the role of RT is indicated in Stage II with unfavourable histology, Stage III and IV, local recurrence and in palliation. RT should be started within 10 days of surgery. Dose recommended is 10Gy to flank + 10Gy boost to gross residual disease (>3crn). In lung metastases, whole lung is irradiated to a dose of 12Gy, liver metastases receive 19.8Gy. Brain mets is treated by WBRT to a dose of 30.6Gy, bone mets receive the same dose with a 3-cm margin. Relapsed cases can receive 12.6–18Gy.
13. Rhabdomyosarcoma (RMS) is a fast-growing, highly malignant soft-tissue sarcoma accounting for 6–8% of childhood tumours that develops in the muscle, mainly in the neck, head, bladder, and testes.
14. RMS patients are risk-stratified according to the pre-treatment TNM staging, surgical grouping, age and histology.
15. Retinoblastoma is the most common eye tumour in children, usually in children <5 years, accounting for 3–5% of childhood cancers.
16. RT in children comes with a specific set of challenges. Immobilization, cast preparation and simulation in a child-friendly environment should be done.
17. In children not getting sedation, communication of the child inside the treatment room with their parents could make them more comfortable. Ketamine and midazolam are the most common anaesthetic agents with Ondansetron given post-RT.
18. Children have lower tolerance to radiation due to growing tissues and likely to suffer more damage. Special care should be given to growing bones, pituitary, thyroid, heart, lungs and cognitive function.
19. Sexual maturity can be affected by RT, risks of which can be reduced by reducing dose to the gonads, oophoropexy should be done where relevant. Fertility preservation is also important, usually by GnRHa.

nating or reducing the dose to gonads, oophoropexy in females to position ovaries away from the RT portal, and avoiding or reducing the total dose of alkylating agents in males.

Secondary cancers may occur months or years after treatment (Table 17) (Fig. 7). These are usually a consequence or side effects of the initial cancer treatment. For example, a patient with breast cancer or Hodgkin's disease may develop acute leukaemia years after completion of therapy. Paediatric cancer patients are especially vulnerable to second cancer, given the likely long-term survival probability after primary treatment of many malignancies. More prolonged survival gives a more extended opportunity for secondary cancers to manifest.

Most antineoplastic drugs can produce acute toxicities (i.e. nausea, vomiting, mucositis and alopecia), generally reversible once the chemotherapy is completed (within 2–4 months) [54]. Some anticancer drugs are associated with delayed toxic effects, which can become evident even many years after the chemotherapy (5, 6) [55]. Therefore, as the number of survivors from childhood cancers is increasing, late effects are now becoming significant concerns, highlighting the importance of long-term follow-up.

Fertility preservation. Pharmacological treatment with GNRH agonists (GnRHa) has become an alternative, non-invasive, and well-tolerated approach, especially for those who cannot access cryopreservation options due to clinical and/or logistic issues. Nevertheless, at present, only very limited evidence from randomized clinical trials on the use of GnRHa in adolescents with cancer is available [56]. Evidence is accumulating that for childhood cancer survivors, late effects, including cardiotoxicity, chronic health conditions, and neurocognitive and behavioural functioning, can hurt their quality of life.

Late effects are a common occurrence in adults who have survived childhood cancer. Their prevalence increases as the time from cancer diagnosis elapses. Many multi-institutional and population-based studies have shown excess risk of morbidity among childhood and young adult cancer survivors compared with age/sex-matched controls. There is some evidence that this risk is disproportionately high among survivors of racial and ethnic minority populations.

Among adults who were treated for cancer during childhood, late effects contribute to a high burden of morbidity. It has been seen that

- 60% to more than 90% of survivors develop one or more chronic health conditions.
- 20% to 80% of survivors experience severe or life-threatening complications during adulthood. [57]

Acknowledgments Dr. Vikas Taneja, Head Department of Paediatrics, Manipal Hospital, Delhi.

Multiple Choice Questions

1. Childhood tumours differ from adult tumours in all of the following except:
   (a) Rare
   (b) Low cure rates
   (c) Special requirements in treatment
   (d) High burden of late effects
2. The most common childhood tumour is:
   (a) Leukaemia
   (b) Neuroblastoma
   (c) Wilms tumour
   (d) Rhabdomyosarcoma
3. The PENTEC provides:
   (a) Qualitative evidence-based dose/volume/risk guidelines.
   (b) Describe physics and dosimetric issues relevant to pediatric radiotherapy.
   (c) Both (a) and (b)
   (d) None of the above
4. The most common extracranial tumour in children is
   (a) Leukemia
   (b) Neuroblastoma
   (c) Nephroblastoma
   (d) Rhabdomyosarcoma
5. Syndromes associated with Neuroblastoma (NB) include(s):
   (a) Hirschsprung's disease
   (b) NF-1
   (c) Noonan syndrome
   (d) All of the above
6. The most common molecular driver seen in NB is
   (a) NMYC amplification
   (b) ATRX inactivating mutation
   (c) TERT re-arrangement
   (d) ALK amplification
7. Rapid myogenic jerks, dancing eye movement with or without ataxia are features of
   (a) Kerner–Morrison's syndrome
   (b) Noonan's syndrome
   (c) Opsoclonus myoclonus syndrome
   (d) Horner's syndrome
8. Favourable prognostic features of NB includes all except
   (a) Below 18 months

(b) Poorly differentiated, intermediate MKI, age below 1.5 years
(c) Nodular ganglioneuroblastoma
(d) Hyperdiploid DNA content

9. Dose recommended in high-risk NB is
(a) 24Gy/12 fractions
(b) 18Gy/12 fractions
(c) 20Gy/12 fractions
(d) 21.6Gy/12 fractions

10. WAGR syndrome is associated with which childhood cancer
(a) Neuroblastoma
(b) Nephroblastoma
(c) Retinoblastoma
(d) Rhabdomyosarcoma

11. Wilms tumour develops due to abnormalities in which stage of development of kidneys?
(a) Pronephric blastema
(b) Mesonephric blastema
(c) Metanephric blastema
(d) None of the above

12. Duration of VAC-D in Stage III and IV Favourable Histology is
(a) 6 weeks
(b) 6 months
(c) 2 months
(d) 2 years

13. Renal sparing surgery is indicated in all of the following except
(a) Horseshoe kidney
(b) Tumour thrombus in renal vein
(c) Denys-Drash syndrome
(d) Standard unilateral tumours

14. RT in Wilms tumour is indicated in all except
(a) Stage II favourable histology
(b) Stage III or IV favourable histology
(c) Stage III or IV unfavourable histology
(d) Local recurrence

15. Risk stratification in RMS includes all of the following except
(a) Pre-treatment TNM staging
(b) Site of tumour
(c) Age of the patient
(d) Surgical grouping
(e) None of the above

16. Common anaesthetic agent/s used in children is
(a) Ketamine
(b) Midazolam
(c) Both (a) and (b)
(d) None of the above

Answer Key

1. (b)
2. (a)
3. (c)
4. (b)
5. (d)
6. (a)
7. (c)
8. (c)
9. (d)
10. (b)
11. (b)
12. (b)
13. (b)
14. (a)
15. (e)
16. (c)

References

1. https://gco.iarc.fr/today/online-analysis-multi-bars?v=2020&mode=cancer&mode_population=countries&population=900&populations=900&key=crude_rate&sex=0&cancer=39&type=0&statistic=5&prevalence=0&population_group=0&ages_group%5B%5D=0&ages_group%5B%5D=3&nb_items=10&group_cancer=1&include_nmsc=0&include_nmsc_other=1&type_multiple=%257B%2522inc%2522%253Atrue%252C%2522mort%2522%253Atrue%252C%2522prev%2522%253Afalse%257D&orientation=horizontal&type_sort=0&type_nb_items=%257B%2522top%2522%253Atrue%252C%2522bottom%2522%253Afalse%257DLast. Accessed 10 Jan 2024.
2. Bhakta N, Force LM, Allemani C, Atun R, Bray F, Coleman MP, Steliarova-Foucher E, Frazier AL, Robison LL, Rodriguez-Galindo C, Fitzmaurice C. Childhood cancer burden: a review of global estimates. Lancet Oncol. 2019 Jan;20(1):e42–53.
3. https://seer.cancer.gov/archive/csr/1975_2016/results_merged/sect_28_childhood_cancer.pdf. Last Accessed on 27 Nov 23

4. Magrath I, Steliarova-Foucher E, Epelman S, Ribeiro RC, Harif M, Li CK, Kebudi R, Macfarlane SD, Howard SC. Pediatric cancer in low-income and middle-income countries. Lancet Oncol. 2013;14:e104–16.
5. https://www.ncdirindia.org/All_Reports/PBCR_REPORT_2012_2014/ALL_CONTENT/PDF_Printed_Version/Chapter4_Printed.pdf. Last Accessed on 27 Nov 23
6. https://iicc.iarc.fr/results/comparative-tables/ Last Accessed on 27 Nov 23.
7. Ganguly S, Kinsey S, Bakhshi S. Childhood cancer in India. Cancer Epidemiol. 2021;71:101679.
8. Munshi A, Ganesh T, Mohanti BK. Radiotherapy in India: history, current scenario, and proposed solutions. Indian J Cancer. 2019;56:359–63.
9. Dang-Tan T, Franco EL. Diagnosis delays in childhood cancer: a review. Cancer. 2007;110(4):703–13. https://doi.org/10.1002/cncr.22849.
10. Linabery AM, Ross JA. Trends in childhood cancer incidence in the U.S. (1992–2004). Cancer. 2008;112:416.
11. Pui CH, Campana D, Pei D, et al. Treating childhood acute lymphoblastic leukemia without cranial irradiation. N Engl J Med. 2009;360:2730–41.
12. Weber DC, Habrand JL, Hoppe BS, Hill Kayser C, Laack NN, Langendijk JA, MacDonald SM, McGovern SL, Pater L, Perentesis JP, Thariat J, Timmerman B, Yock TI, Mahajan A. Proton therapy for pediatric malignancies: fact, figures, and costs. A joint consensus statement from the pediatric PTCOG, PROS, and EPTN subcommittee. Radiother Oncol. 2018;128(1):44–55. https://doi.org/10.1016/j.radonc.2018.05.020. Epub 2018 Jun 21
13. https://www.ptcog.site/index.php/facilities-in-operation-public. Last Accessed on 30 Nov 23.
14. Tinkle CL, Fernandez-Pineda I, Sykes A, et al. Nonrhabdomyosarcoma soft tissue sarcoma (NRSTS) in pediatric and young adult patients: results from a prospective study using limited-margin radiotherapy. Cancer. 2017;123:4419–29.
15. Merchant TE, Schreiber JE, Wu S, et al. Critical radiation dose and volume combinations predict intelligence quotient and academic achievement scores after craniospinal irradiation in children with medulloblastoma. Int J Radiat Oncol Biol Phys. 2014;90:554–61.
16. Lucas JT, Holmes JA. Acute and long-term side effects of radiation therapy in pediatric cancer treatment. In: Lakhoo, K., Abdelhafeez, A.H., Abib, S. (eds). Pediatric Surgical Oncology. Springer, Cham 2025.
17. Morton LM, Onel K, Curtis RE, et al. The rising incidence of second cancers: patterns of occurrence and identification of risk factors for children and adults. Am Soc Clin Oncol Educ Book. 2014:e57–67.
18. Constine LS, Marks LB, Milano MT, Ronckers CM, et al. A user's guide and summary of pediatric normal tissue effects in the clinic (PENTEC): Radiation dose-volume response for adverse effects after childhood cancer therapy and future directions. Int J Radiat Oncol Biol Phys. 2024;119:321–37. https://doi.org/10.1016/j.ijrobp.2023.09.005.
19. Rhee DJ, Akinfenwa CPA, Rigaud B, Jhingran A, Cardenas CE, Zhang L, Prajapati S, Kry SF, Brock KK, Beadle BM, Shaw W, O'Reilly F, Parkes J, Burger H, Fakie N, Trauernicht C, Simonds H, Court LE. Automatic contouring QA method using a deep learning-based auto contouring system. J Appl Clin Med Phys. 2022;23(8):e13647. https://doi.org/10.1002/acm2.13647. Epub 2022 May 17. PMID: 35580067; PMCID: PMC9359039
20. Goodman MT, Gurney JG, Smith MA, Olshan AF. Sympathetic nervous system tumours. In: Cancer incidence and survival among children and adolescents: United States SEER Program, 1975–1995, Ries LA, Smith, MA, Gurney JG, et al (Eds), National Cancer Institute, Bethesda 1999. p.35.
21. Brodeur GM, Hogarty MD, Mosse YP, Maris JM. Neuroblastoma. In: Pizzo PA, Poplack DG, editors. Principles and practice of pediatric oncology. Philadelphia: Lippincott Williams & Wilkins; 2011. p. 886.
22. Cook MN, Olshan AF, Guess HA, et al. Maternal medication use and neuroblastoma in offspring. Am J Epidemiol. 2004;159:721.
23. French AE, Grant R, Weitzman S, et al. Folic acid food fortification is associated with a decline in neuroblastoma. Clin Pharmacol Ther. 2003;74:288.
24. Chow EJ, Friedman DL, Mueller BA. Maternal and perinatal characteristics about neuroblastoma. Cancer. 2007;109:983.
25. Riley RD, Heney D, Jones DR, Sutton AJ, Lambert PC, Abrams KR, Young B, Wailoo AJ, Burchill SA. A systematic review of molecular and biological tumour markers in neuroblastoma. Clin Cancer Res. 2004;10(1 Pt 1):4–12. https://doi.org/10.1158/1078-0432.ccr-1051-2.
26. Viprey VF, Gregory WM, Corrias MV, Tchirkov A, Swerts K, Vicha A, Dallorso S, Brock P, Luksch R, Valteau-Couanet D, Papadakis V, Laureys G, Pearson AD, Ladenstein R, Burchill SA. Neuroblastoma mRNAs predict outcome in children with stage 4 neuroblastoma: a European HR-NBL1/SIOPEN study. J Clin Oncol. 2014;32(10):1074–83. https://doi.org/10.1200/JCO.2013.53.3604. Epub 2014 Mar 3
27. Casey DL, Pitter KL, Kushner BH, Cheung NV, Modak S, LaQuaglia MP, Wolden SL. Radiation therapy to sites of metastatic disease as part of consolidation in high-risk neuroblastoma: Can long-term control be achieved? Int J Radiat Oncol Biol Phys. 2018;100:1204–1209. https://doi.org/10.1016/j.ijrobp.2018.01.008.
28. Schilling FH, Spix C, Berthold F, Erttmann R, Fehse N, Hero B, Klein G, Sander J, Schwarz K, Treuner J, Zorn U, Michaelis J. Neuroblastoma screening at one year of age. N Engl J Med. 2002;346(14):1047–53. https://doi.org/10.1056/NEJMoa012277.
29. Brodeur GM, Pritchard J, Berthold F, Carlsen NL, Castel V, Castelberry RP, De Bernardi B, Evans AE, Favrot M, Hedborg F, et al. Revisions of the

international criteria for neuroblastoma diagnosis, staging, and response to treatment. J Clin Oncol. 1993;11(8):1466–77. https://doi.org/10.1200/JCO.1993.11.8.1466.
30. Cohn SL, Pearson AD, London WB, Monclair T, Ambros PF, Brodeur GM, Faldum A, Hero B, Iehara T, Machin D, Mosseri V, Simon T, Garaventa A, Castel V, Matthay KK, INRG Task Force. The International Neuroblastoma Risk Group (INRG) classification system: an INRG Task Force report. J Clin Oncol. 2009;27(2):289–97. https://doi.org/10.1200/JCO.2008.16.6785. Epub 2008 Dec 1. PMID: 19047291; PMCID: PMC2650388
31. Sokol E, Desai AV, Applebaum MA, Valteau-Couanet D, Park JR, Pearson ADJ, Schleiermacher G, Irwin MS, Hogarty M, Naranjo A, Volchenboum S, Cohn SL, London WB. Age, Diagnostic category, tumour grade, and mitosis-Karyorrhexis index are independently prognostic in Neuroblastoma: an INRG project. J Clin Oncol. 2020;38(17):1906–18. https://doi.org/10.1200/JCO.19.03285. Epub 2020 Apr 21. PMID: 32315273; PMCID: PMC7280049
32. Perez CA, Matthay KK, Atkinson JB, Seeger RC, Shimada H, Haase GM, Stram DO, Gerbing RB, Lukens JN. Biologic variables in the outcome of stages I and II neuroblastoma treated with surgery as primary therapy: a children's cancer group study. J Clin Oncol. 2000 Jan;18(1):18–26. https://doi.org/10.1200/JCO.2000.18.1.18.
33. Twist CJ, Schmidt ML, Naranjo A, London WB, Tenney SC, Marachelian A, Shimada H, Collins MH, Esiashvili N, Adkins ES, Mattei P, Handler M, Katzenstein H, Attiyeh E, Hogarty MD, Gastier-Foster J, Wagner E, Matthay KK, Park JR, Maris JM, Cohn SL. Maintaining outstanding outcomes using response- and biology-based therapy for intermediate-risk Neuroblastoma: a report from the children's oncology group study ANBL0531. J Clin Oncol. 2019;37(34):3243–55. https://doi.org/10.1200/JCO.19.00919. Epub 2019 Aug 6. PMID: 31386611; PMCID: PMC6881103
34. Matthay KK, Perez C, Seeger RC, Brodeur GM, Shimada H, Atkinson JB, Black CT, Gerbing R, Haase GM, Stram DO, Swift P, Lukens JN. Successful treatment of stage III neuroblastoma based on prospective biologic staging: a Children's Cancer Group study. J Clin Oncol. 1998 Apr;16(4):1256–64. https://doi.org/10.1200/JCO.1998.16.4.1256.
35. Coughlan D, Gianferante M, Lynch CF, Stevens JL, Harlan LC. Treatment and survival of childhood neuroblastoma: evidence from a population-based study in the United States. Pediatr Hematol Oncol. 2017;34(5):320–30. https://doi.org/10.1080/08880018.2017.1373315. Epub 2017 Oct 17. PMID: 29039999; PMCID: PMC6764456
36. Ladenstein R, Valteau-Couanet D, Brock P, Yaniv I, Castel V, Laureys G, Malis J, Papadakis V, Lacerda A, Ruud E, Kogner P, Garami M, Balwierz W, Schroeder H, Beck-Popovic M, Schreier G, Machin D, Pötschger U, Pearson A. Randomized trial of prophylactic granulocyte colony-stimulating factor during rapid COJEC induction in pediatric patients with high-risk neuroblastoma: the European HR-NBL1/SIOPEN study. J Clin Oncol. 2010;28(21):3516–24. https://doi.org/10.1200/JCO.2009.27.3524. Epub 2010 Jun 21
37. Kraal KC, Tytgat GA, van Eck-Smit BL, Kam B, Caron HN, van Noesel M. Upfront treatment of high-risk neuroblastoma with a combination of 131I-MIBG and topotecan. Pediatr Blood Cancer. 2015;62(11):1886–91. https://doi.org/10.1002/pbc.25580. Epub 2015 May 15
38. Shusterman S, London WB, Gillies SD, Hank JA, Voss SD, Seeger RC, Reynolds CP, Kimball J, Albertini MR, Wagner B, Gan J, Eickhoff J, DeSantes KB, Cohn SL, Hecht T, Gadbaw B, Reisfeld RA, Maris JM, Sondel PM. Antitumour activity of hu14.18-IL2 in patients with relapsed/refractory neuroblastoma: a Children's Oncology Group (COG) phase II study. J Clin Oncol. 2010;28(33):4969–75. https://doi.org/10.1200/JCO.2009.27.8861. Epub 2010 Oct 4. PMID: 20921469; PMCID: PMC3020698
39. Furman WL, Federico SM, McCarville MB, Shulkin BL, Davidoff AM, Krasin MJ, Sahr N, Sykes A, Wu J, Brennan RC, Bishop MW, Helmig S, Stewart E, Navid F, Triplett B, Santana VM, Bahrami A, Anthony G, Yu AL, Hank J, Gillies SD, Sondel PM, Leung WH, Pappo AS. A phase II Trial of Hu14.18K322A in combination with induction chemotherapy in children with newly diagnosed high-risk neuroblastoma. Clin Cancer Res. 2019;25(21):6320–8. https://doi.org/10.1158/1078-0432.CCR-19-1452. Epub 2019 Oct 10. PMID: 31601569; PMCID: PMC6825564
40. Bellini A, Pötschger U, Bernard V, Lapouble E, Baulande S, Ambros PF, et al. frequency and prognostic impact of *ALK* amplifications and mutations in the European Neuroblastoma Study Group (SIOPEN) high-risk Neuroblastoma trial (HR-NBL1). J Clin Oncol. 2021;39(30):3377–90. https://doi.org/10.1200/JCO.21.00086. Epub 2021 Jun 11. PMID: 34115544; PMCID: PMC8791815
41. Cheung IY, Cheung NV, Modak S, Mauguen A, Feng Y, Basu E, Roberts SS, Ragupathi G, Kushner BH. Survival impact of anti-GD2 antibody response in a Phase II ganglioside vaccine trial among patients with high-risk neuroblastoma with prior disease progression. J Clin Oncol. 2021;39(3):215–26. https://doi.org/10.1200/JCO.20.01892. Epub 2020 Dec 16. Erratum in: J Clin Oncol. 2021 Feb 1;39(4):341. PMID: 33326254; PMCID: PMC8253584
42. Liu KX, Naranjo A, Zhang FF, et al. Prospective evaluation of radiation dose escalation in patients with high-risk neuroblastoma and gross residual disease after surgery: a report from the Children's Oncology Group ANBL0532 study. J Clin Oncol. 2020;38(24):2741–52.
43. Nazmy MS, Khafaga Y. Clinical experience in pediatric neuroblastoma intensity modulated radiotherapy. J Egypt Natl Canc Inst. 2012;24(4):185–9. https://doi.org/10.1016/j.jnci.2012.10.001. Epub 2012 Nov 6

44. Laverdière C, Liu Q, Yasui Y, Nathan PC, Gurney JG, Stovall M, et al. Long-term outcomes in survivors of neuroblastoma: a report from the Childhood Cancer Survivor Study. J Natl Cancer Inst. 2009;101(16):1131–40. https://doi.org/10.1093/jnci/djp230. Epub 2009 Jul 31. PMID: 19648511; PMCID: PMC2728747
45. Children's Oncology Group Long-term follow-up guidelines for survivors of childhood, adolescent, and young adult cancers, version 5.0 (October 2018), Available online at http://www.survivorshipguidelines.org/. Accessed on 10 Feb 2022.
46. Dix DB, Seibel NL, Chi YY, et al. Treatment of stage IV favorable histology wilms tumour with lung metastases: A report from the children's oncology group AREN0533 study. J Clin Oncol 2018;36(16):1564–1570
47. https://www.cancer.gov/types/soft-tissue-sarcoma/hp/rhabdomyosarcoma-treatment-pdq#_1 Last Accessed 10 Jan 2024.
48. Cecchetto G, Bisogno G, De Corti F, et al. Biopsy or debulking surgery as initial surgery for locally advanced rhabdomyosarcomas in children?: the experience of the Italian Cooperative Group studies. Cancer. 2007;110(11):2561–7.
49. Dávila Fajardo R, Magelssen H, Cameron AL, Boterberg T, Mandeville HC. Current and future developments in radiation oncology approach for rhabdomyosarcoma. Cancers (Basel). 2025;17:1618. https://doi.org/10.3390/cancers17101618.
50. Wharam MD, Meza J, Anderson J, et al. Failure pattern and factors predictive of local failure in rhabdomyosarcoma: a report of group III patients on the third Intergroup Rhabdomyosarcoma Study. J Clin Oncol. 2004;22(10):1902–8.
51. Wolden SL, Anderson JR, Crist WM, et al. Indications for radiotherapy and chemotherapy after complete resection in rhabdomyosarcoma: a report from the Intergroup Rhabdomyosarcoma Studies I to III. J Clin Oncol. 1999;17(11):3468–75.
52. Haeberli S, Grotzer MA, Niggli FK, et al. A psychoeducational intervention reduces anesthesia during radiotherapy for young childhood cancer patients. Radiat Oncol. 2008;3:17–22.
53. Turcas A, Boterberg T, Frykholm P, Gaze M, et al; SIOPE working group on pediatric anesthesia in radiation therapy. Anesthesia in pediatric radiotherapy: A systematic literature review by the siop europe working group on pediatric anesthesia in radiation therapy. Pediatr Blood Cancer. 2026; e70090. https://doi.org/10.1002/1545-5017.70090.
54. Ruggiero A, Rizzo D, Catalano M, Coccia P, Triarico S, Attiná G. Acute chemotherapy-induced nausea and vomiting in children with cancer: still waiting for a common consensus on treatment. J Int Med Res. 2018;46(6):2149–56.
55. Ehrhardt MJ, Skinner R, Castellino SM. Renal and hepatic health after childhood cancer. Pediatr Clin N Am. 2020;67(6):1203–17.
56. Hao X, Anastácio A, Viñals-Ribé L, Santamaria Lacuesta A, Diakaki C, Alonso de Mena S, Liu K, Rodriguez-Wallberg KA. Follicle rescue from Prepubertal ovaries after recent treatment with cyclophosphamide-an experimental culture system using mice to achieve mature oocytes for fertility preservation. Front Oncologia. 2021;11:682470.
57. https://www.cancer.gov/types/childhood-cancers/late-effects-hp-pdq Last Accessed 10 Jan 2024.

Online Links

Risk stratification, target volume delineation and management of rhabdomyosarcoma https://www.youtube.com/watch?v=mTr-ZK7N5ao

Neuroblastoma risk stratification and treatment overview https://www.youtube.com/watch?v=Rn-gqAJyRM4

Haematological Malignancies

Vikram Mathews, Pankaj Malhotra, Hasmukh Jain, Siddhartha Laskar, Sangeeta Kakoti, Prasanth Ganesan, Gaurav Prakash, Charanpreet Singh, Akhil Rajendra, and Manju Sengar

1 Introduction

Haematological malignancies are a unique set of neoplasms with marked variation in the clinical presentation from asymptomatic and indolent behaviour to presentation with oncological emergencies and rapidly fatal outcome if not treated urgently. A remarkable progress has occurred over the last decades through well-conducted randomized clinical trials and translational research. This has led to a significantly better understanding of biology and improvement in survival. Appropriate diagnosis and management of these cancers require close interaction between the pathologists, oncologists, radiologists, nursing team and palliative care specialists. The principles of therapy in haematological malignancies have paved the way for other solid tumours too.

In this chapter, we will focus on epidemiology, clinical features, diagnosis and treatment of a few common haematological cancers—acute myeloid leukaemia, acute lymphoblastic leukaemia, Hodgkin and non-Hodgkin lymphomas (including chronic lymphocytic leukaemia), chronic myeloid leukaemia, plasmacytomas and multiple myeloma. The role and technique of radiation have evolved over the last few decades, and the section "evolution of radiotherapy" describes these changes.

2 Acute Myeloid Leukaemia

Acute myeloid leukaemia (AML) represents a group of clonal haematopoietic stem cell disorders, which is characterized by both the failure to differentiate and over-proliferation of the stem cell compartment by non-functional cells called myeloblasts at the expense of the normal cells. AML is rare compared with other cancers but is the most common acute leukaemia in adults. AML affects all age groups; the incidence increases with advancing age and presents at a median age of 67–69 years in the developed world [1].

V. Mathews (✉)
Department of Haematology, Christian Medical College, Vellore, India
e-mail: vikram@cmcvellore.ac.in

P. Malhotra · G. Prakash · C. Singh
Department of Clinical Hematology, Postgraduate Institute of Medical Education and Research (PGIMER), Chandigarh, India

H. Jain · M. Sengar (✉)
Department of Medical Oncology, Tata Memorial Hospital, Mumbai, India

S. Laskar · S. Kakoti
Department of Radiation Oncology, Tata Memorial Hospital, Mumbai, India

P. Ganesan
Department of Medical Oncology, Jawaharlal Institute of Postgraduate Medical Education and Research, Puducherry, India

A. Rajendra
Department of Medical Oncology, Cancer Institute (W.I.A), Adyar, Chennai, India

B. K. Mohanti et al. (eds.), *Radiation Oncology – Principles, Precepts and Practice*,
https://doi.org/10.1007/978-981-95-5171-2_17

2.1 Clinical Features and Diagnostic Workup

Clinical presentation of acute leukaemia is almost always of a very short duration of symptoms and signs, mostly related to cytopenias and susceptibility to infections. Typically, the onset of symptoms is no more than 3 months before diagnosis. The clinical presentation reflects the presence of bone marrow failure, organ infiltration by leukemic cells, and hyperleukocytosis in some. AML is usually a disease that primarily involves the bone marrow and abnormal myeloblasts circulate in the blood. Rarely, AML can present as an extramedullary myeloid tumour (EMMT) without apparent involvement of the blood or bone marrow.

The workup for suspected AML includes complete blood count with peripheral smear, staining for myeloperoxidase, organ function (liver, renal and cardiac), blood grouping, bone marrow aspiration and biopsy with immunophenotyping, conventional cytogenetics, fluorescent-in situ hybridization (FISH) and polymerase chain reaction (PCR) for molecular abnormalities. Patients with EMMT require imaging to assess the extent of involvement. Contrast-enhanced CT can help in delineating the extent of involvement except for patients with central nervous system involvement. PET-CT is useful for response assessment in patients with EMMT. To make a diagnosis of AML, at least 20% blasts must be documented on a bone marrow aspirate smear. A diagnosis of AML with <20% blasts in the bone marrow aspirate can be made in the presence of classical recurrent genetic abnormalities associated with AML [t(15;17), t(8;21), inv (16) or t(16;16) [2]**.

2.2 Prognostication

The most important prognostic factors still remain the age and cytogenetics at diagnosis. Based on the cytogenetics and molecular markers at diagnosis, patients can be divided into three groups: a favourable risk group, an intermediate-risk group and an adverse risk group (summarized in Table 1) [2]**.

Table 1 The 2017 European Leukemia Net (ELN) risk stratification for acute myeloid leukaemia based on genetic abnormalities

Risk category	Genetic abnormality
Favourable	t(8;21)(q22;q22); *RUNX1–RUNX1T1* inv(16)(p13.1q22) or t(16;16)(p13.1;q22); *CBFB–MYH11* Mutated *NPM1* without *FLT3*-ITD or with *FLT3*-ITD[low(c)] Bi-allelic mutated *CEBPA*
Intermediate	Mutated *NPM1* and *FLT3*-ITD[high(c)] Wild type *NPM1* without *FLT3*-ITD or with *FLT3*-ITD[low(c)] (without adverse-risk genetic lesions) t(9;11)(p21.3;q23.3); *MLLT3–KMT2A*[d] Cytogenetic abnormalities not classified as favourable or adverse
Adverse	t(6;9)(p23;q34.1); *DEK–NUP214* t(v;11q23.3); *KMT2A* rearranged t(9;22)(q34.1;q11.2); *BCR–ABL1* inv(3)(q21.3q26.2) or t(3;3)(q21.3;q26.2); *GATA2*, *MECOM(EVI1)* −5 or del(5q); −7; −17/abn(17p) Complex karyotype[a], monosomal karyotype[b] Wild type *NPM1* and *FLT3*-ITD[high] Mutated *RUNX1*[c] Mutated *ASXL1*[c] Mutated *TP53*[d]

Adapted from Döhner et al. [3]

[a]Three or more unrelated chromosome abnormalities in the absence of one of the World Health Organization-designated recurring translocations or inversions (i.e. t(8;21), inv(16) or t(16;16), t(9;11), t(v;11)(v;q23.3), t(6;9), inv(3) or t(3;3); AML with *BCR-ABL1*)

[b]Defined by the presence of a single monosomy (excluding loss of X or Y) in association with at least one additional monosomy or structural chromosome abnormality (excluding core-binding factor AML)

[c]These markers should not be used as an adverse prognostic marker if they co-occur with favourable-risk AML subtypes.

[d]*TP53* mutations are significantly associated with AML with complex and monosomal karyotype

2.3 Principles of Treatment

Therapy for newly diagnosed patients with AML (other than AML-M3) can be considered under the following headings [3].

Induction chemotherapy

Consolidation therapy: Options include

High-dose chemotherapy (Non-myeloablative chemotherapy)

Autologous stem cell transplant

Allogeneic stem cell transplant
Maintenance therapy

Induction chemotherapy Based on earlier studies, the standard induction regimen has consisted of cytosine arabinoside (Ara-C) administered at 100–200 mg/m^2 as a continuous infusion for 7 days and daunorubicin (DNR) administered at 60 mg/m^2 for 3 days (7 + 3 regimen). In the recent past, a number of new molecules have been approved. Addition of Midostaurin to induction and post-remission therapy in FLT3-ITD AML has shown to improve the overall survival. Use of Gemtuzumab Ozogamicin in favourable risk AML has led to improved outcomes for FLT3-ITD. More recently, there has also been interest in the use of lower intensity induction therapy, usually with a combination of hypomethylating agents (HMA) such as azacytidine or decitabine in combination with venetoclax, a BCL-2 inhibitor in patients who are not fit for intensive chemotherapy. Post-induction, response assessment requires bone marrow examination to document a complete response.

Consolidation therapy Following the achievement of complete remission (CR) after induction chemotherapy (achieved in 75–85%), failure to give consolidation therapy will lead to 100% of the patients relapsing. Consolidation therapy is usually done with either repetitive cycles (3–4) of high-dose Ara-C (HiDAC) or an allogeneic haematopoietic cell transplant (alloHCT). Large prospective trials have consistently shown that an alloHCT with a standard myeloablative conditioning regimen is the most potent anti-leukaemia treatment for CR1 AML, with a relapse risk of 25–35% compared to 50–60% with chemotherapy.

Maintenance therapy There is an increased interest in the role of maintenance therapy in the management of AML. Currently, hypomethylating agents (azacytidine) or midostaurin (FLT3 tyrosine kinase inhibitor) have been approved for this purpose in the appropriate clinical setting.

Treatment of elderly AML is based on the comorbidities and frailty. Those who are fit for induction therapy and less than 65 years old can be treated with conventional treatment. Patients who are unfit can be treated with palliative intent with hypomethylating agent with or without venetoclax.

Role of radiotherapy There is a limited role for radiation therapy in AML. It can be used as part of the conditioning regimen (total body irradiation—TBI) prior to an alloHCT or in the setting of EMMT with organ compromise to help shrink the tumour (a hypo-fractionated regimen, usually 6–12 Gy in 1–2 fractions), if it is pressing on vital structures such as the trachea and causing breathing problems, orbit with visual impairment, or if there is extramedullary disease involving the CNS. In patients with isolated EMMT, who achieve a complete response after chemotherapy, there is limited evidence to support the use of radiation. However, in patients with incomplete metabolic response, consolidative radiotherapy to a dose of 24 Gy in conventional fractionation is indicated (ref PMID 30191865). Radiation can also be used rarely to reduce pain in an area of bone that is invaded by leukaemia, if chemotherapy hasn't helped, mostly in the setting of palliative care.

The 5-year OS is 50–60%, 30–40% and 10–15% in good, intermediate and poor risk groups, respectively, when treated with standard chemotherapy. The outcome of elderly AML continues to be poor with 5-year OS of 10–12%.

AML Treatment in India Treatment of AML in India poses its own challenges in a resource-poor setting like India. Outcomes in India are inferior to what is seen in the west due to multiple factors like paucity of centres that could treat AML, non-availability of newer therapeutic agents, lack of finances for the initial phase of the treatment and high induction mortality due to multidrug-resistant infections. In a study by Philips et al. from a non-government non-profit tertiary care hospital in India, the median age of the patients at diagnosis of AML was 40 years, with only 16% patients being ≥60 years. In this study, only 29% patients could proceed to AML induction therapy, 90% of whom were less than 60 years of age, and induction mortality even in this young cohort (all received intensive induction therapy) was a high 23% [4].

3 Acute Lymphoblastic Leukaemia

Acute lymphoblastic leukaemia (ALL) is the commonest cancer in children and characterized by excellent cure rates. Though the condition is rarer among adults, the survival is worse. There is a sharp drop-off in survival when transitioning to the adolescent age groups, and after that, there is a steady decline in older adults. Among patients over 50–60 years of age, the cure rates are abysmal (around 10–15%). The high cure rates in children are due to several factors. One, the disease biology is favourable and highly responsive to chemotherapy. Moreover, children can tolerate the intensive treatment protocols required for this cancer much better than adults [5]. Combination chemotherapy given over multiple phases, such as induction, consolidation, central nervous system (CNS) prophylaxis and maintenance, is the basis of modern ALL treatment. The treatment process is complex and prolonged (usually takes 2.5–3 years), and patient adherence to therapy is an important consideration. This chapter gives an overview of the presentation and principles of childhood and adult ALL treatment. The reader should give attention to ALL described in this chapter, because this disease is not covered in the chapter on Paediatric Tumors of this book.

3.1 Clinical Features and Diagnostic Workup [6]**

ALL involves the proliferation of precursor lymphoid cells (lymphoblasts) in the bone marrow. This leads to compromise of normal haematopoiesis, which manifests as anaemia (fatigue), low numbers of functional white cells (WBC) (infections), and thrombocytopenia (bleeding). The peripheral blood WBC count itself may be normal, increased, or reduced, but a study of the smear reveals the presence of blasts in most cases. Besides the features of pancytopenia, bone pains are common at the time of diagnosis due to infiltration of the bone marrow. Patients may also have fever, myalgias and malaise due to the release of cytokines. Due to infiltration by the blasts, patients have varying degrees of lymphadenopathy or hepatosplenomegaly at presentation. Extramedullary involvement can be present at diagnosis in form of testicular enlargement, cutaneous deposits and central nervous system (CNS) involvement (headache, focal neurological deficits and cranial nerve palsies).

Traditionally, the diagnosis of ALL involved the demonstration of the abnormal lymphoblasts in the peripheral blood and bone marrow. Lymphoblasts are typically large cells with high nuclear-cytoplasmic ratio, scant, agranular cytoplasm, and fine chromatin with rare nucleoli. Expert pathologists can make the morphological differentiation in most cases. However, there may be variations in the appearance of the blasts. Hence, it is common to do thorough immunophenotyping with flow cytometry (FCM) techniques in modern practice. ALL may be of B- (CD19, CD20, CD10+ve) or T-cell (CD3, CD5, CD7+ve) origin and can also rarely have mixed lineage presentation (expressing myeloid markers and lymphoid markers). Baseline FCM-based immunophenotyping is also essential for assessing post-therapy minimal residual disease (MRD), an integral component of current treatment paradigms.

The other investigations at baseline include complete blood counts, liver and renal function tests, assessment for tumour lysis (uric acid, potassium, phosphorus and calcium), cerebrospinal fluid cytomorphology, cytogenetic studies (usually from the bone marrow), and molecular studies. The BCR-ABL translocation is a significant, targetable anomaly. This is rare (<5%) in children but is seen in up to 25% of adults. The molecular studies have important prognostic and therapeutic implications (Table 1). Imaging with

CT or MRI brain may be needed for patients with suspected CNS involvement. Imaging for the detection of extramedullary disease in absence of clinical or laboratory abnormalities is not required.

3.2 Prognostic Factors

Age >35 years, white blood cell count of >30,000/cumm (B-cell) or >100,000/cumm for T-cell, presence of BCR-ABL, t(4;11)/KMT2A rearrangements, low hypodiploidy, near triploidy (60–78 chromosomes), and complex karyotype (≥5 unrelated abnormalities) portend adverse prognosis at diagnosis. In addition, failure to achieve complete remission post-induction, persistent minimal residual disease positive at post induction and consolidation are high-risk features and need intensification of therapy.

3.3 Treatment

The treatment principle is intensive courses of multiagent chemotherapy to achieve disease control, consolidation and maintenance therapy for 2 years. The various treatment components evolved through multiple trials conducted between the 1950s and 1970s (Table 2). Clinical trials conducted in the last three decades have further refined and tailored the treatment approach to reduce long-term and short-term side effects. Combined with improved supportive care (infection-control and transfusions), these studies have improved the survival of childhood ALL to 80–90%. The gains the survival in adults ALL have been more modest. About 50–70% of younger adults are cured with current treatment. However, the cure rates in adults have improved with the addition of targeted agents.

Table 2 Components of treatment in acute lymphoblastic leukaemia [6, 7]**

Phase of treatment	Usual agents	Principle	Duration
Induction of remission	Daunorubicin, Vincristine, Prednisolone, L asparaginase	To achieve remission complete remission	4 weeks
Consolidation	Cyclophosphamide, cytarabine, 6-mercaptopurine, high dose methotrexate	To further reduce the burden of cancer	8–12 weeks
Re-intensification[a]	Doxorubicin, Vincristine, Dexamethasone, L-asparaginase	Similar agents as in induction, to further reduce the burden of disease	4 weeks
CNS prophylaxis[b]	High dose methotrexate or cranial radiation	To achieve blast elimination in the sanctuary site of CNS	4–6 weeks
Maintenance	6-mercaptopurine and methotrexate	To maintain the remission and to eliminate slow-cycling blasts cells	2–3 years
Targeted agents	Imatinib (for BCR-ABL+ve disease), Rituximab (for CD20+ disease), inotuzumab ozogomycin, blinatumomab	Act on specific targets. In these subgroups, the addition of these agents during various components of treatment improves outcomes	Depending on the phase in which it is used.
Allogeneic transplantation	Marrow ablation using high-dose chemotherapy or total body irradiation followed by stem cell rescue from the donor	Improves cure rates in high-risk disease. Must be balanced with the increased risk of mortality due to complications	–

[a]Re-intensification is a usual component of modern paediatric ALL protocols and may not be seen in traditional "adult" type protocols

[b]Most modern paediatric protocols avoid the use of prophylactic cranial radiation except in small subsets with very high risk disease

Induction therapy to achieve complete remission (defined as <5% blasts in the bone marrow with normalization of blood counts and resolution of extramedullary disease) is the first step in managing ALL. However, this doesn't equate to a cure, as most patients will relapse without further therapy. Consolidation and maintenance treatments involve repetitive courses of non-cross resistant agents, which help to reduce the burden of leukemic cells further and thus improve cure rates. CNS is a "sanctuary" site where conventional chemotherapy agents cannot penetrate, and some patients suffer relapses. Traditional ALL-protocols incorporated cranial radiation (CRT) to address this gap. More modern protocols have reduced cranial RT using more refined risk-stratified approaches, and high-dose methotrexate, which crosses the blood–brain barrier. Although no randomized data exists in adult group of patients, extrapolation from paediatric leukaemia studies (ALL BFM trials viz. ALL BFM-90, ALL IC-BFM 2002, ALL BFM-95) have led to reduction in total dose of cranial RT, without compromising its efficacy. At present, 12 Gy of cranial radiation is used for prophylaxis and 18 Gy for patients who have CNS involvement (CNS-2,3). Technique of CRT has been mentioned in detail in subsequent section on evolution of RT in haematological malignancies.

3.4 Relapsed ALL

Unfortunately, at least half of the adults and about quarter of pediatric and young adults with ALL suffer relapse. Salvages are attempted in these patients with repeat intensive chemotherapy agents and consolidation with allogenic transplant. Reasonable success can be expected in younger patients and those with a long remission period before relapse. However, the outcomes with conventional agents and transplant are dismal in those with early relapses. Modern targeted agents (inotuzumab, blinatumomab) as well the introduction of chimeric antigen receptor T cell therapy (CAR-T) has improved the outcomes in these patients [8].

3.5 ALL Survivorship

Most of the ALL patients are children and young adults, and most are cured of the disease. The long-term side effects are an essential consideration in this regard. ALL survivors have an increased risk of multiple other disorders (Table 3) due to chemotherapy and radiation. Hence, it is essential to follow up with these patients in survivor clinics where these can be addressed [9].

Table 3 Long-term toxicities of treatment of ALL [9]

Side effect	Cause	Implications
Second cancers, including leukaemias	Chemotherapy and radiation	Efforts are on to reduce the use of chemotherapy in lower-risk groups
Cardiovascular problems	Multiple chemotherapy agents, especially anthracyclines	Increased risk of heart failure, as well as coronary artery disease and hypertension, have been described in survivors
Endocrine problems	Steroids, cranial radiation affecting the hypothalamus-pituitary axis	Has reduced with lesser use of cranial radiation
Growth retardation	Due to the prolonged treatment with chemotherapy	Addressing the nutritional needs is essential to reduce these effects
Psycho-social issues	Missing school/work due to treatment, financial costs to the family	A multi-disciplinary team is needed to help the patients, including social workers, psycho-oncologists, doctors, and nurses

4 Non-Hodgkin Lymphomas

Non-Hodgkin's lymphoma represents >150 defined entities with differences in biology, clinicopathological features and treatment strategies. The age-adjusted incidence of NHL in India is 1.5–2.9/100,000 population. The median age (54 years) at presentation is a decade younger compared to that reported in the west. Other distinct epidemiological features include male preponderance, higher incidence of diffuse large B-cell lymphoma (DLBCL) and T-cell lymphomas and a greater number of patients presenting with a poor performance status. These features coupled with delays in diagnosis and inadequate treatment has led to relatively inferior survival outcomes [10]. Globally, a similar trend of higher mortality in the lower and middle-income countries is noted when compared to the higher income countries [11].

A specific cause for NHL is not identified in majority of the cases with a few exceptions. In less than 10% cases, a specific factor such as immunodeficiency, infections or autoimmune disorder can be identified. The pathology and clinical behaviour of NHL can be better understood by considering their cell-of-origin in the lymphoid ontogeny (Table 4) [12]**.

Table 4 Common lymphomas and their normal counterparts

	Cell of origin	NHL Subtype
B-lymphocyte	Naïve B cell/ Post Germinal centre B-cell	CLL/SLL
	Pre-Germinal centre/ Antigen-exposed cell (subset)	Mantle Cell Lymphoma
	Germinal centre B cell	DLBCL, Burkitt's lymphoma and follicular lymphoma
	Pre-apoptotic Germinal centre B cell	Hodgkin's lymphoma
	Marginal Zone B cell	Marginal zone lymphoma Lymphoplasmacytic lymphoma
T-lymphocyte	TH1 cells	Peripheral T cell lymphoma NOS (Subset)
	TH2 cells	Subset of PTCL, NOS
	Follicular helper T cells	Angioimmunoblastic T-cell lymphoma PTCL-Follicular helper cell type
	TH17 cells	Anaplastic large cell lymphoma
	Regulatory T cells	Adult- T cell leukaemia/ lymphoma

4.1 Clinical Features and Workup [13]**

The clinical features that help to narrow down the diagnosis include age, extent of adenopathy, aggressive/indolent clinical behaviour and associated manifestations. Even though there are several lymphoma subtypes, the most common subtypes can be suspected based on the above features and are summarized in Table 5.

The workup of these patients can be divided into the following components:

Diagnostic workup Excision biopsy from the most accessible site is the preferred method for diagnosis of lymphoma. This is essential to study the entire nodal architecture, which helps in the correct diagnosis. The nodal region preferred for a biopsy is cervical, axillary and inguinal in descending order. An incisional or core biopsy can be performed when excision is not possible. Fine needle aspiration with flow cytometry can be used to supplement but not as an alternative to establish the diagnosis. The diagnosis is based on morphological assessment and immunohistochemistry. Only a small proportion of cases require molecular studies for confirmation of diagnosis. In certain situations, such as indolent lymphomas with a peripheral blood spill, the diagnosis can be established by flow cytometric evaluation of blood. The WHO classification of NHL is summarized in Table 6 [12].

Table 5 Clinical presentation of common NHL subtypes

Clinical presentation			
Lymphoma subtypes	Extent-localized (L)/ Generalized (G)	Behaviour aggressive (A) Indolent (I)	Other features
DLBCL	L/G	A	Can inolve extranodal sites including GIT, bone and CNS
Burkitt's lymphoma	L/G	A	Involve GIT, bone and CNS
Follicular lymphoma	G	I	Bone marrow, and splenomegaly
Mantle cell lymphoma	G	A/I	GI involvement as extranodal site. Few cases with non-nodal leukemic involvement
Peripheral T-cell lymphoma	G	A	
ALCL	G/L	A	Can have skin and bone lesions
CLL	G	I	Autoimmune haemolytic anaemia
AITL	G	A	Rash, effusions, autoimmune manifestations
NK-T cell lymphoma	L	A	Necrotic lesion in sino-nasal region
Peculiar patterns of involvement			
CNS involvement	Aggressive lymphoma- DLBCL, ALCL, Burkitt's lymphoma T-cell CLPD- ATLL, T-PLL Low-grade lymphoma- Lymphoplasmacytic lymphoma, Dural marginal zone lymphoma		
Orbital involvement	Aggressive lymphoma- DLBCL, NK-T cell lymphoma, Burkitt's lymphoma Indolent lymphoma- MALToma		
Sino-nasal involvement	DLBCL, NK-T cell lymphoma		
GIT	Aggressive- DLBCL, Burkitt's lymphoma, Mantle cell lymphoma, Enteropathy-associated T-cell lymphoma Indolent- MALToma, Follicular lymphoma		
Massive splenomegaly	Splenic marginal zone lymphoma, Hairy cell leukaemia, HCL-variant, T-PLL, Mantle cell lymphoma, Follicular lymphoma, Lymphoplasmacytic lymphoma and Hepatosplenic gamma delta T-cell lymphoma		
Skin	Cutaneous lymphomas, AITL, T-PLL, ATLL and ALCL		

Table 6 WHO classification of NHL [12]**

Mature B cell neoplasms	*Mature T cell neoplasms*
Aggressive neoplasms	*Leukemic or disseminated*
Diffuse large B-cell lymphoma: variants, subgroups, and subtypes T-cell/ histiocyte-rich large B-cell lymphoma Primary DLBCL of the CNS Primary cutaneous DLBCL, leg type	T-cell large granular lymphocytic leukaemia Chronic lymphoproliferative disorders of NK cells T-cell T-cell prolymphocytic leukaemia Adult T-cell leukaemia/lymphoma Aggressive NK-cell leukaemia
Other lymphomas of large B cells	*Extra nodal*
Primary mediastinal large B-cell lymphoma ALK-positive large B-cell lymphoma Plasmablastic lymphoma	Extra nodal NK/T-cell lymphoma, nasal type Enteropathy-type T-cell lymphoma Hepatosplenic T-cell lymphoma Breast implant-associated anaplastic large-cell lymphoma
B-cell lymphoma, unclassifiable, with features intermediate between DLBCL and classical Hodgkin lymphoma	*Cutaneous* Mycosis fungoides Sezary syndrome CD30-positive lymphoproliferative disorders Subcutaneous panniculitis-like T-cell lymphoma Primary cutaneous $\gamma\delta$T-cell lymphoma

(continued)

Table 6 (continued)

High-grade B-cell lymphoma, with MYC and BCL2 and/or BCL6 rearrangements High-grade B-cell lymphoma, NOS Burkitt's lymphoma Mantle cell lymphoma	*Nodal* Peripheral T-cell lymphoma (PTCL), NOS Angioimmunoblastic T-cell lymphoma (AITL) Follicular T-cell lymphoma Nodal peripheral T-cell lymphoma with TFH phenotype Anaplastic large-cell lymphoma (ALCL), ALK positive Anaplastic large-cell lymphoma, ALK negative
Indolent lymphomas	
Follicular lymphoma CLL/SLL Lymphoplasmacytic lymphoma B-cell prolymphocytic leukaemia (PLL) Hairy cell leukaemia Marginal zone lymphoma	

Staging workup A contrast-enhanced CT scan of neck, chest, abdomen and pelvis is used for staging in most lymphomas. In FDG-avid lymphomas, a whole body 18F-FDG PET CT scan can be used instead. Bone marrow studies (morphology and flow cytometry) is recommended for staging in most cases except in DLBCL (can be omitted in early stage or if the PET-CT shows bone marrow involvement) or in the presence of peripheral blood spill. Cerebrospinal fluid analysis is performed in situations when there is likely a high incidence of baseline CNS involvement such as Burkitt's lymphoma, lymphoblastic lymphoma, HIV-associated NHL, DLBCL (High CNS international prognostic index or site-specific indications) and primary CNS lymphoma.

Organ function and prognostic markers workup Complete blood count, liver function test, renal function tests are performed a baseline to assess the organ function. Patients with high-grade lymphomas or those with compromised renal function need assessment and prophylaxis for tumour lysis. In addition, a 2D echocardiogram/MUGA scan is performed before anthracycline-based treatment. Patients who would need high-dose methotrexate-based therapy and have factors (age, underlying comorbidities), which can predispose to renal dysfunction should undergo assessment of glomerular filtration rate by DTPA GFR scan.

Based on the subtype of lymphoma, other serum markers like lactate dehydrogenase and beta-2-microglobulin are tested.

It is essential to test for the presence of HIV, Hepatitis B (surface antigen and core Ig G) and Hepatitis C infections since the presence of these infections can influence the treatment plan and warrant the need for concurrent antiviral therapy.

4.1.1 Staging System and Prognostic Indices

The staging system used for lymphoma has undergone several revisions, and the Lugano system is currently in use [14]**. The staging is based on the extent of nodal and extra-nodal involvement. Stage I refers to a single nodal or extra-nodal site, stage II refers to 2 or more nodal groups or 1 extra-nodal site with contiguous nodal involvement, limited to one side of the diaphragm, stage III refers to nodal involvement on either side of the diaphragm and stage IV refers to additional non-contiguous extra-nodal involvement, bone marrow.

In order to prognosticate the patients, risk-stratify and develop personalized therapy, several indices have been developed. These indices such as the International prognostic index (IPI), NCCN IPI, R-IPI etc. are derived from clinical and laboratory parameters. These indices are validated in cohort of patients with specific subtypes of NHL who are treated with a particular type of systemic therapy [14–18]. Hence, one needs to consider the disease subtype and therapy before applying these tools.

4.1.2 Treatment by Subtypes [13]**

The common subtypes of NHL, their unique features and approach to the management are discussed here:

1. Diffuse large B-cell lymphoma (DLBCL) [19]*

DLBCL is the most common subtype of NHL. It can present as either localized or generalized adenopathy, with extra-nodal sites of involvement such as GIT, bones, paraspinal region and breast.

The principles of treatment are as follows:

A. Limited stage disease:
   (a) 4R-CHOP 21 plus 2 R (Rituximab, Cyclophosphamide, Doxorubicin, Vincristine, Prednisolone)
   (b) 4R-CHOP
   (c) 6R-CHOP 21

   Radiation is reserved for residual disease at the end of systemic therapy or those with baseline bulky disease. The dose of radiation can vary from 30–36 Gy in conventional fractionation in these patients.

B. Advanced stage disease
   (a) 6R-CHOP21

   Radiation is reserved for residual disease at the end of systemic therapy or those with baseline bulky disease. The dose of radiation can vary from 30–36 Gy in conventional fractionation in these patients.

C. CNS prophylaxis- There are certain situations where the risk of CNS relapse is >10% and warrants CNS prophylaxis in the form of intrathecal or systemic methotrexate. There has been increasing evidence (retrospective data) against the use of prophylaxis, with debate on identification of truly high-risk patients and the method of prophylaxis. However, at present, the following indications are used for selection of patients.

   Indications:
   (a) Site-specific- Paraspinal, breast, kidney, adrenal, adnexal and testicular involvement.
   (b) CNS IPI- Intermediate or High risk.
   (c) >1 extra-nodal site with elevated serum LDH

   DLBCL is heterogenous at a biological level, with differences in the gene expression profiling and IHC expression. DLBCL characterized by expression of BCL2 and MYC is known as double expressor lymphoma (DEL). On the other hand, the presence of *MYC* gene rearrangement with either *BCL2* rearrangement is called as a Double-hit lymphoma (DHL). While the data is inconsistent about the inferior prognosis of DEL, studies have clearly shown that DHL carries poor prognosis and needs intensive therapy like dose-adjusted infusional R-EPOCH.

2. Primary Mediastinal B-cell Lymphoma (PMBCL) [20]

PMBCL is a subtype of DLBCL that presents with bulky mediastinal mass in young women, with extra-nodal involvement such as GIT, renal, bone marrow or CNS in some patients. The histology is characterized by sheets of large cells with bands of fibrosis. The cells express CD20, CD30 but are CD15 negative. PMBCL is treated with dose-adjusted R-EPOCH regimen, which obviates the need for radiation in most of the patients who achieve complete metabolic response.

3. Burkitt's Lymphoma (BL) [21]

BL is an aggressive type of NHL characterized by extra-nodal involvement such as bowel or bones. There are three subtypes—endemic—seen in equatorial Africa, HIV-associated and sporadic. Pathologically, sheets of small- to medium-sized cells are seen with a starry-sky appearance. The presence of C-Myc translocation is the hallmark of Burkitt's lymphoma, though recently a new subtype with 11q rearrangement has been defined.

The chemotherapy regimens used to treat BL are dose-intense, with alternate cycles of non-cross-resistant drugs, and include an element of CNS prophylaxis. Several regimens are in use such as R-GMALL NHL 2002, CODOX-M/IVAC, CALGB, R-Hyper-CVAD and R-EPOCH protocols.

4. Mantle Cell Lymphoma (MCL) [22]

Mantle cell lymphoma is a B-cell NHL characterized by the presence of t(11:14) which leads to the overexpression of cyclin D1. The clinical and biological behaviour is heterogenous. Tools such as MIPI (Mantle cell lymphoma prognostic index), Ki-67 and molecular profiling are used to prognosticate the patients. Patients, who are asymptomatic, with a leukemic, non-nodal presentation, are kept under observation. For other patients treatment depends on the fitness for autoSCT. In young fit patients, high-dose Ara-C-based intense regimen is used for induction, consolidated with autoSCT followed by Rituximab maintenance. In the elderly patients, options such as Bendamustine-rituximab, VR-CAP (Bortezomib, Rituximab, Cyclophosphamide, adriamycin and prednisolone) or R-CHOP are considered, followed in most cases by Rituximab maintenance. In the relapsed setting, options such as ibrutinib, acalabrutinib, CAR-T cell therapy and Lenalidomide can be considered.

5. Follicular Lymphoma (FL) [23]

FL is the most common type of indolent NHL. This disease is characterized by generalized adenopathy and bone marrow involvement. Pathologically, it is characterized by the presence of a follicular pattern with neoplastic cells expressing CD20, CD10 and Bcl2. The disease is graded based on the morphological features into Grades 1, 2, 3A or B. Cytogenetically, t(14:18) is the hallmark of FL that leads to overexpression of the *BCL2* gene.

Not all patients with follicular lymphoma need therapy. The localized stage disease can be treated with definitive radiation of 24 Gy. Patients with advances stage disease and those with localized disease (stage II—more than one nodal region noncontinguous) can be kept under watchful waiting with periodic clinical follow-up. Other option for low tumour burden patients with advanced stage disease is single agent rituximab; however, it does not improve the overall survival. The treatment indications include cytopenias, B-symptoms, bulky/symptomatic adenopathy or splenomegaly, effusions or bony lesions. For this subgroup chemoimmunotherapy with Bendamustine and Rituximab is the preferred choice given the better tolerance and longer disease control than R-CHOP. In patients who require chemotherapy-free approach Rituximab and lenalidomide can be used. FL grade 3b is treated on the lines of DLBCL.

A small proportion of patients with FL can transform to DLBCL over the years; however, there are no measures to prevent transformation.

6. Chronic Lymphocytic Leukaemia/Small Lymphocytic Lymphoma (CLL/SLL)

CLL/SLL is a chronic lymphoproliferative disorder. The disease is detected incidentally or can present with B-symptoms, generalized lymphadenopathy and paraneoplastic manifestations. Biologically, the disease is heterogenous, those with IgVH unmutated type and P53 mutation/deletion have an adverse outcome. Similar to FL, not all patients with CLL/SLL require therapy. Asymptomatic patients are kept under watchful waiting with close follow-up every 4–6 monthly. Cytopenias, autoimmune manifestations refractory to steroids, bulky/symptomatic adenopathy or splenomegaly, B-symptoms or fatigue would warrant therapy. In those with an indication for treatment, the options include:

(a) IgVH Unmutated/p53 deleted CLL: Bruton Tyrosine Kinase inhibitor (ibrutinib/ acalabrutininb) or Venetoclax with obinutuzumab.
(b) IgVHmutatedCLL:Chemoimmunotherapy regimen such as Bendamustine-Rituximab, FCR (Fludarabine, cyclophosphamide and rituximab) or chlorambucil-rituximab (in unfit and frail patients)

7. Peripheral T-cell Lymphoma (PTCL), NOS

PTCL is the commonest type of T-cell lymphoma characterized by the presence of generalized adenopathy and B-symptoms in elderly patients. Biologically, two subsets are identified based on the gene expression profiling signature and classified into GATA3 or TBX21.CHOP or CHOP-like regimen forms the mainstay of treatment, with 5-year survival outcomes in the range of 30%. Autologous stem-cell transplant is indicated for patients with advanced-stage disease as a consolidation strategy. More recently, the addition of brentuximab-vedotin to CHP has shown better outcomes than CHOP in this subgroup of patients.

8. Angioimmunoblastic T-cell Lymphoma (AITL)

AITL is a subtype of T-cell lymphoma that arises from follicular helper T-cells. The disease presents in elderly with generalized non-bulky adenopathy, skin rash, effusions and autoimmune manifestations. Recently, a strong association between RHOA mutation and AITL was discovered. The treatment of AITL is similar to PTCL NOS with inferior outcomes.

9. Anaplastic Large-Cell Lymphomas (ALCLs)

ALCLs are subtypes of T-cell lymphomas. The disease is characterized by adenopathy and extra-nodal involvement such as skin, bones and CNS. ALCL is classified based on the expression of ALK by IHC testing. ALK positive ALCL is characterized by t(2:5), ALK negative ALCL is further classified based on the presence of *DUSP22* translocation (good prognosis) and p63 expression (poor prognosis). ALCL is treated with CHP plus Brentuximab-vedotin or CHOP regimen. In adolescent and young adults intensive protocols such as ALCL-99 protocols are used. Stem-cell transplant is used in relapsed/refractory setting.

10. Extra nodal NK/T-cell lymphoma, nasal type [24]

NK/T-cell lymphoma is common in the Southeast Asian region characterized by necrotic and ulcerated lesion in the sino-nasal region. The disease can involve other sites such as bone marrow, skin, testes and also present with hemophagocytic lympho-histiocytosis.

Pathologically, there are areas of necrosis and angio-invasion. Tumour cells express CD56 and EBV-LMP1. Localized disease can be treated with chemotherapy, which is given either sequentially or sandwiched with radiation. Upfront radiotherapy followed by chemotherapy is preferred in localized small volume disease (ref PMID: 30128904). The recommended dose of RT is 45–50 Gy in conventional fractionation. Owing to the critical adjacent structures viz. optic nerves, eyeball, etc., Intensity Modulated Radiation Therapy (IMRT) is the preferred technique; however, in selected cases 3-Dimensional Conformal Radiotherapy (3D-CRT) may suffice. Chemotherapy regimens include DeVIC or VIPD regimen. For advanced disease, drugs that are not affected by MDR-efflux mechanisms are preferred. Regimens such as SMILE, L-AspMetDex or P-GemOx are used with excellent outcomes.

11. Mycosis Fungoides [25]

Mycosis fungoides is the commonest form of primary cutaneous lymphoma. The disease is characterized by polymorphous skin lesions in non-sun-exposed areas. The disease generally runs an indolent course and is diagnosed late. A TNM-based staging system is used to define the extent of involvement that takes into consideration the nature of lesion, extent of involvement, nodal involvement and blood spill.

Localized disease is treated with topical steroids. In the presence of extensive/recurrent lesions, skin-directed therapy (SDT) such as PUVA therapy is used.

Advanced disease is treated with a combination of SDT such as PUVA therapy or TSET (Total skin electron therapy, technique and dose details mentioned in the subsequent section on evolution of RT in haematological malignancies) with systemic therapy such as interferons, oral methotrexate, bexarotene or pralatrexate. Erythroderma/Sezary syndrome is recalcitrant to these therapies and responds well to extracorporeal photopheresis. Large cell transformation in these patients is treated with combination chemotherapy such as CHOP regimen or Brentuximab followed by allogeneic stem-cell transplant. Further details about management of skin lymphomas are provided in the chapter (Special Techniques: Total Body Irradiation, T-SET, IORT, and Hyperthermia- Volume 1)

Post-treatment follow-up All patients should be periodically followed up with clinical examination and appropriate blood investigations. There is no role for surveillance PET-CT/CT post-treatment except if there is clinical suspicion for relapse or disease progression.

5 Hodgkin Lymphoma

Hodgkin lymphoma (HL) is a unique malignancy that predominantly occurs in adolescent and young adults. It is characterized by remarkable sensitivity to chemotherapy and radiotherapy, which results in high cure rates. The name HL is given to honour Dr. Thomas Hodgkin, who first described this condition in young individuals who used to succumb to this unique illness characterized by fever, weight-loss and grape-like cervical node enlargement.

Today, HL is a distinct group of four subtypes: (i) HL—Lymphocyte predominant, (ii) HL—Nodular sclerosis, (iii) HL—Mixed cellularity, and (iv) HL—lymphocyte depletion. Another subtype of HL, previously known as nodular lymphocyte predominant HL, has recently reclassified as a subset of B-cell NHL and now it is called as Nodular Lymphocyte predominant B-cell lymphoma.

HL has an annual incidence of 2–3 cases per 1,00,000 people. It is characterized by a bimodal peak of incidence. The first and dominant peak occurs in between 15 and 30 years of age and the predominant subtype in this age group is nodular sclerosis variety of HL. The second and smaller peak is observed in the sixth decade of life and in this cohort, proportion of patients with mixed cellularity HL is higher than that observed in the first peak [26]**.

Most of the cases with HL are idiopathic in origin. In the past few years, evidence has emerged that EBV is causally related with HL in 25–30% of cases [27]. Apart from EBV, there is little evidence regarding distinctive environmental or genetic factors directly linked with oncogenesis in patients with HL.

The pathologic hallmark of HL is the presence of characteristic Reed-Sternberg cells (RS cells) surrounded by extensive inflammatory and immune cell infiltrate. In the beginning of the twentieth century, Dorothy Reed and Carl Sternberg provided first description and to honour their contributions, these unique cells are called as RS cells [28].

A typical RS cell is a large binucleate cell with large nucleoli in the centre of each nucleus. This arrangement leads to the characteristic "owl-eye" appearance of RS cells. In a lymph-node section, RS cells represent the malignant component and they constitute only around 1% of the cells. A classical RS cell express both CD15, CD30 and PAX5 (weak), while it is negative for CD20 and CD45. The RS cells are of B-cell origin.

5.1 Clinical Features

Painless lymphadenopathy is the commonest presentation of HL. The commonly involved sites include cervical, supraclavicular, mediastinal, and axillary lymph nodes. Infra-diaphragmatic lymph-nodes are involved less frequently and they are more commonly seen in patients with MC-HL and LD-HL. The predominant pattern of anatomic distribution of involved lymph nodes in patients with HL is around central axis, which include cervical, supraclavicular, axillary and mediastinal LNs with contiguous spread. As a result, appendicular lymph nodes like epitrochlear and popliteal LNs are rarely involved by HL. Similarly, extranodal site involvement by HL is less common. Lung is the most commonly involved extranodal site in patients with HL and in majority of these cases, it occurs as a result of direct extension from the involved lymph nodes. The other two extranodal sites of involvement are bone and liver. The clinic-pathologic differences between various subtypes of HL are elaborated in Table 7.

5.2 Staging and Workup

Lugano classification is currently used for staging of patients with HL. The staging and prognostication work-up for a newly diagnosed case of HL includes complete blood counts, renal and liver function tests, serum LDH, HIV, HBsAg, Anti-HCV and a whole-body PET-CT scan. As PET-CT has high negative predictive value for

Table 7 Salient clinical and pathological feature of all four subtypes of HL

Subtype of HL	Characteristics pathology	Clinical attributes
Nodular sclerosis	Nodule formation defined by distinct collagen bands	Commonest subtype in adolescent and young adults Female preponderance Higher incidence of a mediastinal mass
Mixed cellularity	RS cells in a mixed inflammatory background, comprising of eosinophils, neutrophils, histiocytes and plasma cells Higher rate of EBV-positive status	More peripheral lymph nodes and intra-abdominal involvement More common in elderly patients
Lymphocyte predominant	RS cells in a background of B-lymphocytes that form nodules Other inflammatory cells, such as eosinophils, are rare in this subtype	Presents with early stage and indolent clinical course BM involvement and B symptoms are uncommon
Lymphocyte depleted	Higher rate of EBV-positive status	More common in older patients and rare in children Higher incidence in HIV+ individuals Presents with advanced stage and aggressive clinical course Common BM involvement Frequent B symptoms

bone marrow involvement, bone marrow aspiration and biopsy is not required for staging. If PET-CT scan facility is not available then a CECT neck, chest and abdomen and bone marrow biopsy can be done as an alternative. As a majority of the patients of HL would need anthracycline based chemotherapy, it is necessary to do an echocardiography for assessment of baseline cardiac function.

Table 8 Classification for patients with classical Hodgkin lymphoma

Early stage (Favourable)
Stage I/II with none of the factors listed in the unfavorable classification
Early stage (Unfavourable)
Stage I/II with one of these factors:
1. Age >50 years[a]
2. ≥Three (Four[a]) lymph node areas involved
3. An erythrocyte sedimentation rate of more than 50 mm/h (without B symptoms) and an erythrocyte sedimentation rate of more than 30 mm/h (with B symptoms)
4. Extranodal disease
5. Bulky mediastinal involvement[b]
Advanced stage
Stage III/IV or Stage IIB with bulky mediastinum and/or extranodal disease

[a]EORTC classification
[b]Defined as greater than a third of the transthoracic diameter at any level of thoracic vertebrae (MMR >0.33)

For treatment planning, patients with stages I and II (non-bulky) are considered early stage disease and patients with stages III and IV are considered advanced stage disease. The early stage HL is further subdivided into favourable and unfavourable subtypes as defined in Table 8.

Risk Stratification for Advanced Stage Hodgkin's Lymphoma

The international prognostic score is based on a combination of seven factors that independently affect the freedom from treatment failure (FFTF) and was developed by Hasenclever et al. These include Males, stage IV, Age ≥45 years, haemoglobin <10.5 g/dL, total WBC count $\geq 15 \times 10^9$/L, absolute lymphocyte count $<0.6 \times 10^9$/L or <8% and albumin <4 g/dL. On the basis of the number of factors present at diagnosis, the IPS identified subgroups of patients with 5-year freedom from progression (FFP) ranging from 42% to 84% [29].

6 Treatment

In the current era, a risk-adapted approach is the mainstay of treatment for HL. There are two main risk stratification systems used in clinical practice for this purpose [30].

6.1 Early-Stage HL

Patients with early-stage HL have excellent outcomes and high cure rates ranging around 90–95%. As a result, the focus of treatment for this cohort has shifted from achieving higher efficacy to minimizing toxicity, specially the long-term toxicity. The issues related to late effects, particularly second malignancies, cardiac toxicities and pulmonary damage, should be considered at the time of treatment planning.

6.1.1 Early Favourable

For patients with early-favourable HL—combined modality treatment with 2 cycles of ABVD followed by involved site RT (ISRT) to a dose of 20 Gy in conventional fractionation is the current standard treatment. In comparison to chemotherapy alone, a combined modality treatment results in better local control. However, there is no difference in overall survival with both treatment approaches. Therefore, individual patient-related factors need to be considered in deciding treatment of early favourable HL. For example, in a young female patient with axillary/mediastinal involvement, a chemotherapy-only regimen can be a reasonable option as omission of RT can reduce risk of breast and lung cancer, in future.

In recent years, the emphasis has shifted on using response-adapted approach to reduce exposure to chemo/radiotherapy. One such PET-CT-based risk-adapted approach was studied in RAPID trial [31]*. In this study, all patients with early stage HL received 3 cycles of ABVD and underwent an FDG-PET scan. The patients in complete remission were randomly assigned to either receive involved-field radiation therapy or observation. The 3-year progression-free survival rates were 94.6% and 90.8% for these two treatment arms, respectively, with an absolute risk difference of −3.8% points (95%CI: −8.8–1.3%). The non-inferiority of the no further treatment strategy could not be proven (noninferiority margin of 7%). Similarly in the EORTC/LYSA H10 trial (favourable group), non-inferiority of omission of RT could not be established [32]. Hence, the incorporation of RT in the early stage Hodgkin's lymphoma is detrimental to the outcomes of the patients.

6.1.2 Early Unfavourable

The combined modality treatment comprising of ABVD- 4 cycles followed by 30 Gy of involved-field/ involved-site radiation therapy is considered standard treatment as it resulted in an impressive progression-free survival of 84% at 10-year follow-up [33]. An alternative approach is to give 6 cycles of ABVD in patients where the potential long-term complications with radiation can outweigh the benefits.

6.1.3 Advanced Stage

The mainstay of treatment for advanced-stage HL is systemic multi-agent chemotherapy with or without radiotherapy. Six courses of ABVD are still considered to be the regimen of first choice for this subset of patients. At present, any of the following options can be used for upfront treatment of advanced stage HL, and the choice of treatment is determined by age and fitness of a patient, prognostic factors, availability and affordability of the component drugs.

6.2 ABVD: (Doxorubicin, Bleomycin, Vinblastine and Dacarbazine)

A total of 6 courses of ABVD regimen is currently the standard of care for patients with advanced stage HL. Approximately 80% of patients with advanced stage HL will attain a complete response after treatment with ABVD, and around 75% of them will achieve long-term progression-free survival [34].

Similar to early stage HL, response-adapted treatment strategy is being increasingly used for patients with advanced HL. In this strategy, there are two approaches (i) escalation of chemotherapy in cases with suboptimal response (less than complete response) after initial treatment. (ii) De-escalation of chemotherapy on attaining complete remission with the initial treatment.

One particular de-escalation trial called RATHL needs special mention in this regard. The RATHL trial randomly assigned patients with PET-negative disease after 2 cycles of ABVD to continued ABVD in one arm and to give only doxorubicin–vinblastine–dacarbazine (AVD) in the other arm. The omission of bleomycin did not lead to reduction in efficacy and it resulted in fewer pulmonary events than in the ABVD group [35]**. As a result, at centres with access to PET-CT, a response-adapted treatment on the lines of RATHL study is becoming a preferred treatment strategy. Patients who do not show optimal response after 2 cycles would need intensification of therapy with escalated BEACOPP.

6.3 BEACOPP Pregimen: [Bleomycin–Etoposide–Doxorubicin–Cyclophosphamide–Vincristine–Procarbazine–Prednisone]

For patients who are young and fit, another option is the escalated BEACOPP regimen, which was developed and more frequently used by the German HL study group. Complete response rates with BEACOPP are approximately 80–95% with 5-year PFS and OS rates of 81% and 92%, respectively [36]. One of the advantages of BEACOPP is the ability to limit the need for radiation, as demonstrated in the HD15 trial. In this trial, consolidative radiation was guided by the PET scan, and given to only those with a PET positive lesion >2.5 cm at the end of chemotherapy. A strategy that could limit the use of radiation to ~10% patients However, BEACOPP has two major concerns, which have led to limited use of this protocol outside Europe: (i) substantial early morbidity and treatment-related mortality and (ii) risk of late effects leading to cardiovascular morbidity and development of secondary malignancies [37].

6.4 BV-AVD (Brentuximab Vedotin–Doxorubicin–Vinblastine–Dacarbazine)

One of the major breakthrough for the treatment of HL is the development of anti CD30 antibody drug conjugate Brentuximab vedotin. The ECHELON-1 trial randomly assigned patients with advanced-stage HL to 6 cycles of ABVD or 6 cycles of BV-AVD. There was a 5% decrease in risk of progression, death, or new lymphoma treatment with AVD-BV compared with ABVD [38].

With respect to practice in India and other developing countries, the major limitations of this regimen are lack of easy availability of BV and very high cost of treatment. In the times to come, the drug is likely to be accessible and we shall see a larger role of this monoclonal antibody in frontline treatment of HL.

6.5 Role of Radiotherapy for Advanced HL

In patients with HL, relapses more commonly occur in the previously involved sites. Addition of radiotherapy leads to reduction in these local relapse rates. At present, the preferred approach is to give either involved-field or involved-site radiotherapy in patients who had bulky disease (>10 cm diameter) at the time of diagnosis or who have a solitary site of residual disease at the end of 6 cycles of ABVD chemotherapy. The preferred modality and radiation dose is 30 Gy of ISRT.

6.6 Table 9 summarises the used of RT in Hodgkins lymphoma as well as non-Hodgkins lymphoma

Table 9 RT dose and fractionation schedules in HD and NHL

Lymphoma type	Clinical situation	GTV and CTV contours	Dose and fractionation
Hodgkin lymphoma (HL)	*Post-chemo (consolidation)*: Most common; used for early-stage or residual advanced disease.	*GTV*: Residual mass post-chemo. *CTV*: Pre-chemo volume (ISRT) restricted to anatomical boundaries	*20–30 Gy* in *1.5–2.0 Gy per fraction* for non-bulky early-stage disease. *30 Gy* in *1.5–2.0 Gy per fraction* for bulky disease. *Residual or PET-positive disease (Deauville 4–5): 36–40 Gy* in conventional fractions
Non-Hodgkin (indolent)	*Upfront (definitive)*: For early stage (I/II). *Post-Chemo*: Less common unless symptomatic	*GTV*: Visible nodes on CT/PET. *CTV*: Involved site (ISRT) or involved field (IFRT) for localized disease	*Definitive RT: 24–30 Gy* in *12–15 fractions* for early-stage indolent NHL. *Post-chemo residual disease: 30–36 Gy* in conventional fractions. *Palliative "Boom-Boom" RT: 4 Gy in two fractions* over 2 days.
Non-Hodgkin (aggressive)	*Post-chemo (consolidation)*: Common for bulky disease or partial response	*GTV*: Post-chemo residual. *CTV*: Pre-chemo involved site, accounting for organ movement	*Complete metabolic response (CR): 30–36 Gy* in conventional fractions. *Partial response (PR) or residual PET-positive disease: 36–40 Gy* in *1.8–2.0 Gy per fraction*

"Boom Boom" RT refers to a low-dose radiation treatment, typically 4 Gy in two fractions in 2 days for NHL, often used for indolent lymphomas like follicular or marginal zone lymphoma, or as a bridging therapy before CAR T-cell therapy, offering high effectiveness with low toxicity for quick, simple treatment
ISRT involved site radiation therapy, *IFRT* involved field radiation therapy

6.7 Indian Experience

A recently published multicentric report shed some light on the patient characteristics and treatment outcome of paints with HL in India in real-world practice. There were 939 newly diagnosed HL patients with a median age of 38 (range 18–99 years). Nodular sclerosis subtype was the commonest subtype with 60% patients. At the time of presentation, 50% patients had B-symptoms and 53% patients had advanced stage disease. The most common first-line chemotherapy was ABVD-based regimen (94%). The overall response rate was 93.5%. Complete response rates among early-stage favourable and unfavourable risk groups were 92.7% and 86.8%, and in those among advanced-stage low- and high-risk groups were 76.6% and 69.8%, respectively. With a median follow-up of 51 months, the 5-year EFS and OS of all patients were 78.2% and 83.6%, respectively [39].

7 Multiple Myeloma and Plasmacytoma

Multiple Myeloma (MM) and Plasmacytomas are a part of a larger subgroup of plasma cell dyscrasias. These disorders are characterized by abnormal proliferation of clonal plasma cells in the bone marrow and other parts of the body, leading to various clinical manifestations. With the development of newer drugs and treatment strategies, numerous options exist for patients even after multiple relapses, enabling patients to live longer with the disease.

MM seems to develop in most individuals from a previous asymptomatic state of Monoclonal gammopathy of undetermined significance (MGUS) and Smouldering Multiple Myeloma (SMM). A large population-based study from Iceland has estimated the Incidence of MGUS and SMM to be approximately 5% and 0.5%, respectively. However, the reported Incidence of MGUS in India is lower, nearly 1.5% [40*, 41]. The risk of progression from MGUS to MM is almost 1% per year, while the risk of progression is much higher in patients with SMM, (patients with high-risk features having a 60% risk of progression to MM in 2 years) [42]**. The crude rate of MM in India is 1.27/100,000 in males and 0.95/100,000 in females (which is lower than the Western population). Most cases were in the seventh decade of life and the highest incidence was seen in North and South India [43].

Solitary Plasmacytomas are rarer compared to MM and constitute around 5–10% of all plasma cell dyscrasia. Plasmacytomas may further be divided based on clonal plasma cells in the bone marrow (plasmacytoma with or without minimal marrow involvement), with risk of progression being higher in patients with minimal marrow involvement. Plasmacytomas may be involving the bone (more common) or other parts of the body (extramedullary plasmacytoma). The rate of progression to MM is higher with bony plasmacytomas than extramedullary plasmacytomas [44].

7.1 Clinical Features and Workup [45]*

The cardinal features of MM are hypercalcemia, renal failure, anaemia, and bony lesions, denoted by the acronym "CRAB". Anaemia and bony lesions are the most common clinical features among the four cardinal features, followed by renal failure and hypercalcemia. Patients with MM may present with a myriad of symptoms secondary to either proliferation of clonal plasma cells or secretion of large amounts of abnormal protein. Symptoms secondary to clonal expansion of plasma cells include anaemia and cytopenias, pathological fractures, hypercalcemia, spinal cord compression and bone pains. Symptoms secondary to increased secretion of abnormal protein include renal failure, hyperviscosity syndrome, and neuropathy. Alternatively, some patients may be relatively asymptomatic and get diagnosed due an abnormal total protein: albumin ratio.

The most common location for bony plasmacytomas is the vertebrae, while extramedullary plasmacytomas are most frequently seen in the head and neck region, involving the upper airways and paranasal sinus.

The diagnostic criteria for MM and Solitary plasmacytoma are given in Table 10.

At baseline, all patients should get a complete blood count with peripheral blood smear examination, renal function test, calcium profile (including total protein and albumin), serum LDH, urine routine, and 24-hour urine protein examination. In addition, patients should have HIV, Hepatitis B, and Hepatitis C serology done at baseline. A baseline serum protein electrophoresis (SPEP), serum immunofixation (SIFE) and serum free light chain assay (SFLCA) is also required for each patient. If there is evidence of proteinuria, patients should undergo a urine protein electrophoresis and a urine immunofixation. Beta-2 microglobulin (B2M) is required for prognostication and staging of MM. All patients should undergo a bone marrow aspiration with biopsy with cytogenetic evaluation for high-risk cytogenetics via FISH. A renal biopsy may be required to better characterize renal involvement in patients with MM with acute kidney injury or isolated proteinuria. Fat-pad FNAC/Biopsy from the abdomen and rectal biopsy may help document the amyloid protein in patients with suspected amyloidosis. In addition, a 2D echo for cardiac involvement should be done for patients with suspected amyloidosis.

All patients with suspected MM should undergo an ultra-low-dose whole-body CT (LDCT) or a whole-body 18FDG PET scan done at baseline. In patients with an inconclusive LDCT, a whole-body MRI may be considered. In patients with a suspected solitary plasmacytoma, a FDG PET is preferred for extramedullary plasmacytomas, and a whole body MRI is the diagnostic modality of choice for a bony plasmacytoma. A MRI of the spine should be done in patients with suspected vertebral involvement, such as back pain or spinal cord compression.

Table 10 Diagnostic criteria for solitary plasmacytoma and multiple myeloma

Solitary plasmacytoma	All four criteria to be met Biopsy-proven solitary lesion of bone or soft tissue with evidence of clonal plasma cells Normal bone marrow with no evidence of clonal plasma cells Normal skeletal survey and MRI (or CT) of spine and pelvis (except for the primary solitary lesion) Absence of end-organ damage such as CRAB features that can be attributed to a lympho-plasma cell proliferative disorder
Solitary plasmacytoma with minimal marrow involvement	All four criteria to be met Biopsy-proven solitary lesion of bone or soft tissue with evidence of clonal plasma cells Clonal bone marrow plasma cells <10% Normal skeletal survey and MRI (or CT) of spine and pelvis (except for the primary solitary lesion) Absence of end-organ damage such as CRAB features that can be attributed to a lympho-plasma cell proliferative disorder
Multiple myeloma	Clonal bone marrow plasma cells ≥10% or biopsy-proven bony or extramedullary plasmacytoma with any one of the following Hypercalcemia >1 mg/dL higher than upper limit of normal or >11 mg/dL Renal insufficiency: CrCl <40 mL/min or serum creatinine >2 mg/dL Haemoglobin >2gm/dL below the lower limit of normal or a haemoglobin value <10gm/dL One or more osteolytic lesions on skeletal radiography, CT, or PET-CT Clonal bone marrow plasma cell ≥60% Involved: Uninvolved serum FLC ratio ≥100 (involved FLC level must be ≥100 mg/L) >1 focal lesion on MRI studies (at least 5 mm in size)

7.2 Staging and Prognostication

The different staging systems for MM are given in Table 11. The R-ISS system incorporates high-risk cytogenetics and serum LDH into the ISS to improve disease prognostication. The mSMART classification stratifies patients based on number of high-risk cytogenetics and introduced the concept of double hit and triple hit myeloma, defined as the presence of 2 and ≥3 high-risk cytogenetics. Patients with double-hit and triple-hit MM have been shown to have a dismal prognosis in multiple real-world data sets [46].

Various clinical and disease parameters also help in the prognostication of MM patients. The presence of renal failure, especially when it persists after the institution of therapy, has been associated with poorer outcomes [47]. Similarly, the presence of extramedullary disease is associated with a poorer prognosis.

Table 11 Different staging systems of multiple myeloma

Staging system	Definitions	Overall survival [48, 49]
ISS	I- Serum albumin ≥3.5 gm/dL and Serum B2M <3.5 mg/L	Median—62 months
	II- Not fulfilling criteria of Stage I and III	Median—44 months
	III- Serum B2M ≥5.5 mg/L	Median—29 months
R-ISS	I- ISS I with normal LDH and no high-risk cytogenetics[a]	At 3 years—83%
	II- Not fulfilling criteria for Stage I and III	At 3 years—69%
	III- ISS III and either elevated LDH or presence of high-risk cytogenetics	At 3 years—45%

[a]High-risk cytogenetics defined as t(4:14), t(14:16) or del (17p)

7.3 Treatment

Solitary Plasmacytoma Radiotherapy is the treatment of choice for patients with a confirmed solitary plasmacytoma. Plasma cells are exquisitely sensitive to radiotherapy, and it can provide reasonable local disease control. A total dose of 40–50 Gy given in conventional fractionation is recommended. IMRT is the preferred modality in lesions adjacent to critical structures (for e.g. spinal cord), whereas 3D-CRT or conventional portals can also be used in suitable patients. During RT planning, Gross Tumour Volume (GTV) includes the clinico-radiologically evident gross lesion, while the Clinical Target Volume (CTV) encompasses possible extent of microscopic disease in the bone and/or adjacent soft tissue. Planning Target Volume (PTV) is generated based on the set-up uncertainties and probable intra-fraction motion of the target. Radiation therapy provides excellent local control of the disease, with 80–90% response rates. In patients with solitary plasmacytoma, surgery and excision are usually reserved for patients with pathological fractures or spinal instability and cord compression. The use of chemotherapy in patients with a solitary plasmacytoma with no marrow involvement is controversial. Most studies have not shown an extra benefit of adding chemotherapy to radiotherapy and hence is not recommended. However, chemotherapy is generally considered in case of large plasmacytoma (>5 cm), if there is evidence of clonal plasma cells on bone marrow examination, or the plasmacytoma does not respond to initial radiation. These patients require regular follow-up with clinical examination and biochemical evaluation for serological response [50]*.

Multiple Myeloma The treatment for MM has undergone a paradigm shift in the last few decades. The different categories of drugs and standard regimens used in MM are highlighted in Table 3. The treatment of MM depends on the status of the disease (Newly diagnosed vs relapsed/refractory), risk stratification (high risk vs standard risk) as well as transplant eligibility of the patient (transplant eligible vs transplant ineligible).

Transplant Eligible Newly Diagnosed Multiple Myeloma The standard therapy for patients with transplant eligible newly diagnosed multiple Myeloma (NDMM) is triplet therapy consisting of steroids, a proteasome inhibitor (usually Bortezomib) and an immunomodulator (usually Lenalidomide). Cyclophosphamide may be considered in place of Lenalidomide in patients with renal failure. Use of more intense regimens such as Carfilzomib, Lenalidomide and Dexathemasone has not shown to have a clear benefit over standard triplet regimens in standard risk patients [51]. The current standard of care includes 4–6 cycles of induction therapy followed by high-dose therapy and autologous hematopoietic cell transplant followed by maintenance with Lenalidomide and or Bortezomib. Long-term data from the IFM 2009 study shows that early transplant is associated with a progression-free survival (PFS) benefit but no overall survival (OS) benefit compared to delayed Transplant [52]. A recently published study from North India reported similar results. Overall, the outcome of NDMM patients is similar in India compared to western literature, with a 5-year OS of 83.1% [53].

Transplant Ineligible Newly Diagnosed Multiple Myeloma Patients may be ineligible for high-dose therapy followed by autologous stem cell transplant due to age and frailty. Management of these patients is based on the assessment of frailty and comorbidities. Patients who are fit can be treated with triplet therapy based on bortezomib, lenalidomide and dexamethasone. The frail patients will need dose reduction or doublet. Multiple studies have evaluated the use of upfront Daratumumab in this group of patients. Use of upfront Daratumumab has been shown to have a PFS benefit and OS benefit.

Radiotherapy in Multiple Myeloma Role of radiation in multiple myeloma is limited to management of painful bone lesions, spinal cord compression and impending fracture. Radiation can be delivered concurrently with ongoing systemic therapy. The radiation dose can vary from 8 Gy single fraction to 20 Gy in 5 fractions.

Supportive Care All patients should receive a bone-modifying agent- bisphosphonates or denosumab. Regular use of bisphosphonates is associated with better bone-related outcomes in patients with multiple Myeloma, with zoledronic acid being the preferred bisphosphonate. Denosumab is non-inferior compared to zoledronate and may be considered for patients with NDMM when presenting with renal failure. All patients receiving an immunomodulator should receive anti-thrombotic prophylaxis with anti-platelet drug or anticoagulants, depending on the presence of other risk factors. All patients receiving a proteasome inhibitor should receive acyclovir for antiviral prophylaxis. These patients are at a high risk of infection and should be considered for pneumococcal vaccination at the time of diagnosis.

8 Chronic Myeloid Leukaemia

Chronic myeloid leukaemia (CML) is a clonal myeloproliferative neoplasm characterized by the presence of Philadelphia chromosome as an acquired clonal cytogenetic abnormality. CML is the commonest leukaemia in adults in India with an incidence of 0.8–2.2 per 100,000 as per the available estimates. The age of onset in India is younger than in the west with median age being 30–40 years.

8.1 Clinical Features and Workup

The presentation can vary from incidental detection to the presence of fever, weight loss, abdominal pain, early satiety, fatigue and bleeding manifestations due to platelet dysfunction. A large majority (>85–90%) of patients present with the chronic phase at diagnosis. Approximately 10–15% of patients may have advanced phase disease—accelerated phase or blast crisis (myeloid being more common).

Evaluation requires documentation of spleen size, any lymphadenopathy or extramedullary disease, complete blood counts, peripheral smear, liver and renal function tests and bone marrow aspiration, biopsy, conventional cytogenetics/FISH and qualitative RT-PCR for BCR-ABL. Peripheral smear shows a shift to left and basophilia. Documentation of blast percentage in bone marrow and blood, basophil percentage and presence of clonal abnormalities other than Philadelphia chromosome are important to identify the advanced phase disease. In case of blasts crisis (peripheral blood or bone marrow blasts >20%), immunophenotyping is recommended to identify myeloid or lymphoid subtype. Conventional cytogenetics may not be able to identify Philadelphia chromosome in patients with complex/atypical translocations or may fail due to lack of metaphases. FISH is helpful in these cases for identification of BCR::ABL1 translocation for confirmation of diagnosis.

8.2 Prognostication and Treatment

Several prognostic indices like Sokal, Hasford, EUTOS, and now ELTS have been developed and validated over the years. As most patients do not die of CML now due to effective treatment, ELTS is more relevant in the present era. The advent of tyrosine kinase inhibitors (TKI) has changed the outcome of patients with CML with feasibility of survival similar to age-matched general population. The first-line treatment is imatinib in patients with chronic phase disease. Patients with high-risk disease or those who are desirous of treatment-free remission (young female who are not married or have not completed family) can be started on second-generation TKI (dasatinib, nilotinib). The second-generation TKI induce faster and deeper responses; however, there is no improvement in overall survival as compared to imatinib. The selection of second-generation TKI in adults should be based on the presence and type of comorbidities and goal of therapy. Development of pleural effusion, pulmonary arterial hypertension (dasatinib), cardiovascular events, dyslipidemia, pancreatitis, peripheral vascular disease (nilotnib) are some of the adverse events, which should be kept in mind while prescribing these drugs. The response to treatment should be assessed at month for haematological response and then periodically (3–6 months). After achievement of complete cytogenetic response, RQ-PCR for BCR::ABL1 is recommended once in 3–6 months. In case of lack of defined response imatinib or second-generation TKI should undergo mutation analysis to identify the cause for resistance and selection of appropriate second-line drugs. Often the poor compliance is the cause of treatment failure. The use of allogeneic stem cell transplant is now limited to those with advanced phase disease (blast crisis), lack of response to TKI or those who experience significant cytopenias, which does not allow treatment continuation.

9 Evolution of Radiation Therapy in Haematological Malignancies

Definitive radiation therapy (RT) alone with large extended fields (e.g. *Total Lymphoid Irradiation (TLI), Sub-total Lymphoid irradiation (STLI), Mantle field & Inverted Y field)* involving treatment of both supra- and infra-diaphragmatic lymph nodal regions has been successfully used for treatment of Hodgkin's lymphomas in 1950s. Although these treatments resulted in cure of disease in a significant proportion of patients, they were associated with significant long-term toxicities. Use of systemic chemotherapy along with smaller radiation portals, restricted to the involved nodal region only (*Involved field Radiotherapy, IFRT*) came into practice, ensuring optimal treatment efficacy with minimal morbidity.

IFRT involves irradiation of the diseased lymph nodal region. It was often practiced by 2-dimensional planning using bony anatomical landmarks of nodal regions. However, it was noticed that most of the failures in unirradiated patients tend to occur at the initial extent of the disease and thus it was not imperative to irradiate the whole nodal region. Consequently, delineation of the target structure based on the pre-chemotherapy nodal disease extent, by co-registration of the planning CT structures with the baseline PET CT was advocated. This was termed as *Involved Nodal radiotherapy (INRT).*

There were technical challenges in the planning of INRT. Registration of the baseline PET CT with planning CT was not always accurate, due to difference in patient positioning and consequent change in the anatomy of the nodal levels (for e.g. arm position has notable impact on the anatomical extent in CT of axillary nodal levels). Acquisition of the baseline PET CT in radiotherapy planning position, to avoid that inaccuracy, has logistic challenges especially in high-volume centres. This introduced the concept and practice of *Involved Site Radiation therapy (ISRT)*, in which the target volume consists of the pre-chemotherapy disease extent as defined by the co-registered PET CT, with a surrounding safety margin of 1.0–1.5 cm.

Presently, ISRT continues to be the standard of care for consolidative radiotherapy for both HL & NHL [54]. In addition, TLI or STLI still has an important role in treatment of patients with relapsed/refractory lymphomas unsuitable for salvage systemic therapy.

10 Special Radiotherapy Techniques

10.1 Prophylactic and Therapeutic Cranial Irradiation (PCI & TCI)

Cranial irradiation is usually planned using bilateral opposing portals, which includes the reflection of the leptomeninges and the spaces that potentially harbour cerebrospinal fluid (CSF), commonly described as the 'German Helmet' technique. The portals generally are as following: superiorly in air, anteriorly including posterior half of the globe, inferiorly up to the C1/2 junction and posteriorly in air. Shielding is done to avoid irradiation to the anterior half of the globes and oral cavity. Efforts are underway to assess if use of IMRT is superior to conventional portals in preserving neurocognitive functions in patients after cranial irradiation. Dosimetric benefits in terms of hippocampal sparing are encouraging, however mature studies and evidence about clinical implications of the same is still awaited, to recommend routine use of IMRT for cranial irradiation in these patients.

10.2 Total Body Irradiation (TBI)

TBI is an important and commonly used conditioning regimen for allogenic hematopoietic stem cell transplantation, with the aim of myeloablation and/or immune-suppression. The doses and techniques for TBI differ according to its indication. In TBI aiming only at immune-suppression (non-myeloablative), lower doses (2–4 Gy) are used, and hence shielding of lungs are not required. In contrast, in myeloablative TBI, doses of 10–16 Gy are used, usually in twice daily regimens of 1.3–1.5 Gy per fraction, and this requires partial

Table 12 Comparison of TBI, TMLI and TMI

Feature	TBI (total body irradiation)	TMLI (total marrow and lymphoid irradiation)	TMI (total marrow irradiation)
Target volume	Entire body	Bone marrow + major lymphoid tissues (LN, spleen, thymus)	Bone marrow only
Radiation technique	Conventional LINAC (AP/PA fields)	IMRT/VMAT/ tomotherapy	IMRT/VMAT/ tomotherapy
Typical total dose	10–14 Gy	12–20 Gy	12–20 Gy
Common fractionation	12 Gy/6 fx	12–15 Gy/6–10 fx	12–15 Gy/6–10 fx
Dose per fraction	1.5–2 Gy (usually two fractions per day 6–8 h apart)	1.5–2 Gy (usually two fractions per day 6–8 h apart)	1.5–2 Gy (usually two fractions per day 6–8 h apart)
Primary purpose	Myeloablation + immunosuppression	Myeloablation + enhanced immunosuppression	Myeloablation
Organ-at-risk exposure	Full prescription dose to all organs	Significantly reduced	Lowest
Ability to escalate dose	Limited by toxicity	Moderate–good	Best
Acute/late toxicity	Highest	Reduced as compared to TBI	Lowest
Typical indications	ALL (classic), selected AML, historical use in lymphoma	High-risk or relapsed ALL/AML, MDS, lymphoma, reduced-intensity conditioning	AML, MDS, marrow-dominant disease where organ sparing is critical
Current clinical trend	Declining but still useful as reference	Increasing in specialized centres	Increasing in specialized centres

From Ref. [55]

Note: Non-myeloablative conditioning (NMA) with low-dose TBI (total body irradiation, often 2 Gy) is a less intensive pre-stem cell transplant regimen that causes minimal bone marrow suppression, allowing for quicker immune recovery and fewer severe side effects compared to traditional myeloablative approaches, making it ideal for older or sicker patients

shielding of lungs. TBI is a technically challenging procedure, due to the large treatment volume with unequal thickness at various parts. Most of the centres use an extended SSD (source-to-skin distance) technique, AP-PA portals with 6 MV photons, with patient standing upright on a TBI stand, with a beam spoiler to ensure dose deposition to skin and subcutaneous tissues [56]. Other less common techniques used include bilateral portals, translating couch technique etc. Lung blocks are custom-made for each patient, using the radiographic details of the chest. Various methods of pulmonary shielding have been used for patients undergoing myelo-ablative TBI. In our institute, we use a specialized holder/jacket for lung blocks, that is worn by the patient during the treatment duration. Portal films and in-vivo dosimetry are done for quality assurance.

Table 12 shows the comparison between related techniques of TBI (total body irradiation), TMLI (total marrow and lymphoid irradiation), and TMI (total marrow irradiation).

10.3 Total Skin Electron Beam Therapy (TSEBT)

TSEBT is a technique by which radiation therapy is delivered to patients requiring irradiation of the entire skin of the body (mycosis fungoides). The most commonly used technique used for TSEBT is the Modified Stanford technique [57]. Patients are treated with dual angled electron beams (usually 6 MeV, to have Dmax at skin surface), with 6 fields (3 fields in alternating sequence on two successive days). Patients are positioned at an extended SSD (dosimetric calibration preformed for institutional parameters), with a scattering foil in front. In-vivo dosimetry for each patient is performed on the first day of treatment to ensure adequate coverage on all sites. Corneal and nail-bed shields are used throughout the treatment. Although there are recent reports suggesting lower doses of TSEBT (10–12 Gy), doses above 25 Gy are traditionally found to induce durable responses. Further details about management with TSEBT are provided in the chapter (Special Techniques: Total Body Irradiation, T-SET, IORT, and Hyperthermia- Volume 1)

11 Recent Advances in RT

11.1 Residual Volume Radiotherapy

Residual Site Radiation Therapy (RSRT) is an evolving concept in the treatment of lymphomas. In this process, the target volume of RT consists of the morphological residual disease at the completion of planned chemotherapy. This has the potential to significantly reduce toxicities at sites adjacent to critical structures (e.g. mediastinum), in patients who had baseline bulky disease but has significant regression with chemotherapy. It has been found feasible, dosimetrically advantageous and safe in HL [58], PMBCL [59] and DLBCL [60].

11.2 Proton Beam Therapy

The International Lymphoma Radiation Oncology Group (ILROG) recommendation limits the use of proton therapy to patients with mediastinal disease that spans below the origin of the left main stem coronary artery and is anterior to, posterior to, or on the left side of the heart; young female patients in order to reduce breast dose and risk for secondary breast cancer; and heavily pretreated patients who are at higher risk for radiation-related toxicity to the bone marrow, heart, and lungs [61].

11.3 Respiratory Motion Management

Deep Inspiratory Breath-hold (DIBH) is a technique aiming at the movement of heart and lungs away from the irradiation portal, to reduce late toxicities of mediastinal RT. It can be implemented along with IMRT, Butterfly technique of VMAT, full arc VMAT, proton beam therapy, etc. Patients suitable for DIBH include those with disease confined to superior mediastinum. There are a multitude of studies showing dosimetric advantages of DIBH compared to free-breathing technique [62]. However, because these techniques are too new to have adequate follow-up duration of patients, clinical benefits are yet to be compared.

11.4 Total Marrow and Lymphoid Irradiation (TMLI)

Aiming at conformal avoidance of normal structures (oral cavity, liver, kidneys etc.), and thus reduction in treatment-related toxicity seen after TBI, a conformal technique of myeloablation *(Total Marrow & Lymphoid Irradiation, TMLI)* is being tested at multiple centres [56]. TMLI utilizes the basic principles of IMRT in delivering highly conformal radiation while sparing the normal structures. Dosimetric studies have shown the benefit of TMLI over TBI; however, there are scarce data showing translation of the same to clinical benefit.

11.5 Stereotactic Body Radiotherapy (SBRT)

Stereotactic body radiotherapy (SBRT) has been found to be promising in the treatment of metastatic bone lesions, owing to its excellent conformity and lethal biological effects. Centres have tried extrapolating the benefits to bony lesions in Multiple Myeloma as well. Doses of 14–16 Gy have shown excellent and durable pain relief in patients with spinal lesions despite associated vertebral fracture, neural foramina involvement and thecal sac compression [63]. SBRT is a potentially promising technique in the treatment of Solitary Bone Plasmacytomas. A few studies are being undertaken to assess the efficacy, feasibility and benefits of the same.

12 Future Research Areas

There has been remarkable progress in the field of these haematological cancers; however, much is needed to be done, more so in resource-constrained countries.

Important focus in acute leukaemia's remains the induction mortality, which is often due to multidrug-resistant infections. Efforts are needed to search for therapies, which can allow disease control with shorter duration of neutropenia to reduce the risk of infections and antecedent mortality. There is an urgent need to address the multi-drug-resistant gram-negative infections in these patients.

Due to limited availability, access and treatment-related mortality of allogeneic stem cell transplant, we do need to evaluate more effective agents to eradicate the minimal residual disease and maintain the response with safe and effective maintenance therapy.

There is a need for better predictive markers to identify patients at diagnosis who can be given shorter duration of therapy using less-intensive regimens in all the lymphomas. Treatment of PTCL, high-risk DLBCL and role of CNS prophylaxis in DLBCL remain fertile areas for research. Treatment of these malignancies in elderly is another area, which requires considerable amount of research.

13 Summary

1. Diagnostic evaluation of acute myeloid leukaemia should include assessment of risk category with the help of cytogenetics and molecular data.
2. The treatment for acute myeloid leukaemia should be based on the fitness of the patient for intensive chemotherapy and according to risk category.
3. Allogeneic stem cell transplant should be considered as optimal post-remission therapy in fit patients with poor risk features and available donor.
4. All patients with acute lymphoblastic leukaemia should undergo CSF examination at baseline after optimization of thrombocytopenia.
5. Paediatric inspired regimens are preferable for the treatment of adolescent and young-adult patients with ALL.
6. As opposed to paediatric ALL, use of prophylactic cranial radiation in adults is still recommended, especially in high risk patients.
7. All patients with suspected lymphomas should undergo a biopsy—preferably excisional from the representative and accessible node. In cases where excisional biopsy is not feasible, incisional biopsy should be considered. Core biopsy is used for the sites where both excisional and incisional biopsies are not possible.
8. All patients with suspected lymphoma should undergo complete staging work-up as per the subtype except if there are oncological emergencies, which require urgent initiation of therapy.
9. Treatment of non-Hodgkin lymphoma should be based on histopathological subtype. The lymphoblastic lymphomas are treated with acute lymphoblastic leukaemia like therapy.
10. Patients with early stage Hodgkin lymphoma should be considered for combined modality therapy except in situation where the long-term side effects of radiation outweigh the risk of relapse.
11. Post therapy surveillance PET-CT or CT does not improve the outcomes and should be avoided unless there is clinical suspicious of relapse/progression.
12. Solitary plasmacytomas can be adequately treated with radiotherapy.

13. Multiple myeloma can have a varied spectrum of clinical presentation based on the end-organ damage.
14. The treatment of myeloma is required only if the indications of treatment are present.
15. Appropriate institution of supportive care, management of infections and tumour lysis management are key component to improve the outcomes in these haematological cancers.
16. All patients who complete treatment should be monitored for long-term treatment-related complications based on the type of treatment.

Multiple Choice Questions

1. What is not one of the diagnostic criteria for Multiple Myeloma?
   (a) Hb <10 gm/dL
   (b) Creatinine >2 mg/dL
   (c) Calcium >11 mg/dL
   (d) M Band >3 gm/dL
2. Which of the following is not a high-risk cytogenetic abnormality in the R-ISS stagging?
   (a) t(4:14)
   (b) t(11:14)
   (c) t(14:16)
   (d) del (17p)
3. Which of the following currently is not a recommended imaging modality for patients with multiple Myeloma?
   (a) Skeletal Survey
   (b) Whole Body PET CT
   (c) Whole Body MRI
   (d) Low dose whole body CT
4. Which of the following is not a proteasome inhibitor?
   (a) Bortezomib
   (b) Carfilzomib
   (c) Ixazomib
   (d) Lenalidomide
5. Which of the following is not recommended in a patient with newly diagnosed multiple Myeloma on standard triplet therapy?
   (a) Acyclovir prophylaxis
   (b) Anti-thrombotic prophylaxis
   (c) IVIg infusion
   (d) Bisphosphonates
6. Which of the following is the commonest subtype of Hodgkin lymphoma
   (a) HL-Lymphocyte-rich
   (b) HL-Nodular sclerosis
   (c) HL-Mixed cellularity
   (d) HL-Lymphocyte-depleted
7. Which imaging modality, used for staging of a newly diagnosed case of HL, can help in applying a risk-adapted treatment approach
   (a) PET-CT Scan
   (b) CECT-neck, chest and abdomen
   (c) A CECT scan with MRI of the main involved site
   (d) CECT chest with USG abdomen
8. Which of the following drug is not a component of ABVD
   (a) Doxorubicin
   (b) Dacarbazine
   (c) Vincristine
   (d) Bleomycin
9. What will be your preferred choice for management of a 26 year old male patient with stage II HL- nodular sclerosis variety who presented with a 10 cm mediastinal mass
   (a) ABVD 4 cycles alone
   (b) ABVD 2 cycles followed by 16 Gy of IFRT
   (c) ABVD 4 cycles followed by 30 Gy of IFRT
   (d) Only 6 cycles of ABVD
10. Which of the following statement is not true about HL
    (a) Mixed cellularity HL is more common in older patients, and it has higher probability of intra-abdominal involvement
    (b) Response-adapted treatment is increasingly practiced for treatment of HL now
    (c) Overall survival is equal in chemotherapy only approach and combined modality treatment
    (d) Freedom from local failure is equal in chemotherapy only approach and combined modality treatment
11. Workup for a patient with suspected AML includes all except?

(a) Bone marrow aspiration with immunophenotyping
(b) Bone marrow biopsy
(c) PETCT
(d) Cytogenetics

12. Which of the following AML subtypes require >20% blasts in the bone marrow as an essential criteria for its diagnosis?
(a) AML inv 3
(b) AML t(15;17)
(c) AML t(8;21)
(d) AML inv (16)

13. According to the ELN Risk stratification, all of the following fall under the Adverse risk criteria except?
(a) Mutated NPM1 and FLT3 (high allelic ratio)
(b) Wild type NPM1 and FLT3 (high allelic ratio)
(c) Complex karyotype
(d) Monosomal karyotype

14. Allogenic stem cell transplant is an accepted of standard of care for AML patients with the following characteristics except?
(a) MRD positive after 3 + 7 induction
(b) AML with complex karyotype
(c) AML with monosomal karyotype
(d) AML with FLT3-ITD high allelic ratio

15. Which of the following associations of drugs with its mechanism in AML is correct?
(a) Midostaurin—Anti CD33
(b) Venetoclax—BCl2
(c) Ivosedenib—IDH2
(d) Azacytidine—IDH1

16. Which of the following is an approved drug for maintenance in AML?
(a) Sorafenib
(b) Azacytidine
(c) Venetoclax
(d) Ivosedenib

17. Following are B Cell markers except?
(a) CD19
(b) CD20
(c) CD3
(d) CD79a

18. Prevalence of BCR ABL1 positive ALL in children is?
(a) 25%
(b) 50%
(c) <5%
(d) 90%

19. All are an high risk factor at diagnosis for ALL, except?
(a) Age >35 years
(b) TLC >100,000 for B ALL
(c) t(4;11) rearrangement
(d) Hyperploidy

20. All the following are strategies to prevent CNS relapse in treatment of ALL, except?
(a) Intrathecal methotrexate
(b) High dose methotrexate
(c) Cappizzi methotrexate
(d) Cranial irradiation

21. Which of the following targeted agents in ALL and its mechanism is not correct?
(a) Blinatumumab—BiTe
(b) Inotuzumab Ozogamicin—antiCD21 antibody
(c) Rituximab—antiCD20 antibody
(d) Tisagenlecleucel—CAR-T

22. All the following Cell of origin with respect to the lymphomas are correct except?
(a) Pre -Germinal centre B cell—Mantle cell lymphoma
(b) Germinal B Cell—Burkitt lymphoma
(c) Follicular helper T Cell—Follicular lymphoma
(d) Marginal Zone—Marginal Zone lymphoma

23. With regard to lymph node biopsy for establishment of a diagnosis of lymphoma, what would be the preferred method of diagnosis in descending order?
(a) Core biopsy > Excisional biopsy > Incisional biopsy > FNAC
(b) Excisional biopsy > Incisional biopsy > Core biopsy > FNAC
(c) Incisional biopsy > Core biopsy > Excisional biopsy > FNAC
(d) Incisional biopsy > Core biopsy > FNAC > Excisional biopsy

24. A lady presenting with a left sided breast lump.. She does not have any other symptoms. Biopsy from the breast lump reported as Diffuse large B Cell lymphoma. PETCT shows left sided axillary lymph node in addi-

tion to the breast lump. No other sites of disease. Bone marrow biopsy and aspiration is uninvolved. What is the final stage of this patient as per the Lugano classification?
   (a) Stage IE
   (b) Stage IIE
   (c) Stage IV
   (d) Stage IIIE
25. In which of following situations Bone marrow aspiration and biopsy cannot be avoided in patients with DLBCL?
   (a) Stage I DLBCL
   (b) DLBCL with multiple extranodal involvement without BM involvement in PETCT
   (c) DLBCL with PETCT bone marrow involvement
   (d) PMBCL
26. CNS prophylaxis is needed in all the following except:
   (a) DLBCL with testicular involvement
   (b) Burkitt lymphoma
   (c) DLBCL with 1 extranodal site
   (d) PCNSL
27. All the following is true about PMBCL except?
   (a) Common in young females
   (b) Compartmentalizing fibrosis is an hallmark of its histology
   (c) Recommended treatment is 6 cycles of REPOCH (infusional) followed by RT
   (d) IHC profile of PMBCL—CD20+ve, CD30+ve, CD15−ve
28. All the following are false about Burkitt lymphoma except?
   (a) Burkitt lymphoma is an aggressive lymphoma with predominantly nodal and bone marrow involvement
   (b) Current chemotherapy regimens of Burkitt obviate the need for CNS prophylaxis
   (c) Presence of C-Myc translocation is an hallmark of Burkitt's lymphoma
   (d) Endemic Burkitts is more common in the southeast Asian subcontinent
29. All the following are treatment indications for follicular lymphoma except?
   (a) Splenomegaly of 5 cm
   (b) Ascites
   (c) Tumour >7 cm in size
   (d) Involvement in >3 nodes in 3 distinct areas, each >3 cm in diameter
30. All the following regarding CLL is true except?
   (a) IgHV mutated type CLL has better prognosis than unmutated
   (b) TP53 mutated has the worst prognosis
   (c) Autoimmune hemolytic anemia of CLL needs treatment with chemotherapy
   (d) Asymptomatic patients can be kept on watchful waiting
31. Which of the following is correct (in descending order of outcomes)
   (a) ALK+ve ALCL >> DUSP22 rearrangement ALCL >> p63+ve ALCL >> DUSP22−ve and p63−ve ALCL
   (b) ALK+ve ALCL >> p63+ve ALCL >> DUSP22 rearrangement ALCL >> DUSP22−ve and p63−ve ALCL
   (c) ALK+ve ALCL >> DUSP22 rearrangement ALCL >> DUSP22−ve and p63−ve ALCL >> p63+ve ALCL
   (d) ALK+ve ALCL >> p63+ve ALCL >> DUSP22−ve and p63−ve ALCL >> DUSP22 rearrangement ALCL
32. All of the following regarding NK-T Cell lymphoma is correct except?
   (a) Patients can present with hemophagocytic histiocytosis (HLH)
   (b) Association with EBV is established
   (c) Endemic to equatorial Africa
   (d) Inherently resistant to drugs which are removed by MDR efflux

Answer Key

1. (d)
2. (b)
3. (a)
4. (d)
5. (c)
6. (b)
7. (a)
8. (c)
9. (c)

10. (d)
11. (c)
12. (a)
13. (a)
14. (a)
15. (b)
16. (b)
17. (c)
18. (c)
19. (d)
20. (c)
21. (b)
22. (c)
23. (b)
24. (b)
25. (d)
26. (c)
27. (c)
28. (c)
29. (a)
30. (c)
31. (c)
32. (c)

References

1. Juliusson G, Lazarevic V, Hörstedt A-S, Hagberg O, Höglund M, Swedish Acute Leukemia Registry Group. Acute myeloid leukemia in the real world: why population-based registries are needed. Blood. 2012;119(17):3890–9. https://doi.org/10.1182/blood-2011-12-379008.
2. *Arber DA, et al. The 2016 revision to the World Health Organization classification of myeloid neoplasms and acute leukemia. Blood. 2016;127(20):2391–405. https://doi.org/10.1182/blood-2016-03-643544.
3. **Döhner H, et al. Diagnosis and management of AML in adults: 2017 ELN recommendations from an international expert panel. Blood. 2017;129(4):424–47. https://doi.org/10.1182/blood-2016-08-733196.
4. Philip C, et al. Acute myeloid leukaemia: challenges and real world data from India. Br J Haematol. 2015;170(1):110–7. https://doi.org/10.1111/bjh.13406.
5. Cooper SL, Brown PA. Treatment of pediatric acute lymphoblastic leukemia. Pediatr Clin N Am. 2015;62(1):61–73. https://doi.org/10.1016/j.pcl.2014.09.006.
6. **Ganesan P, Kayal S. How I treat adult acute lymphoblastic leukemia in India. Indian J Med Paediatr Oncol. 2021;42(6):584–94. https://doi.org/10.1055/s-0041-1731979.
7. **Ravandi F. How I treat Philadelphia chromosome–positive acute lymphoblastic leukemia. Blood. 2019;133(2):130–6. https://doi.org/10.1182/blood-2018-08-832105.
8. Hunger SP, Raetz EA. How I treat relapsed acute lymphoblastic leukemia in the pediatric population. Blood. 2020;136(16):1803–12. https://doi.org/10.1182/blood.2019004043.
9. Robison LL. Late effects of acute lymphoblastic leukemia therapy in patients diagnosed at 0–20 years of age. Hematol Am Soc Hematol Educ Program. 2011;2011:238–42. https://doi.org/10.1182/asheducation-2011.1.238.
10. Nair R, Arora N, Mallath MK. Epidemiology of non-Hodgkin's lymphoma in India. Oncology. 2016;91(Suppl 1):18–25. https://doi.org/10.1159/000447577.
11. Phillips AA, Smith DA. Health disparities and the global landscape of lymphoma care today. Am Soc Clin Oncol Educ Book Am Soc Clin Oncol Annu Meet. 2017;37:526–34. https://doi.org/10.1200/EDBK_175444.
12. **Swerdlow SH, et al. The 2016 revision of the World Health Organization classification of lymphoid neoplasms. Blood. 2016;127(20):2375–90. https://doi.org/10.1182/blood-2016-01-643569.
13. **Armitage JO, Gascoyne RD, Lunning MA, Cavalli F. Non-Hodgkin lymphoma. Lancet Lond Engl. 2017;390(10091):298–310. https://doi.org/10.1016/S0140-6736(16)32407-2.
14. **Cheson BD, et al. Recommendations for initial evaluation, staging, and response assessment of Hodgkin and non-Hodgkin lymphoma: the Lugano classification. J Clin Oncol. 2014;32(27):3059–68. https://doi.org/10.1200/JCO.2013.54.8800.
15. Ziepert M, et al. Standard International Prognostic Index remains a valid predictor of outcome for patients with aggressive CD20+ B-cell lymphoma in the rituximab era. J Clin Oncol. 2010;28(14):2373–80. https://doi.org/10.1200/JCO.2009.26.2493.
16. Zhou Z, et al. An enhanced International Prognostic Index (NCCN-IPI) for patients with diffuse large B-cell lymphoma treated in the rituximab era. Blood. 2014;123(6):837–42. https://doi.org/10.1182/blood-2013-09-524108.
17. Solal-Céligny P, et al. Follicular lymphoma International Prognostic Index. Blood. 2004;104(5):1258–65. https://doi.org/10.1182/blood-2003-12-4434.
18. Hoster E, et al. A new prognostic index (MIPI) for patients with advanced-stage mantle cell lymphoma. Blood. 2008;111(2):558–65. https://doi.org/10.1182/blood-2007-06-095331.
19. **Susanibar-Adaniya S, Barta SK. 2021 Update on diffuse large B cell lymphoma: a review of current data and potential applications on risk stratification and management. Am J Hematol. 2021;96(5):617–29. https://doi.org/10.1002/ajh.26151.
20. Giulino-Roth L. How I treat primary mediastinal B-cell lymphoma. Blood. 2018;132(8):782–90. https://doi.org/10.1182/blood-2018-04-791566.

21. Crombie J, LaCasce A. The treatment of Burkitt lymphoma in adults. Blood. 2021;137(6):743–50. https://doi.org/10.1182/blood.2019004099.
22. Armitage JO, Longo DL. Mantle-cell lymphoma. N Engl J Med. 2022;386(26):2495–506. https://doi.org/10.1056/NEJMra2202672.
23. Freedman A, Jacobsen E. Follicular lymphoma: 2020 update on diagnosis and management. Am J Hematol. 2020;95(3):316–27. https://doi.org/10.1002/ajh.25696.
24. Wang H, Fu B, Gale RP, Liang Y. NK-/T-cell lymphomas. Leukemia. 2021;35(9):2460–8. https://doi.org/10.1038/s41375-021-01313-2.
25. Dummer R, et al. Cutaneous T cell lymphoma. Nat Rev Dis Primers. 2021;7(1):61. https://doi.org/10.1038/s41572-021-00296-9.
26. **Brice P, de Kerviler E, Friedberg JW. Classical Hodgkin lymphoma. Lancet. 2021;398(10310):1518–27. https://doi.org/10.1016/S0140-6736(20)32207-8.
27. Urayama KY, et al. Genome-wide association study of classical Hodgkin lymphoma and Epstein–Barr virus status–defined subgroups. JNCI J Natl Cancer Inst. 2012;104(3):240–53. https://doi.org/10.1093/jnci/djr516.
28. Harris NL, et al. The World Health Organization classification of hematological malignancies report of the Clinical Advisory Committee Meeting, Airlie House, Virginia, November 1997. Mod Pathol. 2000;13(2):193–207. https://doi.org/10.1038/modpathol.3880035.
29. Hasenclever D, Diehl V. A prognostic score for advanced Hodgkin's disease. International Prognostic Factors Project on Advanced Hodgkin's Disease. N Engl J Med. 1998;339(21):1506–14. https://doi.org/10.1056/NEJM199811193392104.
30. Eichenauer DA, et al. Hodgkin lymphoma: ESMO Clinical Practice Guidelines for diagnosis, treatment and follow-up. Ann Oncol. 2018;29:iv19–29. https://doi.org/10.1093/annonc/mdy080.
31. **Radford J, et al. Results of a trial of PET-directed therapy for early-stage Hodgkin's lymphoma. N Engl J Med. 2015;372(17):1598–607. https://doi.org/10.1056/NEJMoa1408648.
32. André MPE, et al. Early positron emission tomography response–adapted treatment in stage I and II Hodgkin lymphoma: final results of the randomized EORTC/LYSA/FIL H10 trial. J Clin Oncol. 2017;35(16):1786–94. https://doi.org/10.1200/JCO.2016.68.6394.
33. Meyer RM. Limited-stage Hodgkin lymphoma: clarifying uncertainty. J Clin Oncol. 2017;35(16):1760–3. https://doi.org/10.1200/JCO.2017.72.2611.
34. Canellos GP, et al. Chemotherapy of advanced Hodgkin's disease with MOPP, ABVD, or MOPP alternating with ABVD. N Engl J Med. 1992;327(21):1478–84. https://doi.org/10.1056/NEJM199211193272102.
35. **Johnson P, et al. Adapted treatment guided by interim PET-CT scan in advanced Hodgkin's lymphoma. N Engl J Med. 2016;374(25):2419–29. https://doi.org/10.1056/NEJMoa1510093.
36. Federico M, et al. ABVD compared with BEACOPP compared with CEC for the initial treatment of patients with advanced Hodgkin's lymphoma: results from the HD2000 Gruppo Italiano per lo Studio dei Linfomi Trial. J Clin Oncol. 2009;27(5):805–11. https://doi.org/10.1200/JCO.2008.17.0910.
37. Engert A, et al. Reduced-intensity chemotherapy and PET-guided radiotherapy in patients with advanced stage Hodgkin's lymphoma (HD15 trial): a randomised, open-label, phase 3 non-inferiority trial. Lancet Lond Engl. 2012;379(9828):1791–9. https://doi.org/10.1016/S0140-6736(11)61940-5.
38. Connors JM, et al. Brentuximab vedotin with chemotherapy for stage III or IV Hodgkin's lymphoma. N Engl J Med. 2018;378(4):331–44. https://doi.org/10.1056/NEJMoa1708984.
39. Bhurani D, et al. Real-world outcomes of Hodgkin lymphoma: a multi-centric registry from India. Front Oncol. 2021;11:799948. https://doi.org/10.3389/fonc.2021.799948.
40. *Kristinsson SY, et al. Screening for monoclonal gammopathy of undetermined significance: a population-based randomized clinical trial. First results from the Iceland screens, treats, or prevents multiple myeloma (iStopMM) study. Blood. 2021;138(Supplement 1):156. https://doi.org/10.1182/blood-2021-152333.
41. Gupta R, et al. Prevalence of monoclonal gammopathy of undetermined significance in India-a hospital-based study. Clin Lymphoma Myeloma Leuk. 2018;18(9):e345–50. https://doi.org/10.1016/j.clml.2018.06.005.
42. **Mateos M-V, et al. International Myeloma Working Group risk stratification model for smoldering multiple myeloma (SMM). Blood Cancer J. 2020;10(10):10. https://doi.org/10.1038/s41408-020-00366-3.
43. Bora K. Distribution of multiple myeloma in India: heterogeneity in incidence across age, sex and geography. Cancer Epidemiol. 2019;59:215–20. https://doi.org/10.1016/j.canep.2019.02.010.
44. Finsinger P, Grammatico S, Chisini M, Piciocchi A, Foà R, Petrucci MT. Clinical features and prognostic factors in solitary plasmacytoma. Br J Haematol. 2016;172(4):554–60. https://doi.org/10.1111/bjh.13870.
45. **Rajkumar SV. Multiple myeloma: 2020 update on diagnosis, risk-stratification and management. Am J Hematol. 2020;95(5):548–67. https://doi.org/10.1002/ajh.25791.
46. Singh C, et al. Presentation and impact of double and triple hit cytogenetics in patients with multiple myeloma in the real world. Clin Lymphoma Myeloma Leuk. 2022;22(8):e685–90. https://doi.org/10.1016/j.clml.2022.03.005.
47. Sharma R, et al. Lack of renal recovery predicts poor survival in patients of multiple myeloma with renal impairment. Clin Lymphoma Myeloma Leuk. 2022;22(8):626–34. https://doi.org/10.1016/j.clml.2022.04.013.

48. Greipp PR, et al. International staging system for multiple myeloma. J Clin Oncol. 2016. https://doi.org/10.1200/JCO.2005.04.242.
49. Kastritis E, et al. Evaluation of the Revised International Staging System in an independent cohort of unselected patients with multiple myeloma. Haematologica. 2017;102(3):593–9. https://doi.org/10.3324/haematol.2016.145078.
50. *Caers J, et al. Diagnosis, treatment, and response assessment in solitary plasmacytoma: updated recommendations from a European Expert Panel. J Hematol Oncol. 2018;11(1):10. https://doi.org/10.1186/s13045-017-0549-1.
51. Kumar SK, et al. Carfilzomib or bortezomib in combination with lenalidomide and dexamethasone for patients with newly diagnosed multiple myeloma without intention for immediate autologous stem-cell transplantation (ENDURANCE): a multicentre, open-label, phase 3, randomised, controlled trial. Lancet Oncol. 2020;21(10):1317–30. https://doi.org/10.1016/S1470-2045(20)30452-6.
52. Perrot A, et al. Early versus late autologous stem cell transplant in newly diagnosed multiple myeloma: long-term follow-up analysis of the IFM 2009 trial. Blood. 2020;136:39. https://doi.org/10.1182/blood-2020-134538.
53. Yanamandra U, et al. Survival outcomes of newly diagnosed multiple myeloma at a tertiary care center in North India (IMAGe: 001A study). JCO Glob Oncol. 2021;7:704–15. https://doi.org/10.1200/go.20.00625.
54. Specht L, Yahalom J. The concept and evolution of involved site radiation therapy for lymphoma. Int J Clin Oncol. 2015;20(5):849–54.
55. Guo B, Cherian S, Murphy ES, Sauter CS, et al. Dose to circulating blood in intensity-modulated total body irradiation, total marrow irradiation, and total marrow and lymphoid irradiation. Med Phys. 2025;52(7):e17913. https://doi.org/10.1002/mp.17913.
56. Wong JYC, Filippi AR, Dabaja BS, Yahalom J, Specht L. Total body irradiation: guidelines from the International Lymphoma Radiation Oncology Group (ILROG). Int J Radiat Oncol Biol Phys. 2018;101(3):521–9. https://doi.org/10.1016/j.ijrobp.2018.04.071.
57. Hoppe RT. Mycosis fungoides: radiation therapy. Dermatol Ther. 2003;16(4):347–54. https://doi.org/10.1111/j.1396-0296.2003.01647.x.
58. Kriz J, et al. Relapse analysis of irradiated patients within the HD15 trial of the German Hodgkin Study Group. Int J Radiat Oncol Biol Phys. 2015;92(1):46–53. https://doi.org/10.1016/j.ijrobp.2015.01.048.
59. De Sanctis V, et al. Residual site radiotherapy after immunochemotherapy in primary mediastinal B-cell lymphoma: a monoinstitutional retrospective study. In Vivo. 2020;34(3):1407–13. https://doi.org/10.21873/invivo.11921.
60. Fluge Ø, et al. Consolidative radiotherapy to residual masses after chemotherapy is associated with improved outcome in diffuse large B-cell lymphoma. A retrospective, population-based study. Clin Lymphoma Myeloma Leuk. 2018;18(2):125–35.e3. https://doi.org/10.1016/j.clml.2017.12.002.
61. Dabaja BS, et al. Proton therapy for adults with mediastinal lymphomas: the International Lymphoma Radiation Oncology Group guidelines. Blood. 2018;132(16):1635–46. https://doi.org/10.1182/blood-2018-03-837633.
62. Aznar MC, et al. Minimizing late effects for patients with mediastinal Hodgkin lymphoma: deep inspiration breath-hold, IMRT, or both? Int J Radiat Oncol Biol Phys. 2015;92(1):169–74. https://doi.org/10.1016/j.ijrobp.2015.01.013.
63. Miller JA, et al. Spine stereotactic radiosurgery for the treatment of multiple myeloma. J Neurosurg Spine. 2017;26(3):282–90. https://doi.org/10.3171/2016.8.SPINE16412.

For Additional Reading and Viewing

AML 2022 ELN Guidelines https://ashpublications.org/blood/article/140/12/1345/485817/Diagnosis-and-management-of-AML-in-adults-2022

APML 2019 EuropeanLeukemiaNet guidelines https://ashpublications.org/blood/article/133/15/1630/273295/Management-of-acute-promyelocytic-leukemia-updated

ALL 2016 ESMO Guidelines https://www.annalsofoncology.org/article/S0923-7534(19)31639-4/pdf

CML European leukemianet guidelines 2020: https://www.nature.com/articles/s41375-020-0776-2

Talk by Dr Vikram Mathews on the management of APML: https://www.youtube.com/watch?v=0FD5iA1gcYM

Talk by Dr Vincent Rajkumar on the basics of multiple myeloma management: https://www.youtube.com/watch?v=Byksg0SDsZA

Molecular Biology and Genetics in Radiation Oncology Practice

Anusheel Munshi, Indu Bansal,
Meenakshi Ravichandran, and Bidhu K. Mohanti

1 Introduction

Radiotherapy is an important modality in the treatment of cancer patients applied either alone or in combination with other modes of treatment, i.e., surgery or chemotherapy. External beam radiotherapy significantly contributes to cure or palliation of many cancer patients and is utilized in approximately 60% of all cases [1]. During the last 50 years, what we can call as the era of megavoltage radiotherapy, the optimization has focused the efforts on physical and technological aspects for clinical delivery of the dose to the tumor vis-à-vis the normal tissue. Whereas, much less progress has been made to include the individual patient's tumor biological characteristics into treatment approaches [2, 3]. Hence, the molecular and genetic characteristics for radiation oncology is being researched in the recent years.

Cancer is an umbrella term denoting a heterogeneous group of diseases. Cancer is typically characterized by various underlying molecular changes [4]. Tumors with the same pathological features arising from the same anatomical organ can have varied underlying genetic alterations. Also, the response to the same therapeutic modalities can vary dramatically. The same tumor can show different outcomes after treatment in different patients [5]. The availability of next-generation sequencing (NGS) has been a landmark development. It has led to the widespread implementation of genomic and transcriptomic approaches and tools to study human disease [6]. Cancer management has been dramatically changed by the development of personalized treatments to target oncogenic mutations and altered signaling pathways [7]. For many cancers, precision oncology based on genomic and/or transcriptomic profiling at the time of diagnosis or relapse of disease has become a standard of care [8]. In the majority of clinical scenarios, treatment selection for cancer patients without any type of molecular characterization is no longer conceivable. Simultaneously, research work has also highlighted the substantial genetic and microenvironmental differences (i.e., heterogeneity) that can exist within an individual patient's cancer. This certainly complicates the personalized treatment approaches [9].

Nearly 60 percent of patients with cancer receive radiotherapy at some point in their treatment course. However, molecular profile-based personalized treatment in radiation

A. Munshi (✉) · M. Ravichandran
Department of Radiation Oncology, BLK MAX Hospital, New Delhi, Delhi, India

I. Bansal
Department of Radiation Oncology, Paras Hospital, Gurgaon, India

B. K. Mohanti
Department of Radiation Oncology, Bagchi Sri Shankara Cancer Centre & Research Institute, Bhubaneswar, Odisha, India

B. K. Mohanti et al. (eds.), *Radiation Oncology – Principles, Precepts and Practice*,
https://doi.org/10.1007/978-981-95-5171-2_18

oncology has lagged much behind systemic therapy approaches. Very few validated predictors of radiation therapy response are currently available. As a result, even in the present modern era, radiation doses remain uniformly the same across patients for tumors with the same stage and cancer type [10]. Hence, a greater understanding of the microenvironment and immune system of the tumors, which can affect the radiotherapy response, will have the potential to improve the treatment outcomes.

2 Terms and Definitions

There are specific key definitions related to genetics, especially in oncology [11]. The important definitions related to this are given in Table 1.

Table 1 Key terms and definitions explained

Germline mutation	A germline mutation is a change to a gene's DNA sequence, inherited during conception, to produce something different. Genetic variations identified from normal tissues, such as blood, are present in all cells in the body and are referred to as germline variants or germline mutations.
Somatic mutation	The mutation that occurs in the DNA of cell(s) after the conception. Since a tumor develops in a tissue or organ, a mutation identified in a tumor is a somatic mutation and is likely to be found only in tumor cells.
VUS (Variant of uncertain significance)	A variant that can be either benign or pathogenic, as the effect of the variant is not currently known.
Polygenic tests	Tests that incorporate broad genomic information. These tests do not yet exist.
Locus	A specific position on a chromosome
Allele	An allele is one of two or more versions of DNA sequence (a single base or a segment of bases) at a given genomic location. An individual inherits two alleles, one from each parent, for any given genomic location where such variation exists. If the two alleles are the same, the individual is homozygous for that allele. If the alleles are different, the individual is heterozygous.
Allelic imbalance	Both alleles are present, but have different copy numbers (structural genetic variation)
Biallelic inactivation	A pathogenic variant in each of the two copies of a gene resulting in loss of function
Copy number variation	A duplication or deletion that has arisen in the germline
Haplo insufficiency	The situation that occurs when one copy of a gene is inactivated or deleted and the remaining functional copy of the gene is not adequate to produce the needed gene product to preserve normal function. For tumor formation, such haplo-insufficiency, i.e., the presence of the most frequent allele (wildtype) is not sufficient to prevent pathogenicity.
Haplo sufficiency	The presence of the most frequent allele (wildtype) is sufficient to prevent pathogenicity, such that tumor formation is evaded.
Heterozygote	An individual (or tumor) possessing two different alleles at a locus
Homozygote	An individual (or tumor) possessing the same allele at a locus
Loss of heterozygosity (or hemizygosity)	Loss of heterozygosity, LOH. Loss of heterozygosity, LOH, is defined as the loss of one parent's contribution to the cell. It is a common form of allelic imbalance by which heterozygous somatic cells become homozygous because one of the two alleles gets lost. This form of chromosome instability is sufficient to provide selective growth, a major cause of tumorigenesis.
Mutation	A pathogenic variant
Single nucleotide polymorphism	A single nucleotide polymorphism, or SNP (pronounced "snip"), is a variation at a single position in a DNA sequence among individuals. Recall that the DNA sequence is formed from a chain of four nucleotide bases: A, C, G, and T. If more than 1% of a population does not carry the same nucleotide at a specific position in the DNA sequence, then this variation can be classified as a SNP. If a SNP occurs within a gene, then the gene is described as having more than one allele. Although a particular SNP may not cause a disorder, some SNPs are associated with certain diseases. These associations allow scientists to look for SNPs in order to evaluate an individual's genetic predisposition to develop a disease.

Table 1 (continued)

Variant	An alteration in the most frequent DNA nucleotide sequence at the same locus. Variants can be benign, of unknown significance, or pathogenic.
Pathogenic variant	A genetic alteration that increases an individual's susceptibility or predisposition to a certain disease or disorder. When such a variant (or mutation) is inherited, development of symptoms is more likely, but not certain. Also called deleterious mutation, disease-causing mutation, predisposing mutation, and susceptibility gene mutation. (e.g., presence of a disease or syndrome generally when inherited in a homozygous state; or, due to increased radiation toxicity, tumor resistance)
Somatic copy number alteration	A duplication or deletion that occurs during the lifetime of the individual
Somatic homozygosity	A condition where a cell acquires two identical alleles (versions) of a particular gene or a region of a chromosome due to a change that occurs in a non-reproductive (somatic) cell after conception

3 Somatic Versus Germline Mutations

It is critical to appreciate the difference between somatic and germline mutations. Germline DNA refers to the constitutional DNA of an individual resulting from the combination of unique genetic material derived as half from the mother (egg) and the other half from the father (sperm) during conception. The expansion of genomic technologies and the declining costs of next-generation sequencing (NGS) make it often a consideration in everyday clinical practice, similar to our decisions for endoscopy, radiologic scans, immunohistochemical study, etc. [12]. Germline testing is obtained from normal tissues (e.g., blood or saliva), whereas somatic testing relates to and is limited to testing of the tumor.

Genomic tumor instability is a well-known phenomenon. As a consequence of this and other reasons, somatic mutation testing frequently results in a long list of mutations. This is also problematic since determining which somatic mutations are critical for tumor cell growth is still largely empirical. Yet it is clinically proven that even minimal mutations are actionable in terms of having effective therapy, e.g., EGFR mutation in lung cancer and MSI in colorectal cancer. In the absence of evidence for concomitant germline mutations, deleterious tumor mutations only have implications for tumor response and tumor treatment decisions. These mutations do not have implications for normal tissue toxicity or secondary cancers since these are likely to be more affected by germline mutations. In many situations, patients with cancer receive germline genetic testing as a control for their tumor genomic testing.

4 Current Scenarios for Somatic/Germline Testing

Currently, the following may be situations in which somatic or germline testing is done, in order to identify pathogenic or likely pathogenic (P or LP) mutations [13].

1. Clinical history/nomograms/algorithms that assess higher cancer risk to identify otherwise potentially cancerous patients and their family members. Such individuals would become candidates for germline genetic testing. Since frank tumors usually do not exist in such potential patients at this stage, normal body tissue DNA needs to be examined, which would reflect the state of all the cells of the body. Typically, the most accessible sites for assessing normal tissue DNA are saliva or blood. Contamination with microorganisms in saliva has led to blood being the preferred site for sampling.
2. Patients with or without frank risk factors may decide to self-test their normal tissue DNA. Several direct-to-consumer genetic

testing tools are available. It has been recommended that only Clinical Laboratory Improvement Amendments (CLIA) certified tests should be considered in clinical recommendations and discussions with patients.

3. Patients who are diagnosed with cancer may be recommended for tumor biopsy/surgical specimen tissue examination for driver somatic mutations. Driver mutations are responsible for tumor development or growth. Examples include EGFR mutations in lung cancer, BRCA1/2 mutations in the breast, and 1p19q mutations in oligodendroglioma.

Multiple genetic screening panels are available for patients being assessed for germline screening. Typically, for example, in the breast cancer context, these panels include 20–30 specific genes that are associated with an increased risk of cancer. However, panel testing for more genes has been developed. Proportional to the number of tested genes, there is an increase in the number of variants of unknown significance (VUS) found and, less commonly, of pathogenic mutations detected [14–16].

Because the genetic testing is becoming more and more available, even in India and low-and middle-income countries (LMIC), the cost-utility analysis of such tests in routine clinical practice would require careful evaluation [17]. As tumor genomic testing (TGT) is getting more and more prescribed, there is a need to have a clear plan by the treating team or institution, and optimal counselling of the patients before a test is advised. Similarly, the targeted germline genetic testing (GGT) to prevent hereditary cancer is often recommended for those at risk for breast, ovarian, or colorectal cancer. The incremental cost-effectiveness ratios (ICERs; in 2021-adjusted US$) for germline testing versus the standard care option, for quality-adjusted life years (QUALY) saved has shown that for such multigene-cascade screening the ICERs from the payer perspectives were $15,600/QALY, $56,500/QALY, and $69,600/QALY for women in the United Kingdom, Norway, and the United States, respectively [18]. As the field of molecular and genetic tests for any tumor and for decision in any tumor agnostic-management will grow in the future, it is important to develop robust frameworks and guidelines in order to provide sustainable and equitable cancer care.

5 Genetic Alterations and Radiotherapy Side Effects

Genetic alteration in certain pre-existing conditions can carry the risk of increased morbidities and the risk of second cancer (radiation-induced second malignancy, RISM).

Early molecular diagnosis and careful evaluation of treatment risks and benefits are essential for these patients. The risk of RISM is a concern when treating Li-Fraumeni syndrome (LFS) or Li-Fraumeni-like (LFL) patients. Women with Li-Fraumeni syndrome (LFS), a cancer predisposition syndrome caused by germline mutations in TP53, have an over 50% risk of developing breast cancer by age 70 years. Yet it has been observed that, contrary to this lifetime risk of breast cancer, the adjuvant radiotherapy is not shown to carry any increased risk for RISM, and as such, LFS is not a contraindication for radiation therapy in cancer management [19]. Similarly, carriers of pathogenic variants in ataxia-telangiectasia mutated (ATM) have a two- to four-fold increased risk of developing breast cancer. However, adjuvant radiation is safe for most breast cancer patients who harbor ATM variants. The possible exceptions are patients with the variant c5557G>A (rs1801516) and patients younger than 45 years old with certain rare deleterious ATM variants, which may be at higher risk for developing contralateral breast cancer (CBC). These latter patients should be counseled regarding this potential risk, and every effort should be made to minimize the contralateral breast dose. There is increased interest in ATM kinase, which is a key regulator of DNA double-strand breaks and a potential target for radiosensitization. Ongoing research shows the potential that a combination of radiation, ATM inhibitors, and PD-L1 targeted therapy may offer a novel approach to radio-immunotherapy of locally advanced tumors [20].

6 Tumor RNA-Based Genomic Signatures

Most precision medicine approaches in current clinical use are based on the analysis of alterations in DNA (such as mutations) in a few hundred genes. There has been some success with a DNA-based approach, yet those successes are few and far between. The National Cancer Institute (NCI), USA has started research on a new approach where gene expression is measured by examining levels of RNA, the molecular cousin of DNA. For the innovator's first-of-its-kind study, the WINTHER trial, based on RNA approach of targeted drugs, compared to the more established DNA-based targeted therapy, showed 27% response in those cancer patients who did not have any actionable DNA alterations [21]. The WIN consortium has made advancement to apply transcriptomics, RNA expression in tumors compared to normal tissues, for decision to prescribe targeted therapy.

Tumor RNA-based genomic signatures are of interest for predicting the benefit or lack thereof from radiation. There is also interest in using such microRNA (mRNA) signatures of both tumor and normal tissue radiosensitivity within models for genomic-adjusted dose individualization [22]. Preliminary clinical data suggest that gene expression signatures may be useful in predicting clinical outcomes in patients treated with and without radiation therapy [23]. Future clinical trials designed to evaluate genomically guided radiation therapy will ideally compare patients receiving comprehensive genomic-adjusted radiation doses in which a genomic susceptibility for normal tissue toxicity, as well as tumor radiosensitivity, are taken into account with patients in whom genomic factors are not used to alter the standard radiation therapy protocol [24]. In order to improve the response to radiotherapy, studies are conducted to develop genomic and clinical databases based on micro-RNA signatures that would predict the good or poor responders to radiation therapy in some common tumors [25]. Similarly, analysis of RNA expression after radiation exposure has shown alterations not only in mRNAs, but also in ncRNAs (primarily miRNA, circRNA, and lncRNA), implying an important role in cellular stress response. Due to their abundance and stability in serum and other biofluids, ncRNAs also have great potential as minimally invasive biomarkers with advantages over current bio-dosimetry methods. Once thought of as arising from "junk DNA," noncoding RNAs (ncRNAs) have emerged as key molecules in cellular processes and response to stress, including radiation injury [26]. Hence, such genomic studies can pave the way for precision in radiation oncology (Table 2).

Table 2 Key points for determining excess radiation risk due to genetic/molecular alterations

1	Important germline mutations in DNA repair genes such as BRCA1/2 can increase lifetime cancer risk. However, these are not likely to increase radiation-induced cancers or radiation toxicity.
2	BRCA1/2, PALPB2, CHEK2, and RAD50/51 mutations should not affect radiation therapy decisions
3	Mutations that lead to rare radiation sensitivity syndromes are typically obvious before the onset of adulthood. As a corollary, mutations identified in genetic screening in adulthood are not likely to be indicators of severe radiation sensitivity.
4	Deleterious ATMs in younger women may increase contralateral breast cancer risk. Still, the absolute risk remains low. Reasonable to avoid optional radiation for patients with deleterious ATMs. We need to emphasize follow-up screening for contralateral breast cancer after indicated radiation therapy for young patients.
5	Inconsistency of published data limits precise recommendations. This emphasizes the need for further prospective studies. Development of a centralized database cataloging RT outcomes and genetic status is desirable.
6	Heterozygous deleterious ATMs do not increase radiation toxicity risk. At most, they increase it only by a mild measure.

ATM ataxia-telangiectasia mutations

7 Molecular/Biological Imaging for Radiotherapy

Molecular imaging with positron emission tomography and magnetic resonance imaging offers the opportunity to improve diagnostic accuracy. It also allows the integration of tumor biology related to the assessment of tumor cell density, tumor hypoxia, and tumor proliferation into radiotherapy planning. This is, however, not achievable without a correct comprehension of the technical and methodological issues related to image acquisition, reconstruction, and segmentation. There is increasing evidence that imaging modalities like FDG PET and DW MRI have a potential value for delineating the primary tumor GTV, affecting distribution. Since the beginning of twenty-first century, 3-D imaging (CT, MRI) became the key tool to the progress of conformal radiotherapy, such as 3-D CRT and IMRT. In accordance, integrating physical and biological conformality in multidimensional conformal radiotherapy is the emerging new goal in radiation dose planning and delivery [27]. Concepts such as dose painting and allowing heterogeneous dose distribution to the target volume have emerged. PET and multiparametric MRI provide crucial information concerning tumor extent and normal tissue anatomy. Moreover, they are able to visualize biological characteristics of the tumor, which can be considered in the radiation treatment planning and monitoring [28]. Further validation of such approaches is needed before they are adopted in routine clinical practice.

8 The Systemic Effect of Radiotherapy

Radiation therapy is essentially a local modality. In some cases, however, it is noticed that post-radiotherapy effects can happen at a site distant from the actual radiotherapy site. Such effects are classified as "abscopal" effects. Abscopal effects may be related to the radiation dose and fractionation scheme used to induce optimal levels of DNA breaks. The mechanism of these effects is varied. It is well known that RT can upregulate the expression of immune modulatory cytokines and chemokines. The latter controls immune cell differentiation and invasion into the tumor microenvironment. The sporadic events of tumor regression in unirradiated fields, due to such abscopal effect, have been observed for decades. In a systemic review, a total of 46 reported cases have been identified from 1969 to 2014 with a median radiation dose of 31 Gy, median follow-up of 17.5 months, and median documented time to notice the abscopal effect as 2 months [29]. Out of such log-standing knowledge regarding abscopal effect of clinical radiotherapy, the immunological responses to localized irradiation are proposed to be the mediators for systemic effects. The advent of immunotherapy has ushered in further excitement about these effects. It has been seen that the abscopal effect can also be augmented through the combination of RT and immunotherapy [30]. The field of cancer immunotherapy has been aiming for a long time to engage a patient's own immune system to recognize and eliminate tumors. The major stumbling block for these approaches has been the toxicity of these approaches. However, newer agents are showing more promise. These include monoclonal antibodies that block T-cell checkpoint receptors, such as cytotoxic T-lymphocyte antigen-4 (CTLA-4) or the programmed cell death-1 (PD-1) receptor. Since the immune system has a systemic nature, once such a response is induced at a local site, it can trigger an autoimmune tumor response at all disease sites in the body.

Radiotherapy has the potential to interact with the immune system locally. This does initiate the release of tumor-specific antigens, local production of inflammatory cytokines, phenotypic changes in tumor-cell expression of immune-susceptibility markers, vascular effects that enhance immune surveillance, and local eradication of suppressive immune-cell lineages. Reports indicate that the PD-1 ligand (PD-L1) could be upregulated in the tumor microenvironment following radiotherapy [31]. Such approaches are still in the preliminary stage, but if proven effective, can catapult radiotherapy from pure locoregional treatment to a crucial component of systemic therapy.

The Steel hypothesis has described the framework of interaction of radiation and cancer drugs, broadly as five mechanisms: (1) spatial cooperation, (2) temporal modulation, (3) biological cooperation, (4) cytotoxic enhancement, and (5) normal tissue protection [32]. In the molecular era, Steel's framework, which has evolved since 1970s, has the potential to integrate immunotherapy drugs with radiotherapy, giving it the acronym "iRT" for such combined therapy [33]. On a cautionary note, the combination of RT and immune checkpoint inhibitors (ICIs) has demonstrated increased toxicity in some studies. Further, some immunotherapy drugs can cause progression of the tumor at the start of the treatment course before showing a tumor response. It is therefore important to take care in combining the right agents and in the right sequence. The challenges of RT-induced abscopal effects include (a) predicting which tumours are likely to have these effects, (b) identifying biomarkers to predict which patients will have an abscopal effect, and (c) ensuring consistency in response.

9 Biology-Guided Radiotherapy (BgRT)

Biology-guided radiotherapy (BgRT) is broadly characterized as using biological imaging information to guide radiotherapy delivery. BgRT makes use of well-established standards for diagnosing, staging, and monitoring treatment progress for many types of cancer.

The discussion on biology-guided radiotherapy (BgRT) can have several facets. Several research groups have considered giving a spatially non-uniform dose to some regions of the tumor based on biological images, e.g., hypoxic radioresistance regions within a tumor. This is sometimes called biological "dose painting." Imaging technologies in radiotherapy have evolved over several decades and are characterized by constant innovation, mainly with radiographic methods that provide anatomic information, such as 2D planar radiography, cone-beam CT, megavoltage CT, and, most recently, MRI. The evolution of combining anatomical imaging with radiotherapy has enabled progressively more precise delivery of ionizing radiation to targets delineated at finer and finer resolution. This has resulted in significant gains for patients because these technologies improve treatment planning, patient positioning, and sparing of normal tissues, which result in reduced toxicities. Furthermore, these improvements in imaging have allowed for increased dose per fraction, clearing the way for more effective local ablation.

In the context of BgRT, PET/CT images of the tumor are a byproduct of each treatment fraction. It is a new external beam radiotherapy delivery modality combining positron emission tomography-computed tomography (PET-CT) with a 6 MV linear accelerator. The key innovation is the continuous response of the linear accelerator to outgoing tumor PET emissions with beamlets of radiotherapy at sub-second latency. Applying radiomics principles to the interrogation of these images creates the possibility of discovering predictive or prognostic signatures predicated on subtle changes in PET/CT signals observed during the course of radiotherapy. In essence, PET-guided therapy is a novel radiation therapy modality in which a radiolabeled tumor can act as its own fiducial for radiation therapy targeting and real-time delivery of prescribed dose. Biology-guided radiotherapy (BgRT), developed by RefleXion Medical (Hayward, CA, USA), is the first fusion of PET/CT and radiotherapy delivery in a single system, Fig. 1 [34].

FDG is the anticipated workhorse radiotracer for BgRT. However, non-FDG tracers are being investigated for specific clinical indications. For example, FDG may not be suitable for BgRT of brain tumors if the FDG background signal is too high. In addition, some tumor types, such as prostate cancer, may not have adequate FDG uptake. Therefore, new tracers, such as PSMA-targeted tracers for prostate cancer [35] or CA9-targeted tracers for renal cancers [36], may replace FDG in these indications.

One shortcoming of FDG in the context of BgRT is its chemical inflexibility: the FDG molecule cannot be modified to accommodate long-lived PET isotopes, such as 64Cu or 89Zr. Novel tracer designs may improve the flexibility in matching the pharmacokinetic and isotope half-life to the specific clinical indication. As one example, PET tracers targeting fibroblast activa-

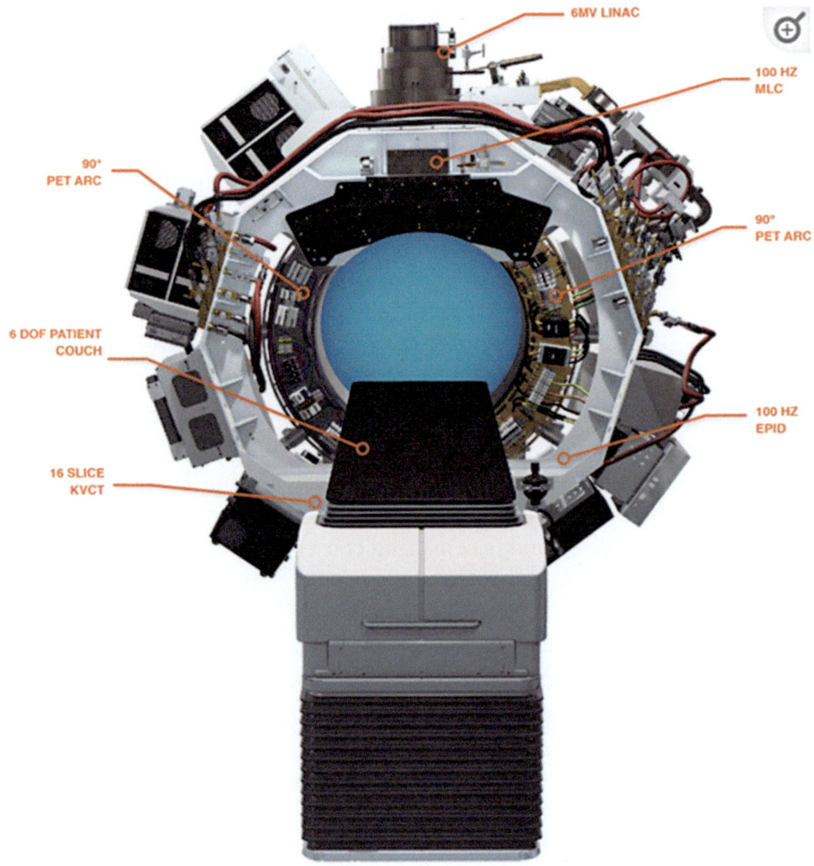

Fig. 1 The RefleXion™ X1 Biology-guided radiotherapy machine

Table 3 Novel RT contouring and planning terms used with BgRT

Biology-guidance margin (BGM)	The term "biology-guidance margin" (BGM) refers to an extension from a GTV/CTV to PTV that takes into consideration localization problems unique to BgRT, such as the residual latency between beamlet delivery and PET emission collection. BgRT produces a tracked dosage distribution, allowing for the expansion of the GTV/CTV at a single time point to define the PTV.
Biology-tracking zone (BTZ)	The BTZ includes the target's motion extent plus an extra margin to account for the biological guidance margin and patient setup errors.
BgRT plan optimization	The BgRT optimization algorithm's objective is to minimize a cost function, which has as inputs target coverage targets set by doctors and OAR restrictions.
Bound dose volume histogram (bDVH)	A bounded DVH (bDVH), which surrounds the DVH line for each volume and OAR with confidence intervals that represent the many variants, is how the BgRT TPS replicates several dose-volume histograms (DVHs) using these potential permutations.

tion protein (FAP) have been created with a host of different isotopes, which might allow investigations of BgRT that combine the versatile injection and uptake schedules of different isotopes with the pan-cancer detection ability of FAP. Lastly, disease-agnostic tracers such as those that highlight hypoxic regions (e.g., FMISO, FAZA) or areas of cellular proliferation (e.g., FLT) may enhance dose delivery tailored to tumor biology.

Some novel contouring and planning terms have come up for biologically guided radiotherapy (Table 3).

10 Liquid Biopsies for Personalized Radiotherapy

The inability to assess the tumor response during a course of radiotherapy has been a long-term lacuna in radiation oncology. The best modality available these days is a cone beam CT, which provides only a gross analysis of tumor dimension change. Onboard MRI in linacs has recently improved this ability.

Unlike imaging parameters, the liquid biopsies of patient's blood samples would show up circulating tumor cells (CTC) and circulating tumor derived DNA (ctDNA) capture the heterogeneity across tumor sites and the evolution of tumor cells and mutations. Effectively, the enumeration of CTC and ctDNA on liquid biopsies would reflect biologically different aspects of disease [37].

Hence, CTC and ctDNA are well poised to transform the way radiotherapy is delivered. These assays enable almost real-time monitoring of the tumor by assessing changes in tumor genotypes and molecular features. Blood-based assays would replace more invasive assays, instilling confidence in the patient and the treating radiation oncologist.

Recent interest has been in interrogating tumor heterogeneity, clonal evolution, and resistance to radiotherapy using liquid biopsies. It is well known that tumors consist of multiple subclones with defined genetic alterations. Tumor biopsies sample a single region of one tumor deposit. As a result, resistant subclones may be missed due to sampling error. In contrast, liquid biopsies may characterize the full extent of intratumoral heterogeneity by sampling circulating tumor DNA released from all of the tumor deposits within a patient. Liquid biopsies can also be repeated at multiple time points, enabling the longitudinal tracking of clonal evolution during radiotherapy and the identification of emergent and expanding tumor subclones that mediate radiation resistance. The advantages and disadvantages of liquid biopsy for cancer management has been analyzed (Table 4).

Table 4 Liquid biopsy (Blood) Advantages verus Disadvantages [38]

Advantages	Disadvantages
1. Non-invasive	1. Low amounts of CTC or ctDNA shed
2. Less expensive than tumor biopsy	2. Reproducibility concerns from different assays/vendors
3. Detect materials shed from multiple tumor sites	3. DNA alterations may be confounded by CHIP
4. Can be assayed serially for cancer screening, therapeutic response, and minimal residual disease	4. Tumor-derived material may not be shed homogenously for all sites
	5. Can be technically challenging (CTC isolation)

11 Prediction of Outcomes through Genetics

Radiation-induced second cancer risks, normal tissue toxicity, and tumor sensitivity have a well-described genetic component [39]. These can be enumerated as of our present knowledge:

1. The current summary is focused on aspects of DNA-based genomic predictors. However, tumor RNA-based genomic signatures are of interest for predicting benefit or lack thereof from radiation as well, and there is also interest in using such mRNA signatures to identify both tumor and normal tissue radiosensitivity for genomic-adjusted dose individualization.
2. As described earlier, preliminary clinical data suggest that gene expression signatures may be useful in predicting clinical outcomes in patients treated with and without radiation therapy [22].
3. Most recently, a large Radiogenomics Consortium led meta-analysis of 6 genome-wide association studies identified 4 new radiotoxicity-associated loci (rs17055178 with rectal bleeding; rs10969913 with decreased urinary stream; and rs11122573 and rs147121532 with hematuria) and provided evidence supporting prior associations [40].

12 Tumour infiltrating lymphocytes (TIL) and Radiotherapy

Radiotherapy (RT) is the major method of treatment for cancer patients and is applied for approximately 60% of all newly diagnosed patients as a frontline therapy. However, despite the increasing precision and effectiveness of RT, recurrences of the neoplastic disease occur. Besides cancer cells, RT also affects the tumor microenvironment (TME): tumor blood vessels and cells of the immune system. It damages endothelial cells and causes radiation-induced inflammation. Damaged vessels inhibit the infiltration of CD8+ T lymphocytes into tumors, and immunosuppressive pathways are activated [41]. Lymphocytes in tumor tissue are called tumor-infiltrating lymphocytes (TILs), and they play a key role in the control and treatment of solid tumors [42]. TILs in the tumor and the surrounding microenvironment are thought to reflect ongoing anti-tumor host immune response. Three main categories of the tumor microenvironment (TME) have been defined across different tumor types: immune-desert ("cold" tumors largely devoid of lymphocytes), immune-excluded (lymphocytes are present in the peritumoral stroma only), and immune-infiltrated/inflamed ("hot" tumors) [43]. The role of TIL density in the outcome of radiotherapy/chemo-radiotherapy for head and neck squamous cell carcinoma (HNSCC) has been studied recently. A significant association of high TIL density with better disease-specific overall survival and improved locoregional relapse-free survival was noted ($p = 0.008$ and 0.02, respectively) [44].

13 Technological Advances Related to BART

Spatially fractionated radiation therapy (SFRT) is an umbrella term that includes GRID, LATTICE RT (LRT), Minibeam RT (MBRT), and Microbeam radiotherapy (MRT). While GRID and LRT use centimeter scale beamlets, MBRT and MRT work with beamlest in the range of hundreds and tens of micrometers, respectively. Also, while a 2 D dose modulation is used for GRID RT, MBRT, and MRT, LRT is based on three dimensional dose modulation characterized by isolated hot spots. Dose heterogeneity is an essential component of SFRT. The generated peaks and troughs of dose have to be spaced immaculately. The spacing and size of peaks and valleys are critical. GRID and LRT are already seeing clinical use, albeit palliative at present. MRT and MBRT are being studied extensively in preclinical studies (Fig. 2).

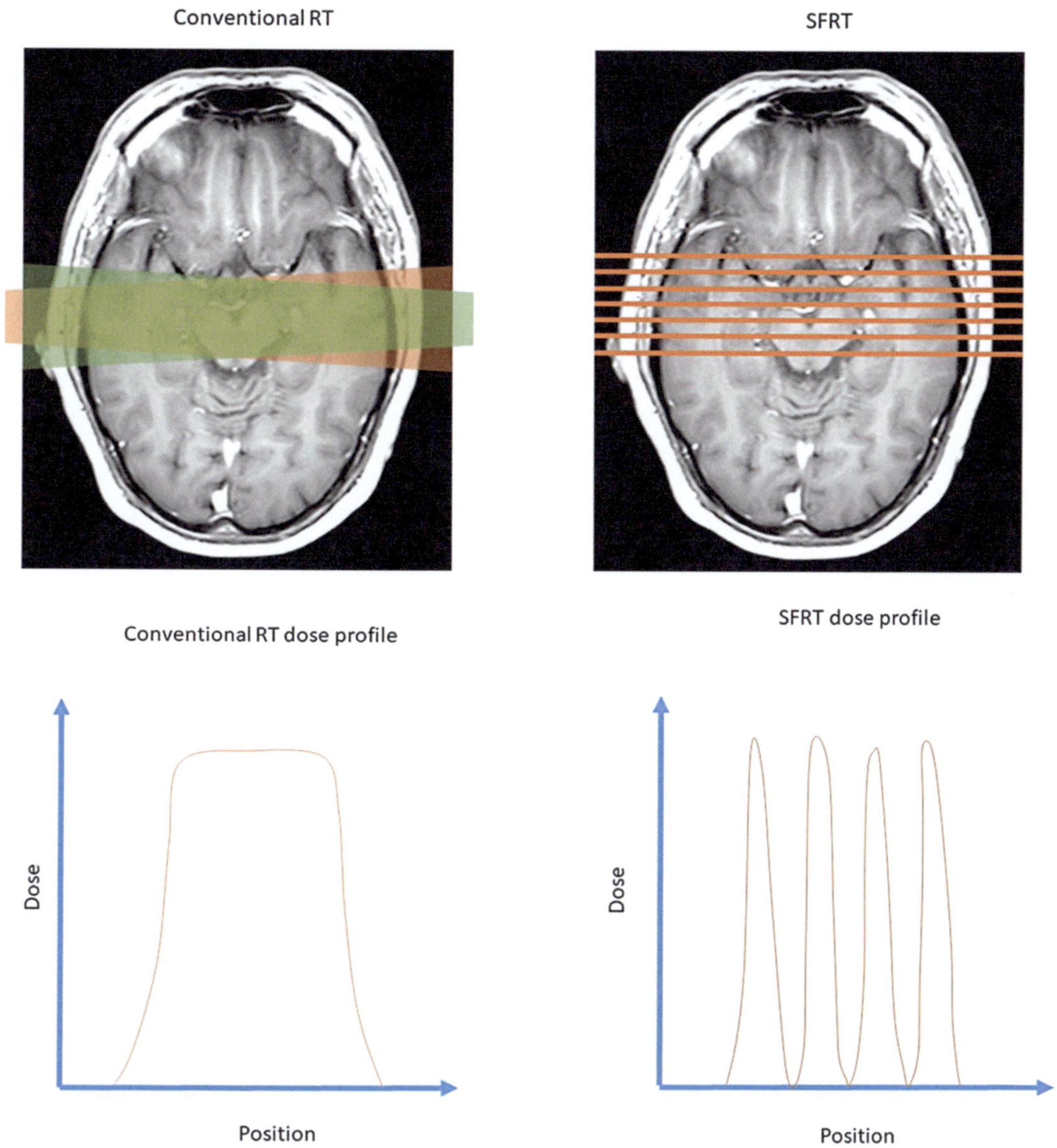

Fig. 2 Conventional RT (left panel) versus SFRT (right panel)

14 GRID Therapy

GRID therapy actually began almost 100 years ago, with the primary goal of skin-sparing for orthovoltage therapy. GRID is a variation of orthovoltage radiation therapy that uses blocking within the beam to create high-dose (>18 Gy) peaks and low-dose valleys in the tumor.

15 LATTICE Therapy

LATTICE therapy has a similar hot/cold-spot goal using image-guided radiation therapy with cone beam computed tomography and volumetric modulated arc therapy. The current use of GRID/LATTICE is now coming to the fore with megavoltage and particle therapy as well.

16 Microbeam Radiotherapy

The initial concept of Microbeam RT involved a Cerrobend grid matrix fitted into the tray holder of available Linacs. There were 256 holes of 7.5 mm diameter in a 16 × 16 cm matrix. The ratio of open to blocked areas was 50:50. However, present-day Microbeam RT has been involved significantly. At present, microbeam radiotherapy has a dose rate of 100 Gy s^{-1} or higher, and the beam is 25 μm (i.e. 0.025 mm) wide [45]. Microbeam is another form of SFRT that can be used in a grid-like pattern for focal ablation of aberrantly functioning nonmalignant tissue.

17 FLASH Radiotherapy

SFRT focuses on spatial modulation of dose, while FLASH RT works on the temporal dose delivery aspects. We all know that the conventional dose rate is around 0.01 Gy/s. FLASH uses an ultrafast dose rate (>40 Gy/s) to deliver treatment in seconds, with preclinical observations improving the therapeutic ratio to date; the mechanisms are being investigated. FLASH-RT is Ultra-fast RT delivery with dose rates generally several thousand times higher than those currently used in routine clinical practice. FLASH-RT versus CONV-RT have been characterized initially using their mean dose rate (>, i.e., 40 Gy/s for FLASH-RT vs. 0.01 Gy/s for CONV-RT). Several other parameters are essential such as repetition rate, pulses (number and width), and total duration of exposure [46]. FLASH effect and sparing of normal tissues seen in various preclinical animal studies/models (mice, rat, zebrafish, pigs/cats).

The postulated mechanisms of action, including oxygen consumption, are still speculative and under investigation. Machines are available and being made to deliver FLASH as electrons, photons, and protons.

In a study in Lung (Mice), the endpoint was radiation-induced pneumonitis/fibrosis. In conventional dose rate RT, the endpoint happened at 17 Gy dose. With the use of FLASH, the endpoint occurred at dose escalation up to 30 Gy. The endpoint in this study was Tumour control/fibrosis. In conventional radiotherapy, around 20% of the 15 Gy irradiated mice free were of the tumor. With FLASH RT, 70% of 28 Gy irradiated mice were free of tumors [47]. The first clinical trial considering FLASH RT with protons for palliative treatment of bone metastasis has recently been reported and has confirmed feasibility of the technique [48]. While FLASH has produced great enthusiasm and excitement, areas of uncertainty remain. These include quality assurance and safeguards for clinical delivery, understanding the FLASH effect when multiple beams are used, and tissue effects where the FLASH dose and dose rate fall off at depth or field margins.

Overall, SFRT faces several questions. These include (a) How fast are we moving in SFRT (b) how long will it take us to implement these in a routine clinical setting (c) What is the role of vendors in this regard (d) what shall be regulatory and reimbursement issues (e) shall we be able to have prescriptions of SFRT that are uniformly understood and implementable at varied centers (Table 5).

Future clinical trials need to be pragmatically designed. These should ideally aim at evaluating patients receiving comprehensive genomic-adjusted radiation doses and comparing them with routine present day standard of care approaches. The end points need to be disease control rates, normal tissue toxicity, as well as tumor radiosensitivity.

Table 5 Critical questions related to biology driven radiotherapy

	How to identify those who will get maximum benefit with …?
A	Existing locoregional treatment alone
B	Additional locoregional treatment (extra dose of RT,/higher dose/#, SRS, SBRT)
C	Modifications in radiotherapy (IGRT, SFRT)
D	Lesser radiotherapy (lower dose/lower dose/#)
E	Addition of chemo/immune therapy
F	No radiotherapy

IGRT image-guided radiotherapy, *SFRT* spatially fractionated radiotherapy, *SRS* stereotactic radiosurgery, *SBRT* stereotactic body radiotherapy

18 Future Challenges

In contrast to systemic therapy, minuscule progress has been made toward molecular biology-driven treatment in radiation oncology. The reasons for this are manifold. Routine tumor genotyping is rarely performed in patients with early-stage localized disease amenable to cure with radiotherapy. Also, local control within the radiation field has not been consistently annotated for most large genomic datasets [49]. Consequently, further analyses correlating radiation sensitivity and underlying molecular aberrations have become technically challenging. Radiotherapy acts through a multipronged mechanism involving both intrinsic and extrinsic effects related to the cell [50, 51]. As a result, the molecular determinants of radiation response are likely to be multifactorial and may vary across tissues and tumor types. Ultimately, a better understanding of these factors will be critical to maximizing the efficacy of radiotherapy while minimizing toxicities. Lack of due support from industry is also a crucial reason for lack of trials and which has impeded the evolution of biology-guided radiotherapy. In contrast, there is ample funding for trials related to medical oncology across body sites.

At the technical level, too, there are multiple challenges in biological-based radiotherapy. Integrating all biological, clinical, imaging, and dosimetric parameters presents a major challenge. Incorporating 4-D motion management in biology-directed treatments/boosts, too is an uphill task. To complicate issues, testing different doses of radiation/combination of RT/Chemotherapy to plan treatments in clinical settings for different tumors and stages require long drawn randomized trials. The final challenge is achieving the optimal toxicity/cure balance.

Despite hurdles and slow progress to integrate molecular- and genetic-based radiation therapy practices, several landmarks have been achieved in the last two decades which can further drive translational and clinical research areas in radiation oncology. Some of those examples are enumerated.

Some examples of evolving clinical scenarios showing how molecular and genetic analysis would be valuable for radiation therapy decisions, dose, and target volumes across different sites:

1.Glioblastoma (Brain):
MGMT promoter methylation and IDH mutation status predict radio sensitivity. Favourable markers support standard-dose RT, while resistant profiles may prompt dose escalation or trial-based adaptive volumes [52].

2.Head & Neck Squamous Cell Carcinoma
HPV (p16) positivity indicates high radio sensitivity. Molecular profiling is enabling radiation de-escalation of dose and elective nodal volumes to reduce long-term toxicity [53].

3.Non–Small Cell Lung Cancer
EGFR or ALK mutations guide integration of targeted therapy with RT. High-risk molecular signatures may justify intensified dose to the primary tumour while sparing uninvolved lung [54].

4.Breast Cancer
Gene-expression assays (e.g., Oncotype DX) identify low-risk disease. Patients with favourable molecular profiles may omit regional nodal irradiation or receive hypo fractionated, reduced volumes [55].

5.Prostate Cancer
Genomic classifiers (e.g., Decipher) stratify local recurrence risk. High genomic risk supports pelvic nodal irradiation and radiation dose escalation to the prostate bed [56].

6.Cervical Cancer
Hypoxia-related gene signatures predict radio resistance. Molecular hypoxia mapping supports focal dose boosting to resistant tumour sub volumes during brachytherapy [57].

7.Rectal Cancer
Mismatch repair deficiency (dMMR) suggests altered radiation response. Molecular profiling

may support selective omission of radiation or reduced dosing in favourable responders [58].

8.Paediatric Medulloblastoma

Molecular subgrouping (WNT, SHH, Group 3/4) defines prognosis. WNT tumours allow reduced craniospinal irradiation dose and smaller boost volumes [59].

9.Lymphoma

Gene-expression and PET-molecular markers identify radiosensitive disease. This further enables involved-site RT with reduced dose and volume instead of extended fields [60].

To summarize, biologic precision radiotherapy remains in its clinical infancy. There remains a role for continued novelty and clinical translation to identify genomic predictors of radiosensitivity and biomarkers to monitor radiation response. Personalized RT is an exciting field of research. There is rapidly emerging data for such approaches. Future work in this area should focus on (1) robust biological validation; (2) building biobanks alongside large radiotherapy randomised controlled trials with dose variance, to demonstrate interaction between radiosensitivity signature and dose; (3) validation of clinical-grade cost-effective assays that are deliverable within current health infrastructure; and (4) an integration with biomarkers of other determinants of radiotherapy response [61]. The next decade could see the start of such approaches in the clinic. Biology-based treatments, in an ideal environment, would require the integration of RT technology, radiobiology, radiology, and targeted therapy.

Percepts Box

1. Precision oncology customizes treatment according to the genetic makeup of the cancer.
2. Mutation testing is done to either assess familial risk or a driver mutation to help with treatment decisions or response prediction, but doesn't predict treatment related toxicities or risk of developing secondary cancers.
3. CBCT and MR based linacs can estimate only the gross response of tumors to RT.
4. Liquid biopsies assess the circulating tumor cells and tumor-derived DNA released by tumor deposits to detect changes in the tumor's molecular features and subclones within the tumor.
5. RT is a local mode of treatment. The abscopal effects are now being studied to explore the possibility of RT working systemically and immunologically.
6. Combining RT and immunotherapeutic agents shows increased response in the tumor microenvironment and depletion of myeloid derived suppressor cells and tumor regression, but at the possible cost of increased toxicity.
7. Biological imaging combines imaging systems like FDG-PET scans or MRI DWI to integrate with the tumor biology, allowing a heterogeneous dose distribution within the target volume.
8. Real-time BgRT uses biological imaging to guide RT delivery. The treatment PET has lesser number of emissions per second, which signal the tumor location throughout the treatment duration, while MRI-DWI uses differential diffusion coefficients of Brownian movements of water molecules.
9. Real-time BgRT also allows us to integrate radiomics of a tumor, such as the texture, heterogeneity, and intensity of dose distribution to help predict prognosis and outcomes of tumors.
10. Spatially fractionated radiation therapy (SFRT) includes GRID, LATTICE RT (LRT), Minibeam RT (MBRT), and Microbeam RT (MRT). These techniques use 3D dose modulation characterized by isolated hot or cold spots.

(continued)

11. FLASH RT is based on the dose delivery rate, usually >40 Gy/s. The 1st clinical trial using FLASH RT has been recently published with promising results. However, studies for QA, regulation, and dose prescriptions need to be done.
12. The Decipher genomic classifier has improved the prognostication of prostate cancer much more than the current variables.
13. The REQUITE study is focusing on integrating databases to identify and validate genetic variants and risk scores for RT induced toxicities.
14. To implement precision oncology in RT, we need a database to compare genomics with tumor outcomes and response to RT. There are technical challenges in integrating biological, clinical, imaging, and dosimetric parameters.
15. Even though the scenario stands at its nascent stages, the findings and progress in last 20 years can further advance the research, and biologic precision radiotherapy could well be the future of RT.

Multiple Choice Questions

1. Germline mutations are typically seen in:
   (a) Tumor cells
   (b) Normal cells
   (c) Both
   (d) Neither
2. Indications of Somatic/Germline testing:
   (a) Identify cancer risk in family members.
   (b) To identify driver mutations
   (c) Self-test normal tissue DNA
   (d) All of the above.
3. Distal effects of RT can be best explained by:
   (a) Stochastic effects
   (b) Non-stochastic effect
   (c) Abscopal effect
   (d) Cannot be explained.
4. Challenges of RT-induced abscopal effects include:
   (a) Predicting which tumors are likely to have these effects
   (b) Identifying biomarkers to predict which patients will have abscopal effects
   (c) Ensuring consistent response
   (d) All of the above.
5. Most common radiotracer in PET scan
   (a) PSMA
   (b) FDG
   (c) CA9
   (d) Cu64
6. Liquid biopsy is most commonly used to diagnose which cancer?
   (a) NSCLC
   (b) SCLC
   (c) Gastric cancers
   (d) GBM
7. Liquid biopsy usually detects:
   (a) Driver mutations
   (b) Circulating tumor DNA or RNA
   (c) IHC
   (d) None.
8. The main categories of tumor microenvironment include
   (a) Immune-desert
   (b) Immune-excluded
   (c) Immune infiltrated
   (d) All of the above
9. Dose painting means
   (a) Specific colors for specific volumes
   (b) Dose prescription is spatially correlated with PET tracer uptake distribution
   (c) Dose over hot or cold spots
   (d) Both (a) and (c)
10. Therapeutic PET varies from diagnostic PET in terms of:
   (a) Tracer used.
   (b) Machine used
   (c) More emissions per second
   (d) Fewer emissions per second
11. The technique that allows us to identify the texture of tumor is called
   (a) Genomics approach

(b) Artificial intelligence
(c) Radiomics approach
(d) Biological approach

12. Spatially fractionated RT includes:
(a) Minibeam RT
(b) Lattice RT
(c) Microbeam RT
(d) All of the above

13. FLASH RT usually delivers dose at:
(a) >40 Gy/s
(b) >100 Gy/s
(c) <40 Gy/s
(d) <10 Gy/s

14. The Decipher genomic classifier has been developed to identify the prognostication of which cancer?
(a) Lung cancer
(b) Prostate cancer
(c) Cervical cancer
(d) Thymoma.

Answer Key

1. (c)
2. (d)
3. (c)
4. (d)
5. (a)
6. (a)
7. (b)
8. (d)
9. (b)
10. (d)
11. (c)
12. (d)
13. (a)
14. (b)

References

1. Delaney G, Jacob S, Featherstone C, Barton M. The role of radiotherapy in cancer treatment: estimating optimal utilization from a review of evidence-based clinical guidelines. Cancer. 2005;104:1129–37.
2. Yaromina A, Krause M, Baumann M. Individualization of cancer treatment from radiotherapy perspective. Mol Oncol. 2012;6(2):211–21.
3. Hirst DG, Robson T. Molecular biology: the key to personalised treatment in radiation oncology? Br J Radiol. 2010;83(993):723–8. https://doi.org/10.1259/bjr/91488645.
4. Hanahan D, Weinberg RA. Hallmarks of cancer: the next generation. Cell. 2011;144:646–74.
5. ICGC/TCGA Pan-Cancer Analysis of Whole Genomes Consortium. Pan-cancer analysis of whole genomes. Nature. 2020;578:82–93. McGranahan N, Swanton C. Biological and therapeutic impact of intratumor heterogeneity in cancer evolution. Cancer Cell. 2015;27:15–26.
6. Koboldt DC, Steinberg KM, Larson DE, Wilson RK, Mardis E. Next-generation sequencing revolution and its impact on genomics. Cell. 2013;155:27–38.
7. Kumar-Sinha C, Chinnaiyan AM. Precision oncology in the age of integrative genomics. Nat Biotechnol. 2018;36:46–60.
8. Walter W, Pfarr N, Meggendorfer M, Jost P, Haferlach T, Weichert W. Next-generation diagnostics for precision oncology: Preanalytical considerations, technical challenges, and available technologies. Semin Cancer Biol. 2022;84:3–15. https://doi.org/10.1016/j.semcancer.2020.10.015. Epub 2020 Nov 7. PMID: 33171257.
9. Turajlic S, Sottoriva A, Graham T, Swanton C. Resolving genetic heterogeneity in cancer. Nat Rev Genet. 2019;20:404–16.
10. Moding EJ, Kastan MB, Kirsch DG. Strategies for optimizing the response of cancer and normal tissues to radiation. Nat Rev Drug Discov. 2013;12:526–42.
11. Bergom C, West CM, Higginson DS, Abazeed ME, Arun B, Bentzen SM, Bernstein JL, et al. The implications of genetic testing on radiation therapy decisions: a guide for radiation oncologists. Int J Radiat Oncol Biol Phys. 2019;105(4):698–712. https://doi.org/10.1016/j.ijrobp.2019.07.026.
12. Cheng HH, Sokolova AO, Schaeffer EM, Small EJ, Higano CS. Germline and somatic mutations in prostate cancer for the clinician. J Natl Compr Cancer Netw. 2019;17(5):515–21. https://doi.org/10.6004/jnccn.2019.
13. Childers KK, Maggard-Gibbons M, Macinko J, Childers CP. National distribution of cancer genetic testing in the United States. JAMA Oncol. 2018;4(6):876–9.
14. Susswein LR, Marshall ML, Nusbaum R, et al. Pathogenic and likely pathogenic variant prevalence among the first 10,000 patients referred for next-generation cancer panel testing. Genet Med. 2016;18:823–32.
15. Tung N, Battelli C, Allen B, et al. Frequency of mutations in individuals with breast cancer referred for BRCA1 and BRCA2 testing using next-generation sequencing with a 25-gene panel. Cancer. 2015;121:25–33.
16. Ricker C, Culver JO, Lowstuter K, et al. Increased yield of actionable mutations using multi-gene panels to assess hereditary cancer susceptibility in an ethnically diverse clinical cohort. Cancer Genet. 2016;209:130–7.
17. Senter L, Veney D, Surplus T, Haynam M, Adams EJ, Hampel H, Toland AE, Presley CJ, Padamsee TJ, Lee

CN, Hovick SR, Stover DG. Patient understanding of tumor genomic testing: a quality improvement effort. JCO Oncol Pract. 2023;19(1):e8–e14. https://doi.org/10.1200/OP.22.00316.
18. Koldehoff A, Danner M, Civello D, Rhiem K, Stock S, Müller D. Cost-effectiveness of targeted genetic testing for breast and ovarian cancer: a systematic review. Value Health. 2021;24(2):303–12. https://doi.org/10.1016/j.jval.2020.09.016.
19. Le AN, Harton J, Desai H, Powers J, et al. Frequency of radiation-induced malignancies post-adjuvant radiotherapy for breast cancer in patients with Li-Fraumeni syndrome. Breast Cancer Res Treat. 2020;181(1):181–8. https://doi.org/10.1007/s10549-020-05612-7.
20. Chiu LY, Sun Q, Zenke FT, Blaukat A, Vassilev LT. Selective ATM inhibition augments radiation-induced inflammatory signaling and cancer cell death. Aging (Albany NY). 2023;15(2):492–512. https://doi.org/10.18632/aging.204487.
21. Rodon J, Soria JC, Berger R, Miller WH, et al. Genomic and transcriptomic profiling expands precision cancer medicine: the WINTHER trial. Nat Med. 2019;25(5):751–8. https://doi.org/10.1038/s41591-019-0424-4.
22. Hall WA, Bergom C, Thompson RF, et al. Precision oncology and genomically guided radiation therapy: a report from the American Society for Radiation Oncology/American Association of Physicists in Medicine/National Cancer Institute Precision Medicine Conference. Int J Radiat Oncol Biol Phys. 2018;101:274–84.
23. Scott JG, Berglund A, Schell MJ, et al. A genome-based model for adjusting radiotherapy dose (GARD): a retrospective, cohort-based study. Lancet Oncol. 2017;18:202–11.
24. Zhao SG, Chang SL, Spratt DE, et al. Development and validation of a 24-gene predictor of response to postoperative radiotherapy in prostate cancer: a matched, retrospective analysis. Lancet Oncol. 2016;17:1612–20.
25. Tang C, Qi J, Wu Y, Luo L, et al. Improving the prediction for the response to radiotherapy of clinical tumor samples by using combinatorial model of MicroRNA expression. Front Genet. 2022;13:1069112. https://doi.org/10.3389/fgene.2022.1069112.
26. May JM, Bylicky M, Chopra S, Coleman CN, Aryankalayil MJ. Long and short non-coding RNA and radiation response: a review. Transl Res. 2021;233:162–79. https://doi.org/10.1016/j.trsl.2021.02.005.
27. Ling CC, Humm J, Larson S, Amols H, Fuks Z, Leibel S, Koutcher JA. Towards multidimensional radiotherapy (MD-CRT): biological imaging and biological conformality. Int J Radiat Oncol Biol Phys. 2000;47(3):551–60. https://doi.org/10.1016/s0360-3016(00)00467-3.
28. Gkika E, Oehlke O, Bunea H, Wiedenmann N, et al. Biological imaging for individualized therapy in radiation oncology: part II medical and clinical aspects. Future Oncol. 2018;14(8):751–69. https://doi.org/10.2217/fon-2017-0465.
29. Abuodeh Y, Venkat P, Kim S. Systematic review of case reports on the abscopal effect. Curr Probl Cancer. 2016;40(1):25–37. https://doi.org/10.1016/j.currproblcancer.2015.10.001.
30. Bristow RG, Alexander B, Baumann M, Bratman SV, et al. Combining precision radiotherapy with molecular targeting and immunomodulatory agents: a guideline by the American Society for Radiation Oncology. Lancet Oncol. 2018;19(5):e240–51.
31. Sharabi AB, Nirschl CJ, Kochel CM, et al. Stereotactic radiation therapy augments antigen-specific PD-1-mediated antitumor immune responses via cross-presentation of tumor antigen. Cancer Immunol Res. 2015;3:345–55.
32. Bentzen SM, Harari PM, Bernier J. Exploitable mechanisms for combining drugs with radiation: concepts, achievements and future directions. Nat Clin Pract Oncol. 2007;4(3):172–80.
33. Zhang Z, Liu X, Chen D, Yu J. Radiotherapy combined with immunotherapy: the dawn of cancer treatment. Signal Transduct Target Ther. 2022;7(1):258. https://doi.org/10.1038/s41392-022-01102-y.
34. Vitzthum LK, Surucu M, Gensheimer MF, Kovalchuk N, et al. BIOGUIDE-X: A first-in-human study of the performance of positron emission tomography-guided radiation therapy. Int J Radiat Oncol Biol Phys. 2024;118:1172–80. https://doi.org/10.1016/j.ijrobp.2023.12.019.
35. Siva S, Udovicich C, Tran B, Zargar H, Murphy DG, Hofman MS. Expanding the role of small-molecule PSMA ligands beyond PET staging of prostate cancer. Nat Rev Urol. 2020;17:107–18.https://doi.org/10.1038/s41585-019-0272-5.
36. Verhoeff SR, van Es SC, Boon E, van Helden E, Angus L, Elias SG, et al. Lesion detection by [89Zr]Zr-DFO-girentuximab and [18F]FDG-PET/CT in patients with newly diagnosed metastatic renal cell carcinoma. Eur J Nucl Med Mol Imaging. 2019;46:1931–9. https://doi.org/10.1007/s00259-019-04358-9.
37. Hench IB, Hench J, Tolnay M. Liquid biopsy in clinical management of breast, lung, and colorectal cancer. Front Med (Lausanne). 2018;5:9. https://doi.org/10.3389/fmed.2018.00009.
38. Nikanjam M, Kato S, Kurzrock R. Liquid biopsy: current technology and clinical applications. J Hematol Oncol. 2022;15(1):131. https://doi.org/10.1186/s13045-022-01351-y.
39. Gopal P, Yard BD, Petty A, Lal JC, et al. The mutational landscape of cancer's vulnerability to ionizing radiation. Clin Cancer Res. 2022;28(24):5343–58. https://doi.org/10.1158/1078-0432.CCR-22-1914.
40. Kerns SL, Fachal L, Dorling L, et al. Radiogenomics consortium genome-wide association study meta-analysis of late toxicity after prostate cancer radiotherapy [e-pub ahead of print]. J Natl Cancer Inst. https://doi.org/10.1093/jnci/djz075. Accessed 16 May 2019.
41. Jarosz-Biej M, Smolarczyk R, Cichoń T, Kułach N. Tumor microenvironment as a "game changer" in cancer radiotherapy. Int J Mol Sci. 2019;20(13):3212. https://doi.org/10.3390/ijms20133212.

42. Li B. Why do tumor-infiltrating lymphocytes have variable efficacy in the treatment of solid tumors? Front Immunol. 2022;13:973881. https://doi.org/10.3389/fimmu.2022.973881.
43. Valenza C, Taurelli Salimbeni B, Santoro C, Trapani D, Antonarelli G, Curigliano G. Tumor infiltrating lymphocytes across breast cancer subtypes: current issues for biomarker assessment. Cancers (Basel). 2023;15(3):767. https://doi.org/10.3390/cancers15030767.
44. Koukourakis IM, Gkegka AG, Xanthopoulou E, Nanos C, Giatromanolaki A, Koukourakis MI. Prognostic and predictive relevance of tumor-infiltrating lymphocytes in squamous cell head-neck cancer patients treated with radical radiotherapy/chemo-radiotherapy. Curr Oncol. 2022;29(6):4274–84. https://doi.org/10.3390/curroncol29060342.
45. Schültke E, Balosso J, Breslin T, Cavaletti G, Djonov V, Esteve F, Grotzer M, Hildebrandt G, Valdman A, Laissue J. Microbeam radiation therapy – grid therapy and beyond: a clinical perspective. Br J Radiol. 2017;90(1078):20170073.
46. Bourhis J, Sozzi WJ, Jorge PG, Gaide O, Bailat C, Duclos F, Patin D, Ozsahin M, Bochud F, Germond JF, Moeckli R, Vozenin MC. Treatment of a first patient with FLASH-radiotherapy. Radiother Oncol. 2019;139:18–22.
47. Favaudon V, Caplier L, Monceau V, Pouzoulet F, Sayarath M, Fouillade C, Poupon MF, Brito I, Hupé P, Bourhis J, Hall J, Fontaine JJ, Vozenin MC. Ultrahigh dose-rate FLASH irradiation increases the differential response between normal and tumor tissue in mice. Sci Transl Med. 2014;6(245):245ra93.
48. Testing proton FLASH RT in bone mets. Cancer Discov. 2022;12(12):2716.
49. Liu J, Lichtenberg T, Hoadley KA, Poisson LM, Lazar AJ, Cherniack AD, Kovatich AJ, Benz CC, Levine DA, Lee AV, et al. An integrated TCGA pan-cancer clinical data resource to drive high-quality survival outcome analytics. Cell. 2018;173:400–416.e11. https://doi.org/10.1016/j.cell.2018.02.052.
50. He L, Lv Y, Song Y, Zhang B. The prognosis comparison of different molecular subtypes of breast tumors after radiotherapy and the intrinsic reasons for their distinct radiosensitivity. Cancer Manag Res. 2019;11:5765–75.
51. Demaria S, Formenti SC. Role of T lymphocytes in tumor response to radiotherapy. Front Oncol. 2012;2:95.
52. Hegi ME, Diserens AC, Gorlia T, et al. MGMT gene silencing and benefit from temozolomide in glioblastoma. N Engl J Med. 2005;352(10):997–1003.
53. Ang KK, Harris J, Wheeler R, et al. Human papillomavirus and survival of patients with oropharyngeal cancer. N Engl J Med. 2010;363(1):24–35.
54. Lindeman NI, Cagle PT, Aisner DL, et al. Updated molecular testing guideline for the selection of lung cancer patients for treatment with targeted tyrosine kinase inhibitors. J Thorac Oncol. 2018;13(3):323–358.
55. Sparano JA, Gray RJ, Makower DF, et al. Adjuvant chemotherapy guided by a 21-gene expression assay in breast cancer. N Engl J Med. 2018;379(2):111–121.
56. Den RB, Feng FY, Showalter TN, et al. Genomic prostate cancer classifier predicts biochemical failure and metastases in patients after postoperative radiation therapy. J Clin Oncol. 2015;33(8):944–951.
57. Höckel M, Vaupel P. Tumor hypoxia: definitions and current clinical, biologic, and molecular aspects. Lancet Oncol. 2001;2(10):593–602.
58. Cercek A, Lumish M, Sinopoli J, et al. PD-1 blockade in mismatch repair–deficient, locally advanced rectal cancer. N Engl J Med. 2022;386(25):2363–2376.
59. Taylor MD, Northcott PA, Korshunov A, et al. Molecular subgroups of medulloblastoma: the current consensus. Acta Neuropathol. 2012;123(4):465–472.
60. Yahalom J, Illidge T, Specht L, et al. Modern radiation therapy for extranodal lymphomas: field and dose guidelines from ILROG. J Clin Oncol. 2015;33(26):3039–3047.
61. Bleaney CW, Abdelaal H, Reardon M, Anandadas C, Hoskin P, Choudhury A, Forker L. Clinical biomarkers of tumour radiosensitivity and predicting benefit from: a systematic review. Cancers (Basel). 2024;16:1942. https://doi.org/10.3390/cancers16101942.

Online Links

https://www.youtube.com/watch?v=wYMm0T2phQw How to interpret a somatic NGS report?

https://www.youtube.com/live/G0admlTmuzo Role of NGS in solid tumours

https://www.youtube.com/live/SDcZyzmftWI Somatic NGS and Molecular Genetic Analysis in Cancer and Precision Oncology

Radiation Therapy for Benign Diseases

Manur Gururajachar Janaki, Arun Rathi, Kishore Singh, Simon Pavamani, and Lithika Lavanya M

1 Introduction

Radiation Therapy (RT) has been used for various benign diseases since as early as 1898, when it was used for pain relief in juvenile arthritis, infection like tuberculosis of the lungs, and in recent time for Covid-19 pneumonia. Soon it was realized that radiotherapy for non-cancer diseases would be associated with a lot of side effects. Again, in the last few decades, newer understanding of cellular and molecular action of radiation at various dose levels, simultaneous development of advanced technology in our field has led to an increase in the use with better outcomes of radiation for benign diseases. The use of RT for benign diseases varies across the globe, with maximum use in Germany [1]. This variation is due to availability of an alternate therapy, acceptance in different countries and awareness of the results of radiation among other specialists. Over the last 20 years, the cases treated have doubled, which means many new diseases are being treated with modern RT practices. Radiation continues to be used for conditions such as Keloids, Graves ophthalmopathy, Heterotopic ossification and benign lesions of the central nervous system. In the eastern world, Keloid is the most common indication for radiation, followed by Juvenile nasopharyngeal angiofibroma [1, 2]. Radiation has found its place for newer indications like ventricular tachycardia, functional disorders like trigeminal neuralgia, and chronic osteoarthritis.

Benign tumours differ from their malignant counterparts in terms of their slow growth, localized nature, lack of invasive capacity and hence hardly spread to distant organs. However, they do cause disfigurement, functional impairment and pressure effects. Radiation is considered when other modalities of tested treatments are either not possible or not effective, mainly due to the fear of radiation-induced late effects in terms of radiation-induced carcinogenesis, growth and fertility issues. Once decided every effort should be made to use the least possible dose, the best technique and careful planning.

M. G. Janaki (✉)
MS Ramaiah Medical College, Bangalore, India

A. Rathi
Radiation Oncology, Maulana Azad Medical College (MAMC), Delhi, India

K. Singh
Department of Radiation Oncology, Subharti Medical College and Swami Vivekanand Subharti University, Meerut, UP, India

S. Pavamani
Department of Radiation Oncology, CMC, Vellore, India
e-mail: simon@cmcvellore.ac.in

L. Lavanya M
Department of Radiation Oncology, MS Ramaiah Medical College, Bengaluru, India

B. K. Mohanti et al. (eds.), *Radiation Oncology – Principles, Precepts and Practice*,
https://doi.org/10.1007/978-981-95-5171-2_19

Very low doses are used for the anti-inflammatory effect, as in covid associated pneumonia, low doses are used for the anti-proliferative effect as in Keloid and high doses of up to 60 Gy are used as in trigeminal neuralgia. It is very important to counsel regarding the treatment modalities available, expected outcome with radiation, possible sequelae and rehabilitation as a part of decision making.

This chapter will focus on conditions that are commonly treated with radiation and lesions such as meningioma, pituitary adenoma, craniopharyngioma, acoustic neuroma and arteriovenous malformations will be discussed in the chapter on central nervous system tumours.

2 Rationale/Radiobiology

Unlike for malignant tumours, decision of radiation as the treatment modality should be done with many important considerations. Firstly, the natural course of the disease has to be understood, and how the available treatments can modify the same has to be studied. Secondly, it is important to explore all other available treatment modalities in terms of the expected results before offering radiation. Thirdly, a detailed counselling stressing on the better outcomes with radiation, importance of advanced technology, possible late side effects in terms of fertility issues, risk of carcinogenesis, especially in younger patients, has to be done and informed consent to be taken. Fourthly, once it's decided to go with radiation, standard protocols in terms of adequate coverage of the tumour with minimal inclusion of normal structures, use of advanced technology, and prescribing lowest possible dose will help in achieving optimal therapeutic ratio. Finally, the patients who are treated with radiation have to be monitored regularly for the related sequelae, and they have to be managed effectively.

Radiation works differently at various dose levels; extensive research is going on, and detailed description is beyond the scope of this chapter and is summarized in Fig. 1. Briefly, it can be understood as follows. The therapeutic range used for benign diseases ranges widely from less than 2 Gy to more than 50 Gy. At very low dose levels of less than 2 Gy, radiation causes immunomodulatory effect which reduces the inflammation and hence finds its place in treating entities such as degenerative conditions such as osteoarthritis, tendinitis, COVID-associated pneumonia, etc. At low dose levels of up to 20 Gy, the predominant effect is antiproliferative and is used for lesions such as Keloid, Dupuytren's contracture and pterygium. At moderate doses of up to 40 Gy, both anti-inflammatory and antiproliferative effects of radiation are exploited to treat Graves ophthalmopathy and orbital pseudotumor. At very high doses of up to 60 Gy, radiation acts on endothelial cells causing stenosis and occlusion of abnormal vessels, as in haemangioma and arteriovenous fistula. Inhibition of cell proliferation and cell kill are also observed at high doses, such as in meningioma and pituitary adenoma [3]. Detailed information is provided at the end of the chapter in Table 2.

3 Radiation-Induced Carcinogenesis

The actual occurrence of radiation-induced cancers (RIC) is very difficult to predict, as these occur after many years of treatment. The number of patients getting radiation for benign conditions is very less; there are varied practices regarding dose fractiontation, techniques and more importantly, not all are reliable for follow-up, the expected latent period is anywhere between 10 and 25 years. The available data is based on older indications, treatment with low energy photons, larger volumes of irradiation and primitive technology which are no longer in practice. However, there is a theoretical possibility, as RIC is stochastic in nature, and there is no threshold below which it does not happen.

Various studies have estimated the risk to be around 0.5–3% at 30 years after radiation compared to lifetime risk of 33–40% for the general population [4]. The chances of RIC depend on the site treated, the dose delivered, inherent genetic susceptibility and, more importantly, the age at which the patient is exposed to radiation. The risk is very low when periphery is treated, lower dose is prescribed, lesser volume is treated and when older individuals are treated compared to children and adolescents. In a study by Trott

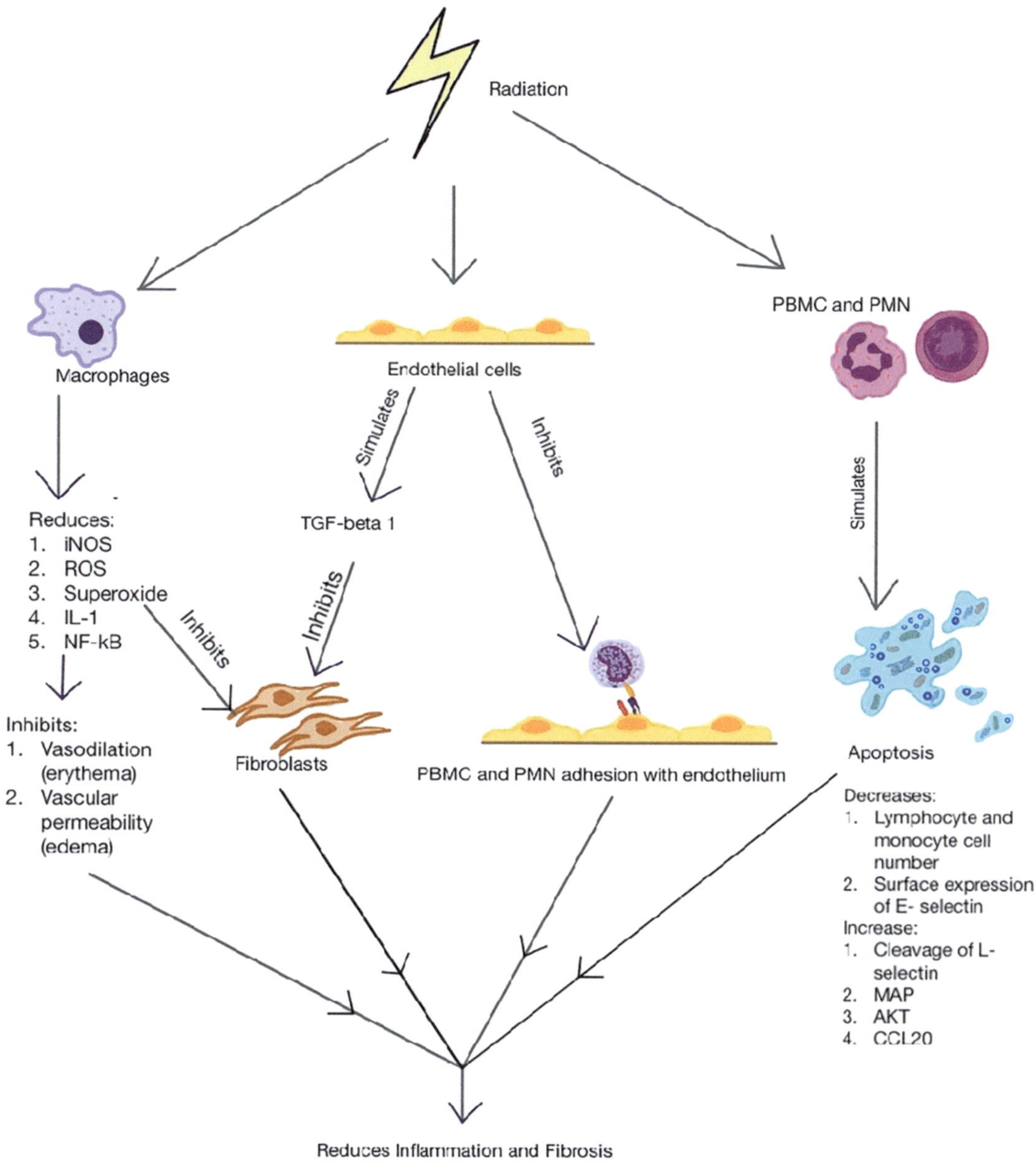

Fig. 1 Flow chart illustrating the effects of radiation on various cellular processes. Radiation impacts macrophages, endothelial cells, and PBMC/PMN. Macrophages reduce iNOS, ROS, superoxide, IL-1, and NF-kB, inhibiting vasodilation and vascular permeability. Endothelial cells stimulate TGF-beta 1, affecting fibroblasts and inhibiting PBMC/PMN adhesion. PBMC/PMN stimulation leads to apoptosis, decreasing lymphocyte and monocyte numbers, and altering surface expression of E-selectin, L-selectin cleavage, MAP, AKT, and CCL20. Overall, these interactions reduce inflammation and fibrosis

et al., it was found that when the breast received one Gy, the chances of breast cancer were around 5% at 10 years when the patient was treated before the age of 35 years while it was 3% between 35 and 45 years and < 1% when the age at treatment was more than 60 years [5]. It is important to weigh the benefits against the theoretical possibility of RIC before taking the decision of starting treatment with radiation.

The risk of developing leukaemia after low-dose radiation goes on for 25 years, and it depends on the age of exposure to radiation, with

Table 2 Summarizing the role of radiation for various benign diseases

Disease [basic pathology]	Treatment options	Mechanism of action of radiation	Radiation dose	Outcome/remarks	Evidence
Heterotopic ossification[bone formation in the soft tissue]	Surgery followed by Physiotherapy Radiotherapy Indomethacin NSAIDs Bisphosphonates	Anti-inflammatory	7 Gy/1 Fr	Reduction in incidence by 40% compared to NSAIDs	Cai et al. [23]
Haemangioma [proliferation of endothelial cells of vessels]	Topical beta blockers Oral propranolol Intralesional steroid injections Transpupillary thermotherapy Photodynamic therapy Surgical resection Laser therapies Radiotherapy	Occlusion of abnormal vessels	15–50 Gy in 2Gy/Fr depends on the site	Pain relief in 87.5% complete response in 45.7%	Alfredo et al. [64]
Keloid [excessive fibroblast proliferation]	Surgery followed by Intralesional corticosteroid injections Radiation Continuous pressure Silicone gel Retinoic acid Silastic sheet coverage NdYaG laser 5-fluorouracil	Anti-proliferative	12-15Gy/3Fr	To be given within 24 h of surgery Either external or brachy can be done	Kalapurmat NM et al. [57]
Graves ophthalmopathy[inflammatory And] Autoimmune	Methyl prednisolone Cyclosporine Azathioprine Radiotherapy Surgery Rituximab	Anti- inflammatory	20Gy/10Fr	RT + glucocorticoid was better compared to RT alone ($p = 0.04$)	Viani et al [42]

Pterygium [fibrovascular proliferation]	Surgery with Strontium brachytherapy or Mitomycin C eye drops 0.02% Or Conjunctival autograft + cyclosporin 0.05% eye drops	Anti-proliferative	25Gy/1Fr (strontium)	Odds ratio for recurrence 0.12 compared to surgery	Zeng et al [47]
Orbital pseudotumor [orbital inflammation]	Systemic corticosteroids Definitive radiotherapy	Anti-inflammatory	20–30Gy/ 10–15Fr	56% stopped and 25% reduced steroids	Matthiesen et al [45]
Glomus tumour [vascular proliferation]	Definitive radiotherapy	Occlusion of abnormal vessels	45–60Gy/ 25–30Fr	Safer compared to surgery	Larner et al [75]
Juvenile nasopharyngeal angiofibroma [highly vascular tumour]	Definitive radiotherapy	Anti-proliferative and occlusion of abnormal vessels	36–46 Gy/18–23Fr	Seen at a young age. Important to counsel regarding late effects	Mallick et al [62]
Langerhans cell histiocytosis [clonal proliferation of langerhans cells]	Observation Intralesional indomethacin/steroids Bisphosphonates Definitive radiotherapy Systemic vinblastine and steroids	Anti-proliferative	10–20 Gy/ 5–10 Fr	71% survival with chemo in multisystem disease	Jan et al [37]
Gynaecomastia [proliferation of breast parenchyma in men]	Reassurance Ultrasonic liposuction Surgical excision of breast tissue and fat Oral tamoxifen 20 mg for 6–12 months Definitive radiotherapy	Anti-proliferative	15Gy/1Fr 12Gy/1Fr Using 6–12 MeV electrons	First line option for bicalutamide-induced	Tunio et al. [48]

(continued)

Table 2 (continued)

Disease [basic pathology]	Treatment options	Mechanism of action of radiation	Radiation dose	Outcome/remarks	Evidence
Peyronie's disease [microtrauma and scarring of tunica albuginea]	Oral anti-oxidants (vitamin E), Pentoxifylline, Analgesics Intralesional injection of collagenase clostridium histolyticum Interferon alfa-2b Verapamil Corticosteroid injections Definitive radiotherapy Surgery Penile traction therapy Extracorporeal shockwave therapy	Anti-inflammatory	Any of the following: 30Gy/15Fr 36Gy/18Fr 32Gy/8Fr 2–3Gy/1Fr Using 50 kV photon	Radiation provides Pain relief, symptom regression and improved penile curvature in 83%, 47% and 49% of patients, respectively	Pietsch et al. [52]
Pigmented villonodular synovitis [focal areas of soft tissue hyperplasia in the synovium]	CSF-1 receptor antagonist (pexidartinib) Partial/total synovectomy with adjuvant radiotherapy Total joint arthroplasty	Anti-proliferative	Any of the following: 26Gy/13Fr 36Gy/18Fr 50Gy/25Fr	Reduces recurrence from 50 to less than 10% compared to surgery alone in gross residual lesions.	Seegenschmiedt MH et al. [50]
COVID pneumonitis [cytokine storm]	Oxygen Supportive care Anti-viral Radiation	Polarization of macrophages, reduction of oxidative burst activity, NK cell activation	70 cGy/1Fr	Giving during the early pulmonary phase reduces O_2 requirement and hospital stay	DN Sharma [85]

a risk of 0.2% for a mean bone marrow dose of 1 Gy [5]. As far as soft tissue sarcoma after radiation, a genetic link is observed between sarcoma and retinoblastoma and the patients are likely to develop sarcoma in the irradiated field.

4 Main Section/Clinical Application and Aspects

4.1 Heterotopic Ossification

Heterotopic ossification (HO) refers to the pathological process of emergence of additional skeletal bone in soft tissues and muscles due to abnormal differentiation of pluripotent mesenchymal cells, where the bone is usually not subsistent [6]. It is still unclear as to what triggers this process, but genetic predisposition has some role to play in fewer cases. Certain mutations, like the ACVR1 and GNAS1 gene mutations, are associated with rare morbid conditions like fibrodysplasia ossificans progressiva and progressive osseous heteroplasia, respectively. Conditions associated with HO are Ankylosing spondylitis, Paget's disease and Diffuse idiopathic skeletal hyperostosis [7]. Most cases have been documented post trauma such as after fractures/fixation, falls and post orthopaedic surgeries like hip arthroplasty. A very high percentage of people suffering from severe burns and traumatic amputations have also shown to develop HO [8]. Common sites of HO are areas exposed to trauma like extremities, pelvis and even head and neck.

4.1.1 Clinical Presentation

The symptoms depend on the phase of the disease process. The initial phase is associated with pain, swelling, tenderness and other signs of inflammation with restricted motion of the affected part, localized swelling (with bone tissue maturation) seen often as the disease transitions into chronic phase [9]. HO can also occur months after any trauma [10, 11]. Brooker staging system has been used to grade the severity of disease, on the basis of imaging (radiographs) of the hip and pelvis [12]. X-rays in the initial phase of the disease might be negative since calcium is missing in the matrix showing signs of ossification and radio-dense mass much later.

CT scans are usually characteristic, showing islands of bone maturation extending from dermis into the deeper layers, and a follow-up scan helps in confirming the diagnosis if it was done too early in the course of disease, as shown in Fig. 2. A three-phase bone scan is ideal and may even detect early ossifications [13]. F [18] NaF PET-CT is an emerging non-invasive and sensitive imaging tool for assessing flare ups in already detected cases of HO [14].

4.1.2 Treatment

There is no definite treatment of this disease since there is no cure: however the focus is on

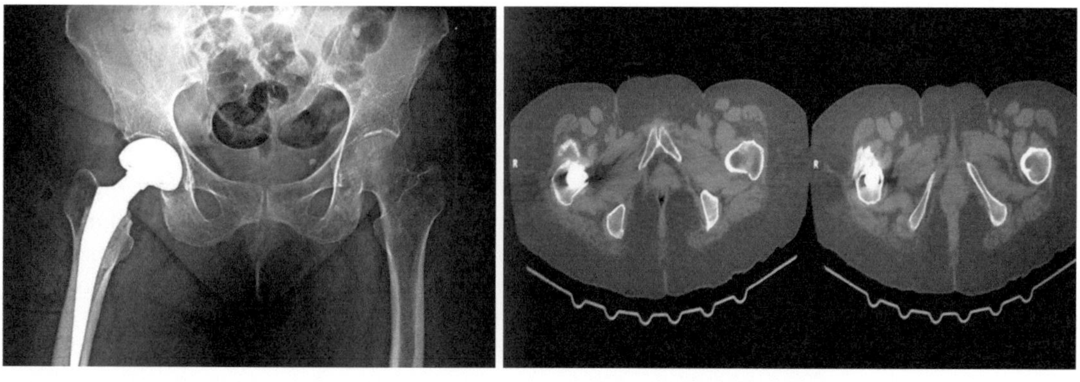

Fig. 2 X-ray of right hip joint (left) in a patient who has undergone partial hip replacement while CT scan (right) around the same time shows ossification in the soft tissue around right hip joint

relief from symptoms and to prevent HO at other sites. Few patients might achieve great results with physiotherapy and may regain range of movements which is the most vital part of treatment [15]. A fraction of patients who develop refractory ankylosis should be assessed for the need of surgery.

Surgery is generally a contraindication since any manipulation leads to a risk of further bone formation and is considered for the possibility of restoration of movements [16]. Prophylaxis for re-development of ossification must commence after surgery. Use of bisphosphonates delays the mineralization of the bone matrix and inhibits the transformation of the active form of calcium in bone. A study has revealed that Etidronate, if administered early, within 3–6 weeks, might help in arresting the progression of disease [17].

NSAIDs have been routinely prescribed for up to 1–6 weeks after surgery for prevention of HO. The gastrointestinal side effects are less commonly observed in selective NSAIDs, but cardiac issues have been noted off late. The lack of sufficient data on cardiac side effects has led to the use of non-selective NSAIDs [18]. They act by altering the prostaglandin-mediated inflammatory pathways and by inhibiting osteoprogenitor cell differentiation [19]. In a Cochrane review, NSAIDs, when used perioperatively, brought down the risk of development of HO by 59% when compared with a placebo [20]*. Indomethacin is the gold standard, prescribed at 75 mg/day up to 6 weeks after surgery. However, other NSAIDs like Brufen and COX inhibitors have also proven to be effective with a lesser side effects profile [21].

4.1.3 Radiation Therapy in HO

Radiation has been mostly used for prevention and sometimes as treatment of HO. It has been compared with NSAIDs and has shown results favouring the former. Pakos et al. conducted a meta-analysis wherein seven randomized trials comprising of 1143 patients were studied, comparing NSAIDs with RT for prevention, irrespective of the type of HO, timing of RT (preoperative vs postoperative), Radiation dose and the equipment used (whether Co-60 or Linear accelerator used) [22]*. Various RT schedules ranging from 1 Gy × 6 Fr, 2 Gy × 5 Fr, 3.5 Gy × 5 Fr to 10 Gy in 5 Fr and 8 Gy in 1 Fr were included. It was concluded that a dose of 6 Gy is more effective in preventing Grade III–IV HO when compared with NSAIDs. Figure 2 shows the meta-analysis of risk review ratio for HO in patients treated with NSAIDs and RT.

In another meta-analysis of 31 studies, four strategies (nonselective NSAIDs, radiation, selective NSAIDs and controls) were compared to avert heterotopic ossification after hip surgery. Radiation was found to be the most efficacious treatment to reduce the probability of HO (all grades of Brooker classification) after total hip arthroplasty [23]**. Pakos et al. reported the probability of HO after radiation treatment was less than 50% of that with NSAIDs. Milakovic et al. found radiation delivered over multiple fractions was found to have more potency than that of single fraction delivery to avert HO progression [24].

4.1.4 Treatment Planning

The patient is simulated in a supine, comfortable and reproducible position using an immobilization device. Conventional two-dimensional techniques or three-dimensional conformal radiation therapy (3D-CRT) technique could be used to treat the hip with the field-specific parameters decided after reviewing the simulation images and are customized for each patient. Anatomically in general, the superior border is about 3 cm above the acetabulum, the caudal border about 3 cm below the lesser trochanter of the femoral head or could include the upper 1/3 of the implant shaft (if used). The multi-leaf collimators are used to shape the radiation field as per tumour anatomy so as to minimally expose the normal tissues to radiation as shown in Fig. 3. Anterior-posterior fields are used to deliver the radiation in an isocentric setup using 6–18 MV photon beams. The acceptable plan criterion is to cover the target with at least 95% of the prescription dose with heterogeneity in the range of −5% – +7% [25]**. Doses ranging from 5–20 Gy in 1–5 Fr have been used as shown in Table 1, but 7 Gy in a single fraction has been found to be effective when compared with higher doses [26].

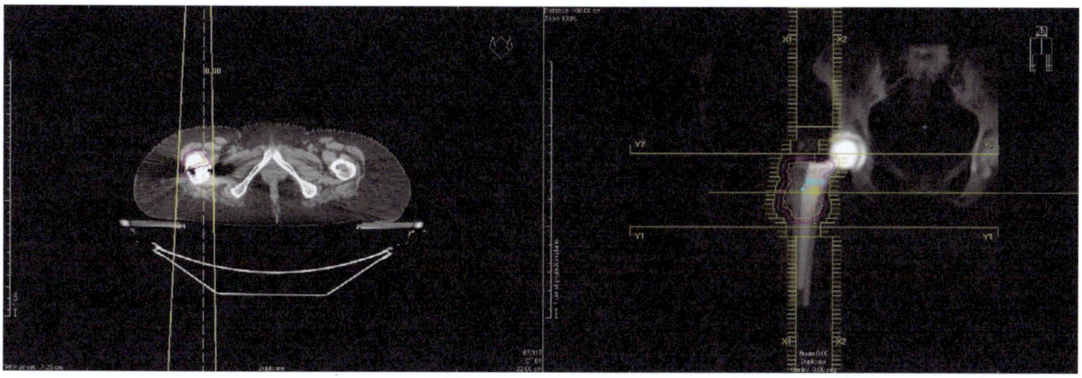

Fig. 3 Showing radiation beam placement on planning CT scan-axial section (left) and beams eye view (right) of the same

Table 1 Heterotopic Ossification: Radiation treatment details and results of established studies

Author	Year	Study	No. hips	Conclusions
Sylvester et al. [29]	1988	20 Gy/10 Fr vs 10Gy/5 Fr	27	Reduced dose effective
Healy [30]	1990	5.5 Gy/ single vs 7Gy/single	147	7 Gy recommended
Pellegrini et al. [31]	1992	8Gy/single Fr vs 10Gy/5Fr	62	Equivalent failure single-dose limited-field radiation is effective
Padgett et al. [32]	2003	5Gy/2Fr vs 10Gy/5Fr	59	10 Gy more efficient
Konski et al. [33]	1990	10Gy/5Fr vs 8Gy/single Fr	37	8 Gy as effective as 10 Gy

Seegenschmiedt et al. reported an equal efficacy of both preoperative (<4 h before surgery) and post-operative (<96 h before surgery) radiation delivered in variable dose fractionation regime. Overall, postoperative radiation appears to have more indications than preoperative radiation, preferring preoperative for III–IV HO [27]. Gregoritch et al. concluded that the results are comparable when the treatment is given 6 h before the surgery to the treatment delivered within 72 h' post-surgery [28]. Follow up with serial X-rays will show varying regression and/or absence of further progression as shown in Fig. 4, correlating with improvement in symptoms.

4.2 Langerhans Cell Histiocytosis (LCH)

Langerhans cell histiocytosis (LCH) or Histiocytosis X (older name) is characterized by clonal proliferation of Langerhans cells. It is mainly a disorder of children and young adults with a wide spectrum of clinical manifestations ranging from single-site, single system, multisite to multi system involvement. It is driven by misguided myeloid differentiation. It is a rare disorder that occurs in approximately 4.6 patients per 10 lakh children, under 15 years of age, with male to female ratio of 1.2: 1. Peak incidence is seen between 1 and 3 years [34, 35].

4.2.1 Clinical Presentation/ Investigations

Bone involvement is the most common presentation. Children most commonly have involvement of vertebral bodies, long bones and mandible in contrast, adults have lesions in cranium and ribs. Laboratory investigations include CBC with ESR, LFT CRP, thyroid function test and urine analysis. One may use ultrasound abdomen for liver and lymph nodes in the abdomen, Chest X-ray and skeletal survey either by bone scan (99mTc) or PET scan. The usual findings on X-ray is a single round or oval lytic bony defect

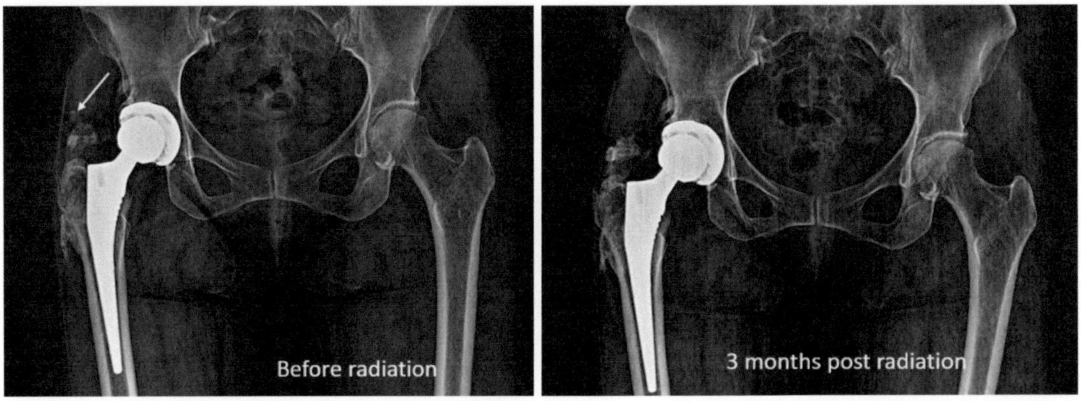

Fig. 4 X-ray images of the hip joint with a prosthetic implant showing HO on the left. The right image, labeled "3 months post radiation," shows peripheral regression of HO

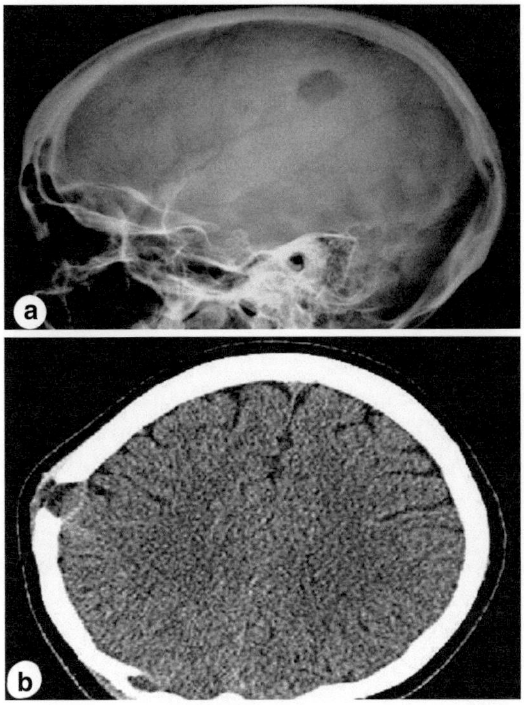

Fig. 5 The image labelled (**a**) shows lateral X-ray of skull, highlighting punched out osteolytic lesion and image labelled (**b**) displays a cross-sectional CT scan revealing skull lesion with normal brain tissue [39]

in the cranium with clear boundaries appearing 'punched out' (Fig. 5). In contrast, rib lesions are often accompanied by pathological fractures, and soft tissue extension may cause extra pleural masses. For histopathological confirmation core needle biopsy is enough, and it differentiates bony diseases from lymphoproliferative disorder or round blue cell diseases. Presence of Langerhans cells is hallmark of LCH and presence of Birbeck granules, Langerin (CD 207) positivity and staining with CD1a and S100 also helps in confirmation of diagnosis [36].

4.2.2 Treatment

Single-site bony lesions can be treated with observation, curettage or intralesional steroids or NSAIDS (Indomethacin). When lesion is progressive, painful or in surgically inaccessible site, low-dose radiation therapy (RT) is used, which is both effective and safe [37].

Multisite bony lesion requires addition of systemic chemotherapy and steroids. Adjuvant RT is needed to control long bone lesions. Addition of bisphosphonate will further enhance stability of bones.

Multisystem disease is mainly treated with vinblastine and prednisolone, which along with RT result in local control rates from 75% to 100%. RT is indicated in isolated unresectable lesions/if resection would significantly compromise anatomic function, e.g. odontoid process, CNS/in recurrent or progressive lesion. Usually, a dose of 10 to 20 Gy (ranging from 1.4 Gy to 45 Gy) is used in adults (Grade C2) [38].

4.2.3 Prognosis

Single-site bony lesions have 100% control and survival at 10 years. In contrast, multisystem disease has 71% survival at 10 years. Organ involvement reduces the survival to 50% at 10 years.

4.3 Graves Ophthalmopathy

Graves's disease (GD) is an autoimmune thyroid disease which presents with thyroid hyperplasia and increased thyroid hormone levels. Graves' Ophthalmopathy (GO) is the major extra thyroidal manifestation of GD and results from infiltration of the orbit by auto-reactive T-lymphocytes, proliferation of orbital fibroblasts and increased orbital fat. This can clinically manifest as classical clinical findings of periorbital oedema, lid retraction and diplopia. Severe cases may have decreased vision. The incidence of GO is around 28% with moderate and severe disease occurring in 15% and 2% respectively [40].

Treatment for GO is based on the clinical activity, severity and duration of the GO. The European Group on Graves' Orbitopathy (EUGOGO) is the most widely followed practice guideline for the treatment of GO.

The EUGOGO determines the activity by using the Clinical Activity Score(CAS), which is a validated scoring system. It comprises seven items, and GO is termed as active if the score is more than equal to 3/7. There is also a ten-item CAS which is used to evaluate recent progression. Severity is graded as mild, moderate to severe, and sight threatening. Both orbital MRI and CT have indications in the management of GO [40].

The cornerstone of the management of GO is referral to a specialized centre with experience of treating patients with GO. Radiotherapy is indicated as a second line treatment for moderate to severe and active GO [40]. First line treatment is steroids i.e. intravenous methyl-prednisolone. If refractory, then there is rechallenge with steroids with the addition of cyclosporine or azathioprine. If there is no response to these therapies, then the patient is referred for surgery. Orbital Radiotherapy is considered if there is a contraindication for surgery in the patient. There has been a decline in the number of patients undergoing radiotherapy in recent years.

A recent survey conducted in India revealed a very low referral rate for orbital radiotherapy [41]. Institutional data have shown only a handful of patients underwent radiotherapy for GO in the past 15 years. Newer agents available now include monoclonal antibodies, namely, Rituximab and Tocilizumab. Delivery of radiotherapy in the past included using conventional techniques using parallel opposed beam arrangements or CT-based three-dimensional conformal radiotherapy to include both the orbits.

However, in the present era, Intensity Modulated Radiotherapy (IMRT) should be employed whenever feasible for superior coverage of the target. The treatment planning begins with immobilization with a thermoplastic mask, acquisition of 2.5 mm slice thickness CT images. The clinical target volume (CTV) would be the origin to insertion of the extraocular muscles and the retro-orbital fatty space with the main bulk. The organs at risk (OAR) would be the lenses, globes, optic nerves and lacrimal glands. Planning Target Volume (PTV) would be generated with a 2 mm expansion of the CTV. Dose delivered would be 20 Gy in 10 fractions [42]. A study with one hundred sixteen patients, treated with IMRT, with a median follow-up of 62 months reported satisfactory symptom control with a favourable side effect profile [43].

4.4 Orbital Pseudotumour

Orbital Pseudotumour, also known as Idiopathic Orbital Inflammatory Syndrome, is described as a nonspecific non-neoplastic inflammatory process of the orbit. It was reported as the commonest orbital inflammatory disease in a series of 6328 patients in South India [44]. The disease presents with periorbital oedema, erythema, proptosis, ptosis, diplopia and pain with eye movements. The differential includes Graves' Ophthalmopathy and Orbital infection. It is an idiopathic tumorous inflammation made up of pleomorphic inflammatory cellular response and a fibrovascular tissue reaction. The aetiology is unknown, but is believed to be caused by an immune-mediated process. Pathologically, the findings are not specific and may only show benign lymphoid hyperplasia, inflammatory cell infiltration and necrotizing vasculitis. The diagnosis is made mainly by exclusion of other orbital diseases with similar presentation. Both CT and MR studies contribute in arriving at the diagnosis.

The mainstay of treatment is systemic corticosteroids, and response is usually seen in a couple of days. The response indicates a correct diagnosis and management.

Radiotherapy is indicated in patients in whom corticosteroids are contraindicated or do not respond to their administration. Recent series have described the usage of both three-dimensional conformal radiation therapy and IMRT. Radiation doses have ranged 20 Gy to 30 Gy [45]. Good response has been reported with a decrease or stoppage of the steroid therapy. Late toxicities include cataracts, chronic dry eye, keratopathy and enophthalmos.

4.5 Pterygium

Pterygium is a degenerative disorder of the conjunctiva characterized by a triangular fleshy fibrovascular proliferation from the bulbar conjunctiva to the cornea. Most commonly seen on the nasal side. The prevalence is more common, 30 degrees north and south of the equator, known as the 'Pterygium belt'. Ultraviolet light exposure is cited as one of the main risk factors for development of pterygium. In India, the prevalence is around 13% in adults.

Surgery is the standard of care and is indicated when there is visual disturbance. The surgery known as the 'Bare Sclera technique' consists of dissecting the head of the pterygium from the cornea and the resection of the conjunctiva and Tenon's capsule. Recurrence after this can range from 30% to 88% [46]. Various adjuvant therapies have been described to reduce the recurrence. Findings of a recent network meta-analysis showed that the following are the best strategies to prevent recurrence after pterygium surgery [47].

1. Bare sclera + Brachytherapy using Strontium applicator 2500 cGy single dose.
2. Bare sclera + Mitomycin C eye drops 0.02%.
3. Conjunctival Autograft + Cyclosporin Eye Drops 0.05%

4.6 Gynaecomastia

Enlargement of a man's breasts is called Gynaecomastia, and it is usually either physiological during puberty or pathological as in hyperthyroidism, hypogonadism, hypopituitarism or germ cell tumour. It could also be seen following hormone therapy, one of it being the use of bicalutamide in prostate cancer patients.

Gynaecomastia associated with puberty will regress without any treatment and needs only reassurance, but the gynaecomastia due to other reasons needs treatment. Hormone therapy-induced gynaecomastia needs prompt treatment as they often result in treatment discontinuation. There are different grades of gynaecomastia, and treatment differs with each type. Various approaches tried are reassurance/ultrasonic liposuction/surgical excision of breast tissue and fat/oral tamoxifen/radiation.

Tamoxifen 20 mg daily for a period of 6 months to 1 year. Radiation is given to a dose of 12 Gy in a single fraction (8–16 Gy in 1–11 fractions) using a 6–12 MeV electron beam targeting a 5 cm diameter circle of tissue around each nipple. Isodose coverage of 90% to skin and chest wall could be accepted [48].

As per the meta-analysis by Tunio et al., radiotherapy should be considered as a first-line treatment option for bicalutamide-induced gynaecomastia [48]. Radiotherapy reduces the incidence of gynaecomastia to a median of 23% with minor self-limiting skin reactions, according to Tyler Safran et al. [49]. Presently, there are no standardized trials comparing tamoxifen and radiotherapy.

4.7 Peyronie's Disease

Peyronie's disease (PD) is a connective tissue disorder of the penile tunica albuginea that occurs in 3–11% of men between the ages of 40 and

70 years. It is characterized by scarring and fibrotic plaques that are assumed to be due to micro trauma during sexual intercourse. The plaques may lead to induration, deviation, pain during sexual intercourse, erectile dysfunction and in turn psychological issues.

Treatment of PD is symptom and severity-directed. In 13% of the cases, PD regresses spontaneously by 18–24 months; hence, reassurance alone is appropriate for patients who have minimal pain/deformity [50, 51]**.

Treatment varies from oral antioxidants (vitamin E), pentoxifylline, analgesics, to intralesional injection of collagenase clostridium histolyticum/interferon alfa-2b/ verapamil/corticosteroids injections and superficial radiotherapy for early PD. In advanced cases and in cases where the curvature interferes with sexual intercourse, surgery is preferred. Penile traction therapy and extracorporeal shockwave therapy are under trial.

Radiotherapy in the form of external photon/electron beam radiation/mold brachytherapy have proven to be an effective and well-tolerated option in early stages presenting with a soft, non-calcified plaque. Doses ranging from 2Gy single fraction to 20 Gy in 200 cGy per fraction. Irradiation using 50 kV superficial X-rays of photons to a total applied dose of 32 Gy in 24 weeks was also used. Bolus use is advised as the lesion is just underneath the skin, and volume consisting of target lesion with a 1 cm margin is irradiated with anterior posterior beams/with lateral opposed beams using an upright fixation technique. Patients must be counselled and protection of testis with lead shield covered with bolus is advised. No grade III adverse event or malignant transformation was observed at any time during treatment or in the follow-up period, even at higher dose range [50]**.

Pietsch et al., showed that 32 Gy in 8 fractions superficial X-ray produced substantial pain relief in 83% of patients, 47% had symptom regression, penile curvature was improved in 49% of patients [52].

4.8 Pigmented Villonodular Synovitis

Pigmented Villonodular Synovitis (PVNS) is a locally aggressive synovial disease presenting with expansion of the synovium, joint effusions, and bony erosions. Commonly affects the knee, hip, ankle joint between 30 and 40 years of age. It is caused by an overexpression of CSF-1 gene, leading to clusters of aberrant cells causing focal areas of soft tissue hyperplasia in the synovial cells lining the joints.

Treatment options available are observation, CSF-1 receptor antagonist (pexidartinib), partial/total synovectomy followed by external beam radiation, and total joint arthroplasty for advanced disease. Treatment depends on joint involved, completeness of resection and type of synovitis [53].

The main treatment is surgical removal of lining tissue, but recurs in 50% of cases post-total synovectomy. Hence, adjuvant irradiation is preferred and it reduces rate of recurrence to 10–20%. A complete resection is based on joint involved, and R0 resection is not possible in 73% of cases only. In such cases, adjuvant radiotherapy is considered, 6–8 weeks post-surgery, and it achieves local control around 95.1% [50]**.

Radiation is also used in recurrence post-surgical procedures as salvage therapy as RT reduces the proliferation of abnormal synovial cells and prevents destruction of the cartilage, bony and soft tissue structures of any affected joint.

Joint can be irradiated using external photon beams to a dose of 26–36 Gy in 2 Gy/ fraction, or 50 Gy in 25 fractions, with both schedules showing equal results. For complete coverage of risk regions, the entire synovial lining of the joint with a 1–2cms margin is irradiated. To achieve accurate delineation, CT and MRI-based planning is done. Intra-articular injection of radioactive isotopes, also known as radiosynoviorthesis, is also tried, but the cost of drug, availability, and need for invasive procedures to inject the drug into the joint space make it sparingly used.

The sequelae of radiation include Grade I dermatitis, joint effusion and minimal restriction of joint movement. No late toxicity or secondary malignancy has been recorded in irradiated patients [54].

4.9 Keloids

Keloid (Keloid scar/Keloid disorder) is characterized by excessive scar formation at the site of trauma. Following trauma, extra collagen deposition in a disorganized pattern causes cosmetic defects, and they differ from hypertrophic scars by their invasion to surrounding normal skin. The word is derived from Greek word 'chele' means 'crab claw', and the suffix -oid, meaning 'like'. In the recently released ICD-11 in 2018, it is grouped under 'fibromatoses and keloids'. Therefore, it is now labelled as a part of 'keloid disorder', different from older versions of 'keloid scar'. Sometimes they are associated with itching or pain, especially when situated in the exposed areas, add to the aesthetic and psychological outlook, making them seek treatment. It is commonly seen among Asians (15 times higher) and reported incidence ranges from 4.5% to 15%. Ladin et al. suggested that keloids may represent a type of incomplete malignancy that has undergone some, but not all tumorigenic changes. Genetic predisposition is considered an important factor for development of keloid. Ramakrishnan et al. described keloid after vaccination in twins [55].

Several treatment options are available; out of them, surgery is the primary modality of treatment, but is associated with a high recurrence rate of more than 50% which is reduced to 30–50% with intralesional corticosteroid injections and addition of immediate post-op radiation reduces the recurrence to 6–27% [56]. The recurrent keloids are always bigger than the prior ones and hence difficult to treat. Various other available treatments are continuous pressure after surgery, silicone gel, intralesional corticosteroid injections and retinoic acid, silastic sheet coverage, NdYaG laser, 5-fluorouracil, and radiation.

Radiation is reserved for adults, mainly to avoid growth sequelae in children. It is most useful for prevention of keloid formation, usually employed in combination with surgery. Both external radiations using superficial X-rays as well as electrons and brachytherapy have been used depending on the availability and the site of keloid. For extensive keloids when skin graft is used, the radiation should be delayed by about a week as the vascularization takes time, however if flaps are used and vascularity is not impaired, radiation should be started within 24 h with subsequent fractions on day 2 and 3 with a total dose of 15 Gy over 3 Fr. The surgery includes complete excision of keloid including healthy skin margin and the wound closed in two layers. Subcutaneous tissue to be closed using absorbable suture, over which a 6F flexible polyethylene brachy catheter could be placed. Skin is closed on top of the tube. The closed end of the tube is to be placed at least 5 mm beyond the wound margin to treat till the edge of the scar.

In a study from India, on 71 keloids from 50 patients, the use of perioperative Cobalt-based HDR brachytherapy of 15 Gy over 3 Fr, the recurrence at 5 months was seen in 2% of patients and only 10% of patients rated cosmesis as unacceptable [57].

In a recent report of efficacy and toxicity of hypo-fractionated radiotherapy (RT) alone in treatment-resistant symptomatic keloids, six out of 13 inoperable and non-responder patients were treated. A total dose of 37.5 Gy by external RT in five fractions was prescribed using 6-MeV electrons in 4 patients and 6-MV photons in 2 patients, and complete response was observed in all patients at sixth month. Only grade II dermatitis was noted in the second week [58]. The procedure of perioperative HDR brachytherapy is as shown in the picture Fig. 6 and Fig. 7.

4.10 Juvenile Nasopharyngeal Angiofibroma

Juvenile nasopharyngeal angiofibroma (JNA) is a benign, vascular and locally aggressive and arises from the posterolateral wall of the nasal cavity. It

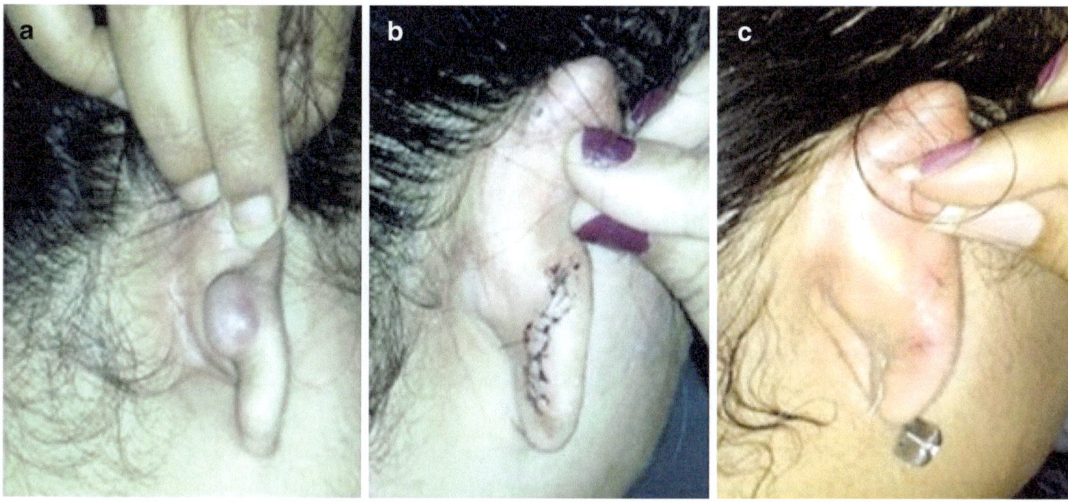

Fig. 6 (**a**) Keloid over ear lobule, (**b**) Immediate post-op and post-brachy and (**c**) Follow-up at 1 year

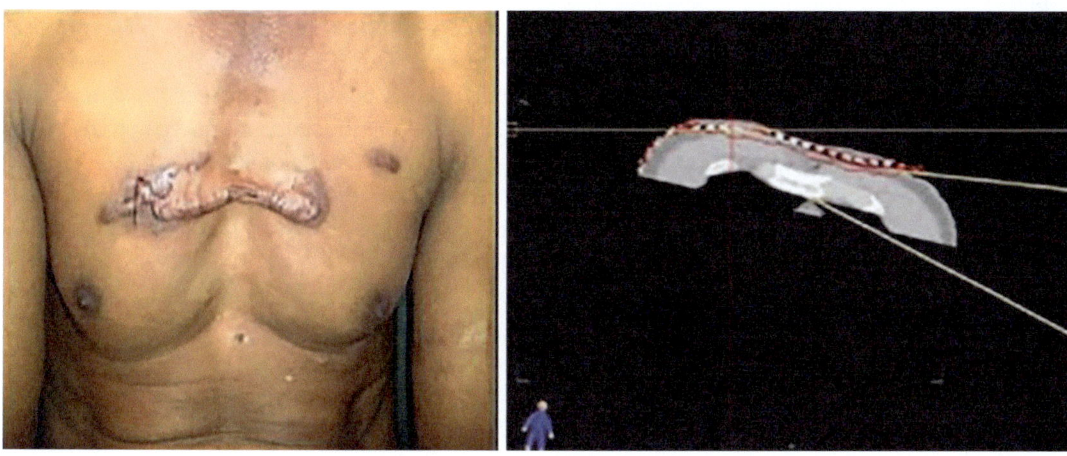

Fig. 7 Showing keloid over chest wall and axial cut end of brachytherapy plan, the red line showing the prescription isodose line

was first described by Chelius in 1847 as a 'fibrous nasal polyp, which commonly occurs in persons around the time of puberty'. The anatomical origin is believed to be from the pterygopalatine fossa and embryologically from a residual vascular plexus, a remnant of the involution of the first branchial arch artery. Also known as juvenile nasopharyngeal angioma, vascular fibroma, juvenile nasopharyngeal haemangiofibroma, juvenile fibroangioma and juvenile fibroma.

JNA, mostly seen in adolescent men and accounts for 0.05% of all head and neck tumours, with an incidence of 1in 150,000. Rarely seen in women and has a higher incidence in the Middle East and India compared to Europe [59]. The common presenting symptoms are nasal obstruction and epistaxis. As the invasion increases, symptoms may include facial numbness, headaches, visual changes and facial deformity. Biopsy to establish a histopathological diagnosis is avoided as it may result in massive bleeding. CT scan is the modality of choice to establish the diagnosis, which typically shows a soft tissue mass involving the bone near the sphenopalatine foramen and extending to the adjacent nasopharynx and pterygopalatine fossa. An MRI study reveals intralesional flow void and increased enhancement after contrast injection, which is suggestive of enlarged blood vessels. An MRI study can also help in detecting intracranial, dural and intracavernous extensions. Staging of the condition is based on the extent of the tumour expansion and intracranial extension. The most widely followed staging system is the one suggested by Radowski et al. in 1996 [60].

Surgery is the preferred treatment modality for JNA [61]. The aim of surgery is to perform a complete resection with minimal morbidity. Both conventional open surgery and endoscopic approaches are acceptable, with the latter being a reasonable option for a surgeon with the expertise to perform the same. Endoscopy can also be combined with trans nasal, trans facial and transcranial approaches. Preoperative embolization of the external carotid artery has been reported to reduce the intraoperative blood loss in patients undergoing endoscopic excision.

Radiotherapy is indicated only for advanced, incompletely resectable lesions and where resection will result in significant morbidity. This is especially true for lesions with significant intracranial extension and encasement of the internal carotid artery. Radiotherapy is usually delivered with IMRT at a dose of 36 Gy in 20 fractions at 1.8 Gy once daily, with a local control in 70.7% at 10 years [62]. Proton Beam therapy may also be used to create more conformal radiotherapy dose distributions. Late effects can include growth retardation, temporal lobe necrosis and the risk of sarcomatous transformation.

4.11 Haemangioma

Haemangiomas are benign vascular anomalies or tumours arising from proliferating endothelial cells of arteries/capillaries/veins. They are often present in childhood and common sites of occurrence are skin, vertebrae, brain, liver and choroidal layer of eye. Different types of haemangiomas are associated with different causes. For example, due to unidentified developmental error of the vascular system/after an injury/with pregnancy/due to genetic abnormalities (e.g., in von Hippel-Lindau disease).

Diagnosis is based on clinical history and physical examination for cutaneous lesions, while imaging with ultrasound or MRI is necessary for visceral haemangiomas. Imaging of local lesions with a screening abdominal ultrasound is recommended for children with five or more multifocal lesions because of an increased risk of concurrent liver haemangioma.

Haemangiomas with symptoms like ulceration, bleeding, vision disturbance, and functional limitations (breathing), disfiguring or associated with underlying syndromes (PHACE syndrome, LUMBAR syndrome) or concerning visceral involvement require intervention.

Treatment options available for haemangioma vary depending on the size, location and proximity to critical structures. The evidence of treatment is often based on retrospective case series. With radiation, the reduction in symptoms varies from 70 to 95% based on site.

In general, the medical treatments include: topical beta blockers, oral propranolol, steroid injections or direct intralesional steroid injections, trans pupillary thermotherapy (TTT), photodynamic therapy (PDT). Surgical resection and laser therapies or antiproliferative effects of radiotherapy may be necessary to optimize long-term outcomes [63].

Vertebral

- In aggressive vertebral haemangiomas with severe spinal cord compression or a vertebral canal encroachment ratio > 40% or with neurologic deterioration, surgery is the option of choice, followed by adjuvant radiotherapy. Radiotherapy is used as a definitive modality in all other cases.
- Radiation of 40 Gy/20 fractions or as hypofractionated RT 25–30Gy/5–6 fractions with RT 2 or 3 days per week; or 18Gy/1 fraction or using proton therapy 50Gy (RBE)/fraction, 25 fractions. Spinal cord received V14 Gy <0.03 cm3; V10 Gy, <0.35 cm3; V7 Gy < 1.2 cm3 [64]. There were no

treatment-related severe acute and late side effects [65].

Hepatic

- If it is a small and asymptomatic liver haemangioma, only periodical imaging is sufficient. Treatment when warranted, surgery is the first choice in resectable cases. Hepatic artery embolization. Radiation of 15 to 30 Gy/15–22 fractions is used in large and/or symptomatic unresectable haemangiomas that do not respond to medications like propranolol, steroids.
- Proton therapy of 28.6Gy (RBE) in 13 fractions has also shown reduction in size with only grade I (elevated AST, ALT) toxicities [66].

Choroidal

- Radiation therapy is recommended for choroidal haemangiomas that do not respond to other non-invasive therapies. It can be either given as photons 16–30 Gy/15 fractions or Gamma knife radiosurgery with 10–26 Gy/1 fraction or protons of 15–30 CGE in 4 fractions or Ruthenium-106/Cobalt-60/Palladium-103/Iodine-125 plaque brachytherapy 25–50 Gy in small non-juxta papillary lesions with extensive retinal detachment [67].

Cavernous

- Cavernous sinus haemangioma treatment of choice is surgery, and risk of worsening cranial neuropathies is still an obstacle for these patients. Due to which, radiotherapy is used either as definitive or in adjuvant setting after incomplete gross resection of tumour.

Patients can receive radiotherapy either as 50–54Gy/25–30 fractions or SRS to a dose of 10–17Gy/ 1 fraction for <5 cm tumour with >3 mm distance with chiasma. The QUANTEC initiative reported expected risks of RION ranging from 3% to 20% [68, 69].

4.12 Coronary Restenosis

The first percutaneous transluminal angioplasty (PTCA) for coronary artery stenosis was performed in 1964, followed by use of bare metal stents (BMS) in the 1980s [70]. This modality of interventional endovascular therapy has been used around the world since then. However, stents were found to have both early and late restenosis. Stent reocclusion is believed to occur due to both acute and late thrombosis as well as late vascular remodelling.

Endovascular brachytherapy (EBVT) was explored to prevent both in-stent thrombosis and restenosis. A randomized control trial by Teirstein et al. in 1997 presented evidence that EBVT could reduce coronary neointimal hyperplasia [71]. This study along with other studies resulted in the U.S. Food and Drug Administration approval in 2001. The availability of drug-eluting stents (DESs), i.e. stents which slowly release a drug, e.g. Paclitaxel, Sirolimus, Evorolimus or Zotarolimus, resulted in the decline of the use of EBVT. These reduced the restenosis rates as compared to EBVT [72]. There is evidence emerging on the role of EBVT for recurrent DES restenosis. The approved radiation sources for EVBT are Iridium 192 (Gamma Irradiation) and Strontium/Yttrium 90(Beta irradiation). The beta emitters are more universally accepted as shielding is not a concern and the delivery can occur during the catheterization.

4.13 Head and Neck Paragangliomas (Glomus Tumours)

Head and neck paragangliomas are benign neuroendocrine tumours arising from the parasympathetic ganglia. They are usually non-secretory in nature. They are highly vascular, slow-growing and originate from neural crest derivatives. Also known as glomus tumours and chemodectomas, which no longer feature in the WHO classification for head and neck tumours. The commonest locations are carotid body (48.1%), Glomus

Jugulare (24.1%), Glomus Tympanicum (11.1%) and Glomus Vagale (11.1%) [73].

A tertiary care centre in India reported the condition to be commoner in women (35:19) with almost half the patients being diagnosed in their thirties and forties. Though most are sporadic, familial predisposition is known to occur. Commonest symptoms at presentation depend on the location and these include diffuse neck swelling, pain, lower cranial nerve and ear discharge. Following a detailed history and physical examination, the mainstay of the diagnostic workup is imaging, which includes computed tomography (CT), Magnetic Resonance imaging (MRI) and Angiography. Staging is performed to determine the location, size and extent.

Surgery has been the mainstay of treatment for the Glomus tumours; however, due to associated neurological and vascular complications, radiation and active surveillance are other approaches adopted. The modality of treatment is adopted based on the location and the outcomes.

Surgery is preferred for Carotid Body tumours. Preoperative morbidity and mortality are stratified using the Shamblin grouping, which is based on the relationship of the tumour to the carotid vessels. These are classified from Type 1 to Type IIIb. This can predict the risk of neurological complications and stroke after surgery [74].

Radiation is preferred for Shamblin Type III and patients with medical comorbidities.

Radiation is preferred for the non-Carotid Body Paragangliomas, i.e. the Vagal and Jugulotympanic Paragangliomas, especially for older patients. Radiation doses can range from 45 to 60 Gy when fractionated in 1.8–2 Gy per fraction [74]. Radiosurgery is a viable alternative when feasible. Radiosurgery dose can range from 12 to 15 Gy for tumour control [75].

4.14 Dupuytrens Disease (DD)

DD comes under the group of fibroproliferative disorders affecting the hands and fingers. The actual cause is unknown; however, probable ones are prior trauma, diabetes mellitus, epilepsy and is usually seen in men beyond fifth decade.

There is a progressive proliferation of the palmar fascia resulting in thickening and shortening to form cords in the early stages, leading to contractures and flexion deformities of the digits in the later stages. This is marked by flexion deformity at metacarpophalangeal and proximal interphalangeal joints, usually of the index and little finger.

The progress of DD is uncertain and varies from patient to patient, so careful follow-up is important to identify patients who progress within a period of 6–12 months should be treated. When given after 24 months, radiation is less likely to help, and hence close monitoring of the symptoms is very essential. There is no cure, and hence the goal is to halt the progression, thereby improving or restoring the function. Various available options include aponeurotomy, fasciectomy, dermatofasciectomy and steroid/collagenase injection into the cords apart from radiation [76].

Radiation works best during early stages or when the degree of contracture is 30 degrees or less. The target volume should include a depth of 5–15 mm and a horizontal margin of 1–2 cm. Superficial X-rays of up to 150 kVp and 6 MeV electrons could be used. A dose of 30 Gy/10 fractions given in two sessions of 5 fractions each with a gap of 6 weeks between two sessions could be used. A dose of 21 Gy /7 fractions could be used on alternate days over 2 weeks [77, 78].

The National Institute for Health and Care Excellence (NICE) guidelines for DD are based on an RCT of 129 patients, including 198 hands. Regression of the disease was seen in 53–56% of patients, and in 37–38%, the disease was stable at 1 year. Progression was seen in 8% of cases, only out of which 3% and 6% needed surgery at 12 and 36 months, respectively. The subjective assessment was even better than the physician assessment, and both schedules of radiation were found to be similar to the observation by Kalila et al. [79]**. Dry desquamation was seen in 20% of patients and skin atrophy was seen in 3%. The NICE concludes that there is limited data for radiation in DD, but there are no serious concerns and hence radiation is safe and effective [77].

Since radiation is used in the initial stages, it is not only effective but economical in terms of maintaining the function of the digits and avoiding various surgical procedures [78].

4.15 Desmoid Tumours

Desmoid tumours (DT) are soft tissue tumours arising from any of the following, such as aponeurosis, muscles, fascia or connective tissues. They are benign in nature but are known for extensive local infiltration, causing disabling symptoms and disfigurement. DTs are either sporadic in occurrence or could be associated with familial adenomatous polyposis [80].

DTs are more common in women, in the age group of 35–40 years, can occur anywhere in the body and are slowly growing. The extremity lesions are diagnosed earlier compared to truncal lesions, and symptoms are due to their locally aggressive nature, such as bowel obstruction or ischemia in mesenteric location and pain in limb lesions. MRI helps in identifying their relationship to the surrounding structures for making treatment decisions.

Asymptomatic patients are best observed, and other modalities used are local therapy in terms of surgery with or without radiation and systemic therapy such as tamoxifen, NSAIDs, low-dose chemotherapy, Imatinib, Sorafenib, etc. Although surgery is the standard treatment, it should be considered only if it is unlikely to lead to severe morbidity because of its association with high rates of local recurrence and functional disability. The 10-year local control rates are in the range of 70% with combined modality of surgery and radiation as per Bishop et al. [81]

Patients who are younger than 30 years, extremity lesions with a size of more than 10 cm have worse outcomes, and various systemic therapies have been tried as first-line therapy [82]. Crago et al. observed that adjuvant radiation in this group is associated with a 15% decrease in the local recurrence rate [83]. A dose of 50.4 Gy in 28 fractions in the adjuvant setting is recommended which would go up to 60 Gy in 30 Fractions for definitive therapy. The choice of the technique depends on the site and relationship to critical structures.

5 Novel Indications

5.1 COVID-Associated Pneumonia

COVID-associated pneumonia has an early and late pulmonary phase. As the virus affects the alveoli between 11th and 14th day of infection, a lot of chemokines are released, which attract the inflammatory cells, such as effector T cells and macrophages from peripheral blood. These, in turn, release cytokines while killing the virus, causing a cytokine storm. Low-dose radiation acts at multiple levels. It suppresses cytokines TNF-α and IL-1, which are proinflammatory, enhances cytokine IL-10, which is anti-inflammatory and in addition reduces the expression of chemokine CCL20. A dose of less than 1 Gy has an anti-inflammatory effect through polarization of macrophages and also reduces oxidative burst activity [84]. In addition, it stimulates cell proliferation by NK cell activation, which in turn kills the cells which are already exposed to cytokines. All these effects are seen following exposure to low-dose radiation, which improves the symptoms when treated during the early pulmonary phase between 11 and 14 days of infection.

A pilot study by Sharma et al. was conducted on 10 patients using a single fraction of 70 cGy using parallel opposed fields with patient in supine position and hands raised above, and bilateral lungs were treated to include costophrenic angles and lung apices. Those who had a respiratory rate of more than 24 and a saturation of less than 94% with oxygen support, otherwise in a stable haemodynamic circulation, were treated, and 9/10 patients had complete recovery in 3–7 days. The only patient who succumbed was having uncontrolled hypertension and developed fungal infection [85].

5.2 Ventricular Tachycardia

With the advent of advanced imaging, the exact site of the pathology in various conditions could be identified, and when the routine treatment fails, radiation would be noninvasive and could be tried under experimental settings. In the last couple of years, Ventricular tachycardia has been treated with radiation. In all these conditions, stereotactic radiation is used, and hence, localized dose can be achieved with minimal side effects.

Ventricular tachycardia after myocardial infarction is due to the scarring, and standard therapy is use of drugs or catheter ablation, which has a 50% recurrence at 6 months [86]. The scar could be identified with contrast-enhanced MRI and electrocardiographic mapping. The rest of the procedure is similar to any SBRT of the thoracic region and a dose of 25 Gy in one fraction is used which resulted in reduction in VT events in all five patients [87].

5.3 Painful Osteoarthritis

The beneficial effects of low dose radiotherapy for painful osteoarthritis (OA) has drawn attention in recent years and is becoming a research topic for clinical immunologists. Several single arm and randomized clinical trials have shown that (a) the pain score is reduced, (b) need for NSAIDs and other drug prescriptions can be scaled down and (c) mobility improvements take place over time. The dose delivered is usually 3 Gy to 6 Gy at 0.5 Gy to 1.0 Gy per fraction, 2 to 3 fractions weekly, over 2 to 3 weeks. RT planning can be 3-D image based or 2-D. For hip, knee and ankle linear accelerator (4 MV to 10 MV photon energies) is suitable, whereas 100-200 KV orthovoltage machine is ideal for regions of fingers and small joints [88].

6 Summary

There are many benign lesions for which radiation forms one of the treatment modalities [89, 90], though, not frequently used, however can definitely be used when other therapies fail/not feasible. The details of these conditions are as shown in Table 2 and 3. Detailed counselling and taking informed consent is a mandatory requirement before starting the treatment.

Table 3 Summarizing the novel role of radiation for newer indications

Site	Condition	Radiation dose (Gy)
Skin	Chronic eczema	4–5
	Hidradenitis suppurativa	10
	Psoriatic nail bed	6–8
	Pilomatrix carcinoma	50
Eye	Dysthyroid ophthalmopathy	20
	Age-related macular degeneration	14.4–20
Glands	Sialorrhoea	10–20
	Lymphorrhea/ lymphatic fistula	3–10
Head and neck	Paragangliomas	12–60
CVS	Coronary stent restenosis	6–40
	Vascular stent restenosis	6–40
Bone and joints	Calcaneal spur	0.5/1/3/6
	Osteoarthritis	3–6
	Rheumatoid arthritis	2/20
	Arthritis tendonitis	2–12
	Aneurysmal bone cyst	30
	Ledderhose disease/ plantar fibromatosis	30
Functional disorders	Epilepsy	12–36
	Gorham stout	36–40

Precept Box

1. The treatment of Benign diseases varies widely across the globe.
2. Awareness of the role of radiation across other specialities is lacking.
3. It's important to discuss the pros and cons of radiation before treating with radiation in a multidisciplinary tumour board.

(continued)

4. Whenever possible, advanced techniques should be used to reduce the side effects of radiation.
5. Radiation has an important role in specific conditions such as HO, JNA, Keloid, LCH
6. Its role in most other lesions is subject to the response to other modalities of treatment.
7. Radiation for Haemangiomas is used in adjuvant more than definitive setting to a dose of 15–54 Gy.
8. Adjuvant radiation for Pigmented Villonodular Synovitis to a dose of 26–50 Gy/13–25 Fr after synovectomy reduces the recurrence by 10–20 %.
9. A single fraction of 2–20 Gy for early Peyronies disease offers good symptom relief.
10. There is an emergence of novel indications such as ventricular tachycardia, inflammatory lesions bone and soft tissue and epilepsy. It is effective and safe in the present era.

Multiple Choice Questions

1. Within how many hours radiation should be delivered to prevent HO post total hip arthroplasty?
   (a) 72 hours
   (b) 6 hours
   (c) 24 hours
   (d) 36 hours
2. Which of the following is true in case of HO?
   (a) Radiation should not be given due to the risk of secondary malignancies
   (b) HO prevention can be achieved at a total dose of 5 Gy of radiation.
   (c) Gastrointestinal toxicities are higher with NSAIDs as compared to radiation.
   (d) None of the above
3. In RT planning for HO, the superior radiation field border should be
   (a) 3 cm above the acetabulum
   (b) 3 cm below the lesser trochanter of the femoral head
   (c) 1.5 cm above the acetabulum
   (d) 1.5 cm below the lesser trochanter of the femoral head
4. What dose of Indomethacin is generally prescribed to a patient?
   (a) 75 mg/day up to 6 weeks
   (b) 45 mg/day up to 6 weeks
   (c) 75 mg/day up to 4 weeks
   (d) 45 mg/day up to 4 weeks
5. What is the risk of HO after radiation in comparison to selective NSAIDs in the study of Cai et al.?
   (a) 40%
   (b) 50%
   (c) 60%
   (d) 70%
6. Web-like ossification extending from dermis into the deeper layers is a characteristic of:
   (a) Fibrodysplasia Ossificans Progressiva
   (b) Progressive Osseous Heteroplasia
   (c) Both
   (d) None of the above
7. Gynaecomastia is commonly seen in prostate cancer patients treated with
   (a) Goserelin
   (b) Degarelix
   (c) Bicalutamide
   (d) Aberateron Acetate
8. First line of therapy in gynaecomastia observed during puberty is
   (a) Surgical excision
   (b) Radiotherapy
   (c) Reassurance
   (d) Tab Raloxifene
9. Gynaecomastia can be treated with
   (a) Tamoxifen 60mg OD for one year
   (b) Modified Radical Mastectomy
   (c) Radiotherapy of 12Gy/1Fr
   (d) Radiotherapy of 40Gy/15Fr
10. Which of the following is the true statement regarding Peyronie's disease
    (a) It is a connective tissue disorder of tunica intima
    (b) Peyronie's disease never regresses spontaneously

(c) Early disease can be treated with intralesional injection of hyaluronic acid.
(d) EBRT, electrons and Brachy are well-tolerated treatment options.

11. Treatment of Peyronie's disease is all of the following except
(a) Radiotherapy 20Gy/10Fr
(b) Radiotherapy 2Gy/1Fr
(c) Radiotherapy 32Gy/8Fr
(d) Intralesional injection of Clostridium perfringes

12. PVNS is commonly seen during
(a) 30–40 years
(b) 60–80 years
(c) 12–18 years
(d) 10–15 years

13. PVNS commonly affects the following joints except
(a) Knee
(b) Elbow
(c) Ankle
(d) Hip

14. Treatment options available for PVNS are all except
(a) Observation
(b) Pexidartinib
(c) Partial/total synovectomy and EBRT
(d) Intralesional injection of interferon

15. Radiation doses tried in PVNS are all of the following except
(a) 36Gy/18Fr
(b) 50Gy/25Fr
(c) 30Gy/15Fr
(d) 60Gy/30Fr

16. As compared to surgery alone, addition of postop radiation reduces the recurrence of keloids to
(a) Less than 5%
(b) 6–30 %
(c) more than 30%
(d) is the same as surgery.

17. Haemangiomas arise from proliferating______.
(a) Endothelial cells
(b) Epithelial cells
(c) Mesenchyme cells
(d) Stromal cells

18. What percentage of vertebral haemangioma patients achieve pain relief with radiation alone?
(a) 40.5%
(b) 57.6%
(c) 87.5%
(d) 99.1%

19. Hepatic haemangioma in the right lobe, 2 × 3 × 3 cms in an asymptomatic patient. What is the intervention of choice?
(a) Surgery
(b) Observation
(c) Surgery followed by radiation
(d) Beta blockers

20. Radiation (photons) dose in choroidal haemangioma is
(a) 10–20Gy
(b) 50–54Gy
(c) 16–30Gy
(d) 50–66Gy

21. What is the minimal distance to be present between optic chiasm and cavernous haemangioma lesion to follow a safe SRS?
(a) 6 mm
(b) 10 mm
(c) 2 mm
(d) 3 mm

Answer Key

1. (a)
2. (c)
3. (a)
4. (a)
5. (a)
6. (b)
7. (c)
8. (c)
9. (c)
10. (d)
11. (d)
12. (a)
13. (b)
14. (d)
15. (d)
16. (b)

17. (a)
18. (c)
19. (b)
20. (c)
21. (d)

References

1. Micke O, Oertel M, Muecke R, Eich HT, Kriz J. 130 Years of radiotherapy for non-malignant diseases: A historical overview. Semin Radiat Oncol. 2026;36:3–17. https://doi.org/10.1016/j.semradonc.2025.11.004.
2. Jan WHL, Paul VH, Jaap D. Indications and treatment schedules for irradiation of benign diseases: a survey. Radiother Oncol. 1998;48:249–57.
3. Fionda B, Lancellotta V, Casà C, Boldrini L, et al. Radiotherapy for benign disorders: current use in clinical practice. Eur Rev Med Pharmacol Sci. 2021;25:3440–3. **
4. Evans DGR, Birch JM, Ramsden RT, Sharif S, et al. Malignant transformation and new primary tumours after therapeutic radiation for benign disease: substantial risks in certain tumour prone syndromes. J Med Genet. 2006;43:289–94. https://doi.org/10.1136/jmg.2005.036319.
5. Trott KR, Kamprad F. Estimation of cancer risks from radiotherapy of benign diseases. Strahlenther Onkol. 2006;182(8):431–6.
6. Naraghi FF, DeCoster TA, Moneim MS, Miller RA, et al. Heterotopic ossification. Orthopedics. 1996;19:145–51.
7. Zhu Y, Zhang F, Chen W, Zhang Q, et al. Incidence and risk factors for heterotopic ossification after total hip arthroplasty: a meta-analysis. Arch Orthop Trauma Surg. 2015;135(9):1307.
8. Garland DE. A clinical perspective on common forms of acquired heterotopic ossification. Clin Orthop Relat Res. 1991;263:13.
9. Sumiyoshi K, Tsuneyoshi M, Enjoji M. Myositis ossificans: a clinicopathologic study of 21 cases. Pathol Int. 1985;35(5):1109.
10. Learning Radiology – Heterotopic, Ossification, HO [Internet]. [cited 2022 Jan 11]. Available from: http://learningradiology.com/archives2007/COW%20240--HO/hocorrect.html.
11. Myositis ossificans. | Radiology Case | Radiopaedia.org [Internet]. [cited 2022 Jan 11]. Available from:. https://radiopaedia.org/cases/myositis-ossificans-14
12. Lee A, Amin NP. Radiation therapy, heterotopic ossification prophylaxis. Stat Pearls; 2018.
13. McCarthy EF, Sundaram M. Heterotopic ossification: a review. Skeletal Radiol. 2005;34
14. Eekhoff EMW, Botman E, Coen Netelenbos J, de Graaf P, et al. [18F] NaF PET/CT scan as an early marker of heterotopic ossification in fibrodysplasia ossificans progressiva. Bone. 2018;109:143.
15. HeterotopicOssification–Physiopedia[Internet].[cited 2022 Jan 11]. Available from: https://www.physio--pedia.com/Heterotopic_Ossification#cite_ref-:0_1-3
16. Pavey GJ, Polfer EM, Nappo KE, Tintle SM, et al. What risk factors predict recurrence of heterotopic ossification after excision in combat-related amputations? Clin Orthop Relat Res. 2015;473(9):2814.
17. Banovac K, Gonzalez F, Wade N, Bowker JJ. Intravenous disodium etidronate therapy in spinal cord injury patients with heterotopic ossification. Paraplegia. 1993;31(10):660.
18. Macfarlane RJ, Ng BH, Gamie Z, el Masry MA, et al. Pharmacological treatment of heterotopic ossification following hip and acetabular surgery. Expert Opin Pharmacother. 2008;9(5):767.
19. Karunakar MA, Sen A, Bosse MJ, Sims SH, et al. Indometacin as prophylaxis for heterotopic ossification after the operative treatment of fractures of the acetabulum. J Bone Joint Surg Br. 2006;88(12):1613–7.
20. Baird EO, Kang QK. Prophylaxis of heterotopic ossification-an updated review. J Orthop Surg Res. 2009;4(1):12.
21. Fransen M, Anderson C, Douglas J, MacMahon S, et al. Safety and efficacy of routine postoperative ibuprofen for pain and disability related to ectopic bone formation after hip replacement surgery (HIPAID): randomised controlled trial. Br Med J. 2006;333(7567):519.
22. Pakos EE, Ioannidis JPA. Radiotherapy vs. nonsteroidal anti-inflammatory drugs for the prevention of heterotopic ossification after major hip procedures: a meta-analysis of randomized trials. Int J Radiat Oncol Biol Phys. 2004;60(3) *
23. Cai L, Wang Z, Luo X, She W, et al. Optimal strategies for the prevention of heterotopic ossification after total hip arthroplasty: a network meta-analysis. Int J Surg (London, England) [Internet]. 2019;62:74–85. [cited 2022 Jan 11]; Available from: https://pubmed.ncbi.nlm.nih.gov/30615954/. **
24. Milakovic M, Popovic M, Raman S, Tsao M, et al. Radiotherapy for the prophylaxis of heterotopic ossification: a systematic review and meta-analysis of randomized controlled trials. Radiother Oncol. 2015;116(1):4.
25. Griem ML. Prescribing, recording, and reporting photon beam therapy. Radiat Res. 1994;138(1):S1–4. **
26. Farris MK, Chowdhry VK, Lemke S, Kilpatrick M, et al. Osteosarcoma following single fraction radiation prophylaxis for heterotopic ossification. Radiat Oncol. 2012;7(1):140.
27. Seegenschmiedt MH, Keilholz L, Martus P, Goldmann A, et al. Prevention of heterotopic ossification about the hip: final results of two randomized trials in 410 patients using either preoperative or postoperative radiation therapy. Int J Radiat Oncol Biol Phys. 1997;39(1):161.

28. Gregoritch SJ, Chadha M, Pelligrini VD, Rubin P, et al. Randomized trial comparing preoperative versus postoperative irradiation for prevention of heterotopic ossification following prosthetic total hip replacement: preliminary results. Int J Radiat Oncol Biol Phys. 1994;30(1):55.
29. Sylvester JE, Greenberg P, Selch MT, Thomas BJ, et al. The use of postoperative irradiation for the prevention of heterotopic bone formation after total hip replacement. Int J Radiat Oncol Biol Phys. 1988;14(3):471.
30. Healy WL, Lo TC, DeSimone AA, Rask B, et al. Single-dose irradiation for the prevention of heterotopic ossification after total hip arthroplasty. A comparison of doses of five hundred and fifty and seven hundred centigray. J Bone Joint Surg Am. 1995;77(4):590–5.
31. Pellegrini VD, Konski AA, Gastel JA, Rubin P, et al. Prevention of heterotopic ossification with irradiation after total hip arthroplasty: radiation therapy with a single dose of eight hundred centigray administered to a limited field. J Bone Joint Surg Am. 1992;74(2):186–200.
32. Padgett DE, Holley KG, Cummings M, Rosenberg AG, et al. The efficacy of 500 centigray radiation in the prevention of heterotopic ossification after total hip arthroplasty: a prospective, randomized, pilot study. J Arthroplasty. 2003;18(6):677.
33. Konski A, Pellegrini V, Poulter C, Devanny J, et al. Randomized trial comparing single dose versus fractionated irradiation for prevention of heterotopic bone: a preliminary report. Int J Radiat Oncol Biol Phys. 1990;18(5):1139.
34. Carlos Rodriguez G, Carl EA. Langerhans cell histiocytosis. Blood. 2020;135(16):1319–31.
35. Carl EA, Miriam M, Kenneth LM. Langerhans-cell Histiocytosis. N Engl J Med. 2018;379(9):856–68. https://doi.org/10.1056/NEJMra1607548.
36. Riccardo H, Milen M, Itziar A, Eva S, et al. Langerhans cell Histiocytosis (LCH): guidelines for diagnosis, clinical work-up, and treatment for patients till the age of 18 years. Pediatr Blood Cancer. 2013;60:175–84. https://doi.org/10.1002/pbc.24367.
37. Jan K, Hans TE, Frank B, Reinhard H, et al. Radiotherapy in Langerhans cell histiocytosis—a rare indication in a rare disease. Radiat Oncol. 2013;8:233.
38. Michael G, Maurizio A, Diego C, Anthony C, et al. Management of adult patients with Langerhans cell histiocytosis: recommendations from an expert panel on behalf of euro-Histio-net. Orphanet J Rare Dis. 2013;8:72.
39. Kakarla S. Imaging approach to unifocal sclerotic bone lesions—a pictorial essay. J Med Sci Res. 2020;8(2):71–81. https://doi.org/10.17727/JMSR.2020/8-10.
40. Bartalena L, Baldeschi L, Dickinson A, Eckstein A, et al. European Group on Graves' Orbitopathy (EUGOGO) consensus statement of the European Group on Graves' orbitopathy (EUGOGO) on management of GO. Eur J Endocrinol. 2008;158:273–85.
41. Pradhan A, Ganguly A, Naik MN, Nair AG, et al. Thyroid eye disease survey: an anonymous web-based survey in the Indian subcontinent. Indian J Ophthalmol. 2020;68(8):1609–14. https://doi.org/10.4103/ijo.IJO_1918_19.
42. Viani GA, Boin AC, De Fendi LI, Fonseca EC, et al. Radiation therapy for graves' ophthalmopathy: a systematic review and meta-analysis of randomized controlled trials. Arq Bras Oftalmol. 2012;75(5):324–32. https://doi.org/10.1590/s0004-27492012000500006.
43. Li YJ, Luo Y, He WM, Li P, et al. Clinical outcomes of graves' ophthalmopathy treated with intensity modulated radiation therapy. Radiat Oncol. 2017;12(1):171. https://doi.org/10.1186/s13014-017-0908-7.
44. Usha RK, Hadi K, William BS, Akash DS. Spectrum of orbital disease in South India: an Aravind study of 6328 consecutive patients. Ophthalmic Plast Reconstr Surg. 2010;26(5):315–22.
45. Matthiesen C, Bogardus C Jr, Thompson JS, Farris B, et al. The efficacy of radiotherapy in the treatment of orbital pseudotumor. Int J Radiat Oncol Biol Phys. 2011;79(5):1496–502. https://doi.org/10.1016/j.ijrobp.2009.12.071.
46. Sánchez-Thorin JC, Rocha G, Yelin JB. Meta-analysis on the recurrence rates after bare sclera resection with and without mitomycin C use and conjunctival autograft placement in surgery for primary pterygium. Br J Ophthalmol. 1998;82(6):661–5. https://doi.org/10.1136/bjo.82.6.661.
47. Zeng W, Liu Z, Dai H, Yan M, et al. Anti-fibrotic, anti-VEGF or radiotherapy treatments as adjuvants for pterygium excision: a systematic review and network meta-analysis. BMC Ophthalmol. 2017;17(1):211. https://doi.org/10.1186/s12886-017-0601-5.
48. Tunio MA, Al-Asiri M, Al-Amro A, Bayoumi Y, et al. Optimal prophylactic and definitive therapy for bicalutamide-induced gynecomastia: results of a meta-analysis. Curr Oncol. 2012;19(4):e280–8. https://doi.org/10.3747/co.19.993.
49. Safran T, Abi-Rafeh J, Alabdulkarim A, Roberge D, et al. Radiotherapy for prevention or management of gynecomastia recurrence: future role for general gynecomastia patients in plastic surgery given current role in management of high-risk prostate cancer patients on anti-androgenic therapy. J Plast Reconstr Aesthet Surg. 2021;74(11):3128–40. https://doi.org/10.1016/j.bjps.2021.03.098.
50. Seegenschmiedt MH, Micke O, Muecke R. Radiotherapy for non-malignant disorders: state of the art and update of the evidence-based practice guidelines. Br J Radiol. 2015;88:20150080. **
51. Eng TY, Abugideiri M, Chen TW, Madden N, et al. Radiation therapy for benign disease: keloids, macular degeneration, orbital pseudotumor, pterygium, peyronie disease, trigeminal neuralgia. Hematol Oncol Clin North Am. 2020;34(1):229–51. https://doi.org/10.1016/j.hoc.2019.09.006. Epub 2019 Oct 31. **
52. Pietsch G, Anzeneder T, Bruckbauer H, Zirbs M, et al. Superficial radiation therapy in peyronie's disease:

an effective and well-tolerated therapy. Adv Radiat Oncol. 2018;3(4):548–51. https://doi.org/10.1016/j.adro.2018.07.009.
53. Kodiyan J, Zlotecki RA, Scarborough M, Reith, et al. The role of radiotherapy in the treatment of pigmented Villonodular synovitis. Hong Kong J Radiol. 2017;20:47–52. https://doi.org/10.12809/hkjr1715385.
54. Lin CS, Kang YM, Lan KL, Wang LW, et al. Treatment and outcome of tenosynovial giant cell tumor/ pigmented villonodular synovitis patients receiving radiotherapy in Taiwan: a single-center experience. Ther Radiol Oncol. 2020;4:14.
55. Mathangi RK, Pothan TK, Sundararajan CR. Study of 1,000 patients with keloids in South India. Plast Reconstr Surg. 1974;53(3):276–80.
56. Ilias GP, Kheeldass J, Eva MR, Thomas Z, et al. Keloid treatment: what about adjuvant radiotherapy? Clin Cosmet Investig Dermatol. 2019;12:295–301. https://doi.org/10.2147/CCID.S202884.
57. Kalapurmat NM, Mysore SV, Ram charith A, Keerthi K, et al. Efficacy of surgical excision and adjuvant high-dose rate brachytherapy in treatment of keloid: our experience. J Cutan Aesthet Surg. 2021;14(3):337–43. https://doi.org/10.4103/JCAS.JCAS_120_16.
58. Yuce Sari S, Yilmaz MT, Yazici G, Uzun H, et al. A hesitated approach: primary radiotherapy for keloids-a case series. Strahlenther Onkol. 2021;197:909–15.
59. Tiwari PK, Teron P, Saikia N, Saikia HP, et al. Juvenile nasopharyngeal Angiofibroma: a rise in incidence. Indian J Otolaryngol Head Neck Surg. 2016;68(2):141–8. https://doi.org/10.1007/s12070-015-0898-4.
60. Marshall AH, Bradley PJ. Management dilemmas in the treatment and follow-up of advanced juvenile nasopharyngeal Angiofibroma. ORL J Otorhinolaryngol Relat Spec. 2006;68:273–8.
61. Mistry RC, Qureshi SS, Gupta S, Gupta S. Juvenile nasopharyngeal angiofibroma: a single institution study. Indian J Cancer. 2005;42:35–9.
62. Mallick S, Benson R, Bhasker S, Mohanti BK. Long-term treatment outcomes of juvenile nasopharyngeal angiofibroma treated with radiotherapy. Acta Otorhinolaryngol Ital. 2015 Apr;35(2):75–9.
63. DeHart A, Richter G. Hemangioma: recent Advances. F1000Res. 2019;8:F1000 Faculty Rev-1926. Published 2019 Nov 18. https://doi.org/10.12688/f1000research.20152.1.
64. Conti A, Starnoni D, Barges-Coll J, Papadimitriou K, et al. Radiosurgery for benign vertebral body hemangiomas of the spine: a systematic review and meta-analysis. World Neurosurg. 2022;164:97–105. ISSN 1878-875.
65. Wang B, Meng N, Zhuang H, Han S, et al. The role of radiotherapy and surgery in the management of aggressive vertebral hemangioma: a retrospective study of 20 patients. Med Sci Monit. 2018;24:6840–50. Published 2018 Sep 27. https://doi.org/10.12659/MSM.910439.
66. Biswal BM, Sandhu M, Lal P, Bal CS. Role of radiotherapy in cavernous hemangioma liver. Indian J Gastroenterol. 1995;14(3):95–8.
67. Turaka K, Turaka A, Koneru BN. Role of radiation therapy for choroidal hemangioma: a brief review. J Clin Res Ophthalmol. 2016;3(1):018–22. https://doi.org/10.17352/2455-1414.000030.
68. Park S, Yoon SM, Lee S, Park JH, et al. Role of fractionated radiotherapy in patients with hemangioma of the cavernous sinus. Radiat Oncol J. 2017;35(3):268–73. https://doi.org/10.3857/roj.2017.00199.
69. Wang X, Mei G, Liu X, Dai J, et al. The role of stereotactic radiosurgery in cavernous sinus hemangiomas: a systematic review and meta-analysis. J Neuro-Oncol. 2012;107:239–45.
70. Scott NA. Restenosis following implantation of bare metal coronary stents: pathophysiology and pathways involved in the vascular response to injury. Adv Drug Deliv Rev. 2006;58(3):358–76. https://doi.org/10.1016/j.addr.2006.01.015.
71. Teirstein PS, Massullo V, Jani S, Popma JJ, et al. Three-year clinical and angiographic follow-up after intracoronary radiation: results of a randomized clinical trial. Circulation. 2000;101(4):360–5.
72. Vivek R, Stanley GR. Coronary restenosis: a review of mechanisms and management. Am J Med. 2003;115(7):547–53.
73. N'da G, Lachgar A, Houessou O, Majjaoui S, et al. Radiation therapy of head and neck Paragangliomas: experience from radiotherapy department at the National Institute of Oncology in Rabat (Morocco). J Cancer Ther. 2021;12:268–78. https://doi.org/10.4236/jct.2021.125025.
74. Erdem H. Does Shamblin classification affect the clinical outcomes following carotid body tumor excision? Cardiovasc Surg Int. 2021;8(2):91–7.
75. Larner JM, Hahn SS, Spaulding CA, Constable WC. Glomus Jugulare tumors. Long term control by radiation therapy. Cancer. 1992;69:1813–7.
76. Chelsea B, Philip B, Nicholas I. Dupuytren contractures: an update of recent literature. J Hand Surg Am. 2021;46(10):896–906.
77. Radiation therapy for early Dupuytren's disease (IPG573). National Institute for Health and Care Excellence (NICE) at https://www.nice.org.uk/ **
78. Eberlein B, Biedermann T. To remember: radiotherapy—a successful treatment for early Dupuytren's disease. J Eur Acad Dermatol Venereol. 2016;30(10):1694–9. https://doi.org/10.1111/jdv.13773.
79. Kalila S, Victoria H, Christine N, Dimitri A, et al. Secondary effects of radiation therapy to the hand for benign conditions. Hand. 2020;15(3):341–7.
80. Maggie YZ, Nam QB, Gregory WC, Pejman G, et al. Current management and recent progress in desmoid tumors. Cancer Treat Res Commun. 2022;31:100562.
81. Bishop AJ, Zarzour MA, Ratan R, Torres KE, et al. Long-term outcomes for patients with Desmoid fibromatosis treated with radiation therapy: a 10-year update and re-evaluation of the role of

radiation therapy for younger patients. Int J Radiat Oncol*Biol*Phys. 2019;103(5):1167–74.
82. Bishop AJ, Landry JP, Roland CL, Ratan R, et al. Certain risk factors for patients with desmoid tumors warrant reconsideration of local therapy strategies. Cancer. 2020;126(14):3265–73.
83. Crago AM, Denton B, Salas S, Dufresne A, et al. A prognostic nomogram for prediction of recurrence in desmoid fibromatosis. Ann Surg. 2013 Aug;258(2):347–53.
84. Kumar R, Haresh KP, Sharma DN, Gupta A, et al. Low-dose radiotherapy for COVID 19: a radio immunological perspective. J Can Res Ther. 2021;17:295–302.
85. Sharma DN, Guleria R, Wig N, Mohan A, et al. Low-dose radiation therapy for COVID-19 pneumonia: a pilot study. Br J Radiol. 2021;94:20210187.
86. Spartalis M, Spartalis E, Tzatzaki E, Tsilimigras DI, et al. Novel approaches for the treatment of ventricular tachycardia. World J Cardiol. 2018;10(7):52–9.
87. Cuculich PS, Schill MR, Kashani R, Mutic S, et al. Noninvasive cardiac radiation for ablation of ventricular tachycardia. N Engl J Med. 2017;377:2325–36.
88. Schlamann A, Yu JB, Rühle A. Low-Dose radiotherapy for osteoarthritis: Current evidence, practical recommendations and future perspectives. Semin Radiat Oncol. 2026;36:39–47. https://doi.org/10.1016/j.semradonc.2025.07.001.
89. McKeown SR, Hatfield P, Prestwich RJ, Shaffer RE, et al. Radiotherapy for benign disease; assessing the risk of radiation-induced cancer following exposure to intermediate dose radiation. Br J Radiol. 2015;88(1056):20150405. https://doi.org/10.1259/bjr.20150405. *
90. Shin HP, Jeong Eun L. Radiotherapy, a new treatment option for non-malignant disorders: radiobiological mechanisms, clinical applications, and radiation. Risk J Rheum Dis. 2017;24(2):74–84.

Online Links

https://www.sciencedirect.com/journal/seminars-in-radiation-oncology/vol/36/suppl/C (RT in Benign Diseases)

https://www.youtube.com/watch?v=1MtkfaCItWY (RT in benign disease)

https://www.youtube.com/watch?v=7aetegmXsWE (RT in benign disease)

https://www.youtube.com/watch?v=bswtDa82Mng (RT in benign skin diseases)

Management of Cancers in Geriatric Population

Punita Lal, Rohini Khurana, and Avinash Poojari

1 Introduction

The increasing global population and life expectancy show the epidemiological projection of 26 million new cancer cases and 17 million associated deaths by the year 2030. The geriatric population will bear a disproportionate global cancer burden, nearly an estimated 50% of all cancer cases. Increasing cancer incidence will occur primarily in low- and medium-income countries (LMIC). Countries, such as China, India, and Bangladesh, are projected to have the highest proportion of geriatric cancer patients and mortality due to certain cancers [1].

The criteria for grouping an individual into elderly age are not clearly defined. It can be an individual above 60 years or 65 years of age [2]. In the modern world, there has been a gradual increase in life expectancy at birth in the world population over the last 60 years. Currently, the overall life expectancy at birth for the world population is 73.2 years, whereas it is 70.42 years in India. In the past decades, there has been a shift in the distribution of a country's population towards older ages, classically known as 'population aging'. With increasing life expectancy and population aging, the likelihood of having age-related medical illness in the geriatric population is expected to increase significantly. Common conditions in the older population include cognitive dysfunction, hearing impairment, cataracts, refractive errors, falls, arthritis, dementia, depression, etc. Hence, the United Nations (UN) General Assembly declared 2021–2030 as the UN Decade of Healthy Aging to improve the lives of older people. Of the overall world's population diagnosed with new cancers, elderly patients (≥65 years) account for more than half the numbers. Despite recent advances in the management of cancer patients, the geriatric age group is often treated with non-standard treatment modalities, often due to multiple factors and associated co-morbidities. Another reason for a lack of standardized treatment for this subset of the population could be due to under representation of these age groups in most of the randomized clinical trials. The geriatric population with cancers, especially with other co-morbidities or non-cancer illnesses, poses a

P. Lal (✉)
Department of Radiotherapy, Sanjay Gandhi Postgraduate Institute of Medical Sciences, Lucknow, India
e-mail: punitalal11@gmail.com

R. Khurana
Department of Radiation Oncology, Dr Ram Manohar Lohia Institute of Medical Sciences, Lucknow, India

A. Poojari
Department of Radiation Oncology, Dr Ram Manohar Lohia Institute of Medical Sciences, Lucknow, India

Department of Radiation Oncology, Vishwabharati Medical College and General Hospital, Kurnool, Andhra Pradesh, India

B. K. Mohanti et al. (eds.), *Radiation Oncology – Principles, Precepts and Practice*,
https://doi.org/10.1007/978-981-95-5171-2_20

significant problem for physicians in deciding the intent of therapy. A significant proportion of patients are being treated with palliative intent treatment rather than definitive intent treatment. Radiotherapy (RT) and surgery are local therapies, whereas chemotherapy, targeted therapy, and immunotherapy are systemic therapies. Among them, RT is a non-invasive local/locoregional therapy. Apart from hospital-based treatment, psychological and social support by caretakers plays a key role in the optimal management of these patients. The current healthcare systems in most parts of the world are poorly prepared to address all the needs of this population due to the altered physiological and functional status of these patients as compared to the non-geriatric population. Beyond 2030, clinical services and research with a focus on geriatric cancers will become a major healthcare parameter for quality cancer management in LMIC.

2 Epidemiology

2.1 Incidence Data

Patients aged ≥65 years comprise more than 50% of the overall cancer burden in the world's population, as per recent global statistical data. The incidence of all cancer rates in age groups more than 65 years was found to be higher in North America and European continents, whereas it was lowest in African countries. Cancers with more than 50% incidence rates in these age groups include cancers arising from the prostate, urinary bladder, pancreas, lung, gall bladder, colorectal, vulva, stomach, esophagus, multiple myeloma, and melanoma of the skin. In India, the cancer incidences in these age groups accounting for more than 50% were of prostate, vulval, vaginal, and bladder cancers [3].

2.2 Mortality Data

Around 60% of deaths due to cancer occurred in this age group of cases worldwide, as compared to 40% in the age group less than 65 years. Among them, prostate cancer is the leading cause of death in this age group, approximately reaching 90%. But in India, mortality rates in this age group are relatively low (38%) as compared to the age group less than 65 years. Nevertheless, prostate cancer remains the leading cause of death in this age group in India.

3 Survival of Cancer Patients Above 65 Years of Age

The 5-year relative survival rate has not significantly changed in the geriatric population in the last 10 years, as per SEER statistics (Fig. 1).

The recent 5-year survival rates were 60% for age ≥65 years as compared to 71% and 82% for ages between 50–65 years and <50 years, respectively.

Physiology and Consequences of Aging With increasing chronological age, various physiological processes occur in almost all the systems of the body, including neurological, cardiovascular, respiratory, gastro-intestinal, renal, blood, endocrine, and musculoskeletal systems. All these aging-related physiological changes may lead to a variety of health-related issues from the accumulation of these damages [4]. A brief summary of the various aging-related changes occurring in various systems of the body is shown in Table 1. The aging process may lead to decreased cardiac output, hypertension, and coronary artery disease (CAD). Other common health conditions related to physiological aging include malnutrition, senile cataract, hearing impairment, cognitive decline, anxiety, depression, risk of falls, renal insufficiency, etc. Also, old age is often associated with comorbidities like diabetes, hypertension, chronic lung disease, chronic kidney disease, and stroke. All these factors may affect potential oncological treatment decisions, prognosis, and quality of life (Table 1).

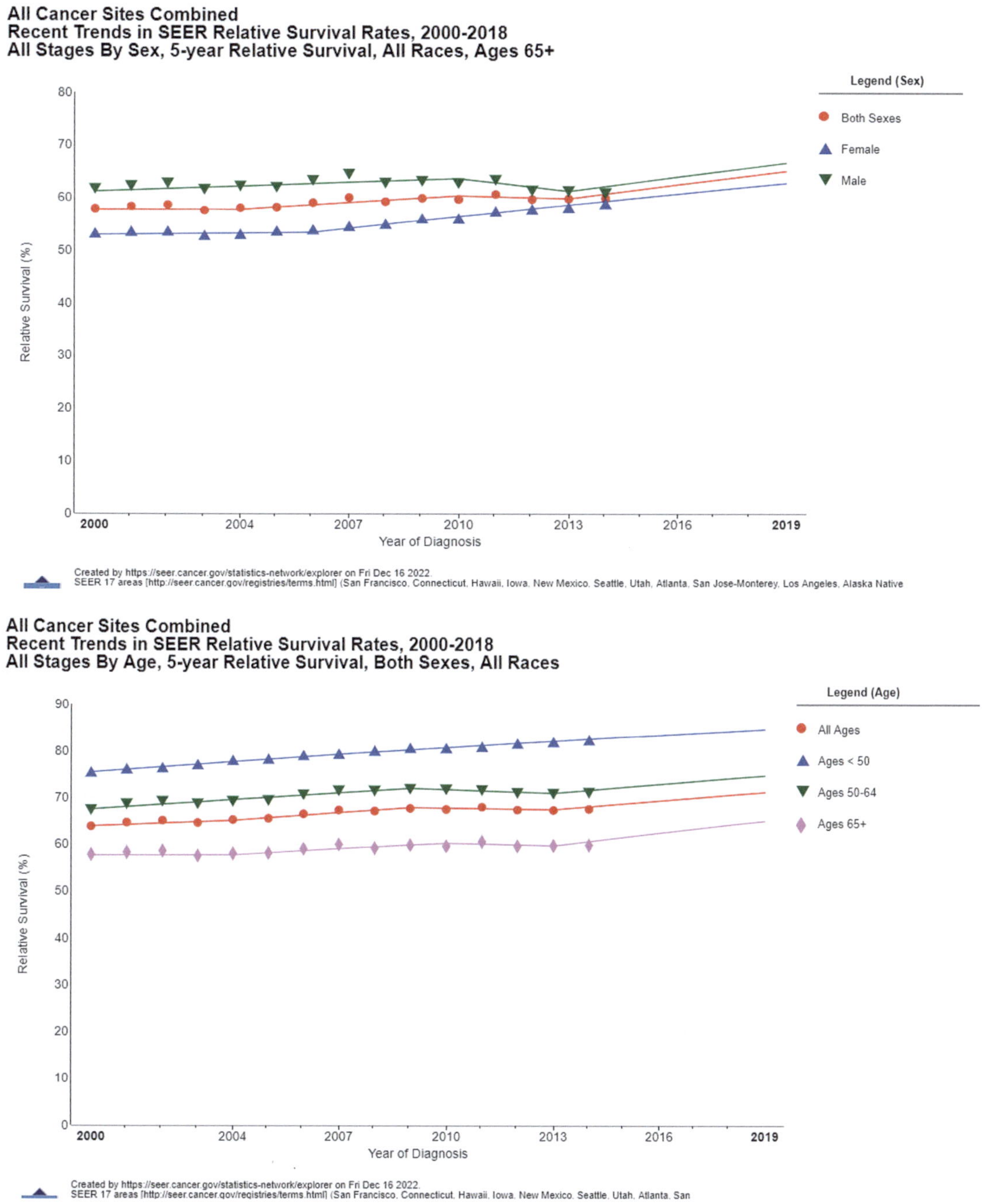

Fig. 1 Recent trends in the 5-year Relative Survival Rates from 2000 to 2018 for elderly patients aged 65 years and above. Top chart displays all cancer sites gender-wise, and bottom chart shows all cancer sites as per different age groups. (Surveillance, Epidemiology, End Results (SEER) Program, 2022).

Table 1 Physiologic changes in various systems of the body with aging and its consequences

S. No.	System	Structural changes	Functional Changes	Metabolic Changes	Clinical Consequences
1	Nervous System	Neuronal cell death, degeneration of myelinated axons, changes in neuronal dendrites and/or synapses resulting in a decrease in loss of grey and white matter. Decreased density of capillaries with/without micro-vessel deformities, cerebral arteritis/atherosclerosis	Increased permeability of the blood-brain barrier	Gradual decrease in dopamine levels, serotonin, and brain neurotrophic factors. Gradual increase in monoamine oxidase levels.	Neuro-cognitive disorders like dementia, Alzheimer's disease, etc.
2	Cardio-vascular system	Gradual decrease in elastin production within the blood vessel system and gradual replacement with less flexible collagen proteins, leading to gradual stiffening of connective tissue within the arteries, veins, and myocardium. Myocyte hypertrophy occurs secondary to arterial stiffening.	Gradual increase in sympathetic nervous system activity resulting in increased release of circulating nor-epinephrine, altered production of nitric oxide from age-related endothelial dysfunction, decreased β-receptor stimulation, impaired baro-receptor function, low vagal tone, and reduced oxygen extraction.		High blood pressures with normal heart rates and ejection fractions but lower left ventricular end-diastolic volumes, stroke volumes, and cardiac outputs, leading to increased incidence of coronary artery diseases.

(continued)

Table 1 (continued)

S. No.	System	Structural changes	Functional Changes	Metabolic Changes	Clinical Consequences
3	Respiratory system	Lung parenchymal changes like decreased elastic recoil, decreased alveolar surface area, and premature closure of smaller airways, leading to atelectasis. Chest wall changes, like reduction in the height of thoracic vertebrae, reduction in muscles mass of respiratory muscles, costo-chondral, and costo-vertebral joint changes, result in decreased compliance of the chest wall. Reduced muscular pharyngeal support in the upper airways.	Altered ventilation/ perfusion ratio affecting gaseous exchange, leading to impaired arterial blood oxygenation.		Reduced VC, low FEV1/FVC ratio, diminished coughing and swallowing mechanisms leading to high vulnerability for infection and aspiration.
4	Gastrointestinal system	Reduction in liver volume due to decreased number of hepatocytes, loss of surface endoplasmic reticulum	Decreased amplitude of esophageal contractions, decreased frequency of peristaltic waves with a standard swallow, and prolonged gastric emptying.	Decreased gastric acid secretion, decreased metabolic activity of hepatic microsomes.	High risk of aspiration during anesthesia or in the post-operative period due to decreased GI contractions, increased toxicity of drugs due to poor metabolism within the liver.
5	Renal and volume regulatory system	Renal arterial changes, like atherosclerosis, medial and intimal thickening, leading to diminished renal blood flow, decreased auto-regulation of volume status. Tubulo-interstitial changes like infarction, scarring, and fibrosis.	Decreased renal plasma flow and tubular functions.	Altered renin-angiotensin-aldosterone, resulting in decreased plasma renin activity.	Decreased GFR and creatinine clearance rates, decreased clearance of pharmacological drugs leading to excess adverse effects, electrolyte disturbances, increased incidences of CKD, and ESRD.
6	Musculoskeletal system	Muscles: mitochondrial dysfunction, primary reduction of muscle mass with age, secondarily due to decreased sex hormones. Bone: decreased bone mass, increased bone turnover, increased osteoclastic, and decreased osteoblastic activities. Cartilage: thickness and tensile strength, decreased chondrocyte activity, and proteoglycan production. Intervertebral disc: breakdown of ECM, increased cell senescence and death, failure to bear weight.			Sarcopenia, Osteoporosis, and postural abnormalities.

(continued)

Table 1 (continued)

S. No.	System	Structural changes	Functional Changes	Metabolic Changes	Clinical Consequences
7	Blood	Decrease in bone marrow cellularity due to reduced numbers of HSCs, a finite number of cell divisions, inability to sufficiently mobilize progenitor cells, lack of hormonal stimulation, or reduced response to hormonal stimulation.			Decreased peripheral blood counts and increased morbidity.

Table 2 Geriatric assessment and relevant tools

Assessment	Tools and procedures
ADL (Activities of daily living)	Katz index, Barthel index
Physical Performance	Short Physical Performance Battery
Cognition	Mini-Mental State Examination, Montreal Cognitive Assessment, Mini-Cog
Depressive symptoms	Geriatric Depression Scale (GDS), Cornell Scale for Depression
Frailty	Clinical Frailty Scale (CFS), Frailty index
Nutrition	Mini-Nutritional Assessment- MNA
Quality of Life (QoL)	Audit of Diabetes Dependent Quality of Life Senior—ADDQoL Senior; SF-36 questionnaire; Older people quality of life questionnaire (OPQOL -35)
Cardiovascular risk assessment	Globorisk score, Atherosclerotic cardiovascular disease (ASCVD) risk calculator. Available at: https://www.globorisk.org/
Comprehensive Geriatric Assessment (CGA)	A multidimensional holistic assessment of an older person, which considers health and wellbeing and formulates a plan to address issues that are of concern to the older person (and their family caregivers). Available at: https://www.cgakit.com/cga

4 Pre-treatment Geriatric Assessment

Older adults with cancer represent a complex patient population, as chronologic age does not necessarily reflect physiologic age. Oncological assessments, throughout the world, are not tailored to the specific needs of the geriatric population, and often physical, social, and cognitive problems are not identified before treatment. There is limited utility of geriatric assessment tools for older adults in oncological decision-making. Hence, geriatric assessment (GA) in older patients with cancer is recommended for a comprehensive cancer care including: (a) identification of undetected diseases and risks for which targeted interventions can be used, (b) to predict the severity of cancer-directed therapy (CDT)-related toxicities, and (c) for better estimation of life expectancy in the context of pre-existing co-morbidities and general health versus severity of the diagnosed cancer. Elderly cancer patients with indications for radiotherapy and chemotherapy will require specific approaches to pre-treatment assessment to predict vulnerabilities and outcomes [5, 6].

GA requires a set of tools to assess a variety of domains that commonly affect older adults, including physical function (Instrumental Activity of Daily Living-IADL), comorbidities (History, Cumulative Illness Rating Score-Geriatrics), nutrition status, cognition (Mini-Cog), and depression (Geriatric Depression Scale-15 item) to guide the oncologist for an optimal cancer treatment selection. As per the statement of Cancer and Aging Research Group (CARG), "A geriatric assessment is utilized to capture information about a patient's medical history as well as functional, cognitive, and psychosocial status, which can then be used by treating physicians to identify the most vulnerable patients (for example, those at high risk for chemotherapy toxicity). The domains that are assessed include functional status, comorbidities, medications, nutritional status, cognitive function, and psychosocial status" [7].

The available scales/tools that can be used for the elderly cancer patients are outlined in Table 2 and Fig. 2.

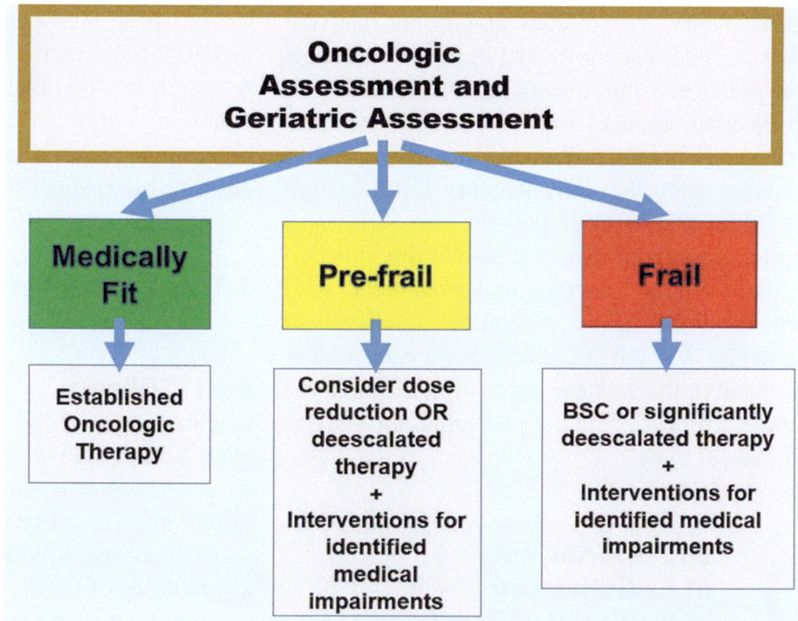

Fig. 2 Oncologic and geriatric assessment. BSC = Best supportive care

A systematic review suggests the beneficial effect of GA on treatment decision-making in older patients with cancer. In this analysis of 65 studies, the oncologic treatment plan was altered in a median of 31% of patients (range 7–56%), with the highest change rates in studies using a multidisciplinary team evaluation [8]. A geriatric assessment can change oncologic treatment plans, lead to non-oncologic interventions, and improve communication about care planning and aging-related issues. More importantly, elderly cancer patients who undergo geriatric assessment before CDT and accordingly chosen for cancer modalities and systemic therapy regimens in an optimized manner, in those the treatment-related toxicities and cancer care costs are much lower. Hence, oncologists and cancer centres should have in place the guidelines for GA, simultaneous with cancer diagnosis for the elderly patients.

5 Under-Representation of These Age Groups in RCTs and Lack of Standard of Care in the Elderly

Cancer is a disease of aging, and as the world's population ages, the number of older persons with cancer is increasing and will make up a growing share of the oncology population in virtually every country. Despite this, older patients are vastly underrepresented in clinical trials that set the standards for the efficacy and safety of cancer treatments [9]. Only 24% of participants in trials registered with the US Food and Drug Administration (FDA) are aged ≥70 years, and <10% of patients in this age group participate in National Cancer Institute (NCI)-sponsored clinical trials. Even when elderly populations are enrolled, they typically have fewer functional impairments or comorbid conditions than the average older patient treated in real-world clinical practice. Consequently, most of what we know about the risks and benefits of cancer therapeutics is based on clinical trials conducted in younger and/or healthier patients. Extrapolation of the results to older patients can sometimes lead to "potential overtreatment" with standard management or "potential undertreatment" with non-standard and/or palliative management strategies. Most of the evidences for cancer management in the geriatric population are obtained from retrospective studies and subgroup analysis of clinical trials.

6 Site-Specific Role of Radiotherapy in the Geriatric Population

6.1 Breast Cancers

Approximately 40% of diagnosed breast cancer patients are in age group >65 years. Adjuvant radiotherapy in breast cancer, following breast conservation surgery (BCS) and for those in high-risk post-mastectomy patients not only reduces the risk of ipsilateral breast cancer recurrence (IBTR) but also improves overall survival [10]. Most often, randomized trials either excluded elderly patients ≥70 years [11, 12] or included limited numbers of aged [13] resulting in limited randomized evidence demonstrating the optimal role of RT in this patient population. Few non-randomized clinical and retrospective studies demonstrate that omission of RT in low-risk (upfront surgery, pT1–T2 and pN0) hormone receptor-positive elderly patients ≥70 years can be done safely after BCS or mastectomy [14–16]. Subsequently, the results from three phase III trials [17–19] evaluating omission of RT in patients aged ≥70 years undergoing BCS found that omission of RT in pT1–T2 (<3 cm), pN0, and hormone receptor positive patients receiving tamoxifen had similar mortality rates as compared to patients receiving RT with tamoxifen, although IBTR rates were relatively higher in the no-RT group. If RT is to be given, partial breast irradiation (PBI, 40–50 Gy in 15–25 fractions) can be preferred over whole breast RT. Avoiding of tumor bed boost, although controversial, can be considered in hormone receptor-positive patients with compromise in expected survival.

6.2 Central Nervous System Tumors

6.2.1 Gliomas

Glioblastoma (GBM) is the most common primary brain tumor in adults. The standard treatment includes maximal safe surgery, which is 'gross total resection' (GTR) based on radiographic images, followed by adjuvant radiotherapy to doses of 60 Gy to the postoperative tumor bed with adequate margins. Current standard therapy should be with or without concurrent plus adjuvant temozolomide based on MGMT methylation status. In elderly GBM patients (≥65 years), adjuvant focal RT up to a dose of 50 Gy by conventional fractionation is superior to best supportive care in survival without increasing adverse effects [20]. The phase III trial showed that hypofractionated RT (HypoRT) (34 Gy in 10 fractions over 2 weeks at 3.4 Gy per fraction once daily), and temozolomide alone improved survival as compared to standard RT in patients ≥70 years of age [21]. Results of the NOA-08 trial [22] have shown that dose dense temozolomide (100 mg/m^2 OD, given for 1 week off) given until disease progression or adverse effects is non-inferior to standard RT. In both the trials [21, 22], median OS improved in the presence of MGMT promoter methylation in patients who received TMZ, but not in patients who received RT, whereas no such benefit was found in unmethylated tumors. In recent years, the focus on treating the elderly as a special group has shown that HypoRT (40 Gy in 15 fractions) plus temozolomide improved survival outcomes as compared to HypoRT alone (40 Gy in 15 fractions), more significantly in those elderly GBM patients with poorer functional status and MGMT promoter methylation [23]. The frail and elderly patients, unfit for temozolomide therapy, can be hypofractionated further to a dose of 25 Gy in 5 fractions (1-week schedule), which has shown similar outcomes as compared to 40 Gy in 15 fractions (3-week schedule) [24]. These developments in the management of gliomas in the elderly should be incorporated into clinical practice.

6.2.2 Brain Metastasis

Brain metastasis is the most common tumor (30–40%) of the central nervous system. The elderly age group has been considered a poor prognostic factor for survival in patients undergoing whole brain RT (WBRT), apart from increased risk of neuro-cognitive dysfunctions. Stereotactic radiosurgery (SRS) in older patients with 1–3 brain metastases versus WBRT plus SRS in patients of all ages shows no significant survival differences between younger and older patients. The risk of neurologic death was similar for SRS group when compared with WBRT plus SRS, with no significant differences between patients <65 years and those ≥65 years [25, 26], but neuro-cognitive function was better with SRS alone. Instead of Recursive Partitioning Analyses (RPA) classes, recently, a diagnosis-specific graded prognostic assessment (DS-GPA) score provides different patterns of diagnosis-specific prognostic factors that might be more appropriate in predicting the outcome that can be expected from the various treatment options in the elderly population [27]. Number of metastases and/or KPS, but not the age, are considered significant prognostic factors as per DS-GPA scores for survival in several cancer types, including cancers of the lung, breast, kidney, gastrointestinal tract, and melanoma. The dose for SRS is given as a single fraction: 20–22 Gy (2.0 cm maximum diameter), 18–20 Gy (2.0–2.9 cm maximum diameter); when WBRT is added, it is prescribed as 30 Gy in 12 fractions (5 fractions/week, with hippocampal avoidance). Protective effects of Memantine hydrochloride, an N-methyl-D-aspartate (NMDA) receptor antagonist, a drug which may enhance cognitive function by binding to and inhibiting channels of receptors located in the central nervous system, along with hippocampal sparing IMRT, have been shown to improve neuro-cognitive functions [26].

6.3 Gastro-Intestinal Cancers

6.3.1 Esophageal Cancer

Esophageal cancer (EC) mostly affects older age groups. Multimodal treatment, including radiotherapy, chemotherapy, and surgery, offers the best chances of curative treatment in the elderly population. Neoadjuvant CTRT followed by definitive surgery is the current standard of care in resectable esophageal cancers [28]. Despite advancements, postoperative morbidity and mortality rates are higher in elderly patients, especially ≥70 years [29], and most patients >80 years often do not undergo definitive surgery. Avoiding the transthoracic approach could be a good treatment alternative for frail elderly patients, if tumor location allows it. Extended transhiatal (abdominal) surgery demonstrated similar long-term survival as compared to transthoracic esophagectomy, although negative resection margins might be more difficult to obtain. Definitive chemoradiation is an alternative option as compared to best supportive care, especially for those in good physical status and yet are unresectable or unfit for surgery. Although the CROSS trial [28] established the utilization of trimodality therapy in EC, the criteria would not fit many elderly EC patients. Careful patient selection continues to be essential in this population. For patients aged >70 years, recent trends from the National Cancer Data Base (NCDB, USA) show that more than 2/3rds of these age groups were treated with definitive CTRT only [30]. Radiation dose delivered with concurrent chemotherapy revealed that low dose (40 Gy) yields similar overall survival (OS) when compared with high dose (50 Gy and above) in the real world NCDB [31]. Despite the progress in chemotherapy and immunotherapy, the omission of RT in these age groups should be decided carefully, because radiotherapy can provide lasting palliation for several months.

6.3.2 Colorectal Cancer

Low- and middle-income countries (LMICs) show increasing rates of colorectal cancer (CRC) incidence in the last decade and lower 5-year survival rates compared to high-income countries

(HICs), where the implementation of screening and treatment services has advanced facilities.

Decision-making for elderly patients with resectable, locally advanced rectal cancer (stage II-III) would depend on (a) underlying patient factors (comorbidities, functional status, geriatric assessments, and overall life expectancy) and (b) the expected tolerance of the standard of care therapy consisting of preoperative chemo-radiotherapy (CTRT) followed by surgery with TME. In elderly patients, rectal cancer is characterized by decreased cancer-related survival rates because of late disease stages at presentation, combined with less aggressive treatment overall [32]. In recent years, elderly patients with locally advanced rectal cancer comprise a large proportion of the patient cohort. Consideration should be given to trimodality therapy in this group, with careful patient selection taking into account biological age, especially in the context of increasing life expectancy and improvement in the management of age-related comorbidities [33]. Although acute toxicities with short-course radiotherapy (SCRT) are relatively low, studies demonstrate that postoperative complications, morbidity rates, and quality of life are worse with SCRT [34]. Surgery in elderly patients was associated with increased mortality. Hence, one has to carefully weigh the risks and benefits of choosing the type of preoperative CTRT in these age groups. In surgically unfit patients but fit for RT, the preferred option would be long-course CTRT to radiation doses of 45–50.4 Gy. Concurrent capecitabine is preferred as it is associated with improved clinical, pathological response rates and disease-free survival rates. Chemotherapy can be tailored based on the CGA scores using appropriate pre-therapy measurements.

6.3.3 Anal Cancer

Anal canal squamous cell carcinomas are relatively uncommon with an annual incidence rate of <1%. Concurrent chemo-radiotherapy (CTRT) with multi-agent chemotherapy, mitomycin-C (MMC) plus 5-FU, with RT doses of 50.4–59.4 Gy is considered standard of care. This regimen is also associated with significant grade 3–4 toxicities, like hematological, skin, and bowel toxicities. Hence, there are reasonable concerns about the utility of this regimen in elderly patients with or without co-morbidities. And, it has been shown to increase mortality in aged ≥65 years [35]. Frequent treatment interruptions and chemotherapy dose reductions/avoidance of chemotherapy were frequently encountered. Replacement of MMC with cisplatin was also tried, but, results were unfavorable [36]. Therefore, elderly fit patients should be offered CTRT with standard regimens. Intensity modulated radiotherapy with bone marrow sparing techniques can be utilized in these patients with encouraging results in terms of treatment compliance and reduced hematological side effects. Patients who are unfit for MMC can be replaced with cisplatin. Patients unfit for standard therapy can be considered for palliative RT.

6.4 Genito-Urinary Cancers

6.4.1 Prostate Cancer

Prostate cancer is frequently found in the geriatric population, as mentioned earlier in this chapter. The screening of frailty using Geriatric-8 (G8) and Mini-COG screening tools is recommended by various international bodies [37]. Elderly localized prostate cancer patients with D'Amico low-to-intermediate risk prostate cancer should be evaluated for life expectancy using validated tools for subsequent decision for either active surveillance (life expectancy >10 years) or watchful waiting (limited life expectancy), when active treatment can be avoided. Fit older patients with D'Amico high-risk group, localized prostate cancer with life expectancy >10 years, are to be treated with curative intent using radical prostatectomy or definitive RT. IMRT is considered the standard of care for radical EBRT in prostate cancer. Dose-escalation (>70 Gy) has shown better outcomes than doses <70 Gy using conventional fractionation [38]. Hypofractionated (Hypo-RT) with decreased treatment time to 4 weeks has proven beneficial as compared to conventional fractionation radiotherapy of 7 weeks or more in low-to-high risk patients by many studies [39, 40]. The proportion of elderly age included in these studies was low. However, late rectal and genitourinary toxicities become significant consideration in low-risk elderly patients. Further decrease in treatment time is possible with permanent seed-based LDR or HDR brachytherapy used as a boost after EBRT or as monotherapy. LDR brachytherapy boost following EBRT to a dose of 46 Gy has provided similar tumor-related outcomes in intermediate and high-risk patients as compared to dose-escalated IMRT [41] in an RCT. This study included a significant number of elderly patients. Although dose-escalation or Hypo-RT is better in terms of overall control rates, it is associated with significant late toxicities. It can be decreased by using rectal spacers during EBRT. SBRT in localized prostate cancers has shown similar outcomes, which is a non-invasive RT technique with fewer treatment visits. Currently, the SBRT dose-fractionation tested in RCT is 36.25 in 5 fractions over 1–2 weeks [42]. Further trials like the HOPE trial are underway. Androgen-deprivation therapy (ADT) is recommended in intermediate and high-risk patients with localized or locally advanced prostate cancer [38]. It is important to observe and manage the side effects of ADT therapy with supportive drugs.

6.5 Gynecological Cancers

6.5.1 Cervical Cancer

Cervical cancers (FIGO stage ≤ IIA) are usually managed with surgery ± adjuvant RT ± chemotherapy. FIGO IIA–IVB stages are usually treated with definitive CTRT with intracavitary brachytherapy (ICBT) with/without interstitial BT (ISBT). In patients unfit for surgery, the preferred treatment is CTRT+ICBT with curative intent. The usual dose prescribed to pelvic RT is 45–50 Gy in 1.8–2 Gy per fraction. Brachytherapy dose schedules vary, but usually prescribed are 5.5–7 Gy per fraction in 3–5 fractions. The survival benefits of cisplatin-based concurrent chemotherapy decline with increasing FIGO stage, showing minimal survival benefit in FIGO stage III-IVA cases [43, 44]. Owing to under-representation of the elderly population with age ≥65 years in most trials, evidence for optimal management in these patients is limited. Most of the elderly patients with cervical cancer are treated with definitive RT plus BT. Concurrent cisplatin was omitted or reduced in dose-intensities in some studies in elderly patients ≥70 years. Despite omission of concurrent chemotherapy, outcomes of these patients with younger age groups seem similar. But, late rectal and hematological toxicities occur at higher rates in these patients due to associated co-morbidities and/or frailty. Therefore, recent advancements, like image-guided IMRT (IG-IMRT), can be used for pelvic RT using bone marrow sparing techniques which significantly reduce acute bowel and hematological toxicities, thereby decreasing treatment interruptions. The image-guided adaptive BT (IGABT) with dose normalization to high-risk clinical target volume (HR-CTV), would reduce doses to bladder and rectum as compared to conventional point A-based brachytherapy (ICBT) . The combination of IG-IMRT with IGABT can reduce the risk of severe acute toxicities, late tissue toxicities, and improve treatment tolerance. MRI-based IGABT is preferred over CT-based planning as the latter overestimates the HR-CTV volumes [45, 46]. In patients of SCC cervix with positive common iliac nodes and/or multiple pelvic nodes and negative para-aortic lymph nodes (PALN), who are fit for RT but unfit for concurrent chemotherapy, prophylactic para-aortic RT improves disease-free survival as compared to pelvic RT alone [47]. However, prophylactic PALN irradiation should not be prescribed routinely for elderly patients. IMRT is the preferred technique while using prophylactic PALN irradiation (Fig. 3).

FIGO stage IVB (and some IVA) patients are treated with palliative intent, where palliative RT (BT or EBRT) dose of 20 Gy in 5 fractions or 30 Gy in 10 fractions(over 1-2 weeks) is frequently used to control bleeding.

6.5.2 Endometrial Cancer

Endometrial cancer mostly occurs in older women, with the median age for diagnosis around 60 years. The standard of care is hysterectomy with bilateral salpingo-oophorectomy plus pelvic lymphadenectomy with para-aortic sampling, and should be considered in medically fit patients. Despite longer operation time, minimally invasive approach like laparoscopic/robotic approaches is relatively safe and feasible with fewer morbidities as compared to the traditional laparotomy approach, which can be preferred [48]. Early-stage, low-grade disease postoperatively can be treated with adjuvant radiotherapy only (EBRT or brachytherapy or both). Intermediate stage or advanced stages require additional adjuvant with/without concurrent chemotherapy [49]. Age alone is found to be an independent prognostic factor. Older women more frequently have high-grade disease, advanced disease, and higher recurrence rates as compared to relatively younger women. IMRT should be the preferred technique for the delivery of adjuvant pelvic RT to a standard dose of 45–50.4 Gy at 1.8–2 Gy/Fr, especially in older as it has been shown to reduce the incidence of small bowel, rectal toxicities, and pelvic bone fractures. Urinary urgency or incontinence are frequently found in older women, which may lead to improper bladder filling during RT delivery; hence, bladder filling protocols can be avoided and can be treated on an empty bladder when IMRT is used. Rectal protocols like daily administration of rectal enemas can be difficult and challenging in this age group, hence, can be preferably avoided.

6.6 Head and Neck Tumors

A significant proportion of head and neck SCC (HNSCC) cases are among those aged ≥70 years. The standard of care in resectable oral cavity SCC is curative surgery followed by adjuvant RT ± chemotherapy based on postoperative pathologic findings. Some elderly patients with resectable oral cavity SCC may not undergo curative surgery due to frailty, co-morbidities, and the risk of higher postoperative morbidities. These patients are either offered definitive radiotherapy ± chemotherapy or treated with palliative intent. Unresectable oral cavity cases (cT4b, some T3 tongue cancers with oropharyngeal extension) are mostly treated with palliative intent only. Pharyngeal and laryngeal cancers are usually treated with radical cisplatin-based CTRT. CTRT has an increased risk of having higher-grade tox-

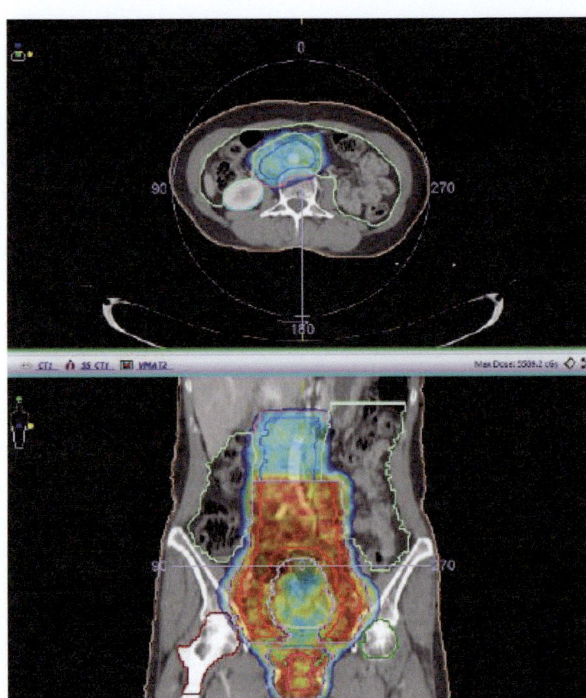

Fig. 3 Volumetric modulated arc therapy (VMAT) planning of prophylactic para-aortic lymph node (PALN) irradiation to a dose of 45 Gy in 25 fractions on a planning computed tomography (**top image**) axial section, and (**bottom image**) coronal CT section showing 95% isodose coverage of PTV-PALN. PTV-Pelvis comprising primary and pelvic nodal groups treated to a dose of 50 Gy in 25 fractions

icities, malnutrition, and morbidity rates. The advantage of CTRT in HNSCC has been shown to decrease with age [50] probably because of the effect of competing risk factors associated with older age on survival. Hence, these patients need to be evaluated for the benefit versus harm of concurrent cisplatin-based chemotherapy, using various GA tools available. Alternatively, hyperfractionated RT (HyperRT) can be used in locally advanced, LAHNSCC patients unfit for concurrent chemotherapy, which has shown survival benefits. Again, the survival benefit with HyperRT decreases with increasing age [51]. Concurrent cetuximab may be used along with definitive RT doses if unfit for cisplatin-based chemotherapy [52], although adverse effects are slightly higher with cetuximab. Nevertheless, radical doses of RT ± chemotherapy with standard IMRT techniques can cause higher-grade dysphagia and aspiration-related toxicities, eventually affecting the nutritional status, quality of life, and mortality rates in elderly people. Recent techniques like dysphagia-aspiration related structures (DARS) sparing IMRT have shown to decrease the doses to deglutition structures, thereby potentially reducing higher grade toxicities to these structures. Human papillomavirus (HPV) infection is frequently associated with oropharyngeal SCC (OPSCC) in younger patients rather than elderly age groups. HPV positive OPSCC cases have better outcomes as compared to HPV negative OPSCC cases, which has led to extensive exploration of various de-intensification strategies in these subgroup of patients. Various de-intensification strategies utilize, (a) reduced radiotherapy dose and treatment volume, (b) modification in systemic chemotherapy drug and/or schedule, (c) adding safe surgery like transoral robotic surgery(TORS) to debulk the tumor, before CTRT. Multiple prospective and retrospective studies have shown that few de-intensification strategies can be employed. Although extensive research on this issue is currently going on, unfortunately, no phase III randomized trials have shown any significant benefit to date. De-escalation of RT includes various strategies like RT dose de-escalation from 70 Gy total dose to 60 Gy by conventional fractionation or decreasing the elective neck node volumes in node-negative patients with the same total dose of 70 Gy. Despite low evidence, de-intensification of therapy might be an option, discussing risks and benefits of these approaches with the elderly patient. Geriatric patients who are unfit for radical RT or with metastatic disease at presentation can be considered for palliative care. RT is an effective modality in the palliation of symptoms in most of the HNSCC cases. Palliative RT is usually hypofractionated RT (HypoRT). An effective palliative RT regimen is yet to be determined, and varies significantly due to many reasons like institutional policy, patient willingness and affordability, volume of the disease, treating physician's choice, etc. Various palliative RT regimens [53] tried and tested so far are: (a) 24 Gy in 3 fractions at 8 Gy/Fr at 0–8–21 days, (b)14–14.8 Gy in four fractions BID separated by a minimum gap of 6-h at 3.5–3.7 Gy/Fr (Quad Shot regimen), (c) 20–25 Gy in five fractions once daily over a week at 4–5 Gy/Fr, (d) 30–36 Gy in 6 fractions once daily over a week at 5–6 Gy/Fr, (e) 40 Gy in 16 fractions at 2.5 Gy/Fr once daily over 5-weeks, and (f) 50 Gy in 16 fractions at 3.12 Gy/Fr once daily over 5-weeks (Christie regimen). The regimens using higher doses (e.g., Christie regimen) have shown better response rates as well as higher ≥ grade 3 toxicities. Therefore, the selection of a palliative regimen should be individualized based on GA scores using appropriate tools. Split-course schedules are preferred by most clinicians as response and toxicities can be tailored after the first/every course of palliative RT sessions. Results of the ELAN-RT trial assessing the effectiveness of HypoRT with split-course versus standard full-dose RT in elderly vulnerable patients are awaited.

6.7 Lung Cancers

6.7.1 Nonsmall Cell Lung Cancer

Management of elderly non-small cell lung cancer (NSCLC) is often challenging. For operable primary tumor, there are no major differences in OS between elderly (≥70 years) and younger patients undergoing surgery for NSCLC, although, quality of evidence is low [54]. The standard of care in clinically early stage (stage I-II, low volume stage IIIA) NSCLC is definitive surgery followed by adjuvant chemotherapy ± adjuvant RT depending on pathological findings. Lobectomy or segmentectomy is the preferred standard surgical procedure, but sub-lobar resections/wedge resections can be considered in elderly patients [55]. Minimally invasive approaches like video-assisted thoracic surgery (VATS) may decrease the perioperative and postoperative morbidity and mortality rates as compared to traditional thoracotomy surgeries [56]. If patients are unfit for surgery (poor lung function, higher expected postoperative morbidity), stereotactic body radiotherapy (SBRT) is a recommended treatment option instead of conventionally fractionated RT in suitable patients [57]. The response rates and toxicities were lower with SBRT. T1-T2N0 (≤5 cm), peripherally located tumors are the most suitable candidates, although tumors >5 cm can also be considered for SBRT. The doses routinely used were 60–66 Gy in 3 divided fractions. Centrally located tumors but within 2 cm of the proximal bronchial tree or ultra-centrally located tumors (within 1 cm from the proximal tracheabronchial tree) can also be treated with SBRT to a dose of 50–60 Gy in 5–8 divided fractions. The latter is associated with higher incidences of central airway necrosis, trachea-esophageal fistulas, or broncho-pulmonary hemorrhages than the former. The tumors with frank endobronchial invasions, hotspots within the endobronchial region, and/or tumors abutting the pulmonary artery are at increased risk of these toxicities. Therefore, these tumors are better treated with conventionally fractionated RT to standard doses of 66 Gy with concurrent chemotherapy. Adjuvant chemotherapy after surgery or RT is preferred over no adjuvant chemotherapy in elderly patients aged ≥65 years as it improves outcomes but can increase side effects. Cisplatin can be replaced with carboplatin in these patient groups, although limited evidence exists. Adjuvant RT after definitive surgery can improve loco-regional rates but not OS in pN1-pN2 cases. Hence, it remains controversial except for positive margins not undergoing revision surgery, in whom RT has shown survival benefits. Recently, targeted therapies like tyrosine kinase inhibitors (TKIs) have been extensively used in NSCLC adenocarcinoma harboring various mutations like EGFR, ALK, and ROS-1 mutations, which showed good-to-excellent response outcomes in patients who failed primary 1st or 2nd line systemic therapies. In elderly locally advanced and/or metastatic settings, TKIs are preferred over chemotherapy in certain patients with good survival rates [58]. Individualization of treatment based on pretreatment CGA scores and expected survival in each patient should be carried out to avoid over- or under-treatment.

6.7.2 Small-Cell Lung Cancer

Small cell lung cancers (SCLC) are aggressive in nature, often with a poor prognosis, with a median age for diagnosis being 65 years. Hence, most trial data reflect the outcomes of the elderly population. Limited stage disease (LS-SCLC) is often treated with CTRT with cisplatin plus etoposide-based chemotherapy to a maximum of 4–6 cycles with prophylactic cranial irradiation (PCI), if no progression on CTRT. But, in older patients, tolerance to CTRT is usually poor. Hence, sequential chemotherapy and RT are preferred. Sequential RT also offers a potential reduction in volumes treated to higher doses. Doses usually used are 45 Gy BID at 1.5 Gy/Fr or 60-66 Gy OD at 2 Gy/Fr to the primary tumor and involved lymph node groups [59].

7 Future Directions

Hypofractionation, stereotactic techniques, particle therapy, along with immunotherapy, targeted therapy, and minimally invasive surgery have expanded the armamentarium to tackle oncological challenges in the vulnerable elderly patients. In majority of cancers in the elderly, radiation therapy has a special role because of short duration treatment course and better tolerability compared to systemic chemotherapy. Comprehensive geriatric score assessment and appropriate representation of this age group in various randomized control trials are vital to answer multiple issues. The socioeconomic issues for cancer care in elderly age can become more pronounced and accordingly the healthcare team should be sensitive to address these hurdles.

Percepts Box

1. The geriatric age population is often treated with non-standard modalities, which could be dictated in part due to factors like co-morbidities, performance status, and in part due to the lack of data available for this population.
2. Pre-treatment geriatric assessment using tools like the cancer aging research group (CARG) tool and chemotherapy risk assessment scale for high-age (CRASH) tool, the Geriatric-8 (G8) scale could help clinicians assess and predict the tolerance of treatment.
3. Certain Phase III trials have shown that the mortality rates of patients >70 years old with early breast cancer (<3 cm tumors), node negative, receptor positive cases receiving RT with tamoxifen are similar to those put on Tamoxifen only.
4. Hypofractionated RT (34 Gy/2 weeks) with Temezolamide (TMZ) in GBM improved survival compared to standard fractionation in patients >70 years according to the Nordic trial.
5. The NOA-08 trial showed that dose-dense TMZ given alone until disease progression was non-inferior to standard RT in the elderly with GBM.
6. SRS is considered non-inferior to WBRT in the elderly with brain metastases in terms of survival. However, SRS is associated with improved neuro-cognition.
7. The CROSS trial in esophageal cancer did not include patients over 75 years. Definitive CTRT can be a good option in these cases, when the elderly is suitably selected.
8. In lower GI cancers, high-age patients may not be deemed fit for surgery. In such cases, standard fractionation courses are preferred.
9. Treatment options for prostate cancers are dictated by the life expectancy and risk stratification. In localized stages, if expected survival >10 years, high-risk patients can be treated by surgery or definitive RT. ADT therapy is well tolerated, yet would require supportive drugs for symptoms of side-effects. Low and intermediate-risk patients can opt for surveillance.
10. Brachytherapy boost in intermediate to high-risk prostate cancer patients can be considered to decrease late toxicities. In low-risk, permanent seed-based LDR or HDR Brachytherapy is a good alternative to an EBRT boost.
11. Gynecological cancer patients can be treated using standard of care approaches, but should be treated using technologies like minimally invasive surgery and IMRT.
12. Late toxicities like rectal and hematological toxicities in cervical cancer can be mitigated by the use of IG-IMRT. IGABT with dose normalization to HR-CTV in brachytherapy can further reduce bladder and rectal toxicities.
13. Standard of care in Head and neck cancers in the elderly is difficult to achieve. RT can also result in a higher rate of toxicities. Hyperfractionated regimens, use of Cetuximab, DARS sparing IMRT, or palliative RT can help mitigate the risk of toxicities. In advanced locoregional stages, palliative radiotherapy can achieve significant symptom relief and growth restraint.
14. HPV positive oropharyngeal tumors have better outcomes than HPV negative tumors, giving rise to a study on de-intensification regimens. This can be an option in older, unfit patients.
15. Treatment options in NSCLC include surgery, SBRT, or conventional fractionation, and targeted therapies. SCLC is associated with a poorer outcome and can be considered for sequential chemotherapy and RT.

Multiple Choice Questions

1. The most common cause of death from cancer in the elderly in India is
   (a) Prostate cancer
   (b) Breast cancer
   (c) Cervical cancer
   (d) Oral cancer
2. Causes for non-standard treatment options offered to the elderly include
   (a) Under-representation in clinical trials
   (b) Age-related changes like comorbidities, performance status
   (c) Lack of psychological and social support
   (d) All of the above
3. Geriatric assessment tools include
   (a) CRASH
   (b) CARG
   (c) VES-13
   (d) All of the above
4. Hypofractionated RT dose in GBM according to the Nordic trial is
   (a) 27 Gy/3 fractions
   (b) 34 Gy/10 fractions
   (c) 40 Gy/15 fractions
   (d) 25 Gy/5 fractions
5. Prognostic factor(s) in assessing the survival according to the diagnosis-specific graded prognostic assessment (DS-GPA) score include
   (a) Age of the patient
   (b) Number of metastases
   (c) KPS
   (d) Both (b) and (c)
6. Factors improving neuro-cognitive functions include all except
   (a) Use of Memantine Hydrochloride
   (b) Hippocampal sparing IMRT
   (c) WBRT
   (d) None of the above
7. Annual incidence rate of Anal cancer is
   (a) <1%
   (b) <2%
   (c) <5%
   (d) <10%
8. The dose fractionation schedule according to the Christie regimen is
   (a) 24 Gy/3 fractions at 0–8–21 days
   (b) 50 Gy/16 fractions over 5 weeks
   (c) 14–14.8 Gy/4 fractions BID separated by at least 6 h
   (d) 30–36 Gy in 6 fractions
9. The dose fractionation schedule according to the Quad shot regimen is
   (a) 24 Gy/3 fractions at 0–8–21 days
   (b) 50 Gy/16 fractions over 5 weeks
   (c) 14–14.8 Gy/4 fractions BID separated by at least 6 h
   (d) 30–36 Gy in 6 fractions
10. The SBRT dose for peripherally located NSCLC is
    (a) 36.25 Gy/5 fractions
    (b) 50–60 Gy/5–8 fractions
    (c) 60–66 Gy/3 fractions
    (d) 27–30 Gy/3 fractions

Answer Key

1. (a)
2. (d)
3. (d)
4. (b)
5. (d)
6. (c)
7. (a)
8. (b)
9. (c)
10. (c)

References

1. Hussain SMA, Sullivan R. Developing geriatric oncology in low- and middle-income countries: what should we do first? J Geriatr Oncol. 2012;3(Supplement 1):S20.
2. OECD Data. Elderly population. 2022. Available from: https://data.oecd.org/pop/elderly-population.htm.
3. Sung H, Ferlay J, Siegel RL, et al. Global Cancer Statistics 2020: GLOBOCAN Estimates of Incidence and Mortality Worldwide for 36 Cancers in 185 Countries. CA Cancer J Clin. 2021;71(3):209–249. https://doi.org/10.3322/caac.21660
4. Alvis BD, Hughes CG. Physiology considerations in geriatric patients. Anesthesiol Clin. 2015;33(3):447–56. https://doi.org/10.1016/j.anclin.2015.05.003.
5. Morris L, Turner S, Thiruthaneeswaran N, O'Donovan A, et al. An international expert Delphi consensus to

develop dedicated geriatric radiation oncology curriculum learning outcomes. Int J Radiat Oncol Biol Phys. 2022;113(5):934–45. https://doi.org/10.1016/j.ijrobp.2022.04.030.
6. Dale W, Klepin HD, Williams GR, Alibhai SMH, et al. Practical assessment and management of vulnerabilities in older patients receiving systemic cancer therapy: ASCO guideline update. J Clin Oncol. 2023;41(26):4293–312. https://doi.org/10.1200/JCO.23.00933.
7. https://www.mycarg.org/.
8. Hamaker M, Lund C, Te Molder M, Soubeyran P, Wildiers H, van Huis L, Rostoft S. Geriatric assessment in the management of older patients with cancer – a systematic review (update). J Geriatr Oncol. 2022;13(6):761–77. https://doi.org/10.1016/j.jgo.2022.04.008.
9. Sedrak MS, Freedman RA, Cohen HJ, Muss HB, Cancer and Aging Research Group (CARG), et al. Older adult participation in cancer clinical trials: a systematic review of barriers and interventions. CA Cancer J Clin. 2021;71(1):78–92. https://doi.org/10.3322/caac.21638.
10. McGale P, Taylor C, Correa C, Cutter D, Duane F, Ewertz M, et al. Effect of radiotherapy after mastectomy and axillary surgery on 10-year recurrence and 20-year breast cancer mortality: meta-analysis of individual patient data for 8135 women in 22 randomised trials. Lancet. 2014;383(9935):2127–35.
11. Veronesi U, Cascinelli N, Mariani L, Greco M, Saccozzi R, Luini A, et al. Twenty-year follow-up of a randomized study comparing breast-conserving surgery with radical mastectomy for early breast cancer. N Engl J Med. 2002;347(16):1227–32.
12. Fisher B, Anderson S, Bryant J, Margolese RG, Deutsch M, Fisher ER, et al. Twenty-year follow-up of a randomized trial comparing total mastectomy, lumpectomy, and lumpectomy plus irradiation for the treatment of invasive breast cancer. N Engl J Med. 2002;347(16):1233–41.
13. Agrawal RK, Aird EGA, Barrett JM, Barrett-Lee PJ, Bentzen SM, Bliss JM, et al. The UK Standardisation of Breast Radiotherapy (START) Trial B of radiotherapy hypofractionation for treatment of early breast cancer: a randomised trial. Lancet. 2008;371:1098–107.
14. Wu N, Tan Q, Su X, Yuan Y, Hou L, Li J. Adjuvant radiation therapy for older women with early – stage breast cancer: a propensity – matched SEER analysis. Clin Transl Oncol [Internet]. Springer International Publishing. 2022. Available from: https://doi.org/10.1007/s12094-022-02967-9.
15. Zhong Y, Xu Y, Zhou Y, Mao F, Lin Y, Guan J, et al. Omitting radiotherapy is safe in breast cancer patients ≥ 70 years old after breast – conserving surgery without axillary lymph node operation. Sci Rep [Internet]. Nature Publishing Group UK. 2020:1–7. Available from: https://doi.org/10.1038/s41598-020-76663-5.
16. Stueber TN, Diessner J, Bartmann CM, et al. Effect of adjuvant radiotherapy in elderly patients with breast cancer. PLoS One. 2020;15(5):e0229518. https://doi.org/10.1371/journal.pone.0229518.
17. Kunkler IH, Williams LJ, Jack WJL, Cameron DA, Dixon JM. Breast-conserving surgery with or without irradiation in women aged 65 years or older with early breast cancer (PRIME II): a randomised controlled trial. Lancet Oncol [Internet]. Elsevier Ltd. 2015;16:266–73. Available from: https://doi.org/10.1016/S1470-2045(14)71221-5.
18. Fastner G, Sedlmayer F, Widder J, Metz M, Geinitz H, Kapp K, et al. Endocrine therapy with or without whole breast irradiation in low-risk breast cancer patients after breast-conserving surgery: 10-year results of the Austrian Breast and Colorectal Cancer Study Group 8A trial. Eur J Cancer. 2020;127:12–20.
19. Hughes KS, Schnaper LA, Bellon JR, Cirrincione CT, Berry DA, McCormick B, et al. Lumpectomy plus tamoxifen with or without irradiation in women age 70 years or older with early breast cancer: long-term follow-up of CALGB 9343. J Clin Oncol. 2013;31:2382–7.
20. Gull HH, Von Riegen AC, Beckmann GT, Ketelauri P, et al. Treatment strategies for glioblastoma in the elderly: what should we focus on compared to younger patients. Cancers (Basel). 2024;16:1231. https://doi.org/10.3390/cancers16061231.
21. Malmström A, Grønberg BH, Marosi C, Stupp R, Nordic Clinical Brain Tumour Study Group (NCBTSG), et al. Temozolomide versus standard 6-week radiotherapy versus hypofractionated radiotherapy in patients older than 60 years with glioblastoma: the Nordic randomised, phase 3 trial. Lancet Oncol. 2012;13:916–26. https://doi.org/10.1016/S1470-2045(12)70265-6.
22. Wick W, Platten M, Meisner C, Felsberg J, Tabatabai G, Simon M, et al. Temozolomide chemotherapy alone versus radiotherapy alone for malignant astrocytoma in the elderly: the NOA-08 randomised, phase 3 trial. Lancet Oncol [Internet]. Elsevier Ltd. 2012;13:707–15. Available from: https://doi.org/10.1016/S1470-2045(12)70164-X.
23. Mazarakis NK, Robinson SD, Sinha P, Koutsarnakis C, et al. Management of glioblastoma in elderly patients: a review of the literature. Clin Transl Radiat Oncol. 2024;46:100761. https://doi.org/10.1016/j.ctro.2024.100761.
24. Roa W, Kepka L, Kumar N, et al. International Atomic Energy Agency Randomized Phase III Study of Radiation Therapy in Elderly and/or Frail Patients With Newly Diagnosed Glioblastoma Multiforme. J Clin Oncol. 2015;33(35):4145–4150. https://doi.org/10.1200/JCO.2015.62.6606
25. Aoyama H, Shirato H, Tago M, Nakagawa K, Toyoda T, Hatano K, et al. Stereotactic radiosurgery plus whole-brain radiation therapy vs stereotactic radiosurgery alone for treatment of brain metastases: a randomized controlled trial. JAMA. 2006;295:2483–91.
26. Brown PD, Gondi V, Pugh S, Tome WA, for NRG Oncology, et al. Hippocampal avoidance during whole-brain radiotherapy plus memantine for patients with brain metastases: Phase III Trial NRG Oncology CC001. J Clin Oncol. 2020;38:1019–29. https://doi.org/10.1200/JCO.19.02767.

27. Sperduto PW, Mesko S, Li J, Cagney D, et al. Survival in patients with brain metastases: summary report on the updated diagnosis-specific graded prognostic assessment and definition of the eligibility quotient. J Clin Oncol. 2020;38:3773–84. https://doi.org/10.1200/JCO.20.01255.
28. Shapiro J, van Lanschot JJB, Hulshof MCCM, van Hagen P, CROSS Study Group, et al. Neoadjuvant chemoradiotherapy plus surgery versus surgery alone for esophageal or junctional cancer (CROSS): long-term results of a randomised controlled trial. Lancet Oncol. 2015;16:1090–8. https://doi.org/10.1016/S1470-2045(15)00040-6.
29. Baranov NS, Slootmans C, van Workum F, Klarenbeek BR, Schoon Y, Rosman C. Outcomes of curative esophageal cancer surgery in elderly: a meta-analysis. World J Gastrointest Oncol. 2021;13(2):131–46. https://doi.org/10.4251/wjgo.v13.i2.131.
30. Verma V, Haque W, Zheng D, Osayande F, Lin C. Patterns of care and outcomes of elderly esophageal cancer patients not meeting age-based criteria of the CROSS trial. Am J Clin Oncol Cancer Clin Trials. 2019;42:67–74.
31. Haque W, Verma V, Butler EB, Teh BS. Radiation dose in neoadjuvant chemoradiation therapy for esophageal cancer: patterns of care and outcomes from the National Cancer Data Base. J Gastrointestinal Oncol. 2018;9:80–9. https://doi.org/10.21037/jgo.2017.09.12.
32. Chang GJ, Skibber JM, Feig BW, Rodriguez-Bigas M. Are we undertreating rectal cancer in the elderly? An epidemiologic study. Ann Surg. 2007;246:215–21.
33. Kang S, Wilkinson KJ, Brungs D, Chua W, Ng W, Chen J, Nasser E, Lee M, Wong K, Bokey L, Winn R, Putnis S, Lee CS, Lim SH. Rectal cancer treatment and outcomes in elderly patients treated with curative intent. Mol Clin Oncol. 2021;15:256. https://doi.org/10.3892/mco.2021.2418.
34. Maas HAAM, Lemmens VEPP, Nijhuis PHA, De Hingh IHJT, Koning CCE, Janssen-Heijnen MLG. Benefits and drawbacks of short-course preoperative radiotherapy in rectal cancer patients aged 75 years and older. Eur J Surg Oncol [Internet]. Elsevier Ltd. 2013;39:1087–93. Available from: https://doi.org/10.1016/j.ejso.2013.07.094.
35. Wang X, Chen H. Clinical characteristics and prognosis of elderly patients with anal cancer. 2022. https://doi.org/10.21203/rs.3.rs-2272276/v1.
36. Gunderson LL, Winter KA, Ajani JA, Pedersen JE, Moughan J, Benson AB, et al. Long-term update of US GI Intergroup RTOG 98-11 Phase III trial for anal carcinoma: survival, relapse, and colostomy failure with concurrent chemoradiation involving fluorouracil/mitomycin versus fluorouracil/cisplatin. J Clin Oncol. 2012;30:4344–51.
37. Mottet N, van den Bergh RCN, Briers E, Van den Broeck T, Cumberbatch MG, De Santis M, et al. EAU-EANM-ESTRO-ESUR-SIOG guidelines on prostate cancer—2020 update. Part 1: screening, diagnosis, and local treatment with curative intent. Eur Urol. 2021;79:243–62.
38. Parker C, Castro E, Fizazi K, Heidenreich A, Ost P, Procopio G, et al. Prostate cancer: ESMO clinical practice guidelines for diagnosis, treatment and follow-up†. Ann Oncol [Internet]. Elsevier Ltd. 2020;31:1119–34. Available from: https://doi.org/10.1016/j.annonc.2020.06.011.
39. de Vries KC, Wortel RC, Oomen-de Hoop E, Heemsbergen WD, Pos FJ, Incrocci L. Hyprofractionated versus conventionally fractionated radiation therapy for patients with intermediate- or high-risk, localized, prostate cancer: 7-year outcomes from the randomized, multicenter, open-label, phase 3 HYPRO trial. Int J Radiat Oncol Biol Phys [Internet]. Elsevier Inc. 2020;106:108–15. Available from: https://doi.org/10.1016/j.ijrobp.2019.09.007.
40. Dearnaley D, Syndikus I, Mossop H, Khoo V, Birtle A, Bloomfield D, et al. Conventional versus hypofractionated high-dose intensity-modulated radiotherapy for prostate cancer: 5-year outcomes of the randomised, non-inferiority, phase 3 CHHiP trial Lancet Oncol [Internet]. Dearnaley et al. Open Access article distributed under the terms of CC BY; 2016;17:1047–60. Available from: https://doi.org/10.1016/S1470-2045(16)30102-4.
41. Rodda S, Tyldesley S, Morris WJ, Keyes M, Halperin R, Pai H, et al. ASCENDE-RT: an analysis of treatment-related morbidity for a randomized trial comparing a low-dose-rate brachytherapy boost with a dose-escalated external beam boost for high- and intermediate-risk prostate cancer. Int J Radiat Oncol Biol Phys [Internet]. Elsevier Ltd. 2017;98:286–95. Available from: https://doi.org/10.1016/j.ijrobp.2017.01.008.
42. Tree AC, Ostler P, van der Voet H, Chu W, Loblaw A, Ford D, et al. Intensity-modulated radiotherapy versus stereotactic body radiotherapy for prostate cancer (PACE-B): 2-year toxicity results from an open-label, randomised, phase 3, non-inferiority trial. Lancet Oncol [Internet]. 2022 [cited 2022 Dec 23];23:1308–20. Available from: https://pubmed.ncbi.nlm.nih.gov/36113498/.
43. Vale C, Tierney JF, Stewart LA, Brady M, Dinshaw K, Jakobsen A, et al. Reducing uncertainties about the effects of chemoradiotherapy for cervical cancer: a systematic review and meta-analysis of individual patient data from 18 randomized trials. J Clin Oncol. 2008;26:5802–12.
44. Datta NR, Stutz E, Gomez S, Bodis S. Efficacy and safety evaluation of the various therapeutic options in locally advanced cervix cancer: a systematic review and network meta-analysis of randomized clinical trials. Int J Radiat Oncol Biol Phys [Internet]. Elsevier Inc. 2019;103:411–37. Available from: https://doi.org/10.1016/j.ijrobp.2018.09.037.
45. Viswanathan AN, Dimopoulos J, Kirisits C, Berger D, Pötter R. Computed tomography versus magnetic resonance imaging-based contouring in cervical cancer brachytherapy: results of a prospective trial and

preliminary guidelines for standardized contours. Int J Radiat Oncol Biol Phys. 2007;68(2):491–8.
46. Viswanathan AN, Beriwal S, De Los Santos JF, Demanes DJ, Gaffney D, Hansen J, et al. American Brachytherapy Society consensus guidelines for locally advanced carcinoma of the cervix. Part II: high-dose-rate brachytherapy. Brachytherapy. 2012;11(1):47–52.
47. Rotman M, Choi K, Pajak TF, Clery M, Marcial V, Grigsby PW, et al. Prophylactic extended-field irradiation of para-aortic lymph nodes in stages IIB and bulky IB and IIA cervical carcinomas: ten-year treatment results of RTOG 79-20. JAMA J Am Med Assoc. 1995;274:387–93.
48. Walker JL, Piedmonte MR, Spirtos NM, Eisenkop SM, Schlaerth JB, Mannel RS, et al. Laparoscopy compared with laparotomy for comprehensive surgical staging of uterine cancer: Gynecologic Oncology Group Study LAP2. J Clin Oncol. 2009;27:5331–6.
49. Duska L, Shahrokni A, Powell M. Treatment of older women with endometrial cancer: improving outcomes with personalized care. Am Soc Clin Oncol Educ B. 2016;36:164–74.
50. Lacas B, Carmel A, Landais C, Wong SJ, Licitra L, Tobias JS, et al. Meta-analysis of chemotherapy in head and neck cancer (MACH-NC): an update on 107 randomized trials and 19,805 patients, on behalf of MACH-NC Group. Radiother Oncol. 2021;156:281–93.
51. Lacas B, Bourhis J, Overgaard J, Zhang Q, Grégoire V, Nankivell M, et al. Role of radiotherapy fractionation in head and neck cancers (MARCH): an updated meta-analysis. Lancet Oncol. 2017;18:1221–37.
52. Bonner JA, Harari PM, Giralt J, Cohen RB, Jones CU, Sur RK, et al. Radiotherapy plus cetuximab for locoregionally advanced head and neck cancer: 5-year survival data from a phase 3 randomised trial, and relation between cetuximab-induced rash and survival. Lancet Oncol. 2010;11:21–8.
53. Shahid Iqbal M, Kelly C, Kovarik J, Goranov B, Shaikh G, Morgan D, et al. Palliative radiotherapy for locally advanced non-metastatic head and neck cancer: a systematic review. Radiother Oncol [Internet]. 2018;126:558–67. Available from: https://doi.org/10.1016/j.radonc.2017.12.011.
54. Sterlacci W, Stockinger R, Schmid T, Bodner J, Hilbe W, Waldthaler C, et al. The elderly patient with surgically resected non-small cell lung cancer – a distinct situation? Exp Gerontol [Internet]. Elsevier Inc. 2012;47:237–42. Available from: https://doi.org/10.1016/j.exger.2011.12.008.
55. Okami J, Ito Y, Higashiyama M, Nakayama T, Tokunaga T, Maeda J, et al. Sublobar resection provides an equivalent survival after lobectomy in elderly patients with early lung cancer. Ann Thorac Surg [Internet]. Elsevier Inc. 2010;90:1651–6. Available from: https://doi.org/10.1016/j.athoracsur.2010.06.090.
56. Wang L, Liu D, Lu J, Zhang S, Yang X. The feasibility and advantage of uniportal video-assisted thoracoscopic surgery (VATS) in pulmonary lobectomy. BMC Cancer [Internet]. 2017;17:1–7. Available from: https://doi.org/10.1186/s12885-017-3069-z.
57. Shinde A, Li R, Kim J, Salgia R, Hurria A, Amini A. Stereotactic body radiation therapy (SBRT) for early-stage lung cancer in the elderly [Internet]. Semin Oncol. Elsevier Inc. 2018. Available from: https://doi.org/10.1053/j.seminoncol.2018.06.002.
58. Vaid AK, Gupta A, Momi G. Overall survival in stage IV EGFR mutation-positive NSCLC: comparing first-, second- and third-generation EGFR-TKIs (Review). Int J Oncol. 2021;58:171–84.
59. Faivre-Finn C, Snee M, Ashcroft L, Appel W, Barlesi F, Bhatnagar A, et al. Concurrent once-daily versus twice-daily chemoradiotherapy in patients with limited-stage small-cell lung cancer (CONVERT): an open-label, phase 3, randomised, superiority trial. Lancet Oncol [Internet]. The Author(s). Published by Elsevier Ltd. This is an Open Access article under the CC-BY 4.0 license; 2017;18:1116–25. Available from: https://doi.org/10.1016/S1470-2045(17)30318-2.

Online Links

https://www.mdcalc.com/calc/10426/g8-geriatric-screening-tool#use-cases G8 Geriatric Assessment Tool (A tool for assessing need for Comprehensive Geriatric Assessment)

https://www.mdcalc.com/calc/10425/chemotherapy-risk-assessment-scale-high-age-patients-crash-score (A tool to predict toxicity related to chemotherapy)

Emergencies in Radiation Oncology

Shikha Goyal, Renu Madan, Ujjwal Gorsi,
Prasanth Ganesan, and Tharmarnadar Ganesh

1 Introduction

Oncology emergencies cover a wide range of issues that require immediate attention; they may be caused by the development of a malignancy already known to exist, occasionally be the first sign of a malignancy that has only recently been discovered or is still undiagnosed, or they may be a side effect of anticancer therapy. Radiation oncologists frequently deal with a number of these clinical situations that must be taken into account, and administering radiation therapy on an emergency basis can save lives.

Since all patients may not exhibit the same symptomss, diagnosing such disorders requires a high index of suspicion. The diagnosis may be simpler in individuals who have known malignancies or are receiving treatment, since some of these symptoms may be predicted. If these issues are the first sign of an underlying illness, it is more difficult to diagnose and treat; multidisciplinary management would still be essential, as would be supportive care, even though radiation therapy is a vital intervention. To achieve the greatest outcomes for their patients, both in terms of lowering morbidity and raising survival, radiation oncologists must learn to recognize, prioritize, and treat these situations. At each stage, emergency management must be balanced with patient and caregiver engagement, proper prognostication, and discussion of life expectancy and quality of life outcomes. Table 1 lists the most common emergencies in oncology.

1.1 Radiology (Diagnosis and Intervention Perspective)

As noted in table 1, emergencies may be classified into three categories: metabolic, hematologic, and structural. Clinical and laboratory data suffice to identify metabolic and hematologic crises, but imaging is necessary to assess structural emergencies. These structural crises may arise from life-threatening bleeding, blockage of ducts, compression and thrombosis of blood vessels, and the mass effect of tumors on the affected and nearby organs [1]. Complications from radiation therapy can also happen. In radiation oncology crises, a variety of radiological modalities can quickly and accurately answer a wide range of

S. Goyal (✉) · R. Madan
Department of Radiotherapy and Oncology, PGIMER, Chandigarh, India

U. Gorsi
Department of Radiodiagnosis, PGIMER, Chandigarh, India

P. Ganesan
Department of Medical Oncology, JIPMER, Pondicherry, India

T. Ganesh
Former Chief Medical Physicist, Manipal Hospitals Dwarka, New Delhi, India

B. K. Mohanti et al. (eds.), *Radiation Oncology – Principles, Precepts and Practice*,
https://doi.org/10.1007/978-981-95-5171-2_21

Table 1 Classification of common oncologic emergencies

Structural	Hematologic	Metabolic
Raised intracranial pressure Spinal cord compression Bone pain Superior vena cava syndrome Malignant effusion Malignant airway obstruction, stridor, or atelectasis Tumor bleed Obstruction (biliary, urinary, bowel)	Hyperviscosity due to dysproteinemia Hyperleukocytosis Disseminated intravascular coagulation	Hypercalcemia Tumor lysis syndrome Syndrome of inappropriate antidiuretic syndrome Febrile neutropenia Hyponatremia

clinical concerns and contribute to the best possible treatment.

The most widely utilized imaging modalities are plain radiography (X-rays), ultrasonography (USG), multidetector computed tomography (MDCT), and magnetic resonance imaging (MRI). In addition, when considering different non-vascular and vascular procedures, fluoroscopy and digital subtraction angiography (DSA) are used. The initial imaging method used to evaluate thoracic crises is often a chest radiograph (CXR), which might show pericardial tamponade, atelectasis, pleural effusion, and/or airway obstruction. If intestinal obstruction or perforation is suspected, an abdominal X-ray can help. An X-ray of the spine can show vertebral body collapse and possibly even indicate spinal cord compression [1].

Most abdominal crises would first be assessed via USG. In several situations, including biliary blockage causing cholangitis and pyonephroses brought on by ureteral obstruction by tumors, USG is generally accessible, inexpensive, and capable of providing a diagnosis. It can identify ascites and hemoperitoneum as well as different abdominal visceral mass lesions. It is beneficial in the early assessment of crises in children and pregnant women since it is radiation-free. However, cross-sectional imaging techniques like MDCT and MRI are often necessary for a full and comprehensive examination.

The preferred imaging technique for assessing thoracic and abdominal crises is MDCT. It is quick, accessible in most emergency rooms, and simple to carry out. Complicated crises that require an immediate diagnosis may be evaluated using volumetric acquisition followed by multiplanar reconstructions in the coronal and sagittal planes. In most cases, intravenous contrast is needed, although oral contrast is skipped when evaluating emergency indications.

By providing excellent anatomical and frequently pertinent functional information, MRI aids in the best evaluation of central nervous system (CNS) and spinal cord crises such as elevated intracranial pressure (ICP), brain herniation, and cord compression. However, it is time-consuming and still not widely accessible. The clinician must make the right imaging requests that will promptly produce an accurate diagnosis. Appropriate radiologic investigations and interventions are discussed further under specific conditions.

1.2 Medical Physicist Perspective

In any modern radiation oncology center, the decision to start emergency radiotherapy services must be taken after careful consideration of several influencing factors and meetings with the stakeholders—viz., radiation oncologists, medical physicists, radiotherapy technologists, nurses, other support staff, radiology team, information technology (IT) personnel, and hospital administrators. The center offering emergency radiotherapy treatments must decide on the personnel required, work out strategies (how to contact them, their transportation, time factor, etc.) to ensure their availability outside regular working hours, and put a duty roster system in place. The duty roster for emergency radiotherapy should contain names of radiation oncologist, medical physicist, radiotherapy technologist, and nurse displayed date-wise, and calendar month-wise at the centre. A standard operating procedure (SOP) for the emergency treatment workflow should be framed. No treatments shall be delivered outside the domain of the department's radiation oncology information system (ROIS), and every treatment must be recorded in the electronic database. Treatment techniques shall be limited to only simple ones like single field, parallel-opposed fields, or 3-dimensional conformal radiotherapy (3DCRT), and should strictly avoid all other advanced techniques in classic emergencies.

The ROIS has a daily backup timeslot which is usually scheduled in the midnight hours. Since the database is locked during this time, the services of the linear accelerator (LINAC) and the treatment planning system become unavailable, and no patients can be treated [2]. In consultation with the vendors, the medical physicist shall keep the stakeholders informed about the exact time and duration of this non-availability slot of treatment services. It should be mentioned in the SOP as well. Although vendors may provide some workaround solutions, it is advisable to avoid patient treatments during these hours since there are high chances for overlooks, and errors, if any, can be severe.

The other challenging task is the independent monitor unit verification (MUV), where the calculated MU for a patient's treatment is verified by employing either a measurement or a calculation before actual treatment delivery [3]. It is a mandatory requirement as per international standards to ensure patient safety. Inside normal working hours, this task is easy to accomplish due to the availability of more than one physicist, but this may not be the case during emergency treatments. According to the American Association of Physicists in Medicine (AAPM) Task Group (TG) Report 40, MUV has to be performed by another authorized individual, other than the one who performed the original calculation, ideally before treatment. If not possible before treatment initiation, it should definitely be completed before the third treatment fraction or before 10% of the dose has been delivered, whichever occurs first [4]. As per the recommendations of the American College of Radiology (ACR)—AAPM, for treatments happening after regular treatment hours, on the weekend, or on a holiday, the institution should have procedures in place for ensuring MUV is performed within one working day after treatment delivery [5]. The AAPM Medical Physics Practice Guidelines require that, for such emergency treatments, the on-call medical physicist reviews the treatment plan remotely or in person. If that is not possible, a radiation oncologist may conduct the initial plan/chart review, and a medical physicist should check the plan on the next working day or before the treatment on the next working day if additional fractions are prescribed [6]. Timely plan/chart review assumes even more importance considering the findings of Gao et al., who warned that the fewer near-miss incidents in emergency treatments in their study may be due to bias in reporting, and when near-misses occur, they can be of greater severity [7].

In summary, emergency services programs should be designed such that all staff are available without causing inconvenience to anyone, patients receive their treatments promptly, an SOP is in place defining the complete workflow, such treatments are not scheduled during ROIS's daily backup timeslot, and an independent MUV is done before delivery of the second treatment fraction.

2 Neurologic Emergencies

2.1 Raised Intracranial Pressure

2.1.1 Clinical Presentation

The most common presenting symptoms are headache and focal neurologic abnormalities. Depending on the location of the lesion and the degree of cerebral edema, the headache may be localized or generalized. Projectile vomiting (which may rarely be accompanied by nausea), seizures, altered sensorium, and even coma may all appear with rising intracranial pressure (ICP). Patients typically have bradycardia and raised blood pressure. Sensorium is variable. Further neurologic deterioration may be prevented with adequate care and prompt identification of the potential cause.

2.1.2 Etiology and Etiopathogenesis

The aforementioned symptoms may indicate the development or progression of brain metastases in a patient with a known systemic cancer once metabolic reasons for altered behavior have been ruled out. Brain metastasis would present as solitary or multiple focal intraparenchymal lesions, dural-based mass, or leptomeningeal dissemination. The three cancers that most frequently metastasize to the brain are melanoma, lung cancer, and breast cancer [8]. Rapid symptom presentation in individuals with known brain tumor would indicate recurrence or progression of a high-grade glioma. ICP elevation can occasionally be caused by hydrocephalus or intratumoral hemorrhage [8, 9]. A tumor's stimulation of vascular endothelial growth factors causes a breach of the blood-brain barrier, increased vascular permeability, vasogenic edema, and raised ICP.

2.1.3 Diagnosis

Imaging is key to diagnosis, especially in a patient with no prior known malignancy. Computed tomography (CT) of the head is usually the first imaging in emergent cases of raised ICP. A non-contrast CT scan can identify a mass lesion, hydrocephalus, herniation, bleed, or mass effect due to edema. If a mass lesion is suspected on plain imaging, a contrast CT or MRI may better define the location and extent of the lesion (or lesions) along with demonstration of any herniation, leptomeningeal enhancement, or obstructive hydrocephalus. MRI is the imaging modality of choice and can identify small metastases and leptomeningeal deposits, and may show abnormalities even when CT is grossly normal [8] (Fig. 1a, b). Perilesional edema causing mass effect may be disproportionate to lesion size in brain metastases (Fig. 1c, d). Imaging features of raised ICP include mass effect on surrounding normal brain due to tumor or surrounding edema, effacement of sulci or cisterns, midline shift, or frank uncial herniation. Immediate biopsy is seldom considered in these clinical and imaging presentations. Only when the clinical findings suggest purely *de novo* CNS disease with equivocal imaging characteristics, then a biopsy would be undertaken after symptomatic management.

2.1.4 Management

Short-term management of raised ICP focuses on symptom relief, followed by definitive management to prevent the recurrence of similar episodes in the future.

Corticosteroids are the cornerstone of symptomatic management and work by reducing vasogenic edema. Depending on the clinical situation, a maximum dose of 16–24 mg dexamethasone (preferred due to negligible mineralocorticoid activity) or equivalent is given in a day divided over 2–3 doses, and subsequently tapered off [10]. Serial monitoring of neurologic status, including sensorium, patient's vitals, and clinical symptoms, would help guide further management over the next 24–72 hours. Other decompressive measures include hyperventilation, diuretics such as mannitol and acetazolamide, or hypertonic saline for short term, and appropriate analgesia and antacid/antiemetics. Those presenting with seizures would also need antiepileptic drugs, although their use as prophylaxis is controversial and not recommended. Patients who undergo surgical resection in the absence of prior seizures also traditionally receive a week of antiepileptics, after which they should be discontinued [11].

For primary glial lesions or lesions causing obstructive hydrocephalus, such as medulloblastomas, primary resection can be done as soon as the patient is stable, offering the best chance of control. Appropriate adjuvant therapy is decided based on the patient's age, disease histology, and extent. For metastatic lesions, the management decision depends on several factors, including primary tumor site and histology, extent of intracranial and extracranial disease, number of lesions within the brain, mass effect, patient's performance status and age, and the expected prognosis in the light of all previous findings. Best supportive care is recommended for patients with poor performance status, extensive disease, and overall poor prognosis with a life expectancy under 3 months. Aggressive management is recommended for the others as it improves longevity. RTOG-derived recursive partition analysis (RPA) divides patients into 3 prognostic groups with different survival, and may serve as a decision-making prognostic tool [12].

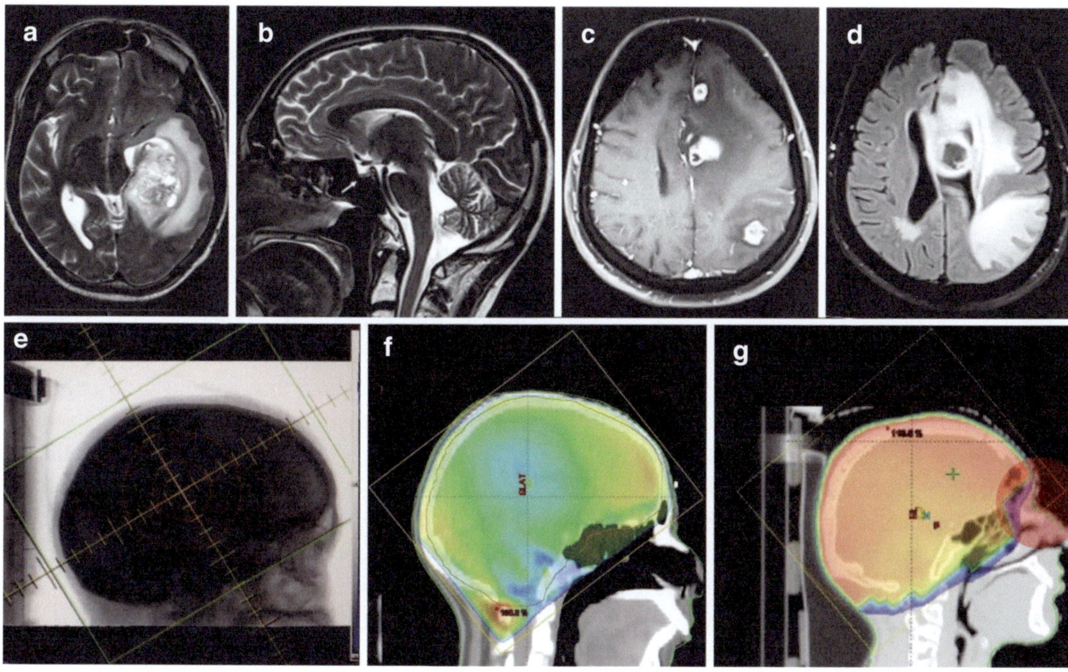

Fig. 1 (**a**) Axial and (**b**) sagittal T2-weighted MR images showing heterogeneous left temporal lobe high-grade glioma with adjoining mass effect and raised intracranial pressure as evidenced by empty Sella (arrow in **b**). (**c**) T1 contrast and (**d**) T2 FLAIR axial images of a patient with renal cell carcinoma who presented with holocranial headache and vomiting. There are multiple enhancing lesions in both cerebral hemispheres with disproportionate edema on FLAIR images. (**e**) Conventional 2-D and (**f**) 3D-CRT field portals (right and left parallel opposed) for whole brain radiotherapy for brain metastases. (**g**) In 3D-CRT, multileaf collimators may be used to shield eyes or other critical structures

For solitary metastases, surgical resection or stereotactic radiosurgery (SRS, as a non-emergency treatment after stabilization of the emergency condition with symptomatic measures) are reasonable options if the lesion size is up to 3 cm. SRS may still be an option for well-preserved patients with up to 4 metastases. Whole-brain radiotherapy is preferred for those with more extensive disease. A dose of 30 gray (Gy) in 10 fractions over 2 weeks is recommended; however, for selected cases, a shorter course of 20 Gy in 5 fractions may be considered (Fig. 1e, f). Based on clinical judgment, SRS boost to gross metastatic disease may be considered. Systemic therapy, as indicated, is initiated based on the patient's age and performance status, primary disease location, extent, and histology.

2.2 Spinal Cord Compression

Spinal cord compression due to epidural malignant disease happens in nearly 5% cancer patients, and may be the presenting feature in almost one-fifth of these. The most common malignancies that result in cord compression are hematologic (multiple myeloma, lymphoma), lung, breast, and prostate cancer [8].

2.2.1 Clinical Presentation

The most common symptom is a backache of variable duration, recent worsening in severity, and aggravation with movement. Neurologic deficits would accompany and may be motor (90%, e.g., paraplegia, gait imbalance, etc.), or sensory (70%, e.g., numbness, tingling, heaviness of limb, perianal numbness), the former being more common [13]. Autonomic dysfunction or cauda equina syndrome may develop in ~40% in the form of altered bowel or bladder habits (urinary incontinence, constipation). Depending on the site of compression, the deficit may be partial (paresis) or complete (paralysis), and may be unilateral or bilateral. Tenderness on palpation is often able to localize the site of the lesion. For those with sensory loss, a sensory level within 2 vertebral levels of the lesion may be discernible. The thoracic vertebrae are most commonly involved [14].

2.2.2 Etiology and Etiopathogenesis

Cord compression most commonly has an extradural origin, secondary to vertebral disease (through either marrow involvement or hematogenous spread). Vertebral lesions may erode cortex, extend into the epidural space, cause spinal canal narrowing, obliterate CSF space, and eventually cause extrinsic compression of the spinal cord or cauda equina, depending on the level of vertebral involvement. Pathologic vertebral fractures may also cause cord compression. Paraspinal mass with extension through neural foramina, leptomeningeal metastases, or intraspinal metastases cause similar symptoms but are far less common. Compression over the spinal cord may lead to loss of neurologic function either directly or due to vascular compromise (due to compression of the epidural venous plexus) and vasogenic intramedullary edema. This would, in time, increase the pressure on small arterioles, causing diminution of capillary vascular flow. If continuing undiminished, this may lead to ischemia and infarction of white matter with permanent damage to spinal cord function at that level.

2.2.3 Diagnosis

History taking and clinical assessment are two core components for initial evaluation. Imaging gives the first clue to the diagnosis. Anterior and lateral views of X-ray spine may hint toward any gross change in vertebral shape or reduction in spinal canal diameter, lytic or sclerotic lesion, collapse, or fracture. It is not possible, however, to visualize the epidural component. A contrast CT scan of the spine or, in stable patients, an MRI (modality of choice) may demonstrate the bony abnormality and the epidural soft tissue component [14]. The entire spine should be imaged, as contiguous or distant vertebral metastases may be seen in nearly 30% patients. Intravenous contrast improves sensitivity and helps diagnose intramedullary metastases and leptomeningeal extension. MRI evaluates the extent of the compressed area and helps in planning radiation therapy. On MRI, tumors that cause cord compression usually are hypointense on T1-weighted images, hyperintense on T2-weighted images, and show enhancement post-contrast. A compressed cord may show a high signal on T2-weighted images due to edema (Fig. 2a, b).

In patients with semi- or non-emergent conditions, other investigations such as bone scan or whole body positron emission tomography—contrast enhanced CT (PET-CECT) may warrant consideration after initial stabilization; however, these are not part of emergency evaluation. CT myelography has reduced in popularity since advent of MRI but may still be considered to identify epidural disease in patients who are not candidates for MRI. A bone scan may estimate the overall extent of metabolic activity but cannot identify epidural cord compression. In selected malignancies, PET-CECT may provide the overall disease extent and activity and can be considered before definitive treatment decisions. Decision-making is tricky for those who have no prior diagnosis of malignancy. If the diagnosis is almost certain based on clinical assessment and imaging is corroborative, the clinical condition warrants immediate anticancer management, and obtaining a biopsy would delay emergency management and its efficacy. A decision to proceed without biopsy may occasionally have to be taken after discussion with oncology peers, and with the patients and their caregivers. All such decisions should be adequately documented and agreed upon. If surgical stabilization is considered part of management, histopathologic proof of malignancy would be easy to obtain in the same sitting.

2.2.4 Management

Corticosteroids should be started promptly for cord compression with present or impending

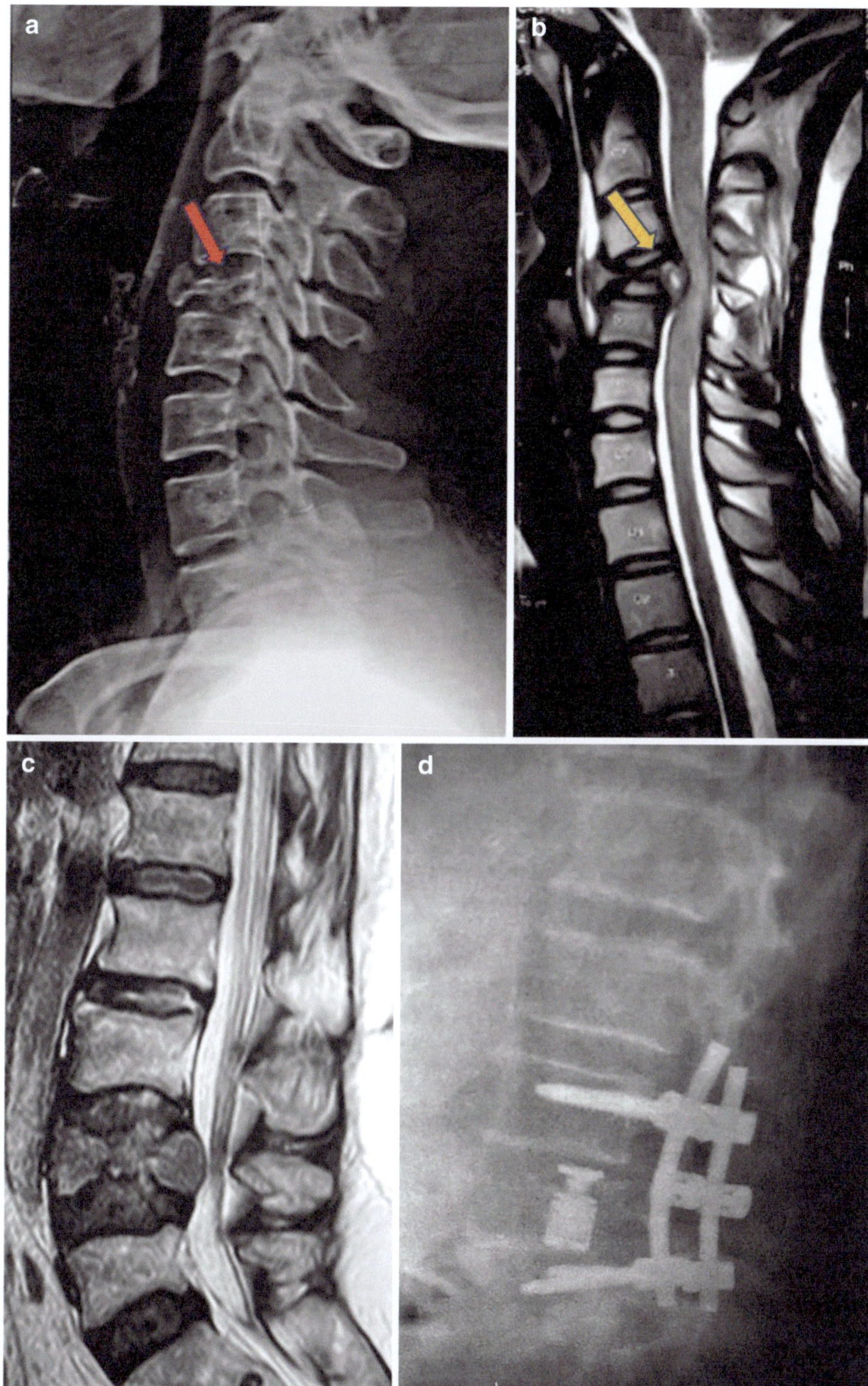

Fig. 2 (**a**) Radiograph of the cervical spine showing collapse of the C4 cervical vertebra (red arrow) in a patient with bronchogenic carcinoma. (**b**) T2-weighted sagittal MR sections of the same patient show cord compression (orange arrow) secondary to a collapsed vertebra. (**c**) Sagittal T2-weighted MRI showing L4 vertebral collapse in a patient presenting with back pain. The patient underwent surgical stabilization, including vertebral prosthesis insertion. (**d**) Lateral spine X-ray showing the surgical hardware (screws, rods, and plates). Biopsy and subsequent workup suggested multiple myeloma, and he received palliative radiotherapy to L3–L5 vertebral (30 gray in 10 fractions)

neurologic deficit and may help prevent further neurologic deterioration. It should ideally be started within 24 hours of the onset of the deficit and preferably within 72 hours. Once the neuro-deficit becomes fixed, reducing vasogenic edema would not help reverse the neurologic compromise. High-dose steroids (dexamethasone 16–24 mg/day or methylprednisolone 1 g/day) are needed, followed by tapering over 1–2 weeks, and often help in improving ambulation as well as relieving pain [15]. Initial intravenous therapy followed by a switch to oral therapy after 1–2 days is well tolerated. Rarely, when lymphomas are suspected, steroids should be given at a lower dose, if necessary, till a prompt biopsy can be obtained.

Improvement in neuro-deficit following steroids indicates that the deficit is reversible and related to mass effect rather than neuronal damage; these patients benefit most from definitive therapy.

The definitive treatment would depend on spinal stability. Patients with unstable spine or fracture fragment impinging on the cord need a brace to reduce spinal movement, such as a neck collar or a thoracolumbar brace, followed by surgical stabilization on an emergency basis (Fig. 2c, d). The NOMS (neurologic, oncologic, mechanical instability, systemic disease) or SINS (spinal instability neoplastic score) criteria may help to standardize decision-making [16, 17] (Tables 2 and 3).

Table 2 Spinal Instability Neoplastic Score (SINS) criteria for assessment of spinal instability status

Component	Criteria	Score
Location	Junctional (O–C2; C7–T2; T11–L1; L5–S1) Mobile spine (C3–6; L2–4) Semirigid (T3–10) Rigid (S2-S5)	3 2 1 0
Mechanical pain	Yes No Lesion is pain-free	3 2 1
Type of bone lesion	Lytic Mixed Blastic	2 1 0
Spine alignment on radiology	Subluxation/translation present Deformity (kyphosis/scoliosis) Normal	4 2 0
Degree of vertebral body collapse	>50% collapse <50% collapse >50% body involved but no collapse <50% body involved, no collapse	3 2 1 0
Involvement of posterolateral elements	Bilateral Unilateral None	3 1 0

Score: Maximum – 18, Minimum – 1
>13: Unstable: Needs surgical stabilization
7–12: Potentially unstable: Surgical consultation and possibly stabilization
<12: Stable: May benefit from radiotherapy or systemic therapy

Patients with radiosensitive tumors should receive palliative radiotherapy to the spine, starting as soon as possible, either upfront (in a stable spine) or after stabilization surgery, to reduce the probability of further neurologic decline. The most straightforward technique that takes minimum time to plan and execute, usually two-dimensional (2D RT) or 3D-CRT, is preferred. Beam arrangement is kept simple, and margins are liberal (one vertebral level above and below the level of compression craniocaudally, lateral extent encompassing the span of transverse processes, depth of prescription is kept such that the epidural soft tissue receives at least 90% of the prescribed dose) so that the requirement of daily image verification is minimized. Patient is treated in the most comfortable position, usually supine, with appropriate neck/knee/foot support. The number of fractions is decided based on the patient's general condition, neurologic status, and extent of compression. Patients with minimal neurologic deficits or those that have improved with steroids, with compression at limited spinal segments and good overall prognosis, are usually planned for a longer course (usually 30 Gy in 10 fractions). Those with an overall poor prognosis, fixed irreversible deficits, inability to lie down, or multiple levels of compression may be considered for shorter courses such as 20 Gy in 5 fractions, or occasionally a single fraction (8 Gy). Retrospective studies have demonstrated similar

Table 3 NOMS criteria for treatment decisions in spinal lesions

Neurologic	Oncologic	Mechanical	Systemic	Recommended therapy
Low-grade epidural spinal cord compression (Bilsky grade 0–1), no myelopathy	Radiosensitive	Stable		Upfront conventional fractionated external beam radiotherapy (EBRT)
		Unstable		Surgical stabilization followed by EBRT
	Radioresistant	Stable		Stereotactic body radiotherapy (SBRT)
		Unstable		Surgical stabilization followed by SBRT
High grade epidural spinal cord compression (Bilsky grade 2–31), with or without myelopathy	Radiosensitive	Stable		Upfront EBRT
		Unstable		Surgical stabilization followed by EBRT
	Radioresistant	Stable	Able to tolerate surgery	Surgical stabilization/ decompression followed by SBRT
			Unable to tolerate surgery	EBRT
		Unstable	Able to tolerate surgery	Surgical stabilization/ decompression followed by SBRT
			Unable to tolerate surgery	Surgical stabilization/ decompression followed by EBRT

post-treatment ambulation with all regimes, ranging from 1 to 20 fractions. However, shorter regimes had higher in-field recurrences [18]. Although stereotactic body radiotherapy (SBRT) also finds a role in managing vertebral metastases with an epidural component in recent times, it is a time-consuming process with a negligible role in an emergency. It can, however, be considered as a non-emergency treatment in a patient with a stable or surgically stabilized spine and minimal neurologic deficits, provided it is possible to wait 2–3 days to initiate radiotherapy after stability has been ensured and the patient can cooperate and comfortably lie down for simulation, image guidance, and therapy for 15–30 min for each fraction.

Prognosis depends on the rapidity of onset of symptoms, pre-treatment ambulatory status, and radiosensitivity of the tumor. Based on time to development of motor deficits, Rades et al. divided patients into 3 groups: A (1–6 days), B (8–14 days), C (>14 days) with respective post-treatment symptom improvement and ambulatory rates of (A) 10% and 35%, (B) 29% and 55%, and (C) 86% [19]. This study underscores the importance of prompt diagnosis and therapy.

2.3 Bone Pain

2.3.1 Clinical Presentation

Patients with metastatic or primary bone disease present with localized pain of varying duration and severity. Bone pain may also be a presenting feature in patients with hematological malignancies such as multiple myeloma or acute leukemias, in which case the pain may be generalized. Other accompanying symptoms may be fever, localized swelling or loss of function, these 'other' symptoms would be specific to the site of origin of malignancy A patient with loss of appetite or weight,or, both together over a short period, usually has advanced disease.

Vertebral localization may produce signs such as tenderness, motor, sensory, or autonomic deficits as discussed earlier in the section on spinal cord compression. If located in the appendicular skeleton, surface changes, such as skin discoloration, localized mass, tenderness, or limitation of joint movement, may be present.

2.3.2 Etiology and Etiopathogenesis

Bone pain may occur in the absence of a fracture at a metastatic site, and the mechanism of the same is not well understood. Disruption of skeletal architecture due to increased osteoclastic activity, bone resorption, and decreased bone density may lead to microfractures involving bony trabeculae and bone distortion [20]. Tumor expansion, bone weakening leading to mechanical stress, entrapment of nerves in periosteum and around blood vessels, direct bone destruction, and nerve infiltration may give rise to mechanical or neurogenic pain. Cytokines responsible for bone resorption may activate pain receptors. Pro-algesic chemicals released within the marrow may produce pain disproportionate to the extent apparent on examination and imaging. Reactive muscle spasm may also contribute to pain. Pathologic fractures may produce severe mechanical pain aggravated with movement for patients with lytic lesions.

2.3.3 Diagnosis

An X-ray of the involved region in appropriate views can demonstrate a lytic/sclerotic lesion or fracture as the cause of pain. CT and MRI are undertaken after initial symptomatic measures to assess the extent of disease, including any soft tissue or marrow involvement. For those with known malignancy, review of prior imaging and disease/treatment details may give adequate clues to diagnosis. Additional assessment should include a review of systems to determine the disease extent, including other sites of metastases, pathologic fracture, or risk of development of the same at the painful site, patient's performance status, relief with conservative measures, and expected prognosis. Patients with known fractures should be assessed for any distal vascular or neurologic compromise, hematoma, and ongoing bleeding. The NOMS framework and SINS criteria have been discussed earlier. Mirels' criteria may help triage patients with pain in long bones according to need for prophylactic surgical fixation based on 4 factors: (a) Site (upper limb, lower limb, trochanteric region), (b) Size of lesion (involving <1/3, 1/3–2/3, >2/3 of cortex), (c) Nature of lesion (blastic, mixed, and lytic), (d) Pain severity (mild, moderate, functional pain) [21]. Based on these factors, scores of 1–3 are given for each factor. A total score of 9 or above indicates the need for prophylactic fixation, while those with 7 or below can be considered for radiotherapy; a score of 8 merits clinical judgment for appropriate therapy. Several prognostic tools that incorporate patient age, performance status, disease histology and extent, prior treatment, and time course of development of bone metastases, such as that devised by Rades and colleagues and RPA developed at Stanford, are available to guide treatment strategies [22, 23] (Table 4).

2.3.4 Management

The initial management consists of pain control with appropriate analgesia. Patients with severe pain or fracture may require narcotics till the cause has been addressed. Emergency orthopedics consultation is needed for appropriate handling and correction/immobilization of the fractured/painful site. Patients with pathologic fractures need prompt correction with external immobilization or internal fixation. Hemodynamic monitoring and management should continue simultaneously. Depending on the primary disease and extent, additional systemic therapies include bone-targeted agents, such as bisphosphonates and, after stabilization, consideration of radionuclides, such as Phosphorus-32, Radium-227, Samarium-153, Strontium-89, Lutetium-177, or Actinium-225-based therapies.

If a decision for radiotherapy has been taken, treatment should be initiated as soon as possible. The patient is appropriately positioned, ensuring comfort and reproducibility at the affected site with proper exposure for radiotherapy field placement. Immobilization devices, such as thermoplastic casts or vacuum cushions can be used for multi-fractionated regimes, with pillow/knee or foot rest as needed for support. Limb position

Table 4 Recursive partitioning analysis for overall survival of patients with bone metastases correlated to tumor origin, performance status, and age

Tumor site	KPS	Age (years)	Overall survival (months)
Breast			35.9
Prostate	≥80		16.9
	<80		4.4
Other	≥80		14.2
	<80		7.5
Lung		<60	8.7
		≥60	3.5
Gastrointestinal	≥80		8.0
	<80		2.3

should be such that it does not interfere with beam entry or exit. Depending upon the clinical situation, manual marking, conventional simulation, or CT-based simulation may be appropriate. Patients with severe pain that may not withstand transfer from one machine to another may be considered for manual marking, while those with less severe pain and tolerant to multiple repositioning sessions may be considered for simulation. The latter may define the disease extent better, and treatment volume may be tailored accordingly. If manual marking is performed, diagnostic images and the extent of tenderness guide the radiation fields. Whatever the target volume determination process, the least time-consuming and simplest treatment should be chosen for easy and least painful reproducible positioning. Symptomatic lesion with 1–2 cm margin should be included within at least 90% isodose of prescribed dose (higher margins for long bones or more mobile sites). Ideally, the edges of treatment fields should coincide with anatomic borders so that subsequent adjacent fields can be matched if future treatments are required. When treating vertebral lesions using conventional methods, the whole vertebra should be included, even for lesions localized to a subpart. When treating long bones, joints should be excluded from the field if uninvolved. If instrumentation precedes radiotherapy, one should discuss the intraoperative findings with the surgeon, and include the entire prosthesis in the long bones, and the entire vertebra with adjacent vertebrae in vertebral lesions. A corridor of normal tissue should be spared to allow adequate lymphatic drainage in limbs; treatments including the entire circumferential extent of the limb should be avoided. For vertebral metastases treated with conventional simulation, the dose is prescribed at the mid-body or posterior body, depending on vertebral and epidural disease. For long bones, the dose is prescribed at midplane. For CT-based 3D-CRT, the gross disease with appropriate planning target volume (PTV) should receive at least 90% of the prescribed dose. A single-field or two-field arrangement may be sufficient for most cases. Electron beam may be used for rib lesions, while 4–6 MV photons suffice for other sites.

Randomized evidence shows that pain control, need for narcotics, and rate of future pathologic fractures were similar with 8 Gy/single fraction, 20 Gy/5 fractions, or 30 Gy/10 fractions [24, 25]. Over 65% response rates are observed with nearly one-third not needing narcotics after 3 months of radiotherapy. However, the durability of pain is lower in low-dose schedules with a higher need for retreatments. The radiation dose may be tailored according to pain severity and stability. For those with painful, uncomplicated bone metastases (~65%, no fracture or compression existing or expected), a single fraction of 8 Gy suffices. For those with painful, complicated (fracture, compression) metastases, patients with good performance status or life expectancy of 1 year or less may be managed with 8 Gy/single fraction, while others may warrant longer treatments (5 or 10 fractions) (Fig. 3a–d). Patients with oligometastases (3 or less) may be considered either for 30 Gy in 10 fractions, or in non-emergency situations where pain is mild to moderate and reasonably controlled with analgesics, a consideration for SBRT can be made.

Patients with extensive metastatic disease involving the entire skeleton may benefit from systemic therapy, including bone-targeted agents, and limited-volume radiotherapy to the most painful sites. However, patients who are unfit for or refractory to systemic agents may be considered for hemi-body radiotherapy, though its use has declined with newer systemic therapy options. Treatment is carried out at an extended source-to-surface distance to encompass the entire target volume. Patient is made to lie supine on the treatment room floor with the couch rotated outside the field and gantry at zero degrees. Radiotherapy is usually delivered in a single fraction of 8 Gy in the lower hemibody and 6 Gy (with lung shield) for the upper hemibody.

3 Tumor Bleed: Upper/Lower Gastrointestinal Tract, Hematuria, Skin/Soft Tissue, and Gynecologic

3.1 Clinical Presentation

Large tumors with aberrant blood vessels, or those that erode into blood vessels during their growth, may cause tumor bleeds that present as emergencies. Oropharyngeal, esophageal, or gastric tumors present with hematemesis, tracheal or pulmonary tumors with hemoptysis, gastrointestinal tumors with melena or fresh rectal bleed, urinary tract malignancies with hematuria, and gynecologic malignancies with vaginal bleeding. Occasionally, tumor bleed is superficial—from skin (squamous cell carcinoma, melanoma), soft tissue (sarcoma) tumors, or fungating lymph nodes. Bleeding episodes range from minimal ooze to large-volume bleeds, which may be life-threatening.

Patients may present with visible bleeding from the surface or into body fluids. Internal bleeding within the viscera may cause progressive severe anemia, deep-seated pain, abdominal distension and shock. Uncontrolled, severe intra-abdominal bleeding in oncology patients is uncommon but life-threatening. Hypervascular tumors like hepatocellular carcinoma (HCC), renal cell carcinoma, and melanoma can produce spontaneous hemoperitoneum [26]. In HCC patients, 10%–15% of patients may present in emergency with intra-abdominal bleed [27]. Lymphoma and leukemia can present with massive abdominal hemorrhage due to spontaneous splenic rupture.

3.2 Etiology and Etiopathogenesis

Atypical neoangiogenesis causes the vasculature of tumors to develop abnormally. These aberrant blood vessels can cause large tumors to hemorrhage and form necrotic regions. Vessels invaded by tumors may bleed, and if a major artery is damaged, the results are catastrophic. In rare cases, bleeding results from tumor regression following radiation or chemotherapy if the initial tumor that was obstructing the vessel has receded. Treatments such as anti-angiogenesis drugs like bevacizumab, anti-inflammatory drugs with antiplatelet action, and anticoagulant drugs for coexisting disorders (cardiac disease, deep venous thrombosis, etc.) can make the bleeding worse. Patients are more susceptible to bleeding if they have thrombocytopenia brought on by a disease (leukemia, myeloma, marrow invasion by solid tumors), chemotherapy, or bone-targeted radionuclides.

3.3 Diagnosis

The route, rate, and volume of bleed, along with the patient's general condition, would determine the source of bleed, whether the bleed is life-threatening or merely a pointer to possible malignancy that needs to be investigated. Symptoms in preceding weeks can indicate the possible origin of internal bleeds. Investigations include complete blood counts (CBC), coagulation profile, renal (KFT) and liver (LFT) function assessment, and other biochemical parameters depending on suspected organ deficit. Contributing factors such

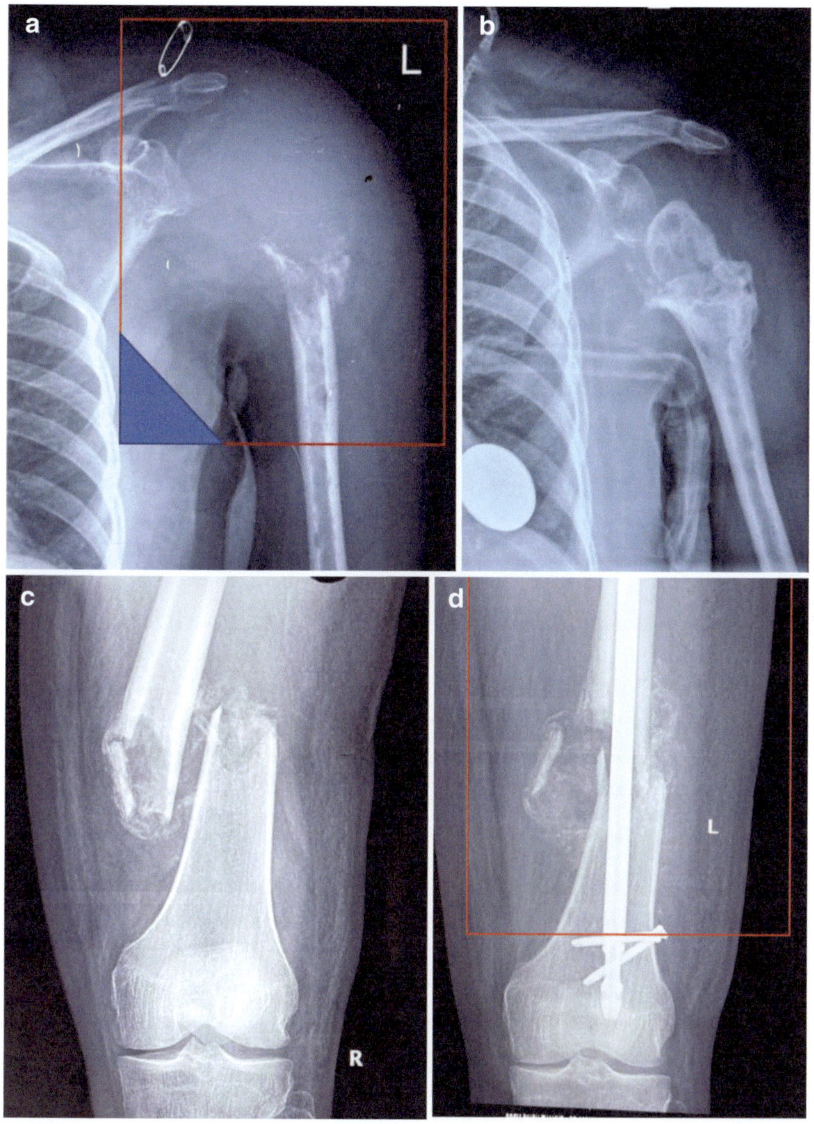

Fig. 3 (**a**) Lytic lesion destroying the head of the left humerus on a left shoulder X-ray in a patient with multiple myeloma, presenting with severe pain and restricted shoulder mobility. She received palliative radiotherapy (20 Gy/5 Fractions, parallel opposed anteroposterior and posteroanterior fields with dose prescribed at midplane, anterior field portal indicated by red outline and corner shield with the blue triangle) with 90% pain relief within a week of RT. (**b**) X-ray of the same patient 2 months after RT with resolution of lytic change and new bone formation. (**c**) A known patient of renal cell carcinoma post-nephrectomy 5 years ago presented with a history of a fall and a displaced pathologic fracture left femur. He underwent open reduction and internal fixation of the fractured limb due to an unstable fracture. (**d**) X-rays 1 month after surgery show callus formation, but the bone is still not united. He has minimal pain and slight gait instability. He received palliative radiotherapy (30 Gy in 10 fractions, parallel opposed anteroposterior and posteroanterior fields with dose prescribed at midplane, anterior field portal indicated by red outline, sparing a strip of lymphatic corridor medially) to the left thigh, followed by systemic therapy

as medication, comorbid conditions, and recent interventions should be elicited in history taking. Imaging the site of bleeding (chest, abdomen, head and neck, limb) should be carried out promptly. Sites such as the urinary tract need endoscopic evaluation. On non-contrast CT, acute intra-abdominal hemorrhage appears as high-attenuation fluid (approximately 30–45 HU). Source of bleeding is identified in some patients by the location of the "sentinel clot," which represents a high-attenuation hematoma. After intravenous contrast injection, active contrast extravasation within the tumor or at peritumoral location suggests ongoing bleed.

3.4 Management

Visible bleeding in the form of ooze may not mandate emergent management but may be disturbing to the patient. It also contributes to anemia and thus needs to be addressed semi-urgently. Patients with known terminal disease need only supportive management without heroic measures, including limiting mobility and appropriate sedation, along with counseling for the eventual outcome.

Catastrophic bleeds are rapidly fatal. If the patient has a salvageable condition, efforts should be made for immediate mobilization of the patient to the hospital. The first and foremost step for unstable patients with torrential bleeding and hemodynamic compromise is stabilization. For patients with upper aerodigestive tract bleeds, securing the airway, ensuring adequate ventilation, and maintaining blood pressure (intravenous fluid or blood transfusion) are needed on an emergent basis.

Discontinuation/dose modification/replacement of responsible/exacerbating agents (e.g., anticoagulants), vitamin K supplementation, blood products or plasma to correct coagulation disorders, and initiation of agents, such as tranexamic acid, help reduce further bleeding episodes. Superficial sites may benefit from local pressure, decreased mobility, non-adherent dressing or packing, or topical agents such as Moh's paste and Monsel's solution in gynecologic tumors [28].

After stabilization, endoscopic assessment (upper gastrointestinal endoscopy, bronchoscopy) would help assess the source and location of the bleed, obtain histologic proof of malignancy if not already available, and, if necessary, plan interventions such as embolization, clipping, LASER, or tumor resection. Large vessel bleeds require emergent interventional procedures, while small vessel or capillary bleeds benefit most from radiotherapy. Imaging (CXR, CT scan) helps estimate tumor size, location, and extensions, and thus guides palliative radiotherapy, which should begin as soon as possible after stabilization of acute bleed [29]. The radiotherapy course and fractionation depend on disease prognosis (based on disease stage and histology) and the patient's performance status. Patients who are stable and have a curable non-metastatic malignancy are considered for curative treatment in standard fractionation (e.g., concurrent chemoradiation with radiation dose of 66–70 Gy at 2 Gy per fraction for a base of tongue carcinoma), as institution of therapy would help control symptoms as well as the disease process. Simple techniques (2D-RT or 3DCRT) with minimum setup requirements and treatment time are instituted for the initial 2–5 fractions and subsequently switched to more advanced but time- and labor-intensive techniques such as intensity modulated radiation therapy (IMRT) if the patient and disease are suitable for the same. Those with metastatic disease, poor performance status, or overall poor prognosis can be treated with hypofractionated regimes such as 8 Gy in a single fraction, 20 Gy in 5 fractions, or 30 Gy in 10 fractions. Retrospective single and multi-institution series have shown a response rate of 70%–85%, with nearly 25% achieving relief immediately on starting therapy [30, 31].

Patients with bleeding from esophageotracheal or gastrointestinal fistulation due to tumor extension need surgical or radiological interventions for stabilization rather than considering radiotherapy. Bleeding due to varices or peptic ulcers does not merit radiotherapy. Palliative or definitive radiotherapy may be instituted for esophageal cancers depending on the overall plan for disease management. Palliative external beam radiotherapy (EBRT) for the esophagus encompasses the entire extent of gross tumor with a 2–3 cm craniocaudal and 1–2 cm radial margin. Treatment is delivered using 2 or 4 fields with appropriate energy. Treatment courses vary from single to 15-fraction schedules. Intraluminal radiotherapy is usually not feasible for patients with active bleeding but is considered for those with bleeding controlled after interventional techniques or initial EBRT. Symptomatic relief, including arrest of bleeding, is seen in over 70% patients. Durability of response depends on total dose delivered and is better for those receiving doses higher than 20 Gy in 5 fractions. Expected lifespan in the light of disease stage and patient's performance status helps treatment decisions of dose and duration of radiotherapy [32]. The role of radiotherapy is less well-defined for bleeding due to gastric cancers. Palliative radiotherapy is an option for patient after failed endoscopic hemostatic techniques or as a consolidating measure in those with advanced incurable disease following successful hemostasis. Regimes with a high biologically effective dose of at least 30 Gy to 39 Gy in 10 fractions are preferred if logistically feasible. A median time of 2–15 days is observed for hemostasis. Palliative radiotherapy helps improve survival in patients with unresectable disease, even in conjunction with other therapies, and responders live longer than non-responders [33]. Similar doses for incurable rectal cancers with bleeding have led to response rates of 80%, with delivered dose determining durability but not the degree of initial response [34].

In genitourinary malignancies presenting with hematuria, the site of disease and source of bleed help determine the need for radiotherapy. Most of these tumors are deemed radioresistant, and alternative measures (e.g., vascular embolization to shrink tumor volume, nephrectomy for renal cell carcinoma, or tumor resection for urothelial malignancies) result in arrest of bleeding. Bladder malignancies with extensive mucosal involvement not controlled with tumor resection and bladder irrigation, patients with castrate-refractory prostate cancer, or patients with poor performance status who are not candidates for surgical resection can be considered for hemostatic radiotherapy. Shorter regimes with high biological doses are as effective as more protracted regimes [35]. Patients with cervical cancer and bleeding respond favorably to supportive measures, including vaginal packing with hemostatic agents such as tranexamic acid and adrenaline. Those with curable disease may be initiated on conventional fractionated curative radiotherapy. Those with advanced disease or poor performance status are offered palliative radiotherapy (1–5 fractions of 3–8 Gy each) and further treatment determined by response and performance status [36].

Skin and soft tissue tumors with bleeding respond well to symptomatic relief of nearly 90%. Various regimes include 1–10 fractions, with dose per fraction ranging from 3 to 10 Gy, and delivered either daily or weekly [37]. The target volume consists of a visible tumor with a 1–2 cm margin radially. The dose is prescribed using electrons or low-energy photons to the tumor depth assessed on palpation or imaging. For bleeding soft tissue sarcomas involving limbs, if other interventions have not succeeded in controlling bleeding and surgery is not being considered immediately, two-field palliative radiotherapy prescribed at midplane helps.

Radiotherapy causes vascular damage and increases the endothelial cell procoagulant activity. Higher secretion of von Willebrand factor (vWf) leads to downstream pathways that mediate radiation response [38].

Patients with ongoing bleeding need emergency embolization or emergent surgical exploration [26]. Minimally invasive image-guided angiography and embolization are the mainstay in the emergency management of uncontrolled malignancy-associated intra-abdominal hemorrhage. Arteries supplying the tumor are selectively cannulated using angiographic catheters and microcatheters under fluoroscopic guidance. Bland embolization is subsequently performed by introducing various embolic agents such as gel foam, polyvinyl alcohol particles, glue, and coils singly or in various combinations into the tumor bed and feeding vessel (Fig. 4a–d). This technique can be used alone as the primary treatment modality or more commonly in combina-

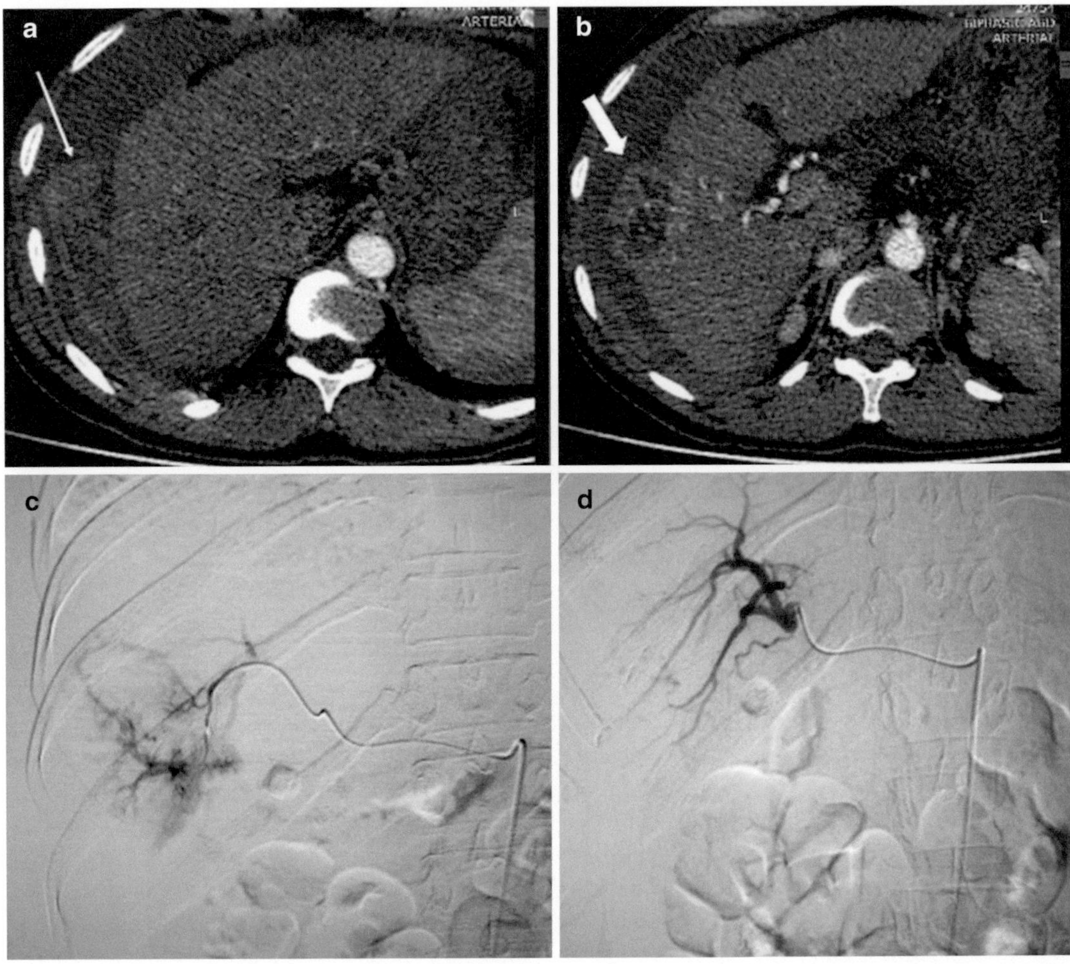

Fig. 4 (**a**) MDCT angiography of the abdomen (**a** and **b**) showing acute intraperitoneal hemorrhage (thin white arrow). (**b**) A transverse section taken inferiorly in the same patient reveals a peripheral hypervascular hepatocellular carcinoma in the background of cirrhotic liver, which has ruptured (thick white arrow). Digital subtraction angiography shows a hyper vascular mass lesion in the right lobe of the liver (**c**), which was embolized using gel foam (**d**)

tion with surgery or percutaneous ablations [39]. In HCC, absence of arterial enhancement on a 4–6 week follow-up scan suggests complete necrosis of the previous viable tumor and hence clinical success of bland embolization [40]. Arterial embolization before the surgery of vascular tumors helps in reducing intraoperative blood loss. Embolization is also used to palliate some inoperable tumors [41].

4 Thoracic Emergencies

4.1 Superior Vena Cava Obstruction

Malignancies most commonly associated with superior vena cava (SVC) syndrome are lung cancer, lymphomas, and metastatic mediastinal tumors.

4.1.1 Clinical Presentation

Usual symptoms are mild to moderate breathlessness, and many patients may have a sense of fullness in the upper body and face, cough, or arm swelling. In severe cases, there may be hypoxia, chest pain, hoarseness of voice (involvement of the recurrent laryngeal nerve), and dysphagia. More severe cases have hoarseness, headache, confusion, and syncope. The manifestations may be due to the underlying etiology, rapidity of onset, and obstruction of the SVC per se [42]. Clinically, there may be evidence of visible veins over the neck and chest wall with plethora of the face. There is often obvious venous distension of the neck and chest wall.

4.1.2 Etiology and Etiopathogenesis

SVC is a thin-walled structure in the mediastinum. Malignancies of the lung and those involving mediastinal lymph nodes can cause compression of the SVC, leading to partial or complete obstruction in blood flow, reduced venous return of head, neck, and upper limb, and consequently the manifestations of SVC syndrome [43]. External compression with or without secondary luminal thrombus leads to backup of blood in this crucial vessel. When the process is slow, there is time for collaterals to develop, and manifestations are subtle [44]. However, in patients with aggressive cancers (lymphoblastic lymphomas, certain germ cell tumors), the presentation is acute with hypoxia and may be rapidly life-threatening.

4.1.3 Diagnosis

SVC syndrome is a clinical diagnosis; however, a CT is required to visualize the lumen of the SVC and brachiocephalic veins and to evaluate associated tumors. CT can provide information regarding tumor size, its characterization and relationship with surrounding structures. CT can accurately delineate the site of obstruction, differentiate between stenosis and occlusion, and between intravascular thrombosis versus extravascular compression (Fig. 5a, b). This information provides a roadmap for subsequent endovascular intervention if planned.

4.1.4 Management

When there are emergency indications for treatment (usually very rare), venovenous stenting can be attempted when possible. Other emergency options are a short course of steroids or radiation. However, steroids or radiation may mask diagnosis, such as lymphomas, and an attempt must be made to establish the diagnosis

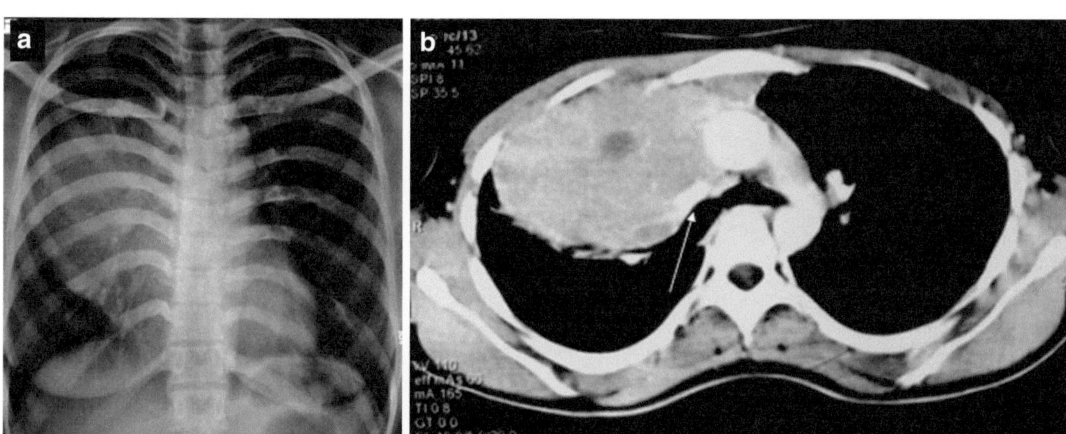

Fig. 5 (**a**) Chest radiograph showing a large mass in the right hemithorax. (**b**) CT scan shows a large anterior mediastinal mass causing compression of the SVC (arrow). True cut biopsy from the lesion revealed the lesion to be high-grade lymphoma

before starting them. In most patients, there is enough time to establish a diagnosis and begin appropriate treatment for the underlying cancer. Investigations that can be done within 1–2 days of presentation in most centers are CXR/CT, serum markers (HCG, AFP for germ cell tumors), guided FNAC/ biopsy from the mass, and blood and marrow investigations (when lymphoblastic etiology is suspected). If a patient has life-threatening SVC syndrome, endovascular thrombolysis and/or recanalization of involved central veins can be done. Access can be taken either from the jugular and femoral vein, and venoplasty of the SVC or brachiocephalic vein with or without stent placement can be done [45] (Fig. 6a–d).

Curable conditions, including non-metastatic lung cancer, lymphomas, germ cell tumors, and thymomas, will require disease-appropriate multi-agent chemotherapy, with local therapy (usually radiation and sometimes surgery) [46] (Fig. 7).

4.2 Hemoptysis

Massive hemoptysis is defined as the expectoration of 300–600 mL of blood over 24 h, and mortality is as high as 60% if massive hemoptysis is secondary to malignancy [1]. Bronchogenic carcinoma is the most common culprit, followed by bronchial carcinoids and endobronchial metastases. In addition, invasive fungal infections such

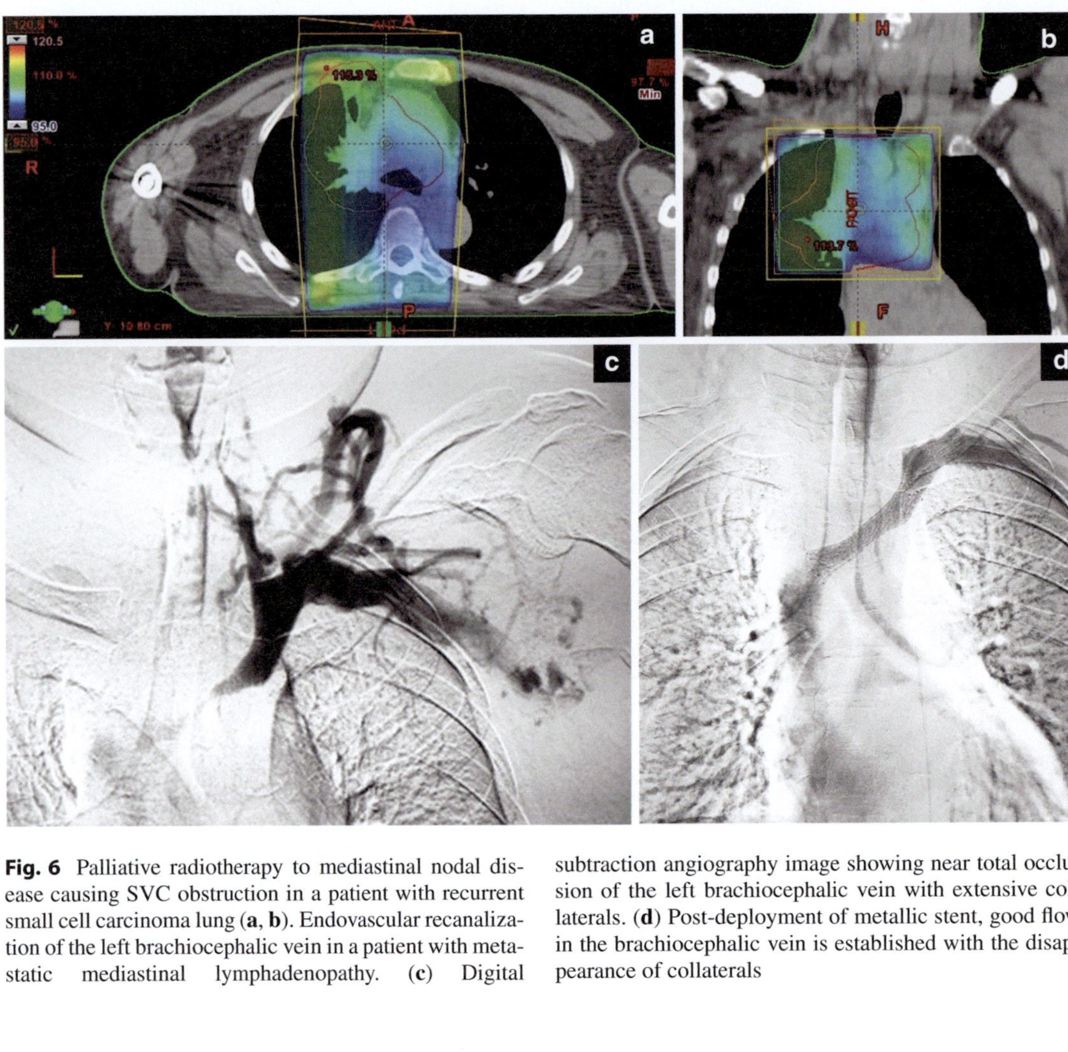

Fig. 6 Palliative radiotherapy to mediastinal nodal disease causing SVC obstruction in a patient with recurrent small cell carcinoma lung (**a**, **b**). Endovascular recanalization of the left brachiocephalic vein in a patient with metastatic mediastinal lymphadenopathy. (**c**) Digital subtraction angiography image showing near total occlusion of the left brachiocephalic vein with extensive collaterals. (**d**) Post-deployment of metallic stent, good flow in the brachiocephalic vein is established with the disappearance of collaterals

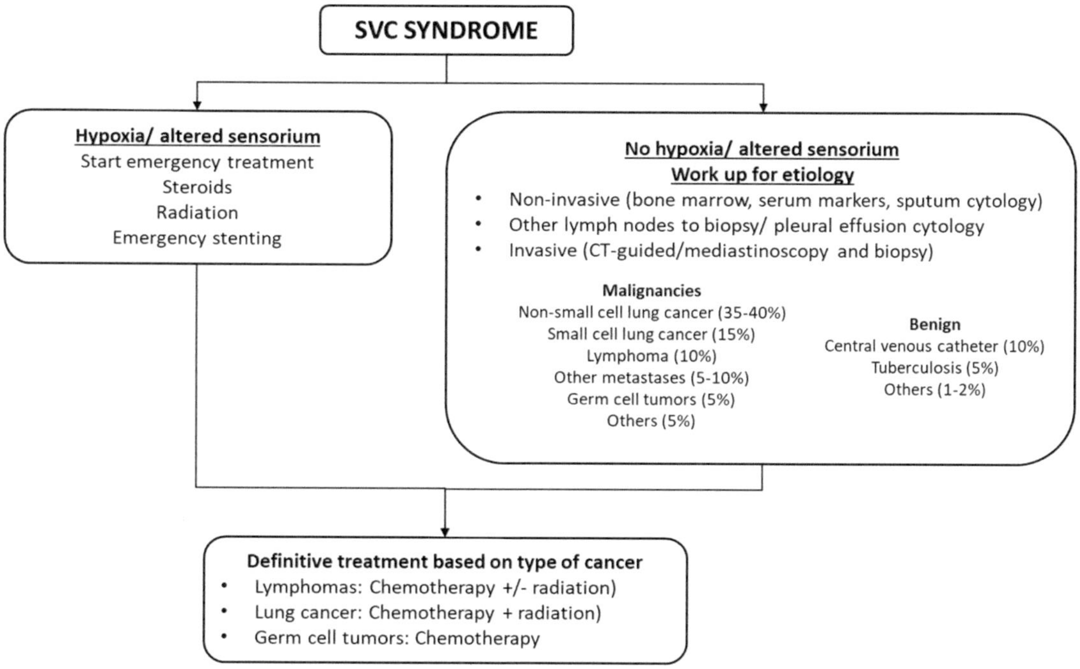

Fig. 7 Approach to a patient with SVC syndrome

as aspergillosis in an immunocompromised oncologic patient can also cause massive hemoptysis [1, 47].

4.2.1 Signs and Symptoms

The patient should be assessed for signs and symptoms of massive bleeding, such as tachycardia, tachypnea, airway obstruction, use of accessory muscles, and cyanosis.

4.2.2 Etiology and Etiopathogenesis

Hemoptysis is defined as expectoration of blood, which can range from mild blood streaking of sputum to gross blood with or without sputum. Hemoptysis in cancer patients can occur due to underlying malignancy or side effects of the treatment. Other possible etiologies include bronchiectasis, tuberculosis, pulmonary aspergillosis, thromboembolism, AV malformation, and certain chemotherapeutic drugs such as bevacizumab. Massive or life-threatening hemoptysis is a rare but lethal condition, but there is no consensus on the definition. Numerous definitions have been proposed to define massive hemoptysis, with blood loss ranging from >100 ml/24 h to >1000 ml/24 h [48]. ACR has graded hemoptysis as minor (<30 ml/24 h), moderate to severe or major (30–300 ml/24 h), and severe (>300 to 400 ml in 24 h) [49] Aspiration, airway obstruction, and hypotension are the major complications of massive hemoptysis, leading to a high mortality rate [50].

4.2.3 Diagnosis

Diagnostic evaluation depends on the grade of hemoptysis. A CXR should be done in all cases and may show tumors, cavities, consolidations, and mediastinal masses. Thin-section CECT chest is needed for recurrence, worsening symptoms, and a high risk of malignancy in stable patients [48]. MDCT can identify the etiology and site and differentiate between bronchial arterial or pulmonary arterial sources of bleeding. MDCT angiography shows the origin, diameter, and course of the bronchial arteries, nonbronchial systemic collaterals, and pulmonary arteries, which may be responsible for hemoptysis. MDCT angiography provides a road map before catheter angiography and facilitates the procedure [1].

Flexible bronchoscopy should be performed if the CT scan is non-contributory [51]. A CT pulmonary angiogram should be done if pulmonary embolism is suspected. Laboratory studies depend on the possible causes and may include CBC, hematocrit levels, coagulation profile, LFT, KFT, sputum culture, and serological testing [52].

4.2.4 Management

Management strategies depend on the degree and severity of hemoptysis. Supportive care includes airway management, oxygenation, ensuring hemodynamic stability, and blood transfusion wherever indicated. The patient should be immediately placed in a decubitus (lying) position; it may be lateral decubitus position where the probable bleeding side is down. Known or suspected bleeding disorders should be corrected.

It is essential to intervene early, as massive hemoptysis can lead to aspiration and complicate airway obstruction. Securing the airway is the most crucial step. In patients with life-threatening bleed, endotracheal intubation using a large-bore endotracheal (ET) tube should be done as a large ET tube can facilitate blood and thrombus extraction and diagnostic bronchoscopy. Bronchoscopic options to manage bleeding include iced saline lavage, infusion of topical vasoconstrictive agents, bronchial blockade device, and balloon tamponade, ablative therapies such as LASER therapy, argon plasma coagulation (APC), or cryotherapy. Surgery is reserved for arterial fistula, pulmonary artery rupture, trauma, and refractory cases. Patients with persistent bleeding despite initial measures should undergo bronchial arteriography for localization and embolization [53]. Radiotherapy is helpful if the hemoptysis is in the setting of airway obstruction due to the presence of a tumor.

EBRT is an effective modality for controlling hemoptysis secondary to tumors. There are no established guidelines for dose fractionation. Various dose fractionation schedules, including 10 Gy in 1 fraction, 17 Gy in 2 weekly fractions, 20 Gy in 5 fractions, or 30 Gy in 10 fractions, have been used [53]. The American Society of Radiation Oncology (ASTRO) recommends that a higher dose fraction (30 Gy in 10 fractions or equivalent) is associated with long-term symptom control in patients with good general condition, while a shorter course (10 Gy in 1 fraction or 17 Gy in 2 weekly fractions) can be used in those with poor general condition [54, 55].

The interventional radiologist can treat oncology patients who present with massive hemoptysis with embolization of the bronchial arteries and non-bronchial systemic collateral arteries using various embolic agents such as polyvinyl alcohol particles, gel foam, and glue [47] (Fig. 8a–f).

Once the cause is identified and the patient is stable, definitive therapy should be directed toward the underlying cause and correction of coagulopathies and thrombocytopenia.

4.3 Malignant Airway Obstruction (MAO)

Central airway obstruction (CAO) is defined as an obstruction in the trachea and mainstem bronchi. Common causes include [56, 57]:

- Lung cancer
- Metastatic mediastinal lymphadenopathy
- Tumors of the esophagus, thyroid
- Mediastinal tumors such as lymphoma, Germ Cell Tumor
- Carcinoid tumors
- Primary malignancies of the trachea

Around 20%–30% of the patients with lung cancer have symptoms of MAO.

4.3.1 Signs and Symptoms

Patients may be asymptomatic or present with variable symptoms such as cough, hemoptysis, and dyspnea, with some presenting to the emergency department with acute respiratory distress, which may be life-threatening [58]. Obstruction of the hypopharynx, larynx, and trachea causes severe respiratory distress, whereas obstruction to the mainstem and lobar bronchi causes dyspnea, cough, and fever due to pneumonitis secondary to obstruction [59].

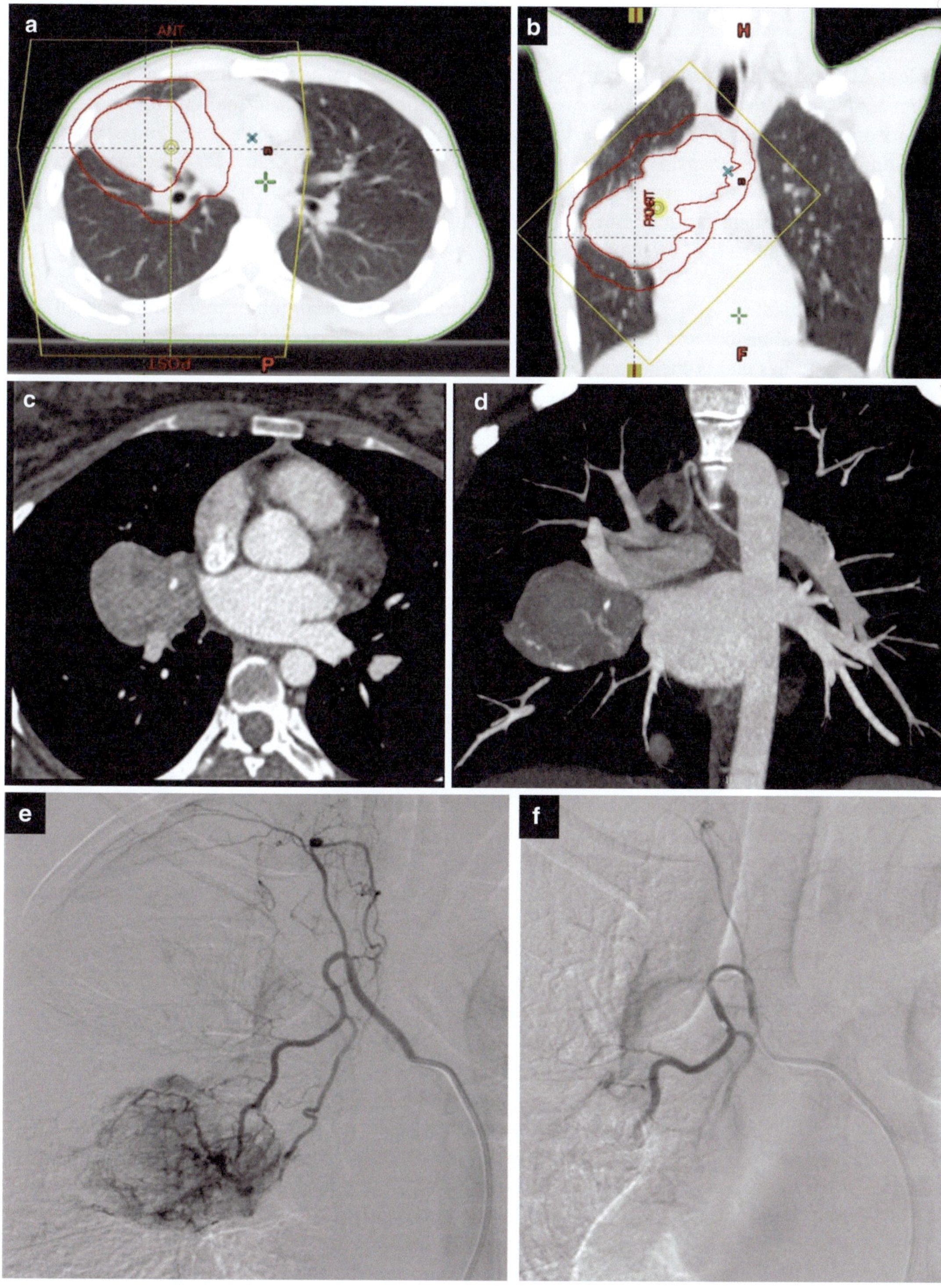

Fig. 8 (**a**, **b**) RT Planning CT showing anterior and posterior parallel opposed field arrangement for palliative radiotherapy for a patient with metastatic nonseminomatous germ cell tumor with progression and presentation with massive hemoptysis. The lung CT showed a large nodal and lung conglomerate mass eroding into the right upper lobar bronchus. MDCT angiography of the chest (**c**) axial and (**d**) coronal views shows a large hyper vascular right hilar mass in a patient who presented with massive hemoptysis. (**e**) Digital subtraction angiography shows extensive vascularity of the lesion derived from the right bronchial artery. (**f**) Post-embolization with polyvinyl alcohol particles, vascularity has disappeared. The lesion turned out to be a Carcinoid tumor on histopathology

4.3.2 Etiology and Etiopathogenesis

Malignancies that involve the tracheobronchial tree, mediastinum, and hila can cause intrinsic (endoluminal) or extrinsic (extraluminal) mechanical compression or invasion of central airways with subsequent luminal narrowing and occlusion, which can be life-threatening.

4.3.3 Diagnosis

Besides the clinical history and detailed examination, imaging studies and bronchoscopy are valuable tools for evaluation. Radiograph of the neck may identify a mass lesion that obstructs the upper airway [1]. CXR is not the ideal modality to detect MAO, but sometimes it is the only modality that a patient with airway obstruction can tolerate. CXR can show mediastinal, hilar, or central lung lesions with associated lung changes such as consolidation and atelectasis. Bronchoscopy is useful in assessing the level of obstruction, taking a biopsy, and removing any impacted foreign body. CT scan can provide valuable information regarding the location and extent of the disease, but it should be done once the patient becomes stable. MDCT delineates the lesion and details the resultant airway compromise (Fig. 9a, b). MDCT with multiplanar reconstructions demonstrates the site, etiology, and severity of airway compromise, along with associated lung parenchymal changes [57, 59] (Fig. 9c, d). MRI is helpful in case of suspected vascular or soft tissue pathology. Pulmonary function test (PFT) should be done in patients with suspected CAO who have subacute symptoms.

4.3.4 Management

Treatment goals include securing the airway and managing the underlying disease. Treatment strategies for CAO depend on the symptomatology and extent of the disease.

Airway management is done using oxygen inhalation, tracheostomy, endotracheal intubation using large-bore ET, or stenting (silicon or metallic stents can be used as a palliative procedure to maintain the airway patency in case of extraluminal obstruction), depending on the extent and level of obstruction [60]. Airway dilation (bronchoplasty) is often used in benign stenosis, but the effect in malignant stenosis is not long-lasting. Bronchoscopic tumor ablation (APC, LASER therapy, or electrocautery for intraluminal obstruction) may provide an immediate response in patients with life-threatening intraluminal obstruction [61, 62].

If feasible, a surgical approach should be considered (i.e., small tumor in a young patient) and includes debulking of the tumor either bronchoscopically or via open surgery.

EBRT is an effective way to relieve symptoms in patients with intraluminal or extraluminal compression by a tumor. However, due to the delayed effect, it is often considered after initial debulking or stent placement. EBRT has a long-standing effect as compared to local ablative techniques. Endobronchial brachytherapy is used occasionally in patients having endobronchial lesions and failed initial EBRT [63, 64]. Similar dose schedules to those mentioned for hemoptysis may be used, with longer schedules preferred for those with better general condition for durable symptom relief [54, 55].

There are no guidelines for concurrent administration of other treatment modalities. In some studies, a combination of local ablative therapies and EBRT has been found useful [65]. Local ablation therapies can be used for immediate relief, followed by EBRT to maintain the patency. Administration of concurrent chemotherapy should be avoided. However, chemotherapy can be given before or after RT for optimal palliation.

4.4 Malignant Pleural Effusion

Patients with malignancies can have pleural infusions, either benign or malignant. They are asymptomatic when small, but when large, they compress the underlying lung parenchyma and cause breathing difficulties. It is one of the most common manifestations of patients with lung cancer. Other etiologies include mesothelioma, breast cancer, lymphoma, and urogenital malignancies. Malignant pleural effusion (MPE) occurs

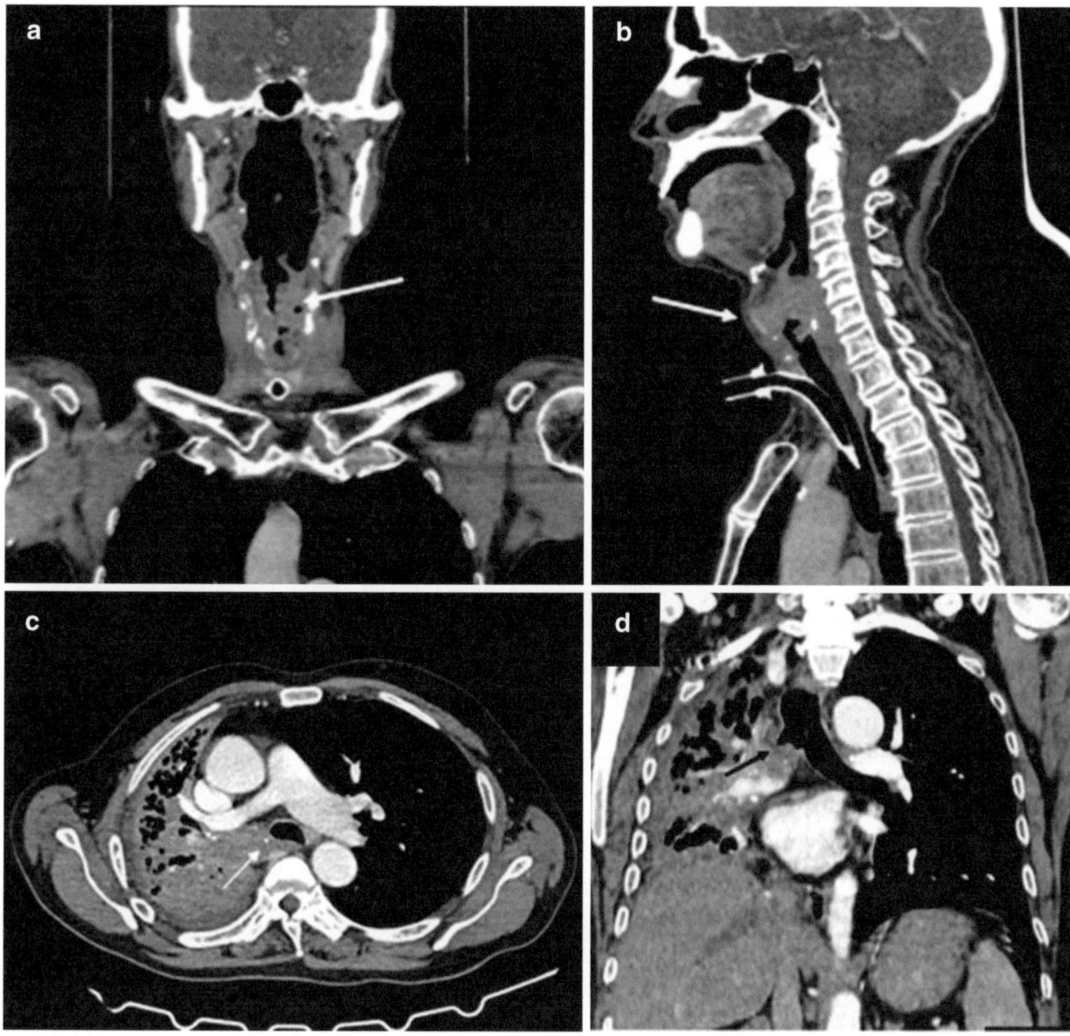

Fig. 9 In a patient with supraglottic carcinoma, (**a**) coronal and (**b**) sagittal orientations of MDCT neck show an obstructive mass lesion (arrows in **a** and **b**) with complete occlusion of the airway. Note is made of the tracheostomy tube in situ. In another patient with bronchogenic carcinoma, (**c**) axial and (**d**) coronal reformation of CT chest shows complete occlusion of the right main bronchus (arrows in **c, white** and **d, black**) due to the mass. Distal to the mass, right lung shows atelectasis and bronchiectatic changes

due to direct invasion of the pleura, and fluid cytology and pleural biopsies are positive for malignancies. Para-malignant pleural effusion (PMPE) is caused by the tumor and/or treatment effects on the surrounding structures and not due to direct cancer cell invasion. Thus in PMPE, the fluid cytology and pleural biopsy are negative for malignancy. The presence of malignant pleural effusion indicates an advanced stage of the disease.

4.4.1 Symptoms

Clinical manifestations range from a mild cough to respiratory distress or acute respiratory failure.

4.4.2 Etiology and Etiopathogenesis

Malignancies arisingwithin thorax or metastatic to the pleura give rise to pleural effusion due to lymphatic obstruction or dissemination (direct or hematogenous) into the pleural cavity, as a consequence of an imbalance between pleural fluid production and resorption. Several tumor and host cell interactions involving secreted mediators such as cytokines, osteopontin, interleukins, tumor necrosis factor (TNF), etc., are implicated.

4.4.3 Diagnosis

Standard posteroanterior/lateral CXR provides ample information about the degree of effusion and contralateral shift. USG and CXR can confirm clinically suspected pleural effusion. USG can be used to guide diagnostic and therapeutic pleural fluid aspiration. CT helps provide additional information on pleural thickening, pneumonia, thromboembolic process, concomitant mass, and obstruction. MDCT is useful to evaluate the underlying lung parenchyma for the presence of infections and malignancies. The presence of nodular or circumferential pleural thickening on MDCT may suggest malignancy [66]. Suspicious areas of pleural thickening can also be biopsied using PET-CECT guided technique [67].

4.4.4 Management

Patients with MPE have a poor prognosis; thus, treatment is directed toward symptomatic relief and improved quality of life. The decision and type of the pleural intervention depend on the following factors:

- Presence of symptoms and extent of effusion
- Expandable or non-expandable lungs
- Responsiveness of underlying malignancy to chemotherapy/radiation therapy
- Expected survival of the patient
- Availability of resources and patient preference

For symptom relief, urgent thoracentesis should be performed in all symptomatic and moderate to large-sized effusions. Prolonged effusion without drainage can result in a non-expandable lung. Therapeutic options include thoracentesis (manual or USG-guided), placement of an indwelling pleural catheter (IPC), also known as a tunnel pleural catheter or chest tube with pleurodesis, thoracoscopy, or thoracic surgery with pleurodesis [68]. Large loculated effusions can be drained using pigtail catheters under USG guidance.

Pleuro-peritoneal shunt and pleurectomy are rarely used in refractory cases [69]. Spontaneous pleurodesis may occur in 27%–70% of patients after IPC drainage. The IPC catheter can be removed if the drain ceases to <50 ml/day for three consecutive days. Irrespective of the drainage, the patient should be treated for the underlying malignancy, as indicated.

Drainage: A simple thoracentesis is performed for those who do not require admission. A needle is inserted through the chest wall in the posterior axillary line into the pleural cavity. Gravity drainage is preferred over repeated manual aspiration to avoid steep fluctuations in pleural fluid pressure and slower lung re-expansion [70]. Large effusions should be drained as much as tolerable by the patients until cough or chest discomfort or end-expiratory pleural pressure under −20 cm H_2O develops [71]. Once the patient develops a cough and chest pressure, further drainage should be discontinued, and the patient should be advised to limit deep breathing and talk in long sentences as further stretching of the lungs can worsen the symptoms. These symptoms resolve spontaneously but occasionally may require non-invasive positive pressure ventilation in severe cases. The American Thoracic Society has given guidelines for pleural effusion drainage, which are summarized in Table 5 [72].

4.5 Stridor

A partially blocked upper airway at the level of the larynx and trachea causes turbulent airflow, which results in an abnormally harsh, melodic, or high-pitched sound [73]. It has to be distinguished from stertorous breathing, a lower-pitched snoring-like sound produced at the level of nasopharynx and oropharynx.

Table 5 Guidance for management of malignant pleural effusion (MPE)

Clinical scenario	Recommendation	Comments
Diagnosed/suspected MPE needing drainage	USG guidance for pleural interventions	Reduces complications such as pneumothorax
Asymptomatic patients with diagnosed/suspected MPE	No intervention	May not need a procedure for 3–10 months
Symptomatic MPE with potentially expandable lung	Large volume paracentesis with pleural manometry Indwelling pleural catheter, or chemical pleurodesis (talc poudrage or slurry)	Need to confirm symptomatic improvement and to identify the presence of nonexpandable lung. Manometry may help predict the success of pleurodesis Use of pleurodesis agent depends on local expertise, need for additional tissue for molecular analysis, and patient factors, such as presence of chest tube
Symptomatic MPE with loculated effusion, poor lung expansion, and failed pleurodesis	Indwelling pleural catheter	Catheters reduce hospital stay Chemical pleurodesis is not effective in a non-expandable lung
Infections associated with an indwelling pleural catheter	Most infections can be treated with suitable antibiotics without removing the catheter Catheter removal is considered only for refractory infections	Consider clinical status, infection type, risk of fluid accumulation after catheter removal, medical and local support availability

4.5.1 Signs and Symptoms

Stridor is a symptom and not a diagnosis; thus patient should be evaluated for the underlying cause. Stridor can be divided into three types depending on its occurrence during the respiratory cycle.

1. Inspiratory stridor: It is the most common and indicates laryngeal obstruction.
2. Expiratory stridor: Indicates tracheobronchial obstruction.
3. Biphasic stridor: Implies a glottic or subglottic malformation.

4.5.2 Etiology and Etiopathogenesis

Stridor is mostly brought on by foreign body aspiration or neoplasms coming from the larynx, trachea, esophagus, or lung, aside from structural and inflammatory/infectious diseases that may coexist. When air moves through a small tube, the lateral pressure keeping it open may abruptly diminish, causing the airway to collapse and cause stridor.

4.5.3 Diagnosis

In stable patients, an anteroposterior and lateral radiograph of the neck can help assess the extent of the retropharyngeal space and the size of the enlarged epiglottis. If a foreign body is detected, a CXR can be acquired [74]. When a patient is stable and the diagnosis is uncertain, a CT scan of the neck and chest is performed. Laryngoscopy and bronchoscopy can directly visualize the airway and offer a conclusive diagnosis.

4.5.4 Management

Management strategies should be tailored based on the rapidity of symptom onset and severity. Non-pharmacological measures consist of head tilt, chin lift, and jaw thrust [75]. Those who present with sudden-onset stridor due to severe airway obstruction are at an increased risk of respiratory failure and death. Emergency interventions involve securing the airway by endotracheal intubation, rigid bronchoscopy, or tracheostomy. Continuous positive pressure ventilation has been used in managing stridor in advanced head and neck cancer patients; however, its efficacy is controversial [76]. Once the diagnosis is confirmed and the patient is stable, the underlying cause is treated. Antibiotics are used if bacterial epiglottitis or tracheitis is suspected. Corticosteroids are used in post-extubation stridors [77]. Surgical management is warranted in cases of laryngeal or tracheal stenosis, for removal of airway foreign bodies, and for excision of airway-compromising tumors. Single or multi-fraction palliative radiotherapy can be used in selected patients with malignancy-related stridor [78]. A tracheostomy can be used before radiotherapy to prevent exacerbation of symptoms.

4.6 Atelectasis

Atelectasis is defined as a loss of lung volume due to the reversible collapse of small airways, leading to impaired gas exchange. It is divided into obstructive and non-obstructive [79]. Obstructive (resorptive) atelectasis results from airway occlusion due to foreign bodies or tumors compressing airways, such as trachea-esophageal or mediastinal neoplasms, resulting in air trapping distal to the obstruction. It is more common after obstruction of the lobar bronchus than the segmental bronchus and frequently occurs in those who breathe a high fraction of inspired oxygen. Non-obstructive atelectasis occurs due to loss of contact between parietal and visceral pleura (passive atelectasis), surfactant dysfunction (adhesive atelectasis), lung tissue scarring (cicatricial atelectasis), infiltrative disease (replacement atelectasis), and strong vertical acceleration force (acceleration atelectasis).

4.6.1 Clinical Presentation

The signs and symptoms depend on the rapidity of bronchial occlusion and the amount of lung affected. The patient may present with chest pain on the affected side, dyspnea, fever, or cyanosis. Hypotension, tachycardia, and shock may occur in severe cases.

4.6.2 Etiology and Etiopathogenesis

The airway collapse may be obstructive (due to lesions within the airway) or nonobstructive (due to lesions causing extrinsic compression of the airway, absorption of alveolar air, or faulty surfactant production), the former being more common in malignancies.

4.6.3 Diagnosis

CXR may show a non-specific area of opacification, segmental or lobar opacities with compensatory hyperinflation, or bilateral lung opacification. Mediastinal shift toward the affected lung helps to distinguish atelectasis from pneumonia and pleural effusion. Chest CT has a better sensitivity than radiograph to evaluate the cause and may help delineate the pleural or parenchymal process. Occasionally, abdominal USG can incidentally detect atelectatic lung as aerated lung cannot be visualized on USG (USG waves cannot penetrate aerated lung; atelectatic lung, however, is a solid and hyperechoic structure). Bronchoscopy can help visualize obstruction by a mucus plug, foreign body, or tumor. Normal CBC may help differentiate atelectasis from pneumonia. Patients may have some degree of hypoxemia depending on the severity and area involved.

4.6.4 Management

The treatment should be directed at symptom control and the treatment of the underlying cause [80].

Chest physiotherapy is the traditional method for treating atelectasis, but little evidence supports its efficacy. Various methods of chest physiotherapy include manual chest physiotherapy, mechanical insufflation-exsufflation, especially in patients with impaired cough clearance, such as Duchenne muscular dystrophy and cerebral palsy, and in patients on mechanical ventilation and intrapulmonary percussive ventilation [81–83].

Inhaled mucolytics, including hypertonic saline, mannitol, acetylcysteine, and DNAase, can help patients with atelectasis who suffer due to abundant secretions. The choice of the agent depends on the underlying cause [84, 85].

Treatment of the underlying cause may include foreign body removal, surgical intervention for compressive atelectasis due to cardiomegaly or tumor, and chemo-radiotherapy for any underlying malignancy. The effectiveness of bronchoscopic insufflation of the lung is not clear, but it is used as a last resort once the non-invasive modalities have failed [86].

5 Febrile Neutropenia

Febrile neutropenia (FN) is one of the most common emergencies in patients with cancer. It is considered an emergency because, without the rapid institution of appropriate antibiotics and supportive drugs, the infection can rapidly disseminate and be fatal.

5.1 Clinical Presentation

Patients may present with high-grade fever, often accompanied by focal symptoms and signs of infection of a specific system, such as pneumonitis, urinary tract infection, or acute gastroenteritis. In patients with pancytopenia from any cause, accompanying pallor, poor general health, and bleeding diathesis may be evident.

5.2 Etiology and Etiopathogenesis

Neutropenia may be due to bone marrow infiltration by cancer (e.g., in leukemias and rarely in solid cancers) or, more often, due to treatment (chemotherapy or rarely radiation). Febrile neutropenia, as a toxicity of systemic anti-cancer therapy, remains a difficult clinical situation causing morbidity and mortality.

5.3 Diagnosis

Febrile neutropenia is defined as a single oral temperature reading ≥38.3 °C or ≥38 °C for ≥1 h with an absolute neutrophil count <500 cells/cmm or expected to fall below 500 cells/cmm during the next 48 hours [87].

A thorough history and examination would help identify the focus of infections and the patient's risk status. Investigations include blood cultures (2 sets) (including from central catheters, if any), CXR, CBC, KFT, and LFT.

Table 6 Risk factors for febrile neutropenia (Multinational Association for Supportive Care in Cancer Risk Index)

Characteristics	Points
Burden of illness: No or mild symptoms Moderate symptoms	 5 (not cumulative) 3
Absence of hypotension	5
Absence of chronic obstructive pulmonary disease	4
Solid tumor or no previous fungal infection	4
Absence of dehydration	3
Outpatient status	3
Age <60 years	2
Maximum score	**26**
Low-risk patients: Total score ≥21 **High-risk patients: Total score ≤20**	

5.4 Management

After drawing cultures, antibiotics should be initiated immediately, followed by treatment as per risk status [88] (Table 6).

All patients can be started on granulocyte-colony stimulating factors till recovery of counts.

Low-risk patients may be managed as outpatients with oral antibiotics, provided the patient is well-aware of the risks and can respond immediately and come for hospital admission in case of worsening status (must be able to travel, stay close enough, and have a reliable caregiver). The preferred drug option is a combination of co-amoxiclav and levofloxacin. One can stop antibiotics with the resolution of symptoms [89].

For high-risk patients (neutropenia expected to last >7 days, comorbidities, unstable, previous fungal infection, leukemia), admission is preferred and antibiotics started (the first line must have a broad spectrum with anti-pseudomonal cover) [90]. Usual options are cefoperazone-sulbactam, cefepime, piperacillin-tazobactam. For higher-risk patients, one may consider carbapenems as the first line. Gram-positive cover (vancomycin) is preferred for patients with mucositis, suspected central venous catheter infection, hypotension, or pneumonia.

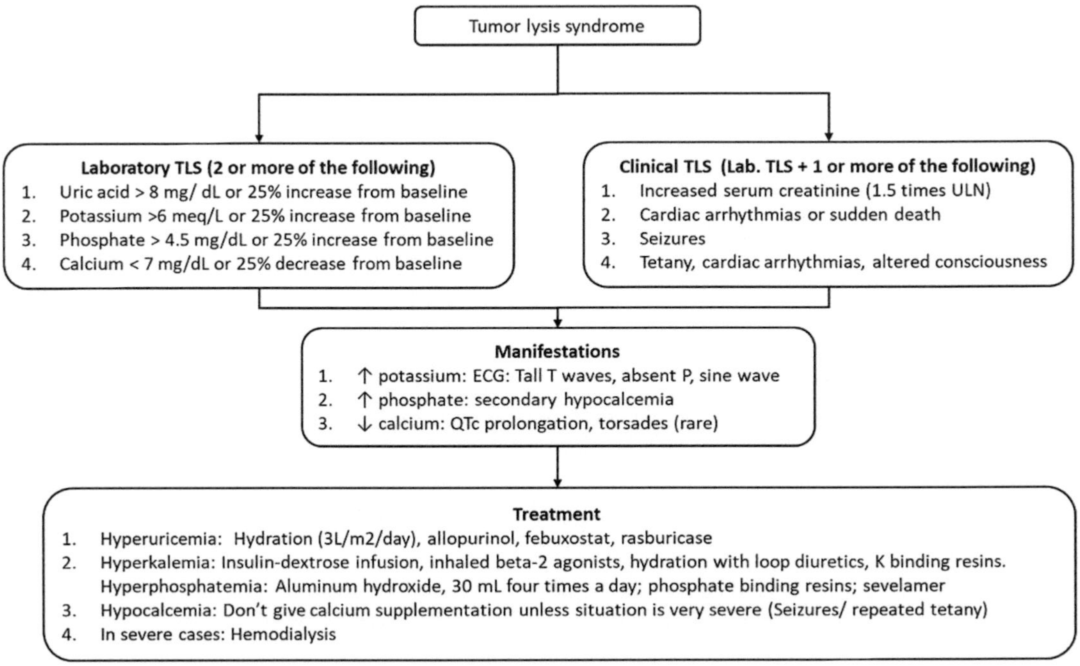

Fig. 10 Management of tumor lysis syndrome

6 Metabolic Disorders

6.1 Tumor Lysis Syndrome

Tumor lysis syndrome (TLS) results from the lysis of cancer cells, usually during the initial treatment with chemotherapy (rarely with radiotherapy), leading to intracellular uric acid, potassium, and phosphate release into the bloodstream. Hypocalcemia is another manifestation that occurs secondary to phosphate binding with circulating calcium. Increased uric acid leads to renal insufficiency and ultimately lactic acidosis. As per the Cairo and Bishop classification, "Laboratory TLS" means abnormal laboratory values without target organ damage or symptoms, and "Clinical TLS" is associated with renal dysfunction, cardiac arrhythmias, or seizures. Thus, patients may be asymptomatic for the manifestations, and only focused investigations may reveal the features. In some very rapidly proliferating tumors such as Burkitt's lymphomas and acute leukemias, spontaneous TLS can occur even before the initiation of therapy [91].

Management: In patients where TLS is anticipated (bulky, aggressive tumors, leukemias, and aggressive lymphomas), hydration (at least 3 liters/m^2/day) is promptly started, with early allopurinol/ febuxostat (to prevent the formation of uric acid), and regular monitoring of TLS parameters. In patients with abnormal biochemistry at diagnosis, 1–2 days of preventive therapy to normalize the values and establish good renal output before starting anti-cancer therapy may be considered. Febuxostat is preferred when there is pre-existing renal dysfunction. When the baseline uric acid load is high and is expected to increase further, rasburicase may be given (usually a single dose and repeated later depending on values) [92, 93]. Cardiac arrhythmias, tetany, and acute renal failure (deposition of insoluble uric acid in the tubules) in severe cases warrant emergent management. Falling urine output and refractory hyperkalemia should trigger immediate consideration for hemodialysis. One must not treat hypocalcemia with calcium supplementation, as this promotes metastatic calcification (Fig. 10).

6.2 Hypercalcemia

Hypercalcemia in cancers is usually a paraneoplastic feature due to the secretion of hormones (parathormone-related protein (PTHrP) and active forms of vitamin D3), leading to osteoclast activation. Rarely, it may occur due to direct bone destruction by metastases [94]. Common cancers causing hypercalcemia are multiple myeloma, cancers of the breast, small cell carcinoma lung, squamous cell carcinomas, and renal cell carcinoma. Though not prognostic in myeloma, hypercalcemia in advanced solid tumors may indicate a poor outcome. Extensive use of bisphosphonates in bone metastases has reduced the severity of hypercalcemia [95]. Hypercalcemia causes osmotic diuresis, nausea, and vomiting, leading to dehydration and worsening renal function.

Management: Aggressive hydration (3 L/m^2/day) corrects the dehydration and establishes a good urine output. This will excrete calcium in the urine. The addition of frusemide after hydration is established can increase urinary calcium elimination. Calcitonin can help in the immediate reduction of calcium, but the effect can be transient (tachyphylaxis), and more permanent solutions like bisphosphonates (zoledronic acid is preferred) need to be instituted. Denosumab (anti-RANKL monoclonal antibody) can be used when hypercalcemia is refractory to zoledronate or when it is contraindicated [96].

6.3 Hyponatremia

Hyponatremia is a fairly common problem in patients with cancer and is defined by a serum sodium level <135 mEq/L. Though many cases are asymptomatic, lower sodium levels may cause neurological symptoms and be life-threatening (Fig. 11). Many studies have also shown that hyponatremia per se may be a poor prognostic factor for survival. The most typical cause is the syndrome of inappropriate secretion of anti-diuretic hormone (SIADH), which may occur in the context of small cell lung cancer (most common) and several other malignancies [97]. In these patients, ectopic secretion of ADH promotes free water retention in the kidneys despite falling plasma osmolality (OsM). Certain drugs may also cause SIADH (vincristine, cyclophosphamide, platinum agents, opioids, and antidepressants). Cisplatin may potentiate hyponatremia by a direct renal tubular injury resulting in sodium loss. Excessive salt wasting may also occur in patients with brain metastasis (cerebral salt wasting). The differentiation of SIADH and salt wasting is essential (both have low sodium with low plasma OsM) because the management is different.

Diagnosis: Demonstration of low serum sodium might trigger a basic workup, which includes calculating serum osmolality and measuring urine sodium. These three factors, along with the clinical picture (edema/ascites signifies hypervolemia, while orthostatic hypotension, reduced skin turgor, and dry mucosa suggest hypovolemia), can pinpoint the diagnosis in the majority of cases.

Treatment: If the patient has symptoms, require prompt treatment to raise sodium in a controlled manner (12 mEq/L in 24 h and <18 mEq/L in 48 h), especially when it is chronic [98]. Either normal saline or hypertonic saline may be used to correct symptomatic patients, depending on the severity, with stopping hypertonic saline once symptoms resolve. When asymptomatic, simpler measures like free-water restriction (500 ml less than the average urine output) and added salt in the diet may suffice. Vasopressin receptor antagonists can produce selective water diuresis without electrolyte loss. Oral tolvaptan can be initiated in an admitted patient and continued after discharge in patients with asymptomatic or mildly symptomatic chronic hyponatremia. These patients should have regular monitoring of liver function, and the usage of tolvaptan should not usually exceed 30 days.

Figure 11 shows an approach to the diagnosis and management of hyponatremia in malignancies.

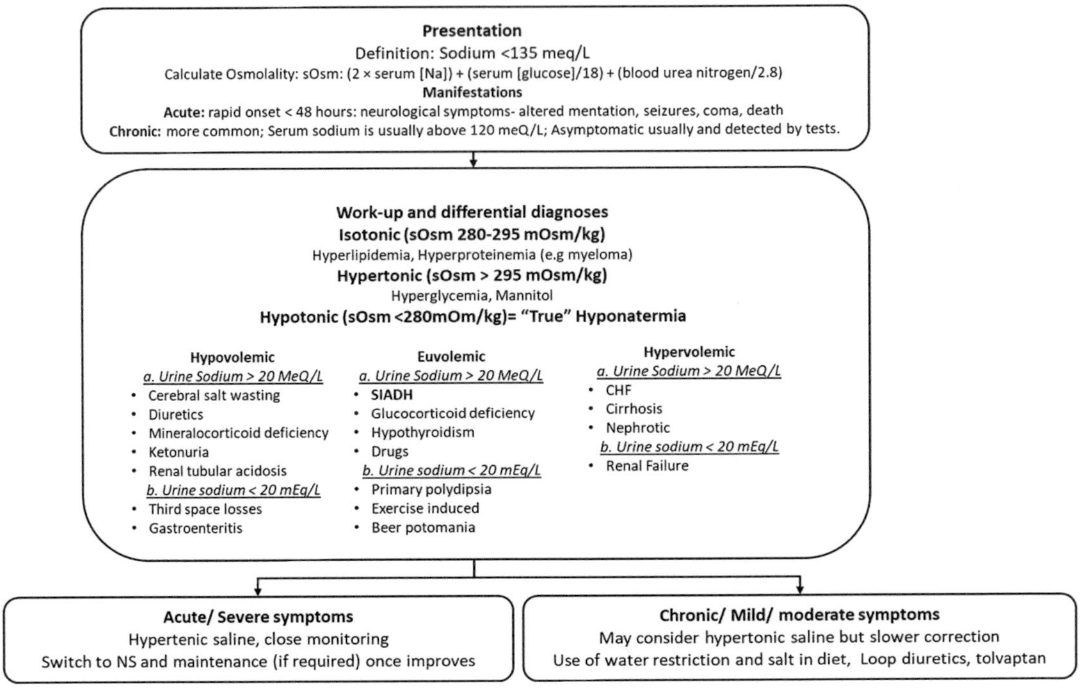

Fig. 11 Approach to diagnosis and management of hyponatremia in malignancies

7 Obstruction of Tubular Structures

7.1 Biliary Obstruction

Biliary obstruction in oncologic patients can be due to diffuse liver metastatic infiltration with resultant small intrahepatic bile ducts obstruction or can occur due to compression or involvement of the main bile ducts due to malignant tumors such as carcinoma gall bladder, cholangiocarcinoma, periampullary tumors, or metastatic lesions [99].

Imaging should demonstrate the presence or absence of biliary obstruction, the level of obstruction, and the cause of obstruction. USG is usually the first method used in suspected biliary obstruction and depicts dilatation of the intrahepatic and extrahepatic biliary dilatation.

Endoscopic retrograde cholangiopancreatography (ERCP) is also used to evaluate the bile ducts, and tissue can also be obtained for histopathological examination. However, this is more invasive and complex than CT or MRI. The second line test is commonly MDCT, as it provides information about biliary dilatation and primary tumor and can also show local and distant metastasis. MRI also visualizes tumors and magnetic resonance cholangiopancreatography (MRCP) sequences, which use heavily T2-weighted MR sequences to show biliary ductal anatomy in detail [100].

Patients with biliary obstruction frequently require drainage. Drainage can be achieved by ERCP or by percutaneous transhepatic biliary drainage (PTBD). Indications for PTBD in a patient with malignant obstruction are severe cholangitis, pruritus, and to decrease raised serum bilirubin so that chemotherapy can be initiated. PTBD involves selective cannulation of a peripheral biliary duct under USG or fluoroscopic guidance, passing a guidewire, serial track dilatation, and then placement of a catheter or stent to facilitate internal or external drainage of bile to achieve decompression of the biliary system [101] (Fig. 12).

Pre-procedure, all patients are administered prophylactic antibiotics, and contrast volume is

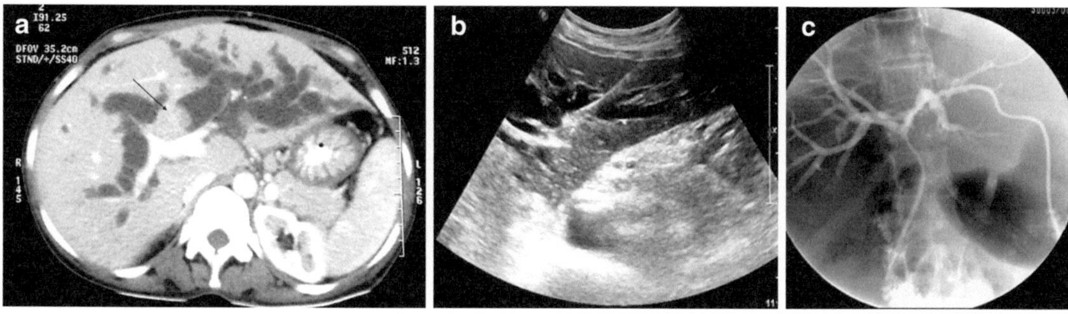

Fig. 12 (**a**) Axial CECT showing hilar mass with resultant bilobar biliary dilatation in a patient of hilar cholangiocarcinoma. (**b**) Dilated biliary system is assessed under ultrasound guidance, and (**c**) biliary drainage is. established subsequently under fluoroscopy guidance with the tip of the drainage catheter in the duodenum

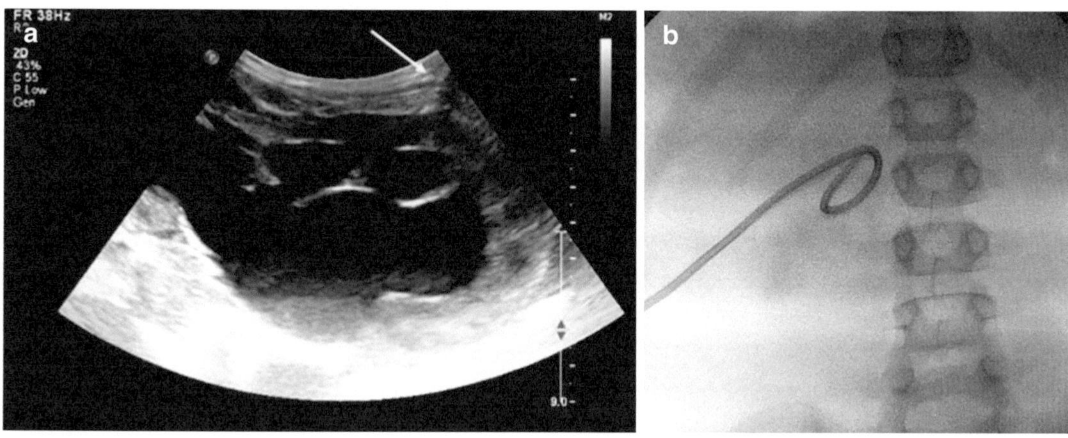

Fig. 13 (**a**) Ultrasound shows hydronephrosis left kidney in a patient of pelvic malignancy (not shown). Dilated pelvicalyceal system was assessed under ultrasound guidance using18G needle (arrow), and (**b**) percutaneous nephrostomy was done under fluoroscopy guidance

kept minimum during cholangiography to minimize septic complications.

7.2 Urinary Tract Obstruction

Malignant urinary tract obstruction can occur in patients with urological (urinary bladder, prostate) or gynecological (cervix, endometrium, ovaries) cancers. Additionally, retroperitoneal or pelvic tumors can compress and invade the ureters, leading to urinary obstruction [102].

USG is the first investigation to detect hydronephrosis. It can also show mobile debris and urothelial thickening, which might suggest the presence of pyonephrosis. MDCT with coronal and sagittal reformatting determines the site of the obstruction, mainly when a retroperitoneal or pelvic mass lesion is present, which may not be apparent on clinical examination. CT will show a mass lesion with upstream unilateral or bilateral hydroureteronephrosis [103]. In patients with deranged renal function, non-contrast MR urography may be used.

Indications for percutaneous nephrostomy (PCN) in the emergent setting in oncology patients include suspected urinary tract sepsis, pyonephrosis, deteriorating renal function, or electrolyte disturbances. The pelvicalyceal system may be assessed with USG or fluoroscopy, followed by insertion of a drainage catheter (Fig. 13). PCN not only drains the contents but also provides access for subsequent uroradiological intervention if needed [104, 105].

Precepts Box

1. Oncologic emergencies may be related to malignancy or complications of anticancer therapies. A high index of suspicion is required for diagnosis.
2. Metabolic and hematologic emergencies are diagnosed based on clinical evaluation and laboratory findings, while structural emergencies (mass effect, vascular or ductal obstruction, bleeding) need radiological investigations for diagnosis. Depending on the site to be evaluated, X-ray, CT, USG, or MRI may be needed.
3. Each radiation oncology department should have a standard operating procedure for stakeholders and department personnel involved in emergency radiotherapy procedures; the simplest and least time-consuming techniques should be used to facilitate ease of delivery.
4. Raised intracranial pressure presents with headache, vomiting, altered sensorium, focal neurologic deficits or seizures, and clinical findings of hypertension and bradycardia. Management includes medical decompression, serial monitoring of sensorium, and definitive local therapy (palliative radiotherapy or surgery) based on disease extent and prognosis.
5. Spinal cord compression presents with pain and neurologic deficits (motor > sensory > autonomic). Local management (radiotherapy or surgery) depends on symptoms, disease extent, spinal stability, and radiosensitivity, using NOMS or SINS criteria.
6. Tumor-related bone pain stems from tumor expansion, neural compression, fracture, decreased bone density, or muscle spasm. Mirels' criteria aid in triage of patients needing surgical stabilization. For stable lesions needing radiotherapy, a single fraction of 8 gray (Gy) is as effective as longer courses but has less durable pain control. For extensive lesions, systemic therapy or hemibody irradiation is preferred.
7. Superior vena cava (SVC) obstruction arises from mediastinal compression and presents with breathlessness, cough, facial swelling, plethora, confusion, and prominent veins over the neck and upper body. Management includes symptom control (steroids, bronchodilators), tumor markers and FNAC/biopsy, and definitive treatment with palliative radiotherapy, systemic therapy (for chemoresponsive tumors), or SVC stenting (uncommon).
8. Febrile neutropenia is common following myelosuppressive chemotherapy. Low-risk patients can be managed on an outpatient basis with oral antibiotics, but high-risk patients need admission, broad-spectrum antibiotics, and G-CSF support.
9. Tumor lysis syndrome is seen during early phases of treatment (usually systemic therapy) in large tumors (lymphomas, leukemias, germ cell tumors) and may be symptomatic or asymptomatic. Clinical manifestations include renal failure, arrhythmias, or seizures, while investigations may show hyperuricemia, hyperphosphatemia, hypocalcemia, and hyperkalemia.
10. Hypercalcemia of malignancy denotes poor prognosis. Aggressive hydration with loop diuretics helps calcium elimination, while bisphosphonates and anti-RANKL agents help in long-term control against bone resorption.

Multiple Choice Questions

1. A 65-year-old woman with a previous history of locally advanced breast cancer and currently on hormone therapy presents with worsening holocranial headache for 2 weeks and early morning vomiting. Which of the following clinical findings would NOT indicate possible brain metastases?
   (a) High blood pressure.
   (b) Left-sided limb weakness.
   (c) Gait imbalance.
   (d) Rapid heart rate.
2. An 15-year-old schoolgirl who was recently diagnosed with acute leukemia is admitted for starting chemotherapy. She reports fatigue and lethargy. Laboratory evaluation reveals pancytopenia, hyperkalemia (K 6.8 mEq/L), hyperuricemia (uric acid 11 mg/ml), hyperphosphatemia (8 mg/ml), and hypocalcemia (calcium 5.5 mg/dl). A diagnosis of tumor lysis syndrome was made. Which of the following is NOT an appropriate management strategy?
   (a) Hydration with loop diuretics.
   (b) Phosphate binding resins.
   (c) Calcium supplementation.
   (d) Insulin-dextrose infusion.
3. A 75-year-old chronic smoker with a history of progressive dyspnea for 2 months presents to the emergency with sudden worsening of dyspnea, inability to lie down flat due to breathing difficulty, plethora over the face, prominent veins over the neck and upper body. He seems disoriented and hypoxic. CXR shows right hilar shadow and mediastinal widening. What is the probable diagnosis?
   (a) Acute coronary syndrome.
   (b) Superior vena cava syndrome.
   (c) Constrictive pericarditis.
   (d) Chronic obstructive airway disease.
4. Hemostatic radiation therapy is indicated for all of the below scenarios EXCEPT:
   (a) Patient with locally advanced cervical carcinoma cervix and profuse vaginal bleed not controlled with local pressure/packing.
   (b) Patient with hepatocellular carcinoma and portal hypertension presenting with hematemesis.
   (c) Patient with a squamous cell carcinoma lesion of size 7 × 7 cm over the thigh with continuous ooze and anemia.
   (d) Patient with a diagnosis of metastatic bronchogenic carcinoma presenting to the emergency with an episode of bloody sputum of around 50 ml.
5. Which of the factors is LEAST important when considering palliative radiotherapy:
   (a) Time taken for planning and delivery of the first fraction.
   (b) Determining the radiosensitivity of the tumor.
   (c) High conformality of radiation planning and delivery.
   (d) Training of all radiation oncology staff on standard operating procedures during emergencies.
6. Which of the following patients with bone metastases would benefit MOST from emergency palliative radiotherapy?
   (a) Known case of breast cancer with progressive backache for 3 weeks and sudden onset of paraplegia within the last 8 hours. CT shows an osteoblastic lesion in D11-D12 vertebrae with a soft tissue component and cord compression.
   (b) Patient with multiple myeloma with generalized bone pains for 2 months, no specific site of tenderness, and preserved neurologic function. CT shows multiple lytic bony lesions, no cortical breach, and no soft tissue component.
   (c) Known case of renal cell carcinoma presenting with sudden onset of pain in the right arm. X-ray shows a lytic lesion with a displaced fracture of the right humerus shaft.
   (d) Known case of castrate resistant prostate cancer with worsening backache. MRI spine shows multiple bone metastases involving almost all bones and degenerative changes with spinal canal narrowing and osteophytes impinging on the cord at multiple levels.

7. A 25-year-old patient on BEP chemotherapy regimen for germ cell tumor presents with high-grade fever for 24 hours (103 °F) and loose stools after a week of chemotherapy. CBC in emergency confirms the diagnosis of febrile neutropenia with an absolute neutrophil count of 300 cells/cmm. What of the following statements is true regarding management?
   (a) Antibiotics should be started immediately in an emergency, and blood cultures, renal function, chest X-ray, and urine culture should be sent after admission and stabilization.
   (b) Only antipyretics and antidiarrheals should be started immediately. Antibiotics should be started once the blood culture returns positive.
   (c) Vancomycin can be started as empirical therapy after sending a blood sample for culture.
   (d) Broad-spectrum antibiotics and G-CSF support should be given after sending blood samples for culture.
8. All of the following are interventions for hypercalcemia of malignancy EXCEPT:
   (a) Normal saline infusion with loop diuretics.
   (b) Bisphosphonate administration.
   (c) Definitive therapy for the tumor.
   (d) Milk-free diet.
9. A 55-year-old, otherwise fit, male patient with ALK-positive adenocarcinoma lung presents with headache, vomiting, and gait imbalance. His vitals and electrolytes are normal, but the CT head shows a 5 cm cerebellar lesion with compression of the fourth ventricle. Which of the following is appropriate management after medical decompression?
   (a) Excision of the cerebellar lesion to reduce mass effect.
   (b) ALK-targeted systemic therapy only.
   (c) Whole brain radiotherapy.
   (d) SRS to cerebellar lesion.
10. Which of the following patients with spinal cord compression and paraparesis is likely to benefit MOST from a course of palliative radiotherapy?
   (a) Renal cell carcinoma with D12 vertebral body lesion and epidural soft tissue component.
   (b) Renal cell carcinoma with D12 vertebral body lesion with fracture fragment impinging on the spinal cord.
   (c) Renal cell carcinoma with intramedullary metastases at D12 vertebral level.
   (d) Renal cell carcinoma with D12 vertebral body lesion with wedging and collapse >50%.

Answer Key

1. (d)
2. (c)
3. (b)
4. (b)
5. (c)
6. (a)
7. (d)
8. (d)
9. (a)
10. (a)

References

1. Katabathina VS, Restrepo CS, Betancourt Cuellar SL, Riascos RF, Menias CO. Imaging of oncologic emergencies: what every radiologist should know. Radiographics. 2013;33:1533–53.
2. Siochi RA, Balter P, Bloch CD, Santanam L, et al. A rapid communication from the AAPM Task Group 201: recommendations for the QA of external beam radiotherapy data transfer. AAPM TG 201: quality assurance of external beam radiotherapy data transfer. J Appl Clin Med Phys. 2011;12:170–81.
3. Stern RL, Heaton R, Fraser MW, Murty Goddu S, et al. Verification of monitor unit calculations for non-IMRT clinical radiotherapy: report of AAPM Task Group 114. Med Phys. 2011;38:504–30.
4. Kutcher GJ, Coia L, Gillin M, Hanson WF, et al. Comprehensive QA for radiation oncology: report of AAPM radiation therapy committee task group 40. Med Phys. 1994;21:581–618.
5. American College of Radiology. ACR-AAPM technical standard for the performance of radiation oncology physics for external beam therapy. 2015. https://www.acr.org/-/media/ACR/Files/Practice-Parameters/Ext-Beam-TS.pdf.
6. Xia P, Sintay BJ, Colussi VC, Chuang C, et al. Medical Physics Practice Guideline (MPPG) 11.

a: plan and chart review in external beam radiotherapy and brachytherapy. J Appl Clin Med Phys. 2021;22:4–19.
7. Gao W, Nyflot MJ, Novak A, Sponseller PA, et al. Can emergent treatments result in more severe errors?: an analysis of a large institutional near-miss incident reporting database. Pract Radiat Oncol. 2015;5:319–24.
8. Law M. Neurological complications. Cancer Imaging. 2009;9:71–4.
9. Provenzale JM. Imaging of traumatic brain injury: a review of the recent medical literature. Am J Roentgenol. 2010;194:16–9.
10. Vecht CJ, Hovestadt A, Verbiest HB, van Vliet JJ, van Putten WL. Dose-effect relationship of dexamethasone on Karnofsky performance in metastatic brain tumors: a randomized study of doses of 4, 8, and 16 mg per day. Neurology. 1994;44:675–80.
11. Glantz MJ, Cole BF, Forsyth PA, Recht LD, et al. Practice parameter: anticonvulsant prophylaxis in patients with newly diagnosed brain tumors. Report of the Quality Standards Subcommittee of the American Academy of Neurology. Neurology. 2000;54:1886–93. https://doi.org/10.1212/wnl.54.10.1886.
12. Agboola O, Benoit B, Cross P, Da Silva V, et al. Prognostic factors derived from recursive partition analysis (RPA) of Radiation Therapy Oncology Group (RTOG) brain metastases trials applied to surgically resected and irradiated brain metastatic cases. Int J Radiat Oncol Biol Phys. 1998;42:155–9. https://doi.org/10.1016/s0360-3016(98)00198-9.
13. Prasad D, Schiff D. Malignant spinal-cord compression. Lancet Oncol. 2005;6:15–24.
14. Schiff D. Spinal cord compression. Neurol Clin. 2003;21:67–86.
15. Sorensen S, Helweg-Larsen S, Mouridsen H, Hansen HH. Effect of high-dose dexamethasone in carcinomatous metastatic spinal cord compression treated with radiotherapy: a randomised trial. Eur J Cancer. 1994;30A:22–7.
16. Barzilai O, Laufer I, Yamada Y, Higginson DS, et al. Integrating evidence-based medicine for treatment of spinal metastases into a decision framework: neurologic, oncologic, mechanicals stability, and systemic disease. J Clin Oncol. 2017;35:2419–27.
17. Fourney DR, Frangou EM, Ryken TC, Dipaola CP, et al. Spinal instability neoplastic score: an analysis of reliability and validity from the spine oncology study group. J Clin Oncol. 2011;29:3072–7.
18. Rades D, Stalpers LJ, Veninga T, Schulte R, et al. Evaluation of five radiation schedules and prognostic factors for metastatic spinal cord compression. J Clin Oncol. 2005;23:3366–75.
19. Rades D, Heidenreich F, Karstens JH. Final results of a prospective study of the prognostic value of the time to develop motor deficits before irradiation in metastatic spinal cord compression. Int J Radiat Oncol Biol Phys. 2002;53:975–9.
20. Mercadante S. Malignant bone pain: pathophysiology and treatment. Pain. 1997;69:1–18. https://doi.org/10.1016/s0304-3959(96)03267-8.
21. Mirels H. Metastatic disease in long bones. A proposed scoring system for diagnosing impending pathologic fractures. Clin Orthop Relat Res. 1989;249:256–64.
22. Rades D, Haus R, Schild SE, Janssen S. Prognostic factors and a new scoring system for survival of patients irradiated for bone metastases. BMC Cancer. 2019;19:1156.
23. Liu Y, von Eyben R, Kidd EA. Consideration of patient and disease characteristics in selecting radiation regimens for treatment of bone metastases. Pract Radiat Oncol. 2017;7:403–10.
24. Bone Pain Trial Working Party. 8 Gy single fraction radiotherapy for the treatment of metastatic skeletal pain: randomised comparison with a multifraction schedule over 12 months of patient follow-up. Radiother Oncol. 1999;52:111–21.
25. Hartsell WF, Scott CB, Bruner DW, Scarantino CW, et al. Randomized trial of short- versus long-course radiotherapy for palliation of painful bone metastases. J Natl Cancer Inst. 2005;97:798–804.
26. Heller MT, Khanna V. Cross-sectional imaging of acute abdominal conditions in the oncologic patient. Emerg Radiol. 2011;18:417–28.
27. Lubner M, Menias C, Rucker C, Bhalla S, et al. Blood in the belly: CT findings of hemoperitoneum. Radiographics. 2007;27:109–25.
28. Eleje GU, Eke AC, Igberase GO, Igwegbe AO, Eleje LI. Palliative interventions for controlling vaginal bleeding in advanced cervical cancer. Cochrane Database Syst Rev. 2019;3:CD011000.
29. Razazi K, Parrot A, Khalil A, Djibre M, et al. Severe hemoptysis in patients with nonsmall cell lung carcinoma. Eur Respir J. 2015;45:756–64.
30. Simpson JR, Francis ME, Perez-Tamayo R, Marks RD, Rao DV. Palliative radiotherapy for inoperable carcinoma of the lung: final report of a RTOG multi-institutional trial. Int J Radiat Oncol Biol Phys. 1985;11:751–8.
31. Fairchild A, Harris K, Barnes E, Wong R, et al. Palliative thoracic radiotherapy for lung cancer: a systematic review. J Clin Oncol. 2008;26:4001–11.
32. Walterbos NR, Fiocco M, Neelis KJ, van der Linden YM, et al. Effectiveness of several external beam radiotherapy schedules for palliation of esophageal cancer. Clin Transl Radiat Oncol. 2019;17:24–31.
33. Kawabata H, Hitomi M, Motoi S. Management of bleeding from unresectable gastric cancer. Biomedicine. 2019;7:54. https://doi.org/10.3390/biomedicines7030054.
34. Cameron MG, Kersten C, Vistad I, Fosså S, Guren MG. Palliative pelvic radiotherapy of symptomatic incurable rectal cancer - a systematic review. Acta Oncol. 2014;53:164–73.
35. Duchesne GM, Bolger JJ, Griffiths GO, Trevor Roberts J, et al. A randomized trial of hypofraction-

ated schedules of palliative radiotherapy in the management of bladder carcinoma: results of medical research council trial BA09. Int J Radiat Oncol Biol Phys. 2000;47:379–88.
36. Smith SC, Koh WJ. Palliative radiation therapy for gynaecological malignancies. Best Pract Res Clin Obstet Gynaecol. 2001;15:265–78.
37. Vuong W, Lin J, Wei RL. Palliative radiotherapy for skin malignancies. Ann Palliat Med. 2017;6:165–72.
38. Jahroudi N, Ardekani AM, Greenberger JS. Ionizing irradiation increases transcription of the von Willebrand factor gene in endothelial cells. Blood. 1996;88:3801–14.
39. Cabrera R, Nelson DR. Review article: the management of hepatocellular carcinoma. Aliment Pharmacol Ther. 2010;31:461–76.
40. Brown DB, Cardella JF, Sacks D, Goldberg SN, et al. Quality improvement guidelines for transhepatic arterial chemoembolization, embolization, and chemotherapeutic infusion for hepatic malignancy. J Vasc Interv Radiol. 2009;20(7 Suppl):S219–26. S226.e1–10.
41. Hague J, Tippett R. Endovascular techniques in palliative care. Clin Oncol. 2010;22(9):771–80. O'Neill SB, O'Connor OJ, Ryan MF, Maher MM. Interventional radiology and the care of the oncology patient. Radiol Res Pract. 2011;1:160867.
42. Straka C, Ying J, Kong FM, Willey CD, Kaminski J, Kim DW. Review of evolving etiologies, implications and treatment strategies for the superior vena cava syndrome. Springerplus. 2016;5:229.
43. McCurdy MT, Shanholtz CB. Oncologic emergencies. Crit Care Med. 2012;40:2212–22.
44. Cheng S. Superior vena cava syndrome: a contemporary review of a historic disease. Cardiol Rev. 2009;17:16–23.
45. Yu JB, Wilson LD, Detterbeck FC. Superior vena cava syndrome: a proposed classification system and algorithm for management. J Thorac Oncol. 2008;3:811–4.
46. Dubashi B, Cyriac S, Tenali SG. Clinicopathological analysis and outcome of primary mediastinal malignancies - a report of 91 cases from a single institute. Ann Thorac Med. 2009;4:140–2.
47. Wang GR, Ensor JE, Gupta S, Hicks ME, Tam AL. Bronchial artery embolization for the management of hemoptysis in oncology patients: utility and prognostic factors. J Vasc Interv Radiol. 2009;20:722–9.
48. Radchenko C, Alraiyes AH, Shojaee S. A systematic approach to the management of massive hemoptysis. J Thorac Dis. 2017;9(Suppl 10):S1069–86.
49. Ketai LH, Mohammed TL, Kirsch J, Kanne JP, Expert Panel on Thoracic Imaging, et al. ACR appropriateness criteria® hemoptysis. J Thorac Imaging. 2014;29:W19–22.
50. Ibrahim WH. Massive hemoptysis: the definition should be revised. Eur Respir J. 2008;32:1131–2.
51. Kang MJ, Kim JH, Kim YK, Lee HJ, et al. 2018 Korean clinical imaging guideline for hemoptysis. Korean J Radiol. 2018;19:866–71.
52. Ittrich H, Bockhorn M, Klose H, Simon M. The diagnosis and treatment of hemoptysis. Dtsch Arztebl Int. 2017;114:371–81. https://doi.org/10.3238/arztebl.2017.0371.
53. Yoon W, Kim JK, Kim YH, Chung TW, Kang HK. Bronchial and nonbronchial systemic artery embolization for life-threatening hemoptysis: a comprehensive review. Radiographics. 2002;22:1395–409.
54. Rodrigues G, Videtic GM, Sur R, Bezjak A, et al. Palliative thoracic radiotherapy in lung cancer: an American Society for Radiation Oncology evidence-based clinical practice guideline. Pract Radiat Oncol. 2011;1:60–71.
55. Lester JF, Macbeth FR, Toy E, Coles B. Palliative radiotherapy regimens for non-small cell lung cancer. Cochrane Database Syst Rev. 2006;4:CD002143.
56. Ernst A, Feller-Kopman D, Becker HD, Mehta AC. Central airway obstruction. Am J Respir Crit Care Med. 2004;169:1278–97.
57. Zhao W, Yang Z, Chen LA. Etiological diagnosis and treatment of central airway obstruction: report of 40 cases and review of the literature [in Chinese]. Zhonghua Jie He He Hu Xi Za Zhi. 2011;34:590–4.
58. Chen K, Varon J, Wenker OC. Malignant airway obstruction: recognition and management. J Emerg Med. 1998;16:83–92.
59. Quint LE. Thoracic complications and emergencies in oncologic patients. Cancer Imaging. 2009;9:S75–82.
60. Chhajed PN, Somandin S, Baty F, Mehta AJ, et al. Therapeutic bronchoscopy for malignant airway stenoses: choice of modality and survival. J Cancer Res Ther. 2010;6:204–9.
61. Oviatt PL, Stather DR, Michaud G, Maceachern P, Tremblay A. Exercise capacity, lung function, and quality of life after interventional bronchoscopy. J Thorac Oncol. 2011;6:38–42.
62. Amjadi K, Voduc N, Cruysberghs Y, Lemmens R, et al. Impact of interventional bronchoscopy on quality of life in malignant airway obstruction. Respiration. 2008;76:421–8.
63. Mallick I, Sharma SC, Behera D. Endobronchial brachytherapy for symptom palliation in non-small cell lung cancer–analysis of symptom response, endoscopic improvement, and quality of life. Lung Cancer. 2007;55:313–8.
64. Goldberg M, Timotin E, Farrell T, Puksa S, Donde B, Sur R. A prospective analysis of high-dose-rate endobronchial brachytherapy in the palliation of obstructive symptoms in lung cancer patients: a single-institution experience. Brachytherapy. 2015;14:655–61.
65. Kvale PA, Selecky PA, Prakash UB, American College of Chest Physicians. Palliative care in

lung cancer: ACCP evidence-based clinical practice guidelines (2nd edition). Chest. 2007;132(3 Suppl):368S–403S.
66. Abramowitz Y, Simanovsky N, Goldstein MS, Hiller N. Pleural effusion: characterization with CT attenuation values and CT appearance. Am J Roentgenol. 2009;192:618–23.
67. Kaifi JT, Toth JW, Gusani NJ, Kimchi ET, et al. Multidisciplinary management of malignant pleural effusion. J Surg Oncol. 2012;105:731–8.
68. George M, Campagna M, Babber P, Faiz SA. Pulmonary and airway emergencies. In: Manzullo EF, Gonzalez CE, Escalante CP, Yeung SJ, editors. Oncologic emergencies, MD Anderson cancer care series. New York: Springer; 2016. p. 93–111. https://doi.org/10.1007/978-1-4939-3188-0.
69. Genc O, Petrou M, Ladas G, Goldstraw P. The long-term morbidity of pleuroperitoneal shunts in the management of recurrent malignant effusions. Eur J Cardiothorac Surg. 2000;18:143–6.
70. Lentz RJ, Shojaee S, Grosu HB, Rickman OB, Interventional Pulmonary Outcomes Group, et al. The impact of gravity vs suction-driven therapeutic thoracentesis on pressure-related complications: the GRAVITAS multicenter randomized controlled trial. Chest. 2020;157:702–11.
71. Feller-Kopman D, Berkowitz D, Boiselle P, Ernst A. Large-volume thoracentesis and the risk of reexpansion pulmonary edema. Ann Thorac Surg. 2007;84:1656–61.
72. Reddy CB, De Camp MM, Diekemper RL, Gould MK, et al. Summary for clinicians: clinical practice guideline for management of malignant pleural effusions. Ann Am Thorac Soc. 2019;16:17–21.
73. Pransku SM, Francis CL. Stridor in infants and children. In: Schoem SR, Darrow DH, editors. Pediatric otolaryngology. Itasca: American Academy of Pediatrics; 2012. p. 323–52.
74. Goodman TR, McHugh K. The role of radiology in the evaluation of stridor. Arch Dis Child. 1999;81:456–9.
75. Meier S, Geiduschek J, Paganoni R, Fuehrmeyer F, Reber A. The effect of chin lift, jaw thrust, and continuous positive airway pressure on the size of the glottic opening and on stridor score in anesthetized, spontaneously breathing children. Anesth Analg. 2002;94:494–9.
76. Lee J, Naing K, Yeo ZZ, Chong PH. The use of continuous positive airway pressure ventilation in the palliative management of stridor in a head and neck cancer patient. J Pain Symptom Manag. 2019;58:e3–5.
77. Khemani RG, Randolph A, Markovitz B. Corticosteroids for the prevention and treatment of post-extubation stridor in neonates, children, and adults. Cochrane Database Syst Rev. 2009;3:CD001000.
78. Mohanti BK, Umapathy H, Bahadur S, Thakar A, Pathy S. Short-course palliative radiotherapy of 20 Gy in 5 fractions for advanced and incurable head and neck cancer: AIIMS study. Radiother Oncol. 2004;71:275–80.
79. Woodring JH, Reed JC. Types and mechanisms of pulmonary atelectasis. J Thorac Imaging. 1996;11:92–108.
80. Schindler MB. Treatment of atelectasis: where is the evidence? Crit Care. 2005;9:341–2.
81. Miske LJ, Hickey EM, Kolb SM, Weiner DJ, Panitch HB. Use of the mechanical in-exsufflator in pediatric patients with neuromuscular disease and impaired cough. Chest. 2004;125:1406–12.
82. Terzi N, Prigent H, Lofaso F. Mechanical insufflation-exsufflation to improve secretion clearance during invasive ventilation. Respir Care. 2018;63:1577–8.
83. Lauwers E, Ides K, Van Hoorenbeeck K, Verhulst S. The effect of intrapulmonary percussive ventilation in pediatric patients: a systematic review. Pediatr Pulmonol. 2018;53:1463–74.
84. Chang AB, Fortescue R, Grimwood K, Alexopoulou E, et al. European Respiratory Society guidelines for the management of children and adolescents with bronchiectasis. Eur Respir J. 2021;58:2002990.
85. Donaldson SH, Bennett WD, Zeman KL, Knowles MR, Tarran R, Boucher RC. Mucus clearance and lung function in cystic fibrosis with hypertonic saline. N Engl J Med. 2006;354:241–50.
86. Abu-Hasan MN, Chesrown SE, Jantz MA. Successful use of bronchoscopic lung insufflation to treat left lung atelectasis. Pediatr Pulmonol. 2013;48:306–9.
87. NCCN Clinical Practice Guidelines in Oncology. Prevention and treatment of cancer-related infections. Version 3.2022. 28 Oct 2022. Accessed from: https://www.nccn.org/professionals/physician_gls/pdf/infections.pdf on 23 Jan 2023.
88. Klastersky J, Paesmans M, Rubenstein EB, Boyer M, et al. The Multinational Association for Supportive Care in Cancer risk index: a multinational scoring system for identifying low-risk febrile neutropenic cancer patients. J Clin Oncol. 2000;18:3038–51.
89. Kumar A, Biswas B, Chopra A, Kapil A, Vishnubhatla S, Bakhshi S. Early discontinuation versus continuation of antimicrobial therapy in low risk pediatric cancer patients with febrile neutropenia, before recovery of counts: a randomized controlled trial (DALFEN study). Indian J Pediatr. 2021;88:240–5.
90. Averbuch D, Orasch C, Cordonnier C, Livermore DM, On behalf of ECIL4, a joint venture of EBMT, EORTC, ICHS, ESGICH/ESCMID and ELN, et al. European guidelines for empirical antibacterial therapy for febrile neutropenic patients in the era of growing resistance: summary of the 2011 4th European Conference on Infections in Leukemia. Haematologica. 2013;98:1826–35.
91. Howard SC, Jones DP, Pui CH. The tumor lysis syndrome. N Engl J Med. 2011;364:1844–54.
92. McBride A, Trifilio S, Baxter N, Gregory TK, Howard SC. Managing tumor lysis syndrome in the

era of novel cancer therapies. J Adv Pract Oncol. 2017;8:705–20.
93. Philips A, Radhakrishnan V, Ganesan P, Ganesan TS, et al. Efficacy of single dose rasburicase (1.5 mg) for prophylaxis and management of laboratory tumor lysis syndrome. Indian J Hematol Blood Transfus. 2018;34:618–22.
94. Stewart AF. Clinical practice. Hypercalcemia associated with cancer. N Engl J Med. 2005;352:373–9.
95. Kuchay MS, Kaur P, Mishra SK, Mithal A. The changing profile of hypercalcemia in a tertiary care setting in North India: an 18-month retrospective study. Clin Cases Miner Bone Metab. 2017;14:131–5.
96. Goldner W. Cancer-related hypercalcemia. J Oncol Pract. 2016;12:426–32.
97. Workeneh BT, Jhaveri KD, Rondon-Berrios H. Hyponatremia in the cancer patient. Kidney Int. 2020;98:870–82.
98. Castillo JJ, Vincent M, Justice E. Diagnosis and management of hyponatremia in cancer patients. Oncologist. 2012;17:756–65.
99. Stroszczynski C, Hunerbein M. Malignant biliary obstruction: the value of findings on imaging. Abdom Imaging. 2005;30:314–23.
100. Yeh TS, Jan YY, Tseng JH, Chiu CT, et al. Malignant perihilar biliary obstruction: magnetic resonance cholangiopancreatographic findings. Am J Gastroenterol. 2000;95:432–40.
101. Saad WEA, Wallace MJ, Wojak JC, Kundu S, Cardella JF. Quality improvement guidelines for percutaneous transhepatic cholangiography, biliary drainage, and percutaneous cholecystostomy. J Vasc Interv Radiol. 2010;21(6):789–95.
102. Guimaraes MD, Bitencourt AG, Marchiori E, Chojniak R, Gross JL, Kundra V. Imaging acute complications in cancer patients: what should be evaluated in the emergency setting? Cancer Imaging. 2014;14:18.
103. Russo P. Urologic emergencies in the cancer patient. Semin Oncol. 2000;27:284–98.
104. O'Neill SB, O'Connor OJ, Ryan MF, Maher MM. Interventional radiology and the care of the oncology patient. Radiol Res Pract. 2011;1:160867.
105. Park BK, Kim SH, Moon MH. Nonvascular interventions of the urinary tract. J Korean Med Sci. 2002;17:727–36.

Online Links

Oncologic Emergencies - The Advanced EM Boot Camp Course. https://youtu.be/l_7xTB537k4.

Managing Oncologic Emergencies. BC Emergency Medicine Network. https://youtu.be/UBU3YaKI2-I.

IROC Session 7 - Radiation oncology emergencies. IROC Session 7 - Radiation oncology emergencies. https://youtu.be/uwAMn_pJD20.

Brain metastases: prognosis, treatment & symptom management - Jerome Graber, M.D., M.P.H. Seattle Science Foundation. https://youtu.be/7coI69CLS4g.

Palliative radiotherapy planning – Webinar. Health Education England—HEE. https://youtu.be/9AW9h71MkRs.

BC Sepsis Guidelines 2022 Webinar - March 10, 2022. BC Emergency Medicine Network. https://youtu.be/2f2GIDudago.

How to manage febrile neutropenia? European Society for Medical Oncology. https://youtu.be/rnN9rlmL3s4.

Metastatic and Oligometastatic Diseases

Anusheel Munshi, Rahul Krishnatry,
Senthil Rajappa, Namita Mohindra,
Dileep R. Hoysal, and Gaurav Agarwal

1 Introduction

Metastasis is the cause of more than 90% of all cancer deaths. While primary tumors can often be controlled by local surgery or radiation, metastasis represents a much more advanced disease state. Nearly all malignancies have the metastatic potential of varying degrees. Common malignancies such as Breast, lung, and gastrointestinal malignancies are well known for developing metastatic disease. Overall, the most common sites of metastatic disease include bone, Lungs, Liver, and brain.

A. Munshi (✉)
Department of Radiation Oncology, BLK MAX Hospital, New Delhi, Delhi, India

R. Krishnatry
Department of Radiation Oncology, Tata Memorial Certre, (HBNI), Mumbai, India

S. Rajappa
Department of Medical Oncology, Basavatarakam Indo American Cancer Hospital and Research Centre, Hyderabad, India

N. Mohindra
Department of Radiology, SGPGI, Lucknow, India

D. R. Hoysal
Department of Endocrine & Breast Surgery, SGPGI, Lucknow, India

G. Agarwal
Department of Endocrine & Breast Surgery, SGPGI, Lucknow, India

Endocrine & Breast Surgery, SGPGIMS, Lucknow, India

There are three major pathways of metastasis. These include (1) the lymphatic system (e.g., neck nodes in head neck primaries), (2) hematogenous (e.g., breast cancer spread to lungs), and (3) across body cavities, such as the peritoneal cavity or within the cerebrospinal fluid (CSF) (e.g., medulloblastoma dissemination within CSF or ovarian tumor dissemination on the peritoneal surface of the intestine).

Typically, any metastatic disease is considered Stage IV disease. Overall, a disseminated metastatic disease for any primary site carries a poor prognosis. Many of these patients, especially those with poor performance status, are suitable only for palliative approaches like palliative radiotherapy and palliative chemotherapy. Early institution of palliative care should be the norm for these patients.

Over the past 30 years, there has been significant interest in treating oligometastases in patients with aggressive local intent. It has become well known that persistent tumors in the local or distant sites can be a source of progression and further metastases. Oligometastasis is derived from Greek word oligo meaning small number and metastasis. Patient outcomes have shown that oligometastatic disease (OMD) and selected polymetastastic disease (PMD) patients will have improved overall survival (OS) with appropriate treatment approaches. Stereotactic ablative radiotherapy (SABR) can provide PF and OS benefits in the OMD state, and it is postu-

B. K. Mohanti et al. (eds.), *Radiation Oncology – Principles, Precepts and Practice*,
https://doi.org/10.1007/978-981-95-5171-2_22

lated that some benefits could extend to the PMD state as well [1, 2].

2 Pathophysiology and Rationale of Treatment for OM and Metastatic Disease

Cancers emerge from an ongoing evolutionary process. Often, multiple competing subclones develop within a single primary tumor. At times, the evolutionary process results in the formation of metastases, which is the cause of 90% of cancer-related deaths. However, despite the immense clinical importance, very little is known about the dissemination of cancer cells to distant organs. The general hypothesis is that each metastasis originates from a single tumor cell. Besides tumor-to-metastasis spread, even metastasis-to-metastasis spread is a frequent phenomenon. This can happen through de novo monoclonal seeding of daughter metastases or by the transfer of multiple tumor clones between metastatic sites [3].

It is imperative for oncologists and cancer scientists to gain foundational knowledge regarding cancer metastasis. Often, cancer originating from certain primary sites have specific natural history of metastasis to specific body sites called metastatic organotropism, which are considered the favorite sites of metastatic disease (Table 1).

Table 1 Metastatic organotropism

Site	Favorite metastatic sites
Ocular melanoma	Liver and lung
Head and neck cancer	Lung and bone
Thyroid cancer	Bone, liver, and lung
Melanoma	Lungs, liver, bones, and brain
Esophageal cancer	Lung, bones, adrenal glands, and brain
Lung cancer	Bone, brain, pleura, diaphragm, liver, adrenal, thyroid, and spleen
Breast cancer	Bone, lung, liver, brain, adrenals, and ovary
Stomach cancer	Liver, lung, and bone
Kidney cancer	Lung, liver, and bone
Pancreatic cancer	Liver, stomach, colon, and peritoneum
Colon cancer	Liver, lung, urinary bladder, and stomach
Bladder cancer	Lung, rectum, colon, prostate, ureter, vagina, bone, peritoneum, pleura, liver, and brain
Prostate cancer	Bone
Testicular cancer	Lung and liver
Uterine cancer	Lung, liver, and ovary
Rectal cancer	Liver, lung, and peritoneum
Ovarian cancer	Diaphragm and peritoneum

Note: Lymph nodes are a common site of metastasis but are considered a part of loco regional disease, unless away from the tumor site

In patients with disseminated metastasis or a scenario where the metastatic disease is evident without a known primary, IHC markers can be of immense help in understanding the primary site. Table 2 provides the IHC markers for potential cancer types.

Patients with metastatic disease can be broadly subdivided into the patients with OM disease, with limited polymetastatic disease, and with disseminated metastatic disease (Fig. 1). In our current state of knowledge, oligometastatic disease is considered an intermediate cancer state with limited metastatic burden, which would be amenable for curative treatments. OMD would need to be evaluated and then suitably classified. In the absence of widespread metastases, the appearance of OMD at limited site(s) is called 'De Novo OMD'- synchronous (within 6 months) and metachronous. With previous history of systemic metastases (PMD), when there is appearance of limited metastasis, this is called "Induced OMD". Such a pictorial representation is provided to understand different states of OMD and PMD (Fig. 1), in order to make multi-disciplinary decision regarding curative or palliative treatment approaches.

As shown in Fig. 2, each of these classes has a survival curve different from the others. With modern-day local and systemic approaches, the aim is to move the curves toward superior outcomes, especially for patients with OM disease.

A further rationale for treatment in a limited metastasis scenario is the presence of sensitive diagnostic modalities in the modern era. These

Table 2 Immunohistochemistry (IHC) markers for identifying primary site of origin

Immunohistochemical marker	Potential cancer type
Pan-cytokeratin and/or EMA	Carcinoma
Desmin, Vimentin, S100, αSMA, myoD1, CD34, KIT and/or CD99	Sarcoma
CD 45/LCA	Lymphoma
S100, HMB45 and/or Melan-A	Melanoma
Detecting broad types of carcinoma	
CK5/6 and/or p63	Squamous cell carcinoma
CK7 and/or CK20	Adenocarcinoma
Chromogranin, synaptophysin, and/or CD56	Neuroendocrine carcinoma
PLAP, OCT4, AFP and/or hCG, CKIT	Germ-cell carcinoma

Categorizing carcinomas into subgroups according to CK7 and CK20 expression

CK7+/CK20−	CK7+/CK20+	CK7−/CK20+	CK7−/CK20+
Lung adenocarcinoma Breast carcinoma Pancreatic adenocarcinoma Gastric adenocarcinoma Endometrial adenocarcinoma Endocervical adenocarcinoma Ovarian (serous) carcinoma Cholangiocarcinoma Small cell lung carcinoma Mesothelioma Thyroid carcinoma Salivary gland tumors Kidney (papillary) Urothelial carcinoma	Urothelial carcinoma Cholangiocarcinoma Bladder adenocarcinoma Pancreatic adenocarcinoma Ovarian mucinous carcinoma Gastric adenocarcinoma	Colorectal adenocarcinoma Gastric adenocarcinoma Merkel cell carcinoma	Prostate adenocarcinoma Renal (clear cell) Hepatocellular carcinoma Small cell lung carcinoma Gastric adenocarcinoma Non-seminoma germ cell tumors Mesothelioma

Site-specific origins for adenocarcinoma	
CA-125, WT1 and/or PAX-8	Ovarian cancer (serous papillary)
ER, GCDFP-15 and/or mammaglobulin (CK7+ and CK20−), GATA 3	Breast carcinoma
PSA, PSMA, NKX 3.1 (CK7− and CK20−)	Prostate carcinoma
CA-125 and/or ER (CK7+ and CK20−), WT-1	Endometrial carcinoma
CA-125, CA 19.9, CEA and/or mesothelin (CK7+ and CK20±)	Pancreatic adenocarcinoma
CDX2 and SATB-2 (CK7− and CK20+)	Colon carcinoma
TTF1 (CK7+ and CK20−), NAPSIN-A	Non-small-cell lung cancer (lung adenocarcinoma)
Hep Par-1, AFP, polyclonal CEA, CD10 and/or CD13, Arginase-1, Glypican-3. (CK7− and CK20−)	Hepatocellular carcinoma
TTF1 and/or thyroglobulin (CK7+ and CK20−)	Thyroid carcinoma
CD10 (CK7− and CK20−)/RCC	Renal cell carcinoma
CK7+, CK 20+, GATA-3	Urothelial carcinoma

CA cancer antigen, *CDX* caudal type homeobox, *SMA* smooth muscle actin, *AFP* α-fetoprotein, *CEA* carcinoembryonic antigen, *CK* cytokeratin, *CLA* cutaneous lymphocyte-associated antigen, *CUP* cancer of unknown primary, *EMA* epithelial membrane antigen, *ER* estrogen receptor, *GCDFP* gross cystic disease fluid protein, *hCG* human chorionic gonadotropin, *Hep Par* hepatocyte-specific antigen, *myoD* myoblast determination protein, *OCT* octamer-binding transcription factor, *PAP* prostatic acid phosphatase, *PAS* periodic acid Schiff, *PGP* protein gene product, *PLAP* placental alkaline phosphatase, *PSA* prostate-specific antigen, *SCC* squamous-cell carcinoma, *TTF* thyroid transcription factor, *WT* Wilms tumor protein

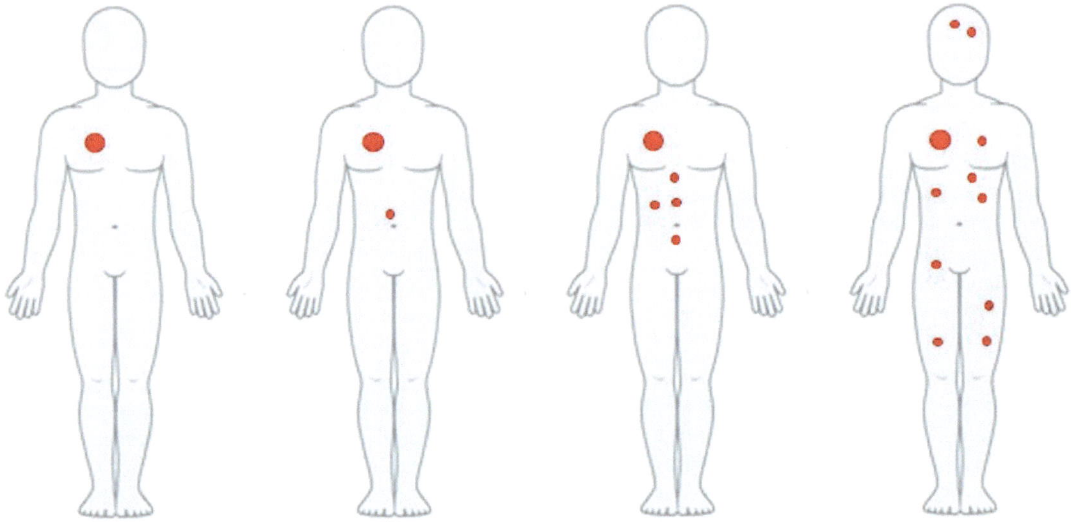

Fig. 1 Spectrum of metastatic disease (to classify OMD and PMD): Left 2 figures limited OMD, next figure represents oligoclonal progression in abdomen, right corner figure represents PMD in chest, abdomen, brain, lymph nodes and extremities

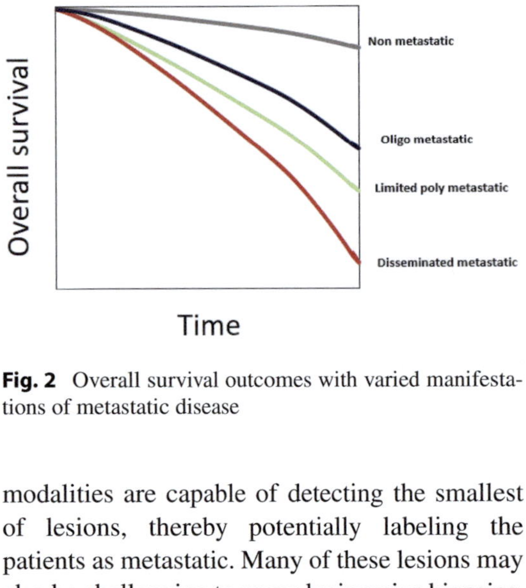

Fig. 2 Overall survival outcomes with varied manifestations of metastatic disease

modalities are capable of detecting the smallest of lesions, thereby potentially labeling the patients as metastatic. Many of these lesions may also be challenging to prove by invasive biopsies, given their small size and accessibility issues. As such, it may be prudent to continue with curative treatment(s) in such situations [1, 2].

3 Radiology Aspects

Imaging is vital to diagnose and define local disease, poly-metastatic or oligo-metastatic status (≤ 5 metastases in ≤ 3 organs). CT or MRI assesses baseline tumor features (size/extent, volume, and metabolism). Even in the absence of symptoms of distant metastasis, "risk assessment" for the probability of metastasis is done based on the baseline tumor features, histological type, and/or genetic profile. Other features, such as angiogenic capability and functional imaging-based tumor properties, such as maximum standardized uptake value (SUV_{max}) are being investigated as biomarkers for predicting the prognosis (risk of recurrence and metastasis) [4].

Tumor types that are predisposed to oligometastasis include lung, prostate, colorectal, sarcoma, and renal cancer [4]. The most typical sites of metastasis are the liver, lung, and skeletal system. Liver and lung evaluation is done by organ-specific imaging, whereas skeletal and nodal evaluation requires whole-body imaging (Table 3).

- Liver metastasis: CT and MRI are robust tools for diagnosing liver metastasis. MRI is considered more accurate for characterization (including lesions <10 mm in size) and also in cases with fatty liver changes [5].
- Lung metastasis: The modality of choice is CT.
- Skeletal metastasis: 18F NaF-PET/CT has the highest sensitivity (100%) and specificity

Table 3 Imaging modalities commonly used for detecting metastasis

Imaging targeted to particular areas	CT	Organ-specific MRI	Whole-body MRI with DWI	18F FDG-PET	PET-MRI	Skeletal scintigraphy
Lung	Widely available, relatively low cost	–	–	PET/CT is superior to PET/MRI for the detection of lung lesions [5]	–	–
Liver	Widely available, relatively low cost	More accurate than CT for characterization (including lesions <10 mm in size) [5]. Hepato-biliary specific contrast agents have higher sensitivity and specificity	–	–	PET/MRI shows superior performance to PET-CT for the detection of brain and liver metastases	–
Skeletal system [6]	Sensitivity 74%, specificity 56%. Can monitor treatment response as the appearance of sclerotic changes	–	Sensitivity 95%, specificity 90%. Can assess treatment response earlier than non-quantitative assessment	Sensitivity 98%, specificity 56%	Sensitivity 95%, specificity 90%	Sensitivity 78%, specificity 48% Limitations: false positive in benign lesions; poor spatial resolution (~1 cm); false negative in lesions with low tracer uptake, e.g., metastasis from RCC
Nodal disease evaluation	Size and morphology used for detection		Good diagnostic performance for some sites (porta hepatis); not good for cervical, mediastinal supraclavicular or mesenteric regions [7]	Higher sensitivity and specificity than CT/MRI	Higher sensitivity for head, neck, and pelvis	–

(97%). Other useful modalities are MRI, SPECT, ^{18}FDG PET, CT, and bone scintigraphy [6].

- Nodal disease: FDG-PET-CT and MRI-based tumor ADC values are useful to predict positive nodal status. Size-based assessment by CT or MRI has low sensitivity and specificity.

Skeletal scintigraphy is most commonly done using the osteotropic agent, methylene diphosphonate (99mTc-MDP) due to its low cost, effectiveness, wide availability, and favorable dosimetry.

SPECT (Single-photon emission CT) imaging of the skeleton also uses 99mTc-MDP; however, images are acquired in cross-section instead of planar orientation. Sensitivity 87%, specificity 91% [6].

18F FDG-PET is a functional imaging modality and is commonly used because of the high glucose uptake in viable tumor cells. Sensitivity varies among different histologies—uptake is limited in tumors with low metabolic activity [6].

18F Na F-PET/CT (18F labeled sodium fluoride) is an osteotropic compound that has a higher first-pass extraction rate than 99mTc-MDP. Sensitivity 100% and specificity 97%. Requires a cyclotron for production, limiting its availability [6].

Whole body MRI (with DWI): has good diagnostic performance for detecting lesions in the liver, bone marrow, and some lymph-nodal sites (porta hepatis). However, it is not very good for the lungs and other lymph-nodal regions (cervical, mediastinal, supraclavicular, or mesenteric regions) [7].

Amongst the hybrid imaging techniques (PET/CT and PET/MRI): PET/CT is superior to PET/MRI for the detection of lung lesions, whereas PET/MRI shows superior performance for the detection of brain and liver metastases [8].

The selection of imaging modalities also depends upon the site of tumor and its propensity to metastasize to a particular area. Colorectal malignancies usually metastasize to the liver, so they should be evaluated by CT or MRI with liver-specific contrast agents. For sarcomas, high-resolution CT should be done.

Lung cancer: FDG PET combined with CT is the standard method for baseline staging and radiation treatment planning [9]. Lung cancer frequently metastasizes to the brain, for which MRI is better than CT.

The sensitivity and specificity of PET imaging are optimized by using disease-specific tracers.

Prostate cancer: PSMA-MR is most specific for loco-regional staging of prostate cancer. ^{68}Ga PSMA PET-CT shows the best detection rates for the assessment of nodal, bone, and visceral metastases, especially for smaller lesions at low PSA levels [10].

For well-differentiated neuroendocrine tumors, [^{68}Ga]Ga-DOTA-peptide PET/CT is the technique of choice.

Limitations of imaging: According to the RECIST criteria, lesions <5 mm (~65 mm^3) are undetectable. The spatial resolution of MRI ranges from 0.5 mm^3 (for organ-specific imaging) to 50 mm^3 for whole body techniques. The spatial resolution of PET CT is 5–7 mm (for ^{18}F). Sensitivities and specificities of modalities vary, and none are high enough to validate an OM status with certainty [4].

4 Radiotherapy in Metastatic and OM Disease

Conventionally, palliative radiotherapy has been employed for symptomatic relief for widespread diseases causing local distress, such as pain, bleeding, obstruction of the airway or food pipe, etc. There are various dose schedules, from single fraction 8–10 Gy to multiple fractionated simple treatments (20 Gy in 5 or 30 Gy in 10 fractions given daily) to offer quick treatment and relief. Most patients with bone metastases have multiple sites of involvement. As many as 76% of those receiving local field to the symptomatic site would require additional treatment for pain at other locations within 1 year. Historically, wide-field radiotherapy, such as hemibody radiotherapy (upper, middle, or lower), is used for some distinct advantages. These include decreased needs for retreatments, more rapid onset of symptom relief (24–48 h), and some benefits for occult metastatic disease. The disadvantage of choosing a patient for hemibody treatments is the need for premedication with steroids and antiemetics. Most patients experience acute gastrointestinal toxicity, with nausea, vomiting, and diarrhea persisting for 24–48 h, but seldom need hydration or admission if appropriate premedication is provided. Myelosuppression is also commonly observed but is rarely of clinical significance. Radiation pneumonitis is rare at doses below 7 Gy to the lungs; restricting the upper hemibody dose to 6 Gy or using lung blocks with 8 Gy is useful.

Apart from hemibody radiotherapy, systemic radionuclides such as Strontium-89 can be used to treat bone metastases (Table 4). Selective absorption into bone metastases limits irradiation of normal tissues and increases the therapeutic ratio. Administration as a single intravenous injection in the outpatient clinic is a further advantage for many patients. This can be specifically considered in patients with widespread bone metastasis disease as an adjuvant to radiotherapy or as first-line therapy. However, it should be avoided when there is imminent epidural cord compression, pathological fracture, or mechanical instability, and poor bone marrow reserve (WBC < 2400, Platelet <100,000).

There is a merging of borders between the locoregional disease to the metastatic state by the invention of the term "oligometastatic disease" (OMD). The OMD has a variety of definitions depending on tumor site, biology, thorough investigations to stage accurately, and the natural history associated and understood today. On similar lines, the scope and goals of palliative radiotherapy have been expanding, thereby blurring with curative treatments. Conventionally, it used to be a symptom-oriented therapy to improve QOL by alleviating symptoms. It has slowly moved to symptom prevention therapy, focusing on avoiding future symptoms or deterioration of QoL, as the patient may be asymptomatic in the current state.

While conventional symptom-related treatment would need single or fewer simple treatments, radical palliation may necessitate long protracted treatment with or without chemotherapy and or targeted therapy or complex short-course treatments, such as stereotactic body radiation therapy (SBRT). Table 5 compares SBRT with other competing/complementary techniques for treating metastatic disease.

SBRT indications, its competing modalities, the prognostic factors affecting SBRT and future outcomes related to SBRT are summarized in Fig. 3.

5 Important Sites of Metastasis

5.1 Bone and Spine

Bone metastases are a frequent complication of cancer (Fig. 4). They occur in up to 70% of patients with advanced breast or prostate cancer and in approximately 15–30% of patients with primary lung, colon, gastrointestinal, stomach, bladder, thyroid, or kidney carcinoma sites. Bone metastasis can be osteolytic, osteoblastic, or mixed. Osteolytic metastases are distressing, for they can mechanically cause pain, spinal cord compression, nerve compression, and pathologic fractures. Metabolically, they can cause life-threatening hypercalcemia. Even patients with osteoblastic metastases can have bone pain and pathologic fractures because of the poor quality of bone produced by the osteoblasts. Overall, bone metastasis is a severe complication of cancer.

For a long time now, conventional radiotherapy has been used as an efficient and cost-effective solution for the palliation of pain and treatment of spinal cord compression. Traditionally, moderately hypofractionated external beam radiotherapy (EBRT) has been the standard of care for metastatic spine disease and has been associated with an overall and complete pain response rate of 70% and 20%, respectively [11]*.

An emerging paradigm in treating bone and vertebral metastasis is SBRT. This is essentially an external beam radiotherapy (EBRT) method that accurately delivers a high radiation dose to an extra-cranial target/tumor in one or a few treatment fractions [12, 13]. SBRT is used to treat various sites, such as the lung, liver, spine, bone, etc., and is usually delivered within one to five sessions.

SBRT is now being increasingly used to manage the OM disease, especially in vertebral metastasis and selected bony sites. The predominant limitation to radiotherapy dose delivery for vertebral metastasis is the spinal cord and cauda equina radiation tolerance. The steep dose fall-off seen with SBRT enables a sharp fall-off towards

Table 4 General features for various commonly used systemic radionuclides

	Half-life	Energy	Distribution	Excretion	Toxicity	Remarks
Strontium-89	50.6 days	Beta: 1.46 MeV	Bone mineral matrix (calcium)	Urine	Hematological	Used in prostate cancer
Samarium-153	46.3 h	0.81 MeV (20%), 0.71 MeV (30%), and 0.64 MeV (50%) and gamma photons of 103 keV (28%)	Chelated to a phosphonate (ethylenediamine tetramethylene; EDTMP) to produce a bone-seeking complex	Urine	Hematological	Man-made A flare of bone pain occurred in 12% of patients. The overall pain relief rate was 74%, with a median duration of palliation of 2.6 months. In responders, relief was obtained promptly within 7–14 days of treatment. Response rates were significantly higher with 2.5 mCi/kg than 1.0 mCi/kg
Rhenium-186	3.8 days	Beta particles of 1.07 MeV and a 137-keV gamma-ray	Complexed into a bone-seeking phosphonate, hydroxyethylene diphosphonic acid (HEDP)	Urine	Hematological	Prostate, breast, colon, and lung. A pain flare occurs in 10% of patients 2–3 days after treatment and resolves within 1 week

Table 5 Comparison of Stereotactic body radiotherapy (SBRT), Surgery and Radiofrequency ablation (RFA)

Characteristic	SBRT	Surgery	RFA
Precision	Excellent	Excellent	Excellent
Tolerability	Good	Depends on PS	Good
Ability to do nonuniform intensity treatments across the disease volume	Yes	No	No
Need for GA	No	Usually GA	No
Post-procedure recovery	Not an issue	Usually takes weeks	Not much issue
Tissue diagnosis	Not available	Available	Not available
Cost	Lower	May be higher	Lower
Complications	Yes, related to RT effects	Yes, related to surgery	Yes, related to RFA
Need for a good performance score (PS) of patient	Fair PS needed	Good PS needed	Fair PS needed

the cord. At the same time, it maintains high doses in the vertebra, increasing the probability of long-term tumor control and adequate pain control. Since spinal SBRT evolved after cranial SBRT, many of the published series of spine SBRT have used single-fraction regimens. Tables 6 and 7 provide the series of patients with spine and bone (non-spine) metastasis undergoing SBRT.

Suitable patients for spinal SBRT include (1) localized spine metastasis from C1 to L5, solitary metastasis or, (2) individual spine levels, such as cervical, thoracic, lumbar, or, (3) separate sites of spine. Each of the separate sites must have a maximal involvement of two contiguous vertebral bodies. (2) Spinal compression (only if there is a gap of >3 mm between the spinal cord and edge of the epidural lesion). (3) Paraspinal mass (<5 cm) contiguous with spine metastasis. (4) Intractable pain [14] Typical dose fractionations for spinal SBRT include (a) 16–24 Gy in 1# (b) 20–24 Gy in 2# (c) 27 Gy in 3# (d) 30 Gy in 5#. Multiple series support high rates of local control from 80% to 95%, and excellent pain relief (up to 40% complete pain response) [15–17]. It is to be noted that even in radioresistant histologies that previously exhibited poor response with conventional EBRT, high local control rates are observed with SBRT [18]. The rate of vertebral compression fractures (VCF) at 3 years after SBRT to the spine is around 10%, and the rate of plexopathy is around 2%. Figure 5 illustrates a breast cancer patient who had two metastatic bony sites, which were treated by SBRT technique.

5.1.1 Metastatic Spinal Cord Compression (MSCC)

Metastatic spinal cord compression (MSCC) develops primarily in one of four ways: (a) growth into the adjacent epidural space; (b) paraspinal mass causing neural foramina extension; (c) vertebral body collapse with the displacement of multiple bony fragments into the epidural space; or (d) primary hematogenous seeding to the epidural space (rare). Prolonged ischemia finally results in an infarct of white matter and permanent cord damage.

Sitewise, the most common primary tumor types causing MSCC are breast cancer, lung cancer, and prostate cancer. The most common site of MSCC involvement is in the thoracic spine (60–80%), followed by the lumbar (15–30%) and cervical spine (<10%). In up to 50% of patients, it can involve multiple levels. The most common symptom is back pain (80%), followed by weakness (70%), sensory deficits (65%), and autonomic dysfunction (45%).

Management of MSCC generally involves using steroids, radiotherapy, and surgery in appropriate cases. A loading dose of 8–10 mg iv dexamethasone followed by a maintenance dose of 4–6 mg every 6–8 h is considered optimal. Subsequently, patients can be switched to an oral regimen. Simultaneously, the patients should be started on a proton pump inhibitor for GI prophylaxis.

For patients with limited disease, good performance status, and life expectancy >6 months,

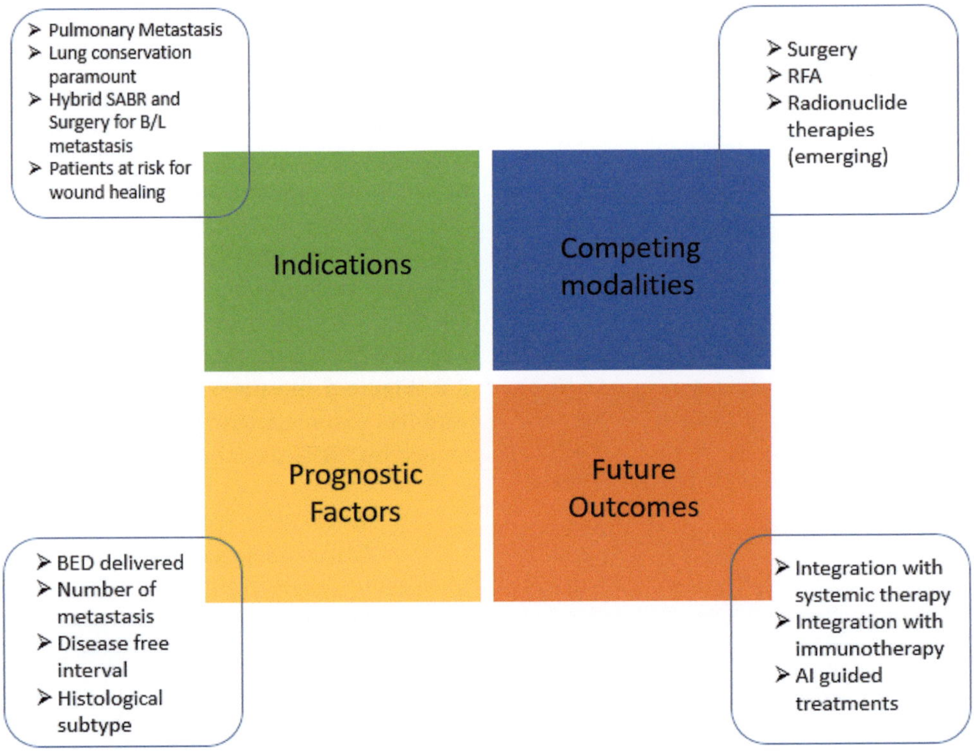

Fig. 3 SBRT in metastatic disease: indications, competing modalities, prognostic factors, and future outcomes

vertebral decompression and stabilization of the spine is a preferable line of management [19].

Palliative radiotherapy has been the standard of care in treating patients with MSCC. A total of 30 Gy in 10 fractions is the most frequently employed fractionation schedule. Other shorter fractionation schedules (8 Gy × 1 or 4 Gy × 5) can be employed in patients with more aggressive disease or with inferior performance status.

Of late, there has been some interest in more aggressive management of limited polymetastatic disease. Randomized data about the usefulness of SBRT in the PM setting is lacking. However, the contraindications for aggressive treatment of polymetastatic disease include patients with (1) poor general condition, (2) poor life expectancy, (3) inability to treat all sites of disease, (4) >5 cm size of metastasis, (5) frank cord compression, (6) impending fractures, and (7) caution to be exerted for patients with ulcerative colitis, Crohn's disease, interstitial lung disease, and lupus.

5.2 Lung Metastasis

Approximately 30% of all patients with cancer will develop pulmonary metastases at some point in the course of their disease. In yesteryears, hematogenous spread of solid organ malignancies to the pulmonary tissue was considered a terminal event, and the role of radiotherapy in disseminated lung metastasis was limited. Low dose RT is occasionally employed as a whole lung bath for malignancies such as Ewing's tumor (Indicated in patients with pleural or pulmonary metastatic disease) on completion of consolidation therapy with reasonable outcomes. Typically, doses of 15–18 Gy in 10–12 fractions (usually 1.5–1.6 Gray per fraction) are used in this scenario.

However, more aggressive local treatment options for limited lung metastasis have been increasingly used in the last few years, including surgery, radiofrequency ablation, and SBRT. After excellent results in the context of

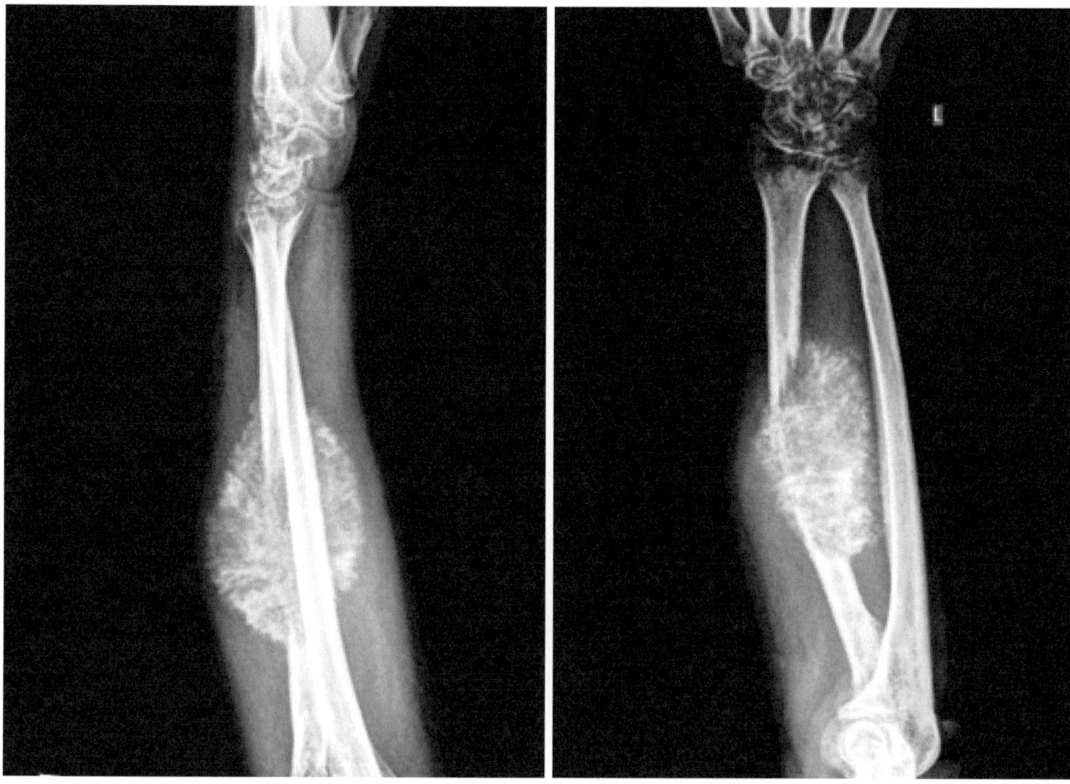

Fig. 4 In a known case of Adenocarcinoma GE junction: X-ray left forearm AP and Lateral views: s/o expansile lytic lesion involving diaphysis (shaft) of the left radius with significant sunburst periosteal reaction. Adjacent soft-tissue swelling is seen

lung cancer, SABR has become an increasingly attractive option in the treatment arsenal for patients with lung metastases. The principles of treatment and planning are nearly the same as for primary lung cancers. While there is no absolute size and number criteria, the typical patients selected have <3–5 metastases, with a size of <3–5 cm each [20, 21].

Different groups have used a variety of treatment fractionations ranging from single-dose RT to hypofractionated RT in 2–4 fractions to treatment in 5–15 fractions (Table 8). Typical dose fractionations used for SBRT for lung metastasis include 18 Gy × 3 and 12 Gy × 5. The target number for SBRT in lung metastasis is also highly variable; hence, a comparison of the different approaches concerning clinical efficacy is challenging. Target volumes are very inhomogeneous in the published data. Furthermore, patient selection will have a significant impact on treatment outcomes.

A (DEGRO) working group pooled analysis included 700 patients from 20 centers with medically inoperable pulmonary metastases [22]. The most significant prognostic factors for OS on multivariable analysis were pretreatment performance status (hazard ratio [HR] 0.972), maximum metastasis diameter (HR 1.118), the number of metastases (single vs. multiple, [HR 0.774]), and the interval between primary tumor diagnosis and treatment (HR 0.968) [23].

Overall, the reported local control rates range from 80% to 95%. The dose significantly influenced local control at the planning target volume (PTV) periphery (HR 1.117), dose to PTV at the isocenter (HR ¼ 0.988), and pretreatment performance status (HR 0.952). There was a trend toward poorer local control with increasing fractions (HR 1.251, $P < 0.052$). Colorectal primary histology has also been variably reported as resistant to ablative radiation.

Table 6 Outcomes for SBRT in spine oligometastatic patients

Study	Patients/ metastasis	Primary tumor site	Dose fractionation	Treatment technique	Median FU	Local control	Overall survival	≥Grade 3 toxicity	Comments
Sprave et al. 2018 [27]	55 patients	Multiple	24 Gy in 1 Fr	SBRT (Tomo/ LINAC-VMAT)	8.1 months	Not reported	Not reported	None	Compared pain responses between high-dose SBRT versus standard 3DCRT. Pain values decreased faster in time period in the SBRT arm (VAS and OMED score)
Tseng et al. 2018 [28]	145 patients/279 spinal mets	Multiple	24 Gy in 2 Fr	SBRT (LINAC)	15 months	1 year-90.3%, 2 year-82.4%	1 year-73.1%, 2 year-60.7% Median OS: 33.3 months	None	VCF at 1 and 2 years was 8.5% and 13.8% respectively. OM: 74.5% patients
Yamada et al. 2017 [29]	657 patients/811 lesions	Multiple	16–26 Gy in 1 Fr	SRS (LINAC)	26.9 months	1-year-99.37% 2-year-97.7% 3-year-97.4% 4-year-96.9% Mean time to LC failure: 26 months (range: 9.7–57)	Median OS: 26.9 months	2 (0.46%)	VCF and pain control: not reported
Germano et al. 2016 [30]	95 patients/143 lesions	Multiple	10–18 Gy in 1 Fr	SRS (LINAC)	16 months	94%	Not reported	None	VCF-21% Pain control-100%
Lee et al. 2016 [31]	79 patients/100 lesions	Multiple	SF-18 Gy/1 Fr fSRS-27 Gy/3 Fr	SRS (LINAC)	29 months	81%	1 year-77.2%, 2 year-49.4%	None	VCF-40.5%
Moussazadeh et al. 2015 [32]	31 patients/36 lesions	Multiple	24 Gy/1 Fr	SRS	6.1 years	91.6%	Not reported	None	VCF-36%
Sellin et al. 2015 [33]	37 patients/40 lesions	RCC	24 Gy/1 Fr 27 Gy/3 Fr 30 Gy/5 Fr	SRS (LINAC)	49 months	57%	Median OS 16.3 months	None	Pain response-41%

Bate et al. 2015 [34]	57 patients/67 lesions	Multiple (common- renal, breast, and lung)	16–23 Gy in 1 Fr	SRS	10 months	94.2% at 1 year	NR	None	21% treated had surgery prior to SRS. VCF-7.2%
Yamada et al. 2008 [35]	93 patients/103 lesions	Multiple (common- RCC, prostate, and melanoma)	18–24 Gy/1 Fr	SRS (IMRT)	15 months	90%	OS- 15 months	None	High rates of efficacy with spine SBRT. Vertebral compression fractures progressed and developed de novo in 4.1% and 3.6%, respectively
Gerstzen et al. 2007 [36]	393 patients/500 lesions	Multiple	15–22.5 Gy/1 Fr	SRS (CK)	21 months	88%	NR	None	Showed the potential of radiosurgery in the treatment of patients with spinal metastases, especially those with solitary sites of spine involvement, to improve long-term palliation.

Table 7 Bone oligometastatic (non spine)

Study	Patients/ metastasis	Primary tumor site	Dose fractionation	Treatment technique	Median FU	Local control	Overall survival	≥Grade 3 toxicity	Comments
Cao et al. 2021 [37]	356 patients/521 lesions	Multiple	15–18 Gy/1 Fr 20–28 Gy/1 Fr 24–31 Gy/2 Fr 24–28 Gy/3–5 Fr 30–35 Gy/3–5 Fr 40–45 Gy/4–5 Fr 50 Gy/5 Fr 50 Gy/10 Fr	SBRT (LINAC)	26.7 months	6 months-83.7%, 1 year-87.4%, 2 year-90.7%	6 months-92.8%, 1 year-83.2%, 2 year-71.3%, 3 year-59.1%	None	Comparably excellent response to SBRT for a balanced distribution of OM NSB and spine lesions. Dose escalation for large and/or radioresistant NSB lesions should be explored
Ven et al. 2019 [38]	131 patients (66 in 3DCRT and 65 in SBRT)	Multiple	8 Gy/1 Fr, 10 Gy/3 Fr, 7 Gy/5 Fr	SBRT (VMAT)	25 months for SBRT	1 year-75%	1 year-85%	None	SBRT to bone metastases did not improve pain response or QoL compared with 3DCRT. Reirradiation was less often needed in the SBRT group
Owen et al. 2014 [39]	74 patients/85 lesions	Multiple	15–50 Gy/1–5 Fr	SBRT (IMRT/ VMAT)	7.6 months	1 year-91.8%	1 year-81.4%	None	Non-spine bone metastases (including sacrum)

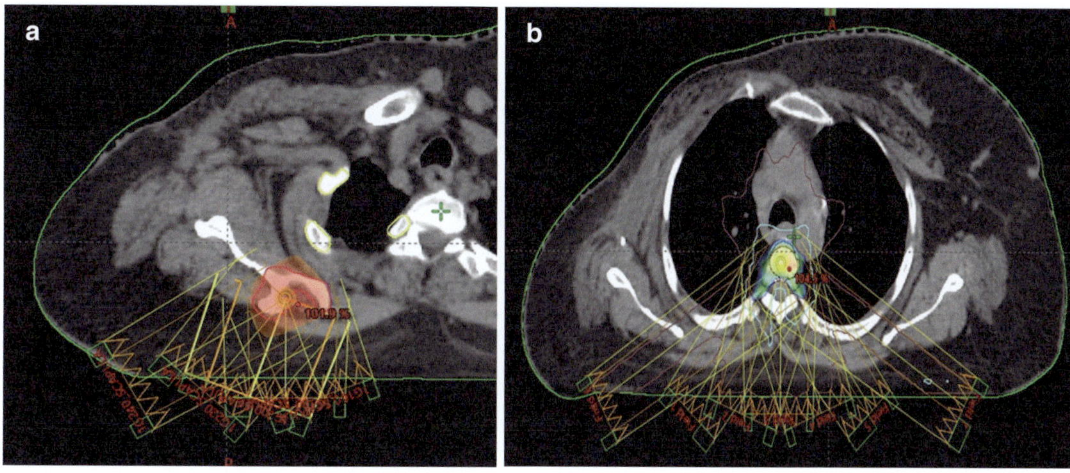

Fig. 5 This breast cancer patient had two OM sites (scapula and spine). The patient received post-mastectomy RT to the chest wall/supraclavicular region followed by SBRT to the OM sites- (A) scapula (B) D4 metastatic site (IMRT beam arrangement and 95% dose wash illustrated)

Combining systemic drug therapies with local stereotactic radiotherapy is of special interest in the era of immunotherapy. This combination, termed iSBRT, can induce pro-immunogenic molecular changes both at the cellular level and within the tumor microenvironment. Preclinical and clinical evidence exists for combining high-dose radiation combined radiotherapy-immunotherapy, making it a fertile field of research with considerable international interest [24, 25].

5.3 Liver Metastases

Liver metastases are a common cause of morbidity and are associated with many cancers, commonly colorectal, breast, and lung. They are usually difficult to treat using conventional systemic therapy because of the natural detoxification function in the liver, and the relative hypoxic state in the organ. 80% perfusion of the normal liver is through the portal venous system, while most liver tumors obtain blood flow almost exclusively through the hepatic arterial system.

Patients with liver metastasis commonly present with nausea, vomiting, changes in bowel habits, distension, and bloating associated with ascites, jaundice, and pain as a result of distension of the liver capsule. Biphasic and triphasic helical CT is the optimal method for detecting liver metastases. During the portal venous phase of the scan, the thickened rind of the metastatic lesion enhances progressively but remains less than adjacent liver. (Primary Hepatocellular lesions typically enhanced on arterial-phase images). Approximately 90% of lesions greater than 1 cm are detected by portal phase images alone; approximately 10% more lesions are seen when the arterial images are combined. An MRI can also help detect liver metastases, but it is expensive and can have motion artifacts. On T1-weighted images, hepatic metastases have low signal intensity, whereas on T2-weighted images, tumors have in homogeneously high signal intensity.

Approximately 70–90% of liver metastases are unresectable, and a safe and effective alternative therapeutic option is necessary. For the management of patients with liver metastasis, the extent of liver involvement and extrahepatic disease remains the critical consideration. Liver metastasis can respond well to chemotherapy and hormone therapy, but most remissions are short-lived. Aggressive local therapies for liver metastases can also provide substantial benefits. Minimally invasive local approaches were introduced as an alternative to surgery, including

Table 8 Lung OM

Study	Patients/ metastasis	Primary tumor site	Dose fractionation	Treatment technique	Median FU	Local control	Overall survival	≥Grade 3 toxicity	Comments
Berkovic et al. 2020 [40]	104 patients/132 lesions	Multiple	60 Gy/3 Fr	SBRT (CK)	22 months	77.8% at 3 years	72.1% at 3 years	4 patients	SBRT is a highly effective local therapy for oligorecurrent lung metastases and could achieve long-term survival in patients with favorable prognostic features
Kalinauskaite et al. 2020 [41]	52 patients/94 lesions	Multiple	22, 24, 25, 26 Gy/1 Fr 12.5 Gy × 3 Fr 15 Gy × 3 Fr 16 Gy × 3 Fr 12 Gy × 4 Fr 9.6 Gy × 4 Fr 5 Gy × 8 Fr	SFRS vs fSBRT (CK)	38 months	1 year-82%, 2 year-70%	1 year-84%, 2 year-71%	None	Single fraction radiosurgery (SFRS) and fractionated SBRT (fSBRT)
Li et al. 2019 [42]	53 patients/105 lesions	Colorectal cancers	75 Gy/10 Fr 63 Gy/9 Fr 60 Gy/10 Fr 60 Gy/8 Fr 50–55 Gy/5 Fr 48–50 Gy/4 Fr 50 Gy/10 Fr	SBRT (VMAT/ IMRT)	14 months	90.4% at 1 year	1 year-95.5%, 2-year-74.5%	None	Both oligomets and oligoprogression
Sharma et al. 2018 [43]	206 patients/327 lesions	Multiple	Peripheral tumors: <3 cm-30 Gy/1 Fr, >3 cm-60 Gy/3 Fr Central tumors: 45–60 Gy/5 Fr Close to the esophagus: 48 Gy/6 Fr or 56 Gy/7 Fr	SBRT	22 months	2 year-85%, 3 year-83%	2 year-63%, 3 year-47%	2%	Factors associated with inferior $LC\text{-}BED_{10} < 100$ Gy, delivery of pre-SBRT chemotherapy, and synchronous metastasis
Osti et al. 2018 [44]	129 patients/166 lesions	Multiple	30 Gy/1 Fr	SBRT (LINAC based)	38 months	3 year-80.1%, 5 year-79.2%	3 year-50.7%, 5 year-37.9%	2 patients (3%)	Lung metastases from colorectal cancer were found to be more radioresistant

Lindsay et al. 2018 [45]	44 patients/144 lesions	Sarcoma	50 Gy/10 Fr 50 Gy/5 Fr 48 Gy/12 Fr 30 Gy/6 Fr 55 Gy/10 Fr 45 Gy/5 Fr 36 Gy/6 Fr	SBRT (IGRT)	14.2 months	Not reported	2 year-82%, 5 year-50%	None	Stereotactic body radiotherapy is an effective and safe treatment for the ablation of pulmonary metastasis from sarcoma
Agolli et al. 2017 [46]	44 patients/69 lesions	CRC	23 Gy/1 Fr 30 Gy/1 Fr 45 Gy/3 Fr (central tumors)	SBRT (LINAC-based)	36 months	1 year-68.8%, 2 year-60.2%, 3 year-54.2%	1 year-82.8%, 2 year-67.7%, 3 year-50.8%	None	CRC with lung mets—local control remains lower compared to other primaries.
Helou et al. 2017 [47]	120 patients/180 lesions	Multiple	48–52 Gy/4–5 Fr, 60 Gy/4 Fr	SBRT (3DCRT/ IMRT/ VMAT)	22 months	1 year-95.6%, 2 year-84.8%	Single metastasis, 1 year-91.49% and 2 year-68.13%. Oligomets-1 year-85.19%, 2 year-74.87% Oligoprogression-1 year-85.19% and 2 year-70.77%	2 patients (<1%)	CRC lung metastases are associated with a higher hazard of LF and require higher SABR doses.
Baumann et al. 2016 [48]	30 patients/39 mets	Sarcoma	50 Gy/4–5 Fr	SBRT (LINAC/ CK)	23 months	1 year-94%, 2 year-86%	1 year-76%, 2 year-43%	None	SBRT is well-tolerated with excellent LC across tumor locations and sizes
Siva et al. 2015 [49]	65 patients/85 lesions	Multiple	26 Gy/1 Fr (peripheral lesions), 18 Gy/1 Fr (central lesions), 48 Gy/4 Fr or 50 Gy/5 Fr (peripheral lesions), and 50 Gy/5 Fr (central lesions)	SBRT (3DCRT/ IMRT/ VMAT)	25 months	2 year-93%	1 year-93%, 2 year-71%	None	Comparable local control, overall survival, and toxicity rates between single-fraction and multi-fraction SABR treatments in patients with FDG-PET-staged pulmonary oligometastases

radiofrequency ablation (RFA) and microwave ablation (MWA). Nevertheless, these techniques have limits, mostly related to lesion size and location (lesions greater than 3–4 cm in diameter or located in the proximity of major blood vessels, biliary tract, gallbladder, or just beneath the diaphragm).

5.3.1 Irradiation Technique and Doses

Radiation techniques for liver metastases include whole-liver radiation, stereotactic liver radiation, and selective internal radiotherapy methods. Radiotherapy is often used to palliate liver-capsule pain and treat patients with chemotherapy-resistant disease. In addition, it can be used on patients with poor liver function who have an expected survival of more than 3 months.

Normal liver has poor tolerance to EBRT if the entire liver is irradiated, and higher doses are not superior to lower doses for palliation. The risk for radiation-induced liver disease (RILD) is low if the whole liver dose is restricted to 30 Gy or less in fractions of 2 Gy or less. Liver radiation for metastatic disease can be of palliative benefit, with proper patient selection and delivery of SBRT to defined lesion(s) by 3-D image-based contouring [26]. Even SBRT dose of 2 fractions (5 Gy × 2 fractions) found improvement at 6 weeks in abdominal pain (63%), distention (30%), night sweats (63%), and nausea (44%).

Patients considered for radioembolization therapy would include (1) unresectable hepatic primary or metastatic cancer, (2) liver-dominant tumor burden, and (3) a life expectancy of at least 3 months. Contraindications for radioembolization therapy may include (1) pretreatment 99m-Tc macro-aggregated albumin (MAA) scan demonstrating the potential of ≥30 Gy radiation exposure to the lung or flow to the gastrointestinal tract resulting in extrahepatic deposition of 99m-Tc MAA that catheter embolization techniques cannot correct, (2) excessive tumor burden with limited hepatic reserve, (3) elevated total bilirubin level (≥2 mg/dL) in the absence of a reversible cause, and (4) compromised portal vein, unless selective or super-selective radioembolization can be performed. Patients with prior radiotherapy involving the liver should be carefully reviewed on a case-by-case basis. It is unclear whether capecitabine chemotherapy treatments represent a contraindication to Y90 treatment.

5.3.2 SBRT for Liver Metastasis

Because the liver's regenerative powers make localized high-dose radiation achievable with minimal toxicity, SBRT has become popular for patients with a limited number of metastases and minimal extrahepatic tumors. As with most SBRT approaches, respiratory arrest or gating is preferred, but four-dimensional CT has also achieved good results. Large and portal lesions can be treated safely, and most studies show local control rates of more than 70%. No clear dose-response has been measured, but all radiation doses and schedules have produced similar results (Table 9).

Although lethal RILD can occur when the median liver dose exceeds 37 Gy in standard fractionation, little or no toxicity is seen when more than 50–70% of the liver is maintained under 30 Gy. Patients primarily report decreased appetite and gastritis; moreover, patients with cirrhosis may experience an exacerbation of hepatitis, and those with subdiaphragmatic tumors can have asymptomatic right pleural effusions. After radiation, tumors often become hypointense on CT scans, and surrounding hepatic damage may correspond to the 37-Gy isodose line. These radiographic changes can be confused with tumor progression because tumors reach a maximum size at 6 weeks to 3 months after irradiation and recover at 6–9 months. The contralateral lobe of the liver commonly hypertrophies to compensate for the lost liver mass; however, total liver volume usually maintains normal levels.

Table 9 Liver oligometastasis (studies >40 patients and follow-up >2 years)

Study	Patients/ metastasis	Primary tumor site	Dose fractionation	Treatment technique	Median FU	Local control	Overall survival	≥Grade 3 toxicity	Comments
Hoyer, Phase II, 2006 [50]	44	Miscl.	45 Gy/3 Fr	SBRT	4.3 years	79% at 2 years	1 year-67% 5 years-13%	48%	High toxicity, due to larger volumes
Fode, Retrospective 2015 [51]	321	Miscl.	BED10 = 72–195 Gy	SBRT	5 years	91% at 1 year	1 year-80% 5 years-23%	4%	Nonspecific rates for liver mets
Goodman, Retrospective 2016 [52]	81	Miscl.	32–60/3–5 Fr	SBRT	2.25 years	96% at 1 year 91% at 4 years	1 year-89.9% 4 years-28%	4.9%	Dose-response relationships
McPartlin, Phase I–II, 2017 [53]	51	Miscl.	22.7–62.1 Gy/6 Fr	SBRT	2.3 years	49.8% at 1 year 26% at 4 years	1 year-63% 4 years-9%	3%	Results worse than surgery and thermo-ablation Suggesting the need for dose escalation above BED 100 Gy Also showed size-response relationships; 3 cm cut off
Joo, Retrospective 2017 [54]	70	Miscl.	45–60 Gy/3–4 Fr	SBRT	2.8 years	93% at 1 year 68% at 3 years	1 year-75%	0%	Dose correlated with outcomes; BED 132 Gy with 2-year local control rates of 89%
Mendez Romero Retrospective, 2017 [55]	40	Miscl.	37.5 Gy/3 Fr 50.25 Gy/3 Fr	SBRT	2.2 years	96% at 1 year 66% at 3 years	1 year-95% 3 years-48%	7.5%	Higher dose correlated with improved outcomes
						90% at 1 year 81% at 3 years	1 year-94% 3 years-65%		
Cozzi Phase II, 2018 [56]	61	Miscl.	75 Gy/3 Fr (82% of lesions) 67.5–52.5 Gy/3 Fr (18% of lesions)	SBRT	6.1 years	94% at 1 year 78% at 5 years	1 year-85.2% 5 years-18%	1%	BED ranging from 144.38 to 262.5 Gy with acceptable toxicity and sustained LCR at 5 years

5.4 Adrenal Gland Metastases

Adrenal gland metastases are a common clinical scenario, particularly in patients with lung cancer, renal cell carcinoma, and melanoma. Postmortem studies of patients with cancer demonstrate an incidence of adrenal metastases between 13% and 27%. The management of symptomatic or OM scenarios is challenging. Generally, surgical resection has been the standard of care. Local ablative procedures, such as radiofrequency ablation, microwave ablation, and cryotherapy, have also been used as an alternative to adrenalectomy. However, it is not feasible in some situations due to patients' medical comorbidities, tumor size, burden of metastatic disease, or preference for noninvasive methods, such as radiotherapy.

While conventional palliative external beam radiotherapy may improve pain, it has a suboptimal local control. There is minimal prospective data on the efficacy of stereotactic radiotherapy in the treatment of adrenal tumors, as the SBRT studies in OM disease included a wide variety of tumor locations. However, multiple retrospective single-institution studies have been published (Table 10). SBRT with 4D or similar motion management technique with appropriate immobilization is employed in all modern series and is highly recommended. While these showed a favorable local control rate and toxicity profile, the studies are small and with a heterogeneous patient population. Although distant metastatic progression remains a concern limiting overall survival, local control of disease may present an important paradigm for a few selected patients with only a site of metastasis or patients in whom effective systemic therapy is available.

5.5 Lymph Nodes

OM involvement of the lymph nodes after treatment of the primary tumor appears in 15–20% of cases, and addressing them with complete resection of retroperitoneal, intra-abdominal, and paraaortic LNs has been known to improve patient survival. Surgical resection of such involvement can often be technically challenging, and R0 resection is difficult. Any previous treatment also increases the risk of surgical complications. Such patients are often indicated for systemic treatment—chemotherapy, targeted therapy, or their combination. SBRT, with its potentially ablative doses of radiation, offers an effective alternative to surgery and may also delay or need in selected patients for instituting systemic therapy. Currently, there is limited but promising data on the use of SBRT in the treatment of lymph node metastases (Table 11). The immobilization technique and motion management to be applied are defined by principles of SBRT for the location of lymph nodes. The dose and fractionation schedule are guided by the surrounding normal tissue and primary histology. Local palliative radiotherapy to lymph nodes in regions such as axilla, groin, retroperitoneum, and mediastinum is often considered for local symptoms of pain, obstruction, or impending fungation are treated with simple fractionation schedules as described before.

The usual organs at risk (OAR's) of concern in SBRT depend on the location being treated and include bronchus/trachea esophagus/great vessels/carotids/spinal cord (Fig. 6).

6 Surgical and Systemic Therapy Approaches for Metastatic and Oligometastatic Disease

6.1 Surgical Treatment

Metastasectomy has been traditionally considered an important tool in the management of metastatic disease. The aim has traditionally been palliation of local symptoms. In the present day, surgical resection of metastasis has been performed with radical as well as palliative aims. Published data on 387 head and neck cancer patients in 11 retrospective studies were analyzed in a meta-analysis. The 5-year overall survival rate was 29% after resection of metachronous pulmonary metastases (most of these patients had single nodules). In the context of Head and neck

Table 10 Adrenal oligometastasis (studies >40 patients)

Study	Patients/ metastasis	Primary tumor site	Dose fractionation BED 10	Treatment technique	Median FU	Local control	Overall survival	≥Grade 3 toxicity	Comments
Shah 2001–2014 [57]	44	Miscl	48 (21–101)	SBRT	5.4 months	97% LC at 1 year	7 months median survival	2% gr 3 gastric ulcer, gr 4–5 tox	Earlier study with historic systemic therapy support and lower SBRT dose
Casamassima 2002–2009 [58]	48	Miscl	79 (60–100)	SBRT	16.2 months	90% 1 and 2 years	40% and 15% 1 and 2 years	2% gr 2 adrenal insufficiency, no gr 3–5 tox	Improved LCR with higher doses
Chance 2009–2015 [59]	43	Miscl	96 (75–113)	SBRT	24 months	74% and 55%	65% and 42%	Gr 1–2 tox common, no gr 3–5 tox	Improved LCR with higher doses, without significant toxicity
Franzese 2011–2015 [60]	46	Miscl	80 (80–80)	SBRT	23 months	66% and 41%	88% and 88%	Gr 2 fatigue and GI tox occurred, no gr 3–5 tox	Time from diagnosis of metastases to SBRT was predictive of LC (HR 1.62, $p = 0.023$)
Figura 2013–2018 [61]	41	Miscl	72 (38–132)	SBRT		96% at 1 year	71% and 51%	2% gr 3 hypertensive crisis, no gr 4–5 tox	No difference in outcomes for oligoprogressive vs non-progressive and metachronous vs synchronous disease

Table 11 Lymph nodes oligometastasis

Study	Patients/ metastasis	Primary tumor site	Dose fractionation	Treatment technique	Median FU	Local control	Overall survival	≥Grade 3 toxicity	Comments
Franzese 2020 [62]	278	Misc	24–54 Gy/3–8 Fr	SBRT	23 months	87.2% (1 year) 76.8% (2 years)	88.4% (1 year) 73.9% (2 years)	1 gr. 3	Better LC was associated with prostate tumor, a small tumor volume, oligorecurrence, and BED10 ≥ 75 Gy
Loi 2018 [63]	91	Misc	40–48 Gy/5–6 Fr	SBRT	24 months	79% (4 years)	43% (4 years)	1 acute No late	Local failure, occurring in 15% of patients, was the only predictor of poor survival (HR: 3.06)
Yeung 2017 [64]	18	GI	31–60 Gy/4–10 Fr	SBRT	34 months	47% (2 years)	74% (2 years)	None	Dose lesser for GI tumors. No chemotherapy.
Jereczek–Fossa 2017 [65]	94	Prostate	Median 24 Gy/3 Fr	SBRT	19 months	84% (2 years)	–	None	Good LC due to primary.
Wang 2016 [66]	22	Misc	Median 39 Gy/5 Fr	SBRT	33 months	91% (1 and 3 years)	79% (1 year) 43% (3 years)	–	–
Ost 2016 [67]	72	Prostate	–	SBRT	21 months	94% (3 and 5 years)	–	None	Relapses after SBRT are often nodal and limited in number
Jereczek–Fossa 2014 [68]	69	Misc	Median 24 Gy/3 Fr	SBRT	20 months	64% (3 years)	50% (3 years)	3 acute 1 late gr. 4	Pattern of failure was predominantly out-field
Bignardi 2011 [69]	19	Misc	24–36 Gy/1–5 Fr	SBRT	12 months	78% (2 years)	93% (2 years)	No acute gr. 3 1 late gr. 3	Good QoL without chemotherapy
Choi 2009 [70]	30	Cervix, corpus	33–45 Gy/3 Fr	SBRT	NR	67% (4 years)	50% (4 years)	6 acute, 1 late.	Mainly para-aortic lymph nodes
Selingerova 2021 [71]		Misc		SBRT	35 months	1, 2, 3, 4 and 5 years is 95%, 75%, 68%, 64%, and 56%, respectively	1, 2, 3, 4 and 5 years is 94%, 79%, 62%, 53%, and 39%		LC was worse for patients with Dmin <30/5# Gy

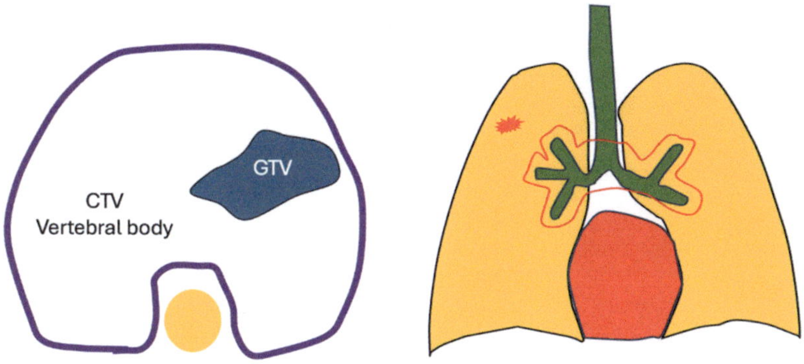

Fig. 6 SBRT is optimally delivered to OM sites as illustrated here. 6.1 to vertebra (protecting the spinal cord), 6.2 to single lung mets (protecting the central lung & mediastinum). For different OM sites, there could be varied dose/toxicity concerns for nearby structures (OARs)

cancers, the poor prognostic factors include the site of the primary tumor in the oral cavity, initial lymph node involvement, the shorter interval from primary diagnosis to pulmonary dissemination (<1 year), incomplete metastasectomy, and multiple pulmonary nodules [72]. Five-year survival after resection of pulmonary and hepatic oligo metastases is approximately similar [73].

Newer surgical techniques have further advanced the cause of metastasectomies. Studies suggest that minimally invasive approaches, such as video-assisted thoracic surgery (VATS) and radiofrequency ablation (RFA) were associated with lower morbidity and similar local control and overall survival compared with an open resection [74]. Finally, the obtained full pathological specimen provides a definitive diagnosis and additional material for immunohistochemical and molecular analyses if needed. In this respect, differentiating a pulmonary metastasis from squamous cell lung carcinoma has been challenging and requires clinical and radiological inputs. In the case of oropharyngeal carcinoma, detection of high-risk HPV infection and not only p16 expression, which can also be found in squamous cell carcinomas originating in the lungs, esophagus, and skin [75, 76]. However, it is to be noted that surgical candidates are usually young, fit patients with good general condition. This needs to be kept in mind in routine clinical practice and also when interpreting the results of available retrospective studies. In patients with frank metastatic disease surgical metastasectomy has the following roles (Table 12).

At presentation, de novo metastatic breast cancer (MBC) is noted in about 3–10% of all breast cancer patients. The benefit of locoregional treatment (LRT) in MBC has long been debated. There have been only a few randomized controlled trials (RCTs) addressing this issue, but it has been studied in many retrospective studies, which may have results influenced by selection bias, making it difficult for a consensus to emerge [83–87]. MBC itself represents a wide spectrum of disease with considerably diverse outcomes—from OM and "bone only" metastatic disease on one end of the spectrum, to widely disseminated visceral disease on the other end. As stated earlier, OM disease has been commonly defined as the presence of ≤5 metastases in ≤3 organs. OM patients have been found to have better overall survival (OS) than patients with disseminated metastasis. Bone only metastasis is largely noticed in hormone receptor positive subtypes and has good outcomes. In an RCT by Badwe et al. [77], no OS benefit was noted in de novo MBC patients who received LRT (Surgery ± radiotherapy), compared to those treated with systemic therapy (ST) alone. Another RCT drew similar conclusions by Khan et al. [79] of the ECOG-ACRIN Research Group (E2108). The study concluded that though there is a 2.5 times higher risk of loco-regional progression without LRT, it did not improve Quality of life (QoL).

Table 12 Palliative surgery/surgical metastasectomy in malignancies

Site	Palliative surgery	Aim
Vertebra	Decompression of extradural compression/ stabilization of spine	Preservation of limb power/pain control
Brain	Resection of large brain metastasis	Rapid decompression of disease, relief of symptoms
Limb	Amputation	Relief from a fungating, non-salvageable metastasis
Bone fracture	Stabilization/nail/implant	Restoration of tensile strength of the area, early return to activity

The ABCSG-28 (POSYTIVE) prospective phase III trial reported by Fitzal et al. [78] did not find an OS benefit from surgical resection of the primary in de novo MBC patients. Conversely, women undergoing surgery had a statistically non-significant trend towards worse progression-free survival (PFS) and OS. Various studies providing level-1 evidence of the impact of LRT on survival in de novo MBC are summarized in Table 11.

In recent years, numerous articles were published on colorectal cancer with liver metastasis, having 10-year survival rates of up to 20–26% after treatment of the primary tumor and the liver metastasis [80].

Stage IV lung cancer occurs in about 40–50% of patients with non-small cell lung cancer (NSCLC). Nearly 7% of these patients show either a solitary or a limited number of metastases after complete evaluation. The international registry of lung metastases reported the outcomes of 5206 patients. All of these underwent resection of lung metastases from a variety of primary cancers and reported a 5-year survival of 36% [81]. Further, the eighth edition of the Lung Cancer TNM Classification and Clinical Staging System reclassified the M Stage descriptor to M1a–M1c. This clearly identifies this subset of the population with single extra-thoracic metastasis, including those with single distant non-regional lymph nodes as M1b.

Lyon et al. recently examined survival outcomes among patients with metastatic renal cell carcinoma (mRCC) treated with or without complete surgical metastasectomy (SM). Of significance, these patients were studied during an era when targeted therapy and checkpoint inhibitors were available [82]. The group reported a greater 2-year cancer-specific survival (CSS) in patients who underwent complete SM than in those who did not (84% vs. 54%, $P < 0.001$). Also, complete surgical metastasectomy was associated with a significantly reduced likelihood of death from RCC. This significance persisted after adjusting for age, sex, timing, number, and location of metastases. They concluded that even in the post-cytokine era, metastasectomy may be considered for appropriately selected patients.

Patients with widely disseminated disease, such as one illustrated in Fig. 7, and poor performance status are least likely to benefit from LRT. Considering patient characteristics like age, performance status, comorbidities, tumor type, and metastatic disease burden, and shared decision-making regarding LRT in de novo MBC would probably lead to more acceptable and better outcomes (Table 13).

6.2 Systemic Therapy Approaches

Systemic therapy forms an extremely important part of improving Quality of life and survival for patients with metastatic and OM disease. Depending on the anatomic site, systemic treatment options include chemotherapy, immunotherapy, targeted therapy, monoclonal antibodies, hormonal therapy to name a few. Table 14 summarizes the systemic therapy options for common cancers.

While there is plenty of evidence supporting the role of systemic therapy in poly metastatic disease, there is a paucity of evidence concerning its effectiveness, timing, and duration in OM disease. While local ablative treatments help to control radiologically detectable metastasis, systemic

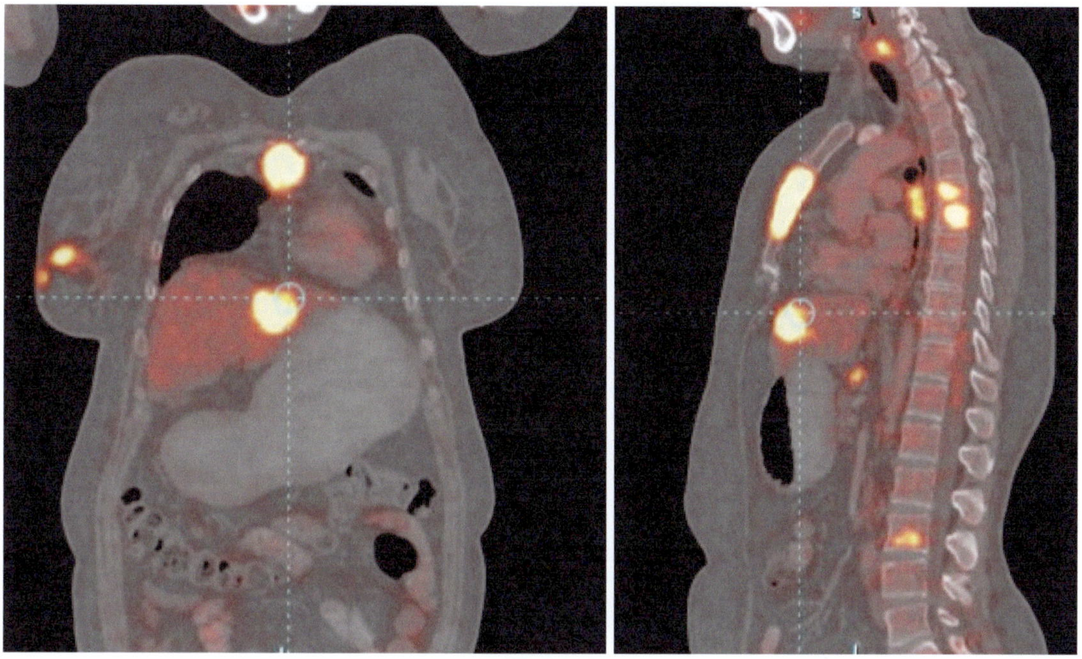

Fig. 7 Whole body 18F-FDG PET scan showing FDG avid multiple right breast tumors, with disseminated metastases in liver, multiple lymph nodes, and multiple skeletal sites

therapy takes care of occult metastatic disease, which remains an important cause of failure and death. Systemic therapies are also likely to have a bearing on the effectiveness of local ablative therapies. Patients whose cancers have effective systemic therapies more often have better benefits from local ablative therapies. Though the optimal timing of local ablative therapies concerning systemic therapy is unknown, the best results are likely to be achieved at the time of maximal response [92, 93].

The role of systemic therapy might vary depending on the type of OM disease. An important scenario is patients with synchronous OM disease after having received local ablative therapies. Barring a few clinical situations (e.g., post metastatectomy and resection of primary from colorectal cancer), most of the evidence for the use of systemic therapies is an extrapolation of results from adjuvant therapy trials [94, 95]. With our recent understanding that OM disease is a distinct clinical entity with unique biology, it is important to answer the question regarding the role of systemic therapy post-ablation of primary and metastatic sites. Subgroup analysis from recent studies in mRCC has shown benefit in the addition of immunotherapy post metastasectomy in OM disease [95].

Systemic therapy, including chemotherapy and targeted therapy, can be used to downstage sites of metastasis (e.g., liver metastasis from colorectal cancer), thereby making these tumors amenable to resection/local ablative therapies [96]. There is increasing use of systemic therapy as an in vivo test of sensitivity and tumor biology in both synchronous and metachronous OM disease. This strategy may help choose patients with good biology for aggressive therapy, resulting in better outcomes.

The proposed systemic therapy approaches to OM disease and polymetastatic disease have been given in Fig. 8a, b, respectively.

In patients with metachronous OM disease, those already on adjuvant systemic therapy will probably need local ablation of the OM and continue the same systemic therapy [97]. However, one may consider a change of systemic therapy if the recurrence is very early during the adjuvant therapy. Early recurrence reflects bad biology, and these patients may benefit from an early

Table 13 Impact of locoregional radiotherapy on survival outcomes in de novo metastatic breast cancer patients: level-1 evidence reported in prospective randomized trials and meta-analyses

Author and year	Study design	*N*	Salient conclusions
Badwe et al. [77], 2015	Prospective randomized trial – Surgery ± RT + ST vs ST alone	350	Median OS was 19·2 months in the LRT group and 20·5 months in the no-LRT group No improvement in OS with LRT
Fitzal et al. [78], 2019	Prospective randomized trial – Surgery + ST vs ST alone	90	Surgery does not improve OS and statistically nonsignificant trend towards worse PFS and OS
Khan et al. [79], 2020	Prospective randomized trial – LRT + ST vs ST alone	256	LRT does not improve OS and does not improve quality of life
Soran et al. [85], 2021	Prospective randomized trial – Surgery + ST vs ST alone	265	At 36-month, no survival advantage was noted with surgery for de novo MBC At 10-year, median 8-month OS benefit noted with surgery. Progression of primary was 14 times higher in the ST group, LRT controls progression of the primary in de novo MBC patients who are expected to survive longer
Gera et al. [88], 2020	Meta-analysis	216,066	Surgical resection in particular, and LRT in any form resulted in a significant 36.2% and 31.8% reduction in mortality respectively
Harris et al. [90], 2013	Meta-analysis	28,693	Surgical excision of the primary tumor in the setting of stage IV breast cancer was associated with a superior survival at 3 years (40% with surgery versus 22% without surgery)
Petrelli et al. [89], 2012	Meta-analysis	29,563	Surgery of an intact primary tumor in de novo MBC, reduces risk of death by 30% Results are independent of age, HER status, type of surgery and margin status, type and extent of metastatic disease
Reinhorn et al. [91], 2021	Meta-analysis	970	LRT in de novo MBC is not associated with improved outcomes

LRT loco-regional therapy, *MBC* metastatic breast cancer, *N* number, *RT* radiotherapy, *ST* systemic therapy, *OS* overall survival, *PFS* progression free survival

change of systemic therapy. In situations where the progression is in a sanctuary site like the brain, where standard chemotherapy is largely ineffective, only local ablative therapies would suffice (e.g., RCC and sarcoma). However, some of the more recent tyrosine kinase inhibitors (e.g., Alectinib, Lorlatinib, and Osimertinib) have excellent CNS penetration and with response rates similar to or even better than radiotherapy [98, 99]. In patients with polymetastatic disease who have oligoprogression, local ablative therapies and the continuation of the same systemic therapy are options. However, if the progression is minimal and not associated with symptoms, continuing the same systemic therapy and reimaging early is an option. There is clinical evidence to show that this strategy might delay the need for a change of systemic therapy by 3–4 months.

The term inducible OM refers to a situation where the patient, to begin with, had polymetastatic disease and, as a result of effective systemic therapy, is left with <5 sites of disease (e.g., mRCC). The duration of systemic therapy post-ablative therapies in this situation remains debatable, i.e., whether to stop after a total duration of 1–2 years or continue indefinitely since the patient primarily had polymetastatic disease. These decisions need to be made on a case-by-case basis, depending on multiple disease and

Table 14 First line systemic therapy in advanced (metastatic) disease for common cancers

Tumor type	First line systemic therapy options
Colorectal cancer	Chemotherapy doublet or triplet (FOLFOX, FOLFIRI, CapeOX, FOLFOXIRI) with monoclonal antibody (Bevacizumab or Cetuximab/Panitumumab). Immunotherapy for MSI high
Non-small cell lung cancer	Immunotherapy ± chemotherapy (based on PDL1 TPS) Targeted therapy for driver mutated tumor
Head and neck cancer	Immunotherapy ± chemotherapy or chemotherapy with Erbitux (based on PDL1 CPS)
Gastric cancer	5FU/Cisplatin or FOLFOX ± immunotherapy (based on PDL1 CPS) or Docetaxel, platinum & 5FU, Trastuzumab Deruxtecan
Hepatocellular cancer	Immunotherapy based therapies
Biliary tract cancer	Gemcitabine, cisplatin, Immunotherapy and Targeted therapy
Pancreatic cancer	FOLFORINOX, Gemcitabine-Nab Paclitaxel
Urothelial cancer	Gemcitabine, cisplatin followed by Immunotherapy maintenance, Enfortumab Vedotin plus Pembrolizumab
Clear cell renal carcinoma	Dual immunotherapy (Intermediate/ poor risk), TKI + Immunotherapy, TKI alone
Epithelial ovarian cancer	Pacltaxel, carboplatin ± Bevacizumab, PARP inhibitor maintenance for HRD high tumors
Endometrial cancer	Paclitaxel, carboplatin, Immunotherapy, TKI
Soft tissue sarcoma	Adriamycin, Ifosfamide, Trabectidin, Eribulin
Melanoma	Immunotherapy or BRAF targeted TKI

FOLFOX 5FU, oxaliplatin, leucovorin, *FOLFIRI* 5FU, irinotecan, leucovorin, *FOLFOXIRI/FOLFORINOX* oxaliplatin/irinotecan, 5FU, leucovorin, *TKI* tyrosine kinase inhibitor, *MSI* microsatellite instability, *TPS* tumor proportion score, *CPS* combined positive score, *PD L1* programmed death-ligand 1

patient-related factors, including toxicity and cost issues. Hopefully, ongoing clinical trials will help answer these questions.

Combining immunotherapy with radiotherapy can be a promising strategy for synergistic enhancement of treatment efficacy. It is well known that radiation delivered to the tumor site affects both tumor cells and surrounding stromal cells. Radiation-induced cancer cell damage exposes tumor-specific antigens. This makes them visible to immune surveillance and promotes the priming and activation of cytotoxic T cells. This is also likely to facilitate the recruitment and infiltration of immune cells. This unique relationship is the Rationale for combining radiation with immune checkpoint blockade. Enhanced tumor recognition and immune cell targeting with checkpoint blockade may unleash the immune system to eliminate the cancer cells. However, challenges remain to be addressed to maximize the efficacy of this promising combination.

7 Supportive Care and Quality of Life

Improvements in medical science and continuing advancement in early detection and treatment have improved the survival of cancer patients remarkably. This has resulted in an increased interest in exploring cancer survivors' health-related Quality of life (HRQoL). Quality of life (QoL) is an umbrella term representing the overall enjoyment of life. QoL has come up as one of the most concerning health issues for oncology patients. It is a combined assessment of patient-reported outcomes (PROs), including the patients' social, financial, psychosocial, and physical activities [100, 101]. This includes the measurement of aspects of an individual's sense of well-being and ability to carry out activities of daily living (ADL). The myriad of symptoms experienced by cancer patients includes sleep disturbance, depression, and poor Quality of life.

Assessing QoL among cancer patients enables designing interventions for improving patients' outcomes. QoL assessment assists patients and clinicians in realizing how anti-cancer treatment, the disease itself, and many other factors impact the QoL. This assessment can also help understand potential beneficial and risky aspects of treatment and assess the impact of a decision. There is a perpetual need to take care of cancer

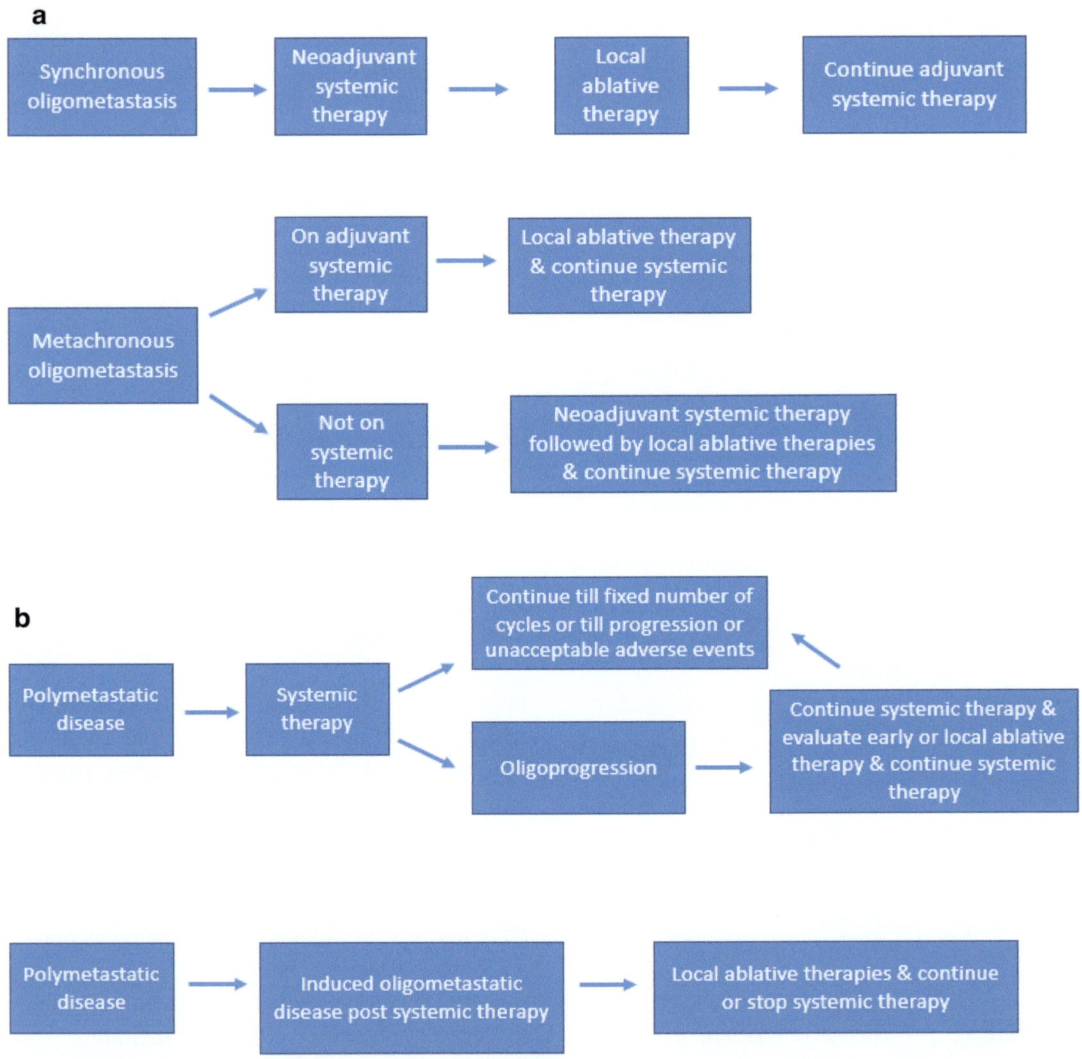

Fig. 8 (**a**) Proposed systemic therapy approach to OM disease. (**b**) Proposed systemic therapy approach to polymetastatic disease

patients' requirements to enable them to live a healthy life.

Again, supportive care is a broad term indicating the care given to improve the QoL of people who have an illness or disease. This includes preventing or treating the disease as early as possible. It also includes addressing the symptoms of the disease and the adverse effects caused by treatment. It includes but is not limited to physical, psychological, social, and spiritual support for patients and their families. Supportive care includes pain management, nutritional support, counseling, exercise, music therapy, meditation, and palliative care. Supportive care may be given with other treatments from diagnosis until the end of life. Indeed, many studies support the initiation of supportive care early in the treatment course of the cancer patient. For more details related to supportive care and QoL, please see vol 1, chapter 21 (Palliative Care in Cancer).

8 Current Ongoing Studies/ Future Research

Several ongoing trials are addressing the issue of metastasis and oligometastasis with respect to radiation therapy (Table 15).

Table 15 Current trials testing management of OM disease

NCT	Disease	Design	Definition (lesions)	Target accrual	Intervention	Outcome
NCT02364557	Breast	Randomized phase II/III	1–4	402	Systemic therapy ± SBRT	Primary: PFS,OS Secondary: presence of CTC (baseline, after treatment); levels of ctDNA
NCT02089100	Breast	Randomized, phase III	≤5	280	SBRT vs best supportive care	PFS
NCT02759783	Breast, prostate, NSCLC	Randomized phase II/III	≤3	245	Standard of care ± SBRT	Primary: PFS Secondary: OS, local control, toxicity
NCT03486431	Mixed	Prospective, phase I	≤3	99	SBRT	Primary: DLT Secondary: median PFS Local control
NCT02581670	Breast Lung/liver metastases	Non-randomized phase II	1–4	40	SBRT	Primary: local control, toxicity Secondary: PFS, OS
NCT03965468	NSCLC	Non-randomized phase II	Oligo (NS)	47	Immunotherapy, chemotherapy, surgery, SBRT	Progression-free survival at 12 months
NCT03070366	Upper aerodigestive	Randomized phase II	Oligo (NS)	78	Chemotherapy, RT, SBRT	OS
NCT03867175	Metastatic NSCLC	Randomized phase III	No strict size or tumor number, patient must have at least one residual site of disease	116	SBRT + Pembrolizumab vs Pembrolizumab	Primary: PFS Secondary: OS, time to progression, rate of failure, number of participants with new site of disease, toxicity
NCT03283605	Metastatic head and neck cancers	Phase I/II	≤10	45	Durvalumab + tremelimumab and SBRT	Primary: acute toxicity, PFS Secondary: LC,OS, PFS, Abscopal events

Immunotherapy with monoclonal antibodies, such as pembrolizumab, may help the body's immune system attack the cancer and interfere with tumor cells' ability to grow and spread. Giving immunotherapy with stereotactic body radiation therapy may work better than immunotherapy alone in treating non-small cell lung cancer patients. This concept also termed as iSBRT, is being actively examined. It is still being studied whether it is appropriate to administer immunotherapy before RT, along with RT (concurrently) or after RT. Ongoing trials include Immunotherapy With or Without SBRT in Patients With Stage IV Non-small Cell Lung Cancer (ClinicalTrials.gov Identifier: NCT03867175), Immunotherapy and SBRT for Metastatic Head and Neck Carcinomas (ClinicalTrials.gov Identifier: NCT03283605).

9 Conclusion

Metastatic disease is a potentially serious event in the course of cancer patients. The traditional approach to this event has considered palliative and supportive care. However, with the development of more and more advancements in surgical, medical, and radiation techniques, many patients with metastatic disease have reasonably good survival outcomes with the preservation of QoL. The key to the overall approach for metastatic disease patients rests on proper patient selection and evidence-based management.

Percepts Box

1. Metastasis is the cause of greater than 90% of cancer deaths.
2. Three main metastasis pathways include the lymphatic system, hematogenous, and across body cavities.
3. Modern imaging modalities such as PET, CT, and MRI have high sensitivity in detecting metastatic disease.
4. Increasingly, more and more patients with limited metastatic disease are being taken for potentially curative treatments.
5. SBRT plays a pivotal role in local control of metastatic disease deposits (overall >80% local control rates) in an OM scenario.
6. SBRT for oligometastatic disease and surgical excision of OM disease are often complementary to each other in overall patient management.
7. Radiotherapy plays a very important role in both disseminated metastatic disease as well as in oligometastatic disease.
8. Systemic therapy, including immunotherapy, is important in the management of frank metastatic disease and also plays a critical role in OM disease.
9. iSBRT is an upcoming modality and is used to denote the combination of immunotherapy and SBRT, suggested to have synergistic and abscopal effects.

Multiple Choice Questions

1. Which is the most common site of metastasis from lung cancer?
   (a) Lung
   (b) Bone
   (c) Brain
   (d) Liver
2. Which of the following treatment modalities can do non-uniform dose intensity treatments across the disease volume in managing oligometastatic disease?
   (a) Surgery
   (b) RFA
   (c) Chemotherapy
   (d) SBRT
3. Which of the following imaging techniques is most sensitive in picking skeletal metastasis?
   (a) Skeletal scintigraphy
   (b) 18 FDG PET/MR

   (c) 18 FDG PET/CT
   (d) 18F NaF-PET/CT
4. The most common site of metastatic spinal cord compression is:
   (a) Thoracic spine
   (b) Dorsal spine
   (c) Cervical spine
   (d) Lumbar spine
5. Which of the following is a contraindication for spinal SBRT?
   (a) Involvement of two contiguous cervical vertebral bodies
   (b) Spinal compression with a gap of <3 mm between the spinal cord and the edge of the epidural lesion
   (c) Paraspinal mass (<5 cm) contiguous with spine metastasis
   (d) Intractable pain
6. Most common cancer-causing metastatic spinal cord compression?
   (a) Breast
   (b) Lung
   (c) Prostate
   (d) Colorectal
7. Which of the following treatment modalities can be used to treat oligometastatic lung lesions locally?
   (a) Surgery
   (b) RFA
   (c) SBRT
   (d) All of the above
8. What are the documented local control rates following SBRT?
   (a) >50%
   (b) >60%
   (c) >70%
   (d) >80%
9. Which of the following diagnostic modalities is best for the characterization of liver lesions?
   (a) Triple phase MRI
   (b) Triple phase CT
   (c) 18 FDG PET CT
   (d) DATA NOC PET CT
10. Which of the following statements is true?
   (a) Immunotherapy with SBRT is known to have synergistic and abscopal effects
   (b) 5 Gy × 4 fractions is the most common palliative external beam radiotherapy schedule for bone metastasis
   (c) Local control rates with SBRT range from 50% to 60%
   (d) PET MR is superior to PET CT for the detection of lung lesions

Answer Key

1. (b)
2. (d)
3. (d)
4. (a)
5. (b)
6. (a)
7. (d)
8. (d)
9. (a)
10. (a)

References

1. Hellman S, Weichselbaum RR. Oligometastases. J Clin Oncol. 1995;13:8–10. *
2. Gutiontov SI, Pitroda SP, Weichselbaum RR. Oligometastatic: past, present, future. Int J Radiat Oncol Biol Phys. 2020;108:530–8.
3. Lambert AW, Pattabiraman DR, Weinberg RA. Emerging biological principles of metastasis. Cell. 2017;168:670–691. https://doi.org/10.1016/j.cell.2016.11.037.
4. deSouza NM, Tempany CM. A risk-based approach to identifying oligometastatic disease on imaging. Int J Cancer. 2019;144:422–30.
5. Karaosmanoglu AD, Onur MR, Ozmen MN, Akata D, Karcaaltincaba M. Magnetic resonance imaging of liver metastasis. Semin Ultrasound CT MR. 2016;37:533–48.
6. Talbot JN, Paycha F, Balogova S. Diagnosis of bone metastasis: recent comparative studies of imaging modalities. Q J Nucl Med Mol Imaging. 2011;55:374–410.
7. Goda HH, Abdallah AEH, Ahmed EA, et al. Whole-body diffusion-weighted MRI in detection of metastasis and lymphoma: a prospective longitudinal clinical study. Egypt J Radiol Nucl Med. 2020;51:141.
8. Mayerhoefer ME, Prosch H, Beer L, Tamandl D, Beyer T, et al. PET/MRI versus PET/CT in oncology: a prospective single-center study of 330

examinations focusing on implications for patient management and cost considerations. Eur J Nucl Med Mol Imaging. 2020;47:51–60.
9. Ung YC, Bezjak A, Coakley N, Evans WK. Positron emission tomography with 18fluorodeoxyglucose in radiation treatment planning for non-small cell lung cancer: a systematic review. J Thorac Oncol. 2011;6:86–97. *
10. Jurgen J, Futterer L, Cristian S, Van den Bergh R, Tsaur I, on behalf of the EAU-YAU Prostate Cancer Working Party. Imaging modalities in synchronous oligometastatic prostate cancer. World J Urol. 2019;37:2573–83.
11. Rich SE, Chow R, Raman S, Liang Zeng K. Update of the systematic review of palliative radiation therapy fractionation for bone metastases. Radiother Oncol. 2018;126:547–57. *
12. Guckenberger M, Andratschke N, Alheit H, Holy R, et al. Definition of stereotactic body radiotherapy: principles and practice for the treatment of stage I non-small cell lung cancer. Strahlenther Onkol. 2014;190:26–33. *
13. Munshi A, Krishnatry R, Banerjee S, Agarwal JP. Stereotactic conformal radiotherapy in non-small cell lung cancer – an overview. Clin Oncol (R Coll Radiol). 2012;24:556–68.
14. Tseng CL, Eppinga W, Charest-Morin R, Soliman H, et al. Spine stereotactic body radiotherapy: indications, outcomes, and points of caution. Global Spine J. 2017;7:179–97.
15. Yamada Y, Bilsky MH, Lovelock DM, Venkatraman ES, et al. High-dose, single-fraction image-guided intensity-modulated radiotherapy for metastatic spinal lesions. Int J Radiat Oncol Biol Phys. 2008;71:484–90.
16. Chang EL, Shiu AS, Mendel E. Mathews LA phase I/II study of stereotactic body radiotherapy for spinal metastasis and its pattern of failure. J Neurosurg Spine. 2007;7:151–60.
17. Gerszten PC, Burton SA, Ozhasoglu C, Welch WC. Radiosurgery for spinal metastases: clinical experience in 500 cases from a single institution. Spine. 2007;32:193–9.
18. Zeng KL, Tseng C-L, Soliman H, Weiss Y, et al. Stereotactic body radiotherapy (SBRT) for oligometastatic spine metastases: an overview. Front Oncol. 2019;9:337.
19. Patchell RA, Tibbs PA, Regine WF, Payne R, et al. Direct decompressive surgical resection in the treatment of spinal cord compression caused by metastatic cancer: a randomised trial. Lancet. 2005;366:643–8. **
20. Tandberg DJ, Tong BC, Ackerson BG, Kelsey CR. Surgery versus stereotactic body radiation therapy for stage I non–small cell lung cancer: a comprehensive review. Cancer. 2018;124:667–78.
21. Videtic GM, Donington J, Giuliani M, Heinzerling J. Stereotactic body radiation therapy for early-stage non-small-cell lung cancer: executive summary of an ASTRO evidence-based guideline. Pract Radiat Oncol. 2017;7:295–301.
22. Rieber J, Streblow J, Uhlmann L, Flentje M, et al. Stereotactic body radiotherapy (SBRT) for medically inoperable lung metastases—a pooled analysis of the German working group stereotactic radiotherapy. Lung Cancer. 2016;97:51–8.
23. Ashworth AB, Senan S, Palma DA, et al. An individual patient data metaanalysis of outcomes and prognostic factors after oligometastatic non-small-cell lung cancer treatment. Clin Lung Cancer. 2014;15:346–55. *
24. Siva S, MacManus MP, Martin RF, Martin OA. Abscopal effects of radiation therapy: a clinical review for the radiobiologist. Cancer Lett. 2015;356:82–90.
25. Reynders K, Illidge T, Siva S, Chang JY. The abscopal effect of local radiotherapy: using immunotherapy to make a rare event clinically relevant. Cancer Treat Rev. 2015;41:503–10.
26. Menichelli C, Casamassima F, Aristei C, Ingrosso G, Borghesi S, et al. Stereotactic radiotherapy for liver oligometastases. Rep Pract Oncol Radiother. 2022;27:32–39. https://doi.org/10.5603/RPOR.a2021.0130.
27. Tseng CL, Soliman H, Myrehaug S, Lee YK, et al. Imaging-based outcomes for 24 Gy in 2 daily fractions for patients with de novo spinal metastases treated with spine stereotactic body radiation therapy (SBRT). Int J Radiat Oncol Biol Phys. 2018;102:499–507.
28. Yamada Y, Katsoulakis E, Laufer I, et al. The impact of histology and delivered dose on local control of spinal metastases treated with stereotactic radiosurgery. Neurosurg Focus. 2017;42:E6.
29. Germano IM, Carai A, Pawha P, Blacksburg S, et al. Clinical outcome of vertebral compression fracture after single fraction spine radiosurgery for spinal metastases. Clin Exp Metastasis. 2016;33:143–9.
30. Lee SH, Tatsui CE, Ghia AJ, Amini B, et al. Can the spinal instability neoplastic score prior to spinal radiosurgery predict compression fractures following stereotactic spinal radiosurgery for metastatic spinal tumor?: a post hoc analysis of prospective phase II single-institution trials. J Neurooncol. 2016;126:509–17.
31. Moussazadeh N, Lis E, Katsoulakis E, Kahn S, et al. Five-year outcomes of high-dose single-fraction spinal stereotactic radiosurgery. Int J Radiat Oncol Biol Phys. 2015;93:361–7.
32. Sellin JN, Reichardt W, Bishop AJ, Suki D, et al. Factors affecting survival in 37 consecutive patients undergoing de novo stereotactic radiosurgery for contiguous sites of vertebral body metastasis from renal cell carcinoma. J Neurosurg Spine. 2015;22:52–9.
33. Bate BG, Khan NR, Kimball BY, Gabrick K, Weaver J. Stereotactic radiosurgery for spinal metastases with or without separation surgery. J Neurosurg Spine. 2015;22:409–15.
34. Yamada Y, Bilsky MH, Lovelock DM, Venkatraman ES, Toner S, Johnson J, et al. High-dose, single-fraction image-guided intensity-modulated radio-

therapy for metastatic spinal lesions. Int J Radiat Oncol Biol Phys. 2008;71:484–90.
35. Gerszten PC, Burton SA, Ozhasoglu C, Welch WC. Radiosurgery for spinal metastases: clinical experience in 500 cases from a single institution. Spine (Phila Pa 1976). 2007;32:193–9.
36. Cao Y, Chen H, Sahgal A, Erler D, et al. An international pooled analysis of SBRT outcomes to oligometastatic spine and non-spine bone metastases. Radiother Oncol. 2021;164:98–103.
37. van de Ven S, van den Bongard D, Pielkenrood B, Kasperts N, et al. Patient-reported outcomes of oligometastatic patients after conventional or stereotactic radiation therapy to bone metastases: an analysis of the PRESENT cohort. Int J Radiat Oncol Biol Phys. 2020;107:39–47.
38. Owen D, Laack NN, Mayo CS, Garces YI, et al. Outcomes and toxicities of stereotactic body radiation therapy for non-spine bone oligometastases. Pract Radiat Oncol. 2014;4:e143–9.
39. Berkovic P, Gulyban A, Defraene G, Swenen L, Dechambre D, Nguyen PV, Jansen N, Mievis C, Lovinfosse P, Janvary L, et al. Stereotactic robotic body radiotherapy for patients with oligorecurrent pulmonary metastases. BMC Cancer. 2020;20:402.
40. Kalinauskaite GG, Tinhofer II, Kufeld MM, Kluge AA, et al. Radiosurgery and fractionated stereotactic body radiotherapy for patients with lung oligometastases. BMC Cancer. 2020;20:404.
41. Li S, Dong D, Geng J, Zhu X, et al. Prognostic factors and optimal response interval for stereotactic body radiotherapy in patients with lung oligometastases or oligoprogression from colorectal cancer. Front Oncol. 2019;9:1080.
42. Sharma A, Duijm M, Oomen-de Hoop E, Aerts JG, et al. Factors affecting local control of pulmonary oligometastases treated with stereotactic body radiotherapy. Acta Oncol. 2018;57:1031–7.
43. Osti MF, Agolli L, Valeriani M, Reverberi C, et al. 30 Gy single dose stereotactic body radiation therapy (SBRT): report on outcome in a large series of patients with lung oligometastatic disease. Lung Cancer. 2018;122:165–70.
44. Lindsay AD, Haupt EE, Chan CM, Spiguel AR, et al. Treatment of sarcoma lung metastases with stereotactic body radiotherapy. Sarcoma. 2018;2018:9132359.
45. Agolli L, Bracci S, Nicosia L, Valeriani M, De Sanctis V, Osti MF. Lung metastases treated with stereotactic ablative radiation therapy in oligometastatic colorectal cancer patients: outcomes and prognostic factors after long-term follow-up. Clin Colorectal Cancer. 2017;16:58–64.
46. Helou J, Thibault I, Poon I, Chiang A, et al. Stereotactic ablative radiation therapy for pulmonary metastases: histology, dose, and indication matter. Int J Radiat Oncol Biol Phys. 2017;98:419–27.
47. Baumann BC, Nagda SN, Kolker JD, Levin WP, et al. Efficacy and safety of stereotactic body radiation therapy for the treatment of pulmonary metastases from sarcoma: a potential alternative to resection. J Surg Oncol. 2016;114:65–9.
48. Siva S, Kirby K, Caine H, Pham D, et al. Comparison of single-fraction and multi-fraction stereotactic radiotherapy for patients with 18F-fluorodeoxyglucose positron emission tomography-staged pulmonary oligometastases. Clin Oncol (R Coll Radiol). 2015;27:353–61.
49. Hoyer M, Roed H, Traberg HA, et al. Phase II study on stereotactic body radiotherapy of colorectal metastases. Acta Oncol. 2006;45:823–30.
50. Chang DT, Swaminath A, Kozak M, Weintraub J, Koong AC, Kim J, Dinniwell R, Brierley J, Kavanagh BD, Dawson LA, Schefter TE. Stereotactic body radiotherapy for colorectal liver metastases: a pooled analysis. Cancer. 2011;117:4060–9.
51. Fairhurst K, Leopardi L, Satyadas T, Maddern G. The safety and effectiveness of liver resection for breast cancer liver metastases: a systematic review. Breast. 2016;30:175–84.
52. Van Cutsem E, Cervantes A, Adam R, et al. ESMO consensus guidelines for the management of patients with metastatic colorectal cancer. Ann Oncol. 2016;27:1386–422.
53. Corsetti M, Comito T, Cozzi L, Clerici E, et al. The challenge of inoperable hepatocellular carcinoma (HCC): results of a single institutional experience on stereotactic body radiation therapy (SBRT). J Cancer Res Clin Oncol. 2015;141:1301–9.
54. Adam R, Chiche L, Aloia T, Elias D, et al. Hepatic resection for non-colorectal nonendocrine liver metastases: analysis of 1452 patients and development of a prognostic model. Ann Surg. 2006;244:524–35.
55. Corsetti M, Comito T, Clerici E, Franzese C, et al. Phase II trial on SBRT for unresectable liver metastases: long-term outcome and prognostic factors of survival after 5 years of follow-up. Radiat Oncol. 2018;13:234.
56. Shah MM, Crow D, Fareed MM, Wen N, et al. Single institution experience treating adrenal metastases with stereotactic body radiation therapy. J Cancer Res Ther. 2019;15(Supplement):S27–32.
57. Casamassima F, Livi L, Masciullo S, Menichelli C, et al. Stereotactic radiotherapy for adrenal gland metastases: University of Florence experience. Int J Radiat Oncol Biol Phys. 2012;82:919–23.
58. Chance WW, Nguyen QN, Mehran R, Welsh JW, et al. Stereotactic ablative radiotherapy for adrenal gland metastases: factors influencing outcomes, patterns of failure, and dosimetric thresholds for toxicity. Pract Radiat Oncol. 2017;7:e195–203.
59. Franzese C, Franceschini D, Cozzi L, D'Agostino G, et al. Minimally invasive stereotactical radio-ablation of adrenal metastases as an alternative to surgery. Cancer Res Treat. 2017;49:20–8.
60. Figura NB, Oliver DE, Mohammadi H, Martinez K, et al. Novel dose escalation approaches for stereotactic body radiotherapy to adrenal oligometastases: a single-institution experience. Am J Clin Oncol. 2020;43:107–14.

61. Franzese C, Badalamenti M, Comito T, Franceschini D, et al. Assessing the role of stereotactic body radiation therapy in a large cohort of patients with lymph node oligometastases: does it affect systemic treatment's intensification? Radiother Oncol. 2020;150:184–90.
62. Loi M, Frelinghuysen M, Klass ND, Oomen-De Hoop E, Granton PV, Aerts J, et al. Locoregional control and survival after lymph node SBRT in oligometastatic disease. Clin Exp Metastasis. 2018;35:625–33.
63. Yeung R, Hamm J, Liu M, Schellenberg D. Institutional analysis of stereotactic body radiotherapy (SBRT) for oligometastatic lymph node metastases. Radiat Oncol. 2017;12:105.
64. Jereczek-Fossa BA, Fanetti G, Fodor C, Ciardo D, et al. Salvage stereotactic body radiotherapy for isolated lymph node recurrent prostate cancer: single institution series of 94 consecutive patients and 124 lymph nodes. Clin Genitourin Cancer. 2017;15:e623–32.
65. Wang Z, Wang J, Zhuang H, Wang P, Yuan Z. Stereotactic body radiation therapy induces fast tumor control and symptom relief in patients with iliac lymph node metastasis. Sci Rep. 2016;6:37987.
66. Ost P, Jereczek-Fossa BA, Van As N, Zilli T, et al. Pattern of progression after stereotactic body radiotherapy for oligometastatic prostate cancer nodal recurrences. Clin Oncol. 2016;28:e115–20.
67. Jereczek-Fossa BA, Piperno G, Ronchi S, Catalano G, Fodor C, et al. Linac-based stereotactic body radiotherapy for oligometastatic patients with single abdominal lymph node recurrent cancer. Am J Clin Oncol. 2014;37:227–33.
68. Burkonn P, Slávik M, Kazda T, Pospisil P, et al. Stereotactic body radiotherapy—current indications. Klin Onkol. 2019;32:10–24.
69. Choi CW, Cho CK, Yoo SY, Kim MS, et al. Image-guided stereotactic body radiation therapy in patients with isolated para-aortic lymph node metastases from uterine cervical and corpus cancer. Int J Radiat Oncol Biol Phys. 2009;74:147–53.
70. Burton P, Selingerova I, Slavik M, Pospisil P, et al. Stereotactic body radiotherapy for lymph node oligometastases: real-world evidence from 90 consecutive patients. Front Oncol. 2021;10:616494.
71. Young ER, Diakos E, Khalid-Raja M, Mehanna H. Resection of subsequent pulmonary metastases from treated head and neck squamous cell carcinoma: systematic review and meta-analysis. Clin Otolaryngol. 2015;40:208–18.
72. Florescu C, Thariat J. Local ablative treatments of oligometastases from head and neck carcinomas. Crit Rev Oncol Hematol. 2014;91:47–63.
73. von Meyenfeldt EM, Wouters MW, Fat NL, Prevoo W, et al. Local treatment of pulmonary metastases: from open resection to minimally invasive approach? Less morbidity, comparable local control. Surg Endosc. 2012;26:2312–21.
74. van Boerdonk RA, Daniels JM, Bloemena E, Krijgsman O, et al. High-risk human papillomavirus-positive lung cancer: molecular evidence for a pattern of pulmonary metastasis. J Thorac Oncol. 2013;8:711–8.
75. Doxtader EE, Katzenstein AL. The relationship between p16 expression and high-risk human papillomavirus infection in squamous cell carcinomas from sites other than uterine cervix: a study of 137 cases. Hum Pathol. 2012;43:327–32.
76. Badwe R, Hawaldar R, Nair N, Kaushik R, et al. Locoregional treatment versus no treatment of the primary tumour in metastatic breast cancer: an open-label randomised controlled trial. Lancet Oncol. 2015;16:1380–8.
77. Fitzal F, Bjelic-Radisic V, Knauer M, Steger G, et al. Impact of breast surgery in primary metastasized breast cancer: outcomes of the prospective randomized phase III ABCSG-28 POSITIVE trial. Ann Surg. 2019;269:1163–9.
78. Khan SA, Zhao F, Solin LJ, Goldstein LJ, et al. A randomized phase III trial of systemic therapy plus early local therapy versus systemic therapy alone in women with de novo stage IV breast cancer: a trial of the ECOG-ACRIN Research Group (E2108). J Clin Oncol. 2020;38(18_suppl):LBA2.
79. Fernandez RAS, Lau RWH, Ho JYK, Yu PSY, et al. Evidence for surgical resections in oligometastatic lung cancer. J Thorac Dis. 2019;11(Suppl 7):S969–75.
80. Pastorino U, Buyse M, Friedel G, et al. Long-term results of lung metastasectomy: prognostic analyses based on 5206 cases. J Thorac Cardiovasc Surg. 1997;113:37–49.
81. Lyon TD, Thompson RH, Shah PH, Lohse CM, et al. Complete surgical metastasectomy of renal cell carcinoma in the post-cytokine era. J Urol. 2020;203:275–82.
82. Lane WO, Thomas SM, Blitzblau RC, Plichta JK, et al. Surgical resection of the primary tumor in women with de novo stage IV breast cancer: contemporary practice patterns and survival analysis. Ann Surg. 2019;269:537–44.
83. Pons-Tostivint E, Kirova Y, Luque A, Campone M, et al. Survival impact of locoregional treatment of the primary tumor in de novo metastatic breast cancers in a large multicentric cohort study: a propensity score-matched analysis. Ann Surg Oncol. 2019;26:356–65.
84. Soran A, Ozmen V, Ozbas S, Karanlik H, et al. Primary surgery with systemic therapy in patients with de novo stage IV breast cancer: 10-year follow-up; protocol MF07-01 randomized clinical trial. J Am Coll Surg. 2021;233:742–51.
85. Soran A, Ozmen V, Ozbas S, Karanlik H, et al. Randomized trial comparing resection of primary tumor with no surgery in stage IV breast cancer at presentation: protocol MF07-01. Ann Surg Oncol. 2018;25:3141–9.
86. Soran A, Spyder A, Ozbas S, Ozmen V, Karanlik H, et al. The role of loco-regional treatment in long-term quality of life in de novo stage IV breast cancer

patients: protocol MF07-01Q. Support Care Cancer. 2021;29:3823–30.
87. Gera R, Chehade HELH, Wazir U, Tayeh S, Kasem A, Mokbel K. Locoregional therapy of the primary tumour in de novo stage IV breast cancer in 216 066 patients: a meta-analysis. Sci Rep. 2020;10:2952.
88. Petrelli F, Barni S. Surgery of primary tumors in stage IV breast cancer: an updated meta-analysis of published studies with meta-regression. Med Oncol. 2012;29:3282–90.
89. Harris E, Barry M, Kell MR. Meta-analysis to determine if surgical resection of the primary tumour in the setting of stage IV breast cancer impacts on survival. Ann Surg Oncol. 2013;20:2828–34.
90. Reinhorn D, Mutai R, Yerushalmi R, Moore A, Amir E, Goldvaser H. Locoregional therapy in de novo metastatic breast cancer: systemic review and meta-analysis. Breast. 2021;58:173–81.
91. Iyengar P, Wardak Z, Gerber DE, et al. Consolidative radiotherapy for limited metastatic non-small-cell lung cancer: a phase 2 randomized clinical trial. JAMA Oncol. 2018;4:1–8.
92. Gomez DR, Tang C, Zhang J, et al. Local consolidative therapy vs. maintenance therapy or observation for patients with oligometastatic non-small-cell lung cancer: long-term results of a multi-institutional, phase II, randomized study. J Clin Oncol. 2019;37:1558–65.
93. National Comprehensive Cancer Network (NCCN). NCCN clinical practice guidelines in oncology. https://www.nccn.org/professionals/physician_gls. Last accessed on 1st June 2022.
94. Choueiri TK, Tomczak P, Park SH, et al. Adjuvant pembrolizumab after nephrectomy in renal cell carcinoma. N Engl J Med. 2021;385:683–94.
95. Masi G, Loupakis F, Pollina L, Vasile E, et al. Long-term outcome of initially unresectable metastatic colorectal cancer patients treated with 5-fluorouracil/leucovorin, oxaliplatin, and irinotecan (FOLFOXIRI) followed by radical surgery of metastases. Ann Surg. 2009;249:420.
96. Weickhardt AJ, Scheier B, Burke JM, et al. Local ablative therapy of oligoprogressive disease prolongs disease control by tyrosine kinase inhibitors in oncogene-addicted non-small-cell lung cancer. J Thorac Oncol. 2012;7:1807–14.
97. Shaw AT, Bauer TM, de Marinis F, et al. First-line lorlatinib or crizotinib in advanced ALK positive lung cancer. N Engl J Med. 2020;383:2018–29.
98. Wu YL, Ahn MJ, Garassino MC, Han JY, et al. CNS efficacy of osimertinib in patients with T790M-positive advanced non-small-cell lung cancer: data from a randomized phase III trial (AURA3). J Clin Oncol. 2018;36:2702–9. *
99. Reale ML, De Luca E, Lombardi P, Marandino L, Zichi C, Pignataro D, et al. Quality of life analysis in lung cancer: a systematic review of phase III trials published between 2012 and 2018. Lung Cancer. 2020;139:47–54. *
100. Vergara N, Montoya JE, Luna HG, Amparo JR, Cristal-Luna G. Quality of life and nutritional status among cancer patients on chemotherapy. Oman Med J. 2013;28:270–4.
101. Bauman GS, Corkum MT, Fakir H, Nguyen TK, Palma DA. Ablative radiation therapy to restrain everything safely treatable (ARREST): study protocol for a phase I trial treating polymetastatic cancer with stereotactic radiotherapy. BMC Cancer. 2021;14:405. *

Online Links

https://www.youtube.com/watch?v=FUuYNlCv79I (palliative radiotherapy for bone metastasis).

https://www.youtube.com/watch?v=KJVJAfsZXAo (oligometastatic prostate cancer).

https://www.youtube.com/watch?v=MOieuFed7aQ (radiotherapy in oligometastatic cancer).

https://www.youtube.com/watch?v=QNQr-uNIyQ4 (imaging for bone metastasis).

https://www.youtube.com/watch?v=WHoPgDVoAhE (oligometastatic breast cancer management).

https://www.youtube.com/watch?v=ZDWF_ZYequM (sbrt for oligometastatic lung cancer).

https://www.youtube.com/watch?v=zhm0din2P6s (sbrt spine in oligometastatic disease).

Resource Appropriate Cancer Management

Praful Pandey, Ranjit Kumar Sahoo, and Bidhu K. Mohanti

1 Introduction

Non-communicable diseases (NCDs)—mainly cardiovascular, cancer, respiratory, and diabetes—are the biggest cause of death worldwide. Approximately 41 million deaths occur (WHO data in 2021), out of which 17 million die prematurely aged between 30 and 70 years. Nearly 80% of such premature deaths, after the NCD diagnosis, happen in low- and middle-income countries (LMIC) [1]. Cancer has emerged as a major contributor to premature deaths in LMIC. Among non-communicable diseases, cancer has a significant health burden in India. Globally, more than seven million people die from cancer annually(in 2020), and cancer deaths account for roughly one-tenth of all deaths in India [2, 3]. This disproportionate mortality stems from a combination of lack of awareness, poor health-seeking behavior, poor access to cancer care facilities, stigma related to the diagnosis of cancer, and affordability issues. Approximately 50–70% of patients present with advanced stages at the index visit and are unable to receive optimal care, given the shortcomings of infrastructure and scarcity of trained manpower in cancer management.

India is among the signatories of the sustainable development goals (SDGs) and has to take steps towards the provision of universal health coverage [4]. The SDGs are a set of 17 goals, which were designed by an assembly of leaders from 193 countries in 2015, and have the ambitious aims to fulfill these goals in 15 years from the conception of SDGs, i.e., by 2030. The United Nations Development Program (UNDP) is one of the leading organizations working to fulfill the SDGs by the year 2030 (Fig. 1) [5]. Within the SDGs, the goal number 3 is for the citizens "good health and well-being". As defined by the World Health Organization (WHO), "Universal health coverage (UHC) means that all people have access to the full range of quality health services they need, when and where they need them, without financial hardship (Fig. 2). It covers the full continuum of essential health services, from health promotion to prevention, treatment, rehabilitation, and palliative care" [6].

The UHC service coverage index (based on 15 key outcome indicators, Fig. 2) has shown gradual improvement in India to achieve the score of 63 (out of 100) in 2021 but still needs significant improvement [6]. Universal health coverage has therefore become a major goal for health reform in many countries, including India, and a priority objective of the WHO.

P. Pandey · R. K. Sahoo
Department of Medical Oncology, All India Institute of Medical Sciences, New Delhi, India
e-mail: drranjitmd@gmail.com

B. K. Mohanti (✉)
Department of Radiation Oncology, Bagchi Sri Shankara Cancer Centre & Research Institute, Bhubaneswar, Odisha, India
e-mail: drbkmohanti@gmail.com

B. K. Mohanti et al. (eds.), *Radiation Oncology – Principles, Precepts and Practice*,
https://doi.org/10.1007/978-981-95-5171-2_23

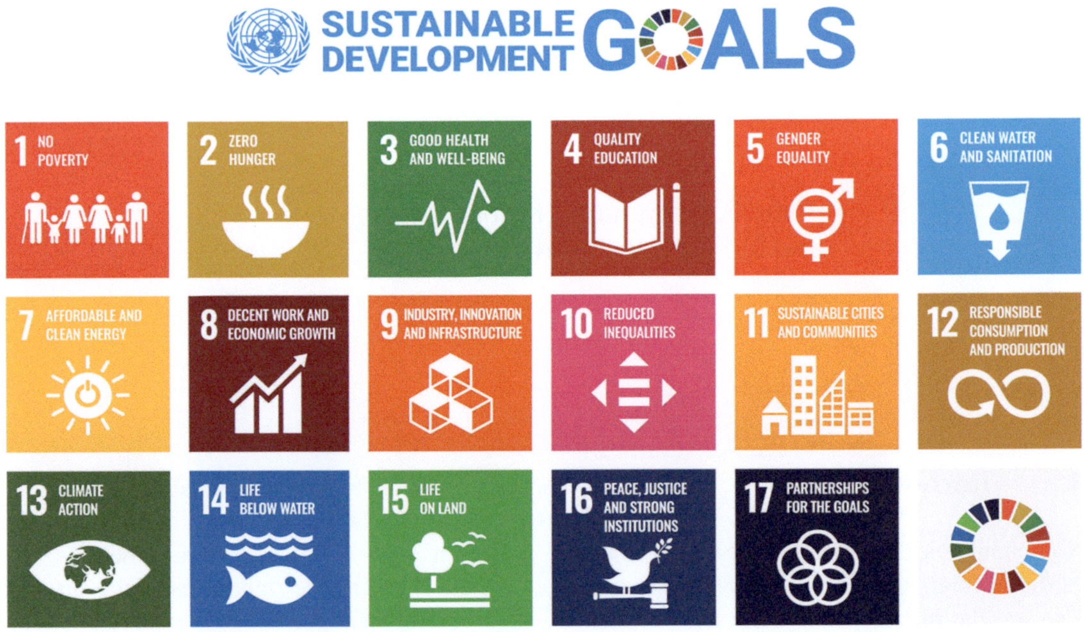
SUSTAINABLE DEVELOPMENT GOALS
1 NO POVERTY
2 ZERO HUNGER
3 GOOD HEALTH AND WELL-BEING
4 QUALITY EDUCATION
5 GENDER EQUALITY
6 CLEAN WATER AND SANITATION
7 AFFORDABLE AND CLEAN ENERGY
8 DECENT WORK AND ECONOMIC GROWTH
9 INDUSTRY, INNOVATION AND INFRASTRUCTURE
10 REDUCED INEQUALITIES
11 SUSTAINABLE CITIES AND COMMUNITIES
12 RESPONSIBLE CONSUMPTION AND PRODUCTION
13 CLIMATE ACTION
14 LIFE BELOW WATER
15 LIFE ON LAND
16 PEACE, JUSTICE AND STRONG INSTITUTIONS
17 PARTNERSHIPS FOR THE GOALS

Fig. 1 Sustainable Development Goals (SDGs) [5]

Health System Attributes	Action domains for UHC
QUALITY	1.1 Regulations and regulatory environment
	1.2 Effective, responsive individual and population-based services
	1.3 Individual, family and community engagement
EFFICIENCY	2.1 System design to meet population needs
	2.2 Incentives for appropriate provision and use of services
	2.3 Managerial efficiency and effectiveness
EQUITY	3.1 Financial protection
	3.2 Service coverage and access
	3.3 Non-discrimination
ACCOUNTABILITY	4.1 Government leadership and rule of law for health
	4.2 Partnerships for public policy
	4.3 Transparency, monitoring and evaluation (M&E)
SUSTAINABILITY AND RESILIENCE	5.1 Public health preparedness
	5.2 Community capacity
	5.3 Health system adaptability and sustainability

Fig. 2 Universal Health Coverage—the attributes and action domains for specific assessments to achieve UHC [5,6]

2 Steps to Create Resource Appropriate Cancer Management

2.1 Priorities

Four key priorities for overall cancer management have been recommended specifically for LMIC [7]:

1. Capacity building in cancer services-facility, manpower, training, research, and planning
2. High-quality cancer data sources—by setting up population-based cancer registry
3. High-quality models of cancer control—specific to cancers in LMIC rather than pursuing HIC models
4. Oncology-related economic evaluations in LMIC

All the above four areas are interrelated. For example, data collected from the cancer registries across India in 2020 would show the cancer burden of major cancer sites/systems as in Table 1 [2].

This kind of cancer data would mean that resource-appropriate management can address 73% of all cancers, i.e., 4 in 5 of all cancers in India. All policy efforts should be targeted towards capacity building, models of cancer control for specific cancer types, and economic aspects of treatment approaches for these specific cancer types. Hence, taking this example of major cancers (Table 1), national and regional priorities can be evolved as short-term and long-term cancer management goals in LMIC. Resource-appropriate cancer management in India, right from cancer awareness and prevention to cancer treatment facilities, should focus upon these 5 major cancer types, so that more than 70% of all cancers can be effectively controlled in the coming decades.

Table 1 Cancer data on major cancers in India, both sexes, 2020

Cancer site/ system	Patients	Cumulative risk	% of total burden
Oral cavity and pharynx	188,969	1 in 60	13.6
Digestive system	273,982	1 in 39	19.7
Breast	210,801	1 in 56	15.1
Genital system	207,524	1 in 54	14.9
Respiratory system	136,032	1 in 74	9.7
All sites	1,392,179	1 in 9	

Adapted from cancer registries of India [2]
Note: The above major sites/systems together accounted for 1,017,308 out of 1,392,179 patients; i.e., 73%

3 Cancer Care Deliveries

Health systems in a country should be geared to meet the needs for cancer control and management. Unlike demands on tertiary and specialized hospitals to diagnose and manage the patients in neurology, cardiology, nephrology, etc., the cancer patient can start the disease management trajectory right from the primary level, near to his or her home. The WHO has emphasized this healthcare delivery mechanism for cancers in LMIC, so that every patient should not always be referred to a cancer center or specialized hospital [8], as shown in Table 2.

For patients with symptoms suspicious of cancer, the clinical assessment approaches to diagnosis can be complex. Yet, a well-placed and sensitive health system can guide the patient from the primary level upward without undue delay and expenditures. Major difficulties noted by cancer patients and their families in LMIC pertain to distances and financial costs, which strongly impact the treatments and survival outcomes [9].

In order to optimize the cancer care deliveries, the health systems from the primary level (near to the suspected or diagnosed cancer patient) and secondary levels would require resource-appropriate provisions of infrastructure, biomedical facilities, and manpower to initiate the cancer management by proper and adequate attention. Similarly, at tertiary and specialized hospital levels, the LMIC must address the comprehensive cancer care access without undue delay. For example, recent studies have highlighted the difficulties in HPV vaccination and getting timely radiotherapy for cervical cancer [10].

Radiotherapy is standard of care for cervical cancer, but major global gaps in access exist,

Table 2 Healthcare service delivery for cancer control and management in LMIC

Health system level	Cancer control and management practices	Requirements	Capacity building
Primary (CHC, PHC, RMP, Field Health Worker, e.g., ASHA staff in India)	1. Cancer awareness 2. Cancer vaccination (e.g., HPV and Hepatitis-B) 3. Clinical assessment 4. Timely referral (to secondary/tertiary levels)	Budget and manpower as per geography	Training Leadership engagement
Secondary (DH;SH)	1. Laboratory tests 2. Imaging and endoscopy 3. Pathology 4. Surgery	1. Dedicated cancer clinic 2. Trained doctors and staff	Training Orientation Cancer management—knowledge and appropriate skills Engagement with non-government organizations and industries
Tertiary (MC&H; SH) and Specialized (cancer center)	1. Nuclear medicine 2. Comprehensive cancer management (diagnosis, surgery, medical oncology, radiation oncology) 3. Palliative care 4. Cancer survivorship program 5. Prevention and screening 6. Specialized laboratories (advanced cancer tests and research) 7. Academic courses, training, manpower building	1. Organised oncology specialties 2. Comprehensive Cancer Centre 3. Qualified and skilled doctors and staff	1. Socio-geographic appropriate cancer care 2. Cost-sensitive cancer diagnosis and treatments 3. Suitable cancer prevention, screening, and health workers training 4. Cancer registration and follow-up 5. Cancer specialty courses, academic and research programs 6. Engagement with non-government organization and industries

Modified from World Health Organization [8]
Note: *CHC* Community Health Centre, *PHC* Primary Health Centre, *RMP* Registered Medical Practitioner, *ASHA* Accredited Social Health Activist, *DH* district hospital, *SH* specialized hospital, *MC&H* medical college/school & hospital

particularly in low- and middle-income countries. A model prepared by Rodin et al. has categorically shown the benefits of a 20-year strategy for scaling up both external beam radiation therapy and brachytherapy resources in LMICs from 2015 to 2035, with an estimated 11.4 million life years saved [11]. The national and regional governments, non-government organizations, industries, and medical societies will need to join hands for improving the equity, affordability, and availability of all cancer care measures, including cancer awareness and prevention.

Because of the well-recognized paucity of facilities and manpower, the cancer centers and oncologists in LMIC can play a significant role at two levels:

1. To identify, enlist, and train doctors, nurses, and paramedics from the primary and secondary health system levels, with due involvement of the local and regional authorities
2. To develop and implement cost-effective diagnostic and treatment practices for the major cancers within the region

However, financial toxicity from cancer care remains rampant. Compared to other diseases, the cost of cancer care is disproportionately high in India, with a consequent risk of financial instability in families not adequately covered by insurance [12, 13]. These challenges pose significant hurdles for India in achieving Universal Health Care (UHC) and mandate the need to develop cancer management protocols synergistic with our healthcare systems and paying capacities.

In this context, we focus on the two main aspects of providing resource-appropriate cancer care: Financial toxicity and its implications; and Universal Health Care with special emphasis on state-funded health insurance schemes in India.

4 Financial Toxicity and Its Implications

4.1 Understanding the Multifaceted Toxicity

Compared to other health-related expenses, cancer patients bear higher out-of-pocket (OOP) medical spending, even in high-income countries like the USA [14, 15]. Non-medical direct expenses such as travel, meals, and accommodation further increase the economic burden. Indirect financial toxicity from loss of job/workdays is an additional source of burden [16–18]. Accrual of these expenses, given the time-consuming nature of most cancer care, leads to significant financial hardship, debt, and mental distress [19, 20]. These findings have alarmed the global cancer community in the last 10 years, more so since 2013. The economic burden on cancer patients to bear the direct cancer treatment costs and simultaneously the non-medical direct expenses, such as travel, meals, and stay at the place of cancer treatments, has been evaluated in India [21]. Thus, there is a greater need for oncologists and health workers in India and LMIC to be sensitized about the financial consequences of the cancer diagnosis and treatments.

4.1.1 Financial Toxicity: Definition

Cancer management, by surgery, chemotherapy, and radiotherapy, has remained a clinical and therapeutic balance or trade-off between disease control and treatment-related toxicities. The physical and psychological morbidities are routinely assessed as disease-related and/or treatment-related toxicities on well-recognized Common Toxicities of Adverse Events (CTCAE) and Quality of Life (QoL) scales. As progress in cancer treatments has advanced in terms of technology, new drugs, and treatment techniques, the costs of cancer care have escalated in the last 20 years. Cancer treatments have become expensive, and much too often expensive cancer drugs and technologies are overutilized with an emphasis on delivering the best of cancer management, not necessarily commensurate with treatment results. This phenomenon has given rise to financial hardship and out-of-pocket expenses (OOPE) for cancer patients globally. In 2013, Zafar and Abernethy from Duke Cancer Institute, USA, first coined the term "financial toxicity". They stated, "Out-of-pocket expenses related to treatment are akin to physical toxicity, in that costs can diminish quality of life and impede delivery of the highest quality care" [22]. Financial toxicity (FT) describes the financial burden and distress that can arise for patients and their family members as a result of cancer treatment. The costs of cancer care can be broadly grouped into direct and indirect costs in an objective and real-world context [23], as shown in Fig. 3.

4.1.2 Features of Financial Toxicity

The multifaceted etiology of financial toxicity (FT) among cancer patients has emerged to appreciate this complex phenomenon. Within the conceptual underpinning of a research framework, FT and its consequences can be classified into three distinctive domains: psychological, behavioral, and material [17]. The psychological manifestations of FT give rise to deleterious effects, encompassing heightened states of anxiety, depression, fatigue, and diminished quality of life [19, 20, 24, 25]. These effects extend their harmful influence not only upon the afflicted patients themselves but also upon their caregivers [26]. Consequently, the psychological repercussions may trigger an escalation in hospital admissions and utilization of emergency services, as the onerous burden of stress and caregiver obligations interferes with optimal clinical management [19, 27]. Moreover, the escalating costs of cancer treatment exert an adverse impact on the patient's compliance with treatments, precipitating instances of chemotherapy or radiotherapy omission, delayed or altogether forsaken medical care, and reduced treatment outcomes [18, 28, 29]. The material dimensions of financial hardship endured by cancer patients, such as the burden of debt and bankruptcy, have been empirically

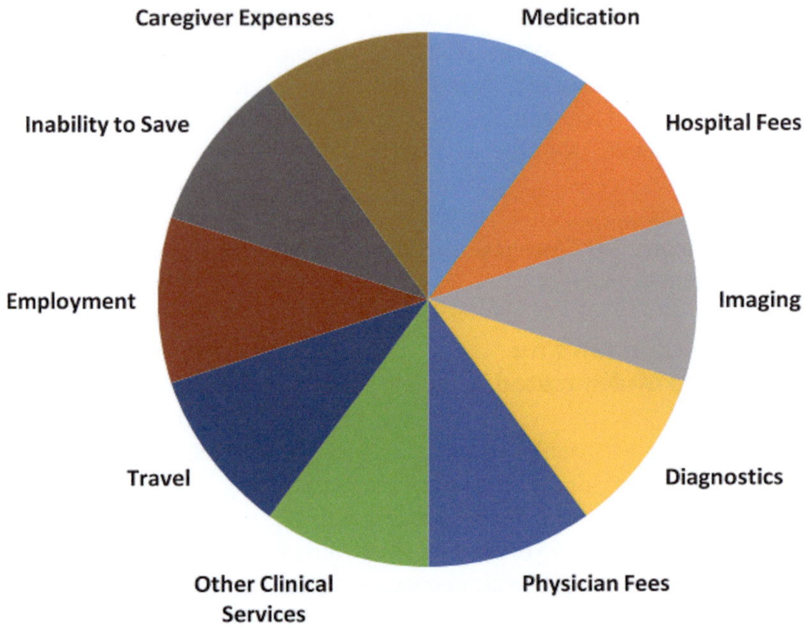

Fig. 3 Identification of the direct and indirect sources of financial burden on cancer patients. (Source: Abrams et al. [23])

linked to deleterious effects on survival rates. Indeed, patients burdened by FT can show increased mortality risk, attributable to suboptimal adherence, loss to follow-up, and heightened incidence of adverse events. The various features of FT stemming from out-of-pocket expenditures are becoming hurdles in LMIC for seeking adequate healthcare services. Thus, FT is becoming a big determinant for access to high-quality cancer care, for which the health policy makers should design clear frameworks.

4.2 Social Determinants of Health (SDoH) and Financial Toxicity

Surveys in the USA have noted that approximately 50% of all cancer patients face personal economic burdens associated with the disease and its treatment [30]. Several studies have consistently identified a correlation between FT and certain socio-economic factors, such as lower household income [31, 32], racial/ethnic minority status [28, 33], rural residency [34], unmarried or unpartnered status [28, 31], and lack of insurance coverage [28, 35]. These factors, collectively known as Social Determinants of Health (SDoH), encompass the environmental conditions and systems that influence individuals' well-being, such as aspects of birth, growth, work, living, and aging [36]. Health-related social needs (HRSN) represent the social and economic needs experienced by patients, including housing and food insecurity, transportation challenges, unemployment, and financial strain [37]. Hence, within a decade of unraveling the financial burden experienced by cancer patients, SDoH, HRSN, and FT are characterized by a continuum of interconnectivity, emphasizing the need for a comprehensive approach to address these factors holistically.

5 Addressing Financial Toxicity

5.1 Professional Organizations and Advocacy

Professional organizations have been keen on shedding light on the issue of financial toxicity (FT) and have earnestly advocated for policy changes to rectify this problem [38]. However, the implementation of these changes has been characterized by sluggishness and a lack of individualization. Nonetheless, it is noteworthy that these policy alterations exert a profound and far-reaching influence. For instance, enhanced social safety nets, regulation of drug pricing, and the broadening of insurance accessibility have demonstrated potential in mitigating FT. Remarkably, the availability of government-funded insurance has demonstrated the capacity to enhance cancer survival rates [39]. Furthermore, insurance design modifications, exemplified by the advent of value-based formulary systems wherein higher-value medications are assigned to lower co-payment tiers, can offer a promising prospect of reducing financial burdens for patients and healthcare systems alike [40]. Although these measures are undoubtedly efficacious in developed countries, oncologists and professional organizations must continue their advocacy at both the health system and government levels to secure improved access to health insurance coverage, lower drug prices, and social programs in LMIC. It is necessary to explore additional measures that can provide timely relief for those cancer patients caught in the plight of FT.

5.2 Implement FT and HRSN Screening into Clinical Care

Identifying at-risk patients vulnerable to financial toxicity (FT) before its onset is not widely recognized and the integration of FT screening into standard practice remains limited across cancer care [22]. Even in prominent Western academic institutions, approximately one in four cancer patients would experience FT. Numerous screening tools are commonly employed, including clinic-specific forms [40, 41]; the National Comprehensive Cancer Network (NCCN) distress thermometer—an assessment tool encompassing concerns about housing, finances, access, and transportation [42, 43]; and the Comprehensive Score for Financial Toxicity Patient-Reported Outcome Measure (COST scale) [44], and a novel five-item FT screening tool [45]. Nevertheless, the performance of these screening tools in resource-constrained developing countries warrants further evaluation.

For practical implementation within cancer management, FT screening tools should be concise, adaptable to varying levels of health literacy, and straightforward for staff to administer. Notably, FT screening should encompass queries aimed at identifying patients experiencing HRSN that may contribute to FT development, such as housing insecurity, transportation expenses, social isolation, or insufficient insurance coverage. Ideally, longitudinal FT screening should be employed since it may develop at a later time point in the cancer care timeline, given its protracted and multifaceted nature.

Upon a positive FT screening result, personalized interventions tailored to the specific needs of individual patients can be initiated. However, it is important to acknowledge that no evidence-based method for mitigating financial toxicity has been established in the existing literature. Sensitivity must be exercised during FT screening, particularly in clinics where caregivers may be acutely aware of the financial constraints that hinder access to optimal care.

5.3 Financial Navigation

Financial navigation is a specialized and comprehensive approach aimed at helping individuals, especially those facing financial challenges due to healthcare expenses, to navigate the complex financial aspects of their medical care [45]. It is particularly relevant in the context of cancer care.

Financial navigation teams, consisting of professionals with expertise in financial matters and healthcare systems, work closely with patients to provide personalized assistance and guidance. They offer a range of services, including:

1. Financial screening
2. Health insurance optimization
3. Health literacy education
4. Referrals to social support services

By offering individualized support and addressing patients' unique financial challenges, financial navigation provides a multitude of benefits. Primarily, it is aimed at reducing out-of-pocket expenses (OOPE). Thus, patients focus on their treatment and recovery rather than being overwhelmed by the financial aspects of their care. Improved oncological outcomes stemming from better compliance and fewer defaults may be possible. Ongoing studies are evaluating the impact of financial navigation on OOPE, institutional healthcare expenses, and outcomes [46, 47].

Financial navigation may be delivered in-person, through remote communications, and via third-party resources. A novel method is the financial toxicity tumor board, a multidisciplinary team of healthcare professionals that assesses and addresses the financial burdens experienced by cancer patients due to the cost of their treatment. The board aims to identify and provide solutions for the economic challenges faced by patients and their families during cancer care, ensuring that financial considerations are integrated into treatment decisions for better patient outcomes [48]. Additionally, the potential of smartphone app-based solutions to identify resources and provide financial assistance based on patient characteristics and electronic health records (EHRs) is being explored [49].

5.4 Discussing Cost Information

Patients want to talk about treatment costs with their oncology teams [50], and in the real world would consider the cost when making decisions about cancer treatments [51]. Patients who discuss costs with their oncology teams have lower out-of-pocket expenses and higher satisfaction without compromising their cancer care [52, 53]. However, even in Western settings, a majority of patients don't have this conversation with the oncologist due to reluctance or a lack of information sharing process related to financial matters [53]. To have more meaningful discussions, oncologists need access to accurate cost information for medical services, prescription drugs, and hospital stays. Integrating pricing information into electronic health records (EHRs) and treatment protocols could give real-time access to out-of-pocket cost details [54]. Oncology care teams need specialized training to feel more comfortable discussing treatment costs [55]. More research is needed to design and implement the best training for clinical care teams to improve confidence in discussing costs with sensitivity.

5.5 Minimize Low-Value Care

Oncologists can make decisions that alleviate financial burden while maintaining effective oncological outcomes [52–55]. This involves using biosimilar or generic drugs when possible, reducing unnecessary hospital visits, repeated laboratory or imaging tests, and selecting cost-effective treatments when equally efficient options exist. Multiple campaigns to minimize costs have gained momentum in the West. In the process, the American Society of Clinical Oncology (ASCO) has also identified ten specific practices in oncology that should be questioned and limited due to their lower-value status [56]. Examples include discouraging routine high-cost imaging for early-stage cancers with low metastatic risk, limiting palliative chemotherapy for patients with poor performance status, and reducing the use of expensive antiemetics except for highly emetogenic treatments. However, the adoption of such measures in cancer care practices has been slow [57]. Practicing cost-conscious care and adhering to evidence-based guidelines can help minimize low-value care to alleviate financial toxicity for patients and optimize resource utilization in oncology practice.

5.6 Leveraging Technology

Telemedicine and remote monitoring can improve access to care and reduce the need for frequent in-person visits, leading to cost savings for patients [58]. Digital health platforms can provide resources and information to help patients manage their financial and health-related social needs more effectively. Artificial intelligence has shown some merit in delineating the population at risk of financial toxicity at an earlier time point [59]. Overall, a multifaceted approach involving policy changes, advocacy efforts, interventions at the provider and health system levels, and the use of technology can help mitigate financial toxicity in cancer care and improve patient outcomes. All these aspects should be addressed for the cancer patients in LMIC.

6 Value-Based Oncology: The Indian Framework

6.1 Existing Framework in India

Three main pillars support the campaign for universal health coverage with regard to cancer care in India: National Health Authority, Ayushman Bharat Pradhan Mantri Jan Arogya Yojana (AB-PMJAY), and the National Cancer Grid.

6.2 National Health Authority

The National Health Authority (NHA) in India is a crucial governing body responsible for the implementation and management of various healthcare initiatives in the country. As an autonomous entity operating under the Ministry of Health and Family Welfare, the NHA plays a central role in shaping India's healthcare landscape. The NHA collaborates with state governments, insurance agencies, and healthcare providers to ensure seamless implementation and reach of PM-JAY to the intended beneficiaries. Through strategic planning, policy formulation, and efficient management, the NHA endeavors to achieve better health outcomes for all citizens and promote a healthier and more resilient nation. As a key player in the Indian healthcare ecosystem, the NHA continues to evolve and adapt to address the diverse healthcare challenges faced by the nation [60, 61].

6.3 Ayushman Bharat Pradhan Mantri Jan Arogya Yojna (PM-JAY)

The Ayushman Bharat Pradhan Mantri Jan Arogya Yojana (AB-PMJAY), commonly known as Ayushman Bharat, is a pioneering and ambitious healthcare scheme in India. Launched by the Government of India, it is one of the largest publicly funded health insurance programs in the world. AB-PMJAY aims to provide financial protection and quality healthcare services to over 500 million vulnerable and poor individuals and families across the country. Under this scheme, eligible beneficiaries can access cashless and paperless treatment for a wide range of secondary and tertiary medical procedures at impaneled hospitals. The coverage includes pre-existing conditions, making it a comprehensive and inclusive healthcare initiative. The scheme operates on a robust technology-driven platform that allows for seamless identification and verification of beneficiaries, ensuring that the benefits reach those who need them the most. AB-PMJAY is a key component of the government's efforts to strengthen the healthcare infrastructure, enhance access to medical services, and reduce the financial burden on vulnerable sections of society. By leveraging the power of health insurance and promoting preventive healthcare, AB-PMJAY aims to contribute significantly to India's journey towards achieving Universal Health Coverage (UHC) and better health outcomes for all its citizens [62, 63]. In line with the Ayushman Bharat, several states in India, such as Andhra Pradesh, Gujarat, Maharashtra, Odisha, Rajasthan, Tamil Nadu, and West Bengal, provide state-specific health coverage for diseases, including cancer. These government health schemes, at national and state levels, are suited for citizens belonging to the poor and lower-middle-class income groups. There is increasing awareness by government and health insurance providers to improve the health coverage for the senior citizens above 60 years of age.

6.4 National Cancer Grid

The National Cancer Grid (NCG) in India stands as a collaborative and transformative initiative in the field of cancer care and research. It brings together over 200 cancer centers, research institutes, and healthcare organizations across the country, creating a unified network with a shared mission. The

NCG's primary objective is to enhance the quality and accessibility of cancer care for patients throughout India. Through seamless knowledge-sharing and collaboration among its member institutions, the NCG seeks to promote best practices, standardize treatment protocols, and facilitate cutting-edge research in the fight against cancer. By leveraging collective expertise, resources, and advancements, the NCG aims to improve cancer treatment outcomes and reduce the burden of cancer on individuals and communities. The initiative not only addresses the clinical aspects of cancer care but also emphasizes cancer education and training for healthcare professionals, contributing to capacity-building and skill development in oncology. More recently, the NCG has entered into collaboration with the NHA to provide context-specific guidelines for the cancer treatment services provided as a part of the PMJAY [64].

6.5 How Are We Improving Cancer Care?

6.5.1 Standardizing and Improving the Quality of Cancer Care Through NCG

The National Cancer Grid (NCG) is dedicated to establishing standardized and evidence-based protocols for cancer prevention, diagnosis, and treatment. It aims to bridge disparities in patient care across different regions of India, promoting cost-effective management strategies accessible to all centers and patients, both in the public and private sectors. The NCG guidelines hold relevance for clinicians, managers, health insurers, and patients alike and are aligned with the Ayushman Bharat Pradhan Mantri Jan Arogya Yojana (AB-PMJAY) scheme, thereby bolstering cancer services delivery and aiding decision-making during disease management and reimbursements. To ensure consistency across groups, the NCG partnered with the National Health Authority (NHA) to develop cancer patient care guidelines under AB-PMJAY. Given variations in cancer epidemiology, resources, access, and affordability, contextualizing guidelines for India is crucial compared to international standards [64–67]. While a multitude of guidelines exist for many tumors, their applicability to Indian settings becomes problematic given the variability in epidemiology, hospital facilities, management skills, patient accessibility, and paying capacity. LMICs are shouldering much of the cancer burden, and more than three-fourths of cancer deaths occur in these countries. Adoption of resource-appropriate clinical practice guidelines (CPG), mainly for common cancers, can improve cancer care and reduce futile expenditures [68]. The NCG employed a "RIGHT Adapt" framework [69], using existing high-quality guidelines and adapting them to the Indian context, expediting guideline development while preserving the validity of recommendations tailored to India's unique healthcare landscape. One example is the CPG for cervical cancer, a common female cancer in LMIC [70].

6.6 Engaging Stakeholders in the Development Process

For developing the National Cancer Grid (NCG) guidelines, stakeholder engagement emerges as an indispensable and well-acknowledged component [71]. This involves healthcare professionals, patients, caregivers, insurers, managers, policymakers, and manufacturers. Justification for involving stakeholders stems from the limitations of available evidence, the need for transparency, democratic values, ownership, and potential policy implications. Accordingly, guideline development must explicitly incorporate the values and preferences of relevant stakeholders, seamlessly integrating them into the recommendations. It is essential to recognize that stakeholders play diverse roles in this process, and their involvement can be intricate, particularly within India's multifaceted healthcare system. The NCG guideline manual furnishes guidance on stakeholder contributions, either as members of the Guideline Development Group (GDG) or via consultation on draft recommendations. The role of the GDG Chair holds particular emphasis, ensuring collaborative work and contributions from all members, with decisions reached through informal consensus or formal voting. Thus, the GDG should diligently identify areas of focus from the outset of guideline development, mindful of the significant task at hand [64, 70]. Given the high cost of cancer management, trade-offs are inevitable to adhere to budget constraints while providing the greatest health outcomes without compromising the standard of care [72]. In LMIC, treatment regimens should further be tailored to local environments with consideration of social and cultural factors and accessible resources that often impact decision-making [73].

6.7 Guideline Development: Navigating Complexity with Elegance

In the process of developing recommendations within the NCG, the Guideline Development Group (GDG) faces challenging tasks: (a) collecting evidence from various sources, and (b) considering factors specific to the Indian health context. To facilitate this decision-making, the WHO-INTEGRATE framework systematically considers the evidence-to-decision with six helpful criteria [74].

These are six criteria are:

1. Balance of health benefits and harms
2. Human rights and sociocultural acceptability
3. Health equity, equality, and non-discrimination
4. Societal implications, financial and economic considerations
5. Feasibility and health system considerations
6. Quality of evidence

Adapting international guidelines entails a careful assessment of multiple factors. Vital to the process is assessing the feasibility of implementing recommendations in practice. GDGs diligently consider the extent of change required in practice, whether at cancer centers, national levels, and taking into account potential health budget impacts. Hence, clinicians treating cancer patients should be encouraged to evaluate factors such as staffing, equipment, services, and infrastructures of the hospital, funding patterns, and policy control, all of which significantly influence the decision-making process [75].

6.8 Crafting Resource-Stratified Recommendations

One key area which would improve resource-appropriate and cost effective cancer care in India and LMIC is targeted at achieving uniform practices for each cancer right from diagnostic tests to treatment approaches and subsequent survivorship follow-up plans. In the process of adapting existing guidelines, the GDG in the NCG meticulously considers various factors to ensure appropriateness to the Indian subcontinent. This includes weighing three options: adopting a recommendation as is, contextualizing it to the Indian context, or updating it as needed. If a priority area identified during scoping is not covered by a source guideline, the GDG may undertake the "de novo guideline development process" to formulate a new clinical/review question and review relevant evidence. The NCG's strength of recommendations is represented as "resource-stratified recommendations," thoughtfully considering clinical evidence, equity, costs, and implementation considerations. These guidelines further categorize recommendations as "essential," "optimal," or "optional," specifically designed for implementation in India and linked to the AB-PMJAY. This classification not only guides clinical practice but also informs preauthorization and claims processing, requiring meticulous documentation. To ensure comprehensive cancer management recommendations, the GDG member selection process involves diverse expertise from different infrastructure settings, effectively stratifying interventions, and establishing the minimum standard of care in the "essential" category [76, 77].

7 Conclusions

Cancer poses a significant health burden in India, with financial toxicity hindering universal health coverage. Initiatives like NCG, NHA, and AB-PMJAY aim to address these challenges. Advocacy, financial screening, and interventions can alleviate financial burdens. Stakeholder engagement, scoping, and contextualizing guidelines ensure resource-stratified recommendations. Technology, like telemedicine and AI, enhances access and reduces costs. Embracing cost-conscious care and adhering to evidence-based guidelines will optimize cancer management practices. Through collaboration, evidence, and technology, India can reduce the cancer burden, improve patient outcomes, and achieve Universal Health Coverage.

Percepts Box

1. Cancer care facilities and cancer incidence registration in LMIC should be strengthened so that cancer prevention and cancer management can reach the rural areas.
2. Costs of cancer treatments are important for every cancer patient and family.
3. Financial toxicity (FT), which consists of out-of-pocket expenditures (OOPE) for the diagnosis and treatments for a cancer patient and family, can become more devastating than the physical toxicity due to morbidities of cancer surgery, radiotherapy, and chemotherapy.
4. From the time of cancer diagnosis and for the lifetime of the cancer patient, the cancer hospitals and health workers should assess the FT by standard measurement tools.
5. Resource-appropriate cancer centers with comprehensive management can improve the patient's comfort and compliance for the treatment duration.
6. Universal health coverage (UHC) should incorporate cancer services, such that insurance schemes like Ayushman Bharat or similar public health insurance will reduce the OOPE.
7. National Cancer Grid (NCG) in India has made it possible for the medical community and smaller hospitals to participate in uniform practices for cancer prevention and management.
8. Approaches to cost-conscious care and adhering to evidence-based guidelines will optimize the cancer management practices. Through collaboration, evidence, and technology, India can reduce the cancer burden, improve patient outcomes, and achieve Universal Health Coverage.

Multiple Choice Questions

1. What multifaceted factor impacts the majority of cancer patients after the cancer diagnosis, leading to suboptimal care?
   (a) Poor health literacy
   (b) Lack of access to cancer care facilities
   (c) Stigma related to cancer diagnosis
   (d) financial toxicity from high cancer care costs
2. Which initiative launched by the Indian government aims to provide financial protection and quality healthcare services to vulnerable and poor individuals through a publicly funded health insurance program?
   (a) National Cancer Grid (NCG)
   (b) Ayushman Bharat Pradhan Mantri Jan Arogya Yojana (AB-PMJAY)
   (c) National Health Authority (NHA)
   (d) National Comprehensive Cancer Network (NCCN)
3. Which three domains are classified as the consequences of financial toxicity among cancer patients, leading to deleterious effects on their well-being?
   (a) Psychological, emotional, and physical
   (b) Behavioral, financial, and medical
   (c) Psychological, behavioral, and material
   (d) Social, economic, and environmental
4. In the context of cancer care, which innovative approach involves a multidisciplinary team of healthcare professionals assessing and addressing the financial burdens experienced by patients and their families during treatment?
   (a) Financial navigation

(b) Financial toxicity tumor board
(c) Health insurance optimization
(d) Financial screening

5. Which healthcare framework emphasizes a comprehensive approach to address the multifaceted challenges of financial toxicity, incorporating the dimensions such as-balance of health benefits and harms, health equity, feasibility, and health system considerations?
   (a) Sustainable Development Goals (SDG)
   (b) World Health Organization (WHO) guidelines
   (c) RIGHT Adapt framework
   (d) National Cancer Grid (NCG) recommendations

Answer Key

1. (d)
2. (b)
3. (c)
4. (b)
5. (c)

References

1. https://www.who.int/news-room/fact-sheets/detail/noncommunicable-diseases.
2. Mathur P, Sathishkumar K, Chaturvedi M, Das P, Sudarshan KL, Santhappan S, et al. Cancer statistics, 2020: report from National Cancer Registry Programme, India. JCO Glob Oncol. 2020;6:1063–75.
3. Sung H, Ferlay J, Siegel RL, Laversanne M, Soerjomataram I, Jemal A, et al. Global cancer statistics 2020: GLOBOCAN estimates of incidence and mortality worldwide for 36 cancers in 185 countries. CA Cancer J Clin. 2021;71(3):209–49.
4. Gera R, Narwal R, Jain M, Taneja G, Gupta S. Sustainable development goals: leveraging the global agenda for driving health policy reforms and achieving universal health coverage in India. Indian J Community Med. 2018;43(4):255–9.
5. UNDP. Sustainable Development Goals. https://www.dev-practitioners.eu/media/key_documents/SDGs_Booklet_Web_En.pdf.
6. WHO. SDG Target 3.8 Achieve universal health coverage (UHC) [Internet]. [cited 2023 Jul 30]. Available from: https://www.who.int/data/gho/data/major-themes/universal-health-coverage-major.
7. Shah SC, Kayamba V, Peek RM Jr, Heimburger D. Cancer control in low- and middle-income countries: is it time to consider screening? J Glob Oncol. 2019;5:1–8. https://doi.org/10.1200/JGO.18.00200.
8. WHO. WHO list of priority medical devices for cancer management. Geneva: World Health Organization; 2017. Licence: CC BY-NC-SA 3.0 IGO.
9. Lubuzo B, Hlongwana KW, Hlongwa M, Ginindza TG. Coordination models for cancer care in low- and middle-income countries: a scoping review. Int J Environ Res Public Health. 2022;19(13):7906. https://doi.org/10.3390/ijerph19137906.
10. Lin LL, Msadabwe SC, Chiao E. Improving access to radiation therapy globally to meet World Health Organization goals to eliminate cervical cancer. Int J Radiat Oncol Biol Phys. 2023;116(2):459–62. https://doi.org/10.1016/j.ijrobp.2022.12.034.
11. Rodin D, Burger EA, Atun R, Barton M, Gospodarowicz M, Grover S, Hanna TP, Jaffray DA, Knaul FM, Lievens Y, Zubizarreta E, Milosevic M. Scale-up of radiotherapy for cervical cancer in the era of human papillomavirus vaccination in low-income and middle-income countries: a model-based analysis of need and economic impact. Lancet Oncol. 2019;20(7):915–23. https://doi.org/10.1016/S1470-2045(19)30308-0.
12. Pramesh CS, Badwe RA, Borthakur BB, Chandra M, Raj EH, Kannan T, et al. Delivery of affordable and equitable cancer care in India. Lancet Oncol. 2014;15(6):e223–33.
13. Singh M, Chauhan A, Rai B, Ghoshal S, Prinja S. Cost of treatment for cervical cancer in India. Asian Pac J Cancer Prev. 2020;21:2639–46.
14. Davidoff AJ, Erten M, Shaffer T. Out-of-pocket health care expenditure burden for Medicare beneficiaries with cancer. Cancer. 2013;119:1257–65.
15. Bernard DS, Farr SL, Fang Z. National estimates of out-of-pocket health care expenditure burdens among nonelderly adults with cancer: 2001 to 2008. J Clin Oncol. 2011;29(20):2821–6.
16. Shankaran V, Jolly S, Blough D. Risk factors for financial hardship in patients receiving adjuvant chemotherapy for colon cancer: a population-based exploratory analysis. J Clin Oncol. 2012;30:1608–14.
17. Tucker-Seeley RD, Yabroff KR. Minimizing the “financial toxicity” associated with cancer care: advancing the research agenda. J Natl Cancer Inst. 2015;108:djv410.
18. Zafar SY, Peppercorn JM, Schrag D. The financial toxicity of cancer treatment: a pilot study assessing out-of-pocket expenses and the insured cancer patient’s experience. Oncologist. 2013;18:381–90.
19. Kale HP, Carroll NV. Self-reported financial burden of cancer care and its effect on physical and mental health-related quality of life among US cancer survivors. Cancer. 2016;122:283–9.
20. Dee EC, Nipp RD, Muralidhar V. Financial worry and psychological distress among cancer survivors in the United States, 2013-2018. Support Care Cancer. 2021;29:5523–35.

21. Mohanti BK, Mukhopadhyay A, Sharma K, Das S, Dash S. The economic burden of cancer. Econ Polit Wkly. 2011;43:112–7.
22. Zafar SY, Abernethy AP. Financial toxicity, part I: a new name for a growing problem. Oncology (Williston Park). 2013;27(2):80–149.
23. Abrams HR, Durbin S, Huang CX, Johnson SF, Nayak RK, Zahner GJ, Peppercorn J. Financial toxicity in cancer care: origins, impact, and solutions. Transl Behav Med. 2021;11(11):2043–54. https://doi.org/10.1093/tbm/ibab091.
24. Longo CJ, Fitch MI, Loree JM. Patient and family financial burden associated with cancer treatment in Canada: a national study. Support Care Cancer. 2021;29:3377–86.
25. Lu L, Gavin A, Drummond FJ. Cumulative financial stress as a potential risk factor for cancer-related fatigue among prostate cancer survivors. J Cancer Surviv. 2021;15:1–13.
26. Sadigh G, Switchenko J, Weaver KE, Elchoufi D, Meisel J, Bilen MA, Lawson D, Cella D, El-Rayes B, Carlos R. Correlates of financial toxicity in adult cancer patients and their informal caregivers. Support Care Cancer. 2022;30(1):217–25. https://doi.org/10.1007/s00520-021-06424-1.
27. Zheng Z, Han X, Zhao J. Financial hardship, healthcare utilization, and health among US cancer survivors. Am J Prev Med. 2020;59:68–78.
28. Kent EE, Forsythe LP, Yabroff KR. Are survivors who report cancer-related financial problems more likely to forgo or delay medical care? Cancer. 2013;119:3710–7.
29. Zullig LL, Peppercorn JM, Schrag D. Financial distress, use of cost-coping strategies, and adherence to prescription medication among patients with cancer. J Oncol Pract. 2013;9:60.
30. Smith GL, Banegas MP, Acquati C, Chang S, et al. Navigating financial toxicity in patients with cancer: a multidisciplinary management approach. CA Cancer J Clin. 2022;72(5):437–53. https://doi.org/10.3322/caac.21730.
31. Banegas MP, Guy GP Jr, Moor JS. For working-age cancer survivors, medical debt and bankruptcy create financial hardships. Health Aff. 2016;35:54–61.
32. Zafar SY, McNeil RB, Thomas CM. Population-based assessment of cancer survivors' financial burden and quality of life: a prospective cohort study. J Oncol Pract. 2015;11:145–50.
33. Jagsi R, Pottow JA, Griffith KA. Long-term financial burden of breast cancer: experiences of a diverse cohort of survivors identified through population-based registries. J Clin Oncol. 2014;32:1269–76.
34. Bremner KE, Yabroff KR, Coughlan D. Patterns of care and costs for older patients with colorectal cancer at the end of life: descriptive study of the United States and Canada. JCO Oncol Pract. 2020;16:e1–e18.
35. Yabroff KR, Han X, Song W. Association of medical financial hardship and mortality among cancer survivors in the United States. J Natl Cancer Inst. 2022;114:863–70.
36. World Health Organization. Social determinants of health. World Health Organization [Internet]; 2021. Available from: https://www.who.int/health-topics/social-determinants-of-health.
37. McPeek Hinz ER, Avery C, Johnson S, Drake C, Spratt SE. Addressing health-related social needs through systematic screening and integration of a social care technology platform. NEJM Catal. 2023;4(5):CAT.22.0324.
38. Khan HM, Ramsey S, Shankaran V. Financial toxicity in cancer care: implications for clinical care and potential practice solutions. J Clin Oncol. 2023;41(16):3051–8.
39. Zhao J, Han X, Nogueira L, Fedewa SA, Jemal A, Halpern MT, Yabroff KR. Health insurance status and cancer stage at diagnosis and survival in the United States. CA Cancer J Clin. 2022;72(6):542–60. https://doi.org/10.3322/caac.21732.
40. Yeung K, Bloudek L, Ding Y. Value-based pricing of US prescription drugs: estimated savings using reports from the Institute for Clinical and Economic Review. JAMA Health Forum. 2022;3:e224631.
41. McLouth LE, Nightingale CL, Dressler EV. Current practices for screening and addressing financial hardship within the NCI Community Oncology Research Program. Cancer Epidemiol Biomarkers Prev. 2021;30:669–75.
42. Khera N, Sugalski J, Krause D. Current practices for screening and management of financial distress at NCCN member institutions. J Natl Compr Cancer Netw. 2020;18:825–31.
43. National Comprehensive Cancer Network. NCCN Guidelines Version 2.2023 Distress Management [Internet]. Available from: https://www.nccn.org/docs/default-source/patientresources/nccn_distress_thermometer.pdf.
44. de Souza JA, Yap BJ, Wroblewski K, Blinder V, et al. Measuring financial toxicity as a clinically relevant patient-reported outcome: the validation of the COmprehensive Score for financial Toxicity (COST). Cancer. 2017;123(3):476–84. https://doi.org/10.1002/cncr.30369.
45. Wheeler SB, Biddell CB, Manning ML, Gellin MS, Padilla NR, Spees LP, et al. Lessening the Impact of Financial Toxicity (LIFT): a protocol for a multi-site, single-arm trial examining the effect of financial navigation on financial toxicity in adult patients with cancer in rural and non-rural settings. Trials. 2022;23(1):839.
46. SWOG Cancer Research Network. A randomized trial addressing cancer-related financial hardship through delivery of a proactive financial navigation intervention (CREDIT) [Internet]. clinicaltrials.gov; 2023 [cited 2023 Aug 4]. Report No.: NCT04960787. Available from: https://clinicaltrials.gov/study/NCT04960787.
47. Henrikson NB, Anderson ML, Dickerson J, Ewing JJ, Garcia R, Keast E, et al. The Cancer Financial Experience (CAFÉ) study: randomized controlled trial of a financial navigation intervention to address cancer-related financial hardship. Trials. 2022;23(1):402.

48. Raghavan D, Keith NA, Warden HR. Levine cancer Institute financial toxicity tumor board: a potential solution to an emerging problem. JCO Oncol Pract. 2021;17:e1433–9.
49. Tarnasky AM, Tran GN, Nicolla J. Mobile application to identify cancer treatment-related financial assistance: results of a randomized controlled trial. JCO Oncol Pract. 2021;17:e1440–9.
50. Zafar SY, Chino F, Ubel PA. The utility of cost discussions between patients with cancer and oncologists. Am J Manag Care. 2015;21:607–15.
51. Greenup RA, Rushing C, Fish L. Financial costs and burden related to decisions for breast cancer surgery. J Oncol Pract. 2019;15:e666–76.
52. Hong YR, Salloum RG, Yadav S. Patient-provider discussion about cancer treatment costs and out-of-pocket spending: implications for shared decision making in cancer care. Value Health. 2020;23:1592–8.
53. de Moor JS, Mollica M, Sampson A, Adjei B, Weaver SJ, et al. Delivery of financial navigation services within National Cancer Institute-designated cancer centers. JNCI Cancer Spectr. 2021;5(3):pkab033. https://doi.org/10.1093/jncics/pkab033.
54. Everson J, Frisse ME, Dusetzina SB. Real-time benefit tools for drug prices. JAMA. 2019;322:2383–4.
55. Su CT, Shankaran V. Defining the role of the modern oncology provider in mitigating financial toxicity. J Am Coll Radiol. 2023;20(1):51–6. https://doi.org/10.1016/j.jacr.2022.10.011.
56. Foundation ABIM. Ten things physicians and patients should question [Internet]. Choosing Wisely, American Society of Clinical Oncology; 2015. Available from: https://www.choosingwisely.org/societies/american-society-of-clinical-oncology/.
57. Nagarajah S, Powis ML, Fazelzad R, Krzyzanowska MK, Kukreti V. Implementation and impact of choosing wisely recommendations in oncology. JCO Oncol Pract. 2022;18(10):703–12. https://doi.org/10.1200/OP.22.00130.
58. Snoswell CL, Taylor ML, Comans TA, Smith AC, Gray LC, Caffery LJ. Determining if telehealth can reduce health system costs: scoping review. J Med Internet Res. 2020;22(10):e17298.
59. Sidey-Gibbons C, Pfob A, Asaad M. Development of machine learning algorithms for the prediction of financial toxicity in localized breast cancer following surgical treatment. JCO Clin Cancer Inform. 2021;5:338–47.
60. National Health Authority [Internet]. [cited 2023 Aug 4]. Available from: https://nha.gov.in/Whos-who.html.
61. India Today. Cabinet to replace National Health Agency with National Health Authority [Internet]. [cited 2023 Aug 4]. Available from: https://www.indiatoday.in/india/story/cabinet-to-replace-national-health-agency-with-national-health-authority-1422677-2019-01-03.
62. Garg S, Bebarta KK, Tripathi N. Performance of India's national publicly funded health insurance scheme, Pradhan Mantri Jan Arogya Yojana (PMJAY), in improving access and financial protection for hospital care: findings from household surveys in Chhattisgarh state. BMC Public Health. 2020;20:949.
63. Kaur S, Jain N, Bhatnagar P. Early trends from utilization of oncology services: insights from Ayushman Bharat Pradhan Mantri Jan Arogya Yojana (PMJAY) [Internet]. 2020. Available from: https://pmjay.gov.in/sites/default/files/2019-11/Working%20paper-4%20(1).pdf.
64. NCG [Internet]. [cited 2023 Aug 5]. Available from: https://tmc.gov.in/ncg/.
65. Woolf SH, Grol R, Hutchinson A, Eccles M, Grimshaw J. Potential benefits, limitations, and harms of clinical guidelines. BMJ. 1999;318(7182):527–30.
66. Institute of Medicine (US) Committee on Standards for Developing Trustworthy Clinical Practice Guidelines. Clinical practice guidelines we can trust [Internet]. Graham R, Mancher M, Miller Wolman D, Greenfield S, Steinberg E, editors. Washington, DC: National Academies Press (US); 2011. Available from: http://www.ncbi.nlm.nih.gov/books/NBK209539/.
67. Fervers B, Burgers JS, Haugh MC, Latreille J, Mlika-Cabanne N, Paquet L, et al. Adaptation of clinical guidelines: literature review and proposition for a framework and procedure. Int J Qual Health Care. 2006;18(3):167–76.
68. Hunter N, Dempsey N, Tbaishat F, Jahanzeb M, Al-Sukhun S, Gralow JR. Resource-stratified guideline-based cancer care should be a priority: historical context and examples of success. Am Soc Clin Oncol Educ Book. 2020;40:1–10. https://doi.org/10.1200/EDBK_279693.
69. Song Y, Alonso-Coello P, Ballesteros M, Cluzeau F, Vernooij RWM, Arayssi T, et al. A reporting tool for adapted guidelines in health care: the RIGHT-Ad@pt checklist. Ann Intern Med. 2022;175(5):710–9.
70. Chopra SJ, Mathew A, Maheshwari A, Bhatla N, et al. National Cancer Grid of India consensus guidelines on the management of cervical cancer. J Glob Oncol. 2018;4:1–15. https://doi.org/10.1200/JGO.17.00152.
71. Armstrong MJ, Mullins CD, Gronseth GS, Gagliardi AR. Impact of patient involvement on clinical practice guideline development: a parallel group study. Implement Sci. 2018;13(1):55.
72. Bilinski A, Neumann P, Cohen J, Thorat T, McDaniel K, Salomon JA. When cost-effective interventions are unaffordable: integrating cost-effectiveness and budget impact in priority setting for global health programs. PLoS Med. 2017;14(10):e1002397.
73. Salek M, Silverstein A, Tilly A, Gassant PY, et al. Factors influencing treatment decision-making for cancer patients in low-and middle-income countries: a scoping review. Cancer Med. 2023;12(17):18133–52. https://doi.org/10.1002/cam4.6375.
74. Rehfuess EA, Stratil JM, Scheel IB, Portela A, Norris SL, Baltussen R. The WHO-INTEGRATE evidence to decision framework version 1.0: integrating WHO norms and values and a complexity perspective. BMJ Glob Health. 2019;4(Suppl 1):e000844.
75. Correa VC, Lugo-Agudelo LH, Aguirre-Acevedo DC, Contreras JAP, Borrero AMP, Patiño-Lugo DF, et al. Individual, health system, and contextual barriers and

facilitators for the implementation of clinical practice guidelines: a systematic metareview. Health Res Policy Syst. 2020;18(1):74.
76. Pramesh CS, Chaturvedi H, Reddy VA, Saikia T, Ghoshal S, Pandit M, et al. Choosing Wisely India: ten low-value or harmful practices that should be avoided in cancer care. Lancet Oncol. 2019;20(4):e218–23.
77. Mehndiratta A, Sharma S, Gupta NP, Sankar MJ, Cluzeau F. Adapting clinical guidelines in India—a pragmatic approach. BMJ. 2017;359:j5147.

Online Links

UNDP Sustainable development goals https://www.dev-practitioners.eu/media/key_documents/SDGs_Booklet_Web_En.pdf.

https://www.youtube.com/watch?v=Wpy_KLRMlOg.

Webinar on Patient Centred Access To Quality Cancer Care https://www.youtube.com/watch?v=3j5QiN79mBA.

MIX
Papier aus verantwortungsvollen Quellen
Paper from responsible sources
FSC® C105338
FSC
www.fsc.org

If you have any concerns about our products,
you can contact us on
ProductSafety@springernature.com

In case Publisher is established outside the EU,
the EU authorized representative is:
Springer Nature Customer Service Center GmbH
Europaplatz 3, 69115 Heidelberg, Germany

Printed by Libri Plureos GmbH
in Hamburg, Germany